Muir's Textbook of Pathology

Tenth Edition

Edited by J. R. Anderson

B.Sc., M.D., F.R.C.P.(Glas.), M.R.C.P.(Lond.), F.R.C.Path., F.R.S. Edin.
Professor of Pathology, University of Glasgow
Pathologist to the Western Hospitals Group, Glasgow
Consultant Pathologist to the Greater Glasgow Area Health Board

Edward Arnold

© J. R. ANDERSON, 1976

First published 1924
by Edward Arnold (Publishers) Ltd.
25 Hill Street, London W1X 8LL

Reprinted, 1924, 1926, 1927
Second edition, 1929
Reprinted, 1930, 1932
Third edition, 1933
Fourth edition, 1936
Fifth edition, 1941
Reprinted, 1944, 1946
Sixth edition, 1951
Reprinted, 1956
Seventh edition, 1958
Eighth edition, 1964
Reprinted, 1968
Ninth edition, 1971
Reprinted, 1972, 1973, 1975
Tenth edition, 1976
Revised reprint, 1978

ISBN 0 7131 4268 5

Filmset in 'Monophoto' Times 10 on 11 pt. by
Richard Clay (The Chaucer Press), Ltd., Bungay, Suffolk
and printed in Great Britain by
Fletcher & Son Ltd., Norwich

Preface

It is with sadness that I record the death, on 13 February 1976, of Professor D. F. Cappell, whose contribution in preparing the 6–8th editions of this book was enormous.

In preparing this edition, the intention has been, as before, to provide an illustrated text in pathology suitable for medical students and yet sufficiently comprehensive to be used by graduate trainees in various branches of medicine, including junior trainees in pathology.

Progress in the biological sciences, including human and experimental pathology, has once again necessitated drastic changes in the text. In order to include the more important recent developments without making the book much bigger, it has been necessary to re-write approximately half of the text and to modify the rest considerably. It has not been my intention to provide the minimum, and the book contains more than will be assimilated readily by most medical students during their formal course in pathology. Methods of teaching have become more varied, and so have the contents of the curricula of different medical schools; students reading this book should receive guidance from their teachers in deciding which aspects of the subject deserve their closest attention.

As before, the text is in two major sections: the first 12 chapters are devoted to the important basic pathological processes—types of cell injury, inflammation, immunological reactions, infections, neoplasia, etc. The remainder of the book consists of 13 chapters, each of which gives an account of the more important pathological changes affecting a particular system—the heart, alimentary tract, skin, etc. The general section has been increased to approximately 300 pages at the expense of shortening some of the systematic chapters, and any increase in size is due mainly to the greater space now allocated to the 1000 or so illustrations, about a quarter of which are new.

Although this book is concerned especially with human pathology, it includes accounts of experimental work which has made important contributions to the understanding of disease processes, and some topics, particularly in the general section, are considered at length mainly because of their basic scientific importance. I believe that this section of the book may be of interest also to non-medical biologists.

In re-writing the systematic chapters, care has been taken to preserve from the previous edition those descriptions of structural changes which are based on a large cumulative personal experience and which are still of importance. Sections on clinico-pathological correlations have also been retained and sometimes extended, and the temptation to expound dogmatic views on subjects which are controversial has, in general, been resisted. Although most of the general chapters were re-written for the 9th edition, the accounts of inflammation, the mononuclear-phagocyte system, the cellular basis of immunity, hypersensitivity reactions and the nature and causation of tumours have been almost completely replaced. Extensive changes have also been made in the systematic chapters, particularly in those on the heart, the respiratory system, the blood and bone marrow, lymphoid tumours, the liver, kidney and endocrine system. A section on those diseases of the eye which are of general importance has been added to the chapter on the nervous system. As before, brief accounts of some of the more important tropical parasitic diseases are included, but for diseases occurring predominantly in tropical countries reference should be made to texts by those with the appropriate experience.

In previous editions, the help of colleagues has been acknowledged in the preface. With increasing specialization the number of contributors has grown steadily, and I have thought it appropriate, in the list of contents which follows, to state who has been mainly responsible for the revision of each chapter. In addition, a number of colleagues have kindly revised or contributed smaller sections: they include Dr. J. Stewart Orr, D.Sc. (the effects of ionising radiations), Dr. Morag Timbury (virus infections), Drs. J. J. Brown, A. F. Lever and J. I. S. Robertson of the M.R.C. Hypertension Research Unit (the renin–angiotensin system; Conn's syndrome), Sir Douglas Black (whose account of oedema has still not required much change), Professor G. P. McNicol (haemostasis, clotting and fibrinolysis) and Professor J. Hume Adams (diseases of muscle). Parts of the chapter on the endocrine system have been revised by Professor R. B. Goudie (thyroid), and Dr. R. N. M. MacSween (endocrine pancreas). For the respiratory system, I have been fortunate to enlist the help of Professor Donald Heath and Dr. J. M. Kay of the Pathology Department of Liverpool University; they have rewritten most of the chapter and have provided a lucid and up-to-date account. I must acknowledge also the work of colleagues who helped with the previous edition but who, for various reasons, have not been involved this time. This includes Drs. R. F. Macadam and J. M. Vetters, Professor W. A. Harland and the late Dr. H. E. Hutchison, much of whose contribution to the haematology chapter has been retained. The book has gained in authority from this multiple authorship, and I am grateful to my colleagues, not only for their contributions, but also for affording me wide editorial licence, which I have used in an endeavour to ensure uniformity of style and nomenclature, to avoid unnecessary overlap between chapters, and hopefully to provide a balanced account. I accept responsibility for errors of fact and judgement.

I am grateful for much useful advice and suggestions provided by Dr. J. Douglas Briggs on the urinary system, Dr. M. J. Davies and Professor N. Woolf on the heart, and Dr. J. W. Kerr on atopic hypersensitivity. I have been helped also by the many useful suggestions made in letters from readers of the 9th edition and hope that this source of advice will continue. I am indebted also to members of the departmental staff and others who have provided illustrations: the latter are acknowledged individually in the legends.

I wish to thank Mr. Robin Callander, F.F.P.A., M.M.A.A. for preparing diagrams, and Messrs. William Carson, F.I.M.L.T. and Norman Russell, F.I.M.L.T. for maintaining the high standard of technical work necessary for the production of suitable material for illustrations, Mr. David McSeveney, F.I.M.L.T. for his outstanding electron microscopy preparations, and Mr. Peter Kerrigan for a very large amount of painstaking and skilful photography. My gratitude is due to various members of staff, and to my wife, for helping with correction of the proofs.

The revision has included much secretarial work: the help of Mrs. Margaret Morton and Miss Helen Scott with communications and correspondence has been invaluable, and they have shared the major task of typing (often from semi-legible manuscripts) with Mrs. Norma McCulloch, Mrs. Anne McLeod, Mrs. Maureen Ralston and Mrs. Pat Bonnar. To all these I express my grateful thanks.

It is a pleasure once again to thank Messrs. Edward Arnold, and particularly Miss Barbara Koster, for their enthusiastic co-operation and determination to overcome delays in publication. Both they and the printers have dealt so successfully and efficiently with the preparation of the new edition that I have been kept under considerable pressure.

Finally, I would like, once more, to thank my wife and family who have faced with sympathetic understanding my preoccupation and bad temper during the revision.

J. R. ANDERSON

Reprinted 10th Edition. I am grateful to the many readers, and particularly to Dr. J. F. Boyd, for helping with the corrections and minor changes which have been made in the reprinted edition.

Contents

Introduction

What is pathology?

Pathology is the study of disease by scientific methods. Disease may, in turn, be defined as an abnormal variation in the structure or function of any part of the body. There must be an explanation of such variations from the normal—in other words, diseases have causes, and pathology includes not only observation of the structural and functional changes throughout the course of a disease, but also elucidation of the factors which cause it. It is only by establishing the cause (*aetiology*) of a disease that logical methods can be devised for its prevention or cure. Pathology may thus be described as the scientific study of the causes and effects of disease.

Methods used in Pathology

These include (*a*) *histology* and *cytology*, in which the structural changes in diseased tissues are examined by naked-eye inspection, or by light and electron microscopy of tissue sections or smears; (*b*) *biochemistry*, in which the metabolic disturbances of disease are investigated by assay of various normal and abnormal compounds in the blood, urine, etc.; (*c*) *microbiology*, in which body fluids, mucosal surfaces, excised tissues, etc., are examined by microscopical, cultural and serological techniques to detect and identify the micro-organisms responsible for many diseases.

These methods may be applied to the study of individuals suffering from a disease, and to animals in which a model of the disease occurs naturally or has been induced experimentally. The development of special techniques to investigate some types of disease has led to further specialisation in pathology. For example, the diagnosis of disorders of the blood involves various quantitative tests on, and morphological examination of, the cells of the blood, assay of the factors involved in clotting, investigation of the metabolism of iron, vitamin B_{12}, etc., the detection of abnormal antibodies to cells of the blood and blood group serology. The many techniques involved have required the establishment of *haematology* laboratories: application of techniques to determine chromosome anomalies has led to the establishment of *cytogenetics* laboratories, and microbiology has divided into *bacteriology* and *virology*. Finally, *immunology*, a subject of enormous interest in biology and of increasing clinical significance, now requires special laboratory facilities. It will be apparent that pathology covers a wide spectrum of techniques, both in the diagnosis of patients and in research into the causes of various diseases. The relative importance of the various branches of pathology varies for different types of disease. In some instances, for example in diabetes mellitus, biochemical investigations provide the best means of diagnosis and are of the greatest value in the control of therapy. By contrast, recognition of the nature of many diseases, for example tumours, and so the choice of the most appropriate therapy, depend very largely on examination of the gross and microscopic features. For most diseases, diagnosis is based on a combination of pathological investigations. To give an example, biochemical tests may indicate that a patient is suffering from impairment of renal function, but the nature of the renal disease responsible for this commonly requires histological examination of renal tissue (*renal biopsy*). Another example is provided by the condition of anaemia, which may have many causes. The changes in the cells of the blood and the bone marrow may suggest deficiency of a factor essential for erythropoiesis, and biochemical and physiological tests are then indicated to confirm the deficiency, e.g. of vitamin B_{12} or folic acid.

Alternatively, anaemia may result from blood loss and this may be due to a structural lesion of the gastro-intestinal tract or of the endometrium, diagnosis of which may require histological examination.

Why learn Pathology?

Most medical students are not going to become pathologists. It is nevertheless essential that the medical school curriculum should include a course of pathology which provides a clear account of the causes, where these are known, and of the pathological changes, of the more important diseases. Most disease processes bring about structural changes and these usually provide a logical explanation for the symptoms and signs and commonly also for the biochemical changes. An appreciation of the pathological processes of disease thus aids the doctor in the correct interpretation of the clinical features of the patient's illness. This applies not only to the clinical diagnostician but also to the surgeon who must recognise the nature of the structural changes exposed at operation and act accordingly, and to the radiologist who can only interpret the significance of shadows on an x-ray film on the basis of the structural changes of disease. To the research worker, histopathology and electron microscopy are superb techniques; both can be adapted to enzymic and other chemical investigations (*histochemistry*), including immunohistological techniques which make use of the exquisite specificity of antigen–antibody reactions to detect tissue and cell constituents and abnormal substances (see Fig. 21.18, p. 761 and Fig. 24.1, p. 940).

From what has been said above, pathology is important to the medical student, regardless of the branch of medicine he intends to pursue. The pathologist is concerned mainly in the diagnosis and in elucidating the nature and causes of disease. He must co-operate fully with his clinical colleagues, both in the diagnosis of individual patients, and in the conduct of clinico-pathological meetings for teaching purposes. One of the best places to learn pathology and to correlate the patient's illness with the structural changes of his disease is the post-mortem room, and a well-conducted necropsy, attended by the clinicians who looked after the patient during life, is unsurpassed as a teaching method.

Pathological processes

It was first pointed out by Virchow that all disturbances of function and structure in disease are due to cellular abnormalities and that the phenomena of a particular disease are brought about by a series of cellular changes. Pathological processes are of a dual nature, consisting firstly of **the changes of the injury** induced by the causal agent, and secondly of **reactive changes** which are often closely similar to physiological processes. If death is rapid, as for example in cyanide poisoning, there may be little or no structural changes of either type. Cyanide inhibits the cytochrome-oxidase systems of the cells and thus halts cellular respiration before histological changes can become apparent. Similarly, blockage of a coronary artery cuts off the blood supply to part of the myocardium and death may be immediate, when no myocardial changes will be found: if, however, the patient survives for some hours or more, the affected myocardium shows the structural changes which occur subsequent to cell death and the lesion becomes readily visible both macroscopically (Fig. 14.9, p. 352) and microscopically (Fig. 1.4, p. 4). Reactive changes may be exemplified by enlargement of the myocardium in the patient with high blood pressure (Fig. 3.32, p. 82). In this condition, there is an increase in the resistance to blood flow through the arterioles and consequently the normal rate of circulation can be maintained only by a rise in blood pressure. Reflex stimulation of the heart results in more forcible contractions of the left ventricle, and in accordance with the general principle that increased functional demand stimulates enlargement (**hypertrophy**) and/or proliferation (**hyperplasia**) of the cells concerned, the myocardial cells of the left ventricle increase in size. Although part of a disease state, the reactive hypertrophy of the myocardium in hypertension is closely similar to the physiological hypertrophy of the skeletal muscles in the trained athlete. To give another example, the invasion of the body by micro-organisms, in addition to causing injury, stimulates reactive changes in the lymphoid tissues, with the development of immunity. The distinction between the changes due to injury and those due to reaction are not usually so well defined as in the above examples. In many instances where cell injury persists without killing the cells, the cytological changes are complex and those due to injury often cannot be distinguished from those due to reaction. Some examples of the various types of cell injury and reaction are provided in Chapter 1.

In order to facilitate the understanding of pathological processes, it is helpful to group together those which have common causal factors and as a consequence exhibit similarities in their structural changes. For example, bacterial infections have certain features in common, and may with advantage be further sub-divided into acute and chronic infections. The features and behaviour of neoplasms or tumours are sufficiently similar to classify most tumours into two categories, benign and malignant, and to provide a general account of each group. The changes resulting from a deficient blood supply are similar for all tissues. Accordingly, the first twelve chapters of this book are of a general nature and deal with the commoner pathological processes. The remaining chapters are systematic and go on to describe the special features of disease processes as they affect the various organs and systems.

The causes of disease

Causal factors in disease may be of a genetic nature or acquired. *Genetically-determined disease* is due to some abnormality of base sequence in the DNA of the fertilised ovum and the cells derived from it, or to reduplication, loss or misplacement of a whole or part of a chromosome. Such abnormalities are often inherited from one or both parents. *Acquired disease* is due to effects of some environmental factor, e.g. malnutrition or micro-organisms. Most diseases are acquired, but very often there is more than one causal factor and there may in fact be many. Genetic variations may influence the susceptibility of an individual to environmental factors. Even in the case of infections, there is considerable individual variation in the severity of the disease. Of the many individuals who become infected with poliovirus, most develop immunity without becoming ill; some have a mild illness and a few become paralysed from involvement of the central nervous system (Fig. 20.43, p. 698). This illustrates the importance of **host factors** as well as causal agents. Spread of tuberculosis is favoured by poor personal and domestic hygiene by overcrowding,

malnutrition and by various other diseases. Accordingly, disease results not only from exposure to the major causal agent but also from the existence of *predisposing* or *contributory factors*.

Congenital disease. Diseases may also be classified into those which develop during fetal life (congenital) and those which arise at any time thereafter during post-natal life. Genetically-determined diseases are commonly congenital, although some present many years after birth, a good example being polyposis coli, which is transmitted by a dominant abnormal gene (see below) and is characterised by multiple tumours of the colonic mucosa, appearing in adolescence or adult life (Fig. 18.71, p. 592). Congenital diseases may also be acquired, an important example being provided by transmission of the virus of rubella (German measles) from mother to fetus during the first trimester of pregnancy. Depending on the stage of fetal development at which infection occurs, it may result in fetal death, or involvement of various tissues leading to mental deficiency, blindness, deafness, or structural abnormalities of the heart. The mother may also transmit to the fetus various other infections, including syphilis and toxoplasmosis, with consequent congenital disease. Ingestion of various chemicals by the mother, as in the thalidomide disaster, may induce severe disorders of fetal development and growth. Another cause of acquired congenital disease is maternal–fetal incompatibility. Fetal red cells, containing antigens inherited from the father, may enter the maternal circulation and stimulate antibody production: the maternal antibody may pass through the placenta and react with the fetal red cells, causing a haemolytic anaemia.

Genetically-determined disease

As already mentioned, this results from abnormalities in the DNA which forms the genome. In some instances the abnormality consists of gain or loss of a whole chromosome or of part of a chromosome. Such gross abnormalities can now be detected by cell culture techniques: most of them probably arise by non-disjunction of chromosomes in the meiosis which precedes germ-cell formation, and only a few appear to be compatible with life, e.g. an additional chromosome 21, which is the usual cause of Down's syndrome (mongolism).

A very large number of diseases result from the inheritance of an abnormal gene, or combination of genes, from one or both parents, commonly termed *mutations*. The development of abnormal genes (*mutation*) can be provoked by irradiation, mutagenic chemicals and probably by viruses, but in most instances the cause of mutations in man remains unknown. Examples of the many conditions resulting from an abnormal gene are colour blindness, albinism, haemophilia, sickle-cell anaemia, dystrophia myotonica and polyposis coli. The abnormal gene may be dominant, i.e. may induce an abnormality in spite of the presence of a normal corresponding gene from the other parent, or it may be recessive, i.e. causing disease only in the absence of a corresponding normal gene. The latter circumstance arises most usually in abnormalities of genes on the X chromosome, males being thus affected (Fig. 16.50, p. 501), or from the presence of two abnormal corresponding genes, the likelihood of which is enhanced by inbreeding.

In addition to those diseases due to mutations or recognisable chromosomal anomalies, there are many which show a familial tendency, but in which the mode of inheritance has not been elucidated. Examples include diabetes mellitus, chronic thyroiditis (see (6) below), and some of the commoner cancers, e.g. of the breast and of the bronchus. It is likely that both genetic and environmental factors are of causal importance in these conditions.

Acquired disease

The major causal factors may be classified as follows:

(1) Deficiency diseases. Inadequate diet still accounts for poor health in many parts of the world. It may take the form of deficiency either of major classes of food, usually high-grade protein, or of vitamins or elements essential for specific metabolic processes, e.g. iron for haemoglobin production. Often the deficiencies are multiple and complex. Disturbances of nutrition are by no means restricted to deficiencies, for in the more affluent countries obesity, due to overeating, has become increasingly common, with its attendant dangers of arterial hypertension and heart disease.

(2) Physical agents. These include mechanical injury, heat, cold, electricity, irradiation, and rapid changes in environmental pressure. In all instances, injury is caused by a high rate of transmission of particular forms of energy (kinetic, radiant, etc.) to or from the body. Important examples in this country are mechanical injury, particularly in road accidents, and burns. Exposure to ionising radiations cannot be regarded as entirely safe in any dosage. While radiation is used with benefit in various diagnostic and therapeutic procedures, any pollution of the environment with radio-active material is potentially harmful to those exposed to it and probably to subsequent generations.

(3) Chemicals. With the use of an ever-increasing number of chemical agents as drugs, in industrial processes, and in the home, chemically-induced injury has become very common. The effects vary. At one extreme are those substances which have a general effect on cells, such as cyanide (see above) which causes death almost instantaneously, with little or no structural changes. Many other chemicals, such as strong acids and alkalis, cause local injury accompanied by an inflammatory reaction in the tissues exposed to them. A third large group of substances produces a more or less selective injury to a particular organ or cell type, for example the barbiturate drugs affect especially the neurones, paraquat causes severe injury to the lungs (Fig. 15.37, p. 432), while many substances cause death of the cells of the liver and of the renal tubules.

(4) Parasitic micro-organisms. These include bacteria, protozoa, lower fungi and viruses. In spite of the advances in immunisation procedures and the extensive use now made of antibiotics, many important diseases still result from infection by micro-organisms, and the danger of widespread epidemics, e.g. of influenza and cholera, has been enhanced by air travel. The disease-producing capacity of micro-organisms depends on their ability to invade and multiply within the host, and on the possibility of their transmission to other hosts. The features of the disease produced by infection depend on the specific properties of the causal organism. Bacteria bring about harmful effects mainly by the production of chemical compounds termed *toxins*, and the biological effects of these, together with the response of the host, determine the features of the disease. Viruses colonise host cells, and have a direct cytopathic effect: features of virus disease depend largely on which cells are colonised, the rate of viral replication, the nature of the cytopathic effect, and the response of the host. Of the protozoa, the malaria parasite is of enormous importance as a cause of chronic ill health in whole populations.

(5) Metazoan parasites are also an important cause of disease in many parts of the world. Hookworm infestation of the intestine and schistosomiasis are causes of ill health prevalent in many tropical countries.

(6) Immunological factors. Harmful effects, both local and general, can result from the reaction of antibody or sensitised cells with foreign antigenic material. Asthma, hay fever, and skin rashes following exposure to various chemicals are examples of such *hypersensitivity* reactions, but they are many and complex, and hypersensitivity to penicillin and other drugs sometimes causes a fatal reaction. Disease may result also from the development of *auto-immunity*: the immunity system develops antibodies and sensitised cells which react specifically with constituents of normal cells or tissues, and injury results from such reactions. Examples are chronic thyroiditis, commonly progressing to myxoedema, and the excessive destruction of red cells in auto-immune haemolytic anaemia.

In another group of disorders, the immunity system is deficient, and the patient lacks defence against micro-organisms: this may result from abnormalities of fetal development or may be induced by immuno-suppressive therapy.

(7) Psychogenic factors. The mental stresses imposed by conditions of life, particularly in technologically advanced communities, are probably largely responsible for three important and overlapping groups of diseases. First, acquired mental diseases such as schizophrenia and depression, for which no specific structural or biochemical basis has yet been found. Second, diseases of addiction, particularly to alcohol, various drugs and tobacco: these result in their own complications, for example alcohol predisposes to liver damage (Fig. 19.23, p. 620) and causes various neurological and mental disturbances, while cigarette smoking is the major cause of lung cancer (Fig. 15.45, p. 444), and chronic bronchitis, and is concerned also in peptic ulceration and coronary artery disease. The third group of diseases is heterogeneous, and includes peptic ulcer (Fig. 18.23, p. 550), high blood pressure and coronary artery disease (Fig. 14.12, p. 354). In these three important conditions, anxiety, overwork and frustration appear to be causal factors, although their modes of action are obscure.

1

Cell Damage

All metabolic activities of the body are carried out and regulated by the cells of the tissues, and since the time of Virchow cell injury has been recognised as the central problem in pathology. It is clearly important to know what factors cause cell damage and how these lead to the cellular disorders which result in the states we recognise as diseases. Unfortunately our knowledge of this large and important subject is still in its infancy because of the slow development of methods for investigating it, and the extremely complex interrelationship of biological activities within the cell. Nevertheless progress in biochemistry and molecular biology is now bringing the pathology of cell damage within our grasp.

In at least one disease, sickle-cell anaemia, we probably know the entire sequence of events leading to cellular destruction and this can be taken as an illustration of the kind of understanding which is our object for the future in other forms of cellular injury. The sickle-cell abnormality is an inherited defect characterised clinically by rapid destruction of red blood cells. Apparently an error has occurred in copying one base in the sequence of 146 base triplets in the DNA constituting the gene for the beta polypeptide chain of the protein moiety of haemoglobin. This error, transcribed through messenger RNA, results in the insertion of the amino acid valine instead of glutamic acid in position 6 from the N terminal end of the beta polypeptide chain and the shape of that end of the chain is altered. The change in structure is of no account when haemoglobin is oxygenated, but as the haemoglobin molecule gives up oxygen it expands and the abnormal parts of the two beta chains come to project from the surface of the molecule. Accordingly the beta chains of deoxygenated sickle haemoglobin can unite with alpha chains of adjacent molecules. Masses of long helical fibres of polymerised

deoxygenated haemoglobin form and these impart to the red cells abnormal rigidity and a characteristic sickle shape which make them unduly prone to mechanical injury and subsequent phagocytosis within the spleen. It should be noted that, compared with most cells, red cells have a very simple structure and are easily obtained for study; furthermore, haemoglobin is one of the few proteins whose molecular structure is known in detail.

The mechanism of most other forms of cell damage is much less clear. For example, the mode of action of carbon tetrachloride on liver cells has been the subject of much study. In liver cells of rats poisoned with this substance there are abnormalities of protein, fat and carbohydrate metabolism, and electron microscopy shows damage first to the granular endoplasmic reticulum and later to other cellular organelles. Attempts to establish the primary site of action of carbon tetrachloride by study of liver cell homogenates have not been successful. Several other poisons, e.g. thioacetamide, cause similar effects on liver cells and it is evident that various different injuries lead to a train or trains of common secondary effects preceding cell death. McLean *et al.* (1965) compare the structure and chemistry of a cell to a net. When a net is pulled, all the links are disturbed, and the weaker links will tend to break no matter where the stress is applied. A damaged part of the cell, detected by methods currently available, may likewise be only indirectly related to the cause of the injury.

In the following account only a few of the many possible examples of cellular damage have been selected. The topic is frequently mentioned in later chapters and our superficial treatment of this important subject is merely a reflection of our present basic ignorance.

It is convenient to consider the effects of cellular injury under two main headings: **(1) cell** death or **necrosis**, in which irreversible changes take place in the cell so that no further integrated function such as respiration or maintenance of selective membrane permeability is possible: **(2) lesser forms of damage** (sometimes described as degenerations) in which functions important for the economy of the cell or body are diminished or lost but in which integrated

vital functions such as respiration and selective membrane permeability remain possible. Many lesser forms of cellular damage are reversible when the cause is withdrawn, for example the injury to neurones by anaesthetic drugs given in therapeutic doses. Others, not resulting in cell death, are irreversible, e.g. radiation damage to chromosomes resulting in non-lethal genetic mutation.

Necrosis

Necrosis means the death of cells or groups of cells while they still form part of the living body, and implies permanent cessation of their integrated function. Necrosis may occur suddenly, for example when cells are exposed to heat or toxic chemicals, or cell death may be preceded by gradual and potentially reversible damage in which case the term **necrobiosis** is occasionally used.

Causes of necrosis

(a) Marked impairment of blood supply, usually the result of obstruction of an end-artery (that is, one without adequate collaterals) is a common and important cause of necrosis, the necrotic area being known as an **infarct** (p. 208). Different cells can withstand anoxia resulting from impaired blood flow for different periods, nerve cells, for example, dying after only a few minutes, while fibrocytes survive much longer periods of anoxia.

(b) Toxins. Certain bacteria, plants, and animals such as snakes and scorpions, produce toxic organic compounds which even in very small quantities can cause cell damage amounting to necrosis. Some toxins have identifiable enzyme activity; for example, the causal organism of gas gangrene, *Clostridium welchii*, forms a lecithinase which acts directly on the lipoprotein of cell membranes. Diphtheria toxin appears to inhibit cellular protein synthesis by indirect interference with the transfer of aminoacyl–tRNA to ribosomes. Certain bacterial toxins, including those mentioned above, exert their effects not only in the proximity of the bacteria but also in organs remote from the infection due to dissemination of toxins by the bloodstream and other routes. The necrosis ac-

companying bacterial infection may be partly due to interference with the circulation brought about by severe inflammation in addition to the effect of toxins.

(c) Immunological injury. As will be described in Chapter 5, cell injury results in various ways from immune reactions. This is a feature of many infections, including tuberculosis in which tuberculoprotein, a nontoxic derivative of the tubercle bacillus, evokes an immune reaction which, though possibly protective in function, paradoxically leads to necrosis of cells in the neighbourhood of the organism.

(d) Infection of cells. In certain infections, notably by viruses, the infecting agent proliferates within cells. Many viruses kill infected cells in tissue culture (cytopathic effect) and an analogous destructive effect *in vivo* is probably the cause of necrosis of the anterior horn cells of the spinal cord in poliomyelitis.

(e) Chemical poisons. Many chemicals in high concentration cause necrosis by non-selective denaturation of the cellular proteins (e.g. strong acids, strong alkalis, carbolic acid, mercuric chloride). Cyanide and fluoroacetate are much more selective poisons and in low concentrations quickly cause cell death by interfering with oxidative production of energy from glucose, fatty acids and amino acids. As shown in Fig. 1.1 cyanide inhibits the enzyme cytochrome oxidase, thereby preventing the use of oxygen, while fluoroacetate forms a powerful competitive inhibitor of the enzyme aconitase which normally converts citrate to isocitrate in the Krebs citric acid cycle. Necrosis of liver or other specialised cells results from poisoning with such substances as carbon tetrachloride but detail of the mode of interaction between poison and cell is usually obscure.

(f) Physical agents. Cells are very sensitive to the action of heat and, depending on the origin of the cells, they die after variable periods of exposure to a temperature of 45 °C. Low temperatures are much less injurious and, provided certain precautions are taken, cell suspensions and even whole animals can be frozen without being killed. Necrosis after frostbite is due to

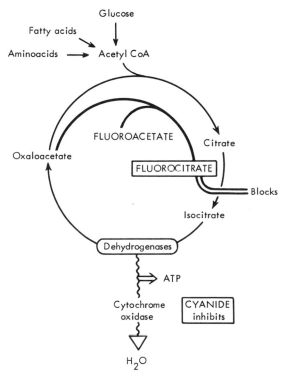

Fig. 1.1 The effects of fluoroacetate and of cyanide on cellular metabolism. Note that fluoroacetate is converted to fluorocitrate which inhibits aconitase.

damage to capillaries which results in thrombosis that may even extend to the arteries. Radiation damage, also a cause of necrosis, is considered on p. 23. Mechanical trauma such as crushing may cause direct disruption of cells. Certain disorders of the nervous system are sometimes accompanied by necrotic lesions in the limbs; these 'trophic' lesions were previously attributed to an ill-defined effect of denervation on tissue nutrition but are now thought to result from unnoticed mechanical trauma consequent upon sensory loss.

The recognition of necrosis

As a rule it is not possible to determine exactly when a particular cell becomes necrotic—i.e. when the disintegration of its vital functions has reached an irreversible stage. Many of the changes by which necrosis is recognised occur *after* cell death and are due to the secondary release of lytic enzymes normally sequestrated within the cell, e.g. in the lysosomes; this process of **autolysis** is described below.

Necrosis of cell suspensions in tissue culture can be studied conveniently by observing changes of permeability of cell membranes to dyes such as neutral red or trypan blue. These dyes are normally excluded from the nucleus but when cells die, the nuclei become stained due to increased permeability of the membranes of the cell (Fig. 1.2). Alternatively, membranous components of the living cells may be labelled with radioisotopes such as Cr^{51} or P^{32};

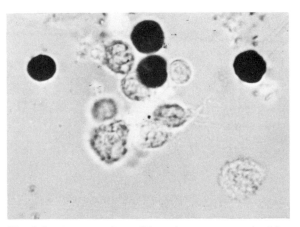

Fig. 1.2 A suspension of lymphocytes treated with cytotoxic iso-antibody and complement. Some of the cells have been killed, and have become stained by trypan blue dye present in the suspending fluid: other cells have survived and are unstained. (Trypan blue.) (Miss Patricia Bacon.)

subsequent severe injury to the cell, probably lethal, is recognised by release of the radioactive label from the cells into the culture medium.

In organised tissues such as liver or kidney, necrosis is usually recognised by secondary changes seen on histological examination. In preparations stained with haematoxylin and eosin, the nuclei may gradually lose their characteristic staining with haematoxylin so that the whole cell stains uniformly with eosin (Fig. 1.3), although the nuclear outline may persist; this change, the result of hydrolysis of chromatin within the cell after its death, is called **karyolysis**. Sometimes the chromatin of necrotic cells, especially those with already dense chromatin such as polymorphonuclear leukocytes, forms dense haematoxyphilic masses (**pyknosis**) and these may break up (**karyorrhexis**) to form granules inside the nuclear membrane or throughout the cytoplasm (Fig. 1.5). In many necrotic lesions the outlines of swollen necrotic cells can be recognised but the cytoplasm is abnormally homogeneous or granular and frequently takes up more eosin than normal. In other tissues, e.g. the central

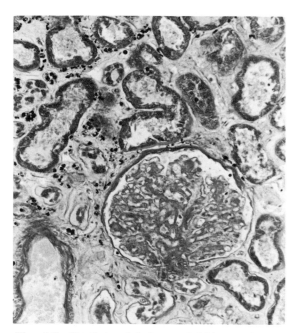

Fig. 1.3 Portion of infarct of kidney, showing coagulative necrosis. A glomerulus and tubules are seen, but the nuclei have disappeared and the structural details are lost. × 172.

nervous system, necrotic cells absorb water and then disintegrate, leaving no indication of the architecture of the original tissue; the lipids derived from myelin etc. persist in the debris of the necrotic tissue. The activities of certain enzymes, e.g. succinic acid dehydrogenase, diminish rapidly after cell death and appropriate tests provide useful indicators of recent tissue necrosis.

Electron microscopy of cells which have undergone necrosis shows severe disorganisation of structure. Gaps are seen in the various membranes and abnormal polymorphic inclusions presumably derived from membranes, lie in the ground substance. Fragmentation and vacuolation of endoplasmic reticulum and

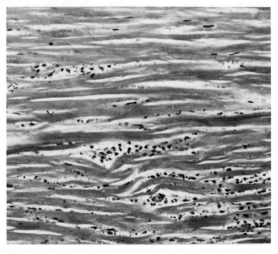

Fig. 1.4 Coagulative necrosis in infarction of heart muscle. The dead fibres are hyaline and structureless; remains of leukocytes are present between them. × 125.

mitochondrial membranes precedes the disappearance of these structures. Curious lamellar structures with concentric whorling form from the cell membrane especially where there have been microvilli. Ribosomes and Golgi apparatus are unrecognisable from an early stage. There is loss of density of the nucleoplasm and large chromatin granules accumulate just inside the nuclear membrane before it disappears.

Less severe injury affecting single cells sometimes leads to **shrinkage necrosis**, a gradual process in which water is lost from the cell so that the nucleus becomes condensed and the cytoplasm appears strongly eosinophilic due to the closely packed organelles. Later the cell breaks into rounded fragments with preservation of ultrastructure and some functional activities which persist until the fragments are phagocytosed and digested by neighbouring parenchymal cells or macrophages. The circular Councilman bodies formed from hepatocytes are examples of this form of necrosis which can be an expression of normal cell turnover in the parenchyma of tissues like liver and adrenal cortex. The term **apoptosis** ('dropping off') has also been used in this context.

Necrosis can often be recognised macroscopically when large groups of cells die. The necrotic area may become swollen, firm, dull and lustreless, and is yellowish unless it contains much blood. This appearance is often found in kidney, spleen and myocardium. Histologically the outlines of the dead cells are usually visible (Figs. 1.3 and 1.4) and the firmness of the tissue may be due to the action of tissue thromboplastins on fibrinogen which together with other plasma proteins has been shown to diffuse through the damaged membranes of necrotic cells. This type of necrosis is appropriately described as **coagulative necrosis.** By contrast, necrotic brain tissue, which has a large fluid component, becomes 'softened' and ultimately turns into a turbid liquid (**colliquative necrosis**) with profound loss of the previous histological architecture.

Certain necrotic lesions develop a firm cheeselike appearance to the naked eye and microscopy shows amorphous granular eosinophilic material lacking in cell outlines; a varying amount of finely divided fat is present and there may be minute granules of chromatin. Because of its appearance this lesion is described as 'caseation'. It is very common in tuberculosis

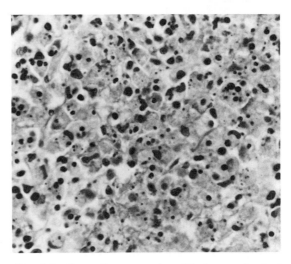

Fig. 1.5 Spreading necrosis with karyorrhexis in lymph node in typhoid fever. Note destruction of nuclei and numerous deeply-stained granules of chromatin. × 412.

but essentially similar changes are occasionally seen in infarcts, necrotic tumours and in inspissated collections of pus.

Necrotic lesions affecting skin or mucosal surfaces are frequently infected by organisms which cause putrefaction, i.e. the production of foul-smelling gas and brown, green or black discoloration of the tissue due to alteration of

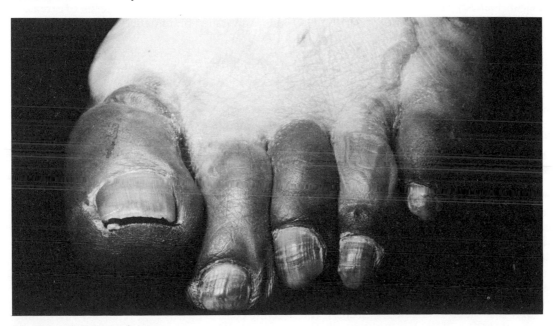

Fig. 1.6 Gangrene of toes.

haemoglobin. Necrosis with putrefaction is called **gangrene** (Fig. 1.6). It may be primarily due to vascular occlusion, e.g. in the limbs or bowel where the necrotic tissue is exposed to putrefactive bacteria, but it may also result from infection with certain bacteria, namely the clostridia which cause gas gangrene (p. 170) or fusiform bacilli which result in **noma** (p. 171).

The special features of **fat necrosis** are described on pages 654 and 926.

Autolysis. The structural disintegration of cells as a result of digestion by their own enzymes is largely responsible for the softening of necrotic tissues and the associated loss of histological structure. In the intact cell, the enzymes concerned do not have general access to the protoplasm. For example, various hydrolytic enzymes are associated with microsomes, mitochondria and lysosomes. The hydrolases confined within the lysosomal membranes include proteases which are most effective at low pH, a state which prevails in necrotic cells due to acid production from anaerobic glycolysis and the action of phosphatases and proteolytic enzymes. The small molecules produced by hydrolysis of macromolecules lead to osmotic swelling of the necrotic cells and their organelles provided that the membranes are sufficiently intact.

It should be noted that when many polymorphonuclear leukocytes are present in necrotic tissue the enzymes from their abundant lysosomes may contribute to the hydrolysis of other cells. This is an important factor in the liquefaction of pus and in the softening seen in infected organs at necropsy.

If tissue is killed by heating, e.g. to 55 °C, or by immersion in fixative such as formalin, the enzymes and other proteins are denatured and the histological features of necrosis attributable to autolysis do not develop. On the other hand if a piece of tissue is deprived of its blood supply by removal from the living body and kept at 37 °C the development of autolysis can be observed, with marked osmotic swelling of membrane-bounded structures.

With the above points in mind consideration must now be given to two practical aspects in the recognition of necrosis. First, morphological signs of necrosis are not apparent until autolysis has developed in the necrotic tissue, and this takes 12–24 hours. Second, following death of the individual (somatic death),

all cells of the body will in time die due to lack of blood supply and post-mortem autolysis will gradually take place. This is particularly marked in the epithelium of the liver and kidney and when seen at necropsy does not necessarily indicate that true necrosis has occurred, i.e. that these cells have died while still part of the living body. This problem is of great importance in electron microscopy which shows ultra-structural evidence of necrosis and of post-mortem autolysis within a very short time.

Somatic death. Though not strictly related to cell necrosis, the interesting subject of somatic death (death of the individual) deserves some consideration. Until recently, somatic death has been defined as complete and persistent cessation of respiration and circulation. For legal purposes the persistence of the state is arbitrarily taken as five or more minutes, by which time irreversible anoxic damage will have developed in the neurones of the vital centres. However, it is now possible to restore the circulatory and respiratory functions of heart and lungs in many cases of somatic death as defined above, and integrated function both of cells and of organs (excluding those of the central nervous system) can then continue for prolonged periods with the aid of special equipment. This fact is of great importance in obtaining organs for transplantation from cadaveric donors and a legal redefinition of somatic death in terms of extensive and irreversible brain damage is now necessary.

Effects of necrosis

By definition, necrotic cells are functionless. The effect of cell necrosis on the general well-being of the body accordingly depends on the functional importance of the tissue involved, the extent of the necrosis, the functional reserve of the tissue, and on the capacity of surviving cells to proliferate and replace those which have become necrotic. For example, the spleen is not an essential organ for health in man and extensive splenic necrosis is apparently of little importance. On the other hand extensive necrosis of renal tubular epithelium results in the serious clinical condition of renal failure which is likely to be fatal unless the patient is kept alive (e.g. by haemodialysis) until there is regeneration of tubules by proliferation of surviving cells. Necrosis of a relatively small number of motor nerve cells may produce severe paralysis which persists because nerve cells cannot proliferate to replace others which are necrotic. Since myocardial cells have not only a contractile but also a conducting function quite small necrotic lesions may result in striking alterations in the electrical activity of the heart.

The breakdown of necrotic cells results in escape of their contents. Enzymes such as transaminases released into the plasma from necrotic liver or myocardial cells form the basis of clinical tests for necrosis in these tissues though it should be emphasised that abnormal enzyme release occurs from cells with damage short of necrosis (e.g. in muscular dystrophy). In poisoning by alloxan, which affects the β cells of the pancreatic islets, discharge of stored insulin from the necrotic cells results in hypoglycaemia which may be fatal (Dunn).

Sequels to necrosis

Neutrophil polymorphs frequently accumulate in small numbers around necrotic cells (Fig. 1.4). Occasionally infarcts and caseous lesions are invaded by large numbers of these cells and this leads to softening as already described. Such softening is a notable feature in a small proportion of myocardial infarcts (which usually show coagulative necrosis) and may lead to rupture of the heart; it is also common in tuberculosis of the lumbar vertebrae where the caseous material liquefies and tracks down beneath the psoas fascia to form a 'cold abscess' in the groin.

Individual cells killed by toxins rapidly undergo autolysis and are absorbed, especially when the circulation is maintained. They may be quickly replaced by proliferation of adjacent surviving cells. When a large mass of tissue undergoes necrosis, e.g. in an infarct, the necrotic material may be gradually replaced by ingrowth of capillaries and fibroblasts from the surrounding viable tissue so that a fibrous scar results. If this process is incomplete the necrotic mass becomes enclosed in a fibrous capsule, may persist for a long time, and may become calcified. Areas of necrotic softening in the brain are usually invaded by microglial phagocytes and eventually become cyst-like spaces containing clear liquid and surrounded by proliferated astroglia.

Old caseous lesions and necrotic fat have a marked affinity for calcium and frequently become heavily calcified.

Cell Damage short of Necrosis

Many forms of injury may cause cellular abnormalities short of necrosis, which may have profound and serious effects on the welfare of the body. Such cellular abnormalities may be detected as disorders of function, i.e. the impairment of a physiological activity such as conduction of a nerve impulse; by chemical or histochemical means (diminished or excessive enzyme activity or storage or depletion of a chemical substance); by structural abnormality revealed by microscopy of one kind or another, or by a combination of these methods. Some of these forms of cellular damage lend themselves to scientific study because they can be accurately, if arbitrarily, defined in contrast to necrosis, the time of onset of which cannot be precisely established.

The following discussion deals with very heterogeneous topics. First we consider damage to the membranes and organelles of the cell, then give examples of damage resulting in abnormal storage of metabolites. Next, the important problem of irradiation damage, both to single cells and cell populations, is discussed and finally, shrinkage of cells (**atrophy**) and alteration of cell structure to a form more resistant to injury (**metaplasia**).

Damage to membranes and organelles

Electron microscopy reveals membranous structures which form the boundary wall around the cell and various compartments (organelles) within. The membranes are composed of lipoprotein (protein combined with phospholipid, predominantly lecithin) and have the general properties of semipermeable membranes. The important definition of cellular compartments depends to a large extent on this property since soluble proteins of different types can thereby be sequestered within the cell; for example, hydrolases, potentially harmful to the cell, are confined within the lysosomes. As a result of the semipermeability of the membrane, the cell and its organelles tend to be subject to swelling and shrinkage depending on the relative osmotic pressures of the solutions in their various compartments and in the extracellular fluid. The membranes are not, however, inert but actively regulate the transport of crystalloids, including electrolytes, by enzymatic action which constantly modifies the chemical structure of the membrane and requires the provision of energy from ATP. Thus although K^+ and to a smaller extent Na^+ can passively diffuse through cell membranes, the intracellular concentration of K^+ is much higher and of Na^+ lower than that of the extracellular fluid; these differences are due to the outward 'pumping' of sodium by the cell membrane.

An additional important function of the membranes of the cell is that they form a cytoskeleton. This to some extent determines the shape of the cell and provides supporting structures for arrays of enzymes which form sequential functional units, such as those involved in the citric acid cycle and the flavoprotein and cytochrome systems of the cristae of the mitochondria.

Cell membranes. It has been shown by microsurgery that cells can survive incision of the surface membrane, and presumably self-sealing gaps develop in membranes when particulate material (e.g. nuclear fragments from normoblasts) is extruded from cells. However, most forms of reversible injury to surface membranes are not associated with demonstrable structural lesions. Blebs and holes in the membranes (Fig. 1.7) due to activation of the esterases of complement by interaction of antibody with antigen associated with cell membrane (p. 115) are followed by lethal osmotic injury to the affected cells.

An indication of surface membrane dysfunction frequently encountered following anoxia and certain poisons is osmotic swelling of the cell with accumulation of water in the cytoplasm and resulting separation of organelles (Fig. 1.8 and 1.9). Such intracellular oedema

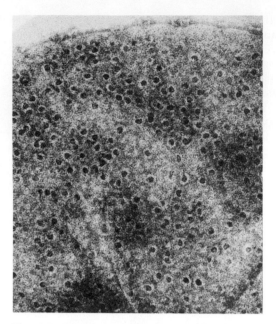

Fig. 1.7 Electron micrograph of part of the cell membrane of *Esch. coli* treated with antibody and complement, followed by treatment with trypsin. Activation of complement at the sites of antigen–antibody reaction has resulted in lesions—apparently holes—in the cell membrane, and these are accentuated by trypsin. × 140 000. (Dr. R. Dourmashkin.)

when reversible is probably in most cases due to increased permeability of the surface membrane to sodium, to failure to remove sodium from the cell consequent upon diminished supply of ATP or to poisoning of the enzymes involved in the sodium pump. Increased cell volume leaves less room for extracellular fluid and this may impair the transport of metabolites between cells and the circulation, with further cell injury. When sodium is taken up by large numbers of cells, for example around extensive burns, there may be severe hyponatraemia (**sick cell syndrome**) which should not be treated by administering sodium.

Hereditary spherocytosis, an anaemia in which the erythrocytes become smaller and more spherical and are unduly prone to destruction in the spleen, illustrates some of the consequences of a lesion of the cell membrane. According to Jacob (1966) the basic defect is an abnormal permeability of the red cell membrane to sodium which tends to accumulate within the cell and stimulates the activity of the sodium pump, the energy being provided by

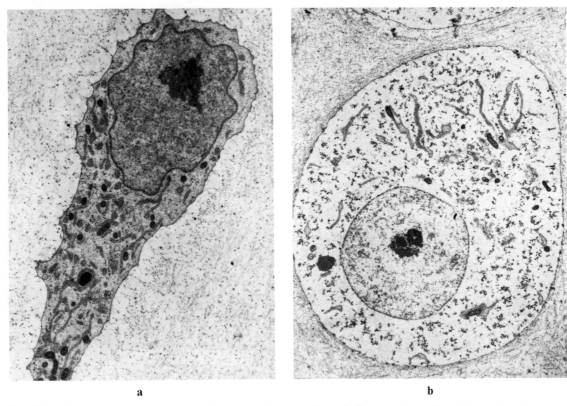

a   b

Fig. 1.8 Electron micrographs of chicken cartilage cells **a** before and **b** after injury by glutamyl-aminoacetonitrile. The damaged cell is swollen due to accumulation of water. × 2500. (Dr. Morag McCallum.)

increased glycolysis. The accelerated sodium transport is effected by cell membrane phospholipid whose metabolism is increased, and this in turn leads to loss of lipid from the cell with diminution of its surface area. The volume of the cell is maintained by its assuming a spherical shape (giving maximum volume for available surface area). The abnormal permeability of the membrane to sodium and the spherical shape of the red cells both contribute to their excessive osmotic fragility in saline *in vitro*, a property long known to be characteristic of hereditary spherocytosis.

Damage to **desmosomes** (the adhesion points of cell membranes which bind epithelial cells together) apparently caused by antibody and complement acting on adjacent intercellular material, is seen in the skin disease pemphigus. The desmosomes of the stratified squamous epithelium of the skin and mucous membranes (the 'prickles' of the prickle cell layer) disappear and the resulting loss of cellular adhesion

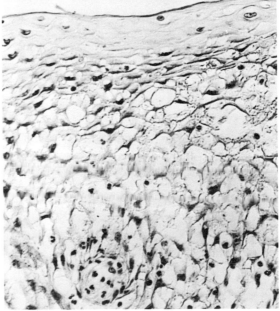

Fig. 1.9 Ballooning of epithelial cells in acute laryngitis. × 250.

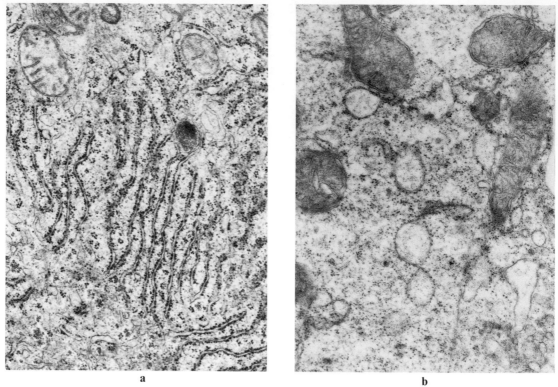

Fig. 1.10 Effect of carbon tetrachloride on the liver cells. **a** Part of normal centrilobular cell of mouse liver: note the regular parallel plates of granular endoplasmic reticulum and discrete clusters of ribosomes. **b** Part of centrilobular mouse liver cell 4 hours after oral administration of carbon tetrachloride. The plates of granular endoplasmic reticulum appear to have segregated into smaller oval vesicles from which many of the ribosomes have become detached and are dispersed singly in the cytoplasmic matrix. Mitochondria show no abnormality. × 21 700. (Dr. Alasdair M. Mackay.)

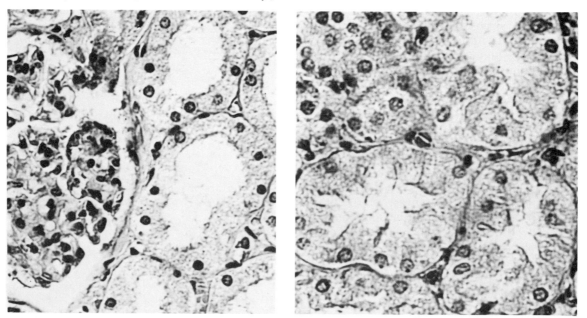

Fig. 1.11 Left, normal kidney. Right, cloudy swelling of renal tubular epithelium, showing cytoplasmic granularity. × 500.

(acantholysis) is expressed in the formation of large intra-epidermal blisters (bullae) containing viable disaggregated prickle cells.

Endoplasmic reticulum. Loss of parallel arrays of endoplasmic reticulum and vacuolation due to accumulation of water within the membrane-lined spaces are frequently encountered as reversible lesions in anoxia and various poisonings, again presumably due to alterations in membrane permeability (Fig. 1.10). The swelling may be so severe in carbon tetrachloride poisoning as to give the cells a ballooned appearance. A marked proliferation of smooth endoplasmic reticulum in liver cells, seen following administration of phenobarbitone for a few days, is interesting in view of the fact that these organelles contain the enzymes responsible for metabolising this drug.

Disaggregation of polyribosomes, presumably associated with decreased production of mRNA, has been noted in ischaemic cell damage and with certain poisons, some of which also cause loss of ribosomal particles from the rough endoplasmic reticulum. The resulting failure of protein synthesis has been corrected in experimental situations by the provision of a synthetic mRNA, but when the outlines of the ribosomal particles, as seen by electron microscopy, become indistinct there is irreversible failure of protein synthesis.

Mitochondria. Diminished oxygen supply quickly interferes with the important mitochondrial function of oxidative phosphorylation— the production of high energy phosphate bonds in ATP by combination of oxygen with hydrogen through the flavoprotein-cytochrome enzyme systems. One minute of ischaemia causes a ten-fold decrease in the ATP:ADP ratio. Mitochondrial function can be restored by a return of adequate oxygenation even after lethal changes have occurred elsewhere in the cell.

Anoxia and many poisons cause reversible osmotic swelling of mitochondria which gives the cell cytoplasm a swollen, cloudy and granular appearance in light microscopy (Fig. 1.11). This change, long known as 'cloudy swelling', is seen especially in metabolically active tissues such as liver, kidney and myocardium, and is exactly the same as that which develops within a few minutes of cessation of the circulation after death of the body or excision of the tissue. For this reason, pathological significance can be

attached to its finding only if pieces of tissue small enough to be permeated rapidly are promptly placed in fixative. Isolated mitochondria can be made to swell and contract *in vitro* by adding calcium ions and ATP respectively to the medium in which the mitochondria are suspended.

Electron microscopy of injured mitochondria, in addition to showing in detail the site of swelling, reveals other abnormalities. A very early indication of anoxic damage is the disappearance of the dense granules occasionally seen in the matrix of normal mitochondria. These bodies are thought to represent lipid-bound calcium which accumulates under the influence of respiration and ATP. A later structural change, characteristic of mitochondrial

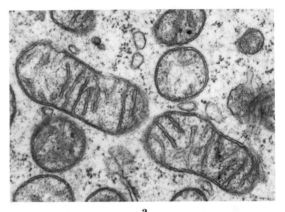

a

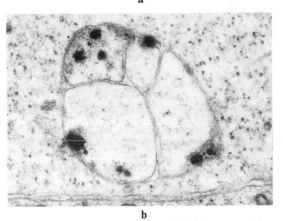

b

Fig. 1.12 Electron micrographs of human erythroblasts. *Above*, mitochondria of normal erythroblast. *Below*, mitochondrion of erythroblast from a patient with sideroblastic anaemia. The mitochondrion is swollen and has an electron-lucent matrix in which lie electron-dense masses of iron-containing material. × 37 400. (Dr. A. M. Mackay.)

damage following various types of cell injury, is development in the matrix of dense poorly defined aggregations of unknown composition. A second type of abnormal mitochondrial inclusion apparently composed of calcium (sometimes as hydroxyapatite) is found in very varied circumstances, e.g. in renal tubular epithelium in nephrocalcinosis due to vitamin D poisoning or to hyperparathyroidism, and in cardiac mitochondria in magnesium deficiency. Dense mitochondrial inclusions (Fig. 1.12) containing iron are found in the red cell precursors in sideroblastic anaemia (p. 486).

Lysosomes. These are cytoplasmic organelles limited by a single membrane. They contain various hydrolase enzymes which act on proteins, fats, carbohydrates, etc. Under the electron microscope they present very varied appearances and can be recognised with certainty only when there is histochemical evidence of acid hydrolase activity. The enzymes have a low pH optimum and become active when the membrane of the **primary lysosome** is altered, e.g. by fusion with a phagocytic vacuole to form a **secondary lysosome** (**phagosome**, or **phagolysosome**).

Lysosomal hydrolases seriously impair the biochemical function and structure of subcellular particles *in vitro* and there has been much speculation on the importance of lysosomal damage in cell injury *in vivo* (see Dingle and Fell, 1973). Damage to the lysosomal membrane leading to release of lysosomal enzymes into the cytoplasm of living cells results in various degrees of cell damage up to necrosis. This happens in certain bacterial infections, e.g. by streptococci, and appears to result from the action of bacterial toxins. It is also encountered in hypervitaminosis A where it is attributed to the surfactant effect of the vitamin on the lysosomal membranes. Another example is the necrosis of macrophages which have ingested silica particles; some of the silica of the particles within phagolysosomes is converted to silicic acid and this forms hydrogen bonds with the phospholipids of the lysosomal membrane which then ruptures and releases the enzymes into the cytoplasm. Some photosensitivity reactions are due to lysosomal membrane damage when certain pigments, e.g. porphyrin, taken up by lysosomes, release energy on exposure to light of appropriate wavelength. Cortisol and chloroquine, drugs known to stabilise lyso-

somal membranes, diminish cell damage in vitamin A poisoning and some photosensitivity reactions. In many forms of cellular injury, however, the 'suicidal' release of lysosomal enzymes into the cytoplasm does not seem to be an important factor. For example, autolysis by lysosomal enzymes in cells injured by hypoxia, carbon tetrachloride and many other poisons occurs only after the cells have become necrotic.

Lysosomes containing membranous structures (e.g. damaged mitochondria) are commonly encountered in cells with focal cytoplasmic damage such as follows irradiation (Fig. 1.13). The damaged parts of the cell are taken into an autophagic vacuole which coalesces with a primary lysosome to form a phagosome, and the activated hydrolases digest the contents of the vacuole. Material resistant to digestion sometimes remains within a lysosome and forms one variety of **residual body** seen on elec-

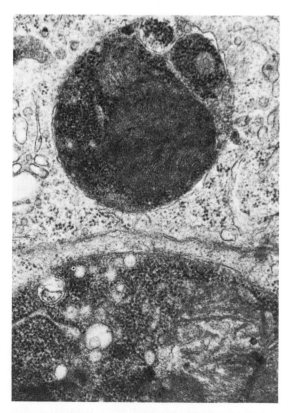

Fig. 1.13 Electron micrograph showing two autophagic vacuoles in adjacent cells of intestinal mucosa of mouse following radiation injury. Mitochondria and glycogen granules can be identified in the large, electron-dense vacuoles. × 57 000.

tron microscopy. Lipofuscin pigment (p. 244) seems to originate from undigested lipid-rich material in this way. The hydrolysis of effete membranous structures and the re-utilisation of the products of digestion are probably of considerable importance in cellular economy.

Several inborn errors of lysosomal function have been described. Most of these involve deficiency of an enzyme and are characterised by progressive accumulation of the appropriate substrate within greatly swollen lysosomes. Some examples of the resulting 'storage diseases' are given on p. 20 and p. 22.

Nuclear damage

The importance of nuclear damage depends on the fact that the cell nucleus contains the genetic information upon which all the vital activities of the cell ultimately depend. Indeed, as already explained, severe nuclear damage indicated by pyknosis and karyolysis are customarily taken as evidence of cell necrosis. It should be remembered, however, that red blood cells, although devoid of a nucleus, maintain selective membrane permeability, produce energy by anaerobic glycolysis and perform their vital specialised function of oxygen transport in the blood for over 100 days in man. Protozoa such as *Amoeba proteus* survive at least for several days following microsurgical removal of their nucleus. Motility and phagocytic activity are arrested but these return together with the ability to reproduce when the nucleus from another amoeba is introduced. It is therefore clear that cells can survive despite total cessation of nuclear function; their metabolic versatility will, however, be greatly reduced and their ability to multiply lost.

Gene mutation. Perhaps the best understood form of nuclear damage is that due to irradiation or to mutagenic chemicals such as nitrogen mustards. These and other unidentified factors may result in errors in the sequence of purine and pyrimidine bases in DNA molecules. If the damage is sufficiently localised, e.g. affecting only one base, it is most unlikely to lead to an alteration in the nucleus demonstrable by available chemical or morphological techniques. Its presence may be inferred if there is an inherited abnormality, e.g. an enzyme deficiency due to incorporation of a 'wrong' amino-acid at a functionally important part of the enzyme

molecule. For example in phenylketonuric oligophrenia, a form of mental deficiency affecting 1 in 20 000 of the population and inherited as a Mendelian recessive, there is deficiency of an enzyme which converts phenylalanine to tyrosine in the liver; in conequence there is a raised concentration of phenylalanine in the blood and cerebrospinal fluid and this results in brain damage. Sickle-cell disease, as already described, is another example of inherited disease due to a single mutation.

In the above examples the mutation has occurred in a germ cell and the resulting abnormality becomes apparent in the descendants of the individual in whom the mutation took place. It is believed that mutation also occurs in cells other than germ cells—**somatic mutation**—but this is likely to be apparent only when the genetically altered cell proliferates to form a large family or clone of similar cells, e.g. when a tumour forms (p. 269) or, in the lymphoid tissues, during stimulation by antigens (p. 104).

Chromosomal abnormalities. Damage to the genetic apparatus more gross than that described above can sometimes be seen when the chromosomes of dividing cells are examined microscopically. An extra chromosome may be found, e.g. three instead of the normal pair of No. 21 chromosomes are commonly present in mongolism (Down's syndrome), (Fig. 1.14), but it is not understood how the chromosome abnormality leads to the physical and mental defects found in this condition. Total absence of one chromosome from all body cells is almost invariably incompatible with survival, with the notable exception of the Y sex chromosome, present in males (XY) but not in normal females (XX). Individuals with one X and no Y chromosome are phenotypically female but have a group of physical abnormalities including dwarfism and failure of ovarian development known as Turner's syndrome. Structural abnormality of chromosomes in the form of deleted portions or added pieces derived from other chromosomes, or unusual shapes such as rings are sometimes found and may be associated with characteristic clinical syndromes (Fig. 1.15). In a familial variety of Down's syndrome the two No. 21 chromosomes are normal but there is an abnormal No. 13 chromosome with an attached extra piece derived from a No. 21. This arises from a

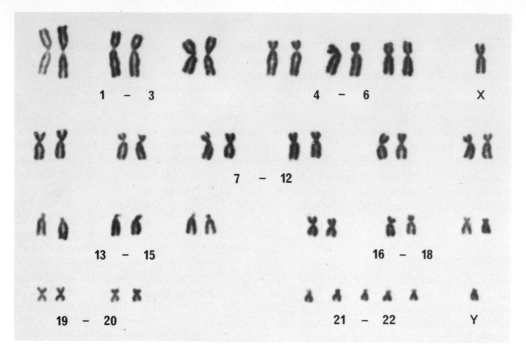

Fig. 1.14 Karyotype in Down's syndrome, showing three No. 21 chromosomes instead of the normal two. (Professor M. A. Ferguson Smith.)

reciprocal exchange of fragments between two chromosomes during meiosis.

As would be expected, the above chromosomal abnormalities affecting all the cells of the body lead to complex abnormalities since many genes must be involved. They arise during meiotic division of germ cells, the presence of an extra chromosome or absence of a chromosome being due to failure of separation of a pair of homologous chromosomes (**non-disjunction**); one of the resulting gametes will have an extra chromosome and the other will be correspondingly defective. Structural chromosomal abnormality is due to chromosome breakage with re-arrangement of fragments during repair. The reciprocal exchange of unequal fragments between non-homologous chromosomes (**translocation**) accounts for the occurrence of abnormally large or small chromosomes.

Abnormal chromosome numbers (**aneuploidy**) and structural chromosomal aberrations are invariably found in the cells of malignant tumours. The best known example of a consistent structural chromosomal aberration in a tumour is the small G chromosomal deletion, the 'Philadelphia' chromosome, present in white and red blood cell precursors in the marrow in chronic myeloid leukaemia (a neoplastic

proliferation of leukocytes). Radiation damage is known to cause chromosomal abnormalities in somatic cells and the frequency of chromosomal breakage has been used to assess exposure to radiation. Aneuploidy and structural abnormalities in individual chromosomes are also found in other circumstances, e.g. in

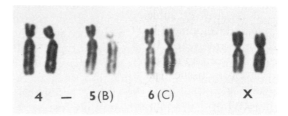

Fig. 1.15 Structural chromosome abnormality; deletion of the short arms of one chromosome 5. (Professor M. A. Ferguson Smith.)

thyroid epithelial cells which have proliferated following stimulation by pituitary thyrotrophic hormone, and in cells damaged by viruses.

The use of staining techniques which demonstrate structural transverse banding patterns is revealing less gross abnormalities and variations in chromosomes and is proving valuable in relating normal and abnormal genes to particular locations on individual chromosomes (**gene mapping**).

Nutritional nuclear damage. An interesting and clinically important form of nuclear damage is encountered in patients deficient in vitamin B_{12} or folic acid. The nuclei are larger than normal but contain less than optimal amounts of DNA for cell division. The chromatin of the large nuclei is arranged in a fine threadlike fashion (Fig. 16.2, p. 451) compared with the condensed masses seen normally (Fig. 16.1, p. 451), and when mitosis occurs the chromosomes in affected individuals are longer and less tightly coiled than normal. These changes occur in many tissues but are best known in the precursors of red cells in the bone marrow which is said to exhibit **megaloblastic erythropoiesis.** In addition to nuclear enlargement in megaloblasts there is increased amount of cytoplasm, cytoplasmic basophilia due to excessive RNA and apparently premature haemoglobinisation as judged by the immature state of the nucleus.

The mechanism of these changes is incompletely understood. Folate plays an essential role in the synthesis of purine bases and of thymine and deficiency of these substances presumably impairs nucleic acid synthesis, especially DNA which, unlike RNA, contains thymine. This could explain the delay of nuclear growth prior to cell division together with prolonged cytoplasmic growth and apparently premature haemoglobinisation. Vitamin B_{12} is thought to influence nuclear structure by affecting folate metabolism (see Chanarin, 1969). Methyl folate is inactive in purine and thymine biosynthesis and one of the main functions of vitamin B_{12} is the transfer of methyl groups from methyl folate for the synthesis of choline. Accordingly, when there is severe vitamin B_{12} deficiency megaloblastic change occurs due to accumulation of methyl folate, and is reversed temporarily by the administration of folic acid, and permanently by life-long administration of vitamin B_{12}.

Abnormal storage of triglyceride fat

Triglycerides (or neutral fats) are glycerol esters of long-chain fatty acids and their storage in excess is a common and conspicuous feature of cell damage. Historically one of the first recognized features of sublethal cellular injury, its mode of development has been a centre of interest for many years. It is important to distinguish between an abnormal increase in the cells of adipose tissue (**pathological obesity**—or, when the condition is localised, **pathological adiposity**) and the accumulation of fat in other types of cell (**fatty change**). The two processes are quite distinct although in pathological obesity fat also commonly accumulates in the liver cells.

Over 95% of the triglyceride in the diet is normally absorbed in the small intestine: much of it is hydrolysed in the gut into free fatty acids and monoglycerides, but these are re-esterified in the jejunal mucosal cells and passed into the lymphatics and thence to the plasma as microscopically visible particles of complex composition termed **chylomicrons.** Reduction in size of the particles, and some hydrolysis, is effected by lipoprotein lipase; the resulting glycerol and fatty acids are removed from the plasma by the cells of various tissues, including the liver. Some of the fatty acid is oxidised to provide energy, but much of it is re-esterified to triglyceride which is combined with protein, phospholipids, cholesterol and cholesterol esters to form the **pre-beta lipoproteins** which are then secreted into the plasma, and provide the means of transporting triglyceride in water-soluble form. These pre-beta plasma lipoproteins rich in triglyceride are of very low density (0·95–1·006): they re-cycle through the liver, but are also taken up by the cells of the fat depots and of other tissues, where the triglyceride is either used for energy or stored. Triglyceride stored in adipose tissue is continuously being hydrolysed, and the fatty acids secreted into the plasma where they are carried in combination with albumin. These so-called **free fatty acids** are taken up by muscle for the production of energy and by the cells of the liver, where they are either oxidised or re-esterified with glycerol to form triglyceride.

The control of these major metabolic processes is influenced by food intake and also by various hormonal and emotional factors: insulin stimulates the deposition of triglyceride in the adipose tissue depots; adrenal hormones (probably catecholamines and corticosteroids acting together) stimulate hydrolysis in the depots and release of fatty acids into the plasma, as does growth hormone and also thyroxine. The rate of uptake of triglyceride and fatty acids by various other tissues, particularly the liver, is dependent on their concentrations in the plasma. Starvation results in release of fatty acids from the depots, and this is suppressed after a fatty meal. In addition to that provided by the diet, triglyceride is synthesised within the body, particularly in the liver and adipose tissues, from glucose, amino acids and fatty acids, and enters the metabolic pathways outlined above.

Fatty change

This is the accumulation of fat in cells other than adipose tissue cells, and was previously subdivided into fatty infiltration and fatty degeneration. It is due to imbalance between fat and fatty acids entering the cell and the rate of utilisation or release of fat by the cell. Probably all parenchymal cells which accumulate an abnormal amount of fat are injured. Even the gross fatty change seen in the liver in obesity (p. 606) can be regarded as a form of injury to the liver cells due to the disturbed fat metabolism resulting from overeating.

Because of its major role in fat metabolism, the liver requires special consideration in fatty change. However, fatty change is seen not only in the liver cells, which are usually most seriously affected, but also in various other organs and tissues. The cells most prone to undergo fatty change are the parenchymal cells of the various organs, and skeletal and heart muscle cells, i.e. the cells which because of their specialised functions have a high metabolic activity. Part of their energy is normally supplied by the oxidation of fatty acids, provided largely by uptake from the plasma of free fatty acids released from the fat depots, and lipoproteins secreted mainly by the liver.

Microscopic appearances. In fatty change of most organs, small droplets, consisting mainly of triglyceride, appear in the cytoplasm of the affected cells. Even in an advanced stage the droplets remain small and discrete, and do not greatly enlarge the cell (Fig. 1.16). In the liver, however, they may fuse to form much larger droplets (Fig. 1.17) and the liver cells may be greatly distended. In most instances, the centrilobular cells are affected first and most severely, but in phosphorus poisoning the change may be very severe and yet confined to

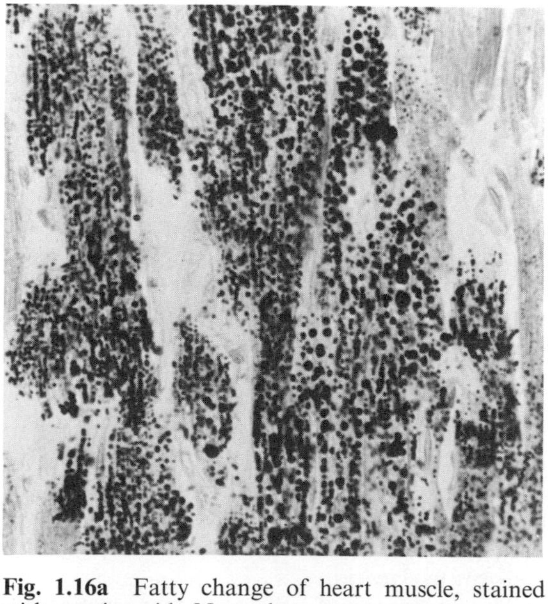

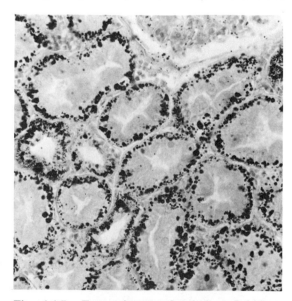

Fig. 1.16a Fatty change of heart muscle, stained with osmic acid. Note the very numerous minute intracellular droplets arranged in rows. × 380.

Fig. 1.16b Fatty change of tubules of kidney, stained with osmic acid. × 325.

the cells in the outer part of the lobules. The distribution of these lesions has not been fully explained.

Electron microscopy shows the fat globules to lie free in the cytoplasmic matrix, without a limiting membrane.

Causes of fatty change. The three major causes of fatty change are (*a*) hypoxia, (*b*) starvation and wasting diseases, and (*c*) numerous chemicals and bacterial toxins.

(a) Hypoxia. The hypoxia resulting from chronic anaemia is a common cause of fatty change in the various organs and tissues. In the liver it occurs especially in the central zone of the lobules, which receives the poorest supply of oxygenated blood, while in the heart it is more marked in parts farthest from the arterioles, that is, it is pararterial in distribution. The change may be seen through the endocardium as a fine mottled pallor ('thrush breast') of the myocardium of the left ventricle and papillary muscles.

Another example of fatty change in hypoxia is in the centrilobular liver cells in chronic venous congestion (p. 194). The fatty change commonly present in the cells of rapidly growing tumours is probably of the same nature, although in both these instances there is inadequate blood supply or flow, and not just hypoxia.

(b) Starvation and wasting diseases. Fatty change is observed in the liver and to a smaller extent in the myocardium and elsewhere in some patients who, previously well nourished, have died of a wasting disease such as gastric carcinoma or pulmonary tuberculosis. In other instances of equally or even more severe wasting, fatty change is not found. This has been explained by Dible and his co-workers (1941) who demonstrated experimentally that fat accumulates in the cells of the liver and other tissues under conditions of near-starvation so long as some adipose tissue remains. Once the fat depots are depleted, the fatty change disappears. The low food intake in wasting diseases leads to excessive lipolysis in the depots and release of fatty acids into the blood: these are taken up in increased amounts by the cells of various tissues and converted to triglyceride. Failure of carbohydrate metabolism resulting from the low caloric intake may also be of importance by interfering with intracellular oxidative breakdown of fatty acids, particularly in the liver.

The fatty change in uncontrolled **diabetes mellitus** is attributable mainly to excessive release of fatty acids from the fat depots and impaired carbohydrate metabolism, both of which are a consequence of deficiency of insulin. The situation is thus similar to that in starvation, and in both conditions oxidation of fatty acids in the liver is incomplete and partial breakdown products, acetoacetic and hydroxybutyric acids, escape into the blood, resulting in ketosis. The subject is discussed more fully on p. 965.

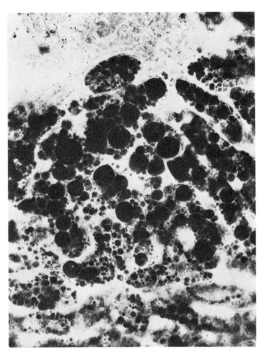

Fig. 1.17 Fatty change of liver. The cells are filled with large globules of fat. (Stained with Sudan IV.) × 190.

Where a wasting disease is attributable to a toxic condition or complicated by severe infection, this may further impair hepatic fat metabolism, as explained below: a good example is provided by infantile gastro-enteritis due to certain strains of *Esch. coli*, in which dietary intake is severely impaired by anorexia, vomiting and diarrhoea, and the liver is subjected to toxins absorbed from the infected gut. The liver usually shows gross fatty change in fatal cases.

(c) Chemical and bacterial toxins. Of the many simple chemicals which can cause fatty change, phosphorus, carbon tetrachloride and puromycin are well-known examples. As in fatty change from other causes, the liver is usually most severely affected, but the changes are widespread, and may involve not only parenchymal cells, but also vascular endothelium and connective tissue cells. Fatty change is also a feature of severe infections, e.g. typhoid, smallpox and septicaemias.

Two factors are involved in the production of fatty change by chemicals and toxins. Firstly, they directly injure the cells; secondly they produce anorexia and often vomiting, and the low calorie intake results, as described above, in increased mobilisation of fatty acids from the depots. The nature of the cell injuries by many chemicals and toxins and the way these cause fatty change is by no means fully understood.

As a result of recent experimental investigations, it has been established that fatty change in the liver is attributable largely to reduced production of lipoprotein. The triglyceride which would normally have been released as lipoprotein thus accumulates in the liver cells. This applies to fatty change induced in rats by administration of chlorinated hydrocarbons, ethionine, phosphorus, puromycin, orotic acid or a diet deficient in choline. The fatty change induced by these agents is preceded by a fall in the very low-density lipoproteins which carry triglyceride and the reduced amount of lipoprotein present in the plasma shows a diminution of protein : fat ratio. The nature of the impaired lipoprotein production has not been established with certainty, but the present evidence suggests that some of the agents responsible, e.g. carbon tetrachloride, phosphorus, puromycin and ethionine, impair the hepatic production of proteins. This has not, however, been demonstrated following administration of orotic acid or a diet deficient in choline, and the mechanisms of fatty change induced by these agents are unknown. There is some evidence that choline deficiency impairs the production of phospholipids, which are an essential constituent of lipoproteins.

It still remains to explain how the various chemicals and toxins which cause fatty change in the liver affect also the cells of various other tissues. With the exception of the intestinal mucosa, which shares with the liver the property of converting fat to lipoprotein, tissue cells in general expend fat mainly by oxidative breakdown. It therefore seems likely that the various chemicals and toxins which produce widespread fatty change interfere in some way with this latter process.

Effects. Fatty change results from cell injury, but there is no constant relationship between fatty change and other signs of cell damage. For example, liver cell necrosis in virus hepatitis is not accompanied by any significant degree of fatty change, but there is severe fatty change associated with liver cell necrosis in phosphorus poisoning. Also the gross fatty change in the liver which may accompany obesity or alcoholism is not itself associated with severely impaired hepatic function.

Fat accumulates less rapidly in the other organs than in the liver, but as in the liver, the important factor is the severity of the cell injury which has caused the fatty change.

Fatty change in the heart may indicate severe myocardial injury, and heart failure may result from any undue strain. For example, in severe anaemia attributable to a lesion requiring surgical intervention, such as recurrent haemorrhage from a peptic ulcer, it is important that, when practicable, the anaemia should be treated and time allowed for the myocardium to return to normal before any major operation is undertaken. The administration of a large volume of blood or packed red cells over a short period carries a risk of overloading the impaired myocardium, especially if followed immediately by major surgery.

Pathological obesity

Obesity, the accumulation of excessive amounts of adipose tissue, is a subject in which it is difficult, if not impossible, to draw a sharp dividing line between the physiological and pathological states. However, there is no doubt that gross obesity is harmful, and must be regarded as pathological.

Basically, obesity is very simply explained, being due to a dietary intake of calories beyond those expended to provide energy for the body's metabolism. It is thus attributable to overeating, particularly of carbohydrates and fats, often combined with lack of exercise. Attempts to demonstrate metabolic differences between fat and thin people, e.g. in efficiency in intestinal absorption or basal metabolic rate have, in general, been unsuccessful and the problem of obesity appears to reside mainly in the elucidation of the factors which result in over-eating, a subject involving psychological factors which will not be discussed here. Despite lack of scientific evidence, however, some individuals seem to be predisposed to obesity more than others, and genetic factors may be involved. It has been observed that when healthy young adults are given a high calorie diet and kept at rest in bed, those who are overweight gain more weight than the thinner subjects. The activity of the thyroid gland, by influencing the rate of general metabolism, has an important influence on energy expenditure, and the pituitary, adrenals and gonads all influence the amount of fat deposited. Damage to the hypothalamus with deficiency of pituitary secretion in early life leads to adiposity along with failure of sexual development, and there is evidence that some forms of obesity in the adult are of similar causation. Extreme degrees of adiposity can be induced in rats by small precisely placed experimental lesions in the tuber cinereum, the mode of action of which appears to be the development of a voracious appetite.

Gross abnormalities of the hypothalamus or of endocrine function have not been demonstrated in the great majority of obese subjects investigated, but it may be that more subtle variations in the functioning of these organs are of importance.

Structural changes. Apart from the increase in size of the normal depots, e.g. the subcutaneous tissue, the omentum, retroperitoneal tissues and epicardium, adipose tissue in obesity may extend to tissue where it is normally absent. For example, in pathological adiposity of the heart, fat extends along the lines of connective tissue through the heart wall (Fig. 1.18), and leads to atrophy of the muscle fibres and consequent weakening of the wall to such an

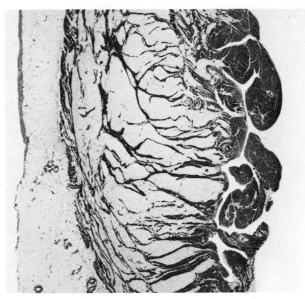

Fig. 1.18 Pathological adiposity of heart. The whole thickness of the wall of the right ventricle is infiltrated with adipose tissue extending from the epicardial layer between the muscle fibres which are consequently atrophied. Even the columnae carneae are involved. × 6.

extent that the right ventricle may rupture. A similar accumulation of stromal fat occurs in the pancreas.

In obese individuals, the liver may be grossly enlarged by accumulation of large droplets of fat in the liver cells. This is discussed on p. 606.

Effects. Apart from the limitations imposed on physical activity by obesity, it has long been recognised, and notably by life insurance companies, that obesity is associated with a reduced expectation of life attributable to an increased incidence of high blood pressure, coronary artery disease, heart failure, chronic bronchitis and respiratory infections, and late-onset diabetes mellitus. The high and increasing incidence of obesity in affluent societies poses a major health problem.

Abnormal storage of other lipids

The lipids of the body other than triglyceride are chemically very heterogeneous and include sterols (cholesterol and its esters), phospholipids and complex lipids (e.g. glycolipids). These substances are frequently united with proteins to form lipoproteins some of which constitute the insoluble membranes of cells while others are soluble and play an important part in the transport of triglyceride in suspension in the plasma. Many diseases are known in which one or some of these substances accumulate in cells in abnormal amounts. By far the most important is **atheroma**, a poorly understood disorder in which various lipids including sterols, phospholipids and triglyceride accumulate in the intima of arteries and cause narrowing or occlusion of the lumen with consequent impairment of blood flow.

Most of the the other disorders are much less common but illustrate interesting principles. Pathological accumulation of lipids other than triglycerides within cells may develop in the following ways.

Inherited deficiency of lysosomal enzymes

Cells may be overloaded following autophagy of their structural lipids or lipids derived from their neighbours. A good example is the rare disease due to inherited deficiency of the lysosomal sulphatase enzyme responsible for the hydrolysis of cerebroside sulphate. As might be expected, the predominant lesions are found in the nervous system where the substrate is particularly abundant. The acid cerebroside sulphate gives a metachromatic reaction with such stains as acidified cresyl violet, and since the lesion is most obvious in the white matter of the brain the disease is known as 'metachromatic leukodystrophy'. Electron microscopy shows lamellated inclusion bodies within lysosomes of affected nerve and glial cells, and similar material lying in extracellular spaces. Other comparable cerebral lipidoses are described on p. 707.

In Gaucher's disease, an inherited deficiency of a lysosomal β-glucosidase leads to intracellular accumulation of glucocerebroside. Neurones and macrophages in the liver and bone marrow are frequently affected but the most striking changes are found in the spleen which may be enormously enlarged probably due to storage of lipid from effete erythrocytes which are removed from the circulation by the spleen as part of its normal function. Gaucher cells present a typical histological appearance (p. 511) and electron microscopy shows large vacuoles containing tubular material. Probably as a result of the lysosomal enlargement, there is a marked increase in acid phosphatase in the spleen and in the serum in this disease.

Metachromatic leucodystrophy and Gaucher's disease illustrate the great differences between lesions due to inherited deficiency of enzymes responsible for intracellular breakdown of lipids and demonstrate some of the reasons for these differences.

Disordered plasma lipid transport

Several inherited abnormalities of plasma lipoproteins are known which lead to massive accumulation of lipid in macrophages. These cells become spherical and enlarged due to the presence of numerous lipid vacuoles which give the cytoplasm a foamy appearance (Fig. 1.19).

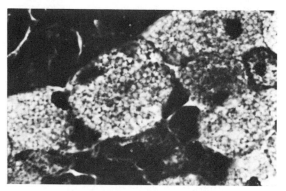

Fig. 1.19 Histiocytes distended with multiple fine droplets of doubly-refractile lipid. Photographed through crossed polarising prisms. $\times$ 500.

The predominant lipids stored are cholesterol esters which are seen to be doubly refractile when viewed under the microscope with polarised light (Fig. 1.20). Large accumulations of these cells (often accompanied by extracellular lipid deposits) may form nodules called **xanthomas** because of their yellow and tumour-like appearance.

In the rare **familial α-lipoprotein deficiency** there is a moderate increase in the plasma level of triglyceride which is associated with β-lipoproteins as unstable complexes. These are phagocytosed by macrophages in the spleen, liver, tonsils and lymph nodes, all of which organs become enlarged due to accumulation of cholesterol esters which are presumably derived from the β-lipoprotein. Great enlargement of the tonsils, orange in colour due to the stored lipid, is a unique finding in this disease.

Familial hyperchylomicronaemia, apparently due to inherited deficiency of serum lipoprotein

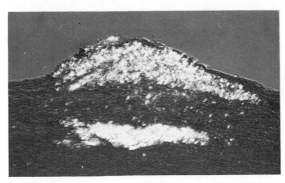

Fig. 1.20 Deposition of doubly-refractile lipid in early atheroma of aorta, photographed by polarised light.

lipase, is characterised by a milky appearance of the serum due to chylomicrons which are not cleared from the plasma at the normal rate. There is lipid storage in the enlarged liver and spleen and xanthomas may be found in the dermis. It is of interest that in both of the above diseases the stored lipid is predominantly cholesterol ester although the main elevation in serum lipid affects the triglycerides. Presumably the latter are broken down following phagocytosis by the macrophages, leaving a steadily increasing residue of less digestible esters of cholesterol. The steroid nucleus cannot readily be broken down and is mainly disposed of by excretion.

Familial hyperbetalipoproteinaemia is a relatively common disorder, inherited as a Mendelian dominant, in which the plasma β-lipoprotein is greatly increased. Cholesterol, an important integral part of the lipoprotein molecule, is correspondingly raised, hence the old name 'familial hypercholesterolaemia'. There is little elevation in triglycerides and the plasma is not milky. Atheroma, fatal even in childhood in rare homozygous individuals, and in many cases xanthomas affecting skin and tendon sheaths, increase with time and parallel in severity the plasma lipoprotein abnormality.

These, and several other inherited lipoprotein disorders, illustrate the varied metabolic abnormalities underlying excessive storage of cholesterol esters in foam cells in different parts of the body. Hyperlipoproteinaemia also develops secondary to other diseases; for example, transitory hyperchylomicronaemia is encountered sometimes when severe diabetes mellitus is inadequately controlled and secondary hyperbetalipoproteinaemia, reversible by thyroxine therapy, is seen in hypothyroidism. These and other disorders (e.g. obstructive jaundice, pancreatitis, alcoholism and nephrotic syndrome) may be associated with various forms of hyperlipoproteinaemia.

Other lipid depositions

Submucosal aggregates of foam cells are often found in the gallbladder giving it a 'strawberry' appearance (Fig. 19.55, p. 646); presumably this results from intracellular storage of part of the cholesterol that is normally reabsorbed from the bile.

The important subject of atheroma will be considered later (p. 312). Suffice it to say here that pressure filtration of lipoprotein from the plasma into the intimal layer of the arteries leads to a difficult problem in disposing of the associated cholesterol by the local population of modified smooth muscle cells. At first the filtered lipid is found within these cells but these are quickly overwhelmed and most of the accumulated lipid eventually lies in an extracellular position. As already indicated, atheroma is particularly prone to develop in individuals with certain of the inherited lipoprotein abnormalities; it seems to result also from modern western dietary habits which lead to alterations in serum lipoproteins and lipids.

Abnormal glycogen storage

The normal human body contains approximately 500 grams of glycogen, present mainly in muscle and liver cells, but also found in small amounts in the other tissues. Glycogen is a water-soluble branched polymer, composed exclusively of glucose units, and is broken down by enzymes (glycogenolysis) when reserves of glucose are needed to meet the body's energy requirements, e.g. during muscular exercise. The depolymerisation is effected mainly by phosphorylase enzymes which liberate glucose 1-phosphate, and this in turn is converted into glucose 6-phosphate which can be used for the intrinsic metabolic needs of the cell. For the maintenance of blood glucose levels during fasting and exercise, glucose 6-phosphate must be converted to glucose before release from the cell, and this happens almost exclusively in the liver, but also in the kidney, both of which contain the necessary enzyme, glucose 6-phosphatase.

Largely as a result of the brilliant biochemical studies of G. E. Cori, at least six distinct inherited **glycogen storage diseases** have been recognised, each associated with a different single enzyme deficiency. In several forms of the disease, the affected organs are enlarged due to an increased content of glycogen. Histological examination of sections stained by haematoxylin and eosin reveals clear unstained material distending the affected cells (Fig. 1.21); histochemical confirmation of the nature of the material is given by Best's carmine, or the periodic acid Schiff (PAS) stain (with and without prior hydrolysis of the section with diastase), and this is most satisfactorily obtained with tissue fixed promptly in alcohol in which glycogen is insoluble. Glycogen also has a characteristic appearance on electron microscopy, occurring as dense particles larger than ribosomes; these sometimes form rosette-like clusters (Fig. 1.22).

In **von Gierke's disease** (Cori Type 1) there is deficiency of glucose 6-phosphatase, an enzyme which is associated with the endoplasmic reticulum. The resulting failure to convert glucose 6-phosphate to glucose for release into the circulation leads to hypoglycaemia and a tendency to increased glycogen storage in liver and kidney, the organs which normally contain glucose 6-phosphatase. As a consequence of the excessive glycogen storage, these organs become enormously enlarged. The disordered carbohydrate metabolism leads to increased lipogenesis and raised serum levels of triglyceride (in the form of low density pre β-lipoprotein), xanthomatosis, obesity, fatty change in the liver and ketoacidosis. The affected children also show retarded growth.

Pompe's disease (Cori Type 2) has recently been shown to result from an inherited deficiency of the lysosomal enzyme acid α-glucosidase which is normally present in all tissues and presumably hydrolyses the small

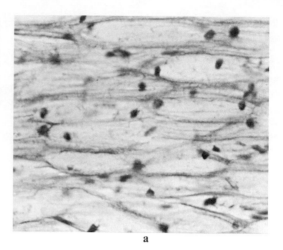

a

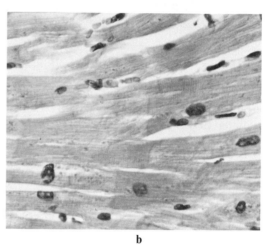

b

Fig. 1.21 Myocardium in Pompe's disease **a**, compared with normal myocardium **b**. The affected muscle fibres are distended with glycogen and appear vacuolated. × 460.

amount of glycogen which enters lysosomes during autophagy. In Pompe's disease, the glycogen taken into α-glucosidase-deficient lysosomes persists and accumulates, being inaccessible to the general cytoplasm with its normal complement of phosphorylase and other enzymes in the major glycogenolytic pathway. Accordingly much of the stored glycogen is seen by electron microscopy to be within greatly enlarged lysosomes, and it seems likely that the serious cellular dysfunction encountered in Pompe's disease is the result of lysosomal rupture and spilling of harmful hydrolases into the general cytoplasm of the cell. This explains most of the features of

Pompe's disease, namely generalised glycogen storage—e.g. in myocardium, skeletal muscle, nervous and lymphoid tissue, and peripheral blood leukocytes—enlargement of organs, cardiac failure, mental deficiency, severe muscle weakness and absence of hypoglycaemia.

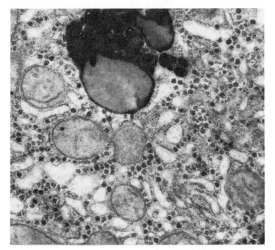

Fig. 1.22 Electron micrograph of normal liver showing the characteristic small, dense, round particles of glycogen. The large dense organelle at the top of the field is a residual body. × 16 000.

Other extremely rare forms of glycogen storage disease include deficiency of muscle phosphorylase (**McArdle's syndrome**) which results in rapid muscle fatigue without hypoglycaemia, and deficiency of liver phosphorylase which causes hepatomegaly and hypoglycaemia.

Of great interest is the deficiency of the enzyme responsible for the branching of the tree-like glycogen molecule during its synthesis: in this condition the stored glycogen has an abnormal structure which impairs the effectiveness of phosphorylase by steric hindrance.

In contrast to the rare disorders described above in which deficiency of a particular enzyme satisfactorily explains most of the observed pathological findings, increased glycogen storage is found in many other disorders but the mechanisms involved are usually obscure. In diabetes mellitus, a serious disorder of carbohydrate metabolism characterised by diminished ability to utilise glucose, there is increased glycogen deposition in cardiac muscle, in Henle's tubules in the kidney, in liver cell nuclei, in polymorphonuclear leukocytes and in the hydropic β-cells seen in acute cases in young subjects in the pancreatic islets; the glycogen content of skeletal muscle is, however, reduced. More glycogen than normal is found in polymorphs in acute inflammation, in recently formed pus and in the peripheral blood when there is a leukocytosis. Glycogen is abundant in embryonic tissues and in some malignant tumours but in these its occurrence is more closely related to the tissue of origin than to the growth activity. It is particularly constant in clear cell carcinoma of kidney.

Cell damage due to ionising radiation

Because of the widespread use of radiation and radioactive materials in industry and medicine the study of their effects on living matter is now of great importance. Of all the branches of radiation biology—molecular, sub-cellular, cellular, organ and whole animal—cellular radiation biology is the most instructive in the present state of knowledge. This is firstly because the measurement of effects in terms of cellular units makes quantitation fairly easy. Secondly, it is mainly by the study and analysis of cellular effects that information can be obtained on molecular and sub-cellular processes in the development and repair of radiation damage. Thirdly, it appears that effects at the level of whole organs or whole animals can often, to a first approximation at least, be described or explained on the basis of cellular injury. This third principle will be illustrated below in terms of the impaired ability of sub-lethally irradiated cells to divide, although the properties which actually characterise a multicellular organism will result in effects which cannot be explained purely by the known properties of individual cells.

Radiation causes its effects by transferring energy to the substance through which it passes. This energy can produce two changes, excitation or ionisation. Excitation is a change in the energy state of some electrons or charged parts of molecules. Radiations which, like ultraviolet light, produce excitations only, are of very low penetrating power and are not discussed in this section. Other radiations produce mixtures of ionisations and excitations.

No widely useful and accurate biological method of measuring radiation dose has so far been developed. This is because the ultimate biological effects produced are very complex. The standard methods of measuring radiation dose are purely physical. The first is based on the application of a voltage to an air-filled chamber through which the ionising radiation passes. This voltage has the effect of separating the positive and negative electric charges produced by the ionisations. The flow of these charges under the influence of the applied voltage constitutes a small electric current which can be measured with great sensitivity and accuracy. The unit of dose measured by ionisation in air is the *roentgen*. This method neglects the excitations produced by the radiation.

The second method of measuring radiation dose is based on the measurement of the total energy absorbed from a beam of radiation by a solid material. The material must be one in which no radiation-produced chemical energy can be stored, all of it being transformed into heat which can be measured by sensitive calorimetry. The unit of absorbed dose is the *rad*.*

Much research has been done on the effects of radiation on aqueous solutions; these are mediated primarily through the decomposition products of the water, and probably reflect the initial damage produced in living biological material. However, this initial damage has never been directly observed. The effects which are observed are the result of an interaction, one side of which is the disruption of the complex of normal biochemical processes arising from the initial molecular damage; the other is the response of the cell or organism in trying to overcome the disruption. From an analysis of these effects much has been learned about the nature of the disruption and repair, but very much more still remains unknown.

Ionising radiations fall into three categories; electromagnetic radiation, charged particles and uncharged particles. The ionisation is caused by

the charged particles—electrons, protons or uncharged particles produce charged particles.

All of these radiations can be administered to animals and human beings externally or internally. External sources include x-ray machines, electron or other charged particle accelerators, high activity γ-ray sources, neutron generators, nuclear reactors and atomic bombs. Internal irradiation arises from the ingestion of any of the hundreds of known radionuclides (radioactive isotopes) many of which are used for medical diagnostic or therapeutic purposes, for commercial non-destructive testing and for irradiating materials for industrial purposes; they are produced in nuclear reactors.† The best known severe radiation damage from accidental ingestion of radioactive material is that produced by radium which was once used extensively in luminising paints. Some sufferers from radium poisoning have been under medical supervision for up to fifty years and the effects are well documented. Today, in spite of strict regulations and control, occasional accidents occur in nuclear reactors, industry and hospitals, which result in significant radiation of personnel. Ionising radiation for diagnosis and therapy, however, has a secure and important place in modern medicine and has been essential for many research purposes.

Cellular radiation effects

The foundation of the quantitative study of cellular radiation effects is the survival curve, based on the ability of cells to produce clones of daughter cells in appropriate environmental conditions. One of the most marked effects of radiation is the destruction of this ability. The number of cells in which the ability survives can be readily measured by counting the number of clones in cultures of the irradiated cells.

The percentage 'survival', that is, the percentage of cells which still retain the ability to produce clones after irradiation, is plotted on a logarithmic scale and the radiation dose is plotted on a linear scale (Fig. 1.23). Since log percentage survival decreases continuously with increasing dosage, the origin is placed in the top

* The *rad* is likely to be replaced by the *gray* (Gy) after a British radiologist who did fundamental work on the oxygen effect described below.

† The dose is measured in *curies*, but these are now to become becquerels (Bq) after the French scientist who discovered radioactivity.

left corner of the figure. The resultant curve usually approximates to a straight line after an initial shoulder. This shoulder shows that an accumulation of sub-lethal damage is necessary before an observable effect is produced. After sufficient dose has been given to reach the straight portion of the survival curve, no further accumulation of sub-lethal damage occurs. If, however, the cells are allowed to recover for some hours, it is found that once again a considerable accumulation of sub-lethal damage is

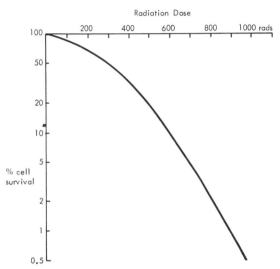

Fig. 1.23 Radiation injury, showing the relationship between percentage cell survival and dose of ionising radiation.

necessary before the radiation effects are produced with maximum efficiency. It appears that the shoulder therefore represents the repair process by which the cells can overcome some of the damage.

The slope of the portion of the survival curve which is almost straight on the log-linear plot of Fig. 1.23—the exponential part—represents the rate at which additional lethal damage is produced as additional dose is administered. The fact that this portion of the curve is almost straight means that, irrespective of the damage already created, a given amount of irradiation always reduces the survival by the same fraction. This kind of relationship is indicative of an effect controlled by probability. In this case it is usually regarded as the probability of the track of ionisations, produced by charged particles, causing damage to small discrete targets in the cells.

The available evidence suggests that, for each type of radiation, no great differences exist in the slopes of survival curves for various types of mammalian cells, unless they are hypoxic when irradiated. The magnitude of the shoulder, however, is dependent on the history, the environment, and the biochemical condition of the cells.

Survival curves referring to different types of radiation have different shapes. The reason for this is that although, for equal doses of different radiations, the total number of ionisations are equal, the geometrical distribution of these ionisations in the cell can vary greatly. These large variations in distribution have a considerable effect on the mean number of ionisations necessary to produce the kind of biological damage which, after complex development, results in a cell losing its ability to continue to divide.

Heavy charged particles moving relatively slowly produce dense columns of ionisations, while electrons produce sparse lines of ionisations with occasional small clumps (Fig. 1.24).

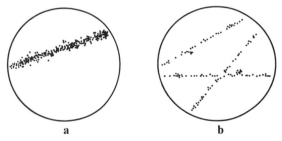

Fig. 1.24 The distribution of ionisations for high LET radiation **a** and low LET radiation **b**.

The average amount of energy deposited per micron of track of a particle or photon is called the linear energy transfer (LET) and can be used to characterise the quality of the radiation. A number of ionisations grouped closely together are more likely to initiate a lethal chain of biological events than the same number of ionisations widely separated. The dense group of ionisations also prevents the cellular repair mechanisms from acting effectively. Thus the survival curves for high LET radiation such as a-particles show no shoulder, and have a steeper slope than those for low LET radiation such as x-rays or electrons (Fig. 1.25). For both these reasons a dose of high LET radiation produces far more biological damage than an equal dose of low LET radiation.

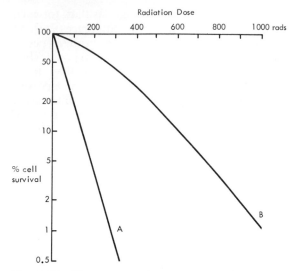

Fig. 1.25 The comparative cytotoxic effects of α particles (A) and electrons (B).

Another factor which has a striking effect on survival curves is the presence or absence of oxygen. Oxygen has the ability to combine with freshly severed ends of molecular structures thus preventing them from rejoining, which they commonly do if the opportunity presents itself. Oxygen thus interferes with a natural recovery process—a different one from that which produces the shoulder—and causes a given dose of radiation to be much more damaging than it would be in hypoxic or anoxic conditions. The ratio of the doses required to reduce the survival to the same level in anoxic

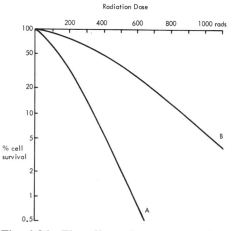

Fig. 1.26 The effect of oxygen on the cytotoxic effect of x-irradiation. A, high oxygen tension; B, low oxygen tension.

and normal conditions is called the oxygen enhancement ratio (OER) (Fig. 1.26).

There are many other radio-sensitisers and radio-protectors which affect different levels of recovery and repair processes. Estimation of the biological damage produced by a given dose of radiation must therefore take into account both the type of radiation, the environment in which it is administered and the time allowed for repair and recovery.

Tissue radiation effects

The effect of radiation in destroying the ability of cells to continue dividing has been discussed above in relation to individual cells. It is important because it plays a major part in causing tissue effects. Cell function which is not related to mitosis and division is relatively insensitive to radiation. Much higher doses of radiation are required to produce gross changes in such function than are required to inhibit cell division. Hence the typical radiation effect on tissues arises from an inhibition of division.

Tissues whose cells are undergoing continuous controlled division, and whose integrity requires a continual flow of new cells are therefore the first tissues to show the effects of radiation. The most obvious are the skin, the intestinal tract, the bone marrow and the immunity system. Similar considerations apply to the therapeutic use of radiation for malignant tumours, in which there is excessive division of cells. The initial effect upon a tissue is a reduction in cell numbers as the supply of new cells falls below the normal rate. The drop in cell numbers leads via homoeostatic feedback mechanisms to a build up of the population of viable stem-cells from which new cells are produced, and to an increase in the rate of cell division. If this compensation is successful, then in due course enhanced production of cells not only restores the depleted population but commonly results in a temporary hyperplasia or overshoot before the cell numbers return to normal (Fig. 1.27).

The fall, rise, overshoot and return to normal of the cell populations exhibiting such behaviour after irradiation can be understood and explained in cellular terms if the appropriate homoeostatic feedback mechanisms are known. The normal cell turnover controls the rate at which the cell population falls following

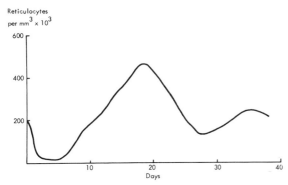

Reticulocytes
per mm^3 × 10^3

Fig. 1.27 Changes in the numbers of reticulocytes in the blood following 200 rads whole-body irradiation.

irradiation. The extent of the fall depends on the percentage of surviving cells and the rate at which they can divide.

If the cell population of a tissue falls below a critical value the tissue can lose its functional effectiveness. In the cases of the intestinal tract and the bone marrow the result is death of the individual. A rapidly administered x-ray dose of about 800 rads to the bone marrow and 1200 rads to the intestinal tract reduces the number of surviving cells to such low levels that the delay before an adequate production of cells can be re-established is long enough to allow the cell population to fall below the critical value.

The cells whose reproductive ability has been destroyed by the irradiation often remain in the tissue for some time. Their abortive attempts to divide or prepare to divide can produce gross abnormalities in cytological appearance (Fig. 1.28). Toxic products of cell disintegration can increase the damage. However, the damaged cells are no longer directly relevant to the course of events leading to permanent damage or repair. This course is determined by the number of surviving cells still capable of division and by the kinetics of proliferation in the tissue. Ultimately, however, if a large enough dose is given (about 1800 rads in a single exposure) a tissue condition described as the *limit of tolerance* is reached. Although the nature of this is not understood, it is the determining factor for radiotherapy, and represents an accumulation of permanent, irreparable damage.

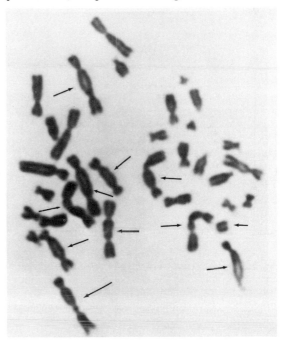

Fig. 1.29 Dividing lymphocyte in peripheral blood culture from a patient with bronchial carcinoma and spinal metastases, treated by five 500 rads of Co^{60} radiation to the lumbar spine. This cell shows the result of extensive chromosome breakage followed by random fusion of broken ends due to radiation. There are nine dicentric chromosomes, one possible tricentric, one acentric fragment and at least three other abnormal chromosomes. 44 centromeres can be counted, indicating elimination of two chromosomes. Aceto-orcein × 2000. (Professor M. A. Ferguson Smith.)

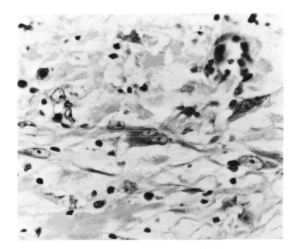

Fig. 1.28 Changes in the sub-epithelial connective tissue of the tongue following irradiation therapy for an epithelial tumour 6 years ago. Note the abnormally large connective tissue cells, one of which is binucleate. × 340.

Tissues whose cells are long-lived and therefore are not normally dividing show very little effect after doses of several hundred rads. Damage has been done, however, and becomes apparent if the cells are stimulated to divide, even after long intervals of time. Examples of such tissue are the adult liver, adult thyroid and long-lived lymphocytes. Again the major effect is that many of the cells are unable to divide when called upon to do so, and in the course of their abortive attempts they show highly abnormal appearances (Fig. 1.29).

Radiation damage to the gonads may lead to infertility due to impairment of germ cell division. Errors also occur in copying the base sequence of DNA in the germ cells, the number of errors—mutations—being related to the

Microscopic appearances. Following a substantial dose of radiation there is a latent interval of hours or days before histological evidence of tissue injury is seen. As already explained, the damage depends on the dose and type of radiation, on the interval following exposure and on the tissue exposed. Early changes in the skin include dilatation of blood vessels and other signs of acute inflammation and these reflect acute tissue injury. With a single dose of 1500 rads mitotic activity of the basal cells is arrested, with subsequent loss of the epidermis and epilation. The walls of the dermal vessels are infiltrated with fibrin; later a characteristic concentric proliferation of intimal fibrous tissue is seen (endarteritis obliterans), followed by replacement with dense homogeneous (hyaline)

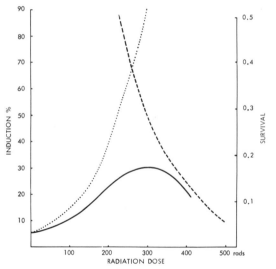

Fig. 1.30 The effect of dosage of radiation on mutation rate in mice. As the dose is increased, the mutation rate rises (dotted line), but the survival rate diminishes (interrupted line). The incidence of mutation-dependent abnormality, in this case leukaemia, is dependent on mutation and survival rates, and is shown by the continuous line.

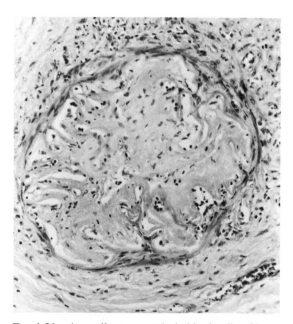

Fig. 1.31 A small artery occluded by hyaline fibrous tissue following radiotherapy. (Same case as in Fig. 1.28.) × 126.

radiation dosage as shown in Fig. 1.30. A given dose of radiation insufficient to cause infertility gives rise to the same total number of mutations irrespective of the number of individuals among whom it is distributed. As a corollary there is no 'safe' level of background radiation. It is known that radiation induces the development of malignant tumours, possibly by causing mutations in somatic cells (p. 259).

collagen (Fig. 1.31). Large bizarre fibrocytic nuclei are present in the dermal connective tissue (Fig. 1.28). With repeated exposure to radiation the dermal collagen becomes very dense and there is a tendency for the dermal connective tissue to become necrotic even years after the exposure; persistent melanin pigmentation and vascular dilatation are also noted. Comparable changes found in other tissues following irradiation are described later in the appropriate chapters; the detailed findings depend, of course, upon the radio-sensitivity of the various types of cells present and the architectural features of the tissue.

Atrophy

By atrophy is meant diminution in size of a cell or reduction in the essential tissue of an organ due to decrease in the size or numbers of its specialised cells. Pathological atrophy has its prototype in the physiological atrophy of old age, which affects all the tissues, and notably the bones, lymphoid tissue, and the sexual organs; and although some of the changes occurring in old age are the result of atrophy of the gonads, this atrophy in its turn cannot be explained. The cause of *senile atrophy* is of course merely part of the larger question of what limits the duration of life. Atrophic specialised epithelial cells tend to lose their special features and to become de-differentiated, as may be seen in local atrophic changes in the liver and kidneys. Senile atrophy is not infrequently accompanied by accumulation of the yellowish-brown pigment lipofuscin and the term *brown atrophy* is then applied. As already indicated (p. 13) lipofuscin represents indigestible lipid which forms residual bodies and is often the product of cellular autophagia.

An organ may be undersized as the result of imperfect development; the term *hypoplasia* is then applied. For example, the hypoplasia of the genital glands which results from deficiency of the pituitary secretion at an early period of life.

Causes of atrophy

1. Defective nutrition. This may be produced locally by arterial disease interfering with the blood supply to a part, when the reduction is not so severe as to cause necrosis. The functioning parenchymatous elements of the tissue then undergo atrophy, and sometimes there is also a concomitant overgrowth of fibrous tissue. This is often seen in the myocardium and in the kidneys, in which small atrophic depressions result from narrowing of the lumina of the small arteries. When there is atrophy of the muscle cells of the walls of arteries, the overgrowth of connective tissue becomes very marked, and this is possibly of compensatory nature since it gives support and minimises dilatation. **General atrophy** is seen in cases of starvation; emaciation depends chiefly upon utilisation of the fat of the adipose tissue but there is also a general wasting of the tissues. The various organs may thus diminish in weight, the liver and spleen are markedly affected, the kidneys and heart to a less though distinct degree, whilst the central nervous system is only slightly affected. In most cases of wasting disease, however, such as malignant tumours of the alimentary tract, chronic tuberculosis or suppuration, other ill-defined factors appear to contribute to the wasting. Various other forms of cellular damage and diminished cell production may thus come to be associated with atrophy; secondary anaemia, for example, is present, although slight or absent in wasting due to starvation alone. The term **cachexia** is often applied to a combination of wasting, anaemia and weakness.

2. Diminished functional activity. It is a general law that diminution in the catabolic processes leads to reduced anabolism and thus to diminution in the size of cells. When the function of a part is in abeyance the blood supply also diminishes. **Disuse atrophy**, as it is sometimes called, is seen when a gland, for example, the pancreas, has its duct obstructed; its functional activity is thus stopped and the exocrine glandular tissue undergoes atrophy. The muscles around a joint which has been immobile for some time undergo marked atrophy and the bones also are affected. Unless such atrophy has become extreme it is reversible and full functional activity may be restored.

3. Interference with the nerve supply. This form of atrophy is seen where there is any destructive lesion of the lower motor neurons or their axons. In this type, **neuropathic atrophy**, there is not only a simple wasting, but also more active degenerative changes in the muscles (Fig. 1.32). For at least a few weeks after nerve

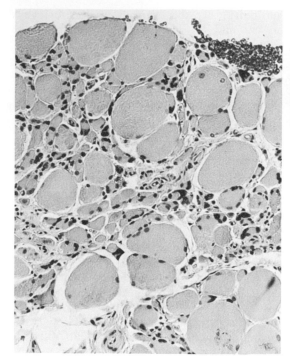

Fig. 1.32 Neuropathic atrophy of skeletal muscle. Note atrophy of groups of fibres and normality or hypertrophy of others. × 200. (Dr. D. Doyle.)

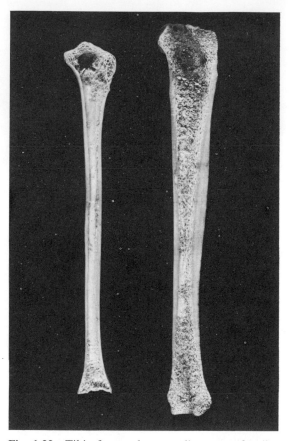

Fig. 1.33 Tibia from a longstanding case of poliomyelitis, showing marked atrophy (*left*). Normal tibia for comparison (*right*). × ⅓.

section, during which the muscle fibre mass may be reduced by half, anabolic processes take place at a normal rate: catabolism due to increased lysosome numbers and activity is greatly accelerated. That this form is different in nature from disuse atrophy is shown by the electrical 'reactions of degeneration' which are given by the muscles and indicate that a complete return to normal is no longer possible. Sometimes marked atrophy occurs also in the bones from the same cause; for example, in cases of poliomyelitis the bones of the limb may become thin and light and this appears to be due simply to inactivity (Fig. 1.33). In some forms of inherited muscular atrophy, however, no nerve lesion is present and the terms *primary myopathy* or *muscular dystrophy* are often applied (p. 871).

4. Deficiency of the endocrine glands. Atrophy of thyroid, gonads and adrenal cortex are seen when destruction of the pituitary results in diminished secretion of trophic hormones. In thyroid deficiency (myxoedema) there occurs marked atrophy of the structures of the skin, hair follicles, sweat glands and sebaceous glands, but structure and function may be restored by oral administration of thyroid hormone.

5. Fever. A good example of atrophy is provided by wasting of the muscles in fevers. No doubt inactivity and interference with nutrition play a part, but the wasting is probably due mainly to utilisation of proteins, as is indicated by the increased excretion of nitrogen. This increased protein catabolism is one of the characteristic features of fever and is generally attributed to toxic action. Other tissues may suffer atrophy in a corresponding way, but in the parenchymatous organs other expressions of cellular injury are more common.

6. Pressure atrophy is also described. The pressure must be continuous, and it acts mainly by interfering with the blood supply and also the functions of a tissue. Thus atrophy of the organs may be brought about by the pressure of benign tumours and cysts. When bone is subjected to pressure there is active absorption by osteoclasts.

Examples of atrophy are provided in the later chapters on diseases of the different systems.

Metaplasia

An interesting cellular response to injury is the phenomenon of metaplasia—the transformation of one type of differentiated tissue into another. An example is provided by the surface epithelium of the bronchi which commonly changes from the normal ciliated pseudostratified columnar type to squamous (Fig. 1.34). In this example it appears that chronic injury or irritation, often due to cigarette smoke, results in adaptive changes in the surface epithelium to a type likely to be more resistant to the cause of the irritation. Similarly stratified squamous epithelium may form as a result of chronic irritation in the mucous membrane of the nose, salivary ducts, gallbladder, renal pelvis and urinary bladder. In some cases

the injurious stimulus is apparent, e.g. when there is a stone in the renal pelvis or in cases of extroversion of the urinary bladder, while in others the cause is obscure. In vitamin A deficiency, in addition to xerophthalmia, stratified squamous epithelium may replace the transitional and columnar epithelia of nose, bronchi, urinary tract, and the specialised secretory epithelia of the lacrimal and salivary glands. In auto-immune chronic gastritis, a condition in which the lymphoid cells attack the mucosa of the fundus of the patient's own stomach, the specialised surface-lining cells and chief and parietal cells of the gastric glands are often replaced by tall columnar cells with striated borders, goblet cells and Paneth cells—*intestinal metaplasia*.

In the connective tissues, metaplasia occurs between fibrous tissue, myxoid tissue, bone and cartilage. Bone formation occasionally follows the deposition of calcium salts in such tissues as arterial walls (Fig. 1.35), bronchial cartilage and the uveal tract of the eye. In healing fractures cartilaginous metaplasia may occur especially when there is undue mobility. The flattened serosal endothelium of the rabbit pleural cavity becomes cubical, columnar, transitional or even squamous following injection of the dye Sudan III with sodium cholate in olive oil and the lining of adjacent alveoli also becomes cubical or columnar. Similar changes, which are rapidly reversible, follow the injection of strontium chloride.

Metaplasia is to be distinguished from a mere loss of the special characters of cells, for example the dedifferentiation which is encountered when there is interference with the function of glands. Developmental epithelial abnormalities, e.g. squamous epithelium within the thyroid, arising from the thyroglossal duct, do not constitute metaplasia nor does encroachment of one tissue upon another. Thus the fatty marrow of the long bones is replaced in certain types of anaemia by red haemopoietic marrow:

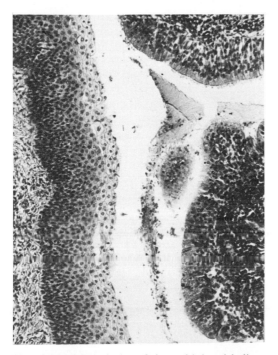

Fig. 1.34 Metaplasia of bronchial epithelium to stratified squamous type is seen on the left side, persistence of columnar ciliated epithelium on the right. × 200.

in this case the haemopoietic tissue has spread by proliferation of haemopoietic stem cells and not by metaplasia of the adipose tissue cells originally present.

It is believed that all nucleated cells carry a complete list of the genetic information required for bodily development, including all types of cellular differentiation and function, but little is yet known about the factors which determine the differentiation of cells in an orderly manner to form the various tissues. The way in which the many different stimuli producing metaplasia act within the cell is correspondingly obscure. It seems likely that a change in gene repression and activation takes place in serosal endothelium when it undergoes metaplasia to squamous epithelium. On the other hand in surfaces lined by columnar epithelium, metaplasia may result from gradual atrophy of the columnar cells and proliferation and maturation of the less well differentiated basal or reserve cells to form squamous epithelium. It is noteworthy that many stimuli which bring about metaplasia are also capable of inducing neoplasia, and indeed tumour formation is relatively common in some metaplastic

epithelia; conversely metaplasia is frequently encountered in malignant tumours. Indeed metaplasia may represent a cellular change in

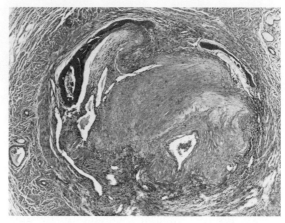

Fig. 1.35 Metaplastic bone formation in the wall of a largely obliterated artery. × 50.

response to injury intermediate between the kind we have been considering earlier in this chapter and that which underlies the development of tumours.

2

Inflammation

Definition and nature of inflammation

Inflammation may be defined as *the series of changes which take place in living tissue following injury*. While commendably brief, this definition is useless without qualification. We have seen in Chapter 1 how tissue cells may be injured, i.e. rendered abnormal, in many ways, and how the effects may range from pathological storage of metabolites to neoplasia. These are not examples of inflammation, and so it is necessary to qualify both the type of injury and the nature of the changes resulting from it.

The injury which causes inflammation may be brought about by: (1) physical agents, such as excessive heating or cooling, mechanical trauma, ultraviolet or ionising radiations; (2) a wide variety of chemical agents, both inorganic and organic, and including the toxins of various bacteria; (3) the intracellular replication of viruses; (4) hypersensitivity reactions, i.e. the reaction of antibody or sensitised lymphocytes with antigenic material such as invasive bacteria or inhaled organic dusts; and (5) necrosis of tissue, which induces inflammation in the surrounding tissue.

The most important cause of inflammation is microbial infection. As indicated above, bacteria produce harmful toxins, viruses injure the host cells which they colonise, and all types of micro-organisms may induce hypersensitivity reactions by the host.

The main features of inflammation. When an appropriate injury, such as excessive heat, is applied to living tissue, an *acute inflammatory reaction* develops. This consists of engorgement with blood of the small vessels in the vicinity of injury, changes in the blood flow through them, and escape of protein-rich fluid and leukocytes from the engorged vessels into the tissue spaces. This reaction is due to changes in the small vessels and, because it includes the escape of blood constituents into the tissues, it is commonly termed *exudative*. When the tissue injury has been slight and brief, the exudative inflammatory reaction is correspondingly mild and soon subsides. However, if the injury persists, the exudative inflammatory reaction can continue for months or even years, as in some persistent bacterial infections, and it is therefore wrong to equate it solely with acute lesions, i.e. those having a short course.

A second type of inflammatory response, sometimes called *productive* or *formative* (to distinguish it from exudative) inflammation, is the production of new fibrous tissue. This occurs particularly in prolonged tissue injury and so is seen especially in *chronic inflammation*. In some instances, both exudative and productive reactions are conspicuous, but in prolonged low-grade injury, fibrous tissue formation is often the more prominent. At first, the young fibrous tissue is highly vascular, soft and gelatinous, and is known as *granulation tissue*. As it ages, it become less vascular, progressively more collagenous, and is thus gradually converted to pale, dense *scar tissue*.

The present account follows tradition in using the terms 'acute inflammation' and 'acute inflammatory reaction' for the exudative process, and 'chronic inflammation' for persistent inflammatory lesions, in which fibrous tissue formation is a prominent feature. It must, however, be emphasised that the two types of reaction commonly occur together.

The inflammatory nature of a lesion is usually indicated by the use of the suffix **-itis**. Thus inflammation of the appendix is appendicitis, inflammation of the meniges, meningitis, and so on.

Inflammation is usually beneficial. It is essential in combating various infections and in limiting the harmful effects of toxic compounds. Like other beneficial processes, it is not without disadvantages: for example, acute inflammatory swelling of the larynx may cause death from asphyxia, and inflammatory reactions caused by hypersensitivity to harmless substances, as in hay fever, appear entirely disadvantageous to the host. Fibrous tissue formed in chronic inflammation may help to wall off bacteria or harmful compounds such as silica particles, but it may also cause disability by distorting and compressing important structures. Inflammatory fibrosis of a hollow viscus, such as the intestine, can cause narrowing of the lumen, and fibrosis occurring in any tissue can constrict blood vessels, nerves, ducts, etc.

We shall now consider in more detail the acute inflammatory reaction and its effects, the special features of chronic inflammation, and the types of cell which participate in inflammatory reactions.

The Acute Inflammatory Reaction

Historical note

Acute inflammation has been recognised since the earliest days of medicine. Celsus (30 B.C. to A.D. 38) gave as its cardinal signs heat, redness, swelling and pain, to which may be added limitation of movement, e.g. of an inflamed limb. These changes are most commonly the result of infection with micro-organisms, but even before the discovery of the pathogenicity of bacteria, inflammation had been produced experimentally, e.g. by Lister (1858), by the application of irritating chemicals to the tissues, and the underlying processes had been studied in detail. Cohnheim (1882) first emphasised the important part played by the small blood vessels in producing the changes of inflammation. It was clear to these early workers that, regardless of the nature of the causal injury, the inflammatory changes were basically the same: this raised the possibility that the changes were mediated by endogenous agents, release or production of which was triggered by the causal injury. Evidence of such mediators was eventually provided by the classical experiments of Lewis and Grant (Lewis, 1927) in which mild inflammation was produced in the skin of the human forearm by firmly stroking with a blunt point or by mild thermal injury. The inflammatory reaction was observed to have three components (triple response), namely a flush (erythema at the site of injury), a flare (erythema of the surrounding skin) and a weal (inflammatory oedema due to exudation of plasma fluid into the tissues) at the site of injury. The flush normally persisted for ten minutes or so, but could be prolonged by interruption of the blood supply to the limb by a tourniquet: it was attributed by Lewis to local release of a chemical endogenous mediator which was removed within ten minutes by the blood and lymph unless this was prevented by obstructing the circulation. Lewis and Grant showed that the same effects could be brought about by pricking histamine into the skin and they called the hypothetical mediator 'H' substance. By experiments on subjects with nerve injuries, it was shown that the flare was dependent on intact sensory nerves, and Lewis attributed it to an axon reflex causing dilatation of arterioles outwith the area of injury (Fig. 2.1).

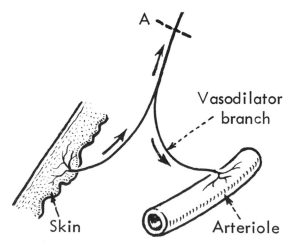

Fig. 2.1 Diagram of peripheral end of sensory nerve fibre with vasodilator axon branch. Stimulation of sensory nerve ending in the skin results in an antidromic reflex along the vasodilator branch, with resulting arteriolar dilatation. Section of the nerve fibre at A does not abolish this reflex until the fibre distal to A has degenerated.

Both the flare and the weal were inhibited by a tourniquet and thus were dependent on either blood flow or intravascular hydrostatic pressure. This work was of great importance in arousing interest in the role of endogenous chemical mediators, but there was little advance until 1940 when Menkin claimed to have shown that the inflammatory exudate produced by an injection of turpentine contained a number of polypeptides with specific pharmacological activities, each mediating a particular component of inflammation. Menkin's findings have lacked confirmation, but they stimulated intensive search for endogenous mediators. Although many substances have been proposed for this role, none of these has so far been shown with certainty to play an important part in the inflammatory response.

Sequential changes of the acute inflammatory reaction

Much of our knowledge of the acute inflammatory reaction is derived from experimental work in which the causal injury, such as heat or chemicals, can be accurately applied and varied at will, and the resulting inflammatory changes can be observed sequentially by methods not applicable to naturally occurring inflammation in man.

As stated above, the macroscopic features of acute inflammation are **reddening**, **swelling**, **warmth**, **pain** and **partial immobilisation**. The explanation of these changes has been provided by microscopic studies, which have revealed that the inflammatory reaction is made up of a number of phenomena, all of which involve the walls of the small blood vessels in the inflamed tissue. In 1882 Cohnheim described the microscopic changes in the living transparent tissues of the frog's tongue and foot-web during inflammation caused by mechanical trauma or chemical irritation. His superb account is a model of accurate observation and the changes he described have subsequently been confirmed by others in mammalian tissues. Since 1924, much use has also been made of the rabbit ear chamber which allows microscopic examination of the inflammatory process in a thin layer of living vascular connective tissue.

When inflammation is produced by heat or various chemicals, there is often an immediate and transient blanching of the injured tissue due to arteriolar contraction: this effect is not of practical importance and is followed within a few minutes by relaxation of the arterioles in and around the injured tissue, so that the capillary network and post-capillary venules become engorged (Fig. 2.2) with rapidly flowing blood (**active hyperaemia**). On inspection, the tissue

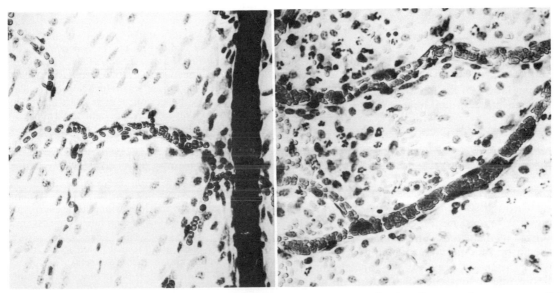

Fig. 2.2 Surface view of stained preparations of guinea-pig omentum showing the normal appearances (*left*) and acute inflammation (*right*). Note engorgement of the small vessels with blood and infiltration of the tissue with neutrophil polymorphs. × 300.

looks red (**erythema**), and in superficial tissue which is normally cool, the increased blood flow of inflammation accounts for the rise in temperature. The onset of active hyperaemia is followed by three phenomena: (*a*) protein-rich fluid, the **inflammatory exudate**, leaks out of the vessels into the surrounding tissue and is largely responsible for the swelling (**inflammatory oedema**) of inflamed tissues; (*b*) the microcirculation remains engorged but the blood flow, at first rapid, becomes progressively slower, and (*c*) phagocytic leukocytes, at first neutrophil polymorphs and later monocytes, adhere to the endothelial surface of venules and migrate through the vessel walls into the tissue spaces (Fig. 2.2).

The relative immobility of acutely inflamed tissues is due to their swelling, and to the increase in tension, and thus pain, caused by attempted movement.

The time of onset and duration of each of these phenomena varies considerably depending on the species, the type and severity of injury, and the tissue subjected to it. The reaction to thermal burns and many irritating chemicals is almost immediate; with ultraviolet irradiation there is a delay of some hours before inflammation of the skin is fully developed, while with ionising irradiations the delay may be 24 hours, or even longer in some tissues.

The major changes of acute inflammation, which will now be considered in more detail are thus:

(1) vascular engorgement and changes in blood flow;
(2) exudation of fluid and solutes;
(3) emigration of leukocytes.

Vascular engorgement and changes in blood flow

Normal microcirculatory control. The flow of blood through a tissue is controlled mainly by changes in the tone of the circular smooth muscle of its arterioles. This is regulated in part by the autonomic nervous system, which largely controls the blood pressure, the cardiac output and to some extent the distribution of blood flow among the various tissues. Superimposed on this overall control are local factors determined by the conditions in individual tissues.

Thus when an organ or tissue is in a resting state of low metabolic activity, many of its arterioles are contracted and blood flow is diminished. When local metabolism increases, for example in the gastric mucosa after a meal, or in an exercising muscle, the arterioles relax and the consequent rise in pressure of blood reaching the capillaries causes them and their draining venules to become engorged with rapidly flowing blood. This engorgement or congestion, due to the force of the heart beat driving blood into and through the capillaries, is termed **active hyperaemia** to distinguish it from the congestion which occurs in other conditions, due to a rise in venous pressure (passive hyperaemia) and which is not accompanied by an increase in blood flow.

It is not known whether this opening up of the microcirculation during increased tissue activity is brought about by local nervous control or directly by humoral agents, such as cell metabolites: current opinion favours the latter.

Although the arterioles and venules are greatly dilated in active hyperaemia, the size of capillaries is restricted by their basement membrane: their diameter is approximately 5–8 μm and in active hyperaemia they become conspicuous not so much by dilatation but because they are filled with whole blood, whereas in the resting tissue state most of them contain slowly flowing plasma with few cells.

In most tissues, the capillaries form an anastomosing network providing routes of various lengths between arterioles and venules. The individual entrances to the network are the *terminal arterioles*, which do not anastomose, and which are the smallest vessels controlled by smooth muscle cells: they function as pre-capillary sphincters and determine the flow of blood through individual capillaries. It is probable that, in resting tissues, the pre-capillary sphincters are so adjusted that blood flows mainly through the shortest capillary routes—the so-called thoroughfare channels—in accordance with the needs of general circulatory control: the pre-capillary sphincters guarding the longer capillary routes are contracted, and most of the capillaries contain only plasma.

The engorgement and rapid flow of active hyperaemia is brought about mainly by relaxation of the arterioles, including most of the pre-capillary sphincters. It is widely assumed that any inherent contractility of the capillaries is weak, and that the amount of blood passing through them depends on the state of the arterioles.

Vascular engorgement and altered blood flow in acute imflammation are local phenomena and are due to predominance of local factors over the general system of arteriolar control. As in physiological activity (see above), the arterioles relax and active hyperaemia develops. The mechanism of the arteriolar relaxation is unknown and is difficult to investigate. It must be assumed that either endogenous mediators or neural factors contribute to the erythema, for this extends beyond the immediate site of the injury. Lewis showed that histamine can induce the mild inflammatory changes of the triple response, but this does not indicate that it is of importance in more severe and prolonged inflammatory changes; indeed, histamine antagonists may delay the erythema of acute inflammation but they do not, in general, depress it significantly. Moreover, all the changes of inflammation may be induced in denervated tissues and Lewis's axon reflex is probably of little practical importance. The list of possible endogenous chemical mediators of inflammatory erythema includes histamine, 5-hydroxytryptamine, kinins, polypeptides and prostaglandins. These and other vaso-active agents can all induce some of the features of inflammation: what is in doubt is their relative importance in the natural process. To complicate matters further, the same group of endogenous compounds appears to be involved in the increased vascular permeability of inflammation and yet the hyperaemia and increased vascular permeability of inflammation do not closely parallel one another either in their timing or in their degree. In inflammation produced in the skin by ultraviolet light, for example, increased permeability may only occur during a short part of the period of hyperaemia.

In experimental inflammation caused by mechanical trauma, heat or chemical irritants, the **rapid blood flow** in the microvessels may persist for up to an hour or so, and is readily explained by the increased hydrostatic pressure of blood resulting from arteriolar relaxation. It is followed by gradual **slowing of blood flow** until, in some vessels, there may be temporary stasis of blood. In severe inflammation, stasis may be prolonged and clotting may occur. Several factors contribute towards the slowing of the blood flow. Firstly, active hyperaemia results in loss of fluid from the blood in capillaries and post-capillary venules, and the cell concentration is thus increased. Secondly, although the exudate is rich in protein, loss of fluid is so much increased that the concentration of proteins in the plasma is actually raised. Both of these changes increase the viscosity of the blood. Thirdly, the increased protein concentration of the plasma and slowing of blood flow result in aggregation of the red cells in rouleaux, with so-called sludging of the blood, and this further increases viscosity. A fourth factor which impairs the blood flow is the adhesion of leukocytes to the walls of post-capillary venules. Not only do the leukocytes adhere to the endothelium but also to one another, and considerable reduction in the effective lumen of venules may result.

Slowing of the blood flow will tend to impair the supply of oxygen, glucose, etc., to the tissues, and also the removal of metabolites, but these effects are diminished by the increased flow of fluid from the plasma into the tissues and increased lymphatic drainage (see below). It is only when the vascular stagnation is extreme that it is likely to impair tissue nutrition seriously and contribute to the necrosis which is commonly observed in severe inflammatory reactions. Such necrosis is more likely to result directly from the injury which has induced the inflammatory response, e.g. bacterial toxic action, thermal injury, etc.

Exudation of fluid and solutes

Microscopic examination of inflamed tissues reveals an accumulation of extracellular fluid, i.e. interstitial oedema (Fig. 2.3). This can only have come from the blood plasma, and since it has been shown that the amount of fluid draining away from inflamed tissues by the lymphatics is also greatly increased, there is obviously a considerable rise in the net amount of fluid leaving the blood vessels. As illustrated in Fig. 2.4, the inflammatory exudate is also much richer in plasma proteins than is normal extracellular fluid or lymph draining from the same tissue, indicating increased permeability of the vessels to macromolecules. These two features of exudation are best considered separately, for the factors involved in the passage of water and small solutes across the walls of

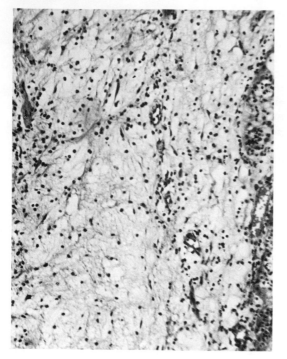

Fig. 2.3 Meso-appendix in acute appendicitis, showing inflammatory oedema with early leukocytic emigration. × 100.

microvessels, in both normal and inflamed tissues, differ from those concerned in the escape of molecules as large as the plasma proteins.

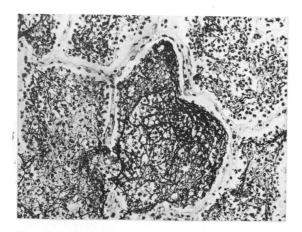

Fig. 2.4 Acute inflammation of the lung in pneumonia. The exudate, which fills the alveoli, is rich in plasma proteins, and this is illustrated by the fine network of fibrin (stained black) which has resulted from the clotting of exuded fibrinogen. (Weigert's fibrin stain) × 150.

Escape of water and micromolecular solutes

In all tissues the capillaries and post-capillary venules are readily permeable to water and micromolecular solutes. For molecules above a molecular weight of 10 000 daltons, the permeability decreases sharply with molecular size, and molecules greater than 40 000 escape from the plasma in relatively small numbers. This applies particularly to the vessels in skeletal muscles, dermis and other connective tissues. In the liver, intestinal mucosa, exocrine and endocrine glands, and the glomeruli, macromolecules escape more readily but still much less so than do micromolecules.

Our understanding of the exchange of water and small molecules between plasma and extravascular fluid is based upon (*a*) the observations of Starling and of Landis on microfiltration, and (*b*) morphological considerations.

(a) Microfiltration theory. Starling regarded the vascular endothelium as behaving like a passive microfilter, across which the movement of fluid and electrolytes was determined by physical forces. He proposed that the main force driving fluid out of vessels was the height of the hydrostatic pressure within the vessels above that in the extravascular space, and that this was opposed by the height of the osmotic pressure of the plasma above that of the extravascular fluid. Thus at the arteriolar ends of capillaries the effective hydrostatic pressure would normally exceed the osmotic pressure and fluid would be forced out. At the venular ends of capillaries the osmotic pressure would exceed the hydrostatic pressure and fluid would be drawn into the capillary (Fig. 2.5). This theory received direct support from the work of an American medical student, Landis (1927), who devised techniques of measuring the hydrostatic pressure in individual small vessels, and of calculating the rate of diffusion of fluid into and out of the vessels. Landis showed that when inflammation was induced in the frog mesentery, there was a rise in the hydrostatic pressure within the microcirculation which upset the balance between hydrostatic and osmotic forces, with a resultant net loss of fluid from the vessels. The escape of plasma proteins from inflamed vessels will tend to reduce the osmotic pressure difference between plasma and extravascular fluid and this may be sufficient to

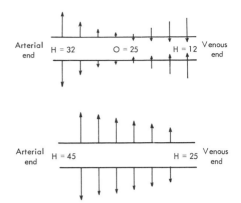

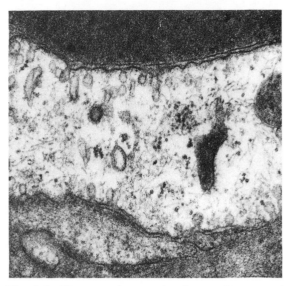

Fig. 2.5 Exchange of fluid across the walls of capillaries and venules. H and O represent the heights of the hydrostatic and osmotic pressures respectively (mm. Hg.) of the plasma above the corresponding pressures of the extravascular space. The arrows indicate the net movement of fluid into and out of the vessels along their length. Upper figure, normal tissue: fluid movement across vessel walls approximates to equilibrium. Lower figure, acute inflammation: much more fluid leaves the vessels than returns to them.

The values of H and O are approximations. In inflammation, H may be less than indicated because of rise of pressure in the extravascular space, and O will also be reduced by escape of plasma proteins into the inflammatory exudate.

accentuate the loss of fluid (Fig. 2.5). These findings have now been confirmed in normal and inflamed mammalian tissues and, while Starling's views have required to be modified in detail to take account of the fluid exchange function of the post-capillary venules, his major suggestion—that the walls of small vessels behave like a passive filter through which the exchange of fluid is determined by opposing haemodynamic and osmotic forces—has been widely accepted.

Acceptance of Starling's microfiltration theory and subsequent studies have suggested the existence in the walls of microvessels of a physiological system of small gaps of sufficient size to allow the escape of water and electrolytes, but impermeable to proteins and other macromolecules (Pappenheimer *et al.*, 1951).

(b) Morphological evidence. There is strong evidence that the basement membrane of small vessels does not form a barrier to water or small molecular solutes and the effective filter thus appears to be in the endothelial layer. Electron microscopy of vascular endothelium suggests

Fig. 2.6 Electron micrograph of part of a normal capillary endothelial cell in which pinocytic vesicles are seen in relation to both the inner and outer surfaces and also lying free in the cytoplasm. The capillary lumen is at the top of the field. × 50 000.

two possible routes of fluid transport across the endothelium. Firstly, endothelial cells appear to engulf fluid and to transport it as droplets (pinocytic vesicles) across the cytoplasm (Fig. 2.6). Secondly, fluid may pass between endothelial cells. Although the relative importance of these two modes of fluid transport is not known, the behaviour of microvessels as passive filters is in favour of the intercellular route, and moreover the number of cytoplasmic vesicles does not increase in inflammation as would be expected if they represented the important transport system. For these reasons, we consider that the important site of fluid and micromolecular exchange across the endothelium is the intercellular junctions, which are seen by electron microscopy as narrow spaces containing amorphous material (Fig. 2.7), and which show constrictions (**zonulae occludentes**) where the adjacent cells are more closely approximated. The endothelial cells of capillaries in the glomeruli, glandular tissues and gut mucosa show zones of extreme cytoplasmic thinning (fenestrae), while those of vascular sinusoids, e.g. in the liver, show relatively large defects. The effects of these features on fluid exchange is not fully understood, but they are likely to account for the relatively high permeability of these vessels to macromolecules.

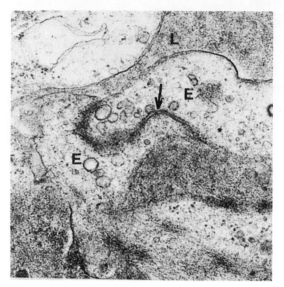

Fig. 2.7 Electron micrograph showing the narrow space (arrow), filled with amorphous material, between adjacent vascular endothelial cells (E). L is the lumen of the vessel. × 45 000.

Leakage of proteins from microvessels

While relatively permeable to water and small solutes, the walls of normal capillaries and venules exert a sieving effect on larger molecules, providing an increasingly effective barrier to macromolecules proportionate to their size. In connective tissues and voluntary muscle there is relatively little loss of albumin and even less of the larger plasma proteins. Nevertheless some protein does escape from the microvessels of all tissues, and physiologists have postulated the existence of a second system of smaller numbers of larger gaps to account for this (Pappenheimer *et al.*, 1951). In an exercised limb, increased pressure and flow of blood through the small vessels of the muscles results in greatly increased flow of lymph, and yet the total protein content of the lymph is not increased. Active hyperaemia does not, therefore, account for the increased protein leakage from the microvessels in acute inflammation, which can be explained only by postulating an increase in permeability of the vascular endothelium. This was substantiated morphologically by Majno *et al.* (1961), who applied histamine and other permeability-increasing agents to striped muscle of animals injected intravenously with colloidal carbon or mercuric sulphide. In

careful electron-microscopic studies, they detected the occurrence of gaps between adjacent endothelial cells (Fig. 2.8). The presence of the injected colloidal material in these gaps indicated that they were indeed the sites of leakage of large molecules. The times at which gaps occur in the endothelium of particular types of vessels (venules or capillaries) have since been shown to correlate closely with the times at which those vessels show increased permeability. The gaps appear to be transient, for injected colloidal material has also been observed deep to normal (i.e. 'tight') endothelial cell junctions in acutely inflamed tissue. Very occasionally, this has been observed in normal (non-inflamed) tissues, suggesting that transient gaps account also for the normal leakage of small amounts of protein.

Although plasma proteins of various molecular sizes appear in the acute inflammatory exudate, a sieving effect persists, the smaller proteins escaping more readily than the larger ones. Since the observed inter-endothelial cell gaps are much larger than the largest protein molecule, it is likely that this sieving effect is a property of the vascular basement membrane.

It is possible that some protein is normally transferred across the vascular endothelium in the pinocytic vesicles (see Fig. 2.6), but these do not increase in inflammation and are unlikely to be an important factor.

In summary, exchange of fluid and micromolecular solutes across the walls of microvessels occurs by passive filtration, probably through the endothelial cell junctions and the increased escape of fluid and electrolytes in inflammation is explained by increased hydrostatic pressure of the blood in active hyperaemia. Leakage of plasma proteins from the microvessels of inflamed capillaries is due to the opening up of transient and relatively large gaps between endothelial cells: this probably accounts also for the leakage of smaller amounts of proteins from normal vessels.

Detection of increased vascular permeability. The increased vascular permeability which allows macromolecules to escape from the small vessels is one of the most important features of the acute inflammatory reaction. It is also more easily detected and measured than some of the other features of the reaction. For these

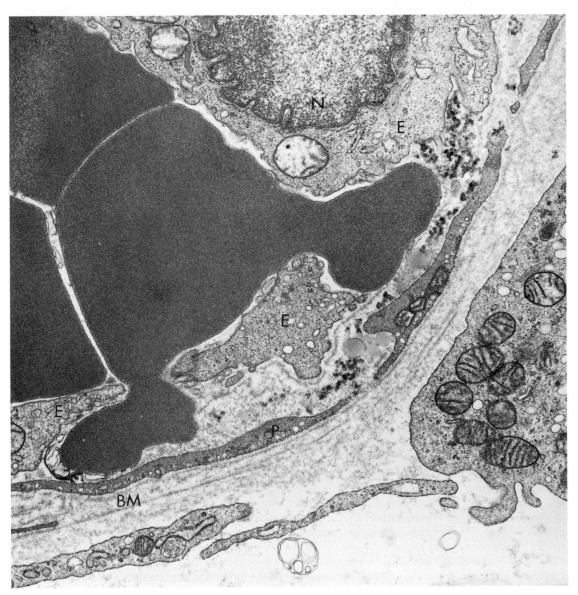

Fig. 2.8 Two gaps caused by histamine in the endothelium (E) of a venule (rat cremaster muscle, 3 min after a local injection of histamine). Red blood cells are very plastic and can easily 'flow' into endothelial gaps; this one is going to have a problem, because it is slipping out of two different gaps! Note the tight folds in the endothelial nucleus (N) (suggestive of cellular contraction). Because the basement membrane (BM) acts as a filter (beyond the endothelial gaps), many blood-borne particles accumulate in the venular wall: the dark granules are carbon black (India ink which had been injected intravenously); the larger, smooth, round bodies are chylomicrons. (P: Pericyte). × 29 700. (Dr. Isabelle Joris.)

reasons, it has been extensively investigated and considerable efforts have been made to identify endogenous chemical mediators responsible for it.

Various methods have been used to detect increased vascular permeability. Plasma proteins have been labelled by dyes such as Evans blue, or by radio-active isotopes, and their leakage into inflamed tissues determined by suitable measuring procedures; intravascularly injected ferritin or colloidal material such as carbon have been used to detect the sites of leakage by light or electron microscopy. Inflamed tissues have also been extracted and analysed for the presence of histamine and other endogenous vaso-active chemicals which may be responsible for increasing vascular permeability.

Phases of increased vascular permeability. Use of procedures such as those described above has shown that the pattern of increased vascular permeability varies greatly, depending on the nature and degree of tissue injury, the type of tissue which is injured, and the species of experimental animal. It has nevertheless been shown that, in inflammation following moderate injury by heat, mechanical trauma or various chemicals, there are often two distinct phases of increased permeability. With more severe injury, the two phases merge into one, while in mild inflammation there may be no second phase. Under suitable conditions, the **early phase** starts almost immediately and subsides within 30 minutes; it is due to leakage of macromolecules from the venules, but not from the capillaries. There is good evidence that this phase is due to release of histamine, for not only has histamine been detected in pharmacologically active concentrations in the early exudate, but prior histamine depletion of the tissues, or administration of histamine antagonists, have been shown to inhibit this early phase of increased vascular permeability. In some animal species, but probably not in man, 5-hydroxytryptamine also appears to play a role.

The **late phase** of increased vascular permeability starts an hour or so after the injury. Except in the mildest of inflammatory reactions, it is much more prolonged and therefore more important than the early phase. The leakage of macromolecules usually occurs from both capillaries and venules, and this poses a problem, for although a number of vaso-active agents have been detected in the late-phase exudate, they all appear to increase the permeability of venules, but not of capillaries. This applies to histamine, 5-hydroxytryptamine, kinins and prostaglandins. In addition to this difficulty, it has not been shown conclusively that specific inhibition of any one of these possible mediators significantly reduces the late

phase of increased vascular permeability: the problem lies in finding inhibitors which are capable of suppressing completely the activity of the suspected mediators and yet have no other effect on the inflammatory reaction.

Hurley (1972) has suggested that the late phase of increased vascular permeability is not due to chemical mediators, but to a direct although delayed effect of the causal injury on the endothelium. He has supported this proposal by demonstrating that, following thermal injury of skin and muscle, the late increase in permeability is localised strictly to the area of injury, and that the intensity of injury of the skin determines whether this phase is restricted to the superficial capillaries or involves also the deeper-lying venules. Although this is convincing evidence, it cannot be assumed to apply to inflammation induced by other agents and in other tissues. In some experimental studies there is strong evidence that the late phase of increased permeability is caused by endogenous mediators, although these have not been identified with certainty. There is also evidence that the small vessels in different tissues vary greatly in their sensitivity to individual endogenous mediators, and it thus seems likely that the mechanism of the late phase of increased permeability differs for different tissues and probably for different types of injury.

Many of the suspected mediators of increased vascular permeability are capable of causing contraction of certain smooth muscle cells, e.g. in the uterus and ileum. Majno (1973) and others have recently demonstrated that vascular endothelial cells contain microfibrils, which may be contractile, and material which antigenically resembles actomyosin. From this and morphological observations, they have suggested that the effect of mediators of increased permeability is to cause contraction of the endothelial cells, thus accounting for the observed gaps, described above, between adjacent cells (Fig. 2.8).

Proof that a particular substance mediates a part of the inflammatory reaction would require (1) the detection of its presence, in biologically active form and effective concentration, in inflamed tissues, and (2) the demonstration of the effectiveness of specifically suppressing its activity without interfering with the inflammatory reaction in any other way. These exacting criteria have not been fulfilled convincingly for any of the suspected mediators except histamine, which is responsible for the brief early phase of increased permeability.

Notes on some endogenous permeability-promoting agents. Since none of the postulated mediators of increased permeability has been proved to be of importance in acute inflammation in man, there is no need to consider them in detail, and the following notes are intentionally brief.

Histamine is stored in an inactive form in the granules of mast cells which are present adjacent to blood vessels in nearly all tissues, and also in basophil and eosinophil leukocytes and platelets. Active histamine is released from these cells by a wide variety of stimuli, including those which elicit an acute inflammatory reaction. In man, mast cells and basophil leukocytes are the major source of stored histamine. Active histamine is probably also synthesised by various other cell types, the amount being controlled by the concentration of cellular histidine decarboxylase. On injection, histamine causes active hyperaemia and increased venular permeability for up to 15 minutes or so. A number of substances, e.g. compound 48/80, are capable of causing histamine release and depletion of mast cells *in vivo*, and there are various inhibitors which compete with histamine for receptor sites on target cells; these vary in specificity and in their effect in animals of different species. However, such agents have not been shown to have important anti-inflammatory effects *in vivo*. The release of histamine, etc. in hypersensitivity reactions is dealt with in Chapter 5.

5-hydroxytryptamine (serotonin) is present in most tissues. Rich sources include the cells of the chromaffin system of the gastro-intestinal tract, the spleen and nervous tissue, mast cells and platelets. On injection, 5-hydroxytryptamine, like histamine, causes a brief increase in venular permeability: it may participate in inflammatory reactions in rats and mice, which are particularly sensitive to it, but in other species, including man, it is unlikely to make an important contribution to inflammation.

The kinin system. Bradykinin is a nonapeptide derived by digestion of kininogen, a plasma glycoprotein, by various proteolytic enzymes, including *kallikrein* which exists as an inactive precursor (prekallikrein) in the plasma and which appears to be activated by a product of activated Hageman factor (p. 198). The system is difficult to investigate because the plasma contains various inhibitors and also kininases which rapidly inactivate bradykinin. On injection, bradykinin causes pain, erythema and increased venular permeability for 10 to 15 minutes. Enzymes with kallikrein activity exist in most tissues and in urine and glandular secretions. In addition to brady-

kinin, there are several closely related peptides with kinin activity.

PF/dil. Diluted human plasma has been shown to be capable of developing the property of increasing vascular permeability and the above term (PF = permeability factor) is applied to the agents responsible. The system can be activated *in vitro* by contact with glass, and the effect of dilution is apparently to render ineffective a plasma inhibitor. There is recent evidence that the system works by activating the kinin system.

Prostaglandins are a group of long-chain hydroxy-fatty acids which are produced by the action of an oxidase (PG-synthetase) on poly-unsaturated-fatty acids such as arachidonic acid. They are rapidly catabolised and are not stored within the body. While they differ greatly in their properties, prostaglandins E1 and E2 have been isolated from inflammatory exudates in man and animals and shown to be capable of causing active hyperaemia, increased vascular permeability and chemotaxis of polymorphs. They are also potent pyrogens when injected into the third ventricle and although small doses intradermally do not cause pain, they lower the pain threshold of nerve endings to histamine, 5-hydroxytryptamine and kinins. Direct evidence that prostaglandins play an important part in inflammation is scanty, but it is of interest that aspirin and related drugs, which have anti-inflammatory, antipyretic and analgesic properties, have been shown to be capable, in low concentrations, of inhibiting the production of prostaglandins, both *in vivo* and *in vitro*, by antagonising prostaglandin synthetase activity.

The complement system: The cascade reaction of this system is not only complex in itself (p. 116) but it is interrelated also with the kinin, coagulation and plasmin systems. The products of complement activation include at least two factors, C3a and C5a, termed anaphylatoxins, which release histamine from mast cells. Their intradermal injection in man results in inflammatory oedema. Normal plasma contains a potent inactivator of C3a and C5a which may also inactivate kinins; it has a molecular weight of 300,000 and so perhaps does not escape from blood vessels in amounts sufficient to inactivate anaphylatoxins or kinins in the extravascular space. The reaction of C2 is also believed to produce a kinin-like peptide.

Apart from its well-known participation in immunological reactions, complement appears to be important in non-immunological inflammatory reactions, for animals in which the complement of the plasma has been depleted by various methods show impaired inflammatory exudation following physical or chemical tissue injury. Since such animals react normally to injected histamine, kinins, etc., complement appears to be of importance either as a source of mediators or by stimulating the production of mediators from other sources.

Peptides. Acutely inflamed tissue contains proteolytic enzymes derived from the plasma, tissue cells and polymorphs, and consequently peptides are formed from digestion of the various proteins in the exudate. It has been shown that, while not as potent as kinins, peptides composed of 8–14 amino-acid residues are capable of increasing vascular permeability.

Conclusions. There is good evidence that increased vascular permeability occurring early in the inflammatory reaction in man and some other species is mediated by histamine. The later and more prolonged and important increase in permeability cannot be attributed with certainty to any one endogenous agent; its mediation seems to vary in different species and in different tissues within a species. With a process as important as increased permeability, it is likely that evolutionary selection has produced complex multi-factorial mechanisms, and that several mediators are involved. There is also evidence that, in some experimental examples of inflammation, direct endothelial-cell injury may contribute to the late phase of increased permeability.

Emigration of leukocytes

The escape of cells from the blood vessels is a prominent feature of inflammation. Escape of erythrocytes is purely passive: they are forced out of capillaries and venules, through gaps between endothelial cells, by the hydrostatic pressure of the blood. Their escape in very large numbers is an indication of severe endothelial injury. By contrast, escape of **neutrophil polymorphs** and **monocytes** is an active process of great importance, and of particular significance in the defence against bacteria. It involves two stages: firstly, the leukocyte becomes arrested on the surface of the vascular endothelium, and secondly it passes through the vessel wall.

In acute inflammatory lesions, neutrophil polymorphs migrate earlier and in much greater numbers than monocytes.

Margination of polymorphs. Arrest of neutrophil polymorphs on the vascular endothelium is often conspicuous in acute inflammation and is known as **pavementing** or **margination** of leukocytes. It is seen mainly in venules and

occurs with the slowing of the blood flow in the dilated vessels. In the earlier stage of rapid flow, blood in the arterioles and venules shows **axial streaming**, the cells being mainly in the central or axial column of blood, separated from the vessel wall by a clear layer of plasma containing only occasional cells. This streaming is dependent on the rapid flow of blood and later, as the rate of flow decreases, axial streaming disappears. In particular, the leukocytes in the venules pass into the peripheral stream, where they can make contact with the endothelium. Neutrophil leukocytes making such contact tend to become arrested momentarily and then become

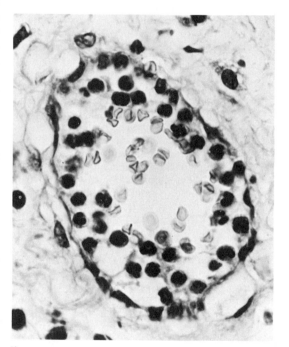

Fig. 2.9 Section of venule in acute inflammation, showing pavementing of polymorphonuclear leukocytes. × 1000.

detached and move on, or roll slowly along the endothelial surface. Eventually more and more of them become arrested for longer periods on the endothelium and they may form an almost continuous layer or may even become heaped up on one another (Fig. 2.9). The nature of adhesion between the leukocytic and endothelial cell surfaces is unknown: changes in the cell surfaces have not been detected by electron microscopy.

In recent studies, vascular endothelial injury

has been caused by a fine laser beam (5–15 μm diameter) in small vessels during perfusion with saline coloured with a dye, and adhesion of leukocytes to the injured endothelium has been observed following restoration of blood flow. Since blood cells and plasma were excluded from the vessel during injury, pavementing can clearly result from enothelial injury alone, and does not require injury to the circulating leukocytes.

Emigration of polymorphs. The 'pavemented' polymorph pushes out cytoplasmic pseudopodia and when one of these encounters the junction between two endothelial cells, it extends between them, disrupting the junction (Fig. 2.10), and the rest of the cell squeezes through: the intercellular junction re-forms rapidly without significant leakage of plasma. The emigrating leukocyte also passes through the basement membrane, which is repaired almost immediately. The mechanisms of disruption and repair of the endothelial cell junction and basement membrane are not known. Emigrated cells wander through the tissues and play a role in digestion and phagocytosis of fibrin, degenerate tissue and cell fragments and, most

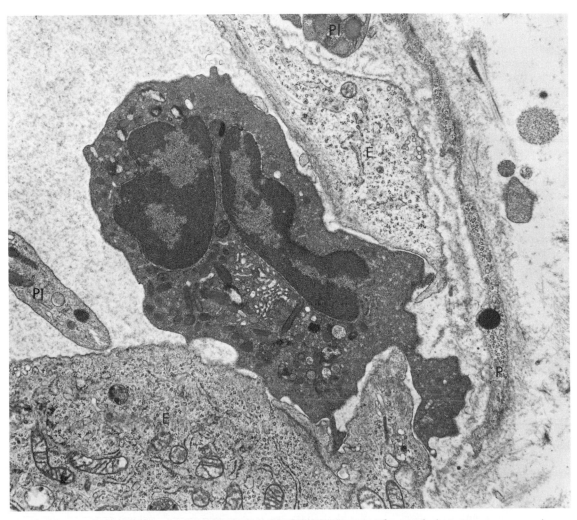

Fig. 2.10 A neutrophil polymorph caught in the act of emigrating out of a venule (rat omentum; experimental inflammation caused by sterile necrotic kidney tissue). Note the many fibrils in the endothelial cell at top; above it, part of a platelet (P1)—which must have slipped out earlier (not necessarily through the gap now being used by the neutrophil). (E: Endothelium; P: Pericyte; Pl: Platelet.) × 24 470. (Dr. Guido Majno.)

important in infections, in the destruction and removal of micro-organisms. The phagocytic function of leukocytes is considered on pp. 51 and 149.

Intensity of leukocyte emigration in acute inflammation depends upon the nature and severity of the tissue injury. It is usually only moderate in physical injury unless infection supervenes. Inflammatory chemicals, including bacterial products, vary greatly in the degree of leukocytic emigration they induce. In the mild inflammatory reaction which occurs around tissue dying from acute ischaemia, i.e. an infarct (p. 208), the degree of polymorph emigration also varies greatly. In myocardial infarction, for example, there may be virtually no polymorph infiltration of the dead muscle, or large numbers may be present, particularly near the margin.

The outstanding examples of intense emigration of polymorphs are provided by bacterial infections: bacteria which, like *Strep. pyogenes*, *Staph. aureus* and *Strep. pneumoniae* are particularly active in this respect, are accordingly termed **pyogenic** (pus inducing) bacteria. Other bacteria, such as, *Salmonella typhi* (the cause of typhoid fever) and *Clostridium welchii* (a cause of gas gangrene), induce far less leukocytic emigration, even though they cause severe inflammation. These special features are considered in more detail below and in Chapter 7, but it is worth noting here that differences between inflammatory reactions are not simply in degrees of severity: the nature of the injurious agent determines to some extent the relative degrees of the various features (exudation, emigration of leukocytes, etc.) of the reaction.

Chemotaxis. The migration of leukocytes through the walls of venules and their subsequent movement in the tissues has been widely assumed to be mediated by chemotaxis, a process in which cells move towards higher concentrations of certain substances termed **chemotactic agents** or **chemotaxins**. Such directed movement is not readily demonstrated *in vivo*, largely because it is difficult to establish and maintain gradients of concentration of test substances in living tissues. Nevertheless, time-lapse cinephotomicrography of inflamed tissues within rabbit's ear chambers has revealed that the movements of polymorphs in pursuit of bacteria appear as purposeful as a dog following a scent. Early attempts to measure the

chemotactic activity of various agents *in vitro* were mostly invalidated by use of serum, which is itself chemotactic, in the culture medium. Reliable methods stem largely from the work of Boyden (1962) who devised a chamber in which a suspension of leukocytes is separated by a millipore membrane from a solution of the substance being tested for chemotactic activity. The

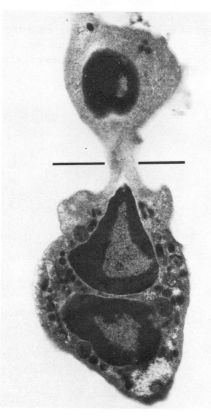

Fig. 2.11 Electron micrograph of a neutrophil polymorph migrating through a millipore membrane in response to a chemotaxin. Most of the organelles have passed into the cytoplasm which, together with two lobes of the nucleus, has moved downwards through a pore, the site of which is indicated by the heavy line. × 14 300. (By courtesy of Dr. P. C. Wilkinson and Churchill-Livingstone.)

number of cells migrating through the membrane (Fig. 2.11) is taken as an index of chemotaxis. In spite of criticisms and subsequent improvements, the technique has proved effective and its use has demonstrated that there is a good correlation between chemotactic activity of a substance *in vitro* and its capacity to promote emigration of leukocytes within an hour of intradermal injection. The time factor is important, because injection of any aqueous solution, even saline, is followed after 2 hours by some leukocytic emigration. Substances with chemotactic properties are numerous but ill defined: they are present (*a*) in extracts of inflamed skin obtained during the period of polymorph migration; (*b*) in saline extracts of neutrophil polymorphs; (*c*) among bacterial products; (*d*) in serum, and particularly serum which has been incubated with homogenates of various organs and tissues. Lysates of polymorphs themselves· are especially potent when incubated with serum.

The nature of these chemotactic and migration-promoting factors is by no means fully established. It has been shown, however, that partial digestion of proteins, including immunoglobulins, by proteases from polymorphs or other cell types, produces chemotactic peptides. It is also known that activation of complement results in chemotactic factors, one of which is the C5a component of reacted complement: this is of importance not only in certain hypersensitivy reactions (p. 124) but also in non-immunological types of inflammation in which there is increasing evidence that activation of complement occurs, probably by the alternate pathway (p. 116). In necrosis of part of the myocardium resulting from experimental ligation of a coronary artery, it has been found that emigration of polymorphs from the blood vessels in the adjacent surviving tissue is largely suppressed by prior depletion of the plasma complement. Apparently the myocardium and some other tissues contain enzymes which are released following necrosis and are capable of splitting C3 and thus of triggering off complement activation.

It may be concluded that chemotaxis is of considerable importance in emigration of leukocytes and that, like mediators of other events of the acute inflammatory response, chemotactic factors are numerous, complex, and largely unidentified.

Emigration of monocytes. Neutrophil polymorphs emigrate earlier and more rapidly than monocytes, so that in short-lived acute inflammation the peak of polymorph emigration has passed before monocytes emigrate in significant numbers. In more prolonged inflammation due to pyogenic bacterial infection, emigration of polymorphs continues until most of the bacteria have been destroyed, and only then do monocytes emigrate in large numbers. It is thus apparent that different factors control emigration of polymorphs and monocytes, and yet most preparations which have been tested for chemotactic activity *in vitro* (see above) have given parallel results with polymorphs and monocytes.

In inflammation due to infection with some bacteria, e.g. *Myco. tuberculosis* and *S. typhi*, emigration of polymorphs is transient or absent, and most of the emigrating cells are monocytes and lymphocytes. The role of cell-mediated immunity in such responses is discussed in Chapter 6, but monocyte emigration also predominates in the experimentally-induced reaction to relatively inert foreign material, such as carrageenan and synthetic polymers, which are unlikely to invoke an immunological reaction. It must therefore be assumed that there are chemotactic factors specific for monocytes, but so far these are largely unrecognised. An exception is a product of *Corynebacterium parvum*, which is chemotactic to monocytes, but not polymorphs, *in vitro*: on intradermal injection, this bacterium calls forth a predominantly monocytic response (Wilkinson, 1973).

The lymphatics in acute inflammation

The smallest lymphatics are blind-ending tubes with a very thin endothelium and a fine, incomplete, i.e. discontinuous, basement membrane. Normally they are partly collapsed, but fine fibrils attach the outer surface of the endothelium to the collagen in the surrounding tissue, and swelling of the tissue by inflammatory exudate tenses these fibrils and distends the lymphatics. The endothelial cells overlap one another and their junctions are very easily separated: they appear to act as valves, allowing fluid to pass in but not out.

These features allow greatly increased lymph drainage from inflamed tissue. Exuded proteins are removed by the lymphatics, and red cells and leukocytes also pass into the lymphatics of inflamed tissue.

The filter function of the lymph nodes in inflammation is described in Chapter 17.

Further stages of acute inflammation

The three common results of the acute inflammatory reaction are:

(*a*) Resolution, i.e. subsidence of the inflammatory changes and return of the tissue to normal.
(*b*) Progression to suppuration.
(*c*) Progression to a chronic phase with fibrosis.

Resolution. Termination of the injury which has caused inflammation is followed by reversal of the inflammatory changes, and provided that there has not been wholesale destruction, the tissue usually returns to normal. Cell and tissue debris are digested by enzymes in the exudate or by phagocytes (Fig. 2.12); pavementing and

away in the lymphatics, and normality is restored.

The most striking example of resolution in clinical medicine is in lobar pneumonia, an acute infection of the lung usually due to *Streptococcus pneumoniae*, in which typically the alveoli throughout a whole lobe become filled with a protein-rich exudate containing a fine network of fibrin and large numbers of neutrophil polymorphs (Fig. 15.24, p. 414). Following destruction of the bacteria, usually after several days, polymorphs and macrophages complete the digestion of fibrin, dead cells and debris, the fluid exudate is removed partly by reabsorption and partly by coughing, and in most cases the lobe returns to normal.

Suppuration. Pyogenic bacteria cause acute inflammation in which emigration of polymorphs is intense, and in which local toxic

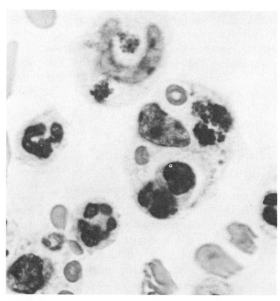

Fig. 2.12 Exudate from peritoneal cavity of guinea-pig in resolving acute inflammation of three days' duration. Note the two macrophages which have phagocytosed red cells and leukocytes. × 1000.

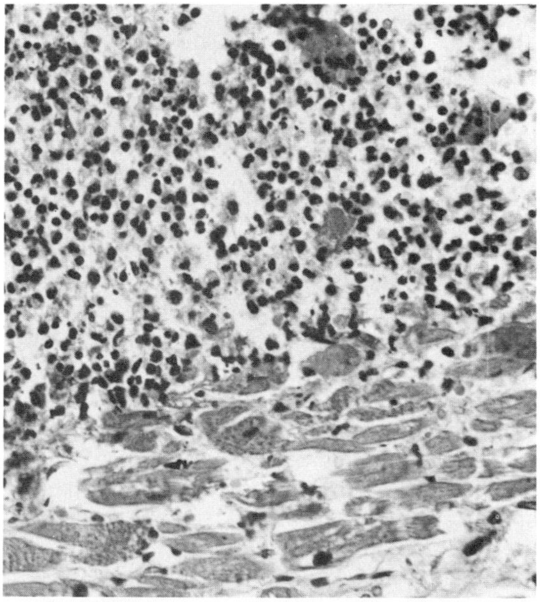

Fig. 2.13 Margin of an abscess cavity in the myocardium. In the upper part of the field the myocardial cells have been killed and digested, leaving a space filled with purulent exudate. × 250.

emigration of leukocytes cease; the vessel walls regain their normal permeability, and blood flow returns to normal. Most of the emigrated polymorphs probably die, while macrophages (emigrated monocytes) may pass to the draining lymph nodes. Inflammatory exudate drains

injury is often severe enough to cause tissue necrosis at the centre of the lesion. The dead tissue is digested by the polymorph enzymes, leaving a space in the tissue filled with inflammatory exudate rich in polymorphs (Fig. 2.13) and containing also bacteria, necrotic tissue and cell debris and fibrin. Such a cavity is termed an **abscess**, and the contained fluid, which may be creamy from its cell content and sticky from its high nucleic acid content (from dead polymorphs) is called **pus** or **purulent exudate**. Return to normal is no longer possible since tissue has been destroyed, and the abscess becomes enclosed in a wall of granulation tissue (the pyogenic membrane) which eventually matures to scar tissue. Pus can also form in a natural body cavity, such as the pleura or peritoneum, without tissue destruction, as a result of pyogenic bacterial infection.

A more detailed account of suppuration and its effects is given in Chapter 7.

Fibrosis in acute inflammation. Although acute inflammatory lesions frequently subside without leaving any significant residual changes, this is by no means always so. Formation of granulation tissue with consequent fibrosis or scarring is a common result. It complicates acute inflammation in the following three circumstances. Firstly, it occurs when the original injury which has brought about the inflammation is severe enough to have caused necrosis of tissue. Secondly, fibrin deposited from the inflammatory exudate may be replaced by fibrous tissue. Thirdly, progression of acute to chronic inflammation is accompanied by fibrosis (p. 53).

Tissue necrosis. Inflammation has been defined as the reaction to injury of *living* tissue, but many injuries, e.g. burns or bacterial infections, bring about necrosis of tissue. Obviously, inflammatory changes cannot occur in necrotic tissue, but inevitably the adjacent, surviving tissue is injured less severely and inflammation occurs in it. Accordingly, necrotic tissue is commonly present in the centre of acute inflammatory lesions. The occurrence of such wholesale necrosis of tissue, as distinct from necrosis of single cells, precludes the possibility of return to normal. If the dead tissue is superficial, as in a burn, it usually becomes detached, leaving a gap in the surviving tissues. If deeper, it may be gradually replaced by granulation tissue (a process termed **organisation**), or it may be digested, as in suppurating infection, leaving an abscess cavity. In all three instances, granulation tissue grows from the adjacent living tissue, and matures to fibrous scar tissue.

It is worth noting that when tissue is excised, leaving a gap, or dies from ischaemia (lack of

blood supply), its place is usually taken by fibrous tissue in the process of healing. The fibrosis which follows necrosis of tissue in acute inflammatory lesions is thus an example of healing.

Organisation of fibrin. The inflammatory exudate contains plasma proteins, including fibrinogen, and frequently this is converted to insoluble fibrin which is deposited in the inflamed tissue. Fine strands of fibrin (Fig. 2.4, p. 38) are readily digested by proteolytic enzymes in the exudate or removed by phagocytosis (see below). Larger deposits of fibrin, however, are not readily removed in this way, but,

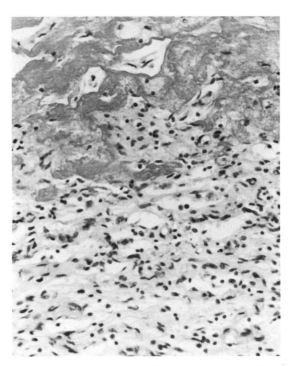

Fig. 2.14 A dense layer of fibrin on the pleural surface, showing organisation, i.e. replacement by vascular granulation tissue, extending from the underlying pleura. × 250.

like dead tissue, are more gradually replaced by granulation tissue (Fig. 2.14) by the process of organisation, with consequent scarring. This is commonly seen in acute inflammation of a serous membrane, such as the pleura or pericardium (Fig. 2.15), when a thick layer of fibrin is deposited on the surface, and its subsequent organisation results in fibrous thickening.

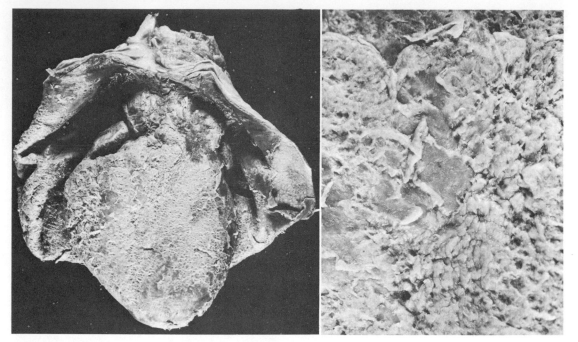

Fig. 2.15 Acute pericarditis, showing a thick, irregular deposit of fibrin on the pericardial surfaces. *Left,* × ⅔; *right,* × 3.

Beneficial effects of acute inflammation

The effects of acute inflammation are due mainly to the flow of exudate through the inflamed tissues and the phagocytic activities of emigrated leukocytes. These two processes both contribute to lessening the harmful effect of toxic agents and to the elimination of infection.

The inflammatory exudate

The fluid exudate is protective in the following ways.

1. Dilution of toxins. When inflammation is caused by toxic chemicals, including bacterial toxins, the exudate diminishes local tissue injury by diluting the toxins and carrying them away by the lymphatics.

2. Protective antibodies. The proteins in the exudate include antibodies which have developed as a result of infection or immunisation and which are present in the individual's plasma. In acute inflammation due to infection, the exudate may thus contain antibodies which react with, and promote destruction of, the micro-organisms, or which neutralise their toxins. Antibodies promote killing of micro-organisms by rendering them susceptible to lysis by complement and destruction by phagocytes. This is described more fully in Chapter 6.

3. Fibrin formation. Fibrinogen in the exudate is converted to solid fibrin by the action of tissue thromboplastin. A network of deposited fibrin is commonly seen in inflamed tissues, and may form a mechanical barrier to the movement and spread of bacteria. It may also aid in their phagocytosis by leukocytes (p. 170).

4. Promotion of immunity. Micro-organisms and toxins in the inflammatory lesions are carried by the exudate, either free or in phagocytes, to the local lymph nodes where they may stimulate an immune response. This provides antibodies and cellular mechanisms of defence which appear within a few days and may be maintained for years.

5. Cell nutrition. The flow of inflammatory exudate brings with it glucose, oxygen, etc., and thus helps to supply the greatly increased numbers of cells: it also carries away their metabolic products.

Phagocytosis

The neutrophil polymorphs in inflammatory lesions are actively phagocytic. The emigrated monocytes are not at first so active, but they rapidly change into the larger, more active macrophages. The process of phagocytosis is similar for both polymorphs and macrophages, and resembles closely the engulfment of food particles by amoebae. First, the surface of the phagocyte attaches to the particle, e.g. bacterium, to be ingested. The cytoplasm then flows around the particle and envelops it in a **phagocytic vacuole**. Finally the plasma membrane enclosing the vacuole breaks away from the cell surface, and the membrane-lined vacuole lies free in the cytoplasm. The subsequent fate of the particle depends on its nature and on the host's response. Adjacent lysosomes fuse with the membrane of the phagocytic vacuole, and pour their contents into it, the vacuole now being termed a **phagolysosome** or **phagosome**. The particle is thus exposed to the lysosomal acid hydrolases, and these include such a wide range of enzymes that most biological material, including red cells, fibrin, collagen and ground substance, dead cells and cell components, are digested. By engulfing and digesting the debris of the inflammatory reaction, the phagocytes act as scavengers (Fig. 2.12). During phagocytic activity, polymorphs and macrophages also release lysosomal enzymes into the surrounding fluid where they contribute to the digestion and so removal of inflammatory debris: the digestion products include peptides, nucleotides, etc. which, by increasing vascular permeability and attracting leukocytes by chemotaxis, may enhance the inflammatory reaction.

Polymorphs and macrophages play a vital protective role in microbial infections. In most bacterial infections, the bacteria are eliminated rapidly by phagocytosis and other protective mechanisms. However, there are exceptions, and some micro-organisms live and even multiply in phagocytes. The factors concerned in these host/parasite relationships are considered in Chapter 6.

Neutrophil polymorphs are highly specialised cells; they are actively motile, rich in lysosomal enzymes, and respond to relatively early chemotactic stimuli in the inflammatory reaction. They have a rich store of glycogen, and enzyme systems which provide the energy required for mobility and phagocytosis by glycolysis. The last property allows polymorphs to function in the low oxygen tension present in highly cellular inflammatory exudates.

The polymorph is an end-stage cell: it is unable to re-synthesise lysosomes and lysosomal enzymes and soon dies following phagocytic activity. The supply of polymorphs is, however, practically unlimited.

Monocytes are less actively motile and phagocytic than polymorphs. They provide a reserve of cells which, on emigration in an inflammatory lesion, change into macrophages: this involves increases in lysosomal enzymes, metabolic activity, motility, and phagocytic and microbicidal capacity. Like polymorphs, they have enzyme systems which supply the energy for this increased activity by anaerobic glycolysis, but they differ in having little stored glycogen and must therefore make use of glycogen released by polymorphs or glucose in the exudate as a source of energy. Macrophages can also produce new lysosomes and synthesise lysosomal enzymes: they are capable of long survival after phagocytic activity, and can divide. These properties suit them particularly to sustained function in prolonged inflammatory reactions.

Chronic Inflammation

In contrast to tissue injury of short duration, which induces a brief or acute inflammatory reaction, prolonged tissue injury causes persistent, or chronic inflammation. There is, however, no generally accepted time limit beyond which an inflammatory lesion is regarded as chronic. To some extent, it depends on the nature of the disease process concerned: for example a whitlow lasting for several weeks might well be regarded as chronic, as compared with the usual short course, while tuberculous lesions showing extensive spread within weeks are regarded as acute in contrast to those which smoulder on for months or years.

An important feature of chronic inflammation is the production of vascular granulation tissue, which matures into fibrous tissue. Such **proliferative changes** are in contrast to the exudative changes of the acute inflammatory reaction, but when acute inflammation fails to resolve and becomes chronic, the two processes are commonly associated. Even in an early stage of acute inflammation, some proliferation of fibroblasts occurs and, in general, the more chronic the inflammatory reaction, the more pronounced are the proliferative changes, and the greater the degree of ultimate fibrous scarring. This is well illustrated in the kidneys, in which an acute bacterial infection produces exudative changes with congestion, inflammatory oedema, and emigration of leukocytes. If the infection is overcome quickly these changes may resolve without residual damage, but if it persists the exudative changes are accompanied by formation of granulation tissue and the kidneys eventually show fibrous scarring (Fig. 21.54, p. 793). Similarly, acute bacterial infection of the gallbladder stimulates an acute inflammatory reaction, but persistent infection results in fibrosis of the wall (Fig. 19.56, p. 647).

Causes of chronic inflammation

The nature and duration of inflammatory lesions depend mainly on the intensity and persistence of the inflammatory stimulus, i.e. the causal injury. Brief but intense injury, such as burning, strong acids or ultraviolet irradiation, causes a short-lived exudative reaction, and unless there has been necrosis or abundant fibrin deposition (p. 49) the tissue soon returns to normal. Acute bacterial infections also are often brief but, as indicated above, the bacteria may be only partially subdued by the host's defence mechanisms, and their persistence in relatively small numbers causes less intense injury with the result that the acute inflammation progresses to a chronic phase with fibrosis.

There are also a number of agents, both physical and chemical and also microbial, which cause relatively low-grade but prolonged injury from the start, and give rise to chronic inflammation which starts insidiously with little or no acute exudative reaction, but with increasing fibrosis. In such lesions, polymorphs are usually scanty, and most of the cells migrating into the injured tissue are mononuclears, i.e. monocytes and lymphoid cells. The causal agents of such 'primary' chronic inflammation fall into the following four main classes.

(a) Bacterial and fungal infections. Various types of bacteria and fungi produce chronic infections in which acute inflammation is minimal, and the most prominent changes are infiltration with mononuclear cells and formation of granulation and fibrous tissue: classical examples are provided by tuberculosis (p. 173) and syphilis (p. 183). The factors which induce the proliferative changes are usually obscure, and while the various micro-organisms concerned may be directly responsible, tissue injury may result also from hypersensitivity reactions to the microbial antigens (see below).

(b) Chemical irritants. Many chemical compounds are mildly irritating, and when they persist within the tissues, chronic inflammatory changes result. Inhalation of certain particulate materials, e.g. silica (quartz), fibrous silicates (asbestos), and dust or fumes of beryllium compounds, produces chronic inflammation of the lungs. Similarly, granulomatous lesions (see p. 54) may result when these and other particulate irritants enter the tissues in dirty wounds; also from suture materials, and from the talc formerly used to lubricate the surgeon's gloves. Chronic inflammation may occur also around organic material, both foreign and endogenous, e.g. cholesterol crystals.

(c) Hypersensitivity reactions. In many chronic infections, a state of hypersensitivity to microbial antigens causes tissue injury and chronic inflammation. This is, for example, a major cause of the lesions of tuberculosis. Hypersensitivity to self-antigens also occurs, and is responsible for chronic 'auto-immune' thyroiditis, gastritis, etc. There is also evidence for a hypersensitivity basis in rheumatoid arthritis, although the antigen has not been identified.

(d) Unknown agents. In some granulomatous reactions, the causal agents remain unknown. One of the most important examples is *sarcoidosis* (p. 182), which produces lesions in the lymph nodes and various internal organs, resembling somewhat those of tuberculosis.

Histological features of chronic inflammation

Chronic inflammation is characterised by formation of new fibrous tissue: in the early stages this may be highly cellular and vascular, the cells being plump spindle-cells (fibroblasts), and the collagen fibres delicate and scanty (Fig. 2.16). As it ages, such young fibrous (granula-

plasma cells and lymphocytes also accumulate in the inflammatory focus (Fig. 2.17), their proportions depending on the nature of the causal agent. In other instances of chronic inflammation, not associated with a marked exudative reaction, polymorphs may be scanty or absent and lymphocytes or plasma cells

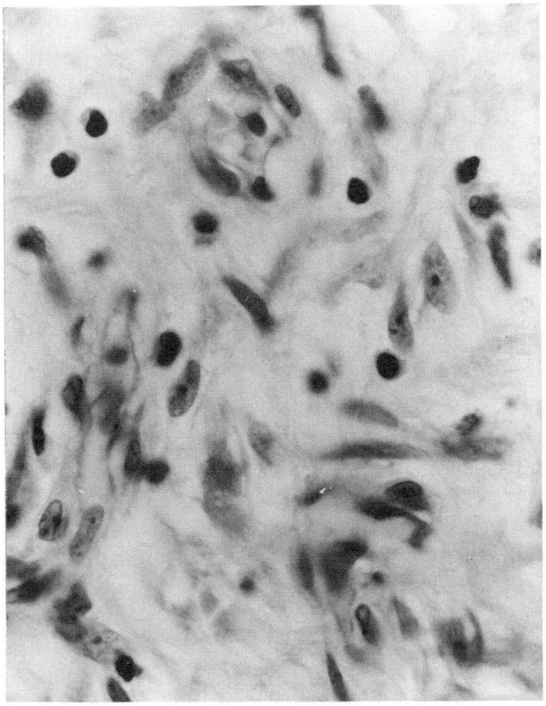

Fig. 2.16 Fibroblasts, capillaries and occasional lymphocytes in young fibrous tissue. × 540.

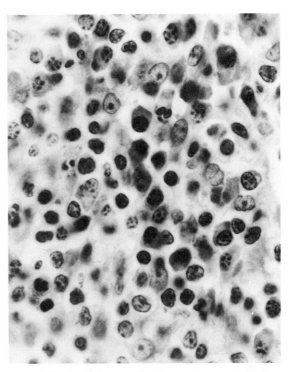

Fig. 2.17 A mixed cellular infiltrate, including plasma cells and lymphocytes, in a chronic inflammatory lesion. × 820.

tion) tissue matures into tougher fibrous tissue: the cellularity and vascularity diminish and thickening of the fibres results from further collagen deposition. When the inflammatory process is very low grade throughout, there may be formation of dense collagen without the preliminary stage of granulation tissue. These processes are described in more detail in relation to healing and repair in the next chapter.

In addition to the above changes, the area becomes infiltrated with leukocytes and macrophages. When the chronic process supervenes on an acute inflammatory lesion, e.g. a persistent pyogenic bacterial infection, polymorphs may continue to emigrate from the blood vessels and there may be foci of suppuration, but

usually predominate. In all instances, macrophages, derived mainly from emigrating monocytes, are present and they may be very numerous (p. 57). They may fuse together to form multinucleated 'giant' cells, as in tuberculosis and in chronic inflammation due to particulate material (Fig. 2.23). These various changes, often accompanied by necrosis, can produce a complex histological picture. Variations in the histological features of chronic inflammation are illustrated by the examples of chronic infections described in Chapter 7. It is often possible to make a provisional diagnosis from the histological features, but there are dangerous pitfalls. For example, several agents can give rise to changes readily mistaken for tuberculosis, and a firm diagnosis usually requires the detection of a specific causal agent, or other procedures such as serological tests for a particular infection. The morphology and staining reactions are, in some instances, sufficiently characteristic for the identification of the causal bacteria or fungi, while examination in polarised light may afford recognition of anisotropic foreign material, e.g. silica, talc, starch, suture material (Fig. 2.18).

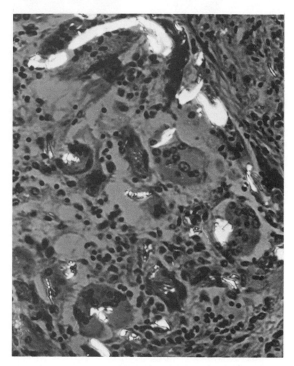

Fig. 2.18 Foreign-body giant cells in a chronic inflammatory reaction to suture material, viewed through partly crossed polarising films to show up the birefringent foreign material. × 250.

Granuloma. The terms *granuloma* and *granulomatous inflammation* or *reaction* have long been used to mean a chronic inflammatory lesion which, because it is in the form of a lump, bears some macroscopic resemblance to a tumour (hence the suffix *-oma*, which is usually reserved for tumours). The terms do not imply particular histological features except that, being chronic inflammatory lesions, granulation tissue is often a prominent feature of granulomas: it may also contain foci of suppuration or necrosis, and any of the various cells seen in inflammatory lesions. There is now an increas-ing tendency to use the terms to mean an inflammatory lesion of any size, composed mainly of macrophages, but to avoid confusion this should be described as a *macrophage granuloma*.

Results of chronic inflammation

The fibrous tissue which is formed in chronic inflammation may induce serious effects by narrowing orifices and tubes—for example, the mitral valve in chronic rheumatic fever or the small intestine in Crohn's disease. Chronic inflammation of internal organs is usually accompanied by loss of parenchymal cells, and this, together with irregular fibrosis, results in shrinkage, irregular scarring and distortion. Commonly the surface becomes uneven, with a fine or coarse granularity: this is particularly well seen in cirrhosis of the liver (Fig. 19.26, p. 622), where the irregularity is accentuated by proliferation and enlargement of surviving liver cells.

In some instances, the fibrous tissue produced in chronic inflammation may have a useful function: for example, weakening of the aorta results from destruction of elastic tissue and muscle of the media in syphilitic aortitis, but fibrous tissue is laid down and may delay or prevent abnormal stretching and rupture.

Other causes of fibrosis. While fibrosis is an important feature of chronic inflammation, it may result from other causes. As stated above, fibrosis is the usual method of repair when tissue has been lost, and occurs in the removal of deposits of fibrin by organisation. Unless it is dissolved by fibrinolytic enzymes, thrombus in blood vessels is also replaced by fibrous tissue. These processes are dealt with in the next chapter.

When the blood supply to a part is gradually diminished by arterial disease, atrophy of the specialised cells may be accompanied by overgrowth of the supporting tissue. Similarly, death of tissue resulting from sudden occlusion of an artery, e.g. by thrombosis, is followed by replacement of the dead tissue by fibrous tissue. Patches of fibrosis of this nature are commonly seen in the myocardium. These effects of deficient blood supply (ischaemia) are described in Chapter 8.

Types of cell in Inflammatory Lesions

Polymorphonuclear leukocytes

Neutrophil polymorphs. The origin and morphology of these cells are described on p. 153 *et seq*. Their migratory activity has already been considered and their roles in the defence against micro-organisms and in Arthus type hypersensitivity reactions are dealt with in later chapters.

Eosinophil polymorphs. The accumulation of these cells in inflammatory lesions is closely associated with hypersensitivity reactions. They are observed particularly in the lesions of bronchial asthma, in the tissues around metazoan parasites, in certain skin diseases, and in various lesions of the gastro-intestinal tract. Intense local accumulation of eosinophils is commonly associated with eosinophil leukocytosis in the blood and there is recent evidence to suggest that this is mediated by an immune response. The thymic-dependent lymphocytes which respond to antigenic stimulation, e.g. by a parasitic worm, in some way stimulate the proliferation of eosinophil precursors in the bone marrow. The function of eosinophil polymorphs is obscure.

Lymphoid cells

Lymphocytes accumulate in chronic inflammatory lesions and their presence in large numbers is suggestive of either a delayed hypersensitivity reaction or possibly of antibody-dependent lymphocyte cytotoxicity. These phenomena are described in Chapters 4 and 5.

The presence of **plasma cells** in inflamed tissues, as elsewhere, is indicative of antibody production: they do not usually appear until about a week after onset of inflammation and are present in greatest numbers in persistent lesions caused by bacteria. Their origin and function are described in Chapter 4.

Macrophages: the mononuclear phagocyte system

The terms **macrophage** and **mononuclear phagocyte** were applied by Metchnikoff, in 1905, to large phagocytic cells, which he distinguished from the smaller phagocytic neutrophil polymorph. In 1924, Aschoff described investigations on tissue cells based on vital staining, i.e. the ingestion of droplets of fluid (micropinocytosis) containing non-toxic dyes bound to protein, and concentration of the dye in the cell cytoplasm. While many cells did this, Aschoff noted particularly intense staining of cells in the lining of vascular and lymphoid sinusoids, reticular cells of the spleen and lymph nodes, and scattered cells lying in connective tissues. He grouped these cells together under the term *reticulo-endothelial system*. From this grouping, the macrophages have emerged as cells which, although widely dispersed through the body, share a common origin and have certain well-defined functions. Accordingly the term 'mononuclear phagocyte system' is being used increasingly for macrophages and their precursor cells. The term 'reticulo-endothelial system' is no longer appropriate: endothelial cells lining blood vessels are quite distinct in their origin and functions, and reticular cells are ill-defined.

Components of the mononuclear phagocyte system. Macrophages may be recognised by their avid phagocytic properties (Fig. 2.19), the

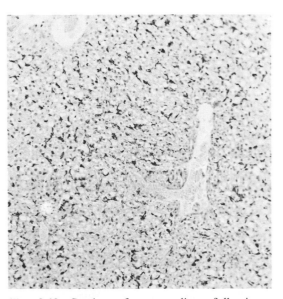

Fig. 2.19 Section of mouse liver following an intravascular injection of colloidal carbon. The hepatic macrophages (Kupffer cells) are black because of the large amount of carbon which they have phagocytosed. × 80.

firmness with which they adhere to a glass surface, both *in vivo* and *in vitro*, and their morphological differences from the other 'professional' phagocyte, the neutrophil polymorph.

Cells of the mononuclear phagocyte system are scattered widely throughout the body. In some sites they are normally inactive and inconspicuous but are capable, on stimulation, of enlargement, increased metabolism, and the active phagocytic role of the macrophage. Cells of the system include the following:

(1) The Kupffer cells, which form part of the lining of the hepatic sinusoids; similar cells in the vascular sinusoids of the bone marrow, spleen, adrenal cortex and adenohypophysis, and in the lymphatic sinuses of lymph nodes.

(2) Cells in the spaces of the network formed by the reticular cells in the medulla of lymph nodes and red pulp of the spleen.

(3) Cells on the surface of the serous cavities. These are particularly numerous in the omentum, where they are aggregated to form the 'milk spots'.

(4) Alveolar macrophages lying free on the surface of, and also within, the alveolar walls.

(5) Histiocytes in connective tissues, osteoclasts in bone, and microglial cells of central nervous tissue.

(6) The monocytes of the blood and their precursors in the bone marrow, the earliest recognisable cell in the system being the promonocyte.

Kinetics of mononuclear phagocytes. In experimental animal studies, it has been shown that the monocytes are produced in the bone marrow, circulate in the blood for a few days, and are the precursors of the cells listed in 1–5 above, which may persist for months or possibly years. The fate of the mononuclear phagocytes is not known. There is some evidence that they may re-enter the blood and pass to the lungs, to be excreted *via* the bronchi.

The kinetics of macrophages in inflammatory lesions have been studied extensively by Spector and others. In various types of granulomatous inflammation, and in various tissues, it has been shown that most of the macrophages are provided by migration of monocytes. Their lifespan in chronic inflammatory lesions has been found to vary depending on the causal agent.

With relatively strong cytotoxic agents, macrophage turnover is rapid, a continuous supply from the blood being necessary to maintain the macrophage population of the lesion. With blander agents, turnover is much slower (i.e. weeks), and mitosis of macrophages in the lesion may be almost sufficient to maintain the population. Curiously, mitosis of inflammatory macrophages is accompanied by a high incidence of chromosomal abnormalities which, by precluding further divisions, must limit their local proliferation.

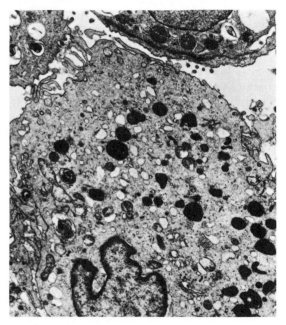

Fig. 2.20   An electron micrograph of part of a macrophage, showing microvilli (*top*) and a portion of the nucleus (*bottom*). The cytoplasmic dense bodies (black) are phagosomes formed by the fusion of lysosomes with phagocytic vacuoles and the 'empty' spaces are dilated endoplasmic reticulum. × 7000.

Morphology of macrophages. Macrophages are motile cells and can assume polarity and various shapes. They have an oval, indented or irregular nucleus, abundant cytoplasm rich in lysosomes, and surface microvilli (Fig. 2.20). Phagocytic vacuoles, if present, are helpful in their recognition. Macrophages vary greatly in size (Fig. 2.21): they are usually larger than monocytes, but in the resting state they may closely resemble lymphocytes (e.g. in the peritoneum), and the distinction cannot always be

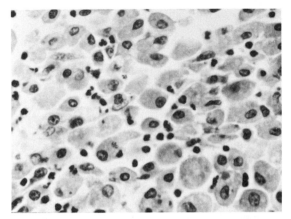

Fig. 2.21 Macrophages of various sizes in the wall of a chronically inflamed gallbladder. Note the ovoid or indented nucleus and abundant cytoplasm. × 405.

made on morphology alone. This may account for some of the claims, which are probably incorrect, of transformation between the two cell types.

Monocytes may be regarded as immature macrophage precursors which, on stimulation, transform to macrophages. The change involves increase in motility, size and phagocytic activity: cytoplasmic RNA and lysosomes increase, and the nucleus becomes larger and less condensed. Similar changes have recently been demonstrated by Spector *et al.* when inflammatory exudate is added to cultures of macrophages (Fig. 2.22).

In chronic inflammatory lesions, macrophages may assume the special features of **epithelioid cells** or of **giant cells**. Change to epithelioid cells (so-called because they have some resemblance to epithelial cells) involves an increase in the amount of cytoplasm and in rough endoplasmic reticulum: epithelioid cells are not actively phagocytic, and they may have a secretory function.

The factors responsible for change of macrophages to epithelioid cells are not fully understood: it is seen in immunological reactions of delayed hypersensitivity type, and may therefore be mediated by lymphoid cells: the same factors may be concerned in formation of Langhans' giant cells (see below) for these are usually associated with epithelioid cells.

Giant cells. It is common to see macrophages with two or more nuclei, but they can fuse together to form very large giant cells with sometimes over 100 nuclei. Such cells are usually classified into **foreign-body giant cells**, which have irregularly scattered nuclei, and **Langhans' giant cells**, in which the nuclei are arranged peripherally (Fig. 2.23). Spector has studied giant-cell formation by monocytes in

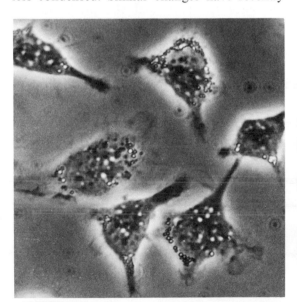
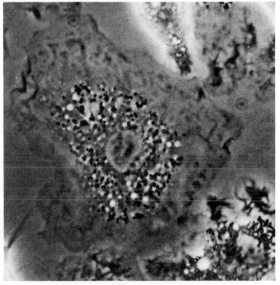

Fig. 2.22 Mouse peritoneal macrophages in culture, viewed by phase-contrast microscopy. Inflammatory exudate has been added to the culture shown on right. Note the increase in size, content of (phase-dense) lysosomes and (phase-lucent) vesicles and extensive cytoplasmic 'ruffling' of the stimulated cell. × 960. (Professor W. G. Spector and Mrs. Katherine M. Wynne.)

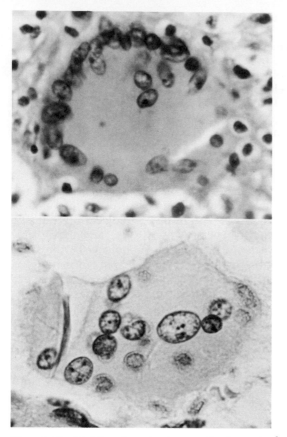

Fig. 2.23 Multinucleated giant cells formed by fusion of macrophages. The upper cell is a Langhans' giant cell in a tuberculous lesion: note the peripheral arrangement of the nuclei and abundant cytoplasm. The lower cell is a foreign-body giant cell: the nuclei vary in size and are irregularly distributed, and the cell has engulfed a fragment of suture material. × 750.

tissue culture. At first, they resemble foreign-body giant cells, but may later develop the features of Langhans' cells.

The *osteoclasts*, which digest bone matrix in the process of bone resorption, appear to be formed by coalescence of monocytes, and thus represent specialised cells within the macrophage system. The influence of the local environment on macrophages is also illustrated by the alveolar macrophages, which require oxygen for full phagocytic activity, whereas macrophages elsewhere can produce the necessary energy solely by glycolysis under anaerobic conditions.

Macrophage functions. The major function of the macrophage is phagocytosis and destruction of micro-organisms and other harmful or unwanted material. The general features of their phagocytic role in inflammation (p. 51) and their protective role in infection (pp. 149–51) are considered elsewhere. Macrophages also have the important physiological role of removing dead or effete cells. For example they are responsible for taking up degenerate erythrocytes: they break down the cell and its haemoglobin, and release the iron, etc. for re-utilisation.

Macrophages are capable of ingesting large amounts of insoluble material (Fig. 2.19), and of retaining it for months or even years. This happens when, for various reasons, abnormal amounts of lipids (p. 20) or iron accumulate in the various tissues, or when dust particles are inhaled in atmospheric pollution. These conditions of abnormal storage are described in later chapters, in relation to the organs and tissues they most affect.

Other functions of the mononuclear phagocytes include participation in immune responses (p. 108), and the production of endogenous pyrogen in pyrexia (p. 156).

Other cells

Serosal cells. In acute inflammation of a serous surface, cells on or near the surface enlarge and often pass into the exudate at an early stage. They include macrophages and endothelial lining cells. In more chronic inflammation, the latter cells may grow in clumps in the fluid exudate in the cavity, and may show nuclear abnormalities and mucin secretion. In aspirated fluid, they are sometimes very difficult to distinguish from cancer cells.

Fibroblasts are seen in most acute inflammatory lesions, but their presence in large numbers is associated with chronic inflammation and repair. They are considered in the next chapter.

3

Healing, Repair and Hypertrophy

Healing and Repair

Reaction of tissues to injury varies greatly in different species of animals and in different tissues. **Regeneration**, i.e. the replacement of a single type of parenchymatous cell by production of more cells of the same kind may be seen in man but different tissues have this ability in varying degree and in some it is lacking. A helpful guide to the expected reaction to damage of any tissue is given by the division of somatic cells into three types.

(*a*) *Labile cells* are those which under normal conditions continue to multiply throughout life and include epidermis, alimentary, respiratory and urinary tract epithelium, uterine endometrium and the haemopoietic bone marrow and lymphoid cells.

(*b*) *Stable cells* normally cease multiplication when growth ceases but retain mitotic ability during adult life so that some regeneration of damaged tissues may occur. This group includes liver, pancreas, renal tubular epithelium, thyroid and adrenal cortex.

(*c*) *Permanent cells* lose their mitotic ability in infancy and the classic example of this group is the neurone.

In many instances healing of an organ or tissue occurs by regeneration, the cells lost being replaced by proliferative activity of those remaining. However, when the injury involves a cell type inherently incapable of this or when other factors, e.g. interruption of blood supply, prevents restoration, healing occurs by the **formation of a fibrous scar** the development of which is best illustrated by the healing of a wound of skin and subcutaneous tissue.

Healing of skin wounds

Healing by first intention (primary union)

Primary union occurs in uninfected surgical incisions and in other clean wounds sutured without undue delay. It is characterised by the formation of only minimal amounts of granulation tissue.

The wound clot and its removal. When an incision is made in the skin and subcutaneous tissue, blood escaping from cut vessels clots on the wound surface and fills the gap between the wound edges which, in sutured wounds, is narrow. The blood clot acts temporarily as a glue which keeps the cut surfaces in close apposition and forms a protective cover. However, excessive and deeply situated blood clot (haematoma) delays healing. During the first 24 hours, there is a mild inflammatory reaction at the wound edges with exudation of fluid and migration of polymorphs and later of monocytes and lymphocytes. Blood clot is digested by enzymes from disintegrated polymorphs and this is aided from about the third or fourth day by macrophages, derived mainly from blood monocytes, which ingest and digest any remaining fibrin, red cells and cellular debris. These changes represent the acute inflammatory (exudative) phase of response to injury and are usually mild unless infection supervenes.

Epithelial regeneration. The first tissue to bridge the incisional gap is the squamous epithelium of the epidermis. Within 24 hours and extending from 3–4 mm around the wound edge there is enlargement and flattening of the basal cells with loss of prominence of rete ridges. Two processes then contribute to the closure of the gap. Close to the cut edge, cells from the deeper part of the epithelium begin to slide over each other, *migrate* out over the wound surface and become flattened to form a continuous advancing sheet. *Proliferation* also occurs, mainly among basal cells in the epidermis and pilosebaceous follicles adjacent to the wound. Mitosis is rarely seen in the migrating cells but occurs later in the new epithelium. While the advancing edge of the sheet of new epidermis consists of a single layer of flat cells, the older part at the periphery of the wound becomes stratified so that there is a gradient of thickness. The cells, which produce proteolytic enzymes, grow beneath the surface clot and also down the cut edges into the dermis (Figs. 3.1 and 3.2). Within 48 hours, and before there is any connective tissue regeneration, the wound may be bridged by epithelium which rapidly becomes stratified but does not form rete ridges (Figs. 3.3, 3.8). Any epithelium which has grown down into the dermis is later resorbed (Fig. 3.1).

Suture tracks. Epithelium also tends to grow down suture tracks, from both ends (Fig. 3.4) and may meet in the deep part of the stitch wound. Often much of the epithelium is avulsed when stitches are removed but some may remain and occasionally gives rise either to a small implantation cyst or to an acute inflammatory reaction to keratin, which may simulate infection. Each suture track is another wound in that there is haemorrhage, death of cells and injury to skin appendages, and in consequence there is a slight inflammatory reaction and

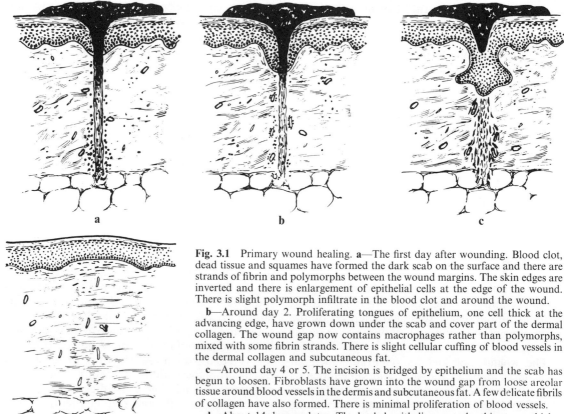

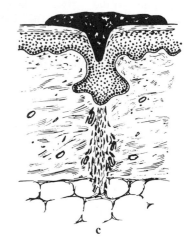

Fig. 3.1 Primary wound healing. **a**—The first day after wounding. Blood clot, dead tissue and squames have formed the dark scab on the surface and there are strands of fibrin and polymorphs between the wound margins. The skin edges are inverted and there is enlargement of epithelial cells at the edge of the wound. There is slight polymorph infiltrate in the blood clot and around the wound.

b—Around day 2. Proliferating tongues of epithelium, one cell thick at the advancing edge, have grown down under the scab and cover part of the dermal collagen. The wound gap now contains macrophages rather than polymorphs, mixed with some fibrin strands. There is slight cellular cuffing of blood vessels in the dermal collagen and subcutaneous fat.

c—Around day 4 or 5. The incision is bridged by epithelium and the scab has begun to loosen. Fibroblasts have grown into the wound gap from loose areolar tissue around blood vessels in the dermis and subcutaneous fat. A few delicate fibrils of collagen have also formed. There is minimal proliferation of blood vessels.

d—About 14 days or later. The healed epithelium may be thinner or thicker than normal, is lacking in rete ridges and slightly raised above the surface. Collagen fibres are now orientated to unite the wound edges. Slightly increased vascularity and cellularity remain to mark the wound site.

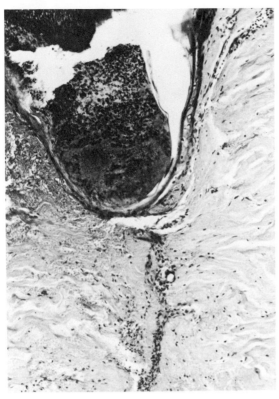

Fig. 3.2 Aseptic abdominal wound showing the stage of healing at five days. The incision is represented merely by a vertical cellular line. The round body on the surface is a small scab beneath which the epithelium has extended down to cover the dermis. × 105.

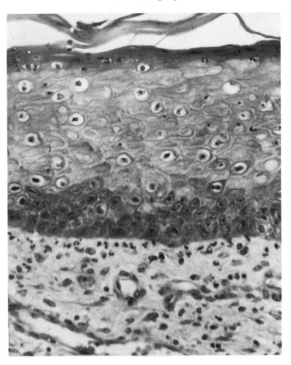

Fig. 3.3 Newly formed epithelium on healed ulcer. The epithelium is several cells thick, but there is little differentiation, and there is no formation of rete ridges. A similar appearance is seen in a healed surgical incision. × 400.

fibroblast proliferation (Fig. 3.4). Because the suture prevents closure of the surface epithelium the track is prone to infection and 'stitch abscesses' are commoner than sepsis of surgical incisions.

Repair of the dermis and subcutaneous tissue. These tissues heal by proliferation of new blood vessels and fibroblasts to form 'granulation tissue'. From about the third day, *vascular proliferation* is seen as capillary sprouts, which grow from blood vessels at the wound margins (Fig. 3.5), and advance up to 2 mm per day into the wound: the capillary sprouts are produced partly by rearrangement and migration of pre-existing endothelial cells and partly by proliferation just behind the advancing tip. The sprouts are at first often solid, but they unite with one another or join a capillary already carrying blood and develop a lumen. These newly formed vessels are more delicate (Fig. 3.12) and

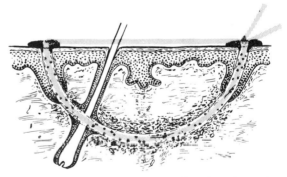

Fig. 3.4 Diagram of suture track a few days after wounding and before removal of sutures. In the centre of the picture the healed epithelium still forms a small projection into the dermis and beneath it the more cellular vertical line of the healing wound is seen.

The surface epithelium and that from a damaged hair follicle have grown along the suture track which is open to the skin surface and contains fibrin and polymorphs. There is more vascular and fibroblastic proliferation around the suture track than around the original wound.

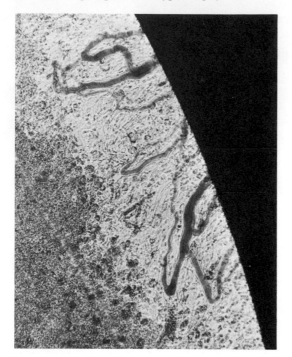

Fig. 3.5 Capillary loops growing into a blood clot in a transparent chamber embedded in a rabbit's ear, photographed *in vivo*. Similar but less marked vascular proliferation is seen in the healing of a simple surgical incision. Note large numbers of macrophages in advance of growing vessels. (The late Prof. Lord Florey.)

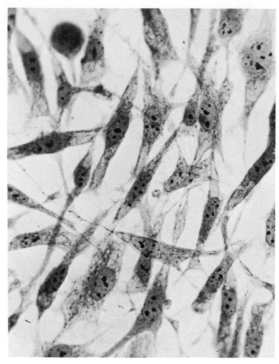

Fig. 3.6a Fibroblasts as seen in tissue culture. (The late Dr. Janet S. F. Niven.)

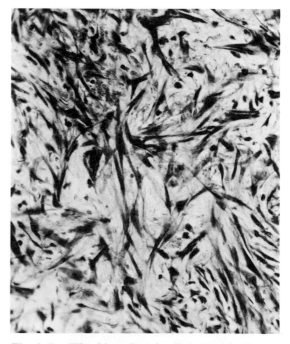

Fig. 3.6b Fibroblasts in a healing wound, showing the characteristic shape and early formation of collagen fibrils. × 350.

behave as if acutely inflamed: they leak protein-rich fluid with some red cells, and polymorphs emigrate from them. It has been observed in rabbits that if blood flow is not soon established through a new vessel then the lumen disappears, the vessel reverting to a solid cord which then breaks and the ends retract by sliding back of endothelial cells to the nearest vessel carrying blood. Within a few days of the establishment of circulation, some of the new vessels differentiate into arterioles and venules by the acquisition of muscle cells either by migration from pre-existing larger blood channels or by differentiation from mesenchymal cells.

Lymphatic channels are re-established in the same manner as blood vessels.

Fibrous tissue proliferation. After the removal of blood, fibrin and dead cells from the wound, and simultaneously with the development of new blood vessels, long, spindle-shaped fibroblasts (Fig. 3.6a and b) in the adjacent tissue begin to proliferate and to move into the incisional area. Within 4 or 5 days fibroblasts mingle in the incision and produce randomly arranged reticulin fibres which are soon converted into the mature collagen which gives scar tissue its physical strength. The fibres come to lie across the incision line and probably unite the cut edges from about the end of the first week after injury. During the second week there is a great increase of both reticulin fibres and mature collagen bundles so that by the third week the total amount of collagen in the wound has almost reached a maximum. In contrast, at this stage the tensile strength of the wound is still low, but it increases over many months by further intermolecular bonding between collagen fibrils and by remodelling of the anatomical configuration of the collagen in response to mechanical stress. Collagen turnover, involving synthesis and lysis, is thought to occur also in resting tissues, the two processes normally being in equilibrium.

While the formation of a collagenous scar is beneficial in restoring the integrity of a skin wound, it may produce undesirable effects, for instance narrowing of a hollow viscus: the most promising attempts to control these unwanted effects have involved the use of chemicals which inhibit intra- and inter-molecular cross-linking of collagen.

It seems likely that fibroblasts are derived chiefly from resting, locally resident fibrocytes or undifferentiated mesenchymal cells in the dermal papillary layer, around blood vessels, and in the deepest layers of the dermis, rather than from the cells of the dense collagenous dermis. On electron microscopy, the fibroblast is seen to contain much endoplasmic reticulum studded with ribosomes and a substantial Golgi apparatus, features characteristic of a secretory cell. Collagen, like other proteins destined for secretion, is synthesised on the polysomes of the rough endoplasmic reticulum as a soluble protein (procollagen). After synthesis is complete, procollagen is modified enzymatically and then probably transferred to the Golgi apparatus before it is discharged through the cell membrane. In the extracellular space (or at the cell surface) procollagen is cleaved by procollagen peptidase to form collagen monomer (tropocollagen). This monomeric collagen spontaneously aggregates laterally and longitudinally to form collagen fibrils which have a characteristic 64 nm banding pattern in the electron microscope (Fig. 3.7). These fibrils become grouped together to form the fibres visible in the light microscope with reticulin stains. The argyrophil reticulin fibres become thicker

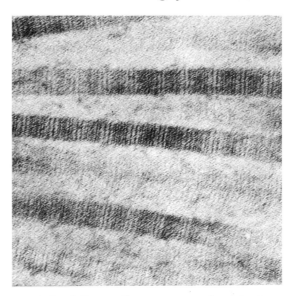

Fig. 3.7 Collagen fibres are seen here in longitudinal section. The characteristic, regular cross banding is evident. × 100 000 approx.

by further accretion of tropocollagen and develop the histological staining reactions of mature collagen. Concomitant with the increase in fibre thickness, cross-links form between and within each collagen molecule in these fibres and it is this process which is partly responsible for the increase in tensile strength of a wound after 14 days.

Events following primary wound healing. Once the wound has healed the young scar is raised above the surface due to the underlying proliferative processes and is red as a result of

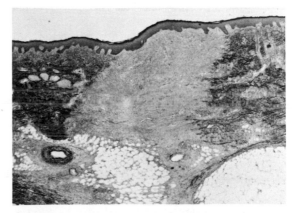

Fig. 3.8 Healed surgical wound of skin of 14 days' duration. The elastic fibres are stained black, and the healed wound is seen in the centre: it is composed of connective tissue in which elastic fibres have not yet formed. × 5.

increased vascularity. The blood vessels gradually decrease in number, probably in the manner already described, and excess fibrous tissue may slowly disappear. *Elastic fibres* are formed much later than collagen (Fig. 3.8). *Sensory nerves* may reach the scar in about three weeks but specialised nerve endings such as Pacinian corpuscles do not re-form. The end result of healing by first intention should be a pale linear scar level with the adjacent skin surface, but sometimes a **hypertrophic scar** or **keloid** forms (p. 291).

Healing by second intention (secondary union)

Healing of an open wound or an infected closed wound occurs by the formation of granulation tissue which grows from the base of the wound to fill the defect. The vascular and fibroblastic proliferation which together make up the granulation tissue are much more abundant than in healing by first intention.

Clean open wounds. As in the closed wound there is haemorrhage and exudation of fibrin from the cut surfaces. This is soon followed by a much greater emigration of polymorphs and subsequently of macrophages: by enzymic action and phagocytosis these cells soften and remove the fibrin and other debris. As in the incised wound, epithelial cells at the margins enlarge and begin to migrate down the walls of the wound in the first day or two after injury. Migration and proliferation together produce a sheet of cells which advances in a series of tongue-like projections beneath any remaining blood clot or exudate on the wound surface. As the single layer of cells moves inwards towards the wound centre, there is stratification of the cells near to the wound margin (Fig. 3.9). Since the denuded area is large, the advancing epithelial sheet does not completely cover the wound until the granulation tissue from the base (see below) has started to fill the wound space. Care should always be taken, in removing dressings from an open wound, that the delicate epithelium, which at first has a tenuous hold on the underlying tissue, is not ripped off. As soon as the wound surface is covered, epithelial cell migration ceases and proliferation, stratification and keratinisation are rapidly completed, though rete ridges are not re-formed.

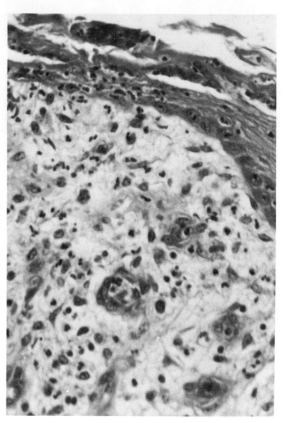

Fig. 3.9 Granulating wound with early growth of epithelium over the surface. The epithelium is growing from the right-hand side and tapers off as a thin layer. × 400.

Delay in epithelial spread occurs in a deep burn in which the cells must burrow their way, helped by the production of collagenases, beneath the thick eschar of dead coagulated dermal collagen. Less delay is occasioned by a thick scab of exudate and as this acts as a barrier against infection and possibly also helps, by becoming drier and so contracting, to reduce the size of the wound, it is usually best left *in situ*. In a superficial wound, a partial thickness ('second degree') burn or the donor site of a 'split thickness' skin graft, re-epithelialisation is relatively rapid as proliferation of epithelium occurs not only from the wound edge but also from the cut mouth of each pilosebaceous follicle. In man, little epithelial regeneration occurs from sweat gland ducts. If skin appendages are destroyed they are not re-formed.

Although epithelium shows the first evidence of reparative activity, within a few days the pre-existing vessels in the wound bed produce vascular sprouts which grow upwards, forming loops and coils at right angles to the wound surface (Fig. 3.10) and giving it a red, granular appearance (Fig. 3.11). From these new, more permeable vessels (Fig. 3.12), small haemorrhages occur and polymorphs migrate, reinforcing those already present in the exudate on the wound surface and helping to keep down bacterial growth. At the same time as the new capillaries form, fibroblasts, some of which are in mitosis, are seen in the base and walls of the wound, often running parallel to the new capillary walls. This fibrovascular granulation tissue continues to proliferate and to fill the wound space only until epithelium grows over its surface, when the exudative inflammatory changes and the migration of polymorphs also subside. Later the fibroblasts become orientated parallel to the wound surface (Fig. 3.13) and about the end of the first week collagen is produced and rapidly increases in amount. If epithelialisation is delayed, e.g. by further trauma or infection, granulations may pout from the wound surface. Following healing, there is gradual retraction and disappearance of some of the new vascular channels and further maturation and remodelling of collagen which, over a period of months, becomes progressively less cellular.

Healing of an open, excised wound is aided by contraction of the surface area, and in ten

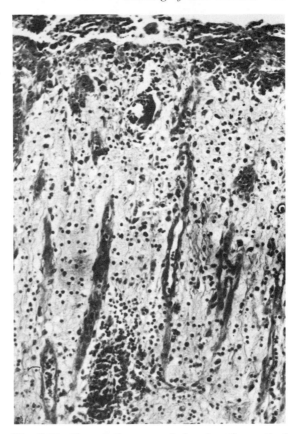

Fig. 3.10 Granulating wound showing the vertical lines of newly formed blood vessels. × 150.

Fig. 3.11 Granulating wound of 12 days' duration. The advancing epithelial margin is seen on the right. Granulation tissue projects from the floor of the wound, and can be seen to contain many small blood vessels. × 10.

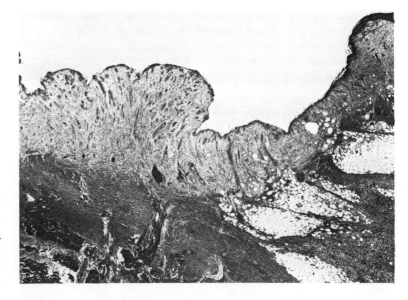

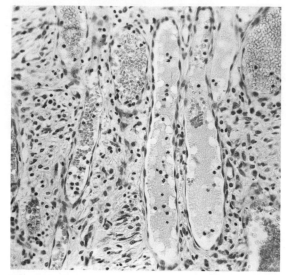

Fig. 3.12   Newly formed thin-walled blood vessels in a granulating wound, the surface of which is to the top. × 150.

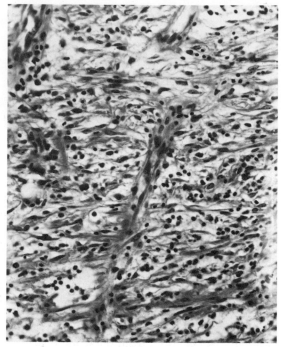

Fig. 3.13   Deeper part of granulating wound. Below, the collagen fibrils are being formed parallel to the surface; above, the vessels are seen running in a vertical direction. × 240.

days it may be reduced to a third of its original size. However, contraction of this degree occurs only in sites where the skin is mobile and loosely attached to underlying tissue. All edges of the wound do not move to the same extent, the degree of contraction being related to skin tension. The movement of the edges towards the centre of the wound is probably brought about by the fibroblasts in granulation tissue which, in addition to producing collagen, contain contractile protoplasm similar to that of muscle cells. These 'myofibroblasts' in granulation tissue appear to be in a state of maximum contraction. The contraction of the healing wound is stabilised by the synthesis of collagen, which maintains the new position of the wound edges. This collagen formation is associated with contracture of the scar which is sometimes unsightly and may be disabling, especially in wounds over flexor surfaces of the joints. Contracture may also follow muscle fibrosis and other, more gross, deep soft tissue damage. Although the myofibroblast in the healing wound is apparently capable of both muscle-like contraction and collagen production, the control of, and relationship between, the two functions is not understood. The former might be amenable to pharmacological control. When desirable, as sometimes in flexures, wound contraction may be inhibited by early full-thickness skin grafting.

Infected wounds. The repair of infected wounds is accomplished by the same processes already described for clean, open wounds; that is, by the production of granulation tissue, but with a more pronounced acute inflammatory reaction, and also by formation of larger and more numerous blood vessels.

Open wounds, apart from those produced under aseptic surgical conditions, are almost always contaminated by bacteria, and for this reason a careful surgical toilet should include removal of devitalised tissue, which promotes bacterial growth; this is an important part of treatment. Granulation tissue provides a good defence against bacteria because, being rich in small blood vessels, it can mount an effective inflammatory response. These local defensive factors may be aided by antibacterial therapy, which may permit early suture or skin grafting. If infection continues, however, more leukocytes pour into the surface exudate, which then becomes purulent. The result of acute infection on the healing processes is to inhibit both epithelial regeneration and proliferation of fibroblasts, so that healing is delayed. This delay and the greater tissue destruction result eventually in increased fibrous tissue and a larger and denser scar (Fig. 3.14).

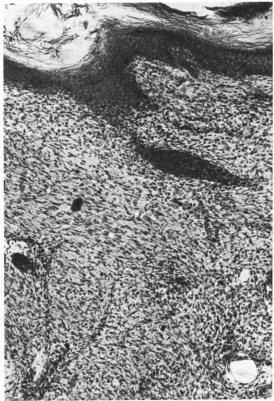

Fig. 3.14 Healed abdominal wound. There has been irritation and healing has been protracted. Note that the line of cellular tissue is much broader than in Fig. 3.2. × 75.

Control mechanisms in healing

While the morphological changes of wound healing are well known, the factors controlling the various observed processes are controversial or unknown.

Control of cell movement. The covering of a wound surface by epithelium cannot be explained simply by movement due to '*growth pressure*'. While a burst of mitoses may displace adjacent cells by a concerted nudge, it is known that healing may occur without cell division and, in the skin, epithelial cell migration over the wound surfaces appears to precede proliferation. There is evidence from tissue culture that virtually all cells have the ability to move along a surface to which they can adhere. If two cultures of fibroblasts are made on a plane surface the cells grow out as a monolayer from each explant until they collide, when movement virtually ceases because the cells will almost never pile upon one another. This is

know as **contact inhibition**. The same phenomenon may govern the covering of the surface of a wound by epithelial cells from around the margin. The concept of contact inhibition in regard to epidermal cells and fibroblasts helps to explain not only initiation of movement but also the direction of cells into the wounded area, especially since there is no evidence that chemotaxis applies to any cell other than leukocytes. Contact inhibition appears to be tissue specific in some degree, for if skin and oesophageal epithelium meet, although both are squamous, cell movement and proliferation continue and cells heap up at the junction.

Explantation of a fragment of adult tissue into a culture medium does not result in rapid migration, although the cells at the free edge of the fragment now lack contact with similar cells. If the tissue is first wounded however, migration is greatly increased and it seems that some factor in addition to loss of contact inhibition may be involved. There is some evidence to suggest that there is a change in the cell surface, causing a diminution of its adhesive properties, thus permitting mobilisation.

The stimulus to migration and proliferation. It has been suggested that the stimulus to wound healing and enhanced mitotic activity is mediated by growth promoters—**trephones** or 'wound hormones'—liberated by damaged cells. Tissue culture studies suggest that there may be a stimulating substance but this has never been shown to initiate cell migration or multiplication *in vivo* and at the moment the existence of a wound hormone derived from damaged cells and promoting healing in animals remains no more than a possibility.

It has been postulated that cells of epidermis and other tissues normally secrete a diffusible tissue-specific depressor of cell mitosis and that a wound, by removing some of this depressor substance or **chalone**, allows an increase in mitotic activity. This possibility is supported by the experimental finding that removal of skin from one side of a mouse's ear provokes a burst of mitotic activity in the intact epidermis of the other side, maximal opposite the middle of the defect rather than opposite the wound edges. There is also tissue culture evidence for the existence of a fibroblast chalone. The acceptance of the validity of this important concept of cell-specific chalones has not been universal because no one has yet purified and biochemically characterised these compounds, although their existence was reported more than a decade ago. The concept of the chalone has interesting implications apart from those related to wound healing. Their inhibitory action on mitoses in skin cultures is apparently potentiated by adrenalin, and the known cyclical fluctuation in adrenal function may thus account for the diurnal mitotic rhythm seen in many organs. The adrenalin-chalone complex appears to act after DNA synthesis is complete, just before prophase in the mitotic cycle. There is some evidence also to suggest that tumour cells (which proliferate abnormally) may fail to synthesise or release adequate concentrations of tissue specific chalones.

Factors which impair healing

Healing may be influenced by local factors. Infection delays healing (p. 66) as does a poor local blood supply; wounds of the relatively avascular shin tend to unite more slowly than those of the highly vascular scalp or face. Defects in collagen formation may result from generalised deficiency of vitamin C or of sulphur-containing amino acids and also from an excess of cortisone. In severe trauma these metabolic disturbances appear to be inter-related.

Deficiency of vitamin C (ascorbic acid) and sulphur-containing amino acids. Man, monkey and guinea-pig are unable to synthesise vitamin C, and in the guinea-pig impaired synthesis of wound collagen occurs after just a few days on a diet lacking the vitamin. In man, however, a much longer dietary deficiency is necessary before collagen formation is depressed, although this may occur before scurvy is clinically apparent (p. 822). Patients with multiple injuries or extensive burns readily become deficient in vitamin C unless intake is increased. Deficiency of the vitamin disturbs the synthesis of collagen at the stage of hydroxylation of amino acids and also arrests the progress of collagen formation from reticulin fibres. As a result the wound is weak and tends to break down after re-epithelialisation and apparent healing: this was a well-known complication of naval surgery on scorbutic sailors. In addition to the reduced amount of collagen formation, capillary endothelial cell proliferation may be diminished so that the blood vessels are fewer and abnormal. Deficient galactosamine may alter the properties of the ground substance. Similar alteration in collagen production with loss of wound strength may be seen in starving animals deficient in the sulphur-containing amino acids such as methionine, which are essential for collagen synthesis. Even when starvation continues, some of the methionine required for wound healing may be obtained from endogenous tissue proteins but wound strength is increased by providing an adequate diet. In well nourished individuals, protein and vitamin supplements will not speed healing or improve wound strength.

Excess of adrenal glucocorticoid hormones. Large doses of glucocorticoids given to susceptible animals have much the same effect on wound healing as ascorbic acid deficiency. In addition to diminished blood vessel formation and ground substance abnormalities, fewer fibroblasts appear in the wound and collagen formation is delayed. The hormone also interferes with the digestive activity of phagocytes. The usual therapeutic doses used in man probably have, however, no appreciable effect on wound healing.

Zinc deficiency. Zinc is necessary for the synthesis of collagen. Oral supplements of zinc may promote wound healing in patients with zinc deficiency, but it is difficult to identify these patients since serum zinc levels may not reflect accurately the overall bodily status of zinc metabolism.

Healing of fractures

Healing by callus formation

Healing in bones bears many resemblances to healing in soft tissues. There is initial haemorrhage and mild acute inflammation, followed by a proliferative or productive stage in which osteogenic cells play a vital part. Continuity between the bone fragments is first established by a mass of new bony and sometimes cartilaginous tissue (**provisional callus**): once continuity is re-established, this undergoes slow remodelling, with resorption and replacement so that, under favourable conditions, firm bony union is achieved. Sometimes restoration is so good that the fracture site is later hardly identifiable.

Early stages. A good deal of force is normally required to break a bone, the fragments are usually displaced, and in addition to a relatively small amount of haemorrhage between the bone ends much blood may seep into the tissues from ruptured vessels of the torn periosteum and adjacent soft tissues. In addition to haemorrhage, local inflammatory changes take place with hyperaemia and exudation of protein-rich fluid from which fibrin may be deposited. Polymorphs are scanty unless there is infection, and this is common only in **compound fractures**, i.e. when a bone fragment has breached the over-lying skin or mucous membrane. Macrophages also invade and phagocytose clot and tissue debris. Red blood cells often disappear rapidly from the fracture site, leaving a homogeneous mass of fibrin between the bone ends. A large amount of clot and debris between the bone fragments delays healing.

Bone necrosis occurs chiefly as a result of tearing of blood vessels in the medullary cavity, cortex and periosteum: the first recognisable histological evidence is observed within a day or two, the haemopoietic marrow cells showing loss of nuclear staining. Fat released from dead adipose marrow may be taken up by macro-

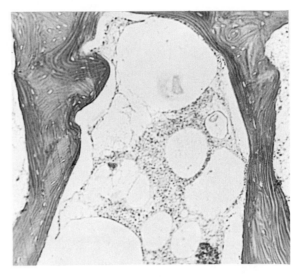

Fig. 3.15 The bone is necrotic and osteocytes have disappeared, leaving empty lacunae. Cell ghosts can be seen in the necrotic haemopoietic marrow. × 100.

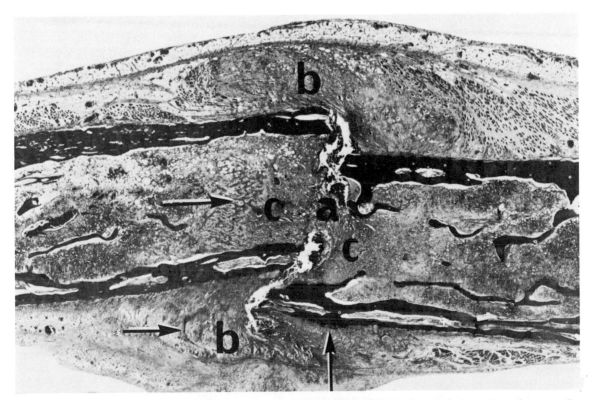

Fig. 3.16 Rib 7 days after fracture. The fracture gap (a) contains fibrin and extends into the adjacent soft tissue. A spindle of highly cellular tissue (b) has formed in the muscle around the fracture site but only a little new subperiosteal bone (arrows) and cartilage have formed as yet. Bone and marrow at the fracture site are dead (c) but there is some early revascularisation of the marrow and a little bony callus is beginning to form in the medullary cavity (arrow). × 10.

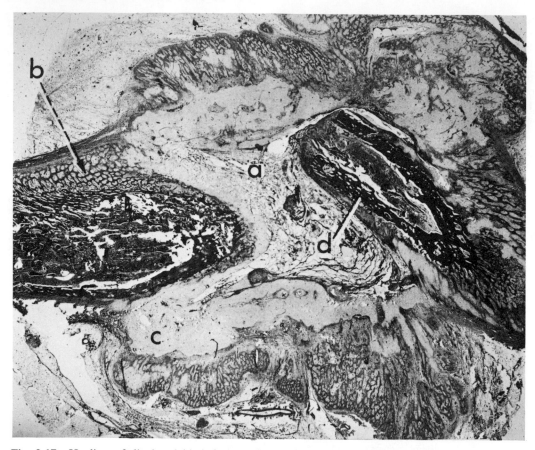

Fig. 3.17   Healing of displaced birth-fracture in the femur of a premature infant. The bone ends are cut obliquely. Bridging periosteal callus has formed but around the bone ends there is still a gap (a) which contains a meshwork of fibrin. The subperiosteal cuff of new bone is well seen at (b). The bridging callus consists partly of woven bone and partly of pale hyaline cartilage (c). The Haversian canals of the living cortex (d) are slightly enlarged by osteoclasis. × 5.

phages, and fat 'cysts' form surrounded by foreign-body giant cells. Damage to the adipose marrow may have serious results when globules enter marrow venules and produce *fat emboli* in the pulmonary bed, brain or kidneys (p. 206). Because of its vascular arrangements the cortical bone usually shows more extensive necrosis than the spongy medullary bone. The amount of bone necrosis depends especially on the local peculiarities of the blood supply; the talus, carpal scaphoid, and femoral head following intracapsular fracture, are particularly liable to undergo extensive ischaemic necrosis. When there is splintering of bone (**comminuted fracture**) some of the fragments may lose their blood supply; they become necrotic and, if small, are eventually resorbed by osteoclasts. Bone death is recognisable histologically by loss

of osteocytes from the bone lacunae (Fig. 3.15) but some cells may remain visible long after their death.

Provisional callus formation. (*a*) *Periosteal reaction.* The cells of the inner layer of the periosteum proliferate in a fairly wide zone overlying the living cortex of each fractured bone end. (Fig. 3.16). A cuff of bone trabeculae is formed around each bone end at right angles to the cortex and anchored to it (Fig. 3.17).

Further woven bone trabeculae (p. 810), less well orientated, form an irregular meshwork whose pattern at this stage is uninfluenced by stress. This formation of new bone is dependent on the blood supply, which derives partly from surviving periosteal vessels but largely from muscle and other surrounding soft tissues. Mixed with this cuff of new bone there are often nodules of hyaline cartilage which usually do not appear until bone formation is well under way (Fig. 3.17). The amount of cartilage which is formed in provisional callus varies greatly from one species to another. Small mammals such as mice, rats and rabbits tend to form chiefly cartilaginous callus while in man the amount, though variable, is less. Cartilage formation is thought to be promoted by a poor blood supply and by shearing strains and stresses so that it is particularly abundant in poorly immobilised fractures: bone gradually replaces the cartilage by endochondral ossification.

The two enlarging cuffs of callus advance towards each other and finally unite to bridge the fracture line leaving a gap between the bone ends (Fig. 3.17). This 'bandage' of *external callus* helps to immobilise the fragments in an unstable or poorly fixed fracture.

The amount of bridging periosteal callus varies greatly in different sites and under different circumstances. In intracapsular fractures, such as subcapital fracture of the femoral neck, the periosteum is lacking and union is almost wholly dependent on *internal callus* formed by osteoblasts lying in the medullary cavity. By contrast, fractures of the diaphysis of large tubular bones, such as the femur and humerus, tend

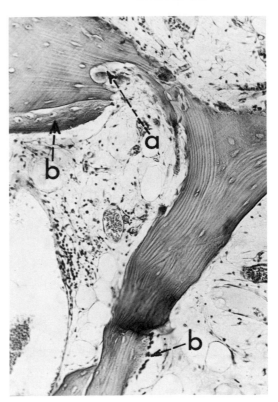

Fig. 3.19 A dead medullary bone trabecula is being removed by osteoclasts at (a) and new bone is being laid down on the surface of dead bone at (b). × 120.

to form much external callus, internal callus in the relatively small medullary cavity not being striking. The formation of bulky external callus probably depends on plenty of surrounding undamaged muscle as a source of blood supply, for one of the causes of the difficulty in healing of fractures of the tibia is that they are partially covered by relatively avascular subcutaneous tissue and tend to form little callus. Poorly aligned fractures and those with much movement at the fracture site (e.g. the ribs and clavicle) are liable to produce abundant external callus, whereas fractures which are well immobilised by external or internal surgical fixation may unite with relatively little callus formation.

(b) Medullary reaction. The first evidence of healing is the advance of capillaries from the viable into the necrotic marrow (Fig. 3.18) closely followed by macrophages, fibroblasts and osteoblasts. The macrophages phagocytose and remove dead material, while osteoclasts begin to resorb dead spongy bone (Fig. 3.19) and the endosteal surface of the necrotic cortex. The osteogenic cells covering the medullary trabeculae

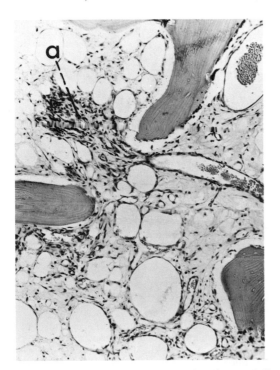

Fig. 3.18 Dead fatty marrow in the medullary cavity is being revascularised. A knot of proliferating capillaries is seen at (a). × 100.

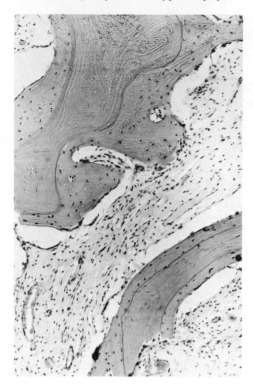

Fig. 3.20 Months after fracture dead bone trabeculae are still recognisable, covered by new living bone. × 70.

and the endosteal surface of the cortex enlarge and produce new woven bone in the marrow spaces: the new bone is deposited partly on the surface of dead trabeculae which, when surrounded by new bone, may remain unresorbed for months or even years (Fig. 3.20).

In contrast with external callus, cartilage is rare in the medullary cavity, perhaps because it is a relatively vascular site and is protected from mechanical stress. It may form, however, when callus formation reaches the fracture gap (see below).

(*c*) *Cortical reaction.* The most striking reaction in the living cortex adjacent to the fracture is an increase in osteoclastic resorption with widening of the canals, presumably partly due to disuse atrophy (Fig. 3.21 and p. 830). This may be followed later by some osteoblastic activity. Similar changes are seen in the dead cortex of the bone ends once there has been revascularisation of the Haversian canals from adjacent vessels in viable bone or from periosteal and medullary vessels. The resorption of necrotic bone may widen the fracture gap.

The fracture gap. The periosteal (external) callus unites the fragments externally but not directly across the bone ends. As already stated, immediately after fracture, blood clot, exuded fibrin and bony debris fill the gap and this is attacked by macrophages and by osteoclasts. The fibrin clot, which usually persists between the bone ends (Figs. 3.16 and 3.17), is finally invaded by blood vessels and cellular tissue containing varying amounts of osteogenic cells and fibroblasts, so that bony union may occur in either of two ways.

(a) Direct ossification is brought about by osteogenic cells spreading from medullary and periosteal callus. Cartilage may also be formed

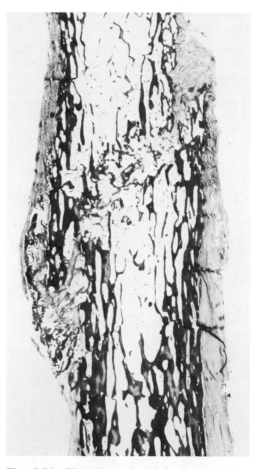

Fig. 3.21 This 12-week-old fracture of the distal fibula in an old man has formed a good deal of external callus medially (on the left). The fracture gap itself is filled with fibrous tissue in which a few trabeculae of metaplastic bone are forming. As a result of immobilisation and disuse the fibula is porotic with enlargement of Haversian canals. × 3.

Fig. 3.22 Pseudarthrosis following fracture of the clavicle. The bone ends have become covered by cartilage. At the top of the picture a split in the cartilage has occurred giving a false joint. There is endochondral ossification of the proliferated cartilage in the lower part of the picture. × 40.

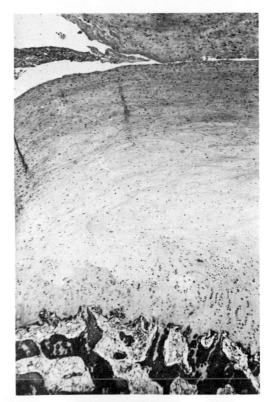

Fig. 3.23 This fracture through the midshaft of the femur united with anterior shift of the proximal fragment. Eighteen months after fracture there is firm bony union. The slab radiograph shows how the provisional callus has become remodelled along lines of stress with buttressing of the posterior and slightly concave part of the fracture line and some retubulation in the medullary canal at the fracture site.

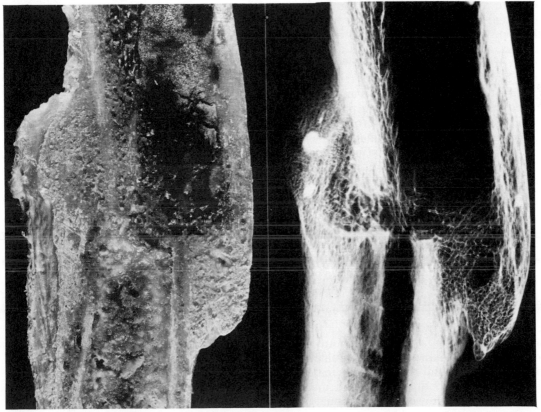

and is converted into bone. This process is relatively rapid and effective.

(b) Fibrous union may occur initially. Fibrous tissue grows in from medulla or periosteum or both, becomes densely collagenised, and only then much more slowly becomes ossified (Fig. 3.21). This slower type of union occurs especially when there is instability, distraction or marked resorption of the bone ends, massive necrosis, a poor blood supply, extensive periosteal damage, comminution or infection. Sometimes conversion to bone following fibrous union is very slow (**delayed union**) and occasionally it fails to occur (**non-union**). In non-union the fibrous tissue may become very dense, hyaline and finally fibrocartilaginous. The appearance of an area of eosinophilic fibrinoid necrosis is followed by a linear split which may enlarge and eventually develop a lining similar to synovium, thus forming a false joint (**pseudarthrosis**) (Fig. 3.22). The bone ends buried in the dense fibrous tissue tend to become very sclerotic.

Later stages: *final remodelling.* Once bony union has occurred and function has been regained, the bone begins to be remodelled in response to mechanical stresses. If the fracture has united at an angle new bone is incorporated on the concave side while resorption occurs on the convex, so that the bone becomes straighter. In any event excessive callus is resorbed, slowly formed lamellar bone begins to replace the hastily laid down woven bone, and any remaining necrotic bone is removed and replaced (Fig. 3.23). The cortex is re-formed across the fracture gap and gradually medullary callus is removed and retubulation of the bone occurs. The whole process may take about a year and is more rapid and complete in children.

Metabolic factors affecting bone healing. Some of the local factors affecting bone healing have already been mentioned but, as in wound healing, general factors are also important. Lack of vitamin C results in depression of both fibroblastic and osteogenic activity so that collagen and bone production are both deficient. Cortisone administered to animals with fractures also delays healing but it seems that it has little effect when given to patients in the usual therapeutic doses. In vitamin D deficiency abundant callus may form, but it fails to calcify, remaining soft until the deficiency is made good.

Primary union

Although primary union of soft tissues is the rule in clean sutured surgical incisions, primary union in fractures is a curiosity. It entails bony union with the formation of only minimal amounts of callus and was first described in compression arthrodesis (i.e. excision of the joint) of the knee, the cancellous surfaces of femur and tibia being held together by compression clamps. Bony union occurs in about 4 weeks and biopsy shows only a thin line of new bone at the contact points of opposing trabeculae. While moderate compression forces may assist union of a fracture, rigid fixation and close apposition of surfaces are probably the major factors. Cortical fractures in dogs, produced by a very fine saw with minimal necrosis, and fixed by a compression plate, have united without periosteal callus. Although union of similarly treated long bone fractures in man occurs quickly and without radiologically apparent periosteal callus, it seems doubtful, in view of the probable amount of bone necrosis, that they can truly be described as undergoing primary union.

Healing of some other tissues

Healing of articular cartilage

There is evidence that articular cartilage remains metabolically active throughout life. Following injury, chondrocytes may proliferate to form cell clusters and there is an increase in synthesis of both chondromucoprotein matrix and collagen. It is, however, exceptional for these intrinsic reactions to produce any significant healing of cartilage defects.

Extrinsic repair may occur by the growth of fibrous tissue onto the articular surface either from the joint margin or, when there is loss of the full depth of the cartilage, from the underlying marrow through cracks in the exposed subchondral bone plate. This collagenous tissue may then acquire a more chondroid matrix, to become fibrocartilage, and is sometimes able to meet biomechanical demands. However, both the amount and quality of new tissue formed by extrinsic repair mechanisms are likely to be functionally inadequate, especially when the defect is large.

Healing of tendon

A good functional result following healing of a severed tendon requires both a strong fibrous union between the ends and retention of a full range of gliding motion. In patients with sutured tendons, repair occurs by ingrowth of fibroblasts and blood vessels from surrounding connective tissue into the fibrin meshwork between the ends. The cells, at first randomly arranged, later become orientated along the line of the tendon and produce reticulin fibres which bond together to form more mature collagen. The amount of collagen synthesised is increased for some weeks after injury and, as in a healing wound, there is subsequent remodelling of the fibrous scar. The extrinsic source of vessels and cells during the healing process makes the formation of adhesions inevitable, but a good range of movement is retained when the adhesions are long and consist of loosely arranged areolar tissue. Restricted movement is associated with short adhesions containing large bundles of collagen fibres. Rough operative handling is thought to promote the formation of such adhesions, but little is known of other factors concerned.

Recent experimental evidence suggests that fibrocytes of tendon are not necessarily inert, but have the intrinsic potential for carrying out repair and remodelling without the formation of adhesions. It may be that it is the surgical suture of the severed ends which, by disturbing the local blood supply, impairs this response and makes healing dependent on extrinsic sources.

Repair and regeneration of muscle

(a) Skeletal muscle. When muscle fibres are damaged, the sarcoplasm of dead fibres disintegrates, and this is followed by phagocytosis of the fragments. Regeneration of muscle occurs

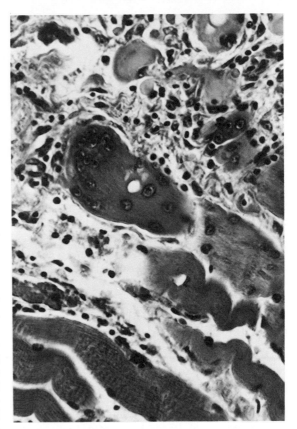

Fig. 3.24 Wounded striped muscle, showing sarcoplasmal sprouts with multiple nuclei. × 200.

in two ways. Firstly, by the formation of multinucleated sprouts (Fig. 3.24) from the surviving ends of injured fibres. It has been estimated that these sprouts advance into the damaged area at a rate of less than 1 mm/day. Secondly, by the growth of mononucleated myoblasts. The origin of these cells is controversial. Regeneration may be complete when the endomysial tube is intact as in **Zenker's hyaline degeneration**. This condition may accompany severe infections and toxaemias, especially typhoid fever, and tends to involve most severely the muscles of the abdominal wall, diaphragm and intercostals. When the connective and supporting tissue in muscle is also destroyed, as in more severe injuries, regeneration is less well orientated and a scar composed of fibrovascular tissue and irregularly orientated muscle fibres is formed. This is seen, for example, in Volkmann's ischaemic contracture (p. 869).

(b) Visceral muscle (smooth, non-striped muscle). The healing of visceral muscle, e.g. in surgical incisions in the bowel, occurs by fibrous repair. Although smooth muscle may be seen in recently differentiated arterioles (p. 62) and in atheromatous plaques (p. 314), its origin is uncertain and it may arise by migration of smooth muscle cells or by differentiation from other mesenchymal cells. Proliferation with mitotic activity is said to occur in the early months of the physiological uterine enlargement of pregnancy.

(c) Cardiac muscle. Destruction of cardiac muscle by infarction is repaired by fibrous tissue (Fig. 14.11, p. 353). Effective regeneration occurs in young patients with Coxsackie virus infections or diphtheria, where there is damage to individual fibres with preservation of the endomysium, a situation similar to that of Zenker's degeneration in skeletal muscle.

Repair and regeneration of nervous tissue and nerves

Central nervous tissue. Once mature nerve cells are destroyed, they are not replaced by the proliferation of other nerve cells. There is also no useful regeneration of axons: indeed when an axon is severed at any point, the entire axon and the nerve cell body degenerate. In contrast, peripheral nerves, because of the presence of Schwann cells, have considerable regenerative capacity. Of the neuroglial cells, proliferation in response to tissue damage is restricted to astrocytes, this being referred to as gliosis (p. 664).

Regeneration of peripheral nerves. When a nerve is transected, the axis cylinders distal to the cut undergo Wallerian degeneration, i.e. the axon and its myelin sheath break down and the debris is absorbed by macrophages. At the same time the Schwann cells proliferate within the neurilemmal sheath to form pathways along which the axons may regrow. Above the level of transection, myelin degeneration extends upwards only to the first or second node of Ranvier and the nerve cell body characteristically shows central chromatolysis (p. 663). Axonal sprouts soon emerge from the proximal ends of the interrupted axis cylinders and, if the cut ends of the nerve are in close apposition, they grow into the distal part of the nerve and along the spaces formerly occupied by axis cylinders and now filled with proliferated

Schwann cells. The axons grow at a rate of about 3 mm per day. These new axons, which at first are very thin, increase in diameter and develop a new myelin sheath. In addition to growth and maturation of the axon, time is also needed for the re-innervation of motor end plates and sensory end organs so that restoration of function is always slow and often imperfect.

The degree of functional recovery in damaged peripheral nerve depends principally on the severity of the injury. If nerve fibres only are disrupted and the other components of the nerve trunk remain intact, as in a crush injury, regenerating axons can grow along their original endoneurial tubes, continuity of which is preserved. If there is considerable disorganisation of the internal structure of individual nerve bundles within the nerve trunk, the continuity of endoneurial tubes is less likely to be preserved: fibrosis then occurs within the damaged segment and provides a barrier to the axons growing from the proximal segment of the damaged nerve. This slows their growth and some axons never traverse the fibrous barrier, while those that do almost never grow along

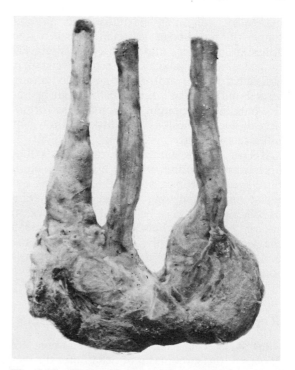

Fig. 3.25 Traumatic neuroma at severed proximal ends of nerves of an amputated arm.

their original endoneurial tubes. Thus many axons fail to reach their original end-organ and an abnormal and incomplete pattern of innervation results. When there is subtotal or complete loss of continuity of the nerve trunk, the proliferation of axonal sprouts, fibroblasts and Schwann cells from the proximal end of the nerve results in the formation of a so-called **traumatic** or **stump neuroma** (Fig. 3.25).

In severely damaged nerves, surgical repair after excision of the involved segment or the traumatic neuroma is often the only means of achieving any functional recovery, but some residual disability almost invariably persists.

Healing of mucosal surfaces

Cells which line mucosal surfaces, are being lost and replaced continuously throughout life and, like all surface epithelia, have a good potential for regeneration (Fig. 3.26). In general, the raw surface is first covered and only later is there differentiation into more specialised cells.

(a) Gastro-intestinal tract mucosa. Physiological replacement of lost surface cells takes place by proliferation of the more protected cells of the mucosal glandular necks. Experi-

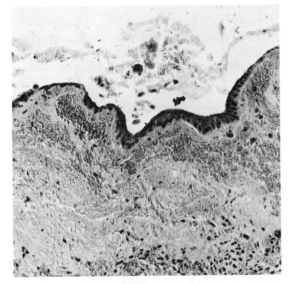

Fig. 3.26 Repair of lining of gallbladder after acute inflammatory desquamation. The epithelial cells extend as a thin flattened layer to reline the viscus. × 150.

mental excision of an area of mucosa, in the stomach for instance, is rapidly followed by re-epithelialisation: epithelial cells of the mucous neck type migrate over the exposed connective tissue, forming first a layer of thin, flattened epithelium, which later becomes cubical or columnar. The epithelium of glands adjacent to the wound undergoes mitosis, as do surface cells, and this proliferation keeps up the supply of migrating cells until the surface is covered. Gland crypts re-form by mucous cells growing down into the underlying granulation tissue and, some weeks later, specialised cells, e.g. parietal cells, differentiate from the mucous cells in the crypts. Failure of re-epithelialisation of chronic peptic ulcers (p. 554) is not fully understood. Wounds of the mucous membranes following surgical anastomoses heal readily, and the line between the two different types of mucosa remains sharp.

The small and to a lesser extent the large bowel mucosae have an excellent capacity for regeneration (Fig. 18.45d, p. 566). Repeated ulceration and repair, as for instance in ulcerative colitis and bilharzial infestation, may lead to overgrowth of the reparative mucosa, producing polypoid projections (Fig. 18.61, p. 579).

(b) Respiratory tract mucosa. The basal cells of the tracheal and bronchial lining epithelium proliferate throughout life and replace loss of the surface ciliated epithelium. Many microbial infections involve the loss of only part of the thickness of the pseudostratified columnar epithelium, and this is readily replaced by basal cell proliferation. Full thickness destruction of the mucosa is followed by the usual pattern of migration and proliferation from surviving cell islands as is seen in the epidermis. Repeated damage, e.g. in chronic bronchitis, may result in less perfect regeneration, the ciliated cells being replaced by columnar non-ciliated, mucus secreting cells, and under very unfavourable circumstances, as in heavy cigarette smoking, metaplasia of the regenerating epithelium to squamous type may be seen.

(c) Urinary tract mucosa. The urinary tract mucosa, like the epidermis, responds to injury by movement and proliferation of cells. The transitional cell epithelium of the bladder has particularly good powers of rapid regeneration, and mitoses may be seen in migrating cells.

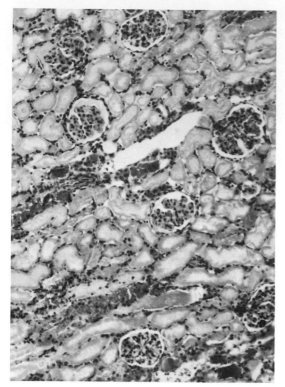

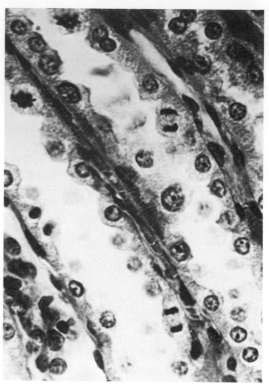

Fig. 3.27a Acute tubular necrosis in the rat. Note the anatomical normality of the glomeruli and the absence of nuclei in the dead tubular epithelial cells. × 150.

Fig. 3.27b Regeneration of renal tubular epithelium following acute tubular necrosis in the rat. Four mitotic figures are present. The adjacent regenerated cells are still of subnormal size. × 450.

Repair and regeneration of kidney

The glomerulus is a highly specialised unit and little effective regeneration follows damage. Lost renal substance is replaced by fibrous tissue. If the basement membrane of the tubules remains intact, damage to tubular epithelium may be followed by proliferation (Fig. 3.27) and slow migration of surviving cells to restore continuity. It is doubtful, however, whether, when the damaged cells are highly specialised, as in the proximal convoluted tubule, the regenerated cells have the same degree of functional efficiency.

Repair and regeneration of the liver

The hepatic parenchymal cells form a fairly stable population, and few mitotic figures are seen in the normal liver. Replacement of normal 'wear-and-tear' cell loss is by division

of neighbouring cells. Some replacement is effected by amitotic division and this probably explains the occurrence of binucleate and multinucleate liver cells, particularly in elderly individuals.

Wounds of the liver are repaired by formation of connective tissue, with minimal replacement of parenchymal cells around the margin of the wound. New liver 'lobules' are never formed.

The outcome of liver cell necrosis depends on the distribution of the cells affected and also upon the presence or absence of an intact vascular system. Occlusion of hepatic arterial branches may be followed by infarction of liver tissue: as in most other tissues, coagulative necrosis occurs and is repaired by organisation, leaving a fibrous scar. Necrosis of individual liver cells scattered throughout the lobules, as in the typical attack of virus hepatitis, is followed by autolysis and disappearance of the dead cells, which are replaced by proliferation

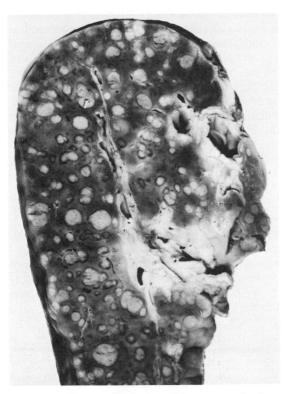

Fig. 3.28 Following extensive liver necrosis there has been proliferation of surviving liver cells. These form the pale rounded nodules lying in a background of scar tissue from which dead liver cells have now disappeared.

of surviving cells with restoration to normal. Even when there is destruction of all the parenchymal cells in the centres or mid-zones of the lobules the more peripheral cells proliferate and extend into the surviving vascular framework so that normality is once again achieved. If, however, there is loss of most or all of the hepatocytes through the whole thickness of the lobules, proliferation of the surviving hepatocytes leads only to irregular nodules of regeneration, the lobular pattern being lost. The vascular framework in the areas depleted of parenchymal cells becomes collapsed and scarred (Fig. 3.28).

The very high regenerative capacity of liver cells has been demonstrated by subjecting animals to excision of various amounts of liver tissue. After excision of two-thirds of the rat's liver, hypertrophy and hyperplasia in the remaining third result in restoration of a normal liver mass in 15–20 days. The capacity of the liver to regenerate in this way is maintained even when partial hepatectomy is performed monthly for up to one year.

The factors which regulate the extent of liver regeneration are not understood. When partial hepatectomy is performed upon one member of a pair of parabiotic rats, hepatocyte proliferation occurs in both animals. This and similar experiments suggest that a humoral mediating factor is responsible for hepatic regeneration, but it is not clear whether proliferation results from release of stimulatory factors or from removal of growth inhibiting chalones. The establishment of a portacaval vascular shunt may impair the rate of regeneration and it thus seems that portal venous flow through the liver has some effect in determining the degree of restoration. Diet, age, hormones and biliary obstruction may modify, but do not specifically impair, the regenerative process.

Organisation

The processes involved in healing are also concerned in the removal, and replacement by fibrous tissue, of inert material such as intravascular thrombus, extravascular blood clot (haematoma) (Fig. 3.29), exuded fibrin in an inflammatory lesion or dead tissue. This is termed organisation and is illustrated by the two following examples.

Organisation of thrombus

Occlusion of a vein by thrombus is followed by the ingrowth from its wall of fibroblasts and macrophages, along with capillaries which probably derive from the plexus of vessels deep to the internal elastic lamina (vasa venorum). This ingrowth of granulation tissue does not

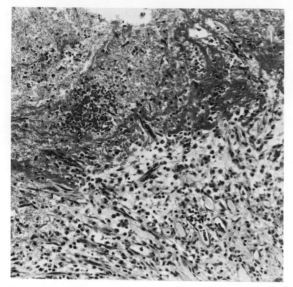

Fig. 3.29 Organisation of a haematoma after 7 days. Capillary sprouts are beginning to grow into the clot and there are also large numbers of macrophages at its margin. × 80.

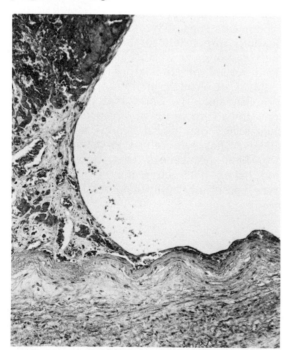

Fig. 3.30 Endothelium has grown over the surface of this partially organised thrombus adherent to an artery wall. × 40.

often occur around the whole circumference of the vessel, usually being confined to sites where thrombosis has caused secondary damage to

the intimal endothelium. Elsewhere around the wall, pockets may form where thrombus has shrunk away as a result of clot retraction and also of local fibrinolysis by plasmin. The cells of the intimal endothelium migrate and proliferate rapidly to cover the free surface of the thrombus (Fig. 3.30), and also penetrate into it. This results in both fragmentation of the thrombus into tiny endothelial covered nodules and in the formation of small capillary channels, many of which are probably blind-ending, while a few link up with capillaries growing into the thrombus from the vein wall. The thrombus is also partially resorbed by the action of macrophages and sometimes the centre is softened by enzymes from groups of dead polymorphs which have migrated from the thin-walled vessels. In this way, by the joining up of pockets, by fragmentation, resorption and softening of thrombus, a lumen may be restored leaving a thickened fibrovascular intimal plaque

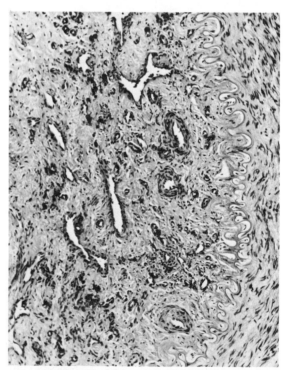

Fig. 3.31 Part of an artery showing the results of organisation of thrombus. The lumen was originally to the left of the internal elastic lamina, which runs vertically near the right margin. The lumen is now filled with vascular fibrous tissue in which some of the new capillaries have enlarged and acquired muscle to become arterioles. × 115.

or a meshwork of fibrous strands marking the site of granulation tissue ingrowth with subsequent fibrosis. Occasionally, however, and perhaps when the thrombus is especially dense and slowly formed, it remains adherent to the whole circumference of the vein: pockets are not formed and significant recanalisation fails to occur. The thrombus is replaced by granulation tissue which becomes increasingly collagenous, the vein eventually being reduced to a solid, shrunken cord without a lumen.

Arteries are less likely than veins to undergo successful recanalisation (Fig. 3.31) and there is some experimental evidence to suggest that, compared with venous, arterial endothelium is a poor source of plasminogen activator.

Mural thrombus. Thrombus may form on a part of the wall of a vessel without extending to fill the lumen. Such mural thrombi are rapidly resurfaced with endothelium from the surrounding intima (Fig. 3.30). Fibrinolysis, fragmentation, resorption and enzymatic break-down probably all play a part in removing some of the thrombus, while granulation tissue grows in from the underlying wall and organises the remainder.

Organisation of exudate

Organisation of fibrinous exudate on a serous surface such as pleura, pericardium or peritoneum follows a similar pattern (Fig. 2.14, p. 49). If the fibrin is abundant and dense, glueing together the visceral and parietal surfaces, capillaries and fibroblasts grow in from the underlying tissue on each side and finally meet, the fibrin being absorbed or phagocytosed by accompanying macrophages. Instead of fibrin, granulation tissue now binds the two surfaces together and gradually this changes to less vascular fibrous tissue. If the fibrin forms a more open meshwork, there may be effective digestion of it by leukocytes with some restoration of the serosal surface.

Hypertrophy

Stimulation of the parenchymal cells of an organ, usually due to increased functional demand or to disturbances of hormonal balance, results in an increase in the total mass of the parenchymal cells. This may be brought about by enlargement of the cells—**hypertrophy** or by an increase in their number—**hyperplasia**. The relative importance of the two processes varies in different organs. In some, e.g. the skeletal muscles, enlargement is purely by hypertrophy, but in most organs hypertrophy and hyperplasia both contribute.

(a) The response to increased functional demand is illustrated by the hypertrophied **muscles** of manual labourers and athletes; the individual fibres increase in thickness and length but not in number. Similarly, when extra work is demanded of the **heart** as a result of valvular disease or high blood pressure (Fig. 3.32), there may be much thickening of the muscular walls affecting those chambers which bear the brunt of the extra work. Narrowing of the mitral valve, for example, produces chiefly left atrial and right ventricular hypertrophy, whereas systemic hypertension gives rise predominantly to left ventricular hypertrophy (Fig. 14.1, p. 347). The heart may increase to twice the normal weight, the degree of hypertrophy being limited by the diffusion of oxygen and nutrients between the capillaries and the thickened fibres. An adequate blood supply is required to allow hypertrophy to occur, but there is no evidence that an increased vascular bed will, of itself and without an increased demand, produce hypertrophy. **Smooth muscle** may also undergo hypertrophy, for example in the wall of the stomach behind a stenosed pylorus, in large bowel proximal to an obstructing tumour (Fig. 18.73, p. 594), or in the bladder when the outflow is narrowed by an enlarged prostate (Fig. 23.11, p. 890). The muscle in arterial walls also hypertrophies in response to long continued high blood pressure (Fig. 13.14, p. 320). The most striking hypertrophy is seen in the pregnant uterus, where a combination of increased functional demand and hormonal stimuli results in enlargement of fibres to more than a hundred times their original volume. In early pregnancy, there may be both hypertrophy and hyperplasia of muscle

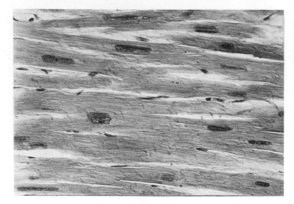

Fig. 3.32a Hypertrophied muscle fibres of heart in a case of arteriosclerosis with high blood pressure. × 250.

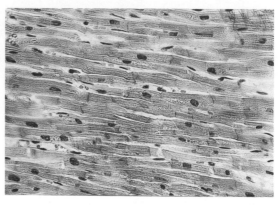

Fig. 3.32b Slightly atrophied heart muscle; to compare with Fig. 3.32a. × 250.

fibres. After parturition, the fibres return to a normal size and this is seen also in hypertrophied heart muscle when the increased work stimulus is removed.

In some instances, the response to an increased demand is by a pure hyperplasia; for instance, blood loss is not followed by enlargement of red cells and leukocytes but by an increase in their production in the haemopoietic marrow (Fig. 16.9b, p. 464).

Compensatory hypertrophy may occur in the survivor of a pair of organs when one is removed. Following nephrectomy, the remaining kidney enlarges and, particularly in young patients, may double its weight. This is not brought about by the formation of new neph-

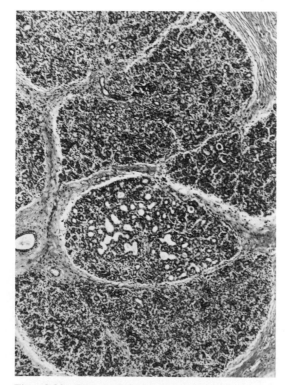

Fig. 3.33 Breast lobule in pregnancy showing marked hypertrophy and hyperplasia. × 50.

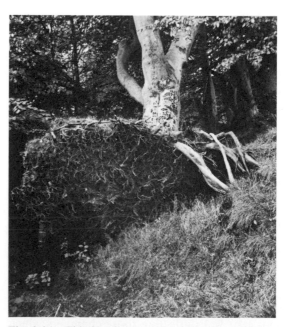

Fig. 3.34 This beech tree was largely uprooted by a gale six years before, and has since leant against its neighbour. It continues to survive because a few roots (on the right) have retained contact with the soil and have become greatly hypertrophied.

rons, but by an increase in nephron size as a result of both hypertrophy and hyperplasia of the component cells of the glomeruli and tubules. Removal of one adrenal leads to hypertrophy of the cells of the opposite cortex, the medulla remaining unchanged. Following removal of a lung, the remaining lung enlarges but this is caused mainly by over-distension, which produces a lasting enlargement of the alveoli; only when it occurs in early life is there any formation of new alveoli. Compensatory hypertrophy is a widespread natural phenomenon, as illustrated in Fig 3.34.

The testes are exceptional in that, in both man and animals, removal of one in adult life is not followed by enlargement of the other, the number of spermatozoa produced being reduced.

(b) Hypertrophy due to hormonal changes. A balanced activity of certain of the endocrine glands is essential for the normal growth and metabolism of the tissues and many of the examples of hypertrophy and hyperplasia already mentioned require the continued physiological action of the growth hormone of the anterior pituitary as well as an adequate blood supply. Excessive secretion of growth hormone (usually due to a tumour of the oxyphil cells of the anterior pituitary) results in adults in acromegaly (p. 944) with bone enlargement and generalised organ and tissue hypertrophy. This is even more strikingly seen when the excess of hormone occurs in adolescence, before the skeleton matures; the result is gigantism (p. 945). An example of physiological hormonal hypertrophy is the enlargement of the breasts in pregnancy, when the formation of mammary gland acini is stimulated chiefly by hormones from the corpus luteum or placenta (Fig. 3.33).

It may be that some examples of unexplained pathological hypertrophy, such as that occasionally seen in the breasts of adolescents and commonly in the prostate gland in the elderly, will ultimately prove to be of endocrine origin.

4

The Immune Response

Introduction

The invasion of the body by living organisms, including viruses, bacteria, and protozoan and metazoan parasites, presents a major threat to the stability of the internal milieu upon which Claude Bernard placed such importance. To counter this threat certain general defence mechanisms have evolved—a relatively impermeable epidermis, methods of ridding the body of noxious material, such as vomiting, diarrhoea and coughing, the dilution of irritants by increased flow of interstitial fluid in inflammatory oedema, and the destruction of particulate matter by phagocytic cells. In addition, there exists in vertebrates a special defence mechanism of immense potential which is mobilised when the body is invaded by foreign organisms and which is expressly and specifically adapted to overcome the effects of the particular invader in question. The special mechanism is called **acquired specific immunity** and its study—the science of **immunology**—is of great importance in the understanding and prevention of disease.

The phenomenon of acquired specific immunity has been recognised for centuries in that individuals who had survived an attack of certain clearly recognisable infectious diseases such as smallpox were known to be much less susceptible to the disease during a later epidemic. Such individuals could be said to show **immunity** (i.e. protection) against the disease, **acquired** inasmuch as it did not apparently exist before the first infection, and **specific** inasmuch as an attack of smallpox protected the individual against a further attack of smallpox but had no bearing on his susceptibility to later attacks of measles, diphtheria, etc.

This knowledge has been applied with great success to the prevention of infectious disease by prophylactic immunisation, a procedure in which a relatively harmless variant, or modified toxin, of a pathogenic organism is purposely introduced into the body, and which results in the development of specific immunity such as would be encountered following recovery from the natural disease. The principle is well illustrated by Edward Jenner's use of fluid from the lesions of cowpox (vaccinia) to vaccinate against smallpox; it was known to Jenner that milkmaids who had had natural cowpox infection had developed not only markedly altered reactivity to re-infection with cowpox but also resistance to a first infection by smallpox, a closely related but much more serious disease. In this case the two viruses are so similar that immunity to one is effective also against the other.

When an individual has become immune following natural infection or prophylactic exposure to a pathogenic organism or its toxin he is said to be **actively immunised** against that organism. Specific resistance to infection can in many instances be conferred upon a non-immune individual by an alternative method, namely the injection of *serum* or *lymphoid cells* from an actively immune individual. The state of **passive immunity** so conferred is not due to transfer of the infecting organism or its toxin but to the transfer of the products of immunisation developed by the actively immunised donor of the serum or lymphoid cells. The *passive transfer* of immunity thus provides a way of analysing the factors which contribute to the immune state, and by transfer experiments it has been shown that in some instances specific immunity results from the presence in the serum of special globulins known as **antibodies**, while in other cases the immune state seems to be mediated directly by **specifically primed (sensitised) lymphocytes** without the participation of serum antibody. Serum containing one or more

84

antibodies produced by active immunisation is termed **antiserum** or **immune serum**.

There is obviously considerable survival advantage in having the ability to acquire specific immunity to pathogenic organisms or their toxins. Unfortunately the specifically altered reactivity produced by an immune response can lead to reactions which result in tissue injury. This can happen following exposure even to relatively harmless substances, such as grass pollen, which on subsequent contact causes a harmful and seemingly unnecessary inflammatory reaction in certain individuals. Such **acquired specific hypersensitivity** has in many cases been shown to be due to reactions of an immunological nature although with its connotation of protection the word 'immune' appears unsuitable. Because of this difficulty and the gradual way in which knowledge of the complex processes involved

has unfolded, an elaborate but imprecise jargon relating to immunology has developed and many authors have used the same terms with different meanings. Von Pirquet, for example, coined the word **allergy** as a unifying term to indicate *altered* specific reactivity of all kinds, including both protective immune responses and also hypersensitivity. Despite this the words allergy and hypersensitivity are frequently used interchangeably.

In this book we follow the current common practice of using the words 'immune' and 'immunity' in two distinct ways: in one they are general terms to embrace all forms of specifically altered reactivity (i.e. allergy in von Pirquet's sense) and in the other they refer to the specific protection against disease; we believe that the meaning implied will be evident from the context.

Antigens

An antigen is a substance capable of evoking an immune response, which may take three main forms.

(1) Antibody production, i.e. the appearance of globulin molecules which have the property of combining specifically with and remaining attached to antigen of the same kind as that which has led to their formation.

(2) Cell-mediated immunity, i.e. the production of specifically primed lymphocytes whose presence can be demonstrated *in vivo* by the development of a local inflammatory reaction appearing about 24 hours after intradermal injection of the antigen a **delayed hypersensitivity reaction**. Most antigenic stimuli evoke both cell-mediated immunity and antibody production. These responses take place in the lymphoid tissues, and their products, specifically primed lymphocytes and antibody, both capable of reacting with the antigen, are released into the bloodstream.

(3) Under certain conditions, an antigenic stimulus may induce a state of **specific immunological tolerance**, i.e. non-responsiveness to subsequent challenge with the same antigen.

The term '*immunological reaction*' should not be confused with '*immune response*' as described

above. An **immunological reaction** is the effect observed when the products of the immune response—antibody or primed lymphocytes—encounter and combine with the appropriate antigen *in vitro* or *in vivo*.

Factors affecting the immune response

The form taken by the immune response depends upon several factors including the nature of the antigen, the genetic constitution of the individual exposed to the antigen, the route by which the antigen enters the body and the dose administered. These factors are discussed below.

The nature of the antigen. It is difficult to define precisely the properties which make a substance capable of evoking an immune response, but in general terms antigens are large molecules, usually of molecular weight exceeding 3000, fairly rigid in structure, and either protein or carbohydrate, with or without associated substances such as lipids. Antigen–antibody reactions appear to be the result largely of stereochemical interactions of molecules of complementary configurations, analogous to the interaction of lock and key.

For this reason floppy molecules such as gelatin are poor antigens. Evidence will be presented later that immune responses follow the binding of antigen molecules to specific receptors on the surface of lymphocytes. It seems likely that, to trigger off an immune response, antigen must form a link between these surface receptors: this explains why most antigens are large molecules.

Although some small molecules, such as para-aminobenzoic acid, are not by themselves antigenic, they may become so if they are attached to larger molecules. Injection of *p*-aminobenzoic acid attached by diazotisation to serum albumin may result in formation of some antibody molecules which combine specifically with the *p*-aminobenzoic acid moiety and not with the albumin carrier protein. In these circumstances, *p*-aminobenzoic acid is said to be a **hapten**, i.e. a substance which is antigenic inasmuch as it can take part in an immunological reaction (in this case antigen–antibody combination) but which cannot by itself evoke an immune response (in this example, the formation of specific antibody) unless it is conjugated with macromolecular material. The existence of such simple haptens suggests that the antigenic specificity of large molecules may be determined by the three-dimensional configuration of small parts of these molecules (**antigenic determinant sites** or **groups**). Study of synthetic polypeptide and polysaccharide antigens has confirmed that specific antigenic determinant sites do consist of a few amino acids or monosaccharides, and it has been shown that macromolecules such as plasma albumin contain several antigenic determinant sites of differing specificity. There is evidence that determinant sites participating in cell-mediated immunity responses are larger than those concerned in antibody production: thus production of cell-mediated immunity to a simple chemical depends not solely upon the specific antigenicity of the chemical, but also on that of the adjacent part of the macromolecular protein carrier to which the chemical is bound.

Genetic constitution of the individual. Inheritance of immunological responsiveness to simple synthetic oligopeptide antigenic determinant groups has been demonstrated in mice and other rodents. For example, some inbred strains of guinea-pigs have a genetically determined inability to respond immunologically to

certain determinant groups which are immunogenic for other strains. This is presumably true also for natural antigens, though less easily demonstrated because of the multiplicity and variety of determinant sites on natural macromolecules.

Genetic factors also play a large part in determining the antigenicity of tissues, and this field has become particularly important in the practice of blood transfusion and of tissue transplantation. The structure of tissues, including potential antigenic sites, is, of course, genetically determined. In general, when tissues are injected or transplanted from one individual to another, the more genetically dissimilar or foreign the two individuals towards one another, the easier it is to induce antibody formation and cell-mediated immunity. For example, human red cells injected into rabbits evoke a wide variety of antibodies reacting with a corresponding variety of antigenic determinants on the human red cell; when, as in this case, the antigen is derived from a species other than that of the immunised animal (and this would include bacteria, etc.), it is called a **hetero-antigen** and the antibodies are **hetero-antibodies**. Injection or transplantation of one human with the red cells or tissue cells of another may result in the formation of antibodies to antigenic groups not shared by both individuals; e.g. human red cells containing the Rhesus antigen D (Rhesus positive cells) into a person whose cells do not contain this antigen (Rhesus negative) may result in the development of antibodies specific for D antigen; antigens which differ within a species are called **iso-antigens** and the corresponding antibodies **iso-antibodies**. In general, iso-antigens are much less numerous and less likely to evoke an immune response than hetero-antigens. Finally it should be noted that injection of an individual with his own cells (**auto-antigen**) results in **auto-antibody** formation or cell-mediated immunity only in exceptional cases; the subject of **auto-immunity** is considered further on p. 132. Unfortunately the prefixes used to indicate the relationship between individuals providing antigen and forming antibody are, by usage, different from those used in the more recent field of tissue transplantation, in which graft rejection is effected mainly by delayed hypersensitivity reactions. Table 4.1 summarises this confusing and irrational situation.

Table 4.1 Terminology of antigens, antibodies and tissue grafts

Relationship between donor and recipient	Genetic terminology	Antibody, antigen	Transplantation terminology
Same animal	—	Auto-antibody Auto-antigen	Autograft
Identical twins and inbred strain	Syngeneic (Isogeneic)	—	Isograft
Same outbred species or different inbred strains	Allogeneic	Iso-antibody Iso-antigen	Allograft (Homograft)
Different species	Heterogeneic Xenogeneic	Hetero-antibody Hetero-antigen	Xenograft (Heterograft)

As stated above, the cells and tissues of an individual are antigenic when injected or grafted into an animal of another species or even into a different individual of the same species, yet with certain exceptions the individual does not react to the antigens of his own cells by the development of auto-antibody or delayed auto-hypersensitivity. Non-reactivity to auto-antigen is a general physiological principle described by Ehrlich as 'horror autotoxicus'. It may reflect absence of lymphoid cells with the genetic coding necessary for the synthetic processes associated with formation of antibody or cell-mediated immunity against 'self' components, analogous to the inherited non-reactivity of certain strains of animals to synthetic polypeptide antigens. Burnet has, however, suggested an attractive alternative explanation, that the various potential antigens in an individual's tissues do act on the cells responsible for immune reactions but that,

instead of causing antibody formation or cell-mediated immunity, they lead during fetal life to specific immunological tolerance. There is recent evidence that 'horror autotoxicus', which is clearly an important safeguard against immunological self-injury, involves 'suppressor lymphocytes' (pp. 107–8; 134–5).

Route of administration of antigen. In most cases antigens elicit an immunological response only when they are introduced parenterally (i.e. not through the alimentary canal) so that their macromolecular state and the configuration of their antigenic determinants are not destroyed by digestion in the gut. Traces of certain proteins, such as those in heterologous milk, may, however, be absorbed from the gut and bring about specific sensitisation, especially in infants. In general, however, antigens introduced via the portal circulation are less immunogenic than when administered by other routes.

Antibodies

Antibody molecules have the special property of combining specifically with antigen or hapten. In so doing they may cover up harmful areas on molecules of toxin, in which case they are said to be **antitoxins**, or their combination with cells such as bacteria may lead (with the help of complement—p. 116) to their dissolution (**bacteriolytic effect**) or phagocytosis by polymorphs and macrophages (**opsonic effect**). Chemically, antibodies belong to the **immunoglobulin (Ig)** proteins of the plasma (sometimes called γ-globulins because of their electrophor-

etic mobility); and there are five classes: IgG, IgM, IgA, IgD and IgE. All immunoglobulins are composed of one or more similar units, each unit consisting of two pairs of identical polypeptide chains (Fig. 4.1); one pair termed the **heavy chains** are about twice the size (molecular weight) of the other pair, which are termed the **light chains**. Digestion of an Ig molecule by papain breaks it into three fragments, of which two are identical and are termed **Fab** (antigen-binding fragments) because each contains a combining site for

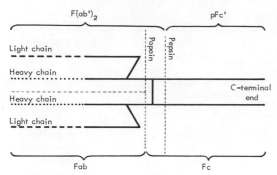

Fig. 4.1 Structure of monomeric immunoglobulin molecule. In any one molecule the two light chains have an identical amino-acid sequence and so also have the heavy chains. Each immunoglobulin class has a distinctive Fc piece (C terminal end of heavy chains). The amino-acid sequence of the interrupted portions of the light chains and dotted portions of heavy chains (the N-terminal ends) vary greatly among immunoglobulin molecules even of the same class and constitute the specific antigen-binding (Fab) sites, of which there are two on each molecule. (The light lines indicate separation of the molecules into an Fc and two Fab fragments by papain digestion, and into F(ab')$_2$ and two pFc' fragments by pepsin.)

antigen. The third fragment consists of the C-terminal ends of the heavy chains, and is termed **Fc** fragment; it is readily obtained in crystalline (hence Fc) form. As shown in Fig. 4.1, digestion of IgG by pepsin frees two Fc' fragments but leaves the two Fab fragments united by part of the Fc fragment as a single fragment—F(ab')$_2$. Heavy chains differ structurally for each class of Ig, and the letters γ, μ, a, δ, ϵ, are used to indicate the heavy chains of IgG, IgM, IgA, etc. respectively. By contrast, there are only two types of light chain, κ and λ, in all Ig classes, and each Ig molecule has either κ or λ light chains. Differences in the behaviour of antibodies of different Ig classes are determined by the properties of their heavy chains.

The combination of antibody with antigen is believed to be achieved by van der Waal's forces which are effective over a very short range and hold separate molecules together only when they fit snugly. The specificity of antigen–antibody union therefore depends on the antibody-combining-site having a complementary shape to the antigenic determinant which permits the necessary close fit. The shape of the combining site is determined by the amino-acid sequence of the N-terminal ends of the heavy and, to a lesser extent, of the light chains. In view of what is now known of protein synthesis this is of great interest and of fundamental importance in elucidating how antigenic stimulation gives rise to specific antibody formation. In contrast to most other proteins, each one of which in a given individual is of uniform amino-acid sequence, the immunoglobulins in a serum show marked heterogeneity at the N-terminal ends (the **variable regions**), the number of variations amounting to millions. This variety allows for the great range of antigens, natural and synthetic, against which antibody may be formed.

Some idea of the specificity of antibody–antigen union can be gained from study of antibody against chemically defined haptens. Landsteiner, for example, showed that antibody raised against para-aminobenzene sulphonic acid does not combine with the ortho- form but gives a weak reaction with meta-aminobenzene sulphonic acid (Fig. 4.2). The latter is called a

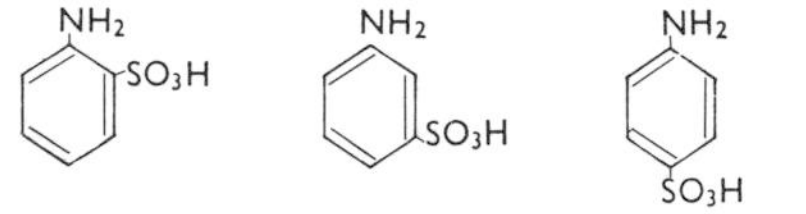

$$NH_2 \qquad NH_2 \qquad NH_2$$

ortho   meta   para

Fig. 4.2 Isomeric forms of aminobenzene sulphonic acid.

cross-reaction and it implies immunological reactivity with an antigen different from that which has led to the production of antibody. It results from the production of some antibody molecules which fit the cross reacting antigen sufficiently well to permit intermolecular attraction by van der Waal's forces. The closeness of fit between the antigen-binding sites of antibody with an antigen of given configuration can thus vary and this affects the firmness of combination; we therefore speak of high or low **affinity** or **avidity** of antibody for a given antigen. Cross reactions are generally of low affinity.

Properties of the immunoglobulin classes

The various immunoglobulin classes have different functions (beyond that of specific combination with antigen, which is common to all) and this is determined by the structure of the part of the heavy chains included in the Fc fragment.

When immunoglobulin of a particular class is injected into animals of another species it acts as an *antigen*, and antibodies specific for the light and for the heavy chains appear in the serum of the injected animal. Combination of the latter antibody with immunoglobulin *in vitro* provides a simple method of demonstrating the class to which a particular immunoglobulin belongs, for example by immunoelectrophoresis (p. 90).

Table 4.2 compares some of the features of

Table 4.2 Size and serum concentrations of immunoglobulins

Class	Molecular weight	Degree of polymerisation	Concentration (normal serum) mg/100 ml
IgG	150 000	Monomer	800–1600
IgM	1 000 000	Pentamer	50–200
IgA	Mainly 150 000	Mono- and polymer	140–400
IgD	185 000	Monomer	0–40
IgE	200 000	Monomer	$2-45 \times 10^{-5}$

the five known immunoglobulin classes. **IgG** is present in the serum in the largest amount and is the most widely studied immunoglobin. IgG antitoxins are of importance because they combine with and neutralise the toxin, thus protecting the individual from its harmful effects. The reaction of IgG antibody with the corresponding antigen can usually be demonstrated *in vitro* (see below): it can cross the human placenta and in this way passive immunity is transferred from mother to child. **IgM**, a macroglobulin consisting of pentamers of the basic four-chain unit (each of which has two antigen-combining sites), is the first Ig class of antibody to be produced following the initial introduction of an antigen. Because of its 10 combining sites, it is usually of high avidity. It is especially effective in activating complement (see below) and in destroying bacterial cells and its reactions are readily demonstrated *in vitro*. The presence of IgM antibody, e.g. to Rubella virus, indicates recent or continuing exposure to that antigen. **IgA** is present in the plasma, and the intestinal mucosa is particularly rich in IgA-producing plasma cells. It is secreted into colostrum, saliva, tears, respiratory-tract mucus and especially into intestinal mucus. The glandular cells concerned in these secretions take up IgA from the extra-

cellular fluid and couple it with a carbohydrate 'transport piece', which may render it resistant to digestive enzymes. The function of IgA is not known, but it may form a protective coating over mucous membranes, and an analogy to 'antiseptic paint' has been made. **IgE** has the special property of attaching to tissue, particularly to mast cells and basophils, by means of its Fc fragment, leaving the specific combining sites (on the Fab fragments) available for union with antigen. If such union takes place, pharmacologically active substances such as histamine are released, with the production of an anaphylactic hypersensitivity reaction within a few minutes (p. 117). The biological properties of **IgD** are unknown, but it appears to act as a lymphocyte surface antigen-receptor in early life.

Demonstration of antigen–antibody reactions

In vivo

Antigen–antibody reactions may be demonstrated *in vivo* in two ways.

(1) A potentially harmful antigenic substance may be rendered harmless by union with antibody and not have the expected effect. For example, in the Schick test, intradermal injection of a small amount of diphtheria toxin into the skin of a non-immune individual results in an area of inflammation. The diphtheria antitoxin present in an immunised individual neutralises the toxin and so suppresses the inflammation.

(2) A normally harmless stimulus may result in tissue injury i.e. a hypersensitivity reaction. For example, inhalation of grass pollen may induce an attack of hay fever or asthma, mediated by its reaction with antibody specific for grass pollen. In this instance, the antibody is usually of IgE class, but hypersensitivity reactions may result from the union *in vivo* of other classes of antibody with antigen: they are of considerable importance in disease processes and are described in Chapter 5.

In vitro

Antigen–antibody combination may be demonstrated *in vitro* in various ways, depending on the nature of the antigen and the type and amount of antibody present.

(1) Visible aggregation of antigen. Since each antibody molecule has at least two combining sites it can bind with two or more antigen molecules. If the antigen molecules contain several antigenic determinants, and if they are in solution, antibody can form cross-linkages between antigen molecules, uniting them in the

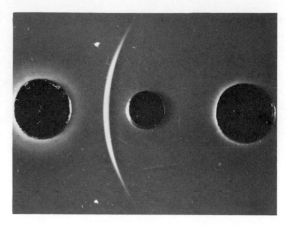

Fig. 4.4 Ouchterlony technique. The central well contains a solution of antigen. The well on the left contains the corresponding antiserum, and that on the right a negative control serum. A white line of precipitate, composed of antigen–antibody complex, has formed between the antigen and antibody wells. In this instance the antigen is thyroglobulin and the test detects auto-antibody to thyroglobulin in the serum of a patient with chronic thyroiditis.

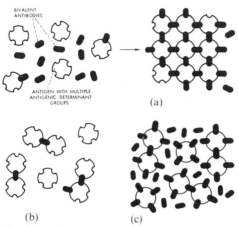

Fig. 4.3 The reaction of antigen and antibody (a) in optimal proportions to form large aggregates: (b) in antigen excess: (c) in antibody excess. In (b) and (c) small complexes are formed. In the case of soluble antigens, large aggregates, as in (a), form precipitates, whereas with particulate antigens, e.g. bacteria, formation of aggregates is termed agglutination.

form of a lattice (Fig. 4.3): if antigen and antibody molecules are present in optimal combining proportions the aggregates will be large (Fig. 4.3a) and visible as an insoluble precipitate (**precipitin reaction**). Lattice formation and therefore precipitation can be inhibited when an excessive amount of antigen saturates the combining sites on all the antibody molecules, and smaller complexes may then be formed (Fig. 4.3b). Conversely, when gross excess of antibody is present (Fig. 4.3c), each antigen combining site may fix a separate antibody molecule, and, once again, the complexes may be too small to form a visible precipitate (**prozone effect**). Optimum antigen–antibody proportions for lattice formation can readily be achieved by allowing antibody and antigen to diffuse towards each other through agar (Ouchterlony technique, Fig. 4.4). The interpretation of agar

diffusion tests involving antiserum raised against a complex mixture of antigens (as when human serum is injected into rabbits) is facilitated by partial separation of the constituent antigens by electrophoresis prior to the precipitin reaction; this method, called immunoelectrophoresis, is illustrated in Fig. 4.5.

When the antigen molecules are associated with a large particle, e.g. the antigenic determinants of the surface of a red cell or bacterium, or are adsorbed artificially on to red cells or latex particles, antibody causes aggregation of the particles (**agglutination reaction**). The visible

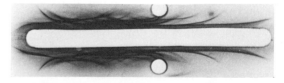

Fig. 4.5 Immunoelectrophoresis. Complex mixtures of antigens have been placed in the circular well in the slab of agar and subjected to electrophoresis. Subsequently an antiserum containing antibodies to the various antigens is placed in the longitudinal trough and discrete lines of precipitate formed by the various reactions can be identified. In this example, the wells contain specimens of human serum and the trough contains antiserum to human serum prepared in a rabbit.

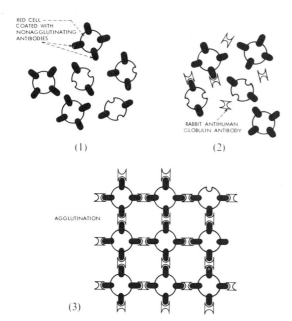

(1)   (2)

AGGLUTINATION

(3)

Fig. 4.6 Antigenic particles sensitised with a non-agglutinating antibody are agglutinated by antibody to immunoglobulin (antiglobulin reagent).

aggregation of large particles such as bacteria can be effected by minute amounts of antibody.

(2) Demonstration of antibody attached to antigen by anti-immunoglobulin reagent. In certain circumstances antibody combines with antigen without causing aggregation. This may occur if the spatial arrangement of the antigen (e.g. the Rhesus antigen on the surface of red cells) prevents the divalent IgG antibody molecule from combining simultaneously with antigenic determinant groups on two different red cells. In these circumstances, exposure of the Rhesus positive red cells to anti-Rhesus antibody merely results in their being coated with IgG. However, the coated cells can be agglutinated by antibody against IgG (**antiglobulin** or **Coombs' reaction**) (Fig. 4.6).

A similar principle is used in the **indirect immunofluorescence (indirect fluorescent antibody) technique** to detect insoluble antigen (e.g. bacterial capsular polysaccharide) in a histological section or smear. When this is exposed to antiserum the antibody combines with antigen without visible effect. The slide is washed to remove the antiserum, leaving only the specific antibody which is, of course, an immunoglobulin, attached to the antigen present in the section. Antibody to immunoglobulin, conjugated with a fluorescent dye such as fluorescein isothiocyanate, is then applied to the section or smear and the site of antigen–antibody combination is visualised by the presence of the fluorescent antiglobulin when the section is examined microscopically with ultraviolet light (Figs. 4.7, 4.8). (In the **direct immunofluorescence technique**

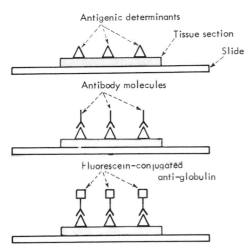

Fig. 4.7 The indirect immunofluorescence technique performed on a tissue section. *Top*, tissue section on slide. *Middle*, section treated with antibody (⅄) to a tissue constituent and washed: antibody molecules adhere to the tissue antigen. *Bottom*, section treated with fluorescein-conjugated antibody (▢) to immunoglobulin: sites of antigen–antibody reaction fluoresce in ultraviolet light.

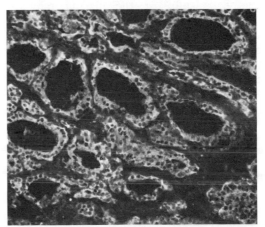

Fig. 4.8 A positive indirect immunofluorescence test for antibody to thyroid epithelium. A frozen section of thyroid tissue has been treated with the serum undergoing test (from a patient with chronic thyroiditis), followed by treatment with fluorescein-conjugated anti-human-IgG. Note fluorescence of the thyroid epithelial cytoplasm. (U.V. microscopy.)

the antibody against the antigen in the histological section or smear is directly conjugated with fluorescent dye and its attachment to the section is demonstrated as above but without the use of an antiglobulin reagent.) More recently, analogous techniques have been introduced in which antibody is labelled with the enzyme *peroxidase* instead of with a fluorescent dye; peroxidase can be localised as a dark deposit by ordinary light microscopy after appropriate histochemical treatment.

(3) **Methods using radioactive antigen.** In the Farr technique, which is valuable in measuring antibody to soluble antigen, excess antigen labelled with radioisotope is added to antiserum; the immunoglobulin (including antigen–antibody complexes) is then precipitated by 50% saturation with ammonium sulphate. Provided that the free antigen (uncombined with antibody) is not salted out by this procedure, the amount of radioactivity precipitated is proportional to the total *antigen binding capacity* of the serum.

In the **antiglobulin coprecipitation technique** the amount of antibody to a given radioactive antigen can similarly be measured by precipitation with class-specific anti-Ig antibody instead of by a salting out procedure.

Numerous very sensitive radioimmunoassays have been devised for the measurement of antigen or antibody. For example, the concentration of insulin in the plasma may be measured by mixing the plasma with anti-insulin and radioactive insulin in standard amounts, and determining how much radioactive insulin is excluded, by the plasma insulin, from combining with antibody.

(4) **Methods involving damage to cells.** Antibody combined with antigen on the surface of intact cells such as bacteria or erythrocytes can damage the cell membrane and cause lysis (partial dissolution) of the cells which is readily demonstrable. The lysis is mediated by a complex group of at least nine factors present in fresh normal serum and known collectively as **complement**. These factors are activated by the Fc portions of antibody molecules which have combined with antigen, and once activated they give rise to a chain of enzyme reactions culminating in digestion of the cell membrane where the antibody is attached. In the course of the reaction complement is used up, or 'fixed'.

(5) **Complement fixation.** Complement is fixed in many antigen–antibody reactions in addition to those involving cell-surface antigens. Invisible antigen–antibody reactions can often be demonstrated indirectly by allowing them to occur in the presence of a measured amount of complement and subsequently adding an indicator system, namely red cells coated with an antibody (haemolysin) which will cause red cell lysis only in the presence of complement. Fixation of complement by the invisible antigen–antibody reaction prevents haemolysis in the indicator system (Fig. 4.9). A more detailed account of complement is given on p. 115.

(6) **Blocking antibody.** In certain circumstances (usually poorly defined), antibody can combine invisibly with antigen which thereby becomes unavailable for participation in a subsequent visible immunological reaction such as agglutination or cytotoxic damage. The presence of blocking antibody in a serum can thus be demonstrated by a two-stage test.

The production of antibody

Injection of an antigen to which an individual has not previously been exposed results in a

	Mix antigen and antibody	Add complement (C)	Add sensitised RBC
Positive test	$Ag^x + Ab^x \longrightarrow Ag^x{-}Ab^x$ (union)	$+ C \longrightarrow Ag^x{-}Ab^x$ $\quad\quad\quad\quad\;\;	$ $\quad\quad\quad\quad\;\; C$ (complement used up)	No lysis
Negative test	$Ag^x + Ab^y \longrightarrow Ag^x + Ab^y$ (no union)	$+ C \longrightarrow Ag^x + Ab^y + C$ (complement not used)	Lysis

Fig. 4.9 The complement fixation reaction depends on the 'fixation' of complement by an antigen–antibody complex (upper line). The fixation of complement is demonstrated by non-lysis of subsequently added red cells coated with a haemolytic antibody. If there is no antigen–antibody reaction (lower line), complement is not used up and lyses the sensitised red cells.

primary antibody response, i.e. the transient appearance in the blood of a small amount of specific antibody of IgM class, about seven days after the injection. Re-injection of the same antigen at a later date leads to a **secondary** or **anamnestic** (remembering) **response** in which large amounts of specific antibody, usually of IgG class, appear in the blood rapidly (in four days or so) and continue to be produced, although in gradually diminishing amounts, for weeks, months or even years. The

of the gut and in the inflammatory lesion which forms around injected antigenic material. **Plasma cells** (Fig. 4.10) are somewhat larger than small lymphocytes, of ovoid shape with a small round nucleus in which granules of chromatin are regularly spaced around the periphery, giving a 'cart-wheel' or 'clock-face' appearance. Their cytoplasm is basophilic and also pyroninophilic, indicating a high content of ribonucleic acid, and electron microscopy (Fig. 4.11) reveals a large amount of complex

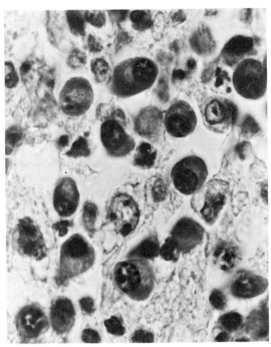

Fig. 4.10 Plasma cells in a lymph node draining a focus of infection. Note the eccentrically-placed, round nucleus with clumping of chromatin, and the deeply-stained (basophilic) cytoplasm showing, in some instances, a crescentic area of pallor alongside the nucleus. × 1000.

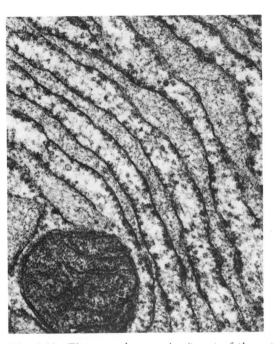

Fig. 4.11 Electron micrograph of part of the cytoplasm of a plasma cell, showing the abundant rough endoplasmic reticulum. Part of a mitochondrion is also included. × 108 000.

greatly enhanced antibody production of the secondary response is the reason for the repeated injections of microbial antigens (vaccines) widely used in prophylactic immunisation.

Most of the antibody found in serum is produced by plasma cells in lymph nodes, spleen and bone marrow but some may also be formed by plasma cells in the lymphoid tissue

granular endoplasmic reticulum of the type found in cells which produce a protein secretion. It has been shown by immunofluorescence that each plasma cell at any given time produces light chains together with heavy chains of only one immunoglobulin class (e.g. IgG or IgM). Furthermore, following stimulation with two distinct antigens (e.g. diphtheria and tetanus toxins) individual plasma cells will produce antibody to one or the other but not to both of these antigens.

Cell-mediated immunity

Many antigenic stimuli lead to the production of lymphocytes which, like antibody, are capable of reacting specifically with the antigen: this is the cell-mediated immune response. It is demonstrated classically by intradermal injection of the antigen, which leads to an indurated erythematous lesion in the dermis maximal 24–72 hours later—the **delayed hypersensitivity reaction**. During development of the lesion there is early emigration of polymorphonuclear leukocytes but this phase is transient, and the polymorphs soon disappear from the site: there follows an increasing accumulation of mononuclear cells (mainly lymphocytes, but with some macrophages), around small veins, hair follicles and sweat glands and accompanied by inflammatory oedema (Fig. 5.8, p. 128). Cell-mediated immunity can also be demonstrated in animals by injecting antigen into the cornea, which results in a similar reaction with corneal opacity 24–48 hours later. These sites are convenient for the elicitation of delayed hypersensitivity reactions, but all tissues are reactive, i.e. the state of cell-mediated immunity is generalised.

Evidence is accumulating that cell-mediated immunity may be demonstrated *in vitro* by observing the effect of the appropriate antigen on living cells from the sensitised individual. For example, it has been shown that tuberculoprotein inhibits the migration from a capillary tube of macrophages obtained from a sensitised guinea-pig. This type of experiment has also been performed using blood leukocytes, and it has been shown that when circulating small lymphocytes from an immunised individual are exposed to the antigen in tissue culture, a small proportion of them *transform* into larger cells with basophilic cytoplasm, synthesise DNA and undergo mitosis. Such tests are being used increasingly to demonstrate cell-mediated immunity to various micro-organisms and other antigens. The mechanism of delayed hypersensitivity reactions is considered in Chapter 5.

A classical example of cell-mediated immunity is that which develops to tuberculoprotein in most individuals who have been infected by *Mycobacterium tuberculosis* or inoculated with BCG. The Mantoux test (p. 127), in which more or less purified tuberculoprotein is injected intradermally, is a classical delayed hypersensitivity reaction. It has been found that injection of protein antigens, which in ordinary circumstances merely evoke an antibody response, can also lead to the development of cell-mediated immunity provided that the antigen is injected emulsified in an oily 'adjuvant' containing *M. tuberculosis* (Freund's adjuvant), other mycobacteria, or a peptidoglycolipid extracted from the cell wall of these organisms. Cell-mediated immunity is also a prominent feature of the immunological response to living allografts and xenografts. When certain simple chemicals, for example picryl chloride, are applied to the skin, they combine with skin proteins to act as haptens and cell-mediated immunity results: on subsequent application to the skin these substances give rise to the lesion known as **contact dermatitis** which is simply a delayed hypersensitivity reaction. It has been suggested by Medawar that delayed hypersensitivity develops when antigen is fixed in the peripheral tissues so that it is encountered mainly by wandering lymphocytes (see p. 98) and is carried only later to the regional lymph nodes in significant amounts. It should be noted that although cell-mediated immunity is usually demonstrated by tests leading to an apparently exaggerated and harmful reaction, there is strong evidence that it plays an important role in the body's defence against infection. Thus in children with congenital hypogammaglobulinaemia, resistance to most virus infections is diminished only when there is co-existing failure of responsiveness of cell-mediated immunity.

The Cellular Basis of the Immune Response

So far, this account has concentrated mainly on describing the usual products of antigenic stimulation, i.e. antibodies and specifically-primed lymphocytes, capable of reacting with the antigen. We must now consider in detail the cellular events involved in these responses.

The cytology of immunological phenomena is complex. Most of the advances have been based on the manipulation of cells and tissues of experimental animals, but the features of immune responses and of naturally occurring immunodeficiency states in man, the effects of therapeutic immunosuppression, and investigation of human lymphocytes *in vitro* all indicate that the same basic rules apply.

The main features of the cellular basis of antibody production and cell-mediated immunity may be summarised as follows.

1. Cell-mediated immunity and antibody production are both attributable to lymphocytes capable of recognising and responding specifically to the stimulus provided by an antigen, i.e. **specifically-responsive lymphocytes**.

2. The specifically responsive lymphocytes which bring about cell-mediated immunity are **thymus-dependent** or **T lymphocytes**. They develop in the thymus, and possibly also in other lymphoid tissues, under the influence of a thymic hormone.

3. On encountering an antigen to which it is specifically responsive, the T lymphocyte proliferates to produce a clone of lymphocytes, all of which are capable of reacting with that antigen—**specifically-primed T lymphocytes**. These are responsible for delayed hypersensitivity reactions.

4. The specifically-responsive lymphocytes which bring about antibody production are **thymus-independent** and are termed **B lymphocytes**.

5. On encountering an antigen to which it is specifically responsive, the B lymphocyte, like the T lymphocyte, proliferates to form a clone of cells capable of reacting with that antigen. Some of these differentiate into plasma cells which secrete antibody reactive with the antigen. The plasma cells are thus derived from B lymphocytes.

6. Some of the lymphocytes produced by antigen-induced proliferation of T and B lymphocytes persist as **memory cells**. In other words, antigenic stimulation increases the number of T and B lymphocytes capable of reacting with that antigen, and some of these lymphocytes

are long-lived and are responsible for a secondary response on subsequent stimulation by the antigen.

7. Although T lymphocytes do not give rise to antibody-producing plasma cells, they co-operate with B cells in antibody responses, and such co-operation is essential to, or enhances, production of antibody to most antigens. T lymphocytes can also have a suppressive effect on immune responses.

8. At some stage in their development, lymphocytes become '**committed**', i.e. capable of responding to a particular antigenic determinant group, or to closely similar determinant groups. Lymphocyte populations thus consist of individual cells which differ in the antigens to which they can respond. No one antigen can stimulate response in more than a small proportion of them.

9. In some circumstances, antigenic stimulation results in neither antibody production nor cell-mediated immunity, but renders the individual specifically unresponsive to subsequent challenge by that antigen. This unresponsive state is termed **acquired immunological tolerance**. It provides an explanation of why we do not usually respond strongly to antigens in our own cells and tissues, and plays an important rôle in successful transplantation of foreign cells and tissues.

These basic features of immune responses are considered more fully below.

The specifically responsive lymphocyte

For the development of specific immunity, it is necessary that cells should recognise specific antigenic determinants, and should respond to them in ways that lead to the production of antibodies and primed lymphocytes, both of which are capable of reacting specifically with the antigen. Much of the credit for demonstrating that these cells—the keystones of the immune response—are lymphocytes, is due to Gowans and his co-workers in Oxford. Gowans used techniques in which lymphocytes were removed from rats by thoracic duct drainage.

By continuous drainage for several days, the fluid being returned to the rat, depletion of a population of small lymphocytes was achieved. The depleted rats were found to be incapable of mounting immunological responses. For example, they failed to reject a skin allograft and made poor antibody responses to injections of sheep erythrocytes or tetanus toxoid. These immunological deficiencies were corrected by injection of thoracic duct small lymphocytes from a second rat, and when the donor had been previously immunised, e.g. by a skin allograft or an injection of sheep erythrocytes, the recipient showed the rapid and intense response to antigenic challenge which is characteristic of the secondary response. These observations suggested that small lymphocytes in thoracic duct lymph are essential for primary immune responses, and showed more conclusively that they included specifically responsive cells resulting from a previous immune response, i.e. immunological memory cells. Gowans' findings have since been confirmed by many other workers and have been shown to apply to several mammalian and avian species. By these and other experimental procedures, it has been established that small lymphocytes include specifically responsive cells. When there has been no previous exposure to a particular antigen, the appropriate specifically-responsive cells are present in small numbers, and are capable of mounting a primary immune response. Previous antigenic challenge leads to the production of increased numbers of specifically responsive '**primed**' or '**memory cells**', so that a second challenge with the same antigen results in the more rapid and enhanced secondary response.

The thymus-dependent or T lymphocytes

The technique of thoracic duct drainage was also used by Gowans to study the kinetics of lymphocytes. By infusing into rats thoracic duct lymphocytes in which the nucleic acid had been labelled *in vivo* with radio-isotopes, he was able to follow the distribution and persistence of the infused cells. He showed that the thoracic duct small lymphocytes were a long-lived population of cells which recirculated continuously between the blood and lymphoid tissues. Thoracic duct lymph also contains larger lymphoid cells, which were found to have a much shorter lifespan and which passed into and remained in various tissues, particularly the mucosa of the gut.

The role of the thymus

Production of lymphocytes. The thymus is a predominantly lymphoid organ, the function of which was for long obscure. It differs in three ways from other lymphoid tissues; firstly, it does not act as a filter for blood or lymph; secondly, it is not a site of significant immune responses to antigenic stimulation; thirdly it is excluded from the pathway, mentioned above, of the recirculating small lymphocytes.

The important clue to thymic function came from the observation, by Good and others, that immunological deficiency states in man were sometimes associated with thymic abnormalities. Experimental thymectomy in adult animals seemed to have little or no effect, but Miller and his co-workers demonstrated that neonatally-thymectomised mice failed to thrive and commonly died of a chronic wasting disease, since shown to be due mainly to infections. Animals which survived long enough for investigation were shown to be deficient in cell-mediated immune responses and in antibody production to some antigens. The thymectomised mice failed to develop the recirculating pool of small lymphocytes described by Gowans, and were deficient in small lymphocytes in the thoracic duct, blood, and parts of the lymphoid tissues. It was thus apparent that the presence of the thymus was necessary for the development of the recirculating pool of long-lived small lymphocytes, which were accordingly termed the **thymus-dependent** or **T lymphocytes** (Fig. 4.12). These findings have been amply confirmed and similar observations have been made in rats, hamsters and chickens. Some mammals, including man, are born in a state of relative immunological maturity, having formed their population of T lymphocytes in fetal life. In man, however, failure of thymic development is accompanied by a deficiency of T lymphocytes.

More direct evidence that T lymphocytes are produced in the thymus has been provided by the demonstration that thymic lymphocytes labelled *in vivo*, by injecting radioactive thymidine into the thymic artery, leave the thymus and join the recirculating small lymphocyte pool.

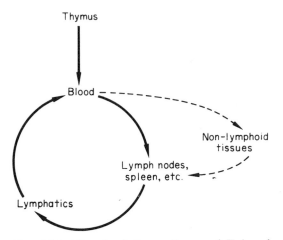

Fig. 4.12 The circulating pathway of T lymphocytes. Although their production is dependent on the thymus, they do not recirculate through it, but through the lymph nodes, spleen and gut-associated lymphoid tissue—the secondary lymphoid tissues. Circulation through the non-lymphoid tissues involves fewer lymphocytes.

In adult animals and man, thymectomy has little effect on immune responsiveness (but see p. 99), the function of the thymus becoming less important with age. The T-lymphocyte pool, which includes the immunological experience of the individual, stored in 'primed' or 'memory' T lymphocytes, becomes largely self supporting. If, however, the T lymphocytes are destroyed, e.g. by x-irradiation, its restoration is dependent on the thymus, and is prevented by previous thymectomy in adult life. The thymus thus remains capable of replenishing the T-lymphocyte population in adult life.

A thymic lymphopoietic hormone. In addition to supplying T lymphocytes, there is evidence that the thymus produces a hormone, '**thymosin**', which stimulates differentiation and proliferation of T lymphocytes. This was first suspected when implantation of thymic tissue enclosed in cell-proof diffusion chambers was found to restore partially the T-lymphocyte population of neonatally thymectomised mice. Subsequently, extracts of thymic tissue have been shown to have a similar effect, and similar activity has been detected in the plasma of normal mice and man, but is absent following thymectomy. According to Bach, the plasma activity in man decreases with age, an observation which accords well with the normal process of thymic involution. It thus seems likely that production of T lymphocytes in the thymus is stimulated by the local effect of thymosin, and that the hormone can also stimulate T-lymphopoiesis in other lymphoid tissues. From electron-microscopic and other observations, the thymic epithelium seems the most likely source of thymosin.

The recirculating pathway of T lymphocytes

As stated above, Gowans investigated the recirculation of small lymphocytes by use of radio-isotopic labelling. Others, and notably Parrott and her co-workers, performed similar experiments, and combined kinetic studies with histological examination of the tissues of neonatally thymectomised mice. By these means, the circulating pathway of T lymphocytes has been elucidated. In the lymph nodes they leave the blood, probably by passing between the columnar endothelial cells of the post-capillary venules in the **deep cortex** (sometimes termed **paracortex**) of the node (Fig. 4.13). They make up the lymphocytic population of the deep cortex,

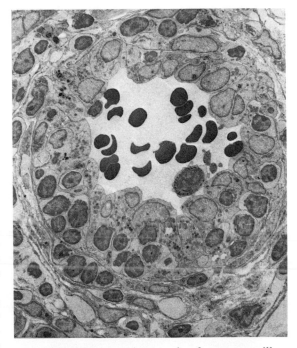

Fig. 4.13 Electron micrograph of a post-capillary venule in a Peyer's patch from a rat, showing a lymphocyte on the luminal surface, several lying between endothelial cells, and others in the surrounding sheath. × 1200. (Dr. Gutta I. Schoefl.)

from where they pass into the medullary sinuses and leave the node by the efferent lymphatic, returning to the blood by the major lymphatics. Similar migration occurs through the gut-associated lymphoid tissues (adenoids, tonsils, Peyer's patches and solitary follicles). In the white pulp of the spleen the lymphocytes leave the blood and enter the lymphoid sheath immediately around the central arteriole, from where they re-enter the blood, presumably via the venous sinuses of the red pulp.

As would be expected, lymph leaving a lymph node by the efferent lymphatic contains many more small lymphocytes than does the lymph in the afferent lymphatics; nevertheless some are present in the afferent lymph, indicating that lymphocytes leave the blood in the non-lymphoid tissues and then enter the tissue lymphatics and pass to the draining lymph nodes (Fig. 4.12). Their number is, however, small when compared to those recirculating as described above. In the rat, the rate of recirculation is such that the time taken for turnover of T lymphocytes in the blood is less than one hour, and there is thus good oppor-

tunity for large numbers of lymphocytes to encounter antigens in almost any part of the body.

Those parts of the lymphoid tissues which normally contain large numbers of recirculating T lymphocytes are known as the **thymus-dependent areas**. In neonatally-thymectomised mice, these areas lack small lymphocytes and are occupied mainly by larger, so-called reticulum cells (Fig. 4.14).

The lymph nodes, spleen and gut-associated lymphoid tissues, which are included in the pathway of the T lymphocytes, are also those in which immune responses take place; they are sometimes known collectively as the **secondary lymphoid tissues**. The thymus is not included in this pathway, and because of its function of producing T lymphocytes, it is sometimes called a primary lymphoid organ. As explained later, the thymus is the only organ of this kind in mammals, although birds have a second primary organ, the **Bursa of Fabricius**, in the wall of the cloaca, where thymus-independent or B lymphocytes are produced.

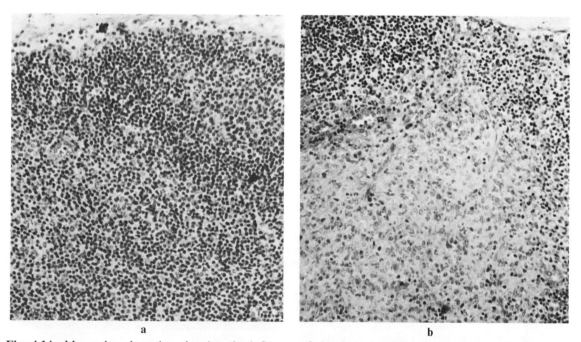

a b

Fig. 4.14 Mouse lymph nodes, showing the influence of the thymus on the histological appearances. **a**, normal lymph node, showing a cortical follicle (top right), and the deep cortex which occupies the lower two thirds of the field. **b**, lymph node from an athymic mouse: the superficial cortex shows little abnormality, but the deep cortex is almost devoid of lymphoid cells and consists largely of 'reticulum cells'. × 150. (Professor D. M. V. Parrott and Dr. M. A. B. de Sousa.)

T lymphocyte function

Following the demonstration of Gowans that removal of lymphocytes by thoracic-duct drainage resulted in depletion of long-lived recirculating lymphocytes and impaired immunological function, and the subsequent discovery of the importance of the thymus in the production of this population of cells, the role of T lymphocytes has been investigated extensively. Use has been made of (*a*) congenitally athymic (nu, nu) mice, (*b*) of animals depleted of T lymphocytes by neonatal thymectomy or administration of anti-lymphocyte globulin (antibody prepared by injection of lymphocytes into an animal of another species), and (*c*) of adult animals subjected to thoracic-duct drainage or treated by thymectomy and whole-body x-irradiation followed by injection of bone marrow cells to restore haemopoiesis and non-thymus-dependent lymphocytes. A regular feature of this deficiency state is an inability to develop cell-mediated immune responses, and this can be corrected by injection of T lymphocytes but not by other types of cells. For example, the T-cell deficient animal fails to reject a skin allograft, but rejection follows the administration of T lymphocytes. Also the lymphocytes of the T-cell deficient animal fail to respond to the antigens of allogeneic cells, either *in vitro* or when injected into suitable allogeneic animals (graft *versus* host reaction). These and other examples demonstrate conclusively that the cell-mediated immune response is a T-lymphocyte function.

The relationship of T lymphocytes to antibody production is more complicated. T-cell deficient animals have normal levels of serum immunoglobulins, and respond to some antigens by normal antibody production: however, the production of antibodies to many antigens is either diminished or absent, and, as will be seen later, T lymphocytes play an indirect but important part in most antibody responses.

Although thymectomy in the adult is without obvious effect on T-lymphocyte function, adolescent mice subjected to thymectomy have been found to exhibit some depression of cell-mediated immunity a year or so later, as judged by their capacity to reject skin allografts. It thus seems that, in this species, in which the life of the T lymphocyte is a few months, thymic function remains of some importance for at least some weeks after birth. There is no firm evidence of immunological deficiency in patients subjected to thymectomy, but, as already stated, the T-lymphocyte pool in man is already present at birth, and moreover there is evidence that human T lymphocytes have a lifespan of many years. This is based on the detection of chromosomal abnormalities incompatible with successful mitosis in the lymphocytes of patients subjected to radiotherapy many years previously.

The response of T lymphocytes to antigenic stimuli. When T lymphocytes encounter an antigen to which they can respond, they transform into larger cells termed **T immunoblasts** or **lymphoblasts**. The nucleus enlarges and the chromatin becomes less condensed: the cytoplasm also increases and becomes basophilic, and electron microscopy reveals abundant ribosomes and polyribosomes, indicating synthesis

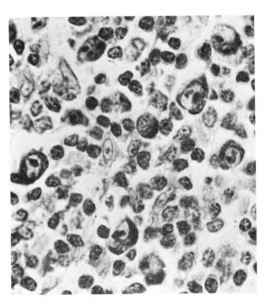

Fig. 4.15 Large lymphoid cells with enlarged nucleus and pyroninophilic cytoplasm (*immunoblasts*) in a human lymph node removed 6 days after a skin allograft. Methyl green pyronin stain. × 480. (Professor D. M. V. Parrott and Dr M. A. B. de Sousa.)

of structural components. Transformation to an immunoblast is accompanied by synthesis of DNA and is a prelude to mitosis. It is seen in the T-dependent areas of the spleen and lymph nodes, etc., during a cell-mediated immune response, and is often most conspicuous in the nodes draining the site of introduction of the antigen, e.g. an allogeneic skin graft (Fig. 4.15) or an application of the hapten, dichloronitro-benzene to the skin. After an unknown number of divisions, the immunoblasts give rise to clones of specifically primed small T lymphocytes which are long-lived memory cells and join the recirculating lymphocyte pool: on subsequent encounter with the appropriate antigen, they themselves transform to immunoblasts, and release the lymphokines (p. 129) which are responsible for the delayed hypersensitivity

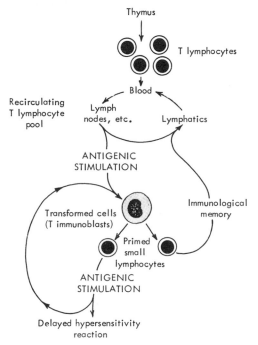

Fig. 4.16 The effects of antigenic stimulation on T lymphocytes.

reaction (Fig. 4.16). Cell-mediated immunity thus involves the development and persistence of T lymphocytes which are specifically primed to react with the antigen: if these cells are present in sufficient numbers, their reaction with antigen can be demonstrated by a delayed hypersensitivity reaction *in vivo*, by their *in-vitro* transformation to immunoblasts or by macrophage migration-inhibition tests (p. 94). In man and some other species, T lymphocytes can be identified by characteristic surface markers, and this has been used to demonstrate that most of the immunoblasts in the responses described above are of T-cell nature.

T-lymphocyte antigen receptors. The specific

response of a cell to an antigen requires of the cell a highly specific recognition process, and the T lymphocyte achieves this by synthesising and inserting into its plasma membrane specific receptors for the antigenic determinant group to which it can respond. The evidence for this is based firstly on the observation that cell-mediated immunity to an antigen is associated with the presence of detectable numbers of recirculating T lymphocytes capable of binding the antigen. Secondly, as already explained, infusion of T lymphocytes will restore cell-mediated immune responsiveness to a T-depleted animal, or to one which has been rendered specifically unresponsive (immunologically tolerant) to a particular antigen. If the T lymphocytes are first exposed *in vitro* to the antigen in insoluble form, some of them adhere to it and may thus be separated from the rest. These adherent cells, which bind specifically to the antigen, have been shown to be responsible for restoring the deficient animal.

The nature of the specific antigen receptors on the surface of T lymphocytes is controversial. Immunoglobulin is not readily demonstrable on the surface of most T lymphocytes, and treatment with antibodies to immunoglobulins does not prevent them from binding antigen. This suggests that the receptors are none of the known classes of Ig, but there are conflicting reports, and it is difficult to visualise specific antigen receptors which are not composed of amino-acid chains. Accordingly, we think they are most likely to consist of the variable parts of the Ig chains, which carry antibody specificity but are not detectable by anti-Ig. Very recently, strong evidence has been produced that the T-lymphocyte receptors are monomeric IgM (as in B lymphocytes), and that the μ chain is buried in the plasma membrane.

The mechanism by which union of antigen with surface receptors stimulates T lymphocytes to enlarge and divide appears to involve the linking of adjacent surface receptors by the antigen molecule. This is supported by the observation that IgG antibody to T lymphocytes, which is, of course, divalent, can stimulate them to proliferate, whereas the univalent Fab fragment of such antibody can react with surface components of the lymphocyte, but is without stimulating effect. The necessity for linkage of antigen receptors would explain why, in general, large molecules with many antigenic determinant sites are strong antigens, whereas single antigenic determinants (i.e. haptens) can only stimulate an immune response if conjugated with protein carriers.

B lymphocytes and antibody production

In birds and some mammals, neonatal thymectomy prevents the formation of the T-lymphocyte population, with consequent deficiency of cell-mediated immune responses; but other lymphocytes appear, and the thymectomised animals have normal serum immunoglobulin levels, and can produce antibodies to some antigens. In birds there is a second primary lymphoid organ, the *bursa of Fabricius*, in the wall of the hind gut, and removal of this at hatching has been found to prevent the appearance of thymus-independent lymphocytes, plasma cells and immunoglobulins. Bursectomised birds can develop cell-mediated immune responses, but cannot produce any antibodies. The bursa of Fabricius is thus essential for the production of a population of non-thymic, or B (for bursa) lymphocytes. In mammals, there is no single organ equivalent to the bursa, and the site of development of B lymphocytes is probably in the secondary lymphoid organs (p. 98) or the haemopoietic marrow.

There is considerable experimental evidence that B lymphocytes are the precursors of plasma cells, and thus responsible for antibody production. For example, the lymphoid cells of mice may be destroyed by total body x-irradiation and the mice then injected with suspensions of B cells and/or thymocytes which can be recognised in the host by chromosomal markers or histocompatibility antigens: the capacity to produce antibodies is restored by B cells, but not by thymocytes, and the antibody-producing plasma cells are derived from the donated B cells. If, in such experiments, the animals are thymectomised before lethal x-irradiation, and then injected with bone marrow cells to restore haemopoiesis, they develop a population of B lymphocytes (from lymphoid stem cells in the haemopoietic tissue) and have been used as 'B' (i.e. T-cell deficient) mice in long-term investigations: they demonstrate well the B cell function of antibody production, but lack cell-mediated immune responses.

The distribution of B lymphocytes in the lymphoid tissues has been deduced from study of animals rendered T-cell deficient (see above) and of humans and animals with congenital T or B cell deficiencies. More recently, it has become possible to recognise and distinguish between T and B cells by their surface characteristics and their distribution has been studied in normal individuals. In the lymph nodes, spleen and gut-associated tissues, B cells are most numerous in and around the lymphoid nodules (follicles): thus in the lymph nodes they populate the superficial cortex, and in the spleen the peripheral part of the Malpighian bodies (white pulp). During antibody responses, B cell proliferation occurs in these areas, with formation of large basophilic cells (**B immunoblasts**), and the subsequent appearance of plasma cells which accumulate in the lymphoid medullary sinuses (Fig. 4.10, p. 93) and in the sinuses of the red pulp of the spleen.

The kinetics of the B lymphocyte population are still obscure. They tend to be more sessile than T cells, i.e. to remain in the lymphoid tissues, but some recirculation does occur, and about 9–14% of human peripheral-blood small lymphocytes are B cells. They also appear to be long-lived (like T cells) unless stimulated by antigens to divide. If an antigenic stimulus is brief, the plasma-cell response is transient, and they are believed to be end-stage cells with a short lifespan.

The reaction of B lymphocytes with antigens. As will be indicated below, techniques are now available for distinguishing between and separating T and B lymphocytes. Use of these, and various manipulations outlined above (e.g. the elimination of T cells in animals) have allowed the effects of antigen on B and T cells to be studied in detail. When B cells are incubated with an antigen, a small proportion of the cells bind the antigen to their surface. By separation techniques similar to those described for antigen-binding T lymphocytes (p. 100), it has been shown that B lymphocytes which bind a particular antigen are stimulated by it to proliferate and produce clones of cells. Some of the cells produced have the morphology of small lymphocytes, and persist as B memory cells. Thus the numbers of B lymphocytes in the blood or lymphoid tissues which can bind the antigen is increased, and if the same antigen is administered a second time, this increase accounts for the rapid and enhanced antibody production of the secondary response. Not all the cells produced by antigenic stimulation of B cells become memory cells: many of them differentiate into plasma cells which synthesise and secrete the appropriate antibody (Fig.

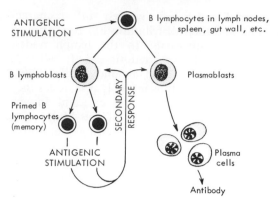

Fig. 4.17 The effects of antigenic stimulation on B lymphocytes.

4.17). This differentiation is evident at the stage of dividing plasmablasts, which differ from T immunoblasts in possessing the rough endoplasmic reticulum characteristic of secretory cells. Presumably the lymphoblast precursors of B memory cells more closely resemble T immunoblasts, but this is uncertain.

It is not known with certainty what factors decide whether the antigen-stimulated B cell clones develop into memory or plasma cells. It may be that recently-divided cells develop into plasma cells, for experiments with labelled cells indicate that plasma cells develop from cells which have divided shortly before antigenic stimulation. The co-operative role of T cells in antibody production (see below) may also be important in this respect.

A characteristic feature of B lymphocytes is the presence of immunoglobulin molecules projecting from their plasma membrane (Fig.

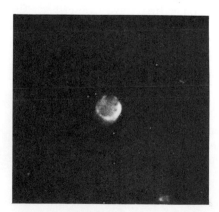

Fig. 4.18 Demonstration of Ig on the surface of human B lymphocyte. The cell has been treated with a rabbit anti-human Ig serum, followed by fluorescein-conjugated anti-rabbit Ig.

4.18). This is predominantly, but not entirely, monomeric IgM (i.e. single molecules with 2 light and 2 heavy μ chains). In the human neonate, the surface Ig of B lymphocytes is predominantly IgD. The Fab parts of the surface Ig molecules project from the surface, and are the specific antigen-receptors. This has been shown by blocking the binding of antigen by treating the cells with anti-Ig, and it has also been observed by the immunofluorescence technique that when B lymphocytes are incubated at 37 °C with an antigen, the binding of antigen leads to aggregation of the surface Ig at one part of the cell surface (**capping**) and finally to its pinocytosis by the cell. On further incubation, the surface Ig is regenerated.

B lymphocytes thus insert into their plasma membrane samples of the antibody which they can synthesise: like T cells, they advertise their wares, and binding of the antigen can stimulate their proliferation to provide more lymphocytes and plasma cells capable of synthesising the same antibody.

It is not known how the binding of antigen stimulates B lymphocytes to proliferate. Linkage of the surface receptors appears to be important, the evidence being similar to that for T lymphocytes (p. 100), and in the case of B cells linkage of the surface Ig by anti-Ig (as by antigen) is stimulating *in vitro*, while binding of the Fab fragment of anti-Ig, which does not link the receptors, is not.

Co-operation of T cells in antibody production

As already stated, T cells are not without effect on antibody production, the primary and secondary responses to most antigens being impaired in T-cell deficient animals. The crucial experiment was carried out by Claman, who showed that antibody responses in mice exposed to x-irradiation were restored much more effectively by injection of both T and B cells than by larger numbers of either T or B cells alone. Without T-cell co-operation, B cells can produce good antibody responses to relatively few antigens, and these are usually of large molecular size with numerous determinant sites, such as might be expected to produce cross-linking of the B-cell surface receptors.

Mitchison and others have shown that antibody response to a hapten coupled to a protein carrier is dependent on cell-mediated immunity to the carrier, i.e. on the presence of a sufficient number of T cells which bind to the carrier molecule. This shows that B cells binding to an antigenic determinant are stimulated by the binding of T cells to a different type of determinant on the same antigen molecule. By aggregating the hapten–carrier molecules on their surface, T cells may present the hapten in a form which stimulates B cells by cross-linking their surface Ig receptors (Fig. 4.19b). There is, however, evidence that T cells which have bound antigen or which have been transformed to immunoblasts by phytohaemag-glutinin (p. 142), can stimulate proliferation of B cells which have bound a second, unrelated antigen (Fig. 4.19c). This 'second stimulus' for B cells is not antigen-specific, for the T and B cells have not bound the same antigen.

To some extent, bacterial endotoxin can take the place of T cells in stimulating B cells to proliferate and produce antibody, but T cells also appear to play some part in the switch-over of B cells from IgM to IgG antibody production.

The roles of T and B cells in immune responses are summarised in Fig. 4.20.

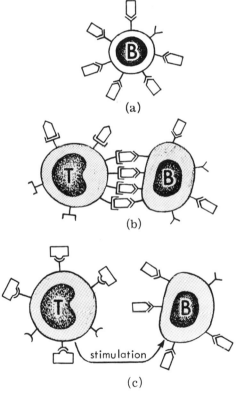

Fig. 4.19 Possible mechanisms of co-operation of T cells in antibody production by B cells. In **a**, a B lymphocyte has bound an antigen by a particular type of determinant, but is not stimulated by it. If a T cell also binds the same antigen by a different determinant, as in **b**, it may effectively cross-link the specific receptors of the B lymphocyte, and thus stimulate it (indicated here by blast transformation of the B cell). However, a T cell which has bound an independent antigen, as in **c**, can also provide a stimulus to the B lymphocyte. In both these forms of co-operation, the stimulating T cell has itself been stimulated to blast transformation, and indeed the second form of co-operation can be provided by a T cell which has been stimulated non-specifically, e.g. by phytohaemagglutinin.

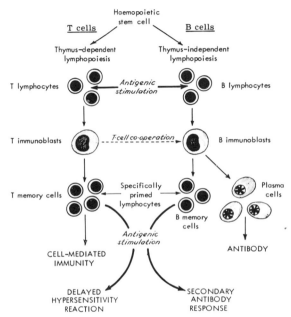

Fig. 4.20 The main cellular events underlying the immune response. T lymphocytes (*left*) are stimulated by antigens to proliferate, producing clones of specifically-primed T lymphocytes, which are responsible for cell-mediated immunity and act as T memory cells. On encountering the antigen, they bring about a delayed hypersensitivity reaction. B lymphocytes (*right*) are stimulated by antigens to produce clones of plasma cells which secrete antibody, and also specifically-primed B lymphocytes (B memory cells) which, on encountering the antigen, produce clones of plasma cells and thus account for the secondary antibody response. Stimulated T cells (T immunoblasts) co-operate with B cells in antibody responses to many antigens.

Lymphoid stem cells

When animals are subjected to a lethal dose of whole-body x-irradiation, death may be prevented by administration of histocompatible bone marrow cells. By use of chromosomal markers to identify cells of donor origin, it has been shown that replenishment of haemopoietic cells in the marrow, thymocytes in the thymus, and T and B lymphocytes in the other lymphoid tissues and the blood, are all of donor origin. There is evidence that the stem cells in the haemopoietic marrow are pluripotential, and capable of differentiating into any of the cell lines required for this repopulation, and that the line taken by any particular stem cell is determined by the micro-environment of the tissue in which it settles (p. 450). Stem cells normally pass from the marrow to the thymus, and possibly to other-lympoid tissues, *via* the blood, and thus maintain a supply of cells for lymphopoiesis.

What determines lymphocyte specificity?

There is now overwhelmingly strong evidence that each functionally mature T or B lymphocyte can respond specifically (i.e. is 'committed' to respond) to only a narrow range of antigenic determinants, and that this restricted responsiveness is passed on to the cell's progeny when it proliferates in response to the appropriate antigenic stimulation. Several indications of such restriction or commitment have been given in the preceding pages. For example, when a suspension of lymphocytes is exposed to an insoluble antigen, only those T and B cells which bind the antigen are capable of mounting an immune response to it. Secondly, when B lymphocytes are incubated with a soluble antigen, the surface Ig of those which bind it is all removed by capping and pinocytosis (indicating that all the Ig consists of receptors of the same specificity). Thirdly, a single plasma cell in culture has been shown to secrete only antibody of a single specificity. Perhaps the strongest evidence is derived from the homogeneous nature of the Ig secreted by myeloma cells. These are plasma cells produced by neoplastic proliferation of a single precursor cell, and the fact that, in each case, all the Ig molecules produced by the tumour clone are identical in the amino-acid sequences in the variable regions of their light and heavy chains indicates that the cell of origin was committed to production of this particular immunoglobulin and no other.

The mechanism of such commitment is not fully understood. It was formerly assumed that it was brought about by encounter between lymphocyte and antigen and that the specific responsiveness of the lymphocyte was determined by the particular antigen first encountered by it (the **instructive theory**), but there are many serious objections to this, and the **clonal selection theory of Burnet** has now been widely accepted. This postulates that the specificity of lymphocyte responsiveness is not determined by encounter with antigen, but by the development, from fetal life onwards, of diversity among lymphocytes, so that each one is programmed to bind, and respond to, a restricted range of antigens (Fig. 4.21). This theory was

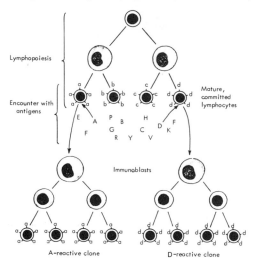

Fig. 4.21 The clonal selection theory of immune response. During lymphopoiesis, each developing T or B cell becomes committed to respond to a narrow range of antigenic determinants: this is reflected by the specificity of the antigen receptors (a, b, c, etc.) on its surface. For example, lymphocytes with hypothetical 'a' receptors can bind an antigen 'A', but not 'B' or 'C', etc. Binding of an antigen stimulates a lymphocyte to proliferate, producing a clone of lymphocytes with identical commitments.

virtually proved by the demonstration that the specific reactivity of antibodies depended on the sequence of amino acids in the variable regions of their heavy and light chains (p. 88), which can only be due to the selection of genes coding for particular sequences. Similarly, it is postulated that each T lymphocyte selects genes coding for the specificity of its surface antigen-receptors (? the variable regions of light and heavy Ig chains—p. 100).

Burnet originally proposed that the diversity of DNA coding for the variable regions of Ig molecules in different cells is due to a high frequency of somatic mutation in the 'variable' components of Ig genes, but recent evidence suggests that every cell in the body contains something like 1000 genes, each coding for a particular sequence of amino acids in the variable part of heavy chains (VH genes) and a similar number coding for the variable parts of light chains (VL genes). Random expression of one VH and one VL gene by each developing lymphocyte would provide about 10^6 different specificities, and thus explain the normal individual's diversity of responsiveness to antigens. It is now believed that such gene expression is brought about by the mechanism illustrated for heavy chain synthesis in Fig. 4.22. By formation and exclusion of loops in

etc), and switching from production of, say, IgM to IgG (as individual plasma cells can do) is probably determined by looping and exclusion of $C\mu$, so that the selected VH gene is now linked to $C\gamma$, and the two operate as a single gene. The same loop mechanism would explain the determination of the amino-acid sequences in the variable part of the light chains, and commitment of T lymphocytes could be similarly explained, except that the T-cell equivalent of the constant parts of the Ig chains has not yet been identified with certainty.

The theory of random selection of genes coding for the parts of Ig which form the specific antigen receptors explains not only the specificity of immune responses, but also the diversity of the antibody produced, even in response to a simple antigen with only one type of determin-

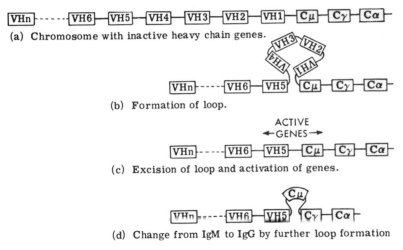

(a) Chromosome with inactive heavy chain genes.

(b) Formation of loop.

(c) Excision of loop and activation of genes.

(d) Change from IgM to IgG by further loop formation

Fig. 4.22 Model of chromosome with genes for the variable region (VH1, VH2 ... VH*n*) and constant region ($C\mu$, $C\gamma$, $C\alpha$) of heavy chains, showing selection of a single VH gene by formation and removal of a DNA loop. In this example, the cell becomes committed to synthesis of heavy chains with a variable region containing the amino-acid sequence determined by VH5. At first IgM is synthesised, but removal of a loop containing $C\mu$ leads to subsequent synthesis of IgG with the same specificity (determined by VH5). A similar mechanism may operate independently for light chains.

the DNA sequences coding for the variable part of the heavy chain, one VH gene is brought into apposition with the gene coding for the constant part ($C\mu$, etc) of the chain. Once this has occurred, the sequence of amino acids in the variable part of the heavy chain of Ig produced by that cell, and its progeny, is irrevocably decided.

Each cell also possesses a gene for the constant part of each class of heavy chain (μ, γ, a,

ant site. The antigen stimulates all those B lymphocytes whose specific surface receptors can bind it sufficiently firmly, and each of these cells gives rise to a clone of plasma cells producing its own distinctive antibody molecules. The result is a mixture of diverse antibodies, some of which can bind the antigen more firmly than others, but the total effect of which is exquisite specificity. If the antigen is administered repeatedly in small doses, it is taken up mainly by those lymphocytes which can bind it most firmly, and as these proliferate, the result predicted would be a progressive increase in the avidity (p. 88) of the antibody, which is indeed what happens.

Control of the immune response

To be effective, the immunity system must be capable of responding, both simultaneously and sequentially, to large numbers of independent antigens. This is achieved very largely by the early commitment of lymphocytes discussed above, for any particular antigenic determinant can stimulate only the small proportion of T or B lymphocytes which are committed to produce antigen receptors capable of binding it, and the remainder are available for responses to other antigens. However, it has been calculated that a stimulated lymphocyte can produce a clone of 10^6 cells, and a plasma cell can produce at least 7×10^6 antibody molecules per hour, and since, as indicated above, an antigen stimulates many different lymphocytes, further controls on the immune response are clearly necessary.

One form of control is exerted by antibody itself. This is illustrated by the prevention of immunisation of Rhesus negative women by the Rhesus antigens of fetal red cells: during labour, some fetal red cells enter the mother's circulation, but development of antibodies can usually be prevented by an injection of IgG Rhesus antibody. The suppressive effect may be partly due to antibody reacting with antigen and thus rendering it non-immunogenic, but this does not appear to be the whole explanation, for in transplantation studies it has been shown that administration of antibody to antigens of the grafted tissue can inhibit the development of an immune response by the host and thus prevent rejection. In this phenomenon, which has been termed **enhancement**, both cell-mediated immunity and antibody production are suppressed by administration of antibody.

While T cells assist in the antibody response to most antigens, they have a suppressing effect on some antibody responses. This is seen in the exaggerated antibody responses of T-cell deficient animals to 'thymus-independent' antigens. In man, the very high antibody titres in patients with lepromatous leprosy, who lack cell-mediated immunity to the antigens of *M. leprae*, may result from failure of T-cell control of antibody production.

Transfer factor

Since 1948, Lawrence has reported investigations which suggest that cell-free extracts of human leukocytes can transfer cell-mediated immunity to non-immunised recipients. In his earlier work, he claimed that incubation of the leukocytes of an immune individual with the appropriate antigen led to release of specific transfer factor. For example, addition of tuberculoprotein to leukocytes from an immunised individual released into the medium a transfer factor which, when injected into a non-immune individual, conferred on him cell-mediated immunity within 12 hours, as indicated by a positive delayed hypersensitivity test: such 'passive' immunity persisted for over a year. These findings were not received with great enthusiasm, firstly because attempts to repeat them in guinea-pigs were unsuccessful, transfer of living cells being required to confer passively cell-mediated immunity. Secondly, Lawrence reported that his transfer factor passed through a dialysis membrane and had a molecular weight of about 3000: this seemed a very small molecule for a factor conferring antigen-specific immunity. In spite of scepticism, Lawrence has extended this work to transfer of specific cell-mediated immunity to fungi, bacteria and allogeneic skin grafts, and other workers have reported confirmatory findings. It now appears that, in addition to the transfer of specific cell-mediated immunity outlined above, extracts of leukocytes disrupted by freezing and thawing (in the absence of antigens) contain 'non-specific transfer factor', which may consist of a mixture of specific transfer factors, but appears to have the effect of non-specifically boosting the recipient's cell-mediated immunity responses.

It is perhaps not surprising that investigations on man, whose cell-mediated immune responsiveness is much greater than that of non-primates, should reveal immunological phenomena not readily detectable in guinea-pigs or mice.

Recently, a number of reports have appeared on the therapeutic use of transfer factor in the treatment of patients with resistant infections due to immunodeficiencies, and with various diseases of obscure causation (e.g. sarcoidosis, disseminated sclerosis, connective tissue diseases and neoplasia). The degree of success achieved has varied greatly, and it is too early to draw conclusions. The existence of human transfer factor is no longer in doubt, although its mode of action is obscure and its antigen-specificity controversial.

Identification of T and B lymphocytes

B lymphocytes may be identified by demonstration, for example by immunofluorescence, of their surface Ig (Fig. 4.18). T lymphocytes do not have readily demonstrable surface Ig, but human T lymphocytes, including thymocytes, have receptors for sheep erythrocytes, and are capable of binding them at 0 °C to form rosettes (Fig. 4.23). In our experience these two

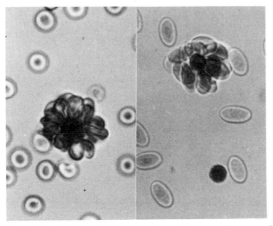

Fig. 4.23 *Left*, a T lymphocyte binding sheep red cells to form a rosette. *Right*, a B lymphocyte binding chicken red cells sensitised with IgG antibody to form a rosette: note also the T lymphocyte, which has not bound the chicken erythrocytes.

tests indicate that approximately 14% of the lymphocytes in the blood are B cells and 70% are T cells. By first removing sialic acid residues from the surface of the sheep erythrocytes by treatment with the enzyme neuraminidase, the proportion of lymphocytes forming rosettes is increased to about 85%, suggesting that the 16% or so of 'null' cells, which have neither surface Ig nor form rosettes with untreated sheep erythrocytes, are T cells.

The detection of surface receptors for the Fc part of IgG has also been used in the identification of lymphocytes. When IgG antibody is allowed to react with antigen, its Fc part is altered in such a way that it can be bound by surface Fc receptors of some lymphocytes (Fig. 4.23). In our experience, approximately 28% of human blood lymphocytes possess Fc receptors, and about half of these are B lymphocytes; we have produced evidence that most of the remainder are 'K' lymphocytes (perhaps a third type of lymphocyte), which are capable of killing target cells sensitised with IgG antibody (p. 123). There is, however, evidence that some stimulated T cells also have Fc receptors. Some B cells also have receptors for the C3b component of activated complement, as indicated by rosette formation with red cells sensitised with IgM antibody and the early components of complement (*immune adherence*). Other cells, for example monocytes and macrophages, also have receptors for C3b, and also for the Fc of IgG.

These techniques and also the response to mitogens (p. 142) and tests involving the use of antisera to T and B cells are now being applied to analyse lymphocyte populations and classify lymphoid neoplasms (p. 519 *et seq.*).

Acquired immunological tolerance

In certain circumstances, administration of antigen does not result in an immune response, but in an unresponsive state in which the recipient is incapable of developing antibody or cell-mediated immunity to that antigen. This is termed acquired immunological tolerance and is antigen-specific, i.e. the unresponsiveness applies to the antigen which has induced it and not to other, unrelated antigens. Acquired tolerance can be abolished by injecting responsive lymphocytes from a normal (non-tolerant) animal of the same inbred strain, indicating that the condition is due to failure of lymphocyte responsiveness, and not to an alteration in the metabolic processing of antigen before it reaches the lymphocytes.

Immunological tolerance is most readily induced in fetal and neonatal animals and lasts only so long as the antigen remains present in the tolerant animal. To give an example, if a neonatal mouse of a hypothetical inbred strain A is injected with living cells of a hybrid, A x B mouse, it becomes tolerant to the histocompatibility antigens of strain B, and will fail to reject grafts of B skin. If, however, it is then injected with lymphocytes from a normal A mouse, it will reject the graft. Tolerance may also be induced to a non-living antigen, e.g. bovine serum albumin (BSA) by injecting it into a neonatal animal, but will persist only until the BSA has been catabolised, and its maintenance requires repeated injections of BSA.

It has been shown by Mitchison that repeated injections of BSA in either very low or very high dosage will induce tolerance in adult mice, and the explanation is that tolerance is readily induced in T lymphocytes, very low doses of antigen being sufficient, while B-lymphocyte tolerance is more difficult to induce and requires much larger amounts of antigen. It follows that 'high dosage' tolerance suppresses both cell-mediated immunity and antibody responses. If the antigen is one for which antibody production requires T-cell co-operation (p. 102), low dosage tolerance prevents both types of immune response, but if it can stimulate a B cell response without the need of T-cell co-operation, there will be antibody production with suppression of cell-mediated immunity, sometimes termed **split tolerance** or **immune deviation**.

The fact that maintenance of tolerance requires continual presence of the antigen suggests that, as maturing lymphocytes become committed (p. 104), they pass through a stage at which encounter with antigen promotes non-responsiveness: if antigen is continuously present, it will 'catch' potentially responsive lymphocytes at this stage and tolerance will persist. Mature lymphocytes are more likely to mount an immune response on encountering the antigen. The corollary is that widely-spaced pulses of antigen should favour an immune response, as indeed they do.

In fact, the situation is more complex than stated above, for any particular antigenic determinant will be bound by many lymphocytes with different specific receptors (p. 104). Some of these cells will have receptors which make a 'good fit' with the antigen and bind it firmly; others will bind it less well because it fits their receptors poorly. These factors will influence not only the amount of antibody

produced, but also its avidity. A concentration of antigen which induces non-responsiveness of strongly-binding cells may stimulate an immune response in those binding the antigen less firmly, with consequent production of a relatively small amount of antibody of poor avidity. The same considerations apply to T lymphocytes, and accordingly tolerance is not an all-or-nothing phenomenon. An antigenic stimulus is likely, in fact, to induce tolerance in some potentially responsive lymphocytes and an immune response in others.

Well-established tolerance to an antigen can sometimes be broken down by administration of a closely related, cross-reacting antigen or by giving the antigen incorporated in Freund's adjuvant. Although tolerance has been widely assumed to result from elimination or suppression of lymphocytes specifically responsive to the tolerance-inducing antigen, there is now evidence that transfer of T cells from a tolerant animal can confer tolerance to the antigen on a normal recipient. This suggests that T cells play an active suppressive role in the tolerant state.

The induction of immunological tolerance to auto-antigens during fetal life is now believed to explain 'horror autotoxicus', i.e. the physiological reluctance of the individual to develop immune responses to self-constituents of his own cells and their products.

The induction of tolerance, particularly in adults, is facilitated by giving immunosuppressive agents together with the antigen. This is probably of importance in clinical renal transplantation, in which the dosage of immunosuppressive drugs can be gradually reduced without rejection of the kidney. Some form of tolerance develops towards the alloantigens of the transplant: this may either be 'classical' tolerance, as described above, or it may be due to production of 'blocking' or 'enhancing' antibody, which suppresses further immune responses, including cell-mediated immunity, to the transplant antigens (p. 106).

Macrophages and the immune response

In attempting to avoid introducing too many of the complexities of the immune response in rapid succession, this account may have given the impression that specifically responsive lymphocytes and the appropriate antigen are the sole ingredients of the immune response. This is an over-simplification, for it has been shown that pure suspensions of lymphocytes respond poorly to most antigens, and that the response is greatly augmented by addition of macrophages. This applies especially to cell-mediated immune responses and to antibody responses which are strongly dependent on T-cell help.

The importance of macrophages in immune responses *in vivo* is suggested by the enhancing effects of Freund's and other adjuvants (p. 94) which stimulate accumulation of macrophages. Use of such adjuvants enhances especially T-cell responses. Also injection of macrophages pre-incubated with the antigen provides a very potent immunogenic stimulus.

The mechanism of macrophage participation in the immune response is not known. It has been shown, however, that while most of the antigen taken up by macrophages is digested and destroyed, some immunogenic material does persist for a long time at the cell surface: this appears to consist of a fraction of the antigen complexed with RNA, and was shown by Askonas to be many times more potent than the original antigen in stimulating an immune response.

The rôle of the dendritic cells in the cortical follicles of lymphoid tissues is considered on p. 112.

Histological features of the immune response

The cellular events of immune responses take place mainly in the secondary lymphoid organs, i.e. the lymph nodes, white pulp of the spleen, tonsils and gut-associated lymphoid tissues. Study of the morphological changes of immune responses is not easy, for the large number of micro-organisms in the alimentary and upper respiratory tracts, and on the exposed mucous membranes, provide continual antigenic stimuli which ensure that the immunity system is never completely at rest. The maintenance of animals in a germ-free environment from birth onwards is helpful, but technically exacting, and does not ensure complete freedom from antigenic stimulation: thus 'germ-free' mice are likely to be infected with mouse leukaemia virus, and do, in fact, show evidence of immune responses in their lymphoid tissues. There is also great regional variation in lymph node responses: when the antigenic stimulus is localised, e.g. in vaccination, the draining lymph nodes usually show the greatest response, but there may be great variations, even between adjacent nodes.

Study of the lymphoid tissues in animals rendered deficient of T cells by neonatal thymectomy, anti-lymphocyte serum or thoracic duct drainage, of fowls rendered B-cell deficient by bursectomy, and in patients with major congenital immunodeficiencies has helped to distinguish between the histological features of the T cell-mediated immune response and those of the antibody (B cell) response.

The thymus

Development. The thymus develops as a paired organ from epithelial ingrowths, probably of endodermal origin, of the 3rd and 4th branchial arches. During fetal development, the two lobes pass medially and caudally to form a single organ. Although initially composed of epithelium, at an early stage of development the thymus becomes converted to a predominantly lymphoid tissue and differentiates further into a lobulated structure in which each lobule has a central core of medullary tissue with finger-like projections, capped by cortical tissue. Both cortex and medulla consist predominantly of small lymphocytes, but their ratio to other cells is far higher in the cortex, and they are much more closely packed there, than in the medulla (Fig. 4.24). The other cells in the thymus include epithelial cells, which are scattered singly as large plump cells in both cortex and medulla, and also macrophages, distinguishable from the epithelial cells only by electron microscopy. The medulla also contains the collections of squamous epithelial cells known as Hassall's corpuscles, which often show central degeneration and cystic change.

Immune responses. As already indicated, the thymus is a site of T lymphopoiesis. It is not an important site of immune responses, but occasional germinal centres and plasma cells are demonstrable in the medulla of the thymus in a

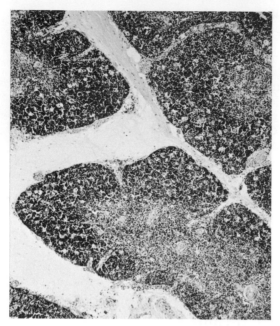

Fig. 4.24   Thymus of child, showing lobulation and division into cortex (darker areas) and medulla. × 50.

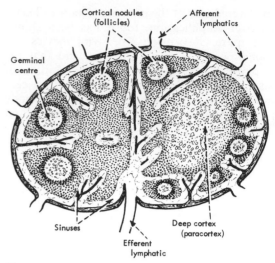

Fig. 4.25   Diagram of a lymph node, portraying the superficial cortex with nodules and germinal centres, and on the right an ill-defined area of deep cortex.

significant percentage of people killed by trauma or dying suddenly or after a short illness, and this suggests that B lymphocytes, presumably entering it from the blood, are capable of mounting an antibody response. Thymic germinal centres are rarely seen in patients dying after a chronic illness, perhaps because there has been increased secretion of adrenal glucocorticoids, which results in thymic and lymphoid atrophy. Thymic germinal centres are, however, numerous in many cases of myasthenia gravis, and occur also in the connective tissue diseases.

Lymph nodes

Normal structure (Fig. 4.25). The lymph node consists of cortex, medulla and lymph sinuses. The cortex occupies the superficial part of the node except at the hilar region: the medulla lies centrally, but extends to the hilium. The framework of the node consists of a network of fine reticulin fibrils which are covered by the cytoplasm of elongated, flat reticulum cells with branching cytoplasmic processes. The mesh of the reticular spaces is 15–30 μm in diam. in the cortex and 5–10 μm in the medulla. The sinuses

are simply channels in the reticular framework, and they also are lined and traversed by reticulum cells. Most of the free cells in the node are lymphocytes, and small lymphocytes usually predominate. In the cortex, the lymphocytes are closely arranged, and in *the superficial part of the cortex* there are foci, termed *primary nodules*, in which lymphocytes are more closely packed. In a stimulated node, as described below, a focus of lymphopoiesis, termed a *germinal centre*, may develop within the primary nodules: nodules in this state are sometimes referred to as secondary, but it now seems inappropriate to use the terms primary and secondary in this context. The *deeper cortex*, sometimes termed the *paracortex*, consists of ill-defined uniform areas of cortical tissue lying between the superficial cortex and medulla (Fig. 4.26): in the stimulated node, there may be intense proliferation of lymphoid cells here, and this may result in one or more large nodules of tissue which compress the medulla of the node.

Lymph arriving at the node by the afferent lymphatics enters the peripheral sinus which surrounds the lymphoid tissue of the node and communicates at the hilum with the efferent lymphatic. From the peripheral sinus, cortical sinuses pass radially inwards to the medulla, running between the superficial cortical nodules and penetrating the deep cortex. In the medulla, the lymph sinuses are numerous, and the lymphoid tissue lies between them as the *medullary*

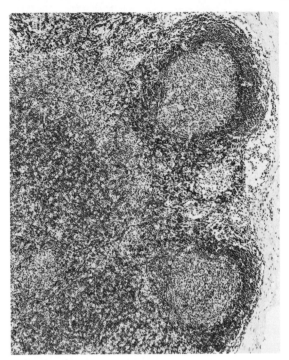

Fig. 4.26 Part of the cortex of a lymph node, showing two large cortical nodules (follicles) with germinal centres. The ill-defined area to the left of these consists of deep cortex. × 40.

cords: the medullary sinuses unite to form the efferent lymphatic.

The lymph nodes have two major functions. One of these is the interception and removal of abnormal or foreign material in the lymph stream passing to them, and is described on pp. 513, 516: the other is the production of immune responses, the histological features of which are described below.

Immune responses in lymph nodes

(a) Cell-mediated immune responses. In lymph nodes draining the site of an antigenic stimulus of a kind which induces this type of response, e.g. an allogeneic skin graft or application to the skin of the hapten dinitrochlorobenzene, the most conspicuous early change is the appearance of large basophilic (and pyroninophilic) lymphoid cells (**immunoblasts**) in the deep cortex of the node. These cells appear two days or so after antigenic stimulation; they multiply rapidly and are maximal at about 5 days. Small lymphocytes also increase in number in the deep cortex, which becomes enlarged and conspicuous, causing appreciable increase in size of the node. If the antigenic stimulation is not prolonged, the immunoblasts disappear after a further few days, the main feature then being an increased number of small lymphocytes in the deep cortex.

As explained on p. 97, the deep cortex is in the pathway of the recirculating T lymphocytes, which are responsible for cell-mediated immune responses, and the appearance of immunoblasts and subsequently small lymphocytes in the deep cortex represents the clonal proliferation of specifically responsive T cells following antigenic stimulation. The responsive cells may have encountered antigen in the tissues and passed to the lymph nodes, or antigenic material, either free or carried by macrophages, may have reached the draining nodes and there stimulated appropriately responsive cells among the recirculating lymphocytes passing through the deep cortex. Only a very small proportion of T cells in the recirculating lymphocyte pool could be specifically responsive to an antigen not encountered previously, and recirculation of small lymphocytes can be seen as a phenomenon providing opportunity for very large numbers of specifically responsive cells to 'inspect' an antigen. The use of tritiated-thymidine labelling has shown that the immunoblasts in the deep cortex proliferate to produce small lymphocytes, and that these appear in the recirculating lymphocyte pool at about the time of development of cell-mediated immunity: recirculation will allow such 'primed' cells to encounter, and react with, the corresponding antigen almost anywhere in the body, a factor of obvious importance in combating infections.

It is not established that *all* the large pyroninophilic lymphocytes which appear in the deep cortex of a node during a cell-mediated immune response are cells which are specifically responsive to the particular antigens. It may be that the responding lymphocytes release a lymphokine which stimulates mitosis in other lymphocytes which are not specifically responsive to that antigen (p. 130).

(b) Antibody production involves the proliferation of B lymphocytes to provide B memory cells and the plasma cells which synthesise and secrete antibody. The main site of cell proliferation observed during antibody responses is in the superficial cortical nodules, which develop

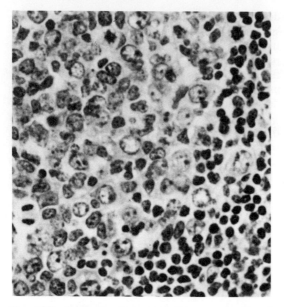

Fig. 4.27 Segment of a germinal centre, showing the appearances of the cells, some of which are dividing. Note the surrounding tightly-packed small lymphocytes. × 850.

large spherical or ovoid germinal centres (Fig. 4.27), consisting of actively dividing, large basophilic blast cells. These are generally believed to be the responding B cells. Plasma cells appear in increasing numbers deep to the germinal centres and in the medullary cords, which are the main site of antibody production. During the early stages of the primary response neither antigen nor immunoglobulins are readily demonstrable in the cells of the germinal centres but, as antibody appears, antigen–antibody complexes become bound to the surface of the large dendritic cells of the germinal centres, and may persist there for many weeks. The nature of the dendritic cells, and the role of their surface complexes in antibody production, are not known; it is tempting to assume that the complexes provide a persistent antigenic stimulus to B cells, with consequent development of plasma cells which pass to the medulla and produce antibody. But this lacks proof, and the complexes could equally represent a homoeostatic mechanism limiting the antibody response. Small numbers of macrophages are also present in the germinal centres and contain ingested pyknotic nuclear material, the significance of which is unknown.

Although the function of the germinal centres is still uncertain, there is no doubt that they are associated with antibody responses, and their presence in individuals with severe T-cell deficiencies indicates that they are not dependent on normal T-cell function. The intensity of mitotic activity in the germinal centres during antibody responses suggests that they are the major site of clonal proliferation of specifically responsive B cells.

During antibody responses, which are often most pronounced in the lymph nodes draining the site of antigen, B immunoblasts leave the node in the efferent lymphatic, and are distributed by the blood to other lymph nodes, etc., to the haemopoietic marrow, the lamina propria of the gut, and to the inflammatory reaction which may develop if antigen persists at the site of its introduction in the tissues (see below). Presumably these migrant cells give rise to both plasma cells and B memory cells.

Although the histological features of cell-mediated immune responses and antibody production are described above separately, it must be emphasised that many antigenic stimuli induce both responses, and indeed the enhancement of many antibody responses by T immunoblasts requires the combined form of response, although the site of T-cell cooperation in the lymphoid tissues is not known.

Immune responses in other lymphoid tissues

Spleen. The structure of the spleen is described briefly on p. 506. Immune responses take place in the white pulp (Malpighian bodies) of the organ, and have been studied in chickens rendered deficient in T or B cells by thymectomy or bursectomy respectively (p. 101). It appears from such investigations, and also from observations in rodents, that the area immediately adjacent to the central arteriole is occupied by T lymphocytes of the recirculating pool, and corresponds to the deep cortex of lymph nodes, while the more peripheral lymphoid tissue corresponds to the superficial cortex of lymph nodes and is the site of formation of germinal centres during antibody production. Antibody-producing plasma cells appear at the periphery of the Malpighian bodies and pass into the adjacent red pulp.

Immune responses in the spleen occur particularly when antigenic material gains entrance to the blood stream, and present morphological appearances similar to those which have been described for the lymph nodes.

Gut-associated lymphoid tissues. The solitary lymphoid follicles and Peyer's patches of the gastro-intestinal tract resemble the lymph nodes and spleen in being sites of cell–mediated immune and antibody responses, and they contain areas corresponding to the superficial and deep cortex of lymph nodes, and also lymph sinuses.

Immune responses in non-lymphoid tissues

When antigenic material persists in the body, e.g. in chronic infections, tissue allografts, and antigen injected in relatively insoluble form, immune responses may occur in the inflammatory lesion which develops around the antigen. T immunoblasts resembling those developing in the deep cortex of the lymph nodes may be observed, and may participate in both the immune response and in a delayed hypersensitivity reaction with the antigenic material. Plasma cells are also commonly present after some days and are presumably derived from precursors produced in the lymphoid tissues, as suggested above: they are responsible for local antibody production. More concrete evidence of the occurrence of all stages of the immune response in the tissues containing the antigen is provided by the development of lymphoid tissue with germinal centres, and the demonstration of antibody in extracts of the tissue.

In intensive and prolonged antibody responses, plasma cells may be widespread in various tissues, including the haemopoietic marrow, which can be an important site of antibody production.

The lamina propria of the gut mucosa, and particularly of the intestinal villi, normally contains plasma cells. There is evidence that many of these produce IgA antibody, and that they are derived from B immunoblasts released from the lymph nodes and spleen during antibody responses.

5

Immunopathology

This chapter is devoted entirely to disease processes which have an immunological basis. It falls naturally into two parts. First, the **hypersensitivity reactions** which are of an immunological nature. It should be noted that this use of the term hypersensitivity is somewhat restricted. It does not include those conditions in which the subject is abnormally sensitive to a drug as a result of genetically determined deficiency of an enzyme system necessary for metabolising the drug or because of failure to excrete the drug or its metabolites, e.g. in diseases of the liver or kidneys: this type of undue responsiveness is termed *idiosyncrasy* and is not dealt with here.

The second main section of the chapter describes the **immunological deficiencies**, i.e. congenital or acquired conditions in which the subject is incapable of the normal range of immunological responses and as a result is unduly susceptible to infection.

Hypersensitivity Reactions

In most instances, hypersensitivity may be defined as a state in which the introduction of an antigen into the body elicits an unduly severe immunological reaction. It follows previous exposure to the antigen and is a consequence of the development of an immune response, i.e. production of antibodies or sensitised lymphocytes reactive with the antigen. It is this reaction between the antigen and products of the immune response which produces the lesions of the hypersensitivity disease processes.

Hypersensitivity reactions may be localised to the site of entry of the antigen, or generalised: the local reactions are mainly of an inflammatory nature, but may also include spasm of smooth muscle. The generalised effects include fever, shock, gastrointestinal and pulmonary disturbances, and sometimes fatal circulatory collapse. One of the earliest examples of hypersensitivity was provided by Richet and Partier (1902) who observed that intravenous injection of small amounts of extracts of sea anemone into dogs was harmless, but a second injection some weeks later was quickly followed by a violent and sometimes fatal reaction with dyspnoea, vomiting, defaecation, micturition and collapse. Since this early report, which illustrates the acute and severe nature of some hypersensitivity reactions, a great deal has been learned, and hypersensitivity reactions may now be classified into four major types (see below).

The definition of hypersensitivity given above refers solely to foreign antigens entering the body from outside. However, the term includes also the conditions commonly known as the *autoimmune diseases*, in which antibodies or sensitised lymphocytes appear which are capable of reacting with a normal cell or tissue constituent *in vivo*, with consequent pathological changes. Hypersensitivity reactions may result also from passive immunisation, for example when antibody is produced in the mother by active immunisation by fetal red cells, and crosses the placenta in a subsequent pregnancy to gain entrance to the fetal circulation. Another special example of hypersensitivity of increasing importance is *the rejection process in heterogeneic or allogeneic tissue transplants*. The increasing diversity and use of drugs has also provided an important group of '*drug hypersensitivities*' and the same applies to the expanding number of chemicals used domestically and in industry.

The four major types of hypersensitivity reactions are described briefly below and then each is dealt with in more detail. They have been elucidated very largely by animal experiments. Hypersensitivity reactions in man, whether they occur naturally, as a result of transplantation, or from administration of a drug, tend to be complex and often involve more than one of the four types.

Anaphylaxis, atopic or type I reactions occur in individuals who are predisposed to develop increased amounts of IgE class antibodies in response to antigenic stimuli. IgE antibody binds to mast cells, and subsequent absorption of the corresponding antigen triggers off release of histamine, etc., from the sensitised mast cells, giving rise to a local inflammatory reaction and smooth muscle spasm, or to a more generalised reaction. Examples include hay fever and asthma.

Cytotoxic antibody or type II reactions occur when antibody develops which is capable of reacting with surface antigens of cells. As a result, the cells are injured by subsequent complement activation, phagocytosis, etc. Examples include destruction of red cells and platelets by auto-antibodies to their surface components.

Immune-complex, Arthus-type or type III reactions are caused by the reaction of antibody, usually of IgG class, with the corresponding soluble antigen. This can occur locally (Arthus reaction) or in the blood. In either case, immune complexes are deposited in the walls of blood vessels, where they activate complement and induce vascular injury.

Delayed hypersensitivity, or type IV reactions occur when the primed T lymphocytes which develop during the cell-mediated immune response encounter the corresponding antigen. The specifically reactive T lymphocytes transform to blast cells and secrete a number of factors (lymphokines) which mediate an acute inflammatory reaction, aggregation of more lymphocytes and monocytes, and sometimes necrosis. The tuberculin skin test is a good example.

It should be noted that type I and II reactions occur in subjects predisposed to unusual immune responses, while types III and IV are the result of normal immune responses.

Before considering types of hypersensitivity in detail, this is a convenient place to give accounts of two systems, the profound importance of which is becoming increasingly apparent. The first is the **complement system**, which was for long regarded as being concerned solely in relation to antigen–antibody reactions, but is now known to participate in many other processes, e.g. in inflammation, blood clotting and fibrinolysis. The second is the **cyclic-AMP system** which plays a central role in most of the functions of animal cells: its role in controlling the release of mast cell products, which is outlined briefly below, is involved in some forms of hypersensitivity, but is only one illustration of its much wider importance.

The properties of complement

The complement system consists of at least 9 enzyme precursors (C1 to C9) in the plasma and, as in the clotting system, they are capable of a sequential reaction in which conversion of each component to the active enzyme (C$\bar{1}$ etc.) results in activation of the next one until all components have been activated. Throughout the reaction, various biologically active factors are produced, and ultimately C8 causes a slow breakdown of the membrane of the cell or micro-organism to which it is attached; this is accelerated by C9. Unfortunately the components are not numbered in the exact order of reaction, C4 being out of place (Fig. 5.1).

Activation of a complement component usually involves its enzymatic cleavage, by the previously activated component, into a larger and a smaller fragment: the larger fragment commonly binds to cells, bacteria, etc., and participates in activation of the next component: the smaller fragment may have various biological activities. For example, C3 is cleaved into C3b, which binds to an adjacent surface and cleaves C5, and C3a (anaphylatoxin) which is released and, by promoting increased vascular permeability, brings about exudation. Because an enzyme molecule can act upon many molecules of its substrate, there is opportunity for amplification of the system at each stage.

The **classical pathway** of complement activation is brought about by antigen–antibody complexes. When IgM or IgG antibodies react with antigen, their Fc parts are altered in such a way that they bind and activate C1: this, in turn, activates C4 and C2 and a complex of $\overline{C42}$ (C3-convertase) activates C3, the reaction then proceeding until finally C9 is activated (Fig. 5.1). At least two closely-adjacent molecules of

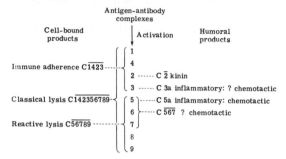

Fig. 5.1 The effects of activation of complement. The components are activated sequentially in the order shown. The properties of some of the free products of activation are shown on the right, and the effects of products binding to antigen–antibody complexes (e.g. antibody-sensitised target cells or bacteria) on the left. Activation at the C1 stage by antigen–antibody complexes (the classical pathway) is illustrated, but activation can also be initiated at the C3 stage (alternate pathway). Note $\overline{C2}$, etc., indicate products of activated C2, etc.: $\overline{C1423}$, etc., indicate complexes of activation products of several complement components. The letters *a* and *b* are used for particular cleavage products of components, e.g. C3a is the smaller fragment produced by activation (which involves enzymic cleavage) of C3.

reacted IgG antibody are required for complement activation, but one molecule of IgM bound, for example, to a red-cell antigen, can activate sufficient complement to lyse the cell.

Activation of C1 is not always due to immune complexes: it can be effected, for example, by plasmin, and probably by other proteolytic enzymes, e.g. in inflammatory reactions.

The **alternate pathway** of complement activation starts at C3, without involvement of C1, 4 or 2. It is brought about by certain bacterial polysaccharides, endotoxin and experimentally by zymosan (yeast cell-wall carbohydrate). These substances activate a series of components known collectively as the **properdin system**, the end-product being an enzyme which, like

C3-convertase, cleaves C3: the reaction then proceeds to completion with final activation of C9. There is also evidence that IgA antibodies, having reacted with antigen, can activate complement at the C3 stage.

The above account is a gross oversimplification. There are a number of factors which modify the activation of complement, e.g. the rapid decay of some of the activated components; $C\overline{1}$-inactivator, an α_2 plasma globulin which unites with and blocks the action of, $C\overline{1}$; and C3b-inhibitor, a β-globulin which breaks down C3b. The system includes feedback mechanisms, for example C3b activates more C3 and so amplifies the later stages of complement activation, but this is limited by the consequent fall in the concentration of C3, and also by C3b-inhibitor which is also termed conglutinogen-activating factor (KAF) because, in inactivating C3b, it converts it into a factor to which auto-antibody (*immunoconglutinin*) develops.

The effects of complement activation. It has long been known that activation of complement can bring about the lysis of bacteria to which antibodies have become bound, and thus help to overcome the infection. This mechanism is not effective in destroying all types of bacteria but the coating of complement components also renders micro-organisms more susceptible to phagocytosis and destruction by polymorphs and macrophages, which have surface receptors for C3b. Activation of complement also provides factors which increase vascular permeability ($C\overline{2}$, C3a and C5a) and are chemotactic to polymorphs and macrophages (C5a and possibly C3a and $\overline{C567}$). The importance of these factors in inflammatory reactions in general has been discussed on p. 43, and their rôle in hypersensitivity reactions and microbial infections will be considered in this and the next chapter respectively. Complement activation is not wholly beneficial: whether activated by the classical or alternate pathways, activated components, e.g. $\overline{C567}$, can bind to tissue cells which have taken no part in the activation: subsequent activation and binding of C8 and 9 leads to the lysis of these innocent bystanders (*reactive lysis*).

Congenital deficiencies of complement components are rare: some of them impair the individual's resistance to infection. Unwanted and harmful activation of complement is seen in individuals lacking C1-inactivator, and gives rise to the features of angio-oedema (p. 217).

Detection of complement components. The measurement of total haemolytic complement activity present in serum is performed traditionally by determining the concentration of serum required to cause lysis of 50% of a suspension of red cells sensitised with antibody (p. 92). Techniques are, however, available to measure individual complement components, and also their activation products: such tests are now in routine use to detect evidence of activation of complement *in vivo* in various diseases, and to distinguish between activation by the classical and alternate pathways.

Cyclic adenosine 3', 5'-monophosphate (Cyclic AMP)

The demonstration of the importance of cyclic AMP in the control of cell behaviour is among the most important biochemical advances of recent years. Cyclic AMP has been shown to be a normal constituent of virtually all types of animal cells, and its intracellular concentration has been shown to exert a major influence on the control of such diverse cell properties as mitosis, differentiation, protein, carbohydrate and lipid metabolism, motility and membrane permeability.

The intracellular concentration of cyclic AMP is controlled mainly by two enzymes: **adenyl cyclase**, which promotes conversion of ATP to cyclic AMP, and AMP-phosphodiesterase, which breaks down cyclic AMP. Adenyl cyclase is present in the plasma membrane and the membranes of various cellular organelles. The effects of most hormones (but probably not steroids) on their target cells is mediated *via* adenyl cyclase: this includes agents with an effect on many types of cell, e.g. catecholamines, histamine, insulin and prostaglandins, and also hormones which affect specific cell types, e.g. TSH, ACTH and parathormone. Many non-physiological compounds, including some bacterial toxins and drugs, also exert their effect through adenyl cyclase. Many pharmacological agents, including some of those listed above, also influence cyclic AMP by exerting an effect on AMP-phosphodiesterase. To complicate the system still further, there is evidence that the adenyl cyclase and AMP-

phosphodiesterase in different parts of the cell differ in their responsiveness to various agents.

While stimulation of adenyl cyclase activity, with consequent increase in cyclic AMP, usually increases the functional activities of most types of cell, there appear to be many exceptions, in which the opposite effect is observed. Technical difficulties, and the complexities of the system, have limited the elucidation of its detailed role in the observed effects of various endogenous and exogenous agents on cells, but investigations on the release of histamine, etc., by mast cells and basophil leukocytes suggest the mechanisms indicated in Fig. 5.2.

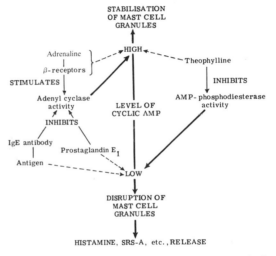

Fig. 5.2 Diagrammatic representation of how various agents which influence the release of mast cell or basophil leukocyte products probably exert their effect *via* the cyclic AMP system. Heavy lines indicate the major features of the cyclic AMP system, light lines show the effects of various factors on this system, and interrupted lines show the outcome of these effects.

Anaphylaxis (atopic, 'immediate' or type I hypersensitivity).

Approximately 10% of the population suffers from this type of hypersensitivity, although in most of these the symptoms are mild and occasional. The commonest manifestations of atopy are **hay fever** and **extrinsic asthma**, which tend to run in families and are sometimes preceded by **atopic eczema** in infancy and childhood. The sufferer from hay fever develops acute inflammation of the nasal and conjunctival mucous membrane with sneezing and nasal and lacrimal hypersecretion within minutes of exposure to an atmosphere containing the causal agent (usually grass or other pollens). Similarly, an acute attack of asthma, with difficult wheezing respiration due to narrowing of the airways by bronchospasm and mucous secretion, develops rapidly when the asthmatic inhales the agent to which he is hypersensitive, e.g. house dust or animal dander. Atopic individuals, particularly in childhood, may also suffer from '**food allergies**' in which absorption of compounds in certain foods, e.g. strawberries, promotes an acute reaction in the gut with colicky pain, vomiting and diarrhoea. Deficiency of secretory IgA in atopic subjects may be a contributory factor to the development of food allergy by allowing food antigens to penetrate into the mucous membrane, with subsequent formation of reaginic antibodies.

In addition to these local disturbances, atopic patients sometimes develop more generalised reactions such as an **urticarial skin rash** and **acute systemic anaphylaxis** (anaphylactic shock) with dyspnoea, urticaria, convulsions, prostration and sometimes death. Generalised reactions occur when the responsible agent is absorbed in sufficient amounts to enter the bloodstream. Fortunately, severe anaphylactic shock is rare, but it sometimes occurs in hypersensitivity to drugs, notably penicillin, and to the venoms of stinging insects.

Demonstration of type I hypersensitivity. This is usually demonstrated by skin testing, in which very small amounts of suspected antigens are injected intradermally. No matter whether the patient suffers from hay fever, asthma or a food allergy, intradermal injection of the responsible agent is followed within a few minutes by an acute inflammatory reaction lasting $1\frac{1}{2}$–2 hours, characterised by itching, erythema and wealing at the injection site (Fig. 5.3). Hence the use of the term *immediate* type hypersensitivity. Pricking small amounts of antigen solution into the skin is preferable to intradermal injection for detecting the antigen(s) to which the patient is hypersensitive, but with both methods reactions are often elicited to antigens not responsible for clinical atopy. Provocation tests, for example bronchial challenge with a controlled inhalation of the suspected antigen by the asthmatic, are said to

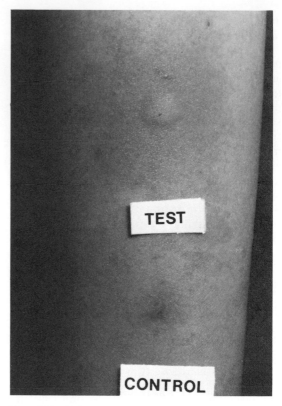

Fig. 5.3 Skin test showing immediate (type I) hypersensitivity reaction. The patient was an asthmatic and the test was performed by intradermal injection of an extract of house dust. Note the oedema and wide zone of reddening. Photograph taken 10 minutes after injection. (Dr. J. W. Kerr.)

be more reliable. In all tests, careful precautions must be taken to avoid a severe reaction.

Passive transfer: the Prausnitz–Küstner reaction. The presence of an antibody-like factor termed **reagin** in the serum of atopic subjects was demonstrated beautifully in the classical investigation of Prausnitz and Küstner (1921). Küstner himself regularly experienced a generalised hypersensitivity reaction after eating fish. Intradermal injection of an extract of cooked fish muscle produced the typical immediate reaction. In attempting passive transfer of the hypersensitivity state, small amounts of Küstner's serum were injected intradermally into Prausnitz, followed 24 hours later by injection of fish muscle extract at the same site: the typical immediate reaction occurred, and was shown to depend on the injection of serum, followed after an interval by fish extract. The experiment was complicated by the fact that Prausnitz had atopic hypersensitivity to pollens, but local hypersensitivity was also induced by passive transfer of Küstner's serum to normal, non-atopic individuals. These findings have since been confirmed repeatedly with serum from subjects with atopic hypersensitivity to various antigens, and it has been shown that the interval between injecting the serum and antigen in the Prausnitz–Küstner reaction may be increased up to 3–4 weeks, thus demonstrating that reagin attaches firmly to some component in the skin. Transient generalised atopic hypersensitivity has also been observed to occur in the recipient of blood from atopic donors. Evidence that reagin sticks to various tissues and not just to skin has been provided by the demonstration that fresh bronchial tissue removed from an atopic subject undergoes contraction of the smooth muscle when exposed to the appropriate antigen, and it has been shown that normal tissues of various types can be sensitised passively by the serum of atopic individuals.

Reaginic antibody: IgE. Isolation of reagin and elucidation of its physical and chemical properties has proved difficult, partly because it is present only in trace amounts in the serum and is less stable than other classes of immunoglobulins, but also because it is *homocytotropic*, i.e. binds to the cells of the same (human) and closely-related (monkey) tissues, but not to those of guinea-pig, rat, etc., and so is demonstrable by its biological effect only in man and monkeys. It was eventually shown by Ishizaka to be due to an immunoglobulin of a different class (IgE) from other antibodies and subsequent investigations were greatly helped by the discovery of a patient with plasma cell myeloma whose myeloma protein was of IgE class, and provided a rich source of IgE. When a solution of IgE or of its Fc component was injected into the skin it was found to block the tissue sites of attachment of reaginic antibody, and so inhibited the elucidation of the Prausnitz–Küstner reaction at the same site. This is strong confirmation that reaginic antibodies are of IgE class, and shows that fixation to tissues is a property of their Fc component. Antibody specific for myeloma IgE is now used to assay the level of IgE in serum and also as the basis of a test for specific IgE antibodies. Raised levels of IgE, and of IgE class antibodies

to the relevant antigens, have been detected in the serum of atopic subjects.

Rôle of the mast cell. Immediate type hypersensitivity has been studied extensively in animals and particularly in the guinea-pig. It has been shown that reagin-like antibody attaches to the mast cells by its Fc component and that subsequent union of antigen with cell-bound antibody results in disruption of the mast cell granules and release of their contents, which include histamine and 5-hydroxytryptamine. Moreover, prior depletion of mast cell granules, for example by compound 48/80, or administration of antagonists of histamine and 5-hydroxytryptamine, inhibit the development of atopic reactions on antigenic challenge of suitably sensitised animals. Mast cell disruption and release of pharmacologically active amines is thus an important mechanism of immediate type hypersensitivity in animals. Experimental hypersensitivity is not, however, strictly comparable with human atopy: for example, in guinea-pigs and rats, the major tissue-binding (homocytotropic) antibody is a sub-class of IgG and not IgE as in man.

There is nevertheless sufficient similarity to suggest that mast cells are involved in human atopic reactions and there is good evidence that human basophil polymorphonuclear leucocytes, which are somewhat similar to, and easier to obtain and study than mast cells, are sensitised by IgE antibody, for subsequent exposure to the appropriate antigen brings about degranulation with release of histamine, etc. It is noteworthy that atopic reactions are partly inhibited by histamine antagonists, indicating histamine as one of the mediators, and that the main sources of tissue histamine in man are the mast cells and basophil leucocytes. From this, and much other indirect evidence, it is likely that anaphylactic reactions in man result from sensitisation of mast cells and basophil leukocytes with IgE homocytotropic antibody and that exposure to antigen triggers off the discharge of the mast cell granules, and release of histamine (Fig. 5.4). Histamine antagonists do not block all the histamine receptors and are not wholly effective in suppressing atopy. Additional chemical mediators are also involved. For example, it has been shown that human lung tissue, removed surgically from an atopic subject who developed a bronchial carcinoma, yielded not only histamine but also a second

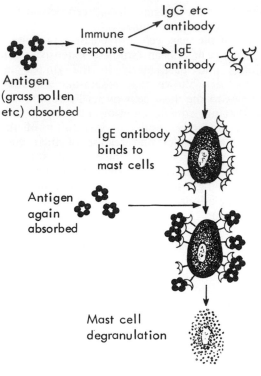

IgG etc
antibody

Immune
response

IgE
antibody

Antigen
(grass pollen
etc) absorbed

IgE antibody
binds to
mast cells

Antigen
again
absorbed

Mast cell
degranulation

Histamine etc.

Fig. 5.4 The mechanism of atopic reactions. IgE antibody to pollens, etc., binds by its Fc component to mast cells (and basophil leukocytes), and subsequently absorbed antigen triggers off the sensitised mast cells (probably by linking together antibody molecules on their surface) to release histamine, etc.

compound, **SRS-A** (the slow reacting substance of anaphylaxis), on perfusion with a solution of the antigen to which the individual was hypersensitive. SRS-A causes an increase in vascular permeability, and more prolonged spasm of the bronchiolar smooth muscle than does histamine. It is apparently a lipid, is formed in many tissues, and may participate in the bronchospasm of asthma and spasm of the gut in food allergies. It is possible that bradykinin and permeability factors derived from plasma components, which may participate in acute inflammation in general, may also act as mediators in anaphylaxis.

The mechanism whereby mast cells are degranulated by an immunological reaction at their surface is not fully elucidated, but there is evidence that the cyclic AMP system is of major importance, as indicated in Fig. 5.2.

Other immunological factors. Although IgE antibody appears to be the important mediating agent of atopy, it may not be the only immunological factor involved. There is recent evidence that a sub-class of IgG antibody can mediate a complement-dependent form of immediate type hypersensitivity. However, it has not yet been proved that this second mechanism plays a significant role in human atopy. It has also been shown that the T lymphocytes of atopic subjects are stimulated *in vitro* by the presence of the responsible antigen, indicating the occurrence of cell-mediated immunity. This may be of some clinical importance because when immediate skin test reactions are suppressed by administration of histamine antagonists, a delayed hypersensitivity reaction appears in some patients, and experimental inhalation of the responsible antigen, e.g. house dust, induces, in over 50% of asthmatic patients, not only an immediate respiratory wheeze, but also a delayed wheezing reaction 6–12 hours after the challenge. In practice, this delayed reactivity often makes it difficult to relate cause and effect.

Atopic hypersensitivity can often be reduced, but seldom abolished, by subcutaneous injection of the responsible antigen in a slowly soluble (e.g. alum precipitated) form. The mechanism of such **hyposensitisation** is not known, but it is popularly believed that slow release of antigen from the depot stimulates the production of antibodies of classes other than IgE and that these have a 'blocking' effect by reacting with any subsequently absorbed antigen, thus preventing its combination with IgE antibody bound to mast cells. Hyposensitisation is not always successful, and the outcome is not predictable. There is, moreover, a possibility that, by stimulating the production of IgG antibody, the procedure may predispose the individual to immune complex disease (p. 213).

Predisposition to atopy. It is not known why atopy tends to run in families. The most likely explanation is a genetic predisposition to develop IgE class antibodies. It is well established that atopic individuals are predisposed to produce more IgE antibody to a wide variety of antigens than are normal individuals. For example, immunisation with diphtheria toxoid results in immediate type hypersensitivity which can be demonstrated by skin testing. It is also not known why, in some individuals and families, hay fever is the dominant atopic manifestation, while in others asthma predominates.

Infestation with parasitic worms tends to promote an IgE antibody response and immediate type hypersensitivity, even in nonatopic individuals. Moreover, when experimental animals are infested with worms, or injected with worm extracts, simultaneous administration of various antigens results in enhanced IgE antibody production. This has raised the possibility that intestinal infestations, which of course may run in families, might predispose to the development of atopic hypersensitivity. However, children in Ethiopia have high IgE levels and little atopic disease, while children in Sweden have low IgE levels and more atopic disease than in Ethiopia. Finally, it has been suggested that immunodeficiency of secretory IgA may predispose to the atopic hypersensitivity by allowing absorption of antigens from mucous membranes.

Patients with atopic diseases show exaggerated reactivity to histamine and other biologically active amines released by mast cells; apparently this is due to an imbalance in the neural control of bronchial smooth muscle. The degree of hyper-reactivity has been shown to be important in determining the severity of the clinical symptoms.

The histological features of atopic lesions are essentially those of acute inflammation, including congestion of microvessels and inflammatory exudation. A distinctive feature is the *accumulation of eosinophil polymorphs*. This is very likely due to a chemotactic factor specific for eosinophils which has been shown to be produced by mast cells. There may also be increased numbers of eosinophils in the blood. It is not known what rôle eosinophil leucocytes play in atopic reactions.

Cytotoxic antibody (type II) reactions

The only distinctive feature of this type of hypersensitivity reaction is that it is mediated by antibodies which cause injury to cells by combining specifically with antigenic determinants on their surface. With few known exceptions, the targets of cytotoxic antibodies are cells of the blood, including platelets. Such injury has been investigated mainly in man, in whom it may occur in the following circumstances.

1. Auto-antibodies may develop which are reactive with normal antigenic constituents on the surface of cells. Such breakdown of self-tolerance is usually unexplained, although it is sometimes associated with lymphocyte neoplasia, and there is some evidence suggesting that it results from a deficiency of suppressor T cells (p. 106).

2. Drug-induced cytotoxic antibodies. Drugs which alter the antigenicity of cell surfaces, either directly by binding to the cell surface, or indirectly by interfering with cell metabolism, may induce the production of antibodies to the altered cell surface antigens.

3. Iso-antibodies can cause injury to cells of the blood following blood transfusion or transplantation of haemopoietic or lymphoid tissue. Maternal iso-antibodies may also pass through the placenta and injure the cells of the fetus.

Cytotoxic antibodies to cells of the blood

Cytotoxic auto-antibodies. The classical example is *auto-immune haemolytic anaemia* in which red cell injury is brought about by auto-antibody reactive with various antigenic determinants inherent in the surface of red cells. The antibody may be of IgG or IgM class, and can be detected on the red cell surface by the anti-globulin test (p. 91). When present in low concentration on the cell surface, IgG may have little or no effect. In higher concentration, it causes agglutination of the cells in places where the circulation is slow, especially in the sinuses of the spleen. Here, the red cells are phagocytosed and destroyed in abnormally large numbers by macrophages, binding to which is facilitated by the macrophage surface receptors for the Fc of IgG (p. 150). IgG antibody can also activate complement and cause intravascular lysis of the cells: this requires pairs of IgG antibody molecules bound to closely adjacent antigenic sites on the red cell surface. IgM antibodies, even in low concentration, often cause red cell destruction by intravascular lysis, single IgM molecules bound to the target cell being capable of activating complement.

Idiopathic thrombocytopenic purpura is caused by auto-antibody which reacts with the surface components of normal platelets, with similarly destructive effects. The frequency with which splenectomy is followed by a rapid rise in the platelet count indicates the importance of the splenic macrophages in the increased platelet destruction.

Auto-antibodies to leukocytes may be a cause of leukopenia (reduced numbers of leukocytes in various diseases), but this has still not been proved.

Drug-induced cytotoxic antibodies. The best known example is the sedative 'Sedormid'* (allyl isopropylacetylurea), which is capable of binding to platelets and acting as a hapten. Antibody is induced against the altered platelet surface membrane and promotes phagocytosis of platelets in the spleen and also fixes complement, resulting in platelet lysis. Patients who develop such antibody are likely to suffer from the effects of platelet destruction after taking the drug, and transfusion of their blood or plasma can confer temporarily the same hypersensitivity state on normal individuals.

Perhaps the commonest example of drug-induced destruction of red cells is that which sometimes results from administration of methyldopa. This drug interferes with the metabolism of red cell precursors in such a way that the red cells have an abnormal surface membrane which can stimulate antibody production. The antibody can also cross-react with the membrane of normal red cells, and the increased red cell destruction, which is usually mild, often persists for weeks or months after stopping the drug.

Cytotoxic iso-antibodies. In blood transfusion, administration of red cells possessing the A or B surface iso-antigens to an individual whose plasma contains the natural anti-A or anti-B iso-antibodies usually results in rapid destruction of the donated red cells. These natural antibodies are of IgM class and so complement fixation and lysis of the incompatible red cells results. There are literally dozens of other red cell iso-antigens, but normally the corresponding antibodies appear in the plasma only after blood transfusion or pregnancy (see below). After the ABO groups, the Rhesus (Rh) system of iso-antigens is of most importance in man. Transfusion of red cells possessing Rh antigens which are not present in the recipient's red cells often results in development of the corresponding Rh antibody, following which the transfused cells are destroyed abnormally rapidly in the spleen. During labour (or abortion) some fetal red cells enter the mother's circulation, and, if Rh-incompatible (which depends on the

* No longer available.

father's Rh group) they sometimes stimulate development of Rh antibodies.

The Rh antibodies are particularly important in pregnancy, because they are usually mainly of IgG class, and so can cross the placenta. If the pregnant woman has developed Rh antibodies, as a result of a previous pregnancy or blood transfusion, they enter the fetal circulation and, if the fetal red cells possess the corresponding Rh antigens, abnormal destruction results in fetal death or anaemia (Fig. 5.5).

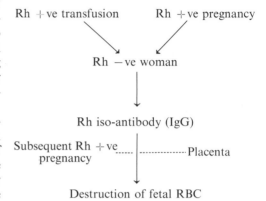

Fig. 5.5 Haemolytic disease of the newborn. Fetal red cell destruction is brought about by maternal isoantibody which has developed as a result of previous Rh +ve pregnancy or transfusion of Rh +ve blood.

Once an individual has developed Rh antibodies, from either pregnancy or transfusion, subsequently transfused Rh-positive red cells are liable to be destroyed rapidly.

In common with tissue cells, the leukocytes and platelets have antigens belonging to the HLA and other 'transplant antigen' systems (p. 137). This is seldom of importance in blood transfusion unless the aim is to supply these cell types to a deficient recipient. Blood transfusion and pregnancy do, however, stimulate the development of HLA and other antibodies, and subsequently transferred platelets or leukocytes may be destroyed rapidly. Such iso-immunisation is of importance if subsequent transplantation, e.g. of a kidney, is performed, and maternal iso-antibodies to platelets may also cause thrombocytopenia in the fetus.

Auto-antibodies to tissue constituents

Auto-antibodies which react with components of tissue cells *in vitro* are demonstrable in the serum of patients with various diseases (p. 132), but the available evidence suggests that they are not usually a major cause of cell injury. In most instances, this is because they react with intracellular, as opposed to surface constitutents, of the target cells. A good example is antibody to deoxyribonucleoprotein, which is present in the plasma of patients with systemic lupus erythematosus: it can react with, and lead to destruction of, the nuclei of dead cells, but does not reach the nuclei of living cells.

One exception is the hyperthyroidism of Graves' disease, in which the serum contains an IgG antibody termed '**long-acting thyroid stimulator**' (**LATS**). On injection into mice or guinea-pigs, LATS stimulates thyroid activity, and temporary hyperthyroidism occurs in newborn infants of mothers with a high serum level of LATS. The antibody reacts specifically with the thyroid epithelial surface receptor for TSH.

Although 'cytotoxic' implies injury to cells, type II hypersensitivity is sometimes extended to include antibody-induced injury to extracellular tissue elements. The best known example of this is the rare type of glomerulonephritis in which auto-antibody develops to glomerular capillary basement membrane. Union of this antibody with the inner surface of the basement membrane is followed by activation of complement, as in the Arthus reaction, and a destructive inflammatory lesion results in the glomeruli.

Antibody-dependent lymphocyte cytotoxicity

When tissue cells or red cells are treated with an IgG class antibody which reacts with their surface membrane, and normal lymphocytes (e.g. from the peripheral blood of a normal individual) are added, some of the lymphocytes bind to the surface of the sensitised cells and by some unknown means bring about their destruction. The nature of the cytotoxic lymphocytes, sometimes called K cells, is unknown (p. 107) and the evidence that they are lymphocytes is mainly morphological.

The importance of this type of cell injury in man is not known, but there is evidence suggesting that it contributes to the destruction of tumour cells in experimental animals.

Immune complex, Arthus-type (type III) reactions

These result from formation of immune complexes by union of antigen with free IgG or IgM antibody with consequent activation (fixation) of complement. This leads, in turn, to acute inflammation with accumulation of polymorphs and aggregation of platelets. The polymorphs phagocytose the immune complexes and release lysosomal enzymes which cause tissue injury and aggravate the inflammatory response. Depending on the distribution of antigen, the reaction may be localised to a particular tissue, and is then termed an Arthus reaction, or immune complexes may form in the blood, producing a generalised reaction commonly known as 'serum sickness' or circulating immune-complex disease.

The local or Arthus reaction

This was described in 1903 by Arthus, who injected rabbits repeatedly with horse serum. When the animals had developed a high level of circulating antibodies to horse serum protein, he noticed that a subcutaneous injection of horse serum induced a local acute inflammatory reaction, developing over a few hours and sometimes progressing to necrosis. It has since been shown that the reaction may be induced by injecting a soluble antigen into various tissues in animals with a high level of the corresponding precipitating antibody in their blood. It can be induced also in animals immunised passively by intravenous injection of precipitating antibody (passive Arthus reaction), or the antigen may be injected intravenously and the antibody locally (reversed passive Arthus reaction).

Histological features. Microscopy of the Arthus reaction shows the typical changes of acute inflammation with congestion of small vessels, inflammatory exudation, and marked pavementing and emigration of neutrophil polymorphs. There may be aggregation of platelets in the small vessels and, depending on the severity, haemorrhages and thrombosis, and necrosis extending from the walls of small vessels to surrounding tissues.

Mechanism. Immunofluorescence techniques have demonstrated precipitates of antigen–antibody complexes in the lesion, particularly in the walls of venules. Fixed components of complement may also be detected in the precipitates. The Arthus reaction is largely suppressed in animals by depletion either of neutrophil polymorphs, e.g. by nitrogen mustard,

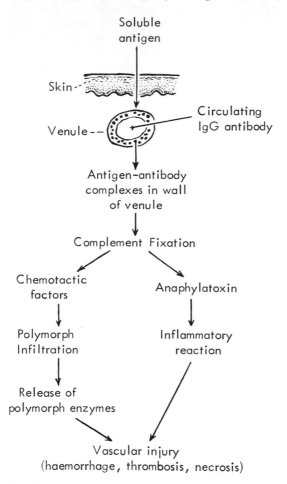

Fig. 5.6 Mechanism of the Arthus reaction. Local injection of soluble antigen into an animal with a high plasma level of the corresponding antibody of IgG class results in union of antigen and antibody in the walls of venules. Complement reacts with the antigen–antibody complexes, and reaction products of complement induce inflammation and polymorph infiltration. The release of polymorph enzymes brings about vascular and tissue injury.

or of complement, e.g. by cobra-venom factor (p. 756); the intensity of the reaction is reduced by administration of corticosteroids. From such evidence it has been deduced that the reaction is

brought about as follows. (See also Fig. 5.6.) Immune complex formation in the walls of venules leads to complement fixation, the products of which include **anaphylatoxins*** (C3a and C5a) which bring about acute inflammation by releasing histamine, etc., from mast cells. C5a, and possibly other complement products, are chemotactic for polymorphs, which consequently migrate into the vessel walls and surrounding tissues in large numbers and phagocytose the immune complexes. In so doing, they release lysosomal enzymes which cause further tissue damage, digest proteins with production of kinins and other vaso-active peptides, and thus aggravate the inflammatory reaction. Platelet aggregation occurs in the damaged vessels and initiates thrombosis with consequent ischaemic necrosis.

The Arthus reaction in man was seen not uncommonly in the days when crude preparations of horse antitoxic globulin or whole antitoxic serum was administered in the prevention and treatment of diphtheria, tetanus, etc. This resulted in the development of precipitating antibodies to horse proteins and a subsequent subcutaneous or intramuscular injection of horse globulin or serum elicited an Arthus reaction. More recently, it has been shown that the Arthus reaction is the basis of 'farmer's lung', in which the farm worker inhales large numbers of the spores of bacteria growing in mouldy hay, and develops precipitating antibody to the bacterial antigens. Subsequent inhalation of the spores induces an acute Arthus reaction in the alveolar walls. It has become apparent that individuals with precipitating antibody in their serum vary greatly in their susceptibility to farmer's lung: there is some evidence suggesting that IgE antibody is also necessary, and that the Arthus reaction is triggered off by an initial atopic reaction which allows escape of antibodies into the vessel walls. As in the rabbit, Arthus reactions in man are inhibited by administration of glucocorticoids.

The local nature of the Arthus reaction depends on all the antigen being complexed around the site of entry. If large doses of antigen are injected, or if the level of antibody in the plasma is not sufficient to complex and precipitate all the antigen locally, then some antigen enters the circulation and immune com-

* The term *anaphylatoxin* is unfortunate, because products of complement fixation do not participate in classical anaphylaxis in man, which is due to IgE antibodies.

plexes form in the blood, with the consequences described below.

Circulating immune-complex disease: serum sickness

In man, antigen–antibody complexes are formed in the plasma, both as a result of administration of foreign proteins and haptenic drugs, and also in a number of natural diseases, particularly infections. Serious effects result from their deposition in the walls of blood vessels, especially in the glomeruli, but also in the skin and the walls of arteries. Local lesions develop at these sites and, depending on the duration of deposition, may be acute and self-limiting, recurrent or chronic.

Experimental basis. The basis of this form of hypersensitivity has been elucidated by Dixon, Cochran and others, mainly in rabbits. After a single injection of a large amount of antigen, e.g. bovine serum albumin, no harmful effects occur until, after several days, antibody is produced. As it appears, it combines with antigen still present in the plasma, forming immune complexes. Initially antigen is present in relative excess and its union with antibody produces small soluble complexes (Fig. 4.3, p. 90). As antibody increases, intermediate-sized soluble, and then large, insoluble complexes are formed, and after a few days free antibody can be detected. The larger aggregates of immune complex are rapidly taken up and destroyed by phagocytic leukocytes and by macrophages in

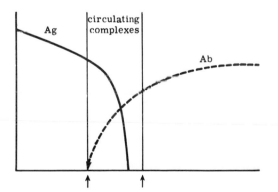

Fig. 5.7 The formation of antigen–antibody complexes in the circulation. Injection of antigen is followed after some days by the appearance of antibody in the plasma: during the next few days, the concentration of antigen falls sharply and antigen–antibody complexes are present in the plasma.

the sinusoids of the liver, spleen, etc. Accordingly, in a rabbit producing a lot of precipitating antibody, complexes disappear from the plasma in a few days (Fig. 5.7). During this period, however, their presence triggers off a series of reactions leading to release of histamine and other vasoactive agents, with consequent increase in vascular permeability. This in turn allows soluble complexes, along with plasma proteins, to leak out between the endothelial cells of various blood vessels. At the sites of leakage, complexes are trapped and accumulate between the endothelium and basal lamina, where their presence results in vascular injury.

The mechanism of increase in vascular permeability, as in inflammation, is complicated, and varies in different species. In the rabbit, in which most of the reservoir of histamine in the blood is in the platelets, histamine release appears to be due mainly to union of antigen with IgE antibody bound to basophil leukocytes (i.e. a type I hypersensitivity reaction): this induces release of a factor which causes the platelets to aggregate and discharge their histamine. Other mechanisms of release of histamine from platelets involve activation of complement by the complexes and participation of neutrophil polymorphs.

In the experiment described above, in which rabbits are given a single injection of an antigen, immune complexes in the blood are deposited deep to the vascular endothelium, particularly in the glomerular capillaries, the small vessels in joints, the heart and focally in various arteries. The deposited complexes continue to fix complement, and, except in the glomeruli, this triggers off an Arthus-type reaction, with acute inflammation, infiltration of polymorphs, and sometimes thrombosis and necrosis. The reaction is particularly intense in the arterial lesions, which may extend to involve the whole thickness of the wall. Activation of complement and polymorphs results in phagocytosis of the deposited complexes within 48 hours, so that, although intense, the reaction is brief. Like the local Arthus reaction, it can be suppressed by prior depletion of polymorphs or complement. In the glomeruli, the deposited complexes fix complement, and yet inflammation is relatively mild and polymorphs are scanty: an obvious explanation is the one-way flow of filtrate from the capillary lumen to the urinary space, which presumably washes away the anaphylatoxins and chemotaxins produced by complement activation. Complexes persist in the glomeruli for many days, and cause glomerular injury by some unexplained mechanism, with resultant proteinuria.

Chronic immune-complex disease can be produced in rabbits by giving daily intravenous injections of soluble antigen in amounts sufficient to provide a period of relative antigen excess over antibody in the plasma after each injection. In contrast to acute serum sickness, the complexes are deposited solely in the glomerular capillaries, where they give rise to lesions resembling various forms of persistent glomerulonephritis in man. Deposition of immune complexes is also influenced by the nature of the antigen and quality of the antibody. Precipitating antibody obviously forms large insoluble complexes which, as stated above, are rapidly phagocytosed and cause little or no injury, so that antigen excess is necessary for formation of smaller, pathogenic complexes. Antibodies which can only react with very few determinant sites on the antigen molecule also form soluble complexes, even when present in relative excess. Accordingly, complex formation with small, simple antigens can produce lesions even when there is a relative excess of antibody in the blood.

Circulating immune-complex disease in man results from injection of heterologous immunoglobulin (now an uncommon cause) and administration of potentially haptenic drugs. It also occurs naturally in systemic lupus erythematosus, in which auto-immune complexes are formed, and in various infections. The formation of immune complexes in the blood may produce both a general reaction, and lesions in the glomeruli and elsewhere resulting from complex deposition in the walls of blood vessels.

The acute generalised reaction of classical serum sickness occurs 7–10 days after the injection of a large amount of heterologous serum or protein, unless the patient has previously been injected with foreign serum of the same species, when it develops much earlier. It is a short febrile illness characterised by intense itching of the skin and urticaria, swelling of peripheral joints, and enlargement of lymph nodes. Histamine antagonists bring partial relief. Examination of the serum reveals immune complexes, a low complement level, and products of complement activation. The polymorph count is at first low, but later raised. After recovery, free antibody appears in the serum. These features indicate that immune complexes form in the blood, activate complement, and trigger off the release of vaso-active agents, including histamine. Phagocytosis of circulating complexes probably results in degeneration and disappearance of most of the polymorphs, and also in the release of endogenous pyrogen and thus the development of fever (p. 156).

The mechanism of release of histamine, etc. is not known. It may involve the anaphylatoxins of complement, release of polymorph lysosomes, activation of Hageman factor and production of kinins. It may also be that, as in the rabbit, basophil polymorphs or mast cells sensitised with IgE antibody are involved. This possibility is supported by the frequency of bronchospasm suggestive of atopy, and the occasional severe circulatory collapse as in generalised anaphylaxis.

The typical attack of serum sickness which followed injection of crude antisera is now uncommon, but similar reactions can follow administration of drugs which can confer antigenicity to plasma proteins, and the severe form of dengue fever is due largely to circulating virus antigen–antibody complexes. In spirochaetal infections, including syphilis, and in lepromatous leprosy and some other chronic bacterial infections, the first dose of treatment by an effective drug may kill very large numbers of micro-organisms and so release microbial antigen, which, depending on the level of circulating antibody and the amount of antigen released, either forms complexes in the blood or induces local Arthus reactions in the lesions. The features of the reaction (*the Jarisch–Herxheimer reaction*) suggest that both phenomena may occur.

Immune-complex deposition is an important cause of glomerulonephritis in man. The typical acute glomerulonephritis following a streptococcal throat infection develops when antibody to streptococcal antigen enters the blood and immune complexes are formed and deposited in the glomerular capillaries, as in acute serum sickness in the rabbit. Other infections and drug hypersensitivities can have the same effect, and more chronic glomerular injury occurs from prolonged or intermittent immune-complex formation in quartan malaria, lepromatous leprosy and some other chronic infections. In systemic lupus erythematosus, auto-antibodies reactive with various cellular constituents develop, and complexes formed in the blood are deposited in small vessels in the skin, glomeruli and elsewhere. The glomerular injury results mainly from deposition of DNA—anti-DNA complexes. In most types of human immune-complex glomerulonephritis, however, the nature of the antigen is unknown. The various patterns of disease depend partly on the size of the circulating complexes and the duration and rate of their deposition.

Arterial lesions due to complex deposition are less common in man, and their nature is usually difficult to prove because, as in the rabbit, the immune complexes are phagocytosed rapidly by polymorphs. Nevertheless, the focal lesions of polyarteritis nodosa and some other forms of arteritis appear to be of this nature, and the Australia antigen of hepatitis virus (p. 614) has been implicated in some cases.

In many patients with immune complex disease, IgM antibodies develop which are capable of reacting with IgG. These antiglobulin factors react most avidly with the IgG in immune complexes, and may cause circulatory disturbances by increasing the viscosity of the blood, or aggravate the injury caused by deposited immune complexes. The IgM–IgG complexes often precipitate in cooled serum, and are termed **cryoglobulins**.

The lesions produced by immune complex deposition in the kidneys and elsewhere are described in more detail in the appropriate chapters.

Delayed hypersensitivity (type IV) reactions

Antibody production and cell mediated immunity are both parts of the normal immune response to most antigens. The union of antibodies with antigens can result in the hypersensitivity reactions described above. Delayed hypersensitivity (DHS) does not involve antibody, but is mediated by the specifically-primed T lymphocytes produced in the cell-mediated immune response. By means of their specific surface receptors, these cells can bind to the antigen which has stimulated their production, and this results in tissue injury characterised by a slowly developing inflammatory reaction—hence *delayed* hypersensitivity.

The reaction of primed T lymphocytes with microbial antigens is an essential defence mechanism against many pathogenic bacteria, viruses and fungi, etc.: the DHS reaction promotes their destruction, and the accompanying tissue injury is the price which must be paid for this protection. Cell-mediated immunity to tumour-cell antigens is known to develop in some cancer patients, and is being intensively investigated in the hope that it may be utilised for the effective destruction of tumours by DHS reactions.

Cell-mediated immunity develops also against harmless foreign antigens, body constituents modified by foreign haptens, against transplanted allogeneic cells or tissues, and sometimes even against the individual's own apparently normal tissue cells. In these circumstances, unwanted DHS reactions occur, resulting respectively in contact dermatitis, rejection of transplants, and auto-immune disease.

Morphological features

The DHS reaction can occur in any part of the body where primed T lymphocytes encounter the corresponding antigen. Its induction in the skin is used as a test for cell-mediated immunity to various antigens, the classical example being **the tuberculin reaction** in which a small amount of tuberculoprotein is applied to the skin or injected intradermally as in the Mantoux test. This has no effect in non-immune individuals, but in subjects who have developed cell-mediated immunity to tuberculoprotein as a result of tuberculosis or immunisation with BCG (attenuated *Mycobacterium bovis*) the typical delayed inflammatory reaction appears in 12–24 hours and persists for 48 hours or more. The skin becomes reddened and a firm central nodule appears. In a highly sensitised individual, necrosis and ulceration may follow. **Microscopically**, the major features are microvascular congestion, accumulation of lymphocytes in and around the small vessels, and swelling of the collagen, apparently due to inflammatory oedema. At the height of the reaction there is intense infiltration with lymphocytes and occasional macrophages, both in and around the capillaries and venules, particularly round the sweat glands and hair follicles (Fig. 5.8). These are the features of the DHS reaction to a soluble protein in man. In

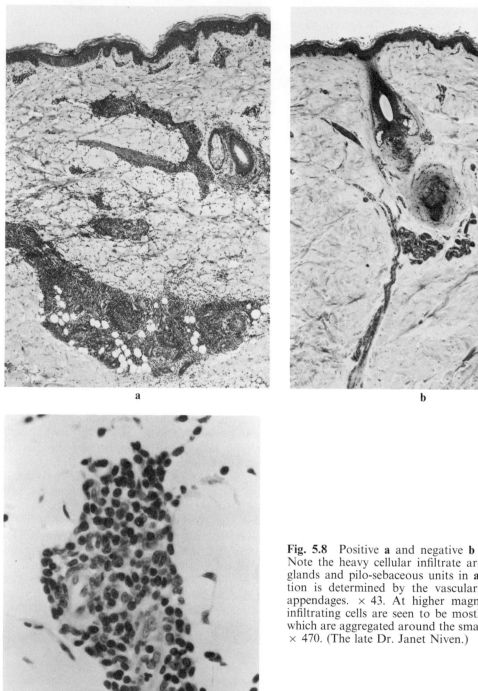

Fig. 5.8 Positive **a** and negative **b** Mantoux tests. Note the heavy cellular infiltrate around the sweat glands and pilo-sebaceous units in **a**. This distribution is determined by the vascularity of the skin appendages. × 43. At higher magnification **c**, the infiltrating cells are seen to be mostly lymphocytes, which are aggregated around the small blood vessels. × 470. (The late Dr. Janet Niven.)

animals, accumulation of polymorphs and macrophages, in addition to lymphocytes, is much more prominent. The morphological features of DHS reactions in infections are complicated by the injuries inflicted directly by the micro-organisms or their toxins and by other types of hypersensitivity reactions. A glance at the microscopic appearances of the lesions of various infections in which DHS is a prominent feature will show considerable differences (e.g. tuberculosis, p. 176, tuberculoid leprosy, p. 181; typhoid fever, p. 573, and contact dermatitis, p. 131). In general, infiltration with macrophages, lymphocytes and lymphoblasts is prominent. The macrophages may also change to epithelioid cells, fuse to form giant cells and undergo necrosis.

Mechanisms of delayed hypersensitivity

Following a cell-mediated immune response, specifically primed T lymphocytes join the recirculating pool (p. 100) and so are present in the blood, lymph nodes, etc., and in thoracic duct lymph. It is widely assumed that subsequent antigenic challenge, e.g. by injection of the antigen or infection with the relevant microbe, results in migration of these specifically primed cells from the blood into the tissues containing the antigen.

Recent animal experiments support this view, but indicate that the primed T cells which emigrate at the antigen site are small lymphocytes which have recently divided and also lymphoblasts. If the cell-mediated response is very recent, such cells will still be present in the blood: if it is more remote, there will be some specifically primed T lymphocytes in the blood, but few or no lymphoblasts, and their production depends on sufficient of the antigen reaching the blood or lymph nodes, etc. to react with and stimulate the relevant primed lymphocytes to proliferate, i.e. to trigger off a 'secondary' cell-mediated immune response. In the case of a previously non-immunised subject, the introduction of a suitable antigen will stimulate a cell-mediated immune response, usually during the next few days, and if antigen is still present at the injection site, a DHS reaction will develop there.

It appears that antigen is not necessarily chemotactic to those T cells capable of reacting with it, for any T lymphoblasts or recently divided T lymphocytes which happen to be in the blood enter the tissues at the antigen site (or the site of injection of an unrelated antigen or of non-specific tissue injury). It thus seems that, in animals, circulating T lymphoid cells migrate into inflammatory lesions of various kinds. This may help to explain why most of the lymphocytes aggregating in DHS reactions are not specifically primed for the particular antigen concerned (but see below).

In pyogenic infections lymphocytes, if present in the exudate, are obscured by the much larger number of polymorphs.

Lymphokines. When suspensions of lymphocytes obtained from a subject who has developed cell-mediated immunity to a particular antigen are incubated with that antigen, the specifically primed T lymphocytes synthesis DNA and transform into immunoblasts (p. 100). During this process, the culture medium acquires biological properties indicating the secretion, by the transformed cells, of soluble factors termed lymphokines. These are capable of inducing at least some features of the DHS reaction, e.g. acute inflammation and accumulation and activation of macrophages.

By a combination of *in-vitro* and *in-vivo* tests on the fluid in which primed T cells have reacted with the corresponding antigen, the following properties of lymphokines have been demonstrated.

1. Induction of acute inflammation. Intradermal injection demonstrates a factor which induces congestion of small blood vessels and inflammatory oedema. This could account for these features in the DHS reaction.

2. Effects on mononuclear phagocytes. These are complex, but there is evidence for the following.

(*a*) *A chemotactic factor.* This induces chemotaxis of monocytes or macrophages *in vitro* and emigration of monocytes *in vivo*: it may account for accumulation of macrophages in DHS reactions.

(*b*) *A macrophage immobilising factor,* demonstrable by its inhibitory effect on the migration of macrophages, e.g. from the open end of a horizontal capillary tube. When the tube is immersed in tissue culture fluid, addition of this factor to the fluid inhibits migration. It may also play a role in the accumulation of macrophages in DHS reactions.

(*c*) *A macrophage activating factor,* which increases the metabolic activity of macrophages and enhances their capacity to kill phagocytosed micro-organisms. This microbicidal effect has been demonstrated *in vitro* and *in vivo.*

(*d*) *A specific macrophage-arming factor* (*SMAF*) has been demonstrated in experimentally-induced cell-mediated immunity to tumour cells. The DHS reaction between primed T cells and tumour cells releases a factor which confers on macrophages enhanced killing properties specific for the tumour cells. This factor differs from (*c*) above in that it is antigen-specific.

3. Other factors. Another factor released when primed T cells react with antigen is cytotoxic for tissue cells, and may contribute to the necrosis commonly seen in DHS reactions. There may also be factors which are chemotactic for, and stimulate mitosis of, non-primed lymphocytes.

Elucidation of these important factors is at an early stage. Their importance as mediators of the changes seen in DHS reactions is suggested by their detection not only in reactions in test tubes, but also in extracts of DHS reaction sites.

Although the major role of specifically primed T cells in DHS reactions has been emphasised above, it has been shown in animal experiments that most of the lymphocytes accumulating in such reactions are not specifically primed. The presence of these non-primed cells is unexplained, and their local effects are unknown. They may be derived from lymphoblasts which appear to migrate 'non-specifically' into inflammatory lesions of various types, or they may be attracted by chemotactic effects of lymphokines.

Man and other primates show, in general, much stronger cell-mediated immune responses and DHS reactions than do lower animals. It is therefore unwise to assume that the findings for guinea-pigs, etc., are applicable to man. **Lawrence's transfer factor** (p. 106) may be important in cellular immunity and DHS reactions in man, in whom it is far more readily demonstrable, and has a much more lasting effect, than any counterpart in guinea-pigs, etc.

Until recently, it was widely assumed that the presence of lymphocytes in a hypersensitivity reaction was a good indication of a DHS component, but it is now known that so-called K cells (p. 123), which have the appearances of small lymphocytes, may bind by surface Fc receptors to target cells sensitised with IgG class antibody and bring about their destruction. The *in vivo* significance of this co-operative cytotoxic effect of antibody and K 'lymphocytes' is not yet known. The presence of macrophages in hypersensitivity reactions is not necessarily indicative of DHS, for in some conditions immune complex formation induces emigration of monocytes rather than polymorphs.

Systemic effects of delayed hypersensitivity reactions

Although this account has concentrated on local DHS reactions, systemic reactions also occur. For example, injection of relatively large amounts of tuberculoprotein into an individual who has developed cell-mediated immunity to it results not only in a severe localised DHS reaction at the injection site, but also fever, malaise and a fall in the level of circulating lymphocytes. If the individual has active tuberculosis, the DHS reaction of the lesion is also aggravated, with extension of necrosis. These effects are known collectively as the *Koch phenomenon* after Robert Koch* who first described them. They are probably attributable to the release of lymphokines following the reaction between tuberculoprotein and specifically primed T cells in the blood, lymphoid tissues and tuberculous lesions. The fever of the Koch phenomenon and of active tuberculosis is probably a secondary effect, due to release of endogenous pyrogen (p. 156) by macrophages activated by lymphokines. The Koch phenomenon is not observed in individuals who have not developed cell-mediated immunity to tuberculoprotein.

Hypersensitivity to drugs and chemicals

Most drugs and chemicals which cause hypersensitivity reactions do so because they or their metabolic products combine with host proteins and act as haptens. At first sight, this seems to contradict the observation that haptens can only stimulate an immune response when combined with *foreign* carrier proteins to which the recipient develops cell-mediated immunity (p. 103). The explanation is that the many drugs

* The German bacteriologist who, in 1882, discovered the tubercle bacillus and showed it to be the cause of tuberculosis.

and chemicals which cause hypersensitivity reactions not only act as haptens, but alter the configuration of the protein molecules with which they combine, thus rendering them 'foreign'.

The type of hypersensitivity reaction which results will then depend on the nature of the immune response, the particular cell or tissue constituent with which the hapten has complexed, the route of administration and dose, etc. In individuals with a tendency to anaphylaxis, reaginic antibodies may develop, and further administration of the hapten can then induce an anaphylactic (type I) reaction, e.g. asthma or hay fever if the hapten is in the form of a gas, vapour, or airborne suspension, an immediate inflammatory reaction if it is applied locally, or a generalised reaction if a large amount of hapten is absorbed by any route. Anaphylactic reactions to penicillin and related compounds are not uncommon, and have resulted in a number of deaths: in most instances the hypersensitivity is directed towards the penicilloyl degradation product of penicillin. The development of IgG class antibody to a haptenic drug or chemical can give rise to local reactions of Arthus type (type III) when the hapten is localised to one particular area within the tissues, or can lead to formation of complexes of hapten and antibody within the plasma, which is liable to produce features closely resembling those of serum sickness.

Thirdly, a drug or its metabolites may bind to a particular type of cell, e.g. red cells, leukocytes or platelets, and cytotoxic antibody may then develop which will destroy the relevant type of cell after taking the drug. Examples of type II reactions of this sort include 'Sedormid purpura' and probably 'amidopyrine agranulocytosis'.

Lastly, cell-mediated immunity may develop towards the hapten–protein complex, and, as described above, subsequent absorption of the haptenic compound gives rise to a delayed hypersensitivity (type IV) reaction. This is seen in *contact dermatitis* in which relatively simple chemicals behave as haptens: they are absorbed into the body, often through the skin, and combine with tissue proteins. Cell-mediated immunity develops against the modified proteins, and subsequent skin contact with the same chemical induces a delayed hypersensitivity reaction (Fig.

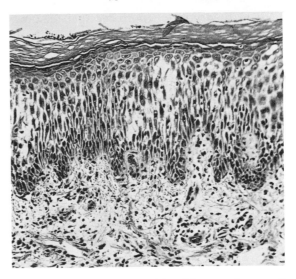

Fig. 5.9 Contact dermatitis. Note oedema of epidermis and perivascular infiltration of lymphocytes in the dermis. The patient had developed hypersensitivity to chromium salts used as a hardener in cement. × 110.

5.9), causing inflammatory lesions with cellular infiltration, predominantly lymphocytic, and oedema which affects both the dermis and epidermis and progresses to formation of vesicles. The substances capable of inducing this condition are very numerous, and include particularly chemicals which combine firmly with proteins, e.g. dyes, chrome salts, formalin and various derivatives of benzene. Reactions which appear to be of this type occur commonly in women in relation to nickel fasteners on underclothes, some of the nickel being dissolved by acid sweat and absorbed presumably as nickel salts which can combine with skin proteins. Contact with poison ivy is another common cause in North America, and cases also occur from the use of hair dyes, such as paraphenylene diamine, which, of course, bind firmly to keratin. Contact dermatitis results also from application of various medicaments to the skin. It is noteworthy that any individual can be sensitised to various chemicals, and contact dermatitis can thus be induced, but nevertheless some people appear to develop it more readily than others. This is seen in the use of various adhesive dressings which usually produce no reaction but in some instances lead to contact dermatitis, and a similar effect may result from wearing rubber face masks.

It is important to appreciate that the above account is an oversimplification. In many instances, hypersensitivity to drugs or chemicals is extremely complex and the clinical features often conflict with the results of the various available tests for hypersensitivity. With the ever-increasing number of chemicals used therapeutically and in industry, it is not surprising that hypersensitivity reactions, particularly those manifested in the skin and mucous membranes, are becoming increasingly common. It is not yet possible to state what properties of a substance are related to the likelihood of its stimulating the development of hypersensitivity, nor to predict which individuals are likely to develop it.

Auto-immunity and auto-immune diseases

Some confusion exists over the definitions of auto-antibodies and auto-immune diseases. **Auto-antibodies** may be defined as antibodies which react with the individual's own *normal* body constituents (which may accordingly be termed **auto-antigens**). This definition excludes antibodies which react only with body constituents which have been altered, for example by a haptenic drug, and so have become 'foreign' to the individual (see 'Sedormid' purpura, p. 122). The definition does not, however, presume that normal body constituents have necessarily stimulated the production of the auto-antibodies. It may be, for example, that a modified constituent has induced the production of antibodies which can cross-react with the normal constituent (see methyldopa-induced haemolytic anaemia, p. 122). Within this definition, auto-antibodies to several cell products or constituents are quite commonly present in the serum of individuals both with and without clinical evidence of disease: they include, for example, antibodies to thyroglobulin, to thyroid epithelial cells, to gastric parietal cells and to the deoxyribonucleoprotein of cell nuclei. These antibodies all react *in vitro* with the individual's own body constituents and with those obtained from others, so that they are acceptable as true auto-antibodies.

Although auto-immunisation occurs without clinical disease, it is strongly associated with a number of diseases. For example, most apparently normal individuals with thyroid auto-antibodies have been shown to have sub-clinical chronic thyroiditis, and patients with more severe, clinically apparent chronic thyroiditis usually have high titres of thyroid antibodies. Similarly, high titres of antibodies to deoxyribonucleoprotein occur especially in patients with the connective tissue diseases, and particularly in systemic lupus erythematosus.

Cell-mediated immunity to particular auto-antigens has also been demonstrated by *in vitro* tests in some diseases. For example thyroid auto-antigens inhibit the migration of leukocytes (p. 94) of patients with chronic thyroiditis.

It is thus apparent that, in some diseases, there is evidence of auto-immunisation against particular auto-antigenic body constituents. These are the so-called **auto-immune diseases**. In most instances, there is still some doubt whether the lesions are due to immunological reactions against the target auto-antigens; in some instances this probability is supported by production of similar lesions by auto-immunisation of animals, or by investigations on naturally-occurring auto-immune diseases in inbred strains of animals.

There are also a number of instances in which auto-antibodies develop as a result of tissue injury and appear to be without pathogenic effect, an example being auto-antibodies to myocardial cells which frequently develop following ischaemic necrosis of the myocardium; presumably antigen is released by the dead muscle cells and stimulates an immune response.

Auto-immune diseases may be classified into: (1) a group of organ-specific diseases affecting glandular tissues; (2) systemic lupus erythematosus and possibly the other connective tissue diseases; and (3) a number of miscellaneous diseases which do not fit readily into either of the above classes.

The organ-specific auto-immune diseases

These are characterised by chronic inflammatory destruction of a particular glandular tissue accompanied by the presence in the plasma of auto-antibodies which react specifically with normal cellular components of the target tissue. The four good examples of diseases in this group affect the thyroid, gastric mucosa, adrenal cortex and parathyroid glands respectively. The main features are exemplified by **chronic auto-immune thyroiditis**, in which infiltration of the thyroid gland by lymphocytes, plasma cells and macrophages is accompanied by glandular epithelial destruction and fibrosis. These changes may be focal and are then sub-clinical and usually non-progressive, or diffuse, giving rise to either thyroid enlargement, sometimes with hypofunction (*Hashimoto's thyroiditis*), or destruction and shrinkage of the gland with gross hypofunction (*primary myxoedema*). Auto-antibodies to normal thyroid constituents are detectable in the serum in virtually all cases of Hashimoto's thyroiditis, and in most cases of primary myxoedema and sub-clinical thyroiditis. They include antibodies reactive with: (1) thyroglobulin, often in sufficient concentration to give a precipitin reaction (Fig. 4.4, p. 90); (2) a second constituent of thyroid colloid; and (3) cell membrane constituents of thyroid epithelium—the so-called thyroid microsomal antibody (Fig. 4.8, p. 91). Chronic thyroiditis occurs much more often in women than in men, and the incidence increases with age. Over 10% of middle-aged or elderly women have one or more thyroid antibodies and some degree of chronic thyroiditis. There is a general correlation between the presence and titres of the serum antibodies and the extensiveness and activity of the thyroiditis, but the correlation is by no means exact for any one antibody or any combination of antibodies.

Chronic auto-immune gastritis, affecting the acid-secreting mucosa of the gastric fundus, has many points of resemblance to chronic thyroiditis. It affects women more often than men, and the incidence increases with age. In most cases, the serum contains 'microsomal' antibody to gastric parietal cells and, in a minority of cases, antibodies to the intrinsic factor essential to absorption of vitamin B_{12}. The affected mucosa is infiltrated with lymphocytes, plasma cells and macrophages, and all grades of destruction of chief and parietal cells are observed. In most cases, the gastritis is mild and sub-clinical, and progresses very slowly, but in some cases it progresses more rapidly to diffuse atrophy of the mucosa (like the thyroid in primary myxoedema) and parietal cell deficiency then results in achlorhydria and lack of intrinsic factor, the latter leading in some cases to B_{12} deficiency and pernicious anaemia.

Auto-immune adrenalitis is a much less common condition; it is, however, the major cause of adrenal cortical atrophy and functional deficiency (Addison's disease). The serum commonly contains 'microsomal' auto-antibody to a cell-membrane constituent of adrenocortical epithelium. **Primary hypoparathyroidism** is rare: specific auto-antibodies are demonstrable in the serum in some cases, and the parathyroid glands are shrunken and extremely difficult to find at necropsy.

In addition to their morphological and serological similarities, each of these diseases tends to have a high familial incidence, and moreover the diseases tend to occur in association, both within affected families and in individuals. For example, patients with Hashimoto's thyroiditis have a high incidence of gastric antibody and a particular tendency to develop pernicious anaemia, while thyroid and gastric antibodies, sometimes associated with the corresponding clinical diseases, are unduly common in patients with auto-immune Addison's disease or primary hypoparathyroidism: even these two latter rare diseases have been found to be particularly associated with one another.

Pathogenesis and aetiology. It has not been proved that these diseases are the result of auto-hypersensitivity reactions, an alternative explanation being that the glandular destruction is due to some other (unknown) agent, and that auto-antibodies develop as a secondary phenomenon. In favour of an auto-immune pathogenesis, auto-antibodies do not, in general, result from destruction of tissue. For example, thyroid injury by large doses of radio-iodine does not stimulate the production of thyroid antibodies, nor does recurrent alcoholic gastritis result in gastric antibodies. Secondly, organ-specific lesions resembling those of the human diseases, but usually reversible, can be induced experimentally in animals by injections of homogenates of the organ (e.g. thyroid or adrenal) incorporated in Freund's adjuvant. The adjuvant enhances immune responses, particularly those dependent on T lymphocytes (p. 94). Skin tests and investigations involving the transfer of these experimental diseases suggest that cell-mediated auto-immunity is important, and that delayed (type IV) auto-hypersensitivity plays an important pathogenic role. In the human diseases, the respective roles of auto-antibodies and cell-mediated immunity are unknown. Leukocyte migration inhibition tests suggest that cell-mediated immunity develops to antigens of the target organ, but the evidence is by no means conclusive. The lesions are typically infiltrated with lymphocytes, which suggests a delayed hypersensitivity reaction, but could also represent an antibody-dependent (type II) cytotoxic reaction (p. 123). Also, there are usually some, and often many, plasma cells in the lesions, and locally produced antibody might have a cytotoxic effect. In spite of the rather flimsy nature of the evidence, there is a fairly general belief that the lesions of these diseases are mediated largely by delayed hypersensitivity reactions.

The familial incidence of the organ-specific auto-immune diseases suggests a genetic predisposing factor, and this is supported by the greater concordance in monozygotic than in dizygotic twins (*i.e.* if one twin has the disease, the other is more likely to develop it if they are monozygotic). The studies on twins also indicate that there must also be environmental predisposing factors, and these have been the subject of speculation, but with little advance. One thyroid auto-antigen, thyroglobulin, is normally present in low concentration in the plasma, and appears to induce 'low-dosage' tolerance of T cells (p. 108): potentially responsive B cells have been demonstrated in normal individuals, but probably they require T-cell co-operation to produce antibody. If this applies to the other auto-antigens in these diseases, then breakdown of T-cell tolerance must be necessary for cell-mediated auto-immunity and auto-antibody production. It has been suggested that T-cell tolerance might be broken by modification of cell constituents by drugs, by microbial products, or by disorders of metabolism, but so far there is no evidence for any of these possibilities in the organ-specific auto-immune diseases. Another possibility is the defective functioning of suppressor T cells (pp. 108, 135).

Systemic lupus erythematosus

This is one of the so-called connective tissue diseases. It is characterised by acute and chronic inflammatory lesions in many organs and tissues, and by the occurrence in the plasma of various auto-antibodies, most of which react with normal constituents common to most types of cell in the body. The sites of lesions include the skin, muscles, joints, glomeruli, heart and blood vessels, but the distribution varies greatly and may be even wider. Auto-antibody to deoxyribonucleoprotein is nearly

always demonstrable in the serum by immunofluorescence tests (Fig. 5.10), and antibodies to DNA, RNA and various cytoplasmic cellular constituents, are commonly present. There may also be cytotoxic auto-antibodies to red cells, platelets and leukocytes and antibodies to clotting factors in the plasma.

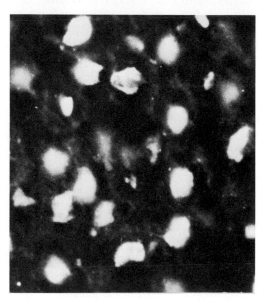

Fig. 5.10 Antibody to deoxyribonucleoprotein demonstrated by the immunofluorescence technique. Note the diffuse nuclear fluorescence. × 775. (Professor J. Swanson Beck.)

The auto-antibodies to nuclear and cytoplasmic constituents are not cytotoxic, and many of them occur in other diseases and, usually in low titre, in some normal subjects. The corresponding auto-antigens may, however, be released by breakdown of cells, and immune-complex (type III) reactions can then result. In fact, disease activity correlates fairly closely with the concentration of anti-DNA in the plasma (measured by DNA binding capacity of the serum) and low levels of serum complement. The glomerular lesions (p. 772) are due to deposition of immune complexes in the glomerular capillary basement membrane and subsequent complement fixation, and this process is responsible also for at least some of the lesions in the skin and elsewhere. Auto-antibodies to native (double-stranded) DNA are virtually specific for SLE and are mainly responsible for the renal lesions. Antibodies to denatured (single-stranded) DNA occur also in other diseases and do not correlate so closely with disease activity.

The familial occurrence of SLE, and of the various auto-antibodies associated with SLE, raises the possibility of genetic factors, and the spontaneous development of a very similar disease in the F1 hybrid of the NZB and NZW inbred strains of mice developed in New Zealand by Bielchowsky, provides a genetically-determined model.

One possibility is that immunological tolerance to DNA and other cell constituents is broken by modification of their antigenicity. For example, exposure to ultraviolet light, which is known to alter DNA, often increases the severity of SLE. Aggravation by various drugs may similarly be due to their combining with DNA and thus altering its antigenicity: there is evidence that some patients with SLE do not acetylate various drugs as rapidly as most normal individuals, and this may allow the drugs to bind with DNA.

There is also circumstantial evidence that a virus infection may be involved in SLE. Virus-like particles have been observed in the renal lesions, and are regularly discernible in the tissues of NZ mice. When maintained in tissue culture, lymphoid cells from these mice release C type RNA virus particles which *in vivo* stimulate the development of antibodies to DNA and RNA. It is possible that this virus, which is responsible for lymphoid neoplasia in mice, modifies the lymphoid cells in some way which predisposes them to auto-immune responses. There is also evidence that the SLE-like disease of NZ hybrid mice is related to thymic deficiency: 'thymic hormone' levels (p. 97) fall at a relatively early age in these mice, and the disease is accelerated by neonatal thymectomy and inhibited by injection of thymocytes from young mice. These observations, and the demonstration that animals rendered immuno logically tolerant to an antigen develop suppressor T cells which are capable, on transfer to a normal animal, of inhibiting the immune response to that antigen (p. 108), raise the possibility that auto-immune responses are normally inhibited by suppressor T cells, and that auto-immune diseases arise particularly in individuals with T-cell deficiencies. This might help to explain the high incidence of the organ-specific auto-immune diseases in elderly people, and also the observed high incidence of auto-antibodies in patients with congenital thymic deficiency (p. 141). In SLE, which occurs most commonly in women of reproductive age, serum antibody levels to some viruses are unusually high, and cell-mediated immune responses are impaired, suggesting that suppressor T-cell function may be deficient.

Other connective tissue diseases. Several other diseases, the most important of which is rheumatoid arthritis, are included in this group. They resemble SLE in that the lesions occur in various tissues, and are associated with some of the auto-antibodies found in SLE. However, in none of them is there good evidence of an auto-immune pathogenesis. Some patients present features of both SLE and one or other of these diseases, but the overlap is slight and undue significance has probably been attributed to it. Because of its high incidence, **rheumatoid arthritis** is the most important of the connective tissue diseases. The main feature is a destructive polyarthritis, in which the synovial membrane is infiltrated with lymphocytes, macrophages and plasma cells. Immune complexes and activated complement components are present in the synovial fluid and are deposited in the synovial membrane. In most cases, the serum contains **rheumatoid factors**: these are immuno-globulins (usually IgM) which behave as antibodies to auto-antigenic components of IgG. Rheumatoid factors react only weakly with native IgG, but strongly with IgG which has been heat-denatured, or with IgG antibody coupled with the corresponding antigen. Experimental evidence suggests that rheumatoid factors develop when IgG antibody forms immune complexes: binding with antigen alters the IgG molecule and renders it auto-antigenic.

The most likely cause of rheumatoid arthritis is an infection of the joints which results in an antibody response and formation of immune complexes in the joint fluid and synovial membrane. This, in turn, activates complement (the level of which is low in affected joints), with consequent inflammation and chemotaxis of phagocytes. Phagocytosis of complexes then results in release of lysosomal enzymes by polymorphs and macrophages, and these cause further tissue injury and bring in various other postulated mediators of the inflammatory reaction. High levels of rheumatoid factors are associated with severe disease, but this may be a secondary effect, due to intense stimulation by immune complexes. The postulated infection is of unknown nature: *Mycoplasma fermentans* has been suggested, but it may well be that different organisms can produce the same effect.

Polyarthritis is not uncommon in SLE, but is seldom so severe or destructive as rheumatoid arthritis. This and other associations do not indicate an auto-immune pathogenesis for rheumatoid arthritis, but merely that common genetic and possibly environmental factors predispose to both conditions.

The other so-called connective tissue diseases are dealt with in the relevant systematic chapters. Apart from the variable occurrence of anti-nuclear and other auto-antibodies, there is little evidence to suggest an auto-immune pathogenesis.

Other auto-immune diseases

Destruction of red cells, leukocytes and platelets by cytotoxic antibodies (p. 121) may occur in isolation, or in association with systemic lupus erythematosus. **Thyrotoxicosis** is another example of a lesion caused by cytotoxic antibody (p. 123) and is associated strongly with auto-immune thyroiditis and the other organ-specific auto-immune diseases.

Other diseases which may lie within the organ-specific group include: (1) some cases of *juvenile-onset diabetes mellitus*, in which auto-antibodies and cell-mediated auto-immunity to cells of the islets of Langerhans have been reported; (2) *ulcerative colitis*, in which the intestinal epithelium may be the target cell of an auto-immune response; and (3) some types of chronic liver disease, notably *primary biliary cirrhosis* and *chronic active hepatitis*, in which there is evidence of auto-immunity to components of bile-duct epithelium and hepatocytes respectively. Various other diseases could be mentioned, but as the list lengthens, the evidence becomes progressively weaker.

Rejection of transplanted tissues

The treatment of burns by skin grafting is a well-established procedure. The epidermis of autologous grafts extends to cover the denuded area and survives indefinitely, while a graft from another individual becomes established, but invariably undergoes necrosis within two or three weeks. Evidence that this rejection process is mediated by an immunological reaction on the part of the host was first provided by

Gibson and Medawar (1943) working in Glasgow. In a series of important experiments, Medawar and his colleagues went on to lay the foundations of transplant immunology. They showed that skin grafts between syngeneic* mice were accepted permanently, while allografts stimulated an immune response in the host and were consequently destroyed ('rejected') 1–3 weeks after grafting. They also showed that mice injected at birth with allogeneic cells would subsequently accept permanently a skin graft from the same donor strain and that this state of unresponsiveness—the first experimental demonstration of acquired immunological tolerance (p. 107)—could be abolished, with consequent rejection of the skin graft, by injection of host-strain lymphocytes from a normal mouse or from one that had previously rejected a graft from the allogeneic strain. Lymphocytes from the latter mouse induced more rapid and intense graft rejection, showing that, as a result of previously rejecting an allograft, it had developed persistent immunity, manifested by the reactivity of its lymphoid cells. This early work suggested the importance of cell-mediated immunity in allograft rejection. It is true that antibodies also developed in the recipients of allografts, but their injection into tolerant animals bearing an appropriate allograft did not result in rejection.

Medawar's major observations and conclusions have been confirmed in experiments involving transplantation of various tissues in many vertebrate species. The mechanism of rejection is complex, but in most situations cell-mediated immunity plays a major role and the graft is destroyed mainly by a delayed hypersensitivity (type IV) reaction, cytotoxic and macrophage-stimulating lymphokines (p. 129) being released by specifically-responsive T lymphoid cells which have reacted with graft antigens. In organs such as the kidney, which are transplanted by connecting the major blood vessels of the graft to host vessels, injury may result also from a cytotoxic antibody (type II) reaction as described below.

Transplant antigens. The cells of probably all vertebrates possess numerous surface iso-antigens, termed transplant antigens. In several species, including man, a major system of strong antigens, characteristic for each species

---

* For terminology, see p. 87.

and determined by multiple alleles at a complex locus, has been demonstrated. In man, this is the HLA system of antigens: each individual inherits HLA antigens from each parent as shown in Fig. 5.11.

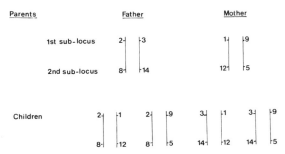

Fig. 5.11 The major histocompatibility complex in man contains at least four allelic genes, situated close together on the same chromosome (No. 6). The diagram shows the mode of inheritance of genes of the first two sub-loci, which code respectively for one antigen of the HLA-A series (antigens 1, 2, 3, 9, 10, 11, 28) and one antigen of the HLA-B series (antigens 5, 7, 8, 12, 13, 14, 17, 27). The individual thus inherits a pair of antigens (one from each parent) in each series. Because of their close linkage, the genes, and so the antigens, are inherited in 'sets', so that siblings with the same antigens in one series (e.g. the same HLA-A antigens) are likely to have the same antigens in the other series. This is shown above for HLA-A and HLA-B antigens, but it applies also to the HLA-C and -D antigens, and explains why there is a 25% chance that two siblings will inherit identical sets of antigens. Transplantation between such siblings is usually highly successful.

In rats and mice, the major transplant antigens are the main factors in determining the intensity of the iso-immune response, and thus of rejection, following transplantation. In human renal transplantation, matching has so far been limited by the availability of suitable antisera and has been restricted largely to HLA-A and -B antigens which (together with HLA-C antigens) are detectable by means of antisera (p. 138). Although the prognosis for well-matched grafts is better than for poorly-matched grafts, there have been many exceptions and it now seems likely that matching for HLA-D antigens (formerly LD antigens) is also important: these antigens are not yet detectable serologically, and matching for them is performed by the mixed lymphocyte reaction in which lymphocytes from the patient requiring a transplant are incubated with lymphocytes

from a prospective donor and examined for DNA synthesis or 'blast' transformation, which indicate incompatibility.

By analogy with the mouse, there is probably also a human system of Ir genes, which exert a genetic influence on immune responsiveness, in the vicinity of the HLA loci.

Graft versus host reaction. If normal lymphoid cells are injected into an allogeneic host, they will be destroyed unless the host is immunologically deficient or tolerant and cannot mount a rejection reaction. In these circumstances, the grafted cells may survive and mount an immune response against the host, with a consequent graft-versus-host (g.v.h.) reaction. This occurs when allogeneic lymphocytes from an adult mouse are injected into neonates or into mice rendered immunodeficient, e.g. by thymectomy and x-irradiation, and when an F1 hybrid mouse is injected with lymphocytes of either parental strain. The g.v.h. reaction is complex and includes splenomegaly, lymph node enlargement, haemolytic anaemia and predisposition to infections. When induced in the neonate, these changes, together with impairment of growth, have been termed *runt disease*. The same condition has occurred in man when lymphoid or bone marrow cells are injected into patients with severe congenital T-cell deficiencies (p. 141) or into patients who have received gross overdosage of x-irradiation or other immunosuppressive agents.

Human renal transplantation

Some thousands of kidneys have been transplanted in the past few years to patients with irreversible renal failure. The major obstacle is immunological rejection of the graft and, except for transplants between identical twins, it is essential to protect the graft by administration of immunosuppressive drugs such as glucocorticoids, azathioprine or actinomycin C. Initially, high dosage is necessary to prevent acute rejection, but the dosage can gradually be reduced, in some cases to very low levels, without rejection occurring. This indicates that the host becomes increasingly less responsive to the graft antigens. One possible explanation is that the continued release of antigens by the graft, together with immunosuppression, results in specific immunological tolerance. Another is that the host develops 'enhancing' antibodies

(p. 106) which protect the graft by suppressing the cell-mediated immune response or by combining with graft antigens and so concealing them from specifically responsive T lymphocytes. Administration of iso-antibodies reactive with antigens of the grafted tissue has been shown to prolong graft survival in animals, and there is preliminary evidence that administration of HLA antibodies may have a similar enhancing effect in human renal transplantation, although such antibodies (presumably in larger amounts) can also cause immediate rejection (see below).

While on large doses of immunosuppressive drugs, transplant patients are very liable to develop infections, both with virulent pathogens and with opportunistic micro-organisms such as cytomegalovirus, *Pneumocystis carinii* and various fungi.

In spite of these problems, approximately 50% of the transplants have done well and are functioning some years later.

Rejection reactions. Immediate rejection, within minutes of renal transplantation, may occur when the kidney donor's ABO blood group is incompatible for the recipient, or when, as a result of pregnancy, blood transfusion or a previous transplant, the recipient has developed HLA antibodies reactive with the donor's cells. In these circumstances, platelet and red cell aggregates occur in the small vessels of the graft; blood flow ceases and, unless removed, the kidney becomes necrotic.

Acute rejection during the month or so following transplantation is usually due to the development of cell-mediated immunity: host lymphoid cells and macrophages accumulate in and around the tubules and bring about destruction of the tubular epithelium. This type of reaction is not often seen in severe form in immunosuppressed patients. Acute rejection may also take the form of necrosis and thrombosis of arterioles, due apparently to the reaction of host antibodies and complement with transplant antigens of the graft. In chronic rejection, vascular obliteration is often prominent (Fig. 5.12) and changes resembling membranous glomerulonephritis may develop, even years after transplantation.

Each of these types of rejection can destroy the transplanted kidney. If it can be detected at an early stage, rejection can sometimes be stopped by more intense therapy with immuno-

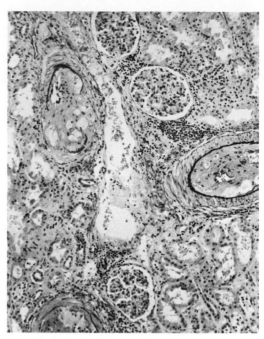

Fig. 5.12 Chronic rejection of a human renal allotransplant. Note the obliterative arterial changes and disruption of the arterial walls. (Professor K. A. Porter.)

suppressant drugs or perhaps antilymphocyte globulin (p. 99). There are, however, no simple and reliable methods of predicting rejection or of distinguishing it from other causes of renal failure. During the first week or two, cadaver renal transplants are often anuric as a result of the ischaemia which precedes their transfer to the patient, and rejection during this period cannot be detected without biopsy of the graft.

Tissue typing. At present, tissue typing is usually performed by a cytotoxicity test, using typing antisera and complement, upon cells of the individual to be typed: if the cells possess the corresponding iso-antigen, they will be killed (Fig. 1.3, p. 4). All tissue cells, leukocytes and platelets (but not red cells) possess HLA antigens, and it is convenient to use blood lymphocytes for typing. HLA antisera are obtained from recipients of blood transfusions or previous transplants, or from parous women, some of whom have developed antibodies to HLA antigens of the fetus. By testing with a panel of lymphocytes of known HLA phenotypes, and suitable absorption to remove unwanted antigens, specific HLA antisera can be provided.

As mentioned above, the HLA-D antigens, detectable by the mixed lymphocyte reaction (p. 137) are likely to be important in clinical renal transplantation. By rendering the donor's lymphocytes unresponsive by treatment with mitomycin C, the reaction of the recipient's lymphocytes to donor HLA-D antigens can be determined (the 'one-way' mixed lymphocyte reaction).

For reasons explained above, it is essential to ensure ABO compatibility in human renal transplantation, and to test the recipient's serum for cytotoxic antibody to donor cells.

Transplantation of other tissues

Infusion of **haemopoietic cells**, which include pluripotent stem cells (p. 104), is a logical treatment for certain immunodeficiency diseases (see below) and for patients exposed to excessive doses of ionising radiations. The depressed immunological status of the recipient helps to protect the donor's cells against rejection, but there is also the danger of fatal graft-versus-host reaction by lymphoid cells derived from the donor's stem cells, and precise HLA matching, which usually means the use of a sibling as donor, is essential.

Successful **corneal allografting** has long been practised without immunosuppression of the recipient. This is because the cornea is avascular and therefore a 'protected site' in which the graft does not induce an immune response in the recipient. If, as sometimes happens, blood vessels extend into the grafted cornea, then rejection occurs.

In allografts of **blood vessels** and **tendon**, the cells either die from ischaemia or are destroyed by a rejection reaction, but the collagen and elastic fibres persist, and are repopulated with host cells and vessels: thus the use of stored vessel or tendon is equally, if not more effective. Similarly, the cells of **bone grafts** die, but the matrix may provide the desired mechanical effect (p. 811). The use of **cartilage grafts** in plastic surgery is of considerable interest: both the cells and the matrix of allografts may survive for long periods without inducing a rejection reaction. This is due to the avascular nature of cartilage, and to the matrix which allows diffusion of nutrients and metabolites between graft chondrocytes and host, but acts as an 'immunological barrier' between them.

Another exception to the general phenomenon of allograft rejection is provided by nature's allograft, **pregnancy**. The trophoblast, of fetal origin, is bathed in maternal blood, and yet it is tolerated for nine months, in spite of the presence of incompatible (paternal) transplant antigens in the fetal cells. There is slight depression of maternal immune responsiveness during pregnancy, but the mother does not develop specific immunological tolerance to the fetus. The most likely explanation of failure to reject the fetus appears to be that the cells of the syncytiotrophoblast are coated with a layer of mucopolysaccharide, which provides an 'immunological barrier'. As already mentioned, pregnancy commonly results in the development of maternal antibodies to the transplant antigens of the fetus, but this is without apparent effect.

Immunological Deficiency States

There are a large number of conditions in which the normal defence mechanisms against invasive micro-organisms are impaired. For most purposes it is useful to classify such deficiencies into two major groups. Firstly, deficiencies of non-specific resistance, as in diabetes mellitus, impaired function of neutrophil polymorphs (p. 459), etc. This miscellaneous group is dealt with under the appropriate diseases: it includes also lesions which impair resistance locally, for example obstruction of hollow viscera, as in the urinary tract or air passages,

and ischaemia of the lower limb leading to gangrene.

In the second major group, which is discussed here, impaired resistance is due to defects in specific immunological responsiveness. These are best classified into primary and secondary types, and also in relation to the type of immunological defect present.

In the group of *primary conditions*, the immunological deficiency becomes manifest usually, but not always, in early childhood, and in most of the conditions there is good evidence that the defect is genetically determined. Other abnormalities, e.g. thrombocytopenia in the Wiskott–Aldrich syndrome, or hypoparathyroidism in the Di George syndrome, may accompany the immunological defect, giving rise to characteristic disease complexes, but the immunological deficiency is not secondary to the other parts of the syndrome. By contrast, the *secondary immunological deficiencies* occur at any age, are not genetically-determined, and the immunological defects are the result of injury to the lymphoid tissues, either by various disease processes, particularly lymphoid neoplasia, or by immunosuppressive agents.

The type of immunological defect present determines the clinical picture and form of therapy required. The division of lymphoid cells into two major classes—thymic-dependent (T) and thymic-independent (B)—has been dealt with in Chapter 4. Its validity in man is demonstrated by the occurrence of immunodeficiency states affecting mainly T-cell function, with depression of cell-mediated immune responses, or mainly B-cell function, with depression of antibody production: combined deficiencies, affecting both T- and B-cell function, are also observed. Such well-defined immunodeficiencies occur as primary, congenital defects, but they are rare. Less serious and less clearly-defined deficiencies also occur, both as congenital and acquired conditions.

Primary immunological deficiencies

(1) Deficiency of B-cell function. This group is exemplified by **infantile sex-linked agammaglobulinaemia**, which was the first to be described and is sometimes known as the **Bruton type of agammaglobulinaemia** after its discoverer. The major abnormality is a virtually complete inability to produce the three major classes of immunoglobulins—IgG, IgM and IgA. In consequence, there is little or no antibody production in response to infections or immunisation procedures, and the normal blood group iso-antibodies are usually not detectable. The condition is observed nearly always in boys, being transmitted by a gene defect in the X chromosome (sex-linked recessive). Symptoms usually arise in the second year of life, protection before that being provided by maternal

antibodies of IgG class transmitted to the fetus. The defect results in unusually frequent and serious bacterial infections, particularly those due to the pyogenic bacteria, and including respiratory and pulmonary infections, meningitis and septicaemia. 'Opportunistic' infections (p. 144), e.g. pneumonia due to the protozoon, *Pneumocystis carinii*, also occur, and candidiasis is common. The infections respond to appropriate antibiotics, and diagnosis depends upon the demonstration of the near-absence of serum IgG (below 50 mg per 100 ml), IgM and IgA (below 3 mg per 100 ml). Deficiency of IgG cannot be demonstrated until the maternal IgG has fallen to a low level—usually by about 8 months old, although very low levels of the other two immunoglobulins are observed before this time, since they do not cross the placenta.

The lymph nodes and tonsils are small, and biopsy reveals an absence of germinal centres and plasma cells, while plasma cells are also absent from the rectal mucosa. The blood lymphocytes are not greatly diminished, but B lymphocytes are virtually absent. The thymus is normal, and cell-mediated immune responses are not impaired. Accordingly, the responses to BCG and vaccinial immunisation are normal and afford protection, and virus infections in general occur with the same frequency and clinical features as in normal children. Chronic polyarthritis, closely resembling rheumatoid arthritis, is of common occurrence.

The effectiveness of regular injections of human IgG in preventing infections has increased the importance of early diagnosis. It is important to distinguish the Bruton type of agammaglobulinaemia, which requires life-long therapy, from **transient hypogammaglobulinaemia**. This latter condition presents similar clinical features and morphological changes in the lymphoid tissues, but is merely a delay, and not a permanent failure, of the capacity to produce immunoglobulins: it is familial, affects both sexes, and the defect disappears within the first three years of life. In most cases, severe immunoglobulin deficiency is limited to IgG, and normal levels of IgM and IgA in the serum may help to distinguish it from the Bruton type.

There are a number of less well-defined conditions which appear to fall within this group. In all of them, there is defective production of one or more classes of immunoglobulins, impairment of antibody production, and relatively normal cell-mediated immune responses. The evidence favouring a genetic predisposition, and a particular mode of genetic transmission, varies in the different types. In some forms, the immunological deficiency does not become manifest until adult life, and yet the disease tends to occur in families, and often exhibits a familial association with other immunological disturbances, e.g. hypergammaglobulinaemia and systemic lupus erythematosus. Some patients with such late-onset immunoglobulin deficiency also develop auto-immune diseases such as pernicious anaemia and connective tissue diseases, but without demonstrable auto-antibodies.

(2) Deficiency of T-cell function. An example of this group is provided by the rare **Di George syndrome**, in which there is almost complete failure of development of the thymus and parathyroids.

In those infants who survive the neonatal period, immunoglobulin production appears normal, although antibody responses, at least to some antigens, are impaired. The lymph nodes contain plasma cells and germinal centres, but the paracortical (thymus-dependent) areas are deficient in small lymphocytes, and the number of circulating lymphocytes, although variable, is low in some cases. The condition may affect infants of both sexes, and there is no evidence for a genetic predisposition. Affected infants suffer from 'opportunistic' infections, e.g. by *Pneumocystis carinii* (p. 420) and fungi and also from severe virus infections. Impairment of cell-mediated immunity is demonstrable by failure to develop contact hypersensitivity to agents such as dinitrochlorobenzene (p. 100) and immunisation with live vaccines is liable to give rise to fatal generalised infections. The condition is fatal: in a few instances life has been prolonged by transplantation of thymic tissue, but the problem here is to prevent rejection of the grafted thymus by the host T lymphocytes which generate under its influence.

(3) Combined immunological deficiency. In **alymphocytic agammaglobulinaemia**, sometimes termed the **Swiss type of agammaglobulinaemia**, both the thymus-dependent and -independent immunity systems fail to develop. The thymus is hypoplastic and deficient in Hassall's corpuscles and small lymphocytes, the lymph nodes are extremely small and lacking in germinal centres, lymphocytes and plasma cells, and circulating lymphocytes are scanty. There is a near-absence of the three main classes of immunoglobulins from the serum, and both antibody production and cell-mediated immunity are grossly defective. The condition is transmitted as an autosomal recessive character, and affected infants show retarded growth, recurrent bacterial and virus infections, and response to antibiotics and chemotherapy is poor. Immunisation with living viruses is likely to prove fatal, and the condition usually results in death during the first or second year. The basic defect appears to lie in the haemopoietic stem cells (p. 450), which fail to undergo lymphopoiesis.

Combined immunological deficiency occurs also in **reticular dysgenesis**, in which there is a deficiency of haemopoietic stem cells, resulting in failure of lymphopoiesis and haemopoiesis: death usually occurs before or shortly after birth.

In both these conditions, the deficiencies are restored by infusion of haemopoietic cells, which include stem cells, but there is a grave risk of fatal graft-versus-host reaction (p. 137).

(4) Other primary immunological deficiencies are mostly of obscure nature. In **ataxia telangiectasia** there are widespread vascular defects resulting in dilatation of small vessels (telangiectases), and an insidiously-developing immunodeficiency with depression of cell-mediated immunity and low levels of IgE and IgA in the blood. The IgG level is also low in some cases. Recurrent infections of the paranasal sinuses and lungs are the most common consequences of the immunological defect. In some instances the thymus has been found to be poorly developed and lacking in Hassall's corpuscles. The condition appears to be determined genetically by an autosomal recessive gene.

Another condition in which immunodeficiency develops insidiously is the **Wiskott–Aldrich syndrome** in which the platelets are abnormal or reduced in number. There is progressive depletion of lymphocytes in the blood and in the T-dependent areas of the lymphoid tissues. The blood levels of IgM and IgA gradually fall and cell-mediated immunity declines. The condition is determined by a sex-linked genetic defect and affects boys, eczema, attacks of diarrhoea and recurrent infections being common features. Recent reports suggest that administration of Lawrence's transfer factor has a restorative effect on the immunodeficiencies in this condition, in which the thymus appears normal or is slightly diminished in size.

Secondary immunological deficiencies

These are conditions in which the immunity system develops and functions normally but becomes defective from the direct or indirect effect of various disease processes or immunosuppressive agents. Causal conditions include malnutrition, certain infections, various forms of cancer and renal failure.

Susceptibility to infections is a well-known feature of malnutrition, but it is only recently that **protein deficiency**, both experimental and in man, has been demonstrated to impair cell-mediated immune responsiveness. Because of its prevalence in many parts of the world, this is probably the most important cause of immunodeficiency.

Depression of cell-mediated immunity may be a feature of various **acute virus infections**, but has been demonstrated most clearly in measles and infectious mononucleosis, in both of which a temporary depression of cell-mediated immunity has been shown by skin tests (e.g. to tuberculoprotein) becoming negative, and by impaired responsiveness of lymphocytes to stimulation *in vitro* by antigens or phytomitogens (see below).

Impaired cell-mediated immunity occurs also in some **bacterial and protozoal infections** in which there is extensive colonisation of the macrophage system, e.g. lepromatous leprosy and leishmaniasis. T-cell function is depressed also in **sarcoidosis**, a condition of unknown cause characterised by tubercle-like granulomas of the lymphoid and various other tissues.

Patients with **advanced cancer** commonly have depression of both T and B cell function: without doubt, this is a result of cancer, although there is evidence that the incidence of cancer (of both the lymphoid and epithelial tissues) is increased in patients who survive with primary immunodeficiencies and in patients on long-term immunosuppressive therapy, e.g. following renal transplantation.

Immunodeficiencies are particularly common in patients with **lymphoid neoplasia (lymphoma)**. In chronic lymphocytic leukaemia, there is very often deficient T and B cell function; this may be due to crowding of the lymphoid tissues, marrow and blood with neoplastic (usually B) lymphocytes. It is, however, of interest that immunosuppression is an early effect of infection

with the oncornaviruses, which induce lymphomas in animals, and it is likely that human chronic lymphocytic leukaemia (and some other lymphomas) are also virus-induced. Depression of antibody levels is a feature of multiple myeloma, a plasma-cell tumour usually confined to the bone marrow; the high levels of Ig secreted by the myeloma cells increase the rate of Ig catabolism and may also depress antibody responses.

In a third lymphoid neoplasm, Hodgkin's disease, the lymphoid tissues are often extensively infiltrated, and T-cell deficiency is then the usual result: tuberculosis or virus infection (e.g. varicella zoster) may prove fatal.

The immunodeficiency of **renal failure** affects T-cell, and probably also B-cell, function. This is important in renal transplantation because it helps initially to prevent rejection of the transplanted kidney.

Assessment of immunological function

In cases of suspected immunodeficiency, information can be obtained from examination of the blood to determine: (*a*) the levels of the various classes of Ig; (*b*) the presence and titres of AB blood group antibodies; and (*c*) the proportions and numbers of T and B lymphocytes. The responsiveness of lymphocytes to stimulation by antigens, e.g. tuberculoprotein, and to phytomitogens, gives some indication of function. Blast-cell transformation occurs when normal blood lymphocytes are cultured in the presence of phytohaemagglutinin (PHA) or concanavalin A (con-A), both of which stimulate T cells, pokeweed mitogen (PWM) which stimulates both T and B cells, and bacterial endotoxin, which stimulates B cells.

Other tests include assay of antibodies against commonly encountered antigens, and cell-mediated immunity may be investigated by skin tests or *in vitro* techniques (p. 94). Finally, antigens may be administered and the responses measured, but live vaccines should not be used for this purpose in subjects who may not be able to eliminate even attenuated microorganisms.

With increasing use of immunosuppressive

and cytotoxic drugs—cortisone, azathioprene, cyclophosphamide, etc., and also radiotherapy, infections due to immunodeficiencies are becoming common, and often limiting factors in renal transplantation and the treatment of various forms of cancer and other fatal diseases. Some of these agents destroy not only lymphocytes, but also polymorphs and macrophages, and thus depress resistance to infection in more than one way.

6

Host–Parasite Relationships

Throughout evolutionary development, many species have adapted to a parasitic existence, living in or on the surface of a host of another species, from which they derive warmth, nourishment and mobility. The relationship is not necessarily harmful to the host, and may be advantageous. For example, various relatively harmless bacteria colonise the skin of man and help to exclude more harmful bacteria, while reabsorption of bile pigment from the gut and the production of vitamin K depend largely on the metabolic activities of the intestinal bacterial flora. These normal inhabitants of the skin and mucous membranes are called **commensals**. Other parasites, termed **pathogens**, are less well adapted and by injuring the host endanger their own survival: they include many species of micro-organisms (microbes) including viruses, bacteria, fungi and protozoa and also metazoa of various sizes. The terms **pathogenicity** and **virulence** are commonly used synonymously to indicate the capacity of a particular micro-organism to cause disease.

Although it is important to distinguish between commensals and pathogens, the distinction is not absolute, for many commensals are only harmless so long as they are kept at bay by the host's defence mechanisms. In immunodeficiency states, for example, various normally harmless microbes may behave as 'opportunistic' pathogens. Similarly, a breach of local defence mechanisms, even in a normal individual, may allow commensals to cause severe infections, an example being *Escherichia coli*, which normally inhabits the gut: this bacterium may be introduced into the urinary tract by catheterisation of the bladder, and may then cause severe acute pyogenic inflammation, even extending into the kidneys. Local abnormalities in the host may also predispose to injury by commensals: for instance, heart valves which have been scarred and distorted by rheumatic

fever are readily colonised by *Streptococcus viridans*, a bacterium which lives in the mouth and finds its way into the blood following tooth extraction, or even when the teeth are brushed vigorously. In normal individuals it is quickly eliminated, but it can settle and multiply in the distorted valve cusps, causing bacterial endocarditis. Because the distinction between pathogens and commensals is not sharp, it is helpful to use the term **infection** to indicate the presence of a particular type of micro-organism in a part of the body where it is normally absent, and where, if allowed to multiply, it is likely to be harmful, i.e. to cause **infective disease**.

As implied above, most infective diseases depend on penetration of the host's tissues by micro-organisms, and the factors concerned in such invasion provide the first major topic of this chapter. Following invasion, the microbes may be eliminated without causing obvious disease (inapparent infection) or clinical disease of any grade of severity may follow: the factors determining these events form a second major topic. Lastly, two important reactions to infection, neutrophil leukocytosis and fever, will be considered.

The subject of infective disease is extremely complex, involving as it does a consideration of the relationships between man and numerous species and strains of micro-organisms. The following account is limited to a brief outline of the subject.

Factors determining invasion

The skin and mucous membranes are exposed to many different types of micro-organisms present in expired droplets in the air, in dust particles, and in food and water. The skin and various mucous membranes on which these organisms settle have properties which render them suitable for the survival and sometimes multiplication of certain organisms, but inhospitable to others. In some instances, the requirements of a particular microbe for growth *in vitro* help to explain its colonisation of particular parts of the surface of the body, but many of the factors determining such colonisation are still unknown, and indeed the predilection of certain bacteria for a particular host species is in most instances quite unexplained. Nevertheless, certain factors are known to be of great importance in limiting or preventing invasion by many types of microbes, and these must be considered briefly.

Barriers to invasion

(a) **Mechanical barriers.** The superficial keratinised layer of the epidermis is an excellent mechanical barrier to microbial invasion, and provided it is kept clean and dry, direct invasion is extremely unlikely. Penetration may however occur when dirt is allowed to accumulate on the skin and particularly in moist warm areas subject to friction, such as the axillae and sub-mammary folds. In many skin diseases which result in exudation with loss or sogginess of the keratin layer, bacterial and fungal infections are common complications. The conjunctival, nasal, oral and gastro-intestinal mucosae, covered as they are by a film of mucous or serous secretion, also present a formidable barrier to most types of micro-organisms.

Wounds and ulcers of the skin and mucous membranes open up pathways for bacterial invasion and are obviously important causes of infection. Burns are particularly liable to become heavily infected because the dead superficial tissue provides a good medium for coliform bacilli, staphylococci, pyocyaneus and many other bacteria. Some parasitic organisms have evolved a life cycle in which they multiply in insect vectors and are introduced to man and other hosts by the insect bite. Examples include the protozoa which cause malaria, the metazoan filarial worms, and the virus of yellow fever, all of which are transmitted by mosquitoes. *Yersinia pestis*, the cause of bubonic plague (the Black Death), is transmitted by the flea of the black rat, and the rickettsiae which cause typhus are spread by ticks, mites and lice.

In the mouth, tooth extraction and tonsillectomy inevitably lead to bacterial invasion, and tonsillectomy has been shown to predispose to invasion by the virus of poliomyelitis in the postoperative period. Vitamin A and C deficiencies also impair the resistance of the mucous membranes and skin to bacterial invasion.

(b) **Glandular secretions.** The secretions of glands opening on to the skin surface play an important role by maintaining the integrity of the skin, and also by providing an environment in which many types of bacteria cannot survive for long. The acidity of the sweat and the long-chain unsaturated fatty acids produced by the action of commensal bacteria on sebaceous secretion both exert a selective bactericidal effect, and consequently the bacterial flora of the skin surface tends to be rather constant: it has been shown that some types of pathogenic bacteria, when placed on the skin, are virtually all destroyed within an hour or two. The secretions of mucous membranes possess similar qualities. **Lysozyme**, an enzyme which digests the mucopeptide of bacterial cell walls, is present in high concentration in the lacrimal gland secretion and probably exerts an important protective effect in the conjunctival sac: it is secreted also by the salivary and nasal glands but in much smaller amounts. **Antibodies of IgA class**, modified by addition of a 'transport piece' so that they are resistant to digestive enzymes, are present in saliva, tears, intestinal contents, respiratory tract mucus, milk and urine (p. 89). Provided that IgA antibody has developed against a particular organism as a result of previous infection, it will be represented in these secretions. This is of importance in preventing invasion by certain viruses, for the virus may encounter the antibody in the surface mucus and be neutralised by it: its significance in relation to bacterial invasion is less certain, although there is evidence that IgA antibody may render bacteria highly susceptible to the lytic action of lysozyme.

The acidity of the gastric juice is effective in killing most types of microbes ingested in food or water; but hypochlorhydria due to chronic gastritis is common, and minor illnesses and even emotional stresses can reduce temporarily the acidity of the juice. In general, those microbes which cause intestinal infections, such as the salmonellae and dysentery bacilli, are relatively acid-resistant. *Entamoeba histolytica,* the cause of amoebic dysentery, produces cysts which resist the gastric juice and pass through the stomach before hatching out and invading the wall of the colon.

The normal acidity of the urine contributes to the defences of the urinary tract against infection. Also there is a mucosal factor which eliminates bacteria in contact with the urinary tract epithelium, for it has been shown that when the mucosa of the rabbit's bladder is exposed and *Esch. coli* placed on its surface, the numbers of living bacteria diminish rapidly.

(c) Secretion currents. The continuous flow of tears over the surface of the conjunctiva has an important effect in the removal of contaminating bacteria, which are carried rapidly into the nasopharynx. In the nose and mouth also, the secretions covering the mucosa flow towards the pharynx and hence to the stomach, carrying with them residual food particles, bacteria, etc. The importance of the saliva is illustrated by the oral infections and severe dental caries which accompany loss of salivary secretion in Sjøgren's syndrome (p. 535). The lacrimal secretion is also diminished, and conjunctival infections result. The importance of removal of contaminating bacteria by the saliva may explain the common occurrence of infection in the crypts of the tonsils and also in the periodontal sulci, for once bacteria gain entrance to these spaces, they are out of the main stream of salivary flow.

In the respiratory tract there is a continuous flow of mucus upwards over the surface of the bronchial and tracheal mucosa: inhaled particles are caught up and removed in this stream, and the air is almost sterile by the time it reaches the respiratory bronchioles. This defence mechanism is dependent on a normal production of mucous secretion and on the integrity of the ciliated respiratory epithelium. The virus of influenza parasitises the respiratory epithelium, interfering with its protective function: as a result, secondary bacterial infection invariably develops, and by extending into the alveoli may give rise to pneumonia. The integrity of the respiratory mucosa is also seriously impaired in chronic bronchitis, most commonly due to cigarette smoking but also to atmospheric pollution: this leads to metaplasia, the ciliated epithelium being replaced by goblet cells or squamous epithelium: there is increase in the amount of secretion, which also becomes more viscous, and this tends to stagnate and become infected.

Intestinal pathogens, such as the salmonellae of 'food poisoning' and the shigellae of bacillary dysentery, induce an acute inflammatory reaction in the intestinal mucosa: diarrhoea results from the increased peristalsis and exudation, and repeated evacuation of the gut helps to get rid of the offending bacteria.

The flow of urine is of importance in preventing growth and spread of any bacteria gaining entrance to the urinary tract by the urethra, and any abnormality resulting in stagnation of urine or incomplete emptying of the bladder, particularly if chronic, e.g. obstruction by an enlarged prostate, predisposes to infection.

(d) Bacterial commensals. In spite of the defence mechanisms described above, the skin, mouth, nasal cavity, conjunctival sac and intestines are all colonised by bacteria of various types. The local environment provided by each of these various surfaces favours the survival of particular types of bacteria and thus each regional surface develops its own flora. In their usual site of colonisation, most of these commensals are non-pathogenic, and they tend to prevent the establishment of other types of microbes, including pathogens, by competing for nutrients and by release of metabolic products which are toxic to other organisms.

In normal circumstances the bacterial florae of the various surfaces are remarkably stable, but if they are disturbed, colonisation by pathogens may result: hence the common occurrence of fungal infections of the pharynx in patients on antibiotic therapy, and the overwhelming growth of resistant staphylococci in the intestines which may arise when the normal flora is depressed by broad-spectrum antibiotics. 'Seeding' of the gut with non-pathogenic bacteria has achieved some success in preventing the overgrowth of pathogens in neonates and in patients treated by antibiotics.

(e) Phagocytes. There is evidence that phagocytic cells migrate on to the surface of various mucous membranes: for example neutrophil polymorphs pass through the thin epithelium lining the depths of the tonsillar crypts, and macrophages pass into the alveoli of the lungs. In both these sites the migrant cells have been shown to phagocytose particles on the surface of the mucosa and this may play a role in preventing invasion.

Invasive capacity of micro-organisms

Micro-organisms vary greatly in their capacity to invade the host's defensive barriers. Most bacteria cause injury only after invading the host's tissues, but some are virtually incapable of invasion and yet can produce disease. For example, *Clostridium tetani*, the cause of tetanus, flourishes only in dead tissue, foreign material and exudate in wounds, but its toxin is absorbed and has serious effects on the nervous system. *Vibrio cholerae* does not invade the mucous membrane of the small intestine, but secretes a toxin which, by disturbing the control of fluid transport across the epithelium, causes severe dehydration. Other organisms, and particularly some viruses, are very highly invasive and infect virtually all individuals who have not previously encountered or been immunised against them, e.g. the viruses of smallpox and poliomyelitis. A great many bacteria lie intermediate between these extremes in their invasive capacity. This applies to the more important pyogenic bacteria which are commonly present in the nose or throat, or on the skin. Their presence is often harmless, but disturbances of defence mechanisms may allow them to invade and cause lesions.

In general, bacteria of high invasive capacity are also highly pathogenic, but there is little correlation between the invasive capacity and pathogenicity of viruses. For example, poliovirus invades readily but only a small proportion of infected individuals develop clinical disease, and non-pathogenic strains are administered orally to produce infection and immunity. Also the protozoon *Toxoplasma gondii* is highly invasive and yet, apart from the lesions it causes in fetal life, it is of low pathogenicity.

Pathogenic effects of micro-organisms

Bacteria which have invaded the host tissues may be destroyed without causing clinically apparent disease, may promote a local inflammatory lesion, or may spread to other parts of the body and produce widespread lesions. The two major ways in which bacteria are known to cause pathological changes are, firstly, by the production of toxins, and secondly by promoting hypersensitivity reactions on the part of the host.

Viruses cause injury by invading the host's cells and utilising the cellular synthetic processes for their own replication. Tissue injury also results from hypersensitivity reactions to virus-induced antigens.

Bacterial toxins

These are of two main types, exotoxins and endotoxins.

Exotoxins are secreted by living bacteria: they are simple proteins, are often extremely potent, and vary considerably in their biological effects upon the host. They are antigenically specific and their biological activity is usually neutralised by union with antibody. Many pathogenic bacteria produce a number of different exotoxins when cultured *in vitro*. Thus *Streptococcus pyogenes* and *Staphylococcus aureus*, two of the most important pyogenic bacteria, produce haemolysins and hyaluronidases. *Strep. pyogenes* also produces a leukocidin which kills leukocytes, and *Staph. aureus* a coagulase which clots fibrinogen. Some exotoxins are injurious to virtually all types of host cell and their effects thus depend on their concentration and distribution. *Corynebacterium diphtheriae*, the cause of diphtheria, secretes such a toxin and at the site of infection, usually the pharynx, it causes local tissue necrosis. Less florid but still severe cell injury is far more widespread and is reflected morphologically in fatty change and necrosis of the parenchymal cells of the various organs: in severe cases, death may result from its effect upon the myocardium (Fig. 6.1). The mechanism of injury by this particular toxin is known (p. 2): other toxins with a similarly widespread effect are produced by many of the pathogenic Gram-positive bacteria but in most instances the mechanism of toxic action is not known. Some have enzymic activity, e.g. phosphatases, proteases, lipases. Some bacteria produce toxins which act specifically on one type of tissue, e.g. the neurotoxins of *Cl. botulinum* interfere with the production of acetylcholine at cholinergic synapses in the peripheral nervous system, and cause a flaccid paralysis, while the neurotoxin of *Cl. tetani* has a contrasting effect on the synapses in the central nervous system, resulting in widespread tetanic

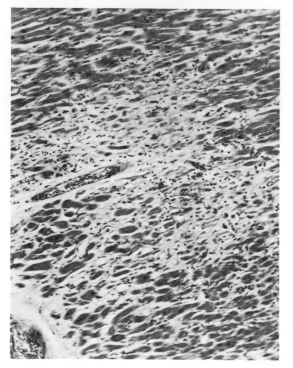

Fig. 6.1 Heart muscle in fatal diphtheria, showing destruction and disappearance of muscle fibres and a light inflammatory cellular infiltrate. × 115.

muscular contractions in response to slight local stimuli.

Attempts to equate the pathogenic effects of a particular micro-organism with its toxins have encountered difficulties: not only are many toxins produced by a single strain of bacteria but different samples of a toxin, even in purified crystalline form, may have different biological properties. Also toxins vary greatly in their effects on hosts of different species, and experimental observations are not necessarily applicable to man. Finally, production or non-production of toxin by bacteria growing *in vitro* does not necessarily indicate a similar behaviour *in vivo*. It is a feature of exotoxins that their biological effects are neutralised by the corresponding antitoxin, and in some instances, e.g. diphtheria and tetanus, prior administration of the antitoxin or active immunisation by injection of *toxoid* (inactivated toxin which maintains its antigenicity) will protect animals against the effects of injection of the toxin and man against the disease. Thus in some instances, particular toxins have been incriminated beyond all reasonable doubt as the pathogenic agents responsible for the disease; in others, it seems most likely that toxins are responsible, but there remains the possibility that the bacteria may have other, at present unknown, pathogenic properties in addition to toxin production.

Endotoxins are structural elements of bacteria and are released only when the bacterium dies. They are constituents of the cell wall of Gram-negative bacteria, and are complexes of phospholipid, polysaccharide and protein. The endotoxins produced by different Gram-negative bacteria are antigenically different but they all have the same biological effects and the active component is believed to reside in the lipid. Endotoxin is responsible for fever, activation of complement by the alternate pathway (p. 116), intravascular conversion of fibrinogen to fibrin, vascular lesions and cellular necrosis in various organs. In small dosage it causes a neutrophil leukocytosis, in large amounts a leukopenia followed by a leukocytosis. In severe Gram-negative bacterial infections, a state of shock develops with some or all of the above features and is termed 'endotoxic shock' (p. 227). Because they produce fever, endotoxins are sometimes termed *pyrogens*. They are heat-stable and unless special precautions are taken are liable to contaminate apparatus and fluids to be used in parenteral therapy.

Hypersensitivity reactions to micro-organisms

Virtually all microbial infections stimulate immune responses by the host, and the reaction of the antibodies or primed T lymphocytes with microbial antigens can result in hypersensitivity of various types. Atopic (type I) reactions, such as urticaria, are a common feature of infestation by parasitic worms, and microbial infections sometimes cause atopic reactions in individuals predisposed to this type of hypersensitivity. Cytotoxic antibody (type II) reactions may, in theory, result from the cross-reaction of microbial-induced antibodies with host cells, a possible example being rheumatic fever, in which antibodies to *Strep. pyogenes* react with heart muscle cells. Immune complex (type III) reactions are important complications of some infections. Local Arthus reactions occur when microbial antigens in infected tissues react with antibodies in the walls of small blood vessels. Circulating immune-complex disease occurs when microbial antigens enter the blood and react with circulating antibodies: an acute generalised reaction may result, or the complexes may be deposited in the tissues, especially in the glomeruli where they are responsible for glomerulonephritis. The acute generalised reaction is seen in the severe form of dengue fever which occurs in people who have had a previous, usually mild infection with the virus. On re-infection, a strong secondary response provides antibody which, by complexing with circulating viral antigen, induces a profound state of shock. Other examples of infections giving rise to immune-complex reactions, and the way in which lesions are produced, are described on pp. 123–7.

Cell-mediated immunity is an important defence mechanism in various infections. The lymphokines released when primed T cells react with microbial antigens (p. 129) are responsible for both destruction of micro-organisms by macrophages and the tissue injury of delayed (type IV) hypersensitivity. Consequently, the two phenomena are commonly associated. The classical example is tuberculosis, in which cell-mediated immunity develops to tuberculo-protein, and is largely responsible for the lesions of this disease. *Myco. tuberculosis* has not been shown to produce toxins and can colonise macrophages in culture without causing apparent injury: addition of primed T lymphocytes reactive with tuberculoprotein results in destruction of macrophages and their ingested micro-organisms. The morphological features of tuberculosis, described in the next chapter, can all be explained on the basis of delayed hypersensitivity. Leprosy is another disease in which delayed hypersensitivity plays a major role. In some cases, cell-mediated immunity is weak or absent and *Myco. leprae* multiply progressively, mostly within macrophages. Like tubercle bacilli, they cause little or no cell injury, and the lesions consist of enlarging nodules composed of macrophages containing large numbers of *Myco. leprae*. In other cases, strong cell-mediated immunity develops, and the bacteria are kept partly in check. Very few are demonstrable in the lesions, but delayed hypersensitivity results in tissue necrosis and fibrosis (p. 127). This is a good example of the dual effect of cell-mediated immunity—it limits the numbers of micro-organisms, but also causes injury of host tissues.

Delayed hypersensitivity reactions are commonly prominent in fungal, viral and chronic bacterial infections. They may be responsible for some of the skin lesions of the acute virus exanthemata (chickenpox, measles, etc.) but firm evidence on the pathogenesis of the skin rashes in these conditions is remarkably scanty.

Defence mechanisms in infections

When micro-organisms have invaded the tissues, there are three major defensive reactions which tend to limit their multiplication and spread, and bring about their destruction: these are the inflammatory reaction, phagocytic activity and specific immune reactions.

The acute inflammatory reaction. The defensive role of this reaction has been considered in Chapter 2. Without doubt, it is of considerable importance, and those infections which are accompanied by acute inflammation at the site of invasion are more likely to remain localised than those in which invasion is accomplished without local injury or reaction. The pyogenic bacteria are a common cause of the former type of infection, while silent invasion is illustrated by *Treponema pallidum*, the cause of syphilis, which spreads widely through the body before the appearance of a local lesion at the site of entry. Other bacteria which may enter the body silently and spread widely include *Neisseria meningitidis*, a cause of acute meningitis, and brucellae, the cause of undulant fever. Many of the parasites transmitted by biting insects, such as the plasmodia which cause malaria, produce generalised infection without a significant local reaction, and many viruses invade the body and produce viraemia without first producing local inflammation.

Chronic inflammatory change also plays a defensive role by surrounding the micro-organisms by a layer of granulation tissue which has been shown to be an effective barrier to bacteria. In the more prolonged infections, such as tuberculosis, surviving micro-organisms may be effectively confined within a zone of dense fibrosis resulting from chronic inflammatory change.

Phagocytosis. A general account of phagocytosis has been given on p. 51, and we are concerned here with factors which determine the capacity of neutrophil polymorphs and macrophages to phagocytose and subsequently kill micro-organisms. Bacteria differ greatly in their resistance to these processes, and such resistance is often an important factor in their pathogenicity. In general, those bacteria which develop a non-protein capsule, e.g. the anthrax bacillus, or smooth strains of *Strep. pneumoniae* or *Haemophilus influenzae*, are not readily phagocytosed. Some bacterial toxins are chemotactic, but *Strep. pyogenes* and some other bacteria secrete toxins which injure phagocytic (and other) cells and so inhibit phagocytosis. Other bacterial products, e.g. the endotoxins of Gram-negative bacteria, enhance the phagocytic activity of polymorphs and macrophages in low concentrations, but inhibit it in higher concentrations.

The inflammatory and immune responses are important host factors favouring phagocytosis and killing of micro-organisms. They help to provide an environment favourable to phagocytosis, render the micro-organism more susceptible to phagocytosis, and increase the phagocytic and killing activities of phagocytes. Emigration of polymorphs and monocytes is part of the inflammatory reaction, and the inflammatory exudate opens up tissue spaces in which the emigrated phagocytes can move. Immunoglobulins and components of complement enter infected tissues in the inflammatory exudate; if specific antibodies are present, they may aid phagocytosis by rendering the micro-organisms more susceptible to phagocytic ingestion (opsonisation), or by neutralising toxins harmful to phagocytes. The reaction of antibodies usually activates complement, which may kill micro-organisms directly, or favour their destruction by enhancing the inflammatory reaction and chemotaxis of phagocytes (pp. 43, 47).

Both polymorphs and macrophages have surface receptors for the Fc component of IgG antibodies, and this facilitates surface binding and subsequent phagocytosis of microbes sensitised with IgG antibodies: they also have surface receptors for the C3b component of reacted complement but, surprisingly, complement fixation by antibody-sensitised bacteria does not directly enhance phagocytosis. IgM antibodies are opsonic, particularly for micro-organisms with a non-protein capsule, but their opsonic effect is not due to specific binding to phagocytes, which do not have surface receptors for Fc of IgM.

Cell-mediated immunity is particularly effective in destroying microbes which invade host cells. The lymphokines released when primed T cells react with antigen include factors which promote inflammation, accumulation of macrophages and lymphocytes, and enhance, both specifically and non-specifically, the phagocytosis and killing of ingested micro-organisms by macrophages (see below).

Once phagocytosed, living micro-organisms are likely to be destroyed but this is no foregone conclusion and many organisms may even multiply within phagocytes, for example the gonococcus, which causes gonorrhoea (Fig. 6.2),

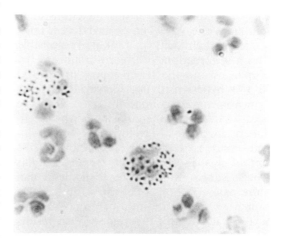

Fig. 6.2 Smear of urethral exudate in acute gonorrhoea. Two polymorphs contain large numbers of gonococci, and show degenerative changes. Other polymorphs contain few or no bacteria and appear relatively healthy. (Gram stain.) × 1200.

while the leprosy bacillus, the brucellae which cause undulant fever, and the protozoon *Leishmania donovani*, the cause of kala azar, all colonise macrophages. In general, those micro-organisms which are less readily phagocytosed, e.g. smooth (capsulated) strains of bacteria, are less readily killed following their phagocytosis. The ways in which phagocytosed bacteria are killed are complex, and probably vary depending on the properties of different bacteria. Unlike phagocytosis, which occurs readily under anaerobic conditions, killing by polymorphs is associated with a burst of aerobic respiration, and the activity of myeloperoxidase and production of hydrogen peroxide appear to be important factors. Polymorphs also synthesise cationic proteins capable of killing some bacteria. Lysozyme may also be contributory but, in general, the lysosomal enzymes of polymorphs and macrophages digest dead bacteria rather than kill live ones. Sensitisation of bacteria by antibody favours their killing by phagocytes.

The immune response. The several ways in which antibodies and cell-mediated immunity help to destroy micro-organisms have been described in this and preceding chapters, and may be summarised as follows. **Antibodies** of IgA class are important in preventing the invasion of mucous membranes by viruses and probably by some bacteria (p. 89). IgM and IgG antibodies can neutralise bacterial toxins, agglutinate and immobilise micro-organisms (p. 89), and prevent cell invasion by viruses: by activating complement, they may cause lysis of microbial cell walls without the intervention of phagocytes (p. 116). Activation of complement also promotes the inflammatory reaction and attracts polymorphs by chemotaxis (pp. 43, 47). Antibodies, particularly those of IgG class, also opsonise micro-organisms, thus favouring their ingestion and destruction by phagocytes (see above).

When the primed T lymphocytes produced by **cell-mediated immune responses** react with microbial antigens, they release lymphokines which induce the inflammatory and other changes of the delayed hypersensitivity reaction (p. 129). In addition to exerting chemotactic and immobilising effects on macrophages, lymphokines include a macrophage-activating factor which increases their killing capacity for ingested micro-organisms, and a second factor—the specific macrophage-arming factor—which enables macrophages to kill allogeneic target cells and may also mediate destruction of micro-organisms

One of the main purposes of this summary is to emphasise the complex relationships and synergism between the inflammatory response, phagocytosis, and immunological reactions, which together provide a closely interwoven system of defence against micro-organisms.

Interferon (p. 161) is probably mainly responsible for arresting virus infections, yet children with congenital T-cell deficiencies tend to develop progressive virus infections, and there is some evidence that interferon is produced by T lymphocytes.

Antibacterial drug therapy

In many types of bacterial infection, antibiotic drugs are capable of killing the bacteria or suppressing their multiplication, and thus tip the balance in favour of the host and terminate the infection. Antibiotic therapy is not, however, without risk. Apart from their toxic side-effects and the induction of hypersensitivity reactions, antibiotics can, as already mentioned, encourage the multiplication of resistant strains of bacteria. Such resistance may be determined by orthodox genetic bacterial inheritance, but one form of resistance can be transmitted from resistant to susceptible bacteria by transfer of *plasmids* (extra-chromosomal genetic factors). Antibiotic therapy has, in some circumstances, resulted in a great increase in the incidence of antibiotic-resistant infections, particularly among hospital patients, and this emphasises the importance of avoiding their indiscriminate use.

Diminished resistance to infection

There is a wide range of individual 'natural' resistance to microbial infections among apparently normal individuals. This is largely unexplained, but there have been suggestions that variations in susceptibility to certain infections are related to the individual's 'transplant' iso-antigens, an example being Reiter's syndrome, which is associated with a high incidence of HLA–B27. In passing, it is worth noting that similar associations with HLA antigens have recently been claimed for many diverse diseases of obscure nature, e.g. disseminated sclerosis, the connective tissue diseases and lymphoid neoplasia. These observations may throw light on genetic factors in disease, and help to explain the nature of 'constitutional' predisposition and resistance.

Impaired resistance to infection can occur in many ways. Defects in local barriers to invasion have been dealt with earlier in this chapter. Normal phagocytic function, immune responsiveness and complement function are all essential factors contributing to the range of protective mechanisms. A serious fall in the number of polymorphs in the blood, as in agranulocytosis, predisposes to bacterial invasion and severe, spreading infections, e.g. of the pharynx and intestine, by both commensals and more highly pathogenic bacteria. Genetically-determined defects of polymorph function also predispose to bacterial infection. These polymorph abnormalities are considered in Chapter 16. There are also many diseases which impair specific immune responses: they include the congenital immunological deficiency states and also acquired diseases which involve the lymphoid tissues and affect their immunological functions.

In other diseases, predisposition to infection is well known but unexplained. A good example is diabetes mellitus, in which boils and urinary tract infections are common and there is a predisposition to tuberculosis: it may be that phagocytic activity, which requires the energy provided by glycolysis, is impaired by the defective carbohydrate metabolism of diabetes.

Two important reactions to infection are leukocytosis and fever, accounts of which follow.

Polymorphonuclear Leukocytosis

The number of neutrophil polymorphs in the blood, normally 2 500–7 500 per mm³ in older children and adults, increases in various pathological conditions. The increase is a controlled reaction and when the cause subsides the leukocyte count returns to the normal level for that individual. This account deals with the causes and mechanisms of such a neutrophil leukocytosis and with the changes in the haemopoietic marrow responsible for increased leukocyte production. The proliferation of leukocytes in myeloid leukaemia appears to be neoplastic rather than reactive and is described in Chapter 16.

Causes

Neutrophil leukocytosis occurs in association with acute inflammatory reactions, tissue necrosis, thrombosis, haemorrhage, acute lysis of red cells, and sometimes cancer. A mild polymorph leukocytosis occurs in pregnancy and also results from strenuous exercise, severe mental stress, and from injection of glucocorticoids, corticotrophin or adrenaline. By far the commonest cause in clinical medicine is inflammation due to bacterial infection, and in general the degree of leukocytosis correlates with the size of the inflammatory lesion and the intensity of polymorph emigration in the infected tissues. Pyogenic infections, due for example to virulent staphylococci, streptococci, pneumococci or coliform bacilli, are accompanied by a brisk leukocytosis, the height of which depends partly on the duration and partly on the extent of the infection. A boil or acute appendicitis may induce a moderate rise, e.g. to 10 000 polymorphs per mm³, while a large abscess, acute bacterial pneumonia or general peritonitis are commonly accompanied by a count of 20 000 or more. In some severe infections with pyogenic bacteria, e.g. streptococcal septicaemia or pneumococcal pneumonia, there may be absence of leukocytosis, or even leukopenia, and this usually indicates overwhelming toxaemia and is a bad prognostic sign. In some severe infections, e.g. gas gangrene due to *Cl. welchii*, polymorph emigration is less intense, and the increase in polymorphs in the blood is less marked, while the acute inflammatory lesions of the intestine caused by the typhoid and paratyphoid bacilli are virtually devoid of polymorphs (Fig. 6.3), and there is actually a fall in the number of polymorphs in the blood. Many virus infections, particularly in the early stages, are also accompanied by a neutrophil leukopenia.

Necrosis of tissue, for example myocardial infarction, causes a slight or moderate neutrophil leukocytosis, and extensive thrombosis, e.g. in the leg veins, or severe haemorrhage, both have a similar effect.

Leukocytosis may develop within a few hours of the onset of a bacterial infection and is of diagnostic value. This early output of polymorphs is due to release of young cells lying in the sinusoids of the haemopoietic marrow. Soon, however, there is an increased rate of

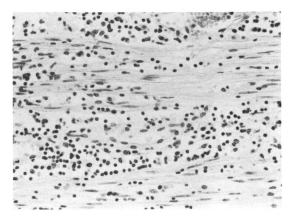

Fig. 6.3 Inflammatory infiltration of the muscular layer of the small intestine in typhoid fever, showing mononuclear cells and absence of polymorphs. × 150.

formation of polymorphs in the marrow and the leukocytosis is thus maintained. The life of the neutrophil polymorph in the blood is probably not more than 3 days, and since there are approximately 5 litres of blood containing about 4 000 polymorphs per mm³, the normal daily production must be at least 7×10^9. In a suppurating infection, ten times this number may be lost daily for weeks or months in the pus discharging from an abscess, while at the same time the blood level may be maintained at 20 000 per mm³ or more. It is thus apparent that output of polymorphs is capable of enormous and sustained increase, and the process responsible for this is hyperplasia of the bone marrow, considered below.

Production of polymorphs (Granulopoiesis)

In the normal adult, production of the granulocyte or myeloid series of leukocytes is restricted to the haemopoietic marrow, where it occurs along with the production of red cells, platelets and monocytes. All these cells, and probably also lymphocytes (p. 103) originate from *haemopoietic stem cells*, which give rise, after an unknown number of divisions, to cells of more restricted potential: some are progenitors of red cells, others of megakaryocytes, while recent observations have demonstrated progenitor cells capable of giving rise to both polymorphs and monocytes (see below).

Because of their basic role in haemopoiesis,

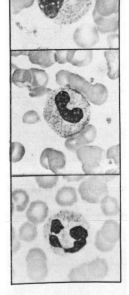

Myeloblast: non-granular (oxidase-negative), basophilic cytoplasm (rich in RNA); nucleus roughly spherical, with dispersed chromatin (euchromatin), and containing 2 or more nucleoli. 10–18 μm diameter.

Promyelocyte: a few primary (oxidase positive) cytoplasmic granules; basophilic cytoplasm; nucleus spherical, still with dispersed chromatin and nucleoli. 12–18 μm diameter.

Myelocytes: cytoplasm less basophilic; primary granules disappear and secondary granules develop—they are strongly oxidase-positive and specific (neutrophil, eosinophil or basophil). Nucleus spherical or ovoid with some condensation of chromatin (heterochromatin). Active mitosis occurs at this stage. 12–18 μm diameter.

Metamyelocyte: cytoplasm only faintly basophilic (poor in RNA), with many specific granules and no primitive granules. Nucleus becoming elongated, smaller and more condensed. 12–15 μm diameter.

Polymorphonuclear leukocyte: cytoplasm as in metamyelocytes; nucleus smaller, and chromatin more condensed, at first horse-shoe shaped, later lobulated. 10–15 μm diameter.

Fig. 6.4 Cells in haemopoietic marrow representing stages of granulopoiesis: from the myelocyte stage, only neutrophil cells are illustrated. Leishman stain × 1000. (Dr. R. Brooke Hogg.)

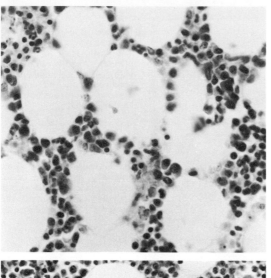

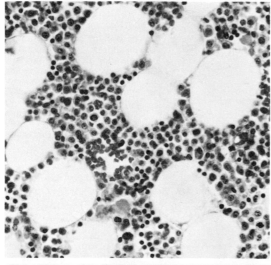

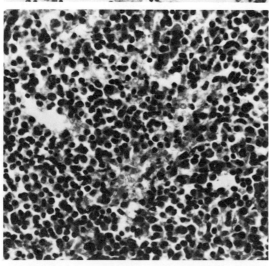

haemopoietic stem cells are dealt with in the chapter on blood (p. 450).

Stages of granulopoiesis. The earliest recognisable granulocyte precursor is termed a myeloblast: small numbers of these are present in normal haemopoietic marrow and they divide to give rise to a population of cells which undergo successive multiplications and form the largest cell population in the marrow. This proliferation is accompanied by a continuous process of differentiation up to the granulocyte stage: representative stages are illustrated in Fig. 6.4. Throughout the process the ratio of cytoplasm to nucleus increases and after initial enlargement up to the early myelocyte stage, diminution in size is a feature of differentiation. In the primitive stages the nucleus is large, ovoid or indented, and the chromatin is finely distributed. Gradually the nucleus shrinks, becoming more deeply staining and eventually it becomes elongated giving the 'band form', followed by division into lobes, the number of which increases during the life span of probably less than 3 days of the polymorph in the blood. In preparations stained by a Romanowsky dye (e.g. Leishman's, Wright's, Jenner's or Giemsa stains), the cytoplasmic changes are as described in Fig. 6.4: from the myelocyte stage, there is not sufficient RNA to impart strong basophilia, and the cytoplasm is pale blue. Lysosomal granules appear in the cytoplasm in the promyelocyte stage: at first they are large and reddish-blue, but in the myelocyte stage these early granules are gradually replaced by the granules specific for neutrophil, eosinophil or basophil polymorphs. In the neutrophil myelocytes the granules are small and have a reddish or purple tint: in the eosinophil they are larger and bright orange, while in the basophil they are large and dark blue. These characteristic granules persist in the three types of mature granulocytes or polymorphs. In an early neutrophil leukocytosis there is an increased proportion of young cells and even myelocytes may appear in the blood.

Fig. 6.5 Sections of haemopoietic marrow illustrating hyperplasia associated with neutrophil leukocytosis. *Top*, normal marrow. *Middle*, marrow showing increased cellularity in a patient with leukocytosis of short duration. *Bottom*, marked hyperplasia of marrow in a patient with prolonged leukocytosis: the fat cells have been replaced by haemopoietic cells. × 315.

Leukocytosis is brought about by hyperplasia, i.e. an increase in the number of cells, in the haemopoietic marrow, and the proportion of myeloid cells, and particularly of myelocytes, is increased. This is termed a *granulopoietic reaction* and is analogous to the erythroblastic reaction in response to an increased requirement of red cells, e.g. after haemorrhage. The fat cells normally present in haemopoietic (red) marrow diminish in number as the cellularity increases (Fig. 6.5) and also foci of haemopoietic tissue arising from stem cells appear in the yellow fatty marrow of the long bones. These foci extend rapidly and in a severe prolonged suppurating infection much of the yellow marrow in the shafts of the femur and other long bones may be replaced by red marrow, the change starting in the upper ends of the bones and extending downwards. All the cellular constituents of normal marrow are present in this newly formed haemopoietic tissue, but myelocytes and later forms predominate (Figs. 6.6, 6.7).

Factors controlling granulopoiesis. It has long been known that many substances promote a neutrophil leukocytosis when injected into animals: they include peptones, digestion products of nucleic acids, and metabolic products and extracts of bacteria. Such observations have not helped much in the elucidation of the mechanisms of leukocytosis, but investiga-

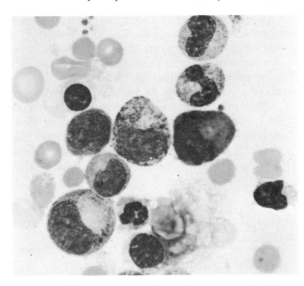

Fig. 6.7 Smear preparation of marrow showing finely granular myelocytes and transitions to polymorphonuclear leukocytes. × 1000.

tions involving the culture of marrow cells *in vitro* have proved more successful. When a suspension of mouse haemopoietic marrow cells is cultured under suitable conditions in semi-solid medium, it has been found that addition of a stimulating factor to the medium results in the proliferation of cells to form discrete colonies. At first, the proliferating cells are mainly or entirely granulocyte precursors, but as the numbers increase some of the cells differentiate into polymorphs and others into monocytes. Since such colonies are derived from single cells, this is good evidence of a common precursor of polymorphs and monocytes. The stimulating factor essential for colony formation (**colony stimulating factor**) can be extracted from most mouse organs and tissues, and is produced by suspensions of various types of cell in culture, including macrophages but not polymorphs. In general, it works best on marrow cells of the same species, but has been demonstrated in extracts of the tissues, serum and urine of other species, including man, using mouse marrow cultures. Increasing use is now being made of human marrow culture, which is likely to have considerable advantages. Bacterial endotoxin *in vivo* increases the amount of colony stimulating factor extractable from tissues and in the serum, and when added to cultures of macrophages it increases the amount of colony stimulating factor released by these cells.

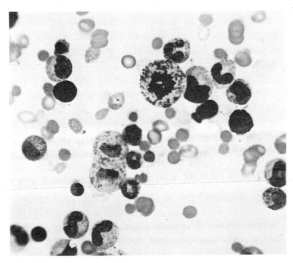

Fig. 6.6 Smear preparation of sternal marrow in leukoblastic reaction. Note granular myelocytes in mitosis and various stages of transition to polymorphonuclear leukocytes. × 600.

A second factor concerned with polymorphonuclear leukocytosis has the property of releasing relatively mature polymorphs from the marrow without stimulating granulopoiesis. This **polymorph releasing factor** appears in the plasma shortly after an injection of endotoxin, before the rise in colony stimulating factor. It may account for the rapid early rise in blood polymorphs in acute infection, etc. **Other factors** of possible importance include a lipoprotein present in normal plasma which, when added to marrow cell cultures, is said to increase the production of monocytes at the expense of polymorphs. A factor is also produced by polymorphs in culture fluid which inhibits proliferation of early polymorph precursors in culture.

Although these recent observations promise considerable advances in our understanding of polymorph production, their relevance to natural neutrophil leukocytosis in man is not known.

Pyrexia (Fever)

In this account, these two terms are used synonymously to mean a rise in the internal temperature of the body ('core temperature') to levels above the normal range. Traditionally, *fever* is also used in the nomenclature of various diseases (usually infections) in which pyrexia is a prominent feature, e.g. typhoid fever, yellow fever and cerebrospinal fever. Doubtless both these usages will continue.

Body temperature is mainly under the exquisite control of a thermo-regulatory mechanism which for practical purposes may be regarded as functioning as a thermostat. The thermo-sensory centre, shown in experimental animals to be in the anterior hypothalamus, responds to variations in the temperature of the blood and, perhaps by secreting prostaglandin (see below) influences the centres in the posterior hypothalamus which, in turn, send out the nervous stimuli which regulate the activity of the physiological processes responsible for heat production and heat loss, thus controlling the temperature.

In considering the many causes of fever, it is important to distinguish disturbances of the thermo-sensory centre (analogous to the thermostat being set high), as in infections, from conditions in which the centre is functioning normally but, for various reasons, heat loss cannot keep pace with heat gain, and so the body temperature rises, e.g. during vigorous exercise in a hot, moist atmosphere.

Disturbances of the thermo-sensory centre

It has long been realised that injection of dead bacteria or bacterial products induces fever. A number of such products, termed **exogenous pyrogens**, have been detected in filtrates of cultures of various bacteria and fungi, but the endotoxins of Gram-negative bacteria have been most extensively investigated. On injection into rabbits, these phospholipid-polysaccharide-protein complexes (p. 147) induce fever in about 1 hour, and this is followed by a refractory period in which further injections of endotoxin are ineffectual. Following injection of endotoxin or other exogenous pyrogen into rabbits, a second pyrogenic factor appears in the plasma; this causes fever in about 20 minutes following injection into a second rabbit, and differs from endotoxin in being pyrogenic in rabbits rendered refractory to endotoxin. This second pyrogen, now called **endogenous** (or **leukocyte**) **pyrogen**, has also been detected in the plasma of animals in the early stages of febrile bacterial and viral infections. It is produced when suspensions of human or rabbit polymorphs or monocytes are stimulated by endotoxin or by readily phagocytosed material such as dead bacteria or antigen–antibody complexes, and when macrophages are activated by lymphocytes in delayed hypersensitivity reactions (p. 129). Synthesis of RNA and protein is necessary for endogenous pyrogen (EP) production, which in polymorphs starts about 2 hours after stimulation: monocytes take longer but secrete much more EP than polymorphs, and the EPs produced by the two cell types differ in their molecular weights. Polymorphs and macrophages obtained from inflammatory exudates produce EP spontaneously when incubated in culture medium, indicating that they have been stimulated *in vivo*.

These various observations suggest that many of the agents capable of inducing fever act by stimulating production of EP. In addition to its production by human leukocytes *in vitro*, EP has been demonstrated in inflammatory exudates in man. Its detection in human plasma during infective fevers has proved difficult, but this is not surprising because fever can be induced in man by injection of amounts of EP too small to provide a detectable level in the plasma. EP has, however, been demonstrated in human plasma at the onset of a bout of malarial fever. Further investigations on EP would be greatly helped by a more sensitive method for its detection than that depending on production of fever in experimental animals.

The fever which accompanies tissue destruction, e.g. myocardial infarction, or necrotic tumours, is probably also mediated by EP released by phagocytes in the inflammatory reaction to the necrotic tissue, although it may be that tissue cells can also release pyrogens.

There is some evidence that EP in some way alters the concentrations of sodium and calcium ions in the hypothalamus, and it has been suggested that the proportions of these ions determine the 'set point' of the sensory centre, sodium predominance being associated with fever.

Effector mechanisms of fever

Although fever cannot be regarded as a physiological reaction, it is nevertheless brought about by stimulation of the physiological mechanisms for heat production and inhibition of those responsible for heat loss. For example, the shivering which accompanies a sharp rise of temperature is the normal response to a cold environment, and is associated with increased catabolic activity and heat production in the skeletal muscles. The coldness and pallor of the skin at the onset of fever are due to cutaneous vasoconstriction and, together with 'gooseflesh' (contraction of the pilo-erector muscles) and inhibition of sweating, are part of the normal heat-saving reaction to cold. Heat production is also increased in fever, as it is in a cold climate, by increased metabolic activity, particularly in

the skeletal muscles (see above) and liver. This is mediated in part by stimulation of the sympathetic system, with increased catecholamine secretion, and eventually thyroid activity may increase. A high caloric diet is necessary to provide the fuel needed to maintain the body at temperatures above normal, failing which catabolism of endogenous fat and protein increases, resulting in a negative nitrogen balance and, especially in children, keto-acidosis. These catabolic activities account for the wasting commonly seen in patients with prolonged fever,* and the metabolic status in fever is, in fact, closely similar to that following injury (p. 229): in both, a warm environment and a high caloric intake, including increased protein, are beneficial.

Not only is the 'thermostat set high' in fever, but it is unstable, so that the temperature commonly fluctuates, and is readily affected by environmental conditions. As described above, a rise of temperature is achieved by increasing heat production and reducing heat loss by physiological mechanisms. Conversely, a fall of temperature, either during or at the end of a fever, is accomplished by reduction in catabolism and by cutaneous vasodilatation and sweating. The skin is flushed, warm and moist, and the patient feels hot. If, during fever, the temperature is fairly steady, the degree of increased metabolic activity, etc. will depend largely on the environmental conditions and, in a chilling environment, on the degree of insulation of the body by clothing.

Heat production and loss are regulated by centres in the posterior hypothalamus, including one which influences activity of the sympathetic system, and a second which appears to control muscle tone and induction of shivering. When injected into the anterior hypothalamus, EP induces fever almost immediately, and accepting that it has a direct action on the thermo-sensory centre analogous to raising the setting of a thermostat, it is still necessary to explain how messages pass from the thermo-sensory centre to those parts of the hypothalamus which control production and loss of heat. The available evidence suggests a neuro-humoral factor, and the most likely mediator appears to be a prostaglandin. Perfusion of the cat's third ventricle with very high dilutions of

---

* The old adage 'starve a fever; feed a cold' had little metabolic justification.

prostaglandin E_1 causes fever, and a threefold rise in prostaglandin-like activity in the cerebrospinal fluid has been demonstrated during fever induced by pyrogens. This might explain the fever associated with induction of labour in pregnant women by an infusion of prostaglandin E_2; it would account also for the antipyretic effect of aspirin and similar drugs, which inhibit the enzyme (prostaglandin synthetase) responsible for production of prostaglandins (p. 43). Cortisone is also antipyretic, but its inhibitory effect on production of EP by leukocytes stimulated by endotoxin, etc., probably accounts for this.

Effects of fever

The ill-effects of fever include general malaise, anorexia and increased catabolism. When the temperature rises to $41 \cdot 6°C$, there is a danger of direct thermal injury to various tissues, and particularly to cerebral neurones. In general, there is no evidence that fever has a beneficial effect, and its reduction by antipyretic drugs or by cooling the body does not seem to influence the course of infections. Apart from the spirochaete of syphilis and gonococcus (the cause of gonorrhoea), micro-organisms in culture do not appear to be adversely affected by moderate rises in temperature. The effects of fever on viruses are complex and require further investigation.

The spontaneous movement of neutrophil polymorphs *in vitro*, and their response to a chemotactic stimulus, are most rapid at $40°C$, and fever may thus enhance the defensive role of these cells in infections.

Other causes of fever

Lesions of the hypothalamus may cause fever by interfering with the functioning of either the thermo-sensory centre or the hypothalamic areas which regulate heat loss and heat production. In experimental animals, injury of the anterior hypothalamus often causes pyrexia, while injury of the posterior hypothalamus may induce hypothermia. In man, haemorrhage in the pons is often accompanied by fever, and lesions between the hypothalamus and upper cervical cord interfere with tracts controlling heat loss and production, rendering the individual less able to respond to environmental temperature changes, etc.

Fever may occur in the absence of any disturbance of the thermo-sensory mechanism in conditions where the physiological mechanisms of heat loss cannot keep pace with heat production. This occurs in *thyrotoxicosis*, in which excess secretion of thyroid hormone stimulates general metabolism and physical activity and thus increases heat production. In normal subjects, vigorous exercise or a hot moist environment may both cause fever, and the combination is particularly likely to do so. Obviously, heat loss is influenced by the temperature and humidity of the atmosphere, air currents and insulation by clothing. These factors affect loss of heat by conduction, convection, radiation and evaporation, and also by the cooling effect of inspired air. Sweating is a major mechanism of heat loss, but is only effective if the sweat evaporates on the skin surface, thus extracting the latent heat of vaporisation. Excessive sweating may, however, cause dehydration and, if water is restored, salt deficiency. Also, marked cutaneous vasodilatation may impair the circulation. These various factors are associated in combinations which give rise to several clinical syndromes, the chief of which are as follows.

1. Heat exhaustion results from physical activity in a hot climate, particularly if the atmosphere is moist. Vasodilatation in the skin and skeletal muscles creates a relative oligaemia, i.e. the filling of the enlarged vascular bed reduces the return of blood to the right side of the heart, and so cardiac output falls. Literally, there is not enough blood to go round. The heart rate increases and the blood pressure falls, giving a fast weak pulse, dyspnoea and other signs of circulatory insufficiency. The skin is hot and damp, and the subject feels tired and becomes confused. Rest and restoration of fluid usually bring rapid improvement.

2. Dehydration exhaustion. When dehydration due to excessive sweating, reduced fluid intake, etc., accompanies heat exhaustion, all the features of circulatory failure are exaggerated by actual, in addition to relative, reduction in the blood volume. The temperature may be very high and collapse and sudden death may occur.

3. Heat stroke. In the two conditions mentioned above, heat-losing mechanisms operate, but are inadequate. In heat stroke, exercise in a hot environment, with consequent fever, leads in some way to a breakdown of the control mechanisms, so that the heat-losing mechanisms remain inactive, and the temperature continues to rise and may reach 43°C. At this temperature, brain injury with coma and convulsions occurs, and death or permanent brain injury results.

4. Heat cramps. Painful cramps in the muscles are the result of salt deficiency. This is liable to occur when there is excessive loss of water and salt by sweating, and only the water is replaced.

5. Malignant hyperpyrexia. This is an unusual complication of general anaesthesia, usually with suxamethonium but also other agents. During the anaesthesia, muscle tone increases and the temperature rises rapidly, often to above 42°C. Cyanosis, shock and keto-acidosis develops and death may occur from cardiac arrest unless the condition is recognised and treated. The underlying predisposition is not understood, but is presumably metabolically determined and in some instances has been shown to run in families.

Hypothermia

This may be defined as a fall in the core temperature of the body to below 35°C. It has no particular relevance to host–parasite relationships and is considered here simply because the processes involved in temperature control, described above in relation to fever, are equally important in hypothermia.

Hypothermia occurs when heat production fails to keep pace with heat loss. In robust adults, this occurs only in conditions of extreme heat loss, such as immersion in the sea or exposure on mountains. However, factors which interfere with heat production predispose to hypothermia in less rigorous environmental conditions. Because of their relatively large surface area and thin layer of insulating fat, infants, particularly if premature, are particularly liable to it. Old people, especially women, living in cold surroundings on an inadequate diet, are especially liable to develop hypothermia in winter. Predisposing diseases include hypothyroidism, generalised skin diseases, psychiatric disturbances and conditions which impair consciousness, metabolic or physical activity, e.g. alcoholism, narcotic drugs, paralysis, severe trauma and general states of disability.

Pathology. In general, metabolic processes decline rapidly below 33°C and the cardiac output, blood pressure and respiratory rate fall. Fluid leaks from the microvessels with consequent haemoconcentration and increased blood viscosity. Blood flow to the tissues is further impaired by peripheral vasoconstriction; hypoxia and CO_2 retention increase and a combination of respiratory and metabolic acidosis develops. Below 25°C, the thermo-regulatory mechanism ceases to function. Death is due to cardiac arrest.

The changes found at necropsy include venous thrombosis, multiple small infarcts in various organs, pulmonary haemorrhages and bronchopneumonia. Acute pancreatitis is a common complication in patients who survive.

Induction of hypothermia to reduce the metabolic requirements of the brain and other organs was formerly practised in surgical procedures involving interruption of the circulation, but it carries a risk of ventricular fibrillation and is now used mainly in association with a pump to maintain the circulation.

7

Types of Infection

Within living memory, infective disease was the major cause of death throughout the world, and the elimination or reduction in the incidence of most of the important infections largely accounts for the greatly increased lifespan in technologically advanced communities. Many factors have contributed to this decline of serious infections: they include improved standards of community and personal hygiene, better nutrition and housing, prophylactic immunisation and antimicrobial therapeutic agents.

In spite of these great triumphs, infective disease is still of considerable importance: it remains the major cause of death in many tropical and subtropical countries where, in addition to bacterial and viral infections, protozoal and metazoal parasites account for a great deal of illness. Even in countries where infections have been greatly reduced, many problems remain. The common cold is as common as ever, and the rise in the volume and speed of world travel has increased greatly the risk of epidemics of influenza, smallpox, cholera, etc. Even antibiotics have not proved an unmixed blessing, for their use has resulted in the spread of resistant pathogenic bacteria, particularly in hospitals. There are, moreover, a number of important diseases which may eventually prove to be due to infections, for example rheumatoid arthritis, multiple sclerosis, ulcerative colitis and sarcoidosis. Virus infections may also prove to be important causal factors of the lymphoid neoplasms, including lymphatic leukaemia, and of other forms of cancer.

This chapter gives a brief account of the various types of infection and describes some of the more important examples. As with other forms of disease, the effects of infection depend not only on the nature of the lesion, but also on its site in the body, and for this reason the special features of infection of the lungs, kidneys, brain, etc., are described in the appropriate systematic chapters.

Virus Infections

Of all the pathogenic organisms which affect man, viruses show the most extreme degree of parasitism. In the extracellular state viruses are metabolically inert and depend absolutely on the metabolism of the host cell for their replication. Basically, all viruses consist of a protein shell or **capsid** which surrounds and protects a single molecule of nucleic acid—which may be either DNA or RNA. The extracellular form (**virion**) of some viruses has an additional outer layer, or **envelope**, partially derived from the plasma membrane of the host cell. When a virus enters a susceptible host cell, the nucleic acid is released from the capsid and becomes function- ally active: it re-directs the synthetic pathways of the host cell to manufacture components for new virus particles. This involves the replication of nucleic acid molecules and the production of proteins which include both the non-structural proteins (e.g. enzymes) necessary for viral replicative processes and also the structural proteins which become incorporated in the capsid of new virus particles.

Apart from those viruses which enter the host by the bite of an insect (e.g. yellow fever), or in the case of rabies virus by the bite of an animal, all parasitic viruses must enter the body by invading the surface epithelial cells of some part of the body. In many instances the site of initial infection is in the alimentary or respiratory tracts. In the case of some viruses the ability to invade and replicate in certain types of host cell appears to depend on the presence of receptor sites on the cell surface to which the protein coat or envelope of the virus can become attached.

In man, most virus infections are mild and are followed by complete recovery. Many infections are entirely symptomless and immunity to reinfection is acquired without serious disturbance at the time of primary infection. Although latent infection with virus may continue for months or occasionally even for years, viruses do not form a non-invasive flora in the way that some bacteria do. A few virus infections, such as smallpox, regularly cause serious disease and even viruses such as *Herpes simplex* or the enteroviruses, which generally cause mild or symptomless infection, may occasionally give rise to severe disease in an unusually susceptible host (Fig. 20.39, p. 695). Viral infections, and especially respiratory virus infections, are extremely common in the community and are, in general, more frequent in childhood than in adult life.

Viruses are structurally simple parasites and do not produce disease by the elaboration of toxins as bacteria do. Lesions in viral infections are due to direct invasion of body tissues with subsequent cell damage due to the effect of viral replication in the host cells. In most clinically-apparent virus infections, replication of the virus is accompanied by death of the infected cell (Fig. 7.1). Some viruses induce fusion between infected and adjacent non-infected cells, with the formation of multinucleated giant cells, e.g. the Warthin–Finkeldey cell of measles pneumonia (Fig. 15.28, p. 420). Such giant cells usually die, at least in tissue culture preparations, but their formation may be important in allowing virus to spread without entering the surrounding medium. There is increasing evidence that the immune response of the host may sometimes play an important role in causing lesions—for example in the development of bronchiolitis due to respiratory syncytial virus, which seems to be due largely to a hypersensitivity reaction in the lungs of the host. In togavirus encephalitis, it has been postulated on the basis of some results of animal experiments that the lesions may be due to virus–antibody

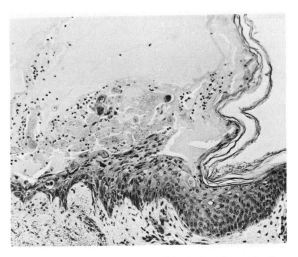

Fig. 7.1 Part of a vesicular skin lesion in varicella, illustrating virus-induced cell injury. The virus has replicated in the epidermal cells, resulting in cell death. The resulting epidermal defect has then become distended with inflammatory exudate, forming the vesicle. Note the swelling and hyperchromatic nuclei of the colonised epidermal cells, lying free in the vesicle and in the underlying epidermis. × 96 (Professor J. A. Milne.)

complexes inducing a type III hypersensitivity reaction rather than to the direct effect of the virus on the cells of the brain.

Unlike some bacterial infections, virus diseases are not usually accompanied by a polymorphonuclear leukocytosis, but a lymphocytosis is common. Most are associated with fever, and rash and lymphadenopathy are quite commonly seen. In the acute phase of virus infection a protein, **interferon**, can be detected in the blood and tissues. Interferon is released from cells in response to virus infection and when taken up by other cells makes them refractory to virus infection. Although the production of interferon is induced by virus, the protein itself is a species-specific cellular protein. It is not virus-specific in its antiviral effect but inhibits virtually all viruses. Interferon production is an important host defence mechanism against virus infection and is probably the major factor in bringing about recovery from acute virus infections. Although specific neutralising antibody is responsible for immunity to re-infection, it begins to appear in the bloodstream only when the acute infection is subsiding. It is notable that infants with immunological deficiencies resulting in impairment of T-lymphocyte function (p. 139 *et seq.*) are prone to develop chronic progressive vaccinia (vaccinia gangrenosa) following vaccination, and chronic infection with measles virus has also been reported.

Distribution of lesions in virus infections

In some instances, the main lesion is at the site of the initial infection. For example, the myxovirus responsible for influenza gives rise to a localised infection which spreads rapidly throughout the epithelial lining of the larger air passages of the respiratory tract. This results in epithelial necrosis of varying extent, and the cell injury and loss results in acute inflammatory oedema, which is the major clinical feature of influenza. The severity of the illness depends on the extent of epithelial necrosis, but secondary bacterial infection of the damaged mucosa is also of importance, especially in major epidemics. Influenza virus may enter the bloodstream, but appears unable to replicate successfully in the cells of other tissues. Other examples of virus infections which remain localised, and produce lesions mostly at the site of initial infection, are molluscum contagiosum (p. 986) and the common cold.

In many other instances, the initial infection is usually clinically silent, but the virus invades various other tissues and organs and produces characteristic lesions in them. Thus in smallpox, the initial infection is probably in the respiratory tract. From there the virus spreads widely, invading the blood (viraemia) and many other tissues and organs. The characteristic vesicular lesions in the skin are due to invasion of the epidermal cells, and are one manifestation of the systemic infection. Suppuration of the skin lesions (pustulation) is due to secondary bacterial infection. The childhood fevers, e.g. measles, mumps, rubella, chickenpox, are other examples of generalised virus diseases which follow initial infection *via* the respiratory tract.

Because of the mode of virus spread in smallpox, the incubation period between initial infection and appearance of symptoms is about 12 days, and it may be even longer in some other exanthemas, e.g. measles and varicella. *Poliovirus* also spreads in a complex fashion within the body: following ingestion of the virus, there is an initial infection of the Peyer's patches in the small intestine. The virus then spreads to the regional lymph nodes, and in some instances produces viraemia. In a few individuals (e.g. about 1% of those infected with poliovirus type 1) the organism invades the anterior horn cells of the spinal cord (Figs. 20.43 and 20.44, p. 698), causing paralytic poliomyelitis. The intestinal infection is clinically silent, but it nevertheless results in the development of antibody in the blood, in the appearance of IgA antibody in the gastrointestinal tract (p. 89), and confers immunity to subsequent infection with the same type of poliovirus.

Persistent virus infections are known to occur in man. Herpes simplex virus, for example, remains latent within the trigeminal ganglion but becomes activated from time to time, e.g. during pneumonia or other febrile illness, to produce vesicles around the mouth. Varicella virus may also remain latent and then multiply within the cells of the dorsal root ganglia to produce an attack of zoster (Fig. 20.42, p. 696).

There is considerable interest at present in **slow virus infections**, which may be defined as virus diseases having a long incubation period, in some instances years, and a prolonged course. Such diseases have been demonstrated to occur in certain animals, e.g. Aleutian disease of the mink, and it seems very likely that kuru (p. 701) and Creutzfeldt–Jakob disease are examples in man. The agent of scrapie, a widespread chronic disease of sheep, is most unusual in its small size and remarkable resistance to heat and viricidal chemicals.

Active immunity can readily be produced by the administration of attenuated viruses, e.g. Sabin poliovirus vaccine, measles and yellow fever vaccines, and also—although somewhat less effectively—by inactivated viruses, e.g. influenza and rabies vaccines. Naturally-acquired immunity after virus infection is generally life-long and is due to the development in the blood of antibodies which neutralise the infectivity of viruses. However, in a few virus diseases, reinfections or repeated infections are common. This may be due to the existence of numerous serologically distinct strains of virus, e.g. the common cold, or to the virus undergoing antigenic variation, e.g. influenza. In the case of certain viruses, and especially herpes simplex and varicella zoster viruses, reactivation of virus in the tissues despite the presence of circulating antibody is not uncommon. The recurrences of infection are probably due to the ability of these viruses to remain latent within cells and to spread on re-activation directly through cell walls to infect neighbouring cells. The presence of antibodies in people who have experienced a virus infection can be demonstrated by various *in vitro* tests such as complement fixation, haemagglutination-inhibition and neutralisation tests.

The possible role of virus infections in neoplasia is considered in Chapter 10.

Acute Bacterial Infections

The several processes which constitute the acute inflammatory reaction have been described in Chapter 2. They are basically the same in all acute inflammatory reactions, including those due to bacterial infections, but they differ in detail depending on the properties of the causal agent and the special features of the tissue involved. In some lesions, for example, inflammatory oedema may be unusually severe, while in others emigration of polymorphs or fibrin deposition may be predominant. In consequence of these variations, some acute inflammatory lesions, usually due to infections, present sufficiently characteristic appearances to warrant the use of the following descriptive terms.

Catarrhal inflammation. Acute inflammation of a mucous membrane is accompanied by glandular secretion, usually of thin watery fluid. Injury to the surface epithelium, together with inflammatory exudation from the superficial underlying vessels, results in detachment of the epithelial cells, either singly or in sheets (Fig. 7.2), and the detached cells are carried away in the mixture of secretion and exudate. When the infection subsides, the epithelium is quickly restored by proliferation of surviving cells, although prolonged or recurrent catarrhal infections may result in formation of granulation tissue and eventually fibrosis, and alteration of the epithelium to a less specialised or sometimes a squamous type.

The best known example of acute catarrhal inflammation—the common cold or coryza—is initiated by virus infection of the nasal mucosa, but various pathogenic bacteria multiply on the inflamed mucosa and aggravate the inflammatory reaction. The mixture of secretion and exudate then becomes increasingly viscid and turbid due to emigration of increasing numbers of polymorphs until it may consist of a mixture of mucus and pus: the inflammation, initially catarrhal, thus becomes *muco-purulent*. Catarrhal bronchitis (Fig. 7.2) is seen in mild influenza and, as in the common cold, the initial virus infection is often complicated by bacterial

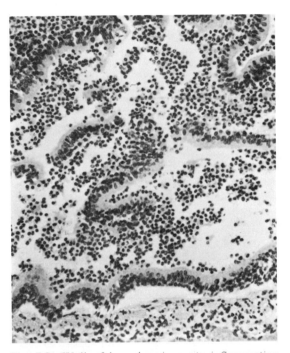

Fig. 7.2 Wall of bronchus in acute inflammation, showing desquamation of epithelium and polymorphonuclear leukocytic infiltration. × 250.

infections, with similar effects. Bacterial infection also induces catarrhal inflammation, for example of the colon in bacillary dysentery of moderate severity, and chemically-induced inflammation, such as that induced by inhalation of formalin or other irritating gases or vapours, may also be catarrhal.

Pseudo-membranous inflammation. This is

usually due to bacteria which have a low invasive capacity but grow on the surface of a mucous membrane and produce exotoxins which cause superficial necrosis, and acute inflammation of the underlying tissue. As the exudate passes to the surface, the fibrinogen in it clots within the necrotic surface layer. The fibrin and dead tissue together form the *false (pseudo-) membrane*, which contains also the causal bacteria, polymorphs and erythrocytes. Eventually the digestive activity of polymorph enzymes at the junction of living and dead tissue results in loosening and detachment of the pseudo-membrane; when the micro-organisms are destroyed, healing occurs, sometimes with some scarring. Examples of this type of inflammation are provided by diphtheria, usually affecting the pharynx or larynx (Fig. 7.3), and in the colon the more severe examples of bacillary dysentery.

Serous inflammation. This consists of acute inflammation in which there is copious fluid exudation but emigration of leukocytes and escape of red cells are minimal. The tissues become grossly oedematous and when the lining membrane of a body cavity, e.g. the pleura, is involved, the 'serous' exudate accumulates in the cavity. Serous inflammation is seen in the early stages of many acute bacterial infections, and particularly in infection by *Clostridium oedematiens*, one of the causal organisms of gas gangrene.

The terms **fibrinous** and **haemorrhagic** are also applied to inflammation, to indicate respectively marked fibrin deposition and escape of red cells.

Two important variants of acute bacterial infections with special features—**pyogenic infections** and **gas gangrene**—are described below.

Pyogenic infections: suppuration

In many acute bacterial infections, emigration of polymorphs is intense, and these cells accumulate in huge numbers in the inflamed tissues. If, as commonly happens, tissue necrosis also occurs, then the dead tissue is digested and a cavity is formed which contains polymorph-rich (**purulent**) exudate, or **pus** (Figs. 7.4, 7.5). Such a cavity is called an **abscess** and

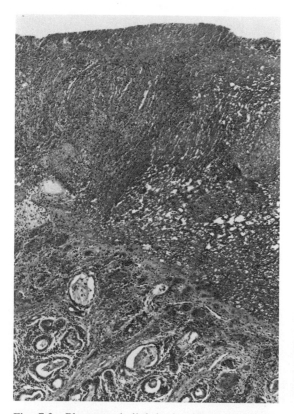

Fig. 7.3 Pharyngeal diphtheria. The mucosal surface (top) is coated with a false membrane composed of dead epithelium and fibrinous exudate. The underlying connective tissue shows acute inflammatory congestion. × 85.

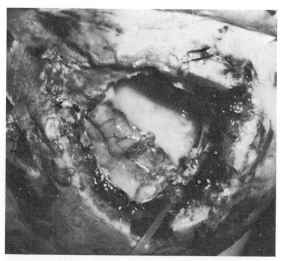

Fig. 7.4 Abscess of brain. Part of the skull has been removed surgically and a cavity containing pus is seen in the brain. (Photographed at necropsy.)

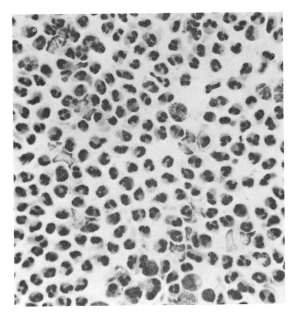

Fig. 7.5 Smear of pus. Most of the cells are neutrophil polymorphs: some are undergoing autolysis. × 400.

the process of abscess formation is termed **suppuration**. The adjective **pyogenic** is applied to bacteria which cause suppuration. Pyogenic bacterial infection of a natural body cavity, such as a joint, the peritoneum or subarachnoid space, results in accumulation of pus in the cavity without the necessity for tissue necrosis and digestion.

Suppuration. Initially, a pyogenic bacterial infection shows the usual features of acute inflammation: as it progresses, local bacterial spread results in enlargement of the lesion, and unless the bacteria are destroyed rapidly, the tissue in the centre of the lesion undergoes necrosis. This is probably due mainly to the high concentrations of powerful toxins produced by pyogenic bacteria, but the pressure of inflammatory oedema, slowing of the blood flow, and sometimes thrombosis due to endothelial injury, may also be important. The central necrotic tissue becomes infiltrated with polymorphs from the surrounding inflamed tissue, and during the process of phagocytosis and subsequent degeneration, these cells release lysosomal enzymes which digest the dead cells and tissue framework. Gradually a space, or abscess cavity, is formed containing fluid exudate rich in polymorphs, fragments of necrotic tissue, sometimes fibrin clots (from fibrinogen in the exudate), red cells and, of course, bacteria.

Necrosis of tissue and abscess formation favour multiplication of the causal bacteria. In acutely inflamed tissue, the continuous flow of exudate from small blood vessels into the tissue spaces and its removal by lymphatics is important in host defence (p. 50). In an abscess, however, the exudate is relatively stagnant: some fluid can exude into the space from the surrounding inflamed tissue, but lymphatic drainage is inadequate. The intense migration of polymorphs into the abscess cavity also increases its contents, and in consequence the hydrostatic pressure in the cavity rises. The stagnant exudate in the abscess is a suitable growth medium for most pyogenic bacteria, and so they multiply and produce toxins which, by devitalisation of the surrounding living tissue, result in extension of the necrosis and enlargement of the abscess. Because of its raised pressure, the pus in an abscess tends to extend along tissue planes of least mechanical resistance; if present, for example, in the kidney, it may extend radially within and around the tubules, and may also burst through the capsule and spread extensively in the loose perinephric fatty tissue. An abscess forming near the skin, a mucous membrane or a serosal cavity, tends to extend towards the surface and rupture and discharge its pus.

If the growth of bacteria is checked, either by the natural defence mechanisms alone or with the help of antimicrobial drugs, the abscess stops enlarging, and becomes enclosed in a layer of granulation tissue (the *pyogenic membrane*) which grows from the surrounding inflamed tissue. Commonly, bacteria persist in the pus for a long time and the granulation tissue extends inwards while its outer part gradually matures to fibrous tissue. A long-standing abscess thus becomes enclosed in dense scar tissue which progressively thickens and, as long as the bacteria persist, is lined on its inner side by a layer of granulation tissue showing the changes of acute inflammation (Fig. 7.6). In the innermost granulation tissue, emigration of polymorphs may be conspicuous, while further out there may be plasma cells, lymphocytes and macrophages.

Extension of an abscess is accompanied by increase in toxaemia, fever and neutrophil

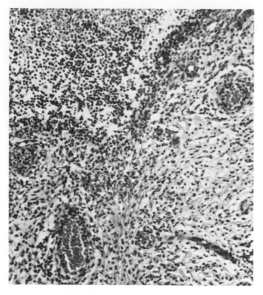

Fig. 7.6 Wall of an abscess. The abscess cavity is seen at the top left. The wall consists of vascular connective tissue showing an inflammatory reaction. × 120.

leukocytosis, and rupture into a serosal cavity may result in extensive infection, e.g. generalised peritonitis or pleurisy. This is sometimes prevented, however, for as the abscess extends towards the cavity, fibrin in the inflammatory exudate glues adjacent viscera to the inflamed serosa, and by the time the abscess reaches the surface, that part of the cavity may be walled off. When an abscess ruptures through the skin or into the alimentary tract, the pus discharges and the release of pressure allows free flow of exudate from the surrounding tissue into the abscess cavity: this favours elimination of the bacteria, not only by their removal in the discharging exudate, but also by the protective mechanisms afforded by a free flow of exudate (p. 50). Accordingly, surgical incision and drainage of an abscess is an important therapeutic measure: by promoting bacterial elimination and destruction, it allows the abscess cavity to heal with minimal scarring. The pressure in an abscess is well illustrated by the spurting out of pus when it is incised, but needs no emphasis for anyone who has experienced the throbbing pain of an apical tooth abscess.

Abscesses which are not drained, and which do not discharge naturally, may persist for months or even years: they become surrounded by dense scar tissue. The bacteria may even-

tually be destroyed, and if the cavity is still small it may be gradually filled by granulation and eventually scar tissue. The pus in larger abscess cavities may be slowly transformed to clear fluid as the cell debris, etc. is removed by macrophages, leaving a cyst-like cavity which cannot collapse because of the surrounding rigid fibrous tissue. Occasionally the pus becomes inspissated to a solid, lipid-rich crumbly material, and deposition of calcium salts converts this into a stony hard mass which may finally be replaced by bone. Even when an abscess is drained or discharges naturally, bacteria may persist in the cavity and drainage track, particularly if sufficient fibrosis has occurred to prevent its collapse.

Perhaps the commonest example of an abscess is a **boil (furuncle)**. It occurs most often in the dense dermal connective tissue at the back of the neck. The causal organism, *Staphylococcus aureus*, invades *via* the hair follicles or sebaceous ducts and sets up an acute inflammatory swelling. It spreads locally in the dermis, and necrosis of a patch of skin at the centre of the lesion results from toxic action and the vascular factors outlined above: polymorphs migrate from the surrounding inflamed tissue and digest the periphery of the necrotic 'core', which thus becomes separated from the lining tissue by a layer of pus. When separation is complete, the core is discharged, leaving an ulcer (Fig. 7.7). This is usually followed by elimination of the staphylococci, and the ulcer heals, leaving a pitted scar. In some instances, particularly in individuals with impaired resistance to infection, e.g. untreated diabetics, the infection may spread extensively in the dermal and underlying soft tissue of the neck, giving rise to a **carbuncle** consisting of a complex loculated abscess, or several separate abscesses, with multiple discharging sinuses (Fig. 7.8).

Suppuration in a serous cavity presents the same general features as an abscess developing in a solid tissue, and the principles of treatment are the same.

Composition of pus. As indicated above, pus consists of an accumulation of inflammatory exudate containing very large numbers of neutrophil polymorphs which give it an opaque appearance. Many of the polymorphs in recently formed pus are living, but the life of polymorphs which have emigrated is probably 24

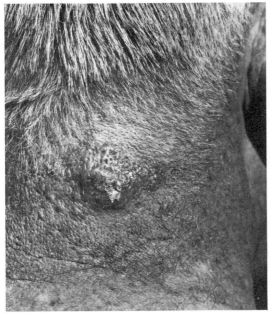 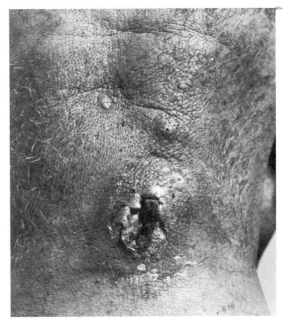

Fig. 7.7   Furuncle ('boil'). *Left*, the centre of the lesion is necrotic and about to be discharged. *Right*, the necrotic core has been discharged, leaving a ragged ulcer. × 1. (Professor J. A. Milne.)

hours or less, and in old pus most of the cells are dead and in various stages of degeneration and digestion. Release of DNA from these cells accounts for the sticky, slimy nature of pus. Some red cells are usually present, particularly in newly formed pus, and also fragments of tissue debris: fibrin may be present as free fragments, or may form a layer lining the wall of the cavity. In old pus, the number of macrophages increases and cholesterol crystals and globules of fat, derived from blood lipids or from degenerated cells, gradually accumulate.

Bacterial infection of the blood

It is customary to classify the presence of bacteria in the blood into **bacteraemia**, **septicaemia** and **pyaemia**. The distinction between the three is not sharp, but they are none the less useful terms. In bacteraemia, bacteria are present in the blood in relatively small numbers but do not multiply significantly. Septicaemia and pyaemia are much more serious conditions in which bacteria, usually of high pathogenicity, multiply in the blood.

Only very rarely are bacteria present in the blood in sufficient numbers to be detected by

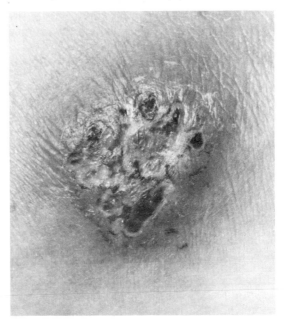

Fig. 7.8   Carbuncle: the foci of suppuration have extended to the overlying skin and discharged pus at several places. × 1. (Professor J. A. Milne.)

direct microscopy, cultivation of the blood being necessary for their detection.

Bacteraemia. Small numbers of bacteria are probably present from time to time in the blood of normal subjects, or in individuals with minor, often subclinical lesions. *Streptococcus viridans* may be cultured from the blood after vigorous brushing of the teeth, particularly if there is dental sepsis, and it is likely that occasional intestinal bacteria enter the portal circulation. Because of its high content of antibodies and complement, and the large numbers of circulating phagocytes and sinus-lining macrophages in the liver, spleen, etc., the blood is a hostile environment to most microorganisms, and although bacteria may multiply in local infections, those entering the blood are usually destroyed rapidly. Even in more serious and extensive localised infections, such as pneumococcal pneumonia or subacute bacterial endocarditis, bacteria can often be detected by blood culture, but usually they fail to multiply significantly in the blood and disappear from it when, or even before, the local infection subsides. This applies also to the bacteria which enter the bloodstream as a regular feature of certain diseases, for example in typhoid fever and brucellosis (undulant fever).

Bacteraemia is of some importance, for whenever they enter the blood, bacteria may settle in various parts of the body and cause lesions, for example suppurative meningitis or arthritis in pneumococcal pneumonia, and periostitis due to *Salmonella typhi* in typhoid fever.

Septicaemia means the multiplication of bacteria in the blood, and is applied especially to the rapid multiplication of highly pathogenic bacteria, e.g. the pyogenic cocci or the plague bacillus, *Yersinia pestis*. The term thus implies a serious infection with profound toxaemia, in which the bacteria have overwhelmed the host defences.

In some instances it is difficult to distinguish between bacteraemia and septicaemia. For example, *Escherichia coli* causes infection of the peritoneal cavity, urinary and genital tracts: blood infection may occur, particularly as a complication of generalised peritonitis, but it is often not clear whether the bacteria are multiplying in the blood or are continuously entering it, e.g. from the infected peritoneum.

Multiple small haemorrhages may occur in septicaemia (Fig. 20.25, p. 683), due either to capillary endothelial damage from the severe toxaemia or to multiple minute metastatic foci of bacterial growth. The number of neutrophil

polymorphs in the blood may be raised, although in overwhelmingly severe septicaemia they may be diminished, and show toxic granulation (p. 458). The spleen is often enlarged and congested, and may contain large numbers of polymorphs. If the septicaemia is not rapidly fatal, foci of suppuration may develop in various parts of the body as a result of haematogenous infection.

Pyaemia. In localised pyogenic infections, toxic injury to the endothelium of veins involved in the lesion may result in thrombosis: bacteria multiply in the thrombus, which then becomes heavily infiltrated by polymorphs and broken down by their digestive enzymes. Small fragments of the softened septic thrombus may then break away and be carried off in the blood (**pyaemia**—literally, pus in the blood). Where they become impacted in small vessels, they cause local injury both by obstructing the vessels and by the release of toxins from their contained bacteria: a combination of necrosis, haemorrhage and suppuration results, with formation of multiple **pyaemic abscesses** in the various tissues, their distribution depending on the site of the original septic thrombosis. Pyaemic abscesses are typically surrounded by a zone of haemorrhage (Fig. 7.9): microscopy of an early lesion may show a central zone of necrosis often

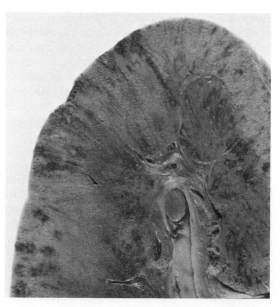

Fig. 7.9 The kidney in pyaemia, showing multiple small abscesses which are seen as pale areas surrounded by dark haemorrhagic zones.

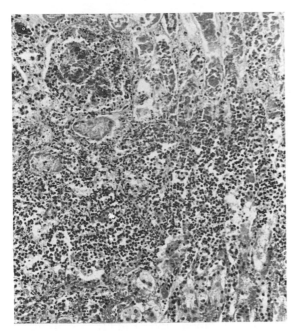

Fig. 7.10 Pyaemic abscess of kidney in a case of staphylococcal pyaemia. Infarcted tissue (*above*) is separated from congested living tissue (*below*) by a zone of suppuration. The dark patches in a glomerulus are masses of staphylococci, and have probably increased after death. × 65.

containing huge numbers of bacteria (Fig. 7.10). This is surrounded by a zone of suppuration and an outermost zone of acutely inflamed, often haemorrhagic tissue. As the lesions progress, the necrotic tissue is digested, and apart from their multiplicity and widespread distribution, they become indistinguishable from non-haematogenous abscesses. In septic thrombosis of major veins, larger fragments may be released into the circulation, and by impacting in arteries give rise to correspondingly larger foci of necrosis and suppuration (**septic infarcts**).

Septic thrombosis of systemic veins results especially, but not exclusively, in pyaemic abscesses in the lungs, while septic thrombosis in pulmonary veins results in pyaemic abscesses mainly in the systemic arterial distribution. In acute bacterial endocarditis, in which septic thrombus forms on the infected valve cusps, the distribution of pyaemic lesions depends on the particular heart valves involved. Septic thrombus of a portal venous tributary, e.g. in acute appendicitis, gives rise to **portal pyaemia**, with abscesses mainly in the liver.

Inevitably, bacteria are released from septic thrombus in pyaemia, and frank septicaemia commonly supervenes.

Septicaemia and pyaemia were formerly most often due to the pyogenic cocci. The incidence has, however, been greatly reduced by antibiotic therapy, and bacterial infections which are less readily eliminated by antibiotics have increased in relative importance, *Escherichia coli* now being the commonest cause of blood infections in general hospital practice. In states of lowered resistance to bacterial infection, e.g. agranulocytosis, immunodeficiencies and therapeutic immunosuppression, blood infection is a particular hazard. Because of impaired defence mechanisms, bacteria normally of relatively low resistance may cause septicaemia and pyaemia in these conditions.

The common pyogenic bacteria

Pyogenic infections in man are most commonly caused by *Staphylococcus aureus* and *Streptococcus pyogenes*. *Staphylococcus aureus* is the usual cause of boils, carbuncles and septic lesions of the fingers: the infection usually remains localised, although suppurating lymphadenitis may occur in the local nodes, and unless treatment is effective, septicaemia and pyaemia may occur. Some types of *Staph. aureus* are resistant to penicillin and sometimes to other antibiotics. Symptomless nasopharyngeal carriers of resistant types are commonly responsible for outbreaks of infection of surgical wounds, burns, etc., in hospital: phage typing has proved of great value in tracing the source of such outbreaks. Staphylococci are also a cause of pneumonia complicating influenza and other virus infections of the respiratory tract, and may produce a fulminating enteritis in patients receiving broad-spectrum antibiotics. The staphylococcal lesion shows the usual features of acute inflammation, and unless checked by antibiotic therapy it frequently progresses to suppuration and discharges a thick creamy pus.

Streptococcus pyogenes commonly produces acute pharyngitis and tonsillitis, 'septic fingers', otitis media and mastoiditis, also extensive inflammation of the subcutaneous connective tissues (*cellulitis*), and *erysipelas*, a spreading infection of the dermis producing a raised, red, painful lesion of the skin, usually of the face, with a well-defined margin. Before the introduction of antiseptics, *Strep pyogenes* was a very common and important cause of fatal peritonitis or septicaemia arising from infection of the genital tract following childbirth. It can also cause fatal septicaemia resulting from a minor injury, e.g. a finger prick sustained by the surgeon or pathologist dealing with a streptococcal infection.

The differences between infections due to staphylococci and streptococci are partly explicable by their toxins (p. 147). Staphylococcal infections show a greater tendency to remain localised, possibly due in part to the production of staphylocoagulase which clots fibrinogen, producing a deposit of fibrin which may help to limit spread of the organism and promote their phagocytosis. Streptococcal lesions tend to spread, possibly due partly to the production of hyaluronidase, which digests hyaluronic acid and thus liquefies the ground substance of connective tissues. *Streptococcus pyogenes* also produces fibrinolysins, and leukocidins which kill polymorphs.

Other pyogenic bacteria include *Strep. pneumoniae* (the common cause of lobar pneumonia) which may be complicated by metastatic blood-borne lesions, e.g. suppurative meningitis or arthritis; *Neisseria meningitidis* (meningococcus) which invades the nasopharynx, often silently, and produces a septicaemia or bacteraemia with the subsequent development of meningitis; *Neisseria gonorrhoeae* (gonococcus), transmitted by coitus and producing an acute urethritis, etc.

The intestinal commensals are important causes of pyogenic infections in the abdomen, e.g. appendicitis, diverticulitis and peritonitis, and in the lungs; they also infect surgical and other wounds, bedsores, burns and ulcers of the skin. They include *Escherichia coli*, *Bacterioides*, anaerobic streptococci, *Proteus*, *Pseudomonas pyocyanea* and *Klebsiella*, and may cause infections singly and in various combinations. These organisms are of particular importance in debilitated and immunosuppressed patients. All of them, but especially *Esch. coli* and *Bacterioides*, give rise to septicaemia and pyaemia, with severe septic shock (p. 227).

Gangrene

Definition. The term gangrene means digestion of dead tissue by saprophytic bacteria, i.e. bacteria which are incapable of invading and multiplying in living tissues. Many types of bacteria, often present in various combinations, may participate, and breakdown of tissue proteins, carbohydrates and fat may result in simple end-products: volatile bodies and gases may be formed, giving the foul odour of putrefaction, and the same changes are observed in putrefaction of meat, etc. Gas production may give rise to emphysematous crackling on palpation. The changes in colour—dark-brown or greenish-brown, and sometimes almost black— are due to changes in haemoglobin, and are most conspicuous when the dead tissue contains a lot of blood.

Gangrene may be either *primary* or *secondary*. In the former, tissue death is caused by the toxins of anaerobic bacteria which then invade the dead tissue and bring about digestive changes in it. In secondary gangrene, tissue death is produced by some other cause (e.g. cutting off the blood supply) and then saprophytic microbial invasion and putrefaction follow.

Primary or gas gangrene. This is caused by a group of anaerobic sporulating bacteria, the *Clostridia*, of which the three most important are *Cl. welchii*, *Cl. oedematiens* and *Cl. septicum*. These organisms are intestinal commensals in man and animals; their spores are widespread, and are liable to contaminate wounds. Being anaerobic and saprophytic, they cannot multiply in living, oxygenated tissue, but they flourish in blood-soaked foreign material and dead tissue in lacerated wounds such as are caused by shrapnel and road accidents. Given such a favourable environment, the *Clostridia* produce exotoxins which diffuse into and kill the adjacent tissues and these in turn are invaded, so that the process spreads rapidly, particularly along the length of skeletal muscles (Fig. 7.11). Gas gangrene is most often due to *Cl. welchii*. Before the muscle and other tissues are killed, they become intensely oedematous, are extremely painful, and appear swollen and pink. Microscopically, emigration of leukocytes is minimal. Among a number of toxins, *Cl. welchii* produces a lecithinase (α toxin) which, by its action on phospholipids, lyses cell and mitochondrial membranes, also hyaluronidase which digests ground substance. *Cl. welchii* ferments sugars, producing CO_2 which collects as bubbles in the dead tissues, rendering them crepitant on palpation. The subcutaneous tissue

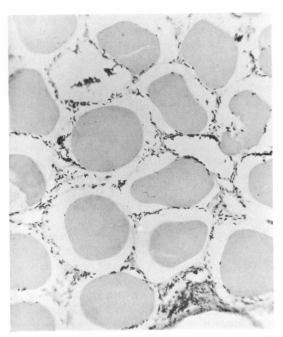

Fig. 7.11 Skeletal muscle in gas gangrene. The muscle fibres are necrotic and their nuclei have disappeared. Large numbers of *Cl. welchii* are present in the dead tissue, mainly in the endomysium. × 400.

and skin are also involved, and the affected area, often a limb, may burst open as a result of the swelling of oedema fluid and pressure of gas. The dead tissues are commonly invaded by a mixture of other organisms, which may play a major role in putrefaction. Gas gangrene may complicate intestinal lesions, e.g. appendicitis or strangulation of the gut (p. 584), clostridia being present in the intestine; it occurs also as a puerperal infection of the uterus from contamination via the perineum.

In addition to the rapidly spreading local lesion, gas gangrene is accompanied by acute haemolysis and a severe toxaemia which affects all the internal organs, and death results from peripheral vascular collapse. At necropsy, all the tissues may contain large numbers of clostridia, with extensive digestive changes. The clostridia of gas gangrene may also cause infection of subcutaneous tissue (cellulitis) without affecting the underlying muscle, or may grow in dirty wounds, producing a foul discharge but without either severe toxaemia or invasion of the surrounding tissues.

If lacerated wounds are treated by early excision of the devitalised tissue, and toxic action is controlled by the use of antitoxic sera, clostridial infections are unlikely to establish themselves. Antibiotics have also contributed greatly to the prevention of gas gangrene by inhibiting the growth of clostridia.

Noma (*cancrum oris*) is a gangrenous condition which occasionally occurs in poorly nourished children and tends to complicate debilitating infections; it begins on the gum margin and spreads to the cheek, where an inflammatory patch of dusky red appearance forms and then becomes darker in colour and ultimately gangrenous. The original necrosis is caused by a characteristic fusiform bacillus (*Fusobacterium fusiforme*); the dead tissues then undergo putrefaction. Deficient intake of the vitamin B complex, especially of nicotinic acid, predisposes to the condition.

Secondary gangrene. Here death of the tissue is produced by deprivation of the blood supply or by necrotising chemicals, and putrefying bacteria then invade the dead part. This occurs wherever the necrosis involves the skin surface or a mucous membrane to which the necessary organisms have access, and two varieties are distinguished, namely dry and moist.

Moist gangrene occurs in the internal organs. When a portion of the bowel has had its blood supply cut off, e.g. by strangulation in a hernial sac, gangrene commonly follows. First there is interference with the venous return, with consequent oedema, haemorrhages, arrest of blood flow and necrosis. Anaerobic intestinal bacteria flourish and digest the dead wall of the gut. Moist gangrene also occurs in thrombosis of the mesenteric blood vessels, and sometimes complicates acute appendicitis and acute pancreatitis. It is seen also when infarction of the lower leg occurs in an oedematous or obese individual.

The occurrence of gangrene is favoured by any condition of depressed resistance to infection. For example in untreated diabetics, pneumonia is apt to be followed by gangrene of the lung. The entrance of putrid fluids into normal tissues may cause both necrosis and putrefaction. For instance, a cancer of the oesophagus may ulcerate into a bronchus and, by allowing access of contaminated food and secretions, may lead to gangrene of the lung.

Gangrene of the leg. Infarction of toes, a foot, or the lower leg is not uncommon as the result of arterial blockage (Fig. 1.6, p. 5), the collateral circulation being insufficient to keep the part alive. This occurs most often in old people (hence the term *senile gangrene*) and is caused by arterial thrombosis complicating advanced atheroma (p. 203), which tends to be marked in diabetes. It may occur also in early or middle adult life, due to thrombo-angiitis obliterans, a disease which affects multiple arterial branches, especially in the lower limbs. Another occasional cause is the symmetrical spasmodic contraction of arteries in Raynaud's disease.

If there is much subcutaneous fat, and particularly when the limb is oedematous, as in congestive heart failure, moist gangrene commonly supervenes in the infarcted tissues, with blebs of fluid in the skin, sometimes gas production, and rapid putrefaction: there is no sharp line of demarcation between dead and living tissue, and indeed gangrene may spread proximally beyond the tissues primarily affected. When infarction occurs in a non-oedematous leg, particularly when there is little subcutaneous fat and when gradual arterial occlusion has preceded the actual infarction, so-called *dry gangrene* is liable to ensue. The skin becomes cold and waxen, the haemoglobin diffuses out of the veins and produces reddish-purple staining of the dead tissues, which then become brownish-red and ultimately almost black, and the dead tissue becomes drier and shrinks (*mummification*).

Use of the term dry gangrene is controversial. Commonly, mummification occurs with little or no putrefaction. Saprophytic organisms are, however, usually present in small numbers, particularly adjacent to the junction with living tissue, where the dead tissue remains moist. If amputation is not performed, putrefaction becomes established at this site, and a process of slow putrefactive ulceration penetrates the soft tissues, ultimately down to the bone.

Anthrax

Anthrax is a fatal epizootic disease of animals, particularly cattle and sheep, caused by a large Gram-positive sporulating bacillus, the spores of which can survive for 50 years or more in soil. In herbivors the disease is contracted by ingestion of spores and causes a severe acute enteritis with a terminal septicaemia: the excreta and secretions are highly infective. More chronic, localised lesions can also occur in animals. In man, *B. anthracis* is of low infectivity, but acute lesions occur in the skin from direct contact with infected material, or more rarely by inhalation or ingestion of spores.

The factors determining the virulence of the bacillus include a capsular polypeptide rich in D-glutamic acid, which renders the organism resistant to phagocytosis, and a complex exotoxin which promotes increased vascular permeability, causing gross inflammatory oedema. Death can result from hypovolaemic shock due to local and generalised exudative loss of plasma fluid.

Cutaneous anthrax (malignant pustule) of man occurs from direct contact with animal material, e.g. carcasses, hides or bristles in shaving brushes. The organism probably enters through a minor abrasion, and a painful papule forms and becomes blistered: it is surrounded by a zone of intense congestion and oedema. Central haemorrhage and necrosis follow, resulting in a black crust (Fig. 7.12). Leukocytic emigration is usually scanty. Spread may occur to the regional lymph nodes, which become enlarged. Although uncommon, the condition is an important example of a serious, sometimes

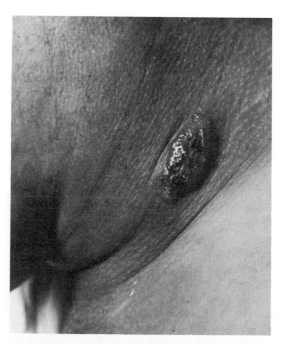

Fig. 7.12   Anthrax pustule on skin of neck. × 1·5.

fatal infection which can be effectively treated if diagnosed early.

Respiratory anthrax occurs from inhaling spores, usually from hides or wool. A localised lesion develops in the lower trachea or larger bronchi: it consists of a patch of haemorrhagic, ulcerated mucosa with intense oedema, involvement of hilar and mediastinal lymph nodes, extension to the lungs and haemorrhagic pleural and pericardial effusions: the prognosis is poor.

Intestinal anthrax is rare in man. It consists of one or more haemorrhagic foci in the wall of the upper small intestine, with central necrosis, gross oedematous swelling and involvement of the mesenteric lymph nodes.

Septicaemia and a haemorrhagic meningitis may occur in man, but are rare.

Chronic Bacterial Infections (Infective Granulomas)*

Under this heading may be included the many infections which give rise to chronic inflammation without a conspicuous exudative reaction, but usually with production of granulation tissue which eventually progresses to fibrosis. The general features of chronic inflammation have been described on pp. 51–4, and a more detailed account of the production of granulation tissue is given on pp. 61–6. The following account describes briefly some of the more important chronic infections. Because of its wide prevalence and tuberculous-like features, sarcoidosis is also included here, although there is no evidence that it is an infection.

Tuberculosis

Formerly one of the great killing diseases of temperate climates, tuberculosis is now much less common in Western Europe and North America. It is, however, prevalent in communities with a poor standard of living, and still ranks among the world's most important diseases. The disease illustrates well various basic features of bacterial infection, and in particular the importance of the reaction of the host in determining the nature of the lesions, and the spread of infection within the body. The causal mycobacteria, or tubercle bacilli, are aerobic Gram-positive bacilli with a waxy cell wall which renders them difficult to stain. Once the stain has penetrated the cell wall, however, it is also difficult to remove, and the mycobacteria are sometimes referred to as acid- and alcohol-fast bacteria, since they resist decolourisation by various strengths of acids and by limited exposure to alcohol. Tubercle bacilli grow slowly in culture; they are highly pathogenic for the guinea-pig, which has been much used for their detection when present in small numbers in sputum, etc. In man, they usually cause chronic disease but can also produce a much more acute and even rapidly fatal infection. In addition to the tubercle bacilli, of which there are two major types causing human disease (see below), the mycobacteria include the lepra bacillus which causes leprosy, and there are also various ill-defined organisms, sometimes termed *anonymous* or *atypical mycobacteria*, which cause lesions in the skin, lymph nodes, lungs and elsewhere.

Epidemiology

The two types of tubercle bacillus mainly responsible for disease in man are the human type, *Mycobacterium tuberculosis*, and the bovine type *Mycobacterium bovis*. The *human type* is the more important: infection with it is usually contracted by inhalation, and the initial or primary lesion is nearly always in the lungs. Patients with chronic pulmonary tuberculosis provide the reservoir of infection and spread the disease by exhaling infected droplets and by coughing up infected sputum. The organism is resistant to drying and can survive for long periods in dust, inhalation of which is the usual method of contracting the disease. Infection of the tonsils or of the intestine can also occur

---

* As stated on p. 54, there is an increasing tendency to restrict *granuloma* to inflammatory lesions consisting of aggregates of macrophages. I have preferred to use *macrophage granuloma* to describe such a lesion, and to use *granuloma* to mean any chronic inflammatory lesion.

from swallowing the human type of tubercle bacillus in contaminated dust, or the bovine type of bacillus in contaminated milk from cows with tuberculous mastitis.

Several factors are responsible for the declining incidence of tuberculosis in Western Europe and North America. Firstly, the rising standards of nutrition and housing: there is no doubt that under-nourishment predisposes to tuberculosis and impairs the resistance of the individual who has contracted the disease. Overcrowding and inadequate personal and domestic hygiene are also of importance in spreading the disease in the home and in public transport and meeting places, etc. The environment of a subject coughing up the organism is likely to be heavily contaminated, and spread within families is especially common, giving rise to both pulmonary and alimentary infections.

Since the 1939–45 war, the use of specific chemotherapeutic bactericidal agents has also helped to reduce the incidence of the disease by diminishing greatly the infectivity of patients with chronic pulmonary tuberculosis. Mass miniature radiography has revealed unsuspected cases of tuberculosis in the community, and protection against infection has been provided by means of BCG vaccination.

In countries where the disease is rife, infants and young children are particularly at risk, and in this country the mortality rate in children contracting the infection before the age of 3 years was formerly very high. Those who overcome the infection develop partial resistance to the organism, but may become re-infected and develop chronic pulmonary tuberculosis in adult life. The bacteria may survive for many years in dormant lesions, without clinical manifestations, and these may become active as a result of malnutrition, as in war or famine, as a complication of other debilitating diseases such as diabetes mellitus, or from administration of corticosteroids or other immunosuppressive agents. In Western Europe, a high proportion of 'new' cases are middle-aged or old and have had dormant lesions for many years from the time when the disease was much commoner: childhood cases are now relatively uncommon. *Mycobacterium bovis* causes mastitis in cattle, and is transmitted to man by consuming infected milk and milk products. Infection results usually by way of the gut or tonsils. In many countries, bovine infection in man has been eradicated by pasteurisation of milk, which kills the organism, and by tuberculin testing of cattle and elimination of infected cows. The avian tubercle bacillus (*Myco. avium*) is a rare cause of disease in man.

Hypersensitivity and immunity

The immune response to the tubercle bacillus provides the classical example of cell-mediated immunity, i.e. the production of specifically primed T lymphocytes which are capable of reacting directly with antigenic protein of the mycobacterium. The mechanism of this type of response, and the state of delayed hypersensitivity which results from it, have been described in Chapters 4 and 5 respectively. It is not understood why cell-mediated immunity is the dominant type of immune response to the tubercle bacillus, but it may be of significance that mycobacteria, living or dead, have a powerful enhancing effect on the cell-mediated immune response to antigens in general, and this forms the basis of their use in Freund's adjuvant (p. 94). Whatever the explanation of its adjuvant effect, infection with tubercle bacilli results, within two weeks or so, in the development of a high degree of cell-mediated immunity to a protein fraction (tuberculoprotein) of the organism* and the subsequent course of the infection and the features of the lesions are profoundly influenced by the hypersensitivity state. The specifically primed T cells react with tuberculoprotein, and release the various factors described on p. 129. The results are both beneficial and harmful. The tubercle bacillus has not been shown to produce any direct toxic effect, and can survive and multiply within macrophages in tissue culture without harm to the cultured cells. Indeed, it is likely that the tissue injury resulting from tuberculous infection is due mainly or entirely to the delayed hypersensitivity reaction against the bacteria. Nevertheless, without an immune response, multiplication of the organism would presumably continue unchecked. The delayed hypersensitivity reaction is therefore to be regarded as protective in reducing or eliminat-

---

* This state of hypersensitivity was demonstrated by Robert Koch (1891), using a crude preparation termed 'old tuberculin'. A more refined preparation is termed 'purified protein derivative' (PPD).

ing the infection, but at the same time injurious to the tissues. Interpretation of the features of the lesions of tuberculosis in terms of delayed hypersensitivity is attempted in the account of structural changes (below).

Although antibodies to mycobacterial antigens develop in tuberculosis, they do not appear to influence the course of the infection, and have not provided a useful diagnostic test.

Tuberculin skin testing. This is carried out by intradermal injection of very small amounts of tuberculoprotein, as in the *Mantoux test*, or by applying tuberculoprotein to the skin in the *patch test*. In individuals who are, or have previously been, infected, a delayed hypersensitivity reaction develops, the features of which are described on p. 127. In some patients with very severe tuberculosis, the test is negative, presumably because the large amount of tuberculoprotein being released from the lesions has overwhelmed the state of hypersensitivity. Tuberculin skin tests give positive reactions in infections with both human and bovine types of tubercle bacillus, and with other types of mycobacteria. For this reason they may be positive in individuals infected with *Mycobacterium leprae*.

Immunisation against tuberculosis. Protective immunisation requires the induction of cell-mediated immunity to tuberculoprotein, and this is most effectively achieved by injecting living mycobacteria. Attenuated strains of the bovine type, e.g. *bacille Calmette-Guérin* (BCG), or other non-human strains such as *Myco. muris* (the vole bacillus), are used for this purpose. Cell-mediated immunity develops, with consequent delayed hypersensitivity reactions at the site of injection and in the draining lymph nodes. The attenuated bacilli are destroyed and the lesions heal, but the cell-mediated immunity persists.

Structural changes

When a guinea-pig is inoculated with *Myco. tuberculosis* there is little reaction during the first day or so apart from local infiltration with neutrophil polymorphs, which soon disappear. During the next few days, macrophages migrate into the area and ingest the bacteria without bringing about their destruction. These very early stages of infection cannot, of course, be observed in man, but the subsequent changes are closely similar in man and the guinea-pig. After ten days or so, lymphocytes begin to appear in the lesion, and macrophages derived mainly from monocytes of the blood aggregate in increasing numbers to form a minute nodule consisting of a macrophage granuloma. The macrophages enlarge and change to **epithelioid cells** (p. 57). Small lymphocytes accumulate around the margin of the nodule, which is then termed a **tubercle** and becomes visible to the naked eye about 3 weeks after the onset. In the central part of the lesion, multinucleated **Langhans' giant cells** (p. 57) are formed by fusion of epithelioid cells (Fig. 7.13). As the

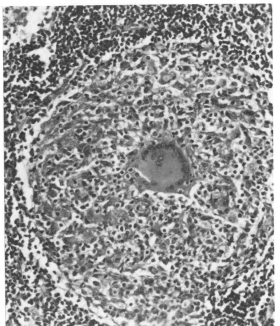

Fig. 7.13 An early tubercle, consisting mainly of epithelioid cells, some of which have fused to form a Langhans' giant cell. Lymphocytes are scattered among the epithelioid cells and are numerous around the periphery. × 174.

tubercle enlarges, the epithelioid and giant cells in the central part undergo necrosis (Fig. 7.14): the cells lose their outline and nuclear staining and become fused into a homogeneous or slightly granular material, which may also contain fibrin from vascular exudation. The tubercle thus comes to consist of a necrotic centre, surrounded by epithelioid and sometimes giant cells (Fig. 7.15), with a peripheral aggregation of small lymphocytes. The necrotic

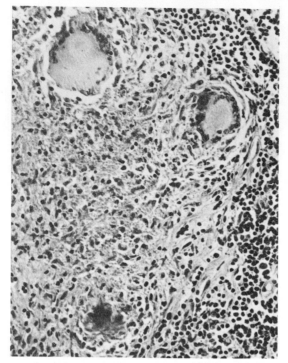

Fig. 7.14 A more advanced tubercle with three giant cells and early necrosis among the most centrally-placed epithelioid cells. × 150.

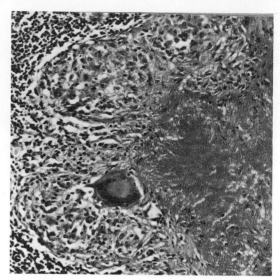

Fig. 7.15 Part of a tuberculous lesion with central caseation (*right*) and surrounding epithelioid cells with giant-cell formation. Note the structureless appearance of the caseous material. × 150.

material is creamy-white, and resembles cream cheese in appearance and consistence—hence the terms **caseation** and **caseous material**.

The initial accumulation of macrophages and phagocytosis of tubercle bacilli occur before there is any immune response and are seen also in the reaction to particles of various non-antigenic foreign materials. Lymphocytic infiltration, however, follows the development of cell-mediated immunity and presumably some of the cells are specifically primed T-cells which, by releasing various lymphokines (p. 129) contribute to the arrival of more macrophages by chemotaxis, and to their arrest around the tubercle bacilli by migration-inhibition factor: macrophage-activating factor may transform the macrophages to epithelioid cells, and may, together with specific macrophage-arming factor, mediate the destruction of phagocytosed bacilli. The T-cell cytotoxic factor presumably accounts for the necrosis of macrophages at the centre of the lesion, although the tubercle follicle is avascular and ischaemia may also be important. It has been shown in animal experiments that many of the lymphocytes in the

tuberculous lesion are not specifically primed cells resulting from the cell-mediated immune response: they may be attracted to the site of infection by a chemotactic lymphokine, but their significance in the lesion is obscure.

The further course of the infection depends on several factors, including the infecting dose and virulence of the organism, and also the

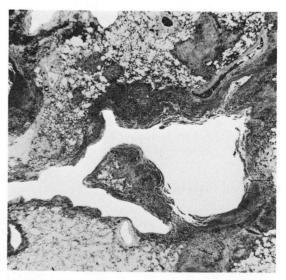

Fig. 7.16 Formation of a tuberculous cavity. The lesion has ulcerated into a bronchus and the caseous material is discharging. × 4.

degree of resistance of the host. What determines virulence in strains of tubercle bacilli is not understood, but the so-called virulent strains are those which are capable of relatively rapid multiplication *in vivo*. If bacterial multiplication is checked, tubercles are replaced by fibrous tissue. If the bacteria continue to multiply in the lesions, they may escape and gain a foothold in the surrounding tissues, with further tubercle formation. A cluster of tubercles may thus arise, and as these enlarge, they become confluent, and the central areas of caseous necrosis eventually unite to give a large caseous patch with tubercles around the periphery. Such lesions may reach several centimetres in diameter. When they arise in the lungs, they seldom reach this size without involving the wall of a bronchus, and the caseous material is then discharged, leaving a tuberculous cavity (Fig. 7.16). In other tissues, and particularly in the kidneys and in lesions of bone extending into the surrounding soft tissues, caseous material may be invaded by neutrophil polymorphs, with resultant liquefaction ('tuberculous pus'). Such a lesion used to be called a **cold abscess**, because it is not accompanied by the acute inflammatory features of a pyogenic abscess. The softened caseous material may track through the tissues and may eventually reach a surface and discharge.

Some tuberculous lesions present more acute features than those described above. For example, rapid dissemination may occur by the air passages throughout the lung, resulting in multiple scattered lesions. Microscopy then shows extensive filling of the alveoli with large rounded macrophages (Fig. 7.17); these cells rapidly undergo fatty change and necrosis, and the lesions enlarge and coalesce with little or no attempt at healing. If it infects the subarachnoid space, usually by way of the bloodstream, the tubercle bacillus multiplies rapidly in the cerebrospinal fluid and the meningitis is of acute exudative inflammatory type with deposition of fibrin and accumulation initially of neutrophil polymorphs and later of macrophages and lymphocytes. Tubercles are usually poorly formed, and involvement of the walls of arteries and veins lying in the subarachnoid space may cause severe narrowing of their lumina by endarteritis (Fig. 20.30, p. 688) or occlusion by thrombosis. The lesions which result from infection of the pleural and peritoneal cavities

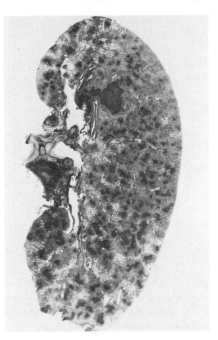

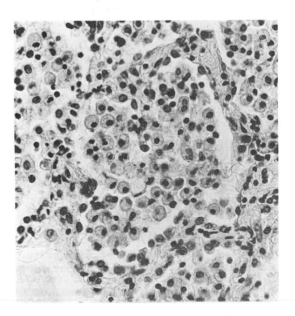

Fig. 7.17 Acute tuberculous bronchopneumonia. *Above*, Primary pulmonary tuberculosis in a child. The infection has spread by the bronchi and has caused widespread lesions which are becoming confluent and have undergone central caseation (dark areas). *Below*, the lesions consist initially of accumulations of macrophages and lymphocytes in the alveoli. The macrophages undergo fatty change and appear 'foamy': necrosis then supervenes. × 370.

are also commonly exudative, with a serous or serofibrinous exudate, and when the pericardium is involved the exudate may be rich in fibrin and is often haemorrhagic, presumably as a result of the mechanical effect of the heart beat.

Primary and reinfection tuberculosis

Infection of an individual who has not been previously infected or immunised gives rise to the **primary lesion** at the portal of entry in the lung, tonsil or small intestine. This usually remains small, and commonly heals without becoming detectable. Early spread of bacteria to the regional lymph nodes is, however, the rule, and their rapid multiplication may occur in the affected nodes, i.e. at the root of the lung (Fig. 15.29, p. 422), in the neck or in the mesentery, depending on the site of the primary lesion. The combination of the primary lesion and enlarged, caseous regional lymph nodes is called the **primary complex**.

Reinfection tuberculosis results from infection of an individual who has overcome a primary infection or been immunised by BCG. The reinfection lesion is usually in the apex of one or other lung and may extend to give a large local lesion with one or more cavities (Fig. 7.18). There is usually little or no involvement of the local lymph nodes. Reinfection lesions occur also in the tonsils, small intestine, pharynx and skin, again without much involvement of the regional nodes, but these are relatively uncommon sites. Individuals with reinfection tuberculosis of the lungs may, however, develop lesions in the larynx, mouth and intestines as a result of endogenous infection by coughing up and swallowing sputum containing tubercle bacilli (Fig. 18.53, p. 575). These metastatic lesions resemble those of reinfection tuberculosis in spreading locally with minimal or no involvement of the local nodes.

The differences between primary and reinfection tuberculosis appear to depend mainly on the multiplication and spread of the bacilli in the early stages of the primary infection, i.e. before the development of delayed hypersensitivity.

Although the term 'reinfection tuberculosis' is commonly used for chronic tuberculosis occurring usually in adults, it may well be that, in some cases, tubercle bacilli have persisted in a healed primary lesion and eventually multiply and produce the 'reinfection'.

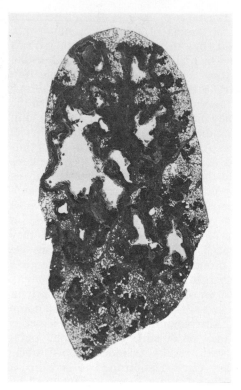

Fig. 7.18　Apical part of the lung showing chronic (reinfection) tuberculosis. The infection has extended to form coalescing lesions with central caseation and peripheral fibrosis. The caseous material in the larger lesions has discharged *via* the bronchi, leaving several cavities with fibrous walls. × $\frac{2}{3}$.

The spread of infection within the body is discussed below, but more detailed accounts of the resulting lesions are given in the chapters on regional pathology, e.g. pulmonary tuberculosis, pp. 421 *et seq.*

Spread of infection

Tuberculous infection is very prone to spread by lymphatics and to produce lesions in lymph nodes. This occurs especially in the early stages of the primary infection, with resulting involvement of the draining lymph nodes and infection may spread from these to adjacent nodes or groups of nodes, e.g. in the mediastinum. In chronic (i.e. reinfection) tuberculosis, lymphatic spread is usually localised to the tissue immediately around the lesions, the draining lymph nodes seldom being severely involved. This limitation of lymphatic spread is probably attributable to the modified behaviour of macrophages which results from delayed hypersensitivity. There is experimental evidence that lymphatic spread results from ingestion and transport of *M. tuberculosis* by macrophages, and the T-cell factors which convert macrophages into 'killer' cells and interfere with their mobility are likely to impede such spread.

Spread also occurs by the bloodstream. This is seen notably in **acute miliary tuberculosis**, in which large numbers of bacteria enter the blood and give rise to multiple scattered tubercles in the various organs. The condition arises most commonly in primary tuberculosis and is due usually to involvement of a vein by the large caseating lymph node lesions of the primary complex—in most cases the pulmonary hilar nodes: the caseating process extends into the wall of an adjacent vein, usually one of the pulmonary veins, and caseous material containing large numbers of mycobacteria is then discharged into the circulation. The resulting lesions are particularly numerous in the lungs, liver, kidneys and spleen. They consist of tubercles of fairly uniform size, and without specific therapy death usually results from tu-

berculous meningitis after about a month, at which time the tubercles are of approx. 1–2 mm diameter (Fig. 15.31, p. 425): they are rather poorly developed, often without giant cells, but with central necrosis (Fig. 7.19) and are termed **miliary tubercles** (latin *milium*—millet seed). In some instances, the bacteria escape into a systemic vein, either directly or by involvement of the thoracic duct, and as a result the number of miliary lesions in the lungs far exceeds those in other organs. When a relatively small number of tubercle bacilli gain entrance to the bloodstream, few tubercles are produced in the various organs, and since the patient may survive much longer than is the case in untreated acute miliary tuberculosis, the lesions may become larger. One or more large metastatic lesions may also occur, for example in the bones, joints, kidneys, epididymes or fallopian tubes, and less commonly in the brain. Although blood-borne lesions arise most commonly as a complication of the primary tuberculous complex, they may also occur in reinfection tuberculosis, particularly in advanced cases: haematogenous lesions are also observed when tuberculosis is complicated by other debilitating diseases, or

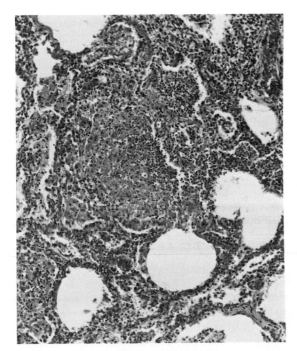 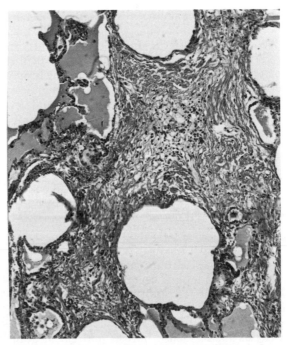

Fig. 7.19 On the left is shown a miliary tubercle of lung with central caseation and acute exudate in the surrounding alveoli from a patient with untreated miliary tuberculosis; on the right a fibrous scar containing a few lymphocytes, the remains of a miliary tubercle after specific chemotherapy. × 100.

as a result of corticosteroid or other immuno-suppressive therapy.

Spread of tuberculous infection occurs also along hollow viscera and in body cavities. In the lungs, spread by the bronchi is of great importance. Mycobacteria coughed up in sputum may settle and give rise to lesions in the larynx and intestine. Spread may occur from the fallopian tubes to the endometrium, and from the kidney to the urinary tract, and dissemination may occur within the pleural, pericardial and peritoneal cavities and within the subarchnoid space and ventricles of the brain.

Healing of tuberculous lesions

The healing of tubercles or larger tuberculous lesions is dependent on the elimination or reduction in numbers of mycobacteria. Healing is brought about by formation of reticulin around the lesions, and by maturation of this into fibrous tissue. If caseation is slight or absent, as in early tubercles, the whole lesion may be gradually replaced by fibrous tissue, leaving a scar (Fig. 7.19), but extensive patches of caseation usually persist and become encapsulated in fibrous tissue. Slow progressive deposition of calcium salts commonly occurs in the caseous material, which eventually may become stony hard and clearly visible in radiographs: in some instances the calcified material may be replaced by bone, which may even develop spaces containing haemopoietic marrow. The course of the disease depends on the balance between bacterial multiplication, with extension and caseation of the lesions, and the reactive processes involved in killing the bacteria, preventing their spread, and promoting a fibroblastic reaction.

The effects of drugs. The course and prognosis of tuberculosis have been radically changed by effective specific chemotherapy, which has also greatly modified the appearance of tuberculous lesions. When healing occurs 'naturally', i.e. without specific chemotherapy, large caseous lesions become walled off first by cellular tubercles and then by new-formed fibrous tissue, which penetrates the outer zone of tubercles and finally encapsulates the central caseous mass. Dense fibrosis and calcification complete the process: there is little resolution. Effective drug therapy is accompanied successively by resolution of the surrounding exudative lesions, increased vascularity, and reversion of the epithelioid cells to foamy macrophages, formation of granulation tissue, absorption of necrotic and caseous material, and finally by healing with the production of minimal amounts of fibrous tissue. Combined therapy thus strikingly modifies the outcome; early lesions may clear up almost completely without residual effects and chronic caseous and fibrotic pulmonary lesions with excavation are transformed to smooth-walled cavities, which may become lined by epithelium.

Because of the spontaneous occurrence of mutant tubercle bacilli resistant to one or more drugs, it is now accepted practice to administer a combination of three drugs, usually isonicotinic acid hydrazide (isoniazid), streptomycin and ethambutol (which has largely replaced para-aminosalicylic acid). Because the tubercle bacillus multiplies relatively slowly, it may take some months for the selective advantage conferred by drug therapy on a resistant mutant to be reflected in clinical deterioration, and repeated bacteriological examinations, e.g. of sputum, are therefore important during treatment.

Leprosy

It is estimated that there are some 10 million people with leprosy throughout the world. The disease now occurs mainly in those tropical and sub-tropical countries with poor living standards, although it was formerly quite common in Europe and North America. The causal organism, *Mycobacterium leprae*, was the first bacterial pathogen to be seen and described in a human disease. It is an acid-fast bacillus, demonstrable by a modified Ziehl–Neelsen staining technique: it has not yet been grown in culture and does not cause natural disease in species other than man, although it is pathogenic for animals in which cell-mediated immunity has been depressed by neonatal thymectomy or anti-lymphocyte serum. Infectivity is low, and although the bacillus is often present in large numbers in the nasal and oral secretions of patients, only a small percentage of long-term close contacts develop the disease.

The leprosy bacillus appears to be highly temperature-dependent, for it produces lesions mainly in colder parts of the body, namely the

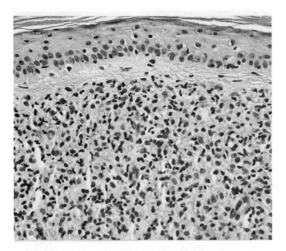

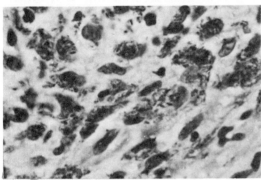

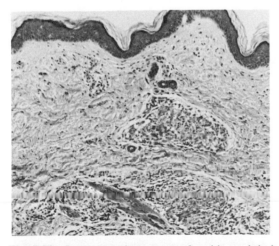

skin, especially of the nose, lobes of the ears and extremities, the anterior part of the eye, the nasopharynx, mouth and upper respiratory tract, superficial lymph nodes and testes. It also has a predilection for nerves; it always involves the small nerve twigs in the skin and often larger superficial nerves.

Host resistance is dependent mainly on the cell-mediated response to *Myco. leprae*. In **lepromatous leprosy** this is depressed, and the lesions progress relentlessly and contain huge numbers of bacilli. A strong response is associated with **tuberculoid leprosy**, in which the lesions contain relatively few bacilli, and may become stationary or subside.

Lepromatous leprosy. The lesions consist of aggregates of macrophages (Fig. 7.20), containing huge numbers of lepra bacilli lying parallel in bundles or aggregated to form large acid-fast masses (globi). In the absence of cell-mediated immunity, the bacilli are not destroyed, and multiply within the macrophages which have ingested them. Like tubercle bacilli, they appear to be non-toxigenic and macrophages containing large numbers of organisms show little evidence of injury apart from fatty change. Lymphocytes are scanty or absent, and tissue injury is probably due mainly to pressure. However, the skin lesions become very extensive and may ulcerate and be secondarily infected with various bacteria. Similar changes are seen in the oral, nasal and upper respiratory lesions. In spite of extensive involvement of superficial nerves, anaesthesia and paralysis are often late features of the disease. The internal organs are rarely seriously involved, although small clusters of macrophages containing lepra bacilli may occur in the liver, spleen, etc.

Tuberculoid leprosy. The lesions resemble those of tuberculosis, consisting of tubercle-like follicles (Fig. 7.20) and more extensive infiltrates of epithelioid cells (modified macrophages), lymphocytes and Langhans' giant-cells. Necrosis is absent or inconspicuous and leprosy bacilli are often difficult to find. Nerve injury occurs early, and patches of hypopigmentation and sensory loss are often presenting features. The internal organs are seldom involved.

Fig. 7.20 Leprosy. *Above*, part of a skin nodule in lepromatous leprosy. The lesion is a macrophage granuloma: lymphocytes are scanty and necrosis has not occurred. × 60.
Middle, part of the same lesion, stained by Triff's method for acid-fast bacilli: the macrophages contain numerous *Myco. leprae*. × 650.
Below, skin lesions in tuberculoid leprosy, composed of epithelioid cells, giant cells and lymphocytes. Such lesions contain few bacilli. × 64. (Professor J. A. Milne.)

Forms of leprosy intermediate between lepromatous and tuberculoid are commonly encountered. In some instances, lesions of both types may be present (**borderline** or **dimorphous leprosy**), and such cases may progress in either direction. Drug therapy helps to convert lepromatous to tuberculoid leprosy, and to cure the latter.

Immunological reactions in leprosy. Intradermal injection of lepromin, an antigenic extract of *Myco. leprae*, elicits a delayed hypersensitivity reaction, resembling the tuberculin reaction, in individuals with tuberculoid leprosy: the reaction occurs also in individuals with cell-mediated immunity to the tubercle bacillus and other mycobacteria. A later granulomatous reaction may develop within 4 weeks: this also is not diagnostic of leprosy. The test is usually negative in lepromatous leprosy, and becomes positive if the patient converts, spontaneously or as a result of drug therapy, to tuberculoid leprosy. These observations are supported by parallel results of *in vitro* tests for cell-mediated immunity, and together with the morphological features of the disease indicate that tuberculoid lesions are modified by a delayed hypersensitivity reaction to the lepra bacilli, whereas lepromatous lesions represent the growth of the bacilli in the absence of delayed hypersensitivity.

Failure of cell-mediated immunity in lepromatous leprosy is not fully explained. The lymph nodes show lymphocyte depletion of the T-dependent zones, i.e. paracortex, and diminution of T lymphocytes in the blood has been reported. A plasma factor which depresses T lymphocyte function has also been described.

There is usually a high titre of antibody to *Myco. leprae* in the serum of patients with lepromatous leprosy, but this seems to afford little protection: drug therapy results in destruction of large numbers of bacilli, and release of antigen may then give rise to an acute Arthus reaction in the lesions (**erythema nodosum leprosum**) or generalised immune complex disease with glomerulonephritis (p. 125). Another complication is amyloid disease.

Sarcoidosis

This disease, which is of unknown causation, is characterised by multiple granulomatous lesions, and may affect lymph nodes, lungs, skin, eyes, salivary glands, liver and the bones, particularly of the hands and feet. It is of world-wide distribution, and is more common in negroes than whites in the U.S.A., and in immigrants than natives in Great Britain. The highest reported incidence is in Sweden.

The disease most commonly gives rise to enlarged mediastinal and pulmonary hilar lymph nodes, often without symptoms, but sometimes accompanied by fever. Other groups of lymph nodes are often affected and minute lesions in the lungs may present an x-ray picture resembling that of miliary tuberculosis. Skin lesions of erythema nodosum are sometimes the earliest clinical feature, but sarcoid lesions also occur in the skin. Microscopically, the lesions consist of tubercle-like follicles composed of epithelioid cells with occasional giant cells and scanty peripheral lymphocytes (Fig. 7.21 and Fig. 17.8, p. 517). The giant cells may contain curious star-shaped or conchoid inclusions (*asteroid* or *Schaumann bodies*). Unlike tuberculosis, the lesions do not undergo caseation although there may be a little central necrosis.

Intradermal injection of a sterile suspension prepared from sarcoid lesions (**Kveim test**) leads to the development of a lesion becoming

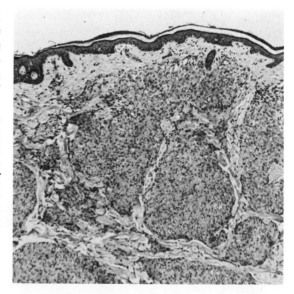

Fig. 7.21 Sarcoidosis of skin. The lesions consist of aggregates of epithelioid cells with relatively few lymphocytes. In contrast to tuberculosis, there is little or no necrosis. × 80.

maximal in about six weeks and having the histological features of sarcoidosis. The test is positive in most cases of sarcoidosis, but conflicting results have been reported in some other conditions, and notably in Crohn's disease (p. 562). During the course of sarcoidosis, tuberculin tests are negative in most cases even when known to have been previously positive. The capacity to produce antibodies is not, however, impaired.

The course of the disease is unpredictable: it may be acute or chronic, and temporary or permanent remission may occur spontaneously. It can cause blindness by involving the uveal tract, and is occasionally fatal, usually as a result of fibrosis of the pulmonary lesions with consequent right ventricular heart failure, or as a result of intercurrent infections. Hypercalcaemia may develop with consequent renal damage.

Disseminated lesions closely resembling those of sarcoidosis can result from inhalation of beryllium, but most cases of sarcoidosis are of unknown cause. Subsequent development of tuberculosis has been observed in some patients, but sarcoidosis seems unlikely to be a modified form of tuberculosis, because depression of delayed hypersensitivity (as in sarcoidosis) would be expected to be associated with a florid form of tuberculosis.

Syphilis

Historical note

It is generally believed that syphilis was introduced into Europe on the return of the Spanish sailors of Columbus from America and that by the end of 1494 it had spread throughout Spain and along the Mediterranean coast into Italy. Within a century it had become widespread throughout Europe, having been carried everywhere by the mercenary troops returning to their own countries after the Siege of Naples (1495). At this time syphilis was clearly recognised as a new disease and its manifestations became so well known that Shakespeare was able to give a remarkably accurate (although anachronistic) account of them in *Timon of Athens* (Act IV, Scene 3). Absence of syphilis from the Old World is supported by the complete lack of evidence of the disease in skeletal remains dating back from 1494, whereas bones found in ancient tombs in Central America bear clear indications of the disease. The name comes from a poem composed in 1530 by Girolamo Frascatoro, a Verona physician, in which Syphilis, a

swineherd, offended Apollo, who inflicted him with the disease.

General features

Formerly common, syphilis is now relatively infrequent in Western Europe: recent reports show some increase, particularly among homosexuals, but the rise is much less than for gonorrhoea. Syphilis is an important **venereal disease**, i.e. it is usually contracted by coitus and the primary lesion is then on the genitals. Extragenital infections occur on the lip, tongue or breast and also on the fingers from handling infective lesions. The causal agent is a small motile spiral micro-organism or spirochaete, *Treponema pallidum*. Infection is usually by direct contact, the presence of a minute abrasion or crack in the skin apparently facilitating invasion. The disease has a distinct incubation period, followed by a primary lesion and then a febrile secondary stage with skin eruptions, and this may be followed by a tertiary stage, with localised lesions, and a late stage with disease of the central nervous system. It is convenient to give a general survey of the course of the untreated disease at this point. The special features of the individual lesions will be considered in the appropriate sections later.

'Stages' of syphilis

The primary sore. The primary sore or chancre (Fig. 7.22) appears usually on the external genitals, after an incubation period of 3–4 weeks, as a small, slowly growing, hard, pale brownish-red, usually painless nodule. The centre ulcerates and there may be some exudate which, in a skin lesion, is usually scanty and forms a crust. When the lesion is on a mucous surface and the part is not kept clean, there may be more extensive ulceration, and various organisms, sometimes including other spirochaetes, are present in addition to *Tr. pallidum*. The ulcer persists for some weeks, during which the inguinal lymph nodes, usually on both sides, become somewhat enlarged and hard (bilateral inguinal 'bubo'). *Treponema pallidum* is often detectable in the exudate of the ulcerated chancre, either by dark-ground microscopy or by fluorescence microscopy, using fluorescein-labelled antibody: if this fails,

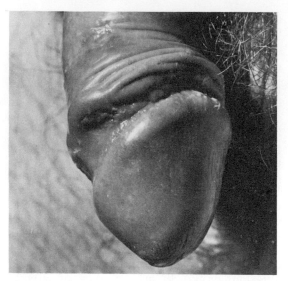

Fig. 7.22 Primary syphilitic chancre of penis. The lesion is seen as a swelling with (in this instance) central necrosis and ulceration: it is situated in the coronal sulcus and involves the reflexion of the prepuce.

it may be demonstrable in fluid withdrawn by puncture of the bubo. Dissemination by the blood takes place before the appearance of the primary lesion, and syphilis has been accidentally transmitted by transfusion of blood withdrawn before the primary lesion had appeared in the donor.

Secondary lesions appear at a variable interval, usually from 2–3 months after infection; they include multiple symmetrical lesions of the skin and squamous mucous membranes. The skin rash may be macular, papular or pustular, the palms of the hands and soles of the feet being commonly involved. Lesions of the hair follicles in the scalp lead to loss of the hair— *alopecia*. In the vulva, anus and perineum, flat raised papules sometimes develop— *condylomata lata*—and are intensely infective: they must not be confused with *condylomata acuminata*, the so-called venereal warts, which are of viral nature. The buccal and pharyngeal mucosa shows white, shining patches caused by thickening of the keratinised layer, and these break down, giving '*snail-track ulcers*'. General slight enlargement of lymph nodes is also common and is most easily detected in the superficial nodes. The secondary lesions are usually accompanied by fever, anaemia and general malaise. After some months all these features

disappear spontaneously and the disease becomes latent.

Tertiary lesions appear irregularly, especially in the internal organs, skin and mucous membranes; they are few in number but usually much larger than the primary and secondary lesions, and lead to serious and permanent damage. They rarely appear within the first few years, and sometimes only after many years. Tertiary lesions are characterised by diffuse chronic inflammation, often with central necrosis, and extensive formation of granulation tissue. If necrosis is present, the lesion is termed a **gumma**. The central necrotic portion is dull yellowish, firm and rubbery; this is surrounded by a more translucent capsule of young connective tissue which has often a very irregular outline (Fig. 23.2, p. 882). Tertiary lesions may occur in any tissue, but especially in the liver, testes and bones. They cause extensive destruction, e.g. in the nasal bones with loss of the bridge of the nose and perforation of the palate, ulceration and destruction of the larynx, creeping ulcers in the skin, etc. Of special importance are the cardiovascular lesions. All tertiary lesions tend to heal eventually, and much distortion of the organs and interference with function may result from scarring.

Neurosyphilis. Lastly, in a small proportion of cases there occur two important nervous diseases, *tabes dorsalis* and *general paralysis*. Since these develop usually only many years after infection they are sometimes called *quaternary* lesions; they are due to the actual presence of the spirochaetes in the central nervous system.

Microscopic appearances

The main feature of the early **chancre** is heavy cellular infiltration of the dermis (Fig. 7.23) with lymphocytes, plasma cells and occasional macrophages, which are mainly responsible for the hardness and swelling. At the periphery, the infiltrating cells lie mainly around the small vessels (periarteritis). Later, ulceration occurs with exudative inflammation and formation of granulation tissue. The histological features are not diagnostic without the demonstration of *Tr. pallidum*, which requires special staining techniques. After a time the cellular infiltration gradually diminishes and only a little thickening of the fibrous stroma remains. There is usually

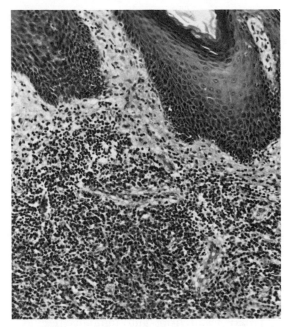

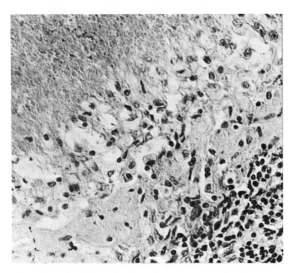

Fig. 7.25 Section of part of a gumma, showing the necrotic centre (*upper left*), bounded by connective tissue heavily infiltrated with lymphocytes. × 250.

Fig. 7.23 Primary syphilitic chancre, showing the heavy cellular infiltration of the dermis. Most of the infiltrating cells (not readily identified at this magnification) are lymphocytes and plasma cells. × 120.

little or no residual scarring unless there has been much ulceration.

In the **secondary lesions** in the skin and mucous membranes the main changes are vascular engorgement and infiltration, mainly

membranes usually subside naturally, i.e. without specific therapy, and without scarring.

The **gumma** of the **tertiary stage** consists of parenchymal necrosis, surrounded by a layer of connective tissue infiltrated with lymphocytes and plasma cells (Fig. 7.25). Eventual healing is accompanied by shrinkage, considerable scarring and distortion. Another common type of lesion is chronic interstitial inflammation or

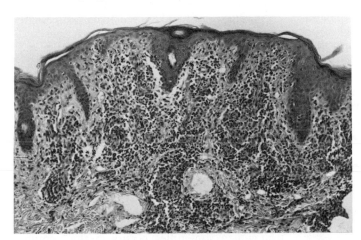

Fig. 7.24 Papular syphilitic rash, showing abundant infiltration of the corium by lymphocytes and plasma cells. Note also the hyperkeratosis. × 115.

of plasma cells, but also lymphocytes and macrophages (Fig. 7.24). Cellular infiltration occurs also around and into the hair follicles, and the hairs may fall out. All these disseminated lesions of the skin and mucous

fibrosis, often spreading extensively, and sometimes containing foci of gummatous necrosis. In the necrotic tissue, the structural outlines may be preserved for a long time, the cells not having the same tendency to fuse into amorphous material as is seen in caseous tuberculosis. Giant cells may be present in the granulation tissue at the periphery, but they are usually smaller than in tuberculosis, and there are no well-formed follicles. Nevertheless the histological diagnosis between the two diseases may be difficult. The important **vascular lesions** of syphilis are described later: those in the larger arteries are due to the presence of spirochaetes in the adventitial sheath and media: they give rise to cellular infiltrations like those described above, and some medial necrosis may follow.

The number of spirochaetes in gummatous lesions is small, and the necrosis seems to be due either to ischaemia resulting from endarteritis of small vessels, or to a hypersensitivity reaction, possibly of delayed type.

Congenital syphilis

The first pregnancy after infection is likely to terminate prematurely with a stillborn macerated fetus, in the tissues of which spirochaetes are abundant. The parenchymatous organs show diffuse proliferation of fibroblasts with minute foci of necrosis—miliary gummas, and there is severe damage to the liver, lungs, pancreas, etc. In subsequent pregnancies the effects are progressively less severe. The next child may be born alive with lesions of congenital syphilis, namely a papular rash around mouth and nose, on the buttocks, palms of hands and soles of feet. Disease of the nasal bones and mucosa leads to 'snuffles' and interference with feeding. Syphilitic hepatitis with jaundice, splenomegaly, and lesions in the bones are also common. Later a characteristic deformity appears in the incisor teeth, which are peg-shaped with notched edges (Hutchinson's teeth) and there is also pitting of the first permanent molars. Still later, interstitial keratitis produces corneal opacity and blindness. Pregnancy has a curiously ameliorating effect on syphilitic lesions in the mother, who may appear healthy in spite of producing syphilitic offspring.

Immunology of syphilis

A number of antibodies develop in syphilis, and their detection in the serum is of considerable diagnostic value. The older tests are based on the detection of antibodies reactive with antigenic phospholipids of mitochondrial membranes. Alcoholic extract of beef heart muscle ('*cardiolipin*') is employed as antigen, but extracts of various normal animal and human tissues may also be used. Antibody is demonstrable by various precipitation (flocculation) techniques, e.g. the Kahn, Klein or Hinton tests, or by the Wassermann test which is based on complement fixation (p. 92). These are the so-called **standard tests for syphilis**: they are useful screening tests, antibody being detectable from an early stage, but are not specific for syphilis, **false positive reactions** occurring in various conditions, including malaria, infectious mononucleosis, systemic lupus erythematosus and occasionally in apparently normal individuals, particularly during pregnancy. There is evidence that, in syphilis, antibodies develop to phospholipids of *Tr. pallidum*, and cross-react with mitochondrial phospholipids, but the false positive reactions are unexplained, and may result from auto-immunisation as a result of tissue destruction and release of cellular constituents.

Confirmatory tests for syphilis depend on the demonstration of antibody specific for *Tr. pallidum*. In the treponemal immobilisation test the patient's serum is added to a suspension of living *Tr. pallidum* and antibody is indicated by immobilisation of the treponemas. A more recent test is based on the fluorescent antibody technique (p. 91), and if group treponemal antibodies are first absorbed from the patient's serum, this provides a test of high sensitivity and specificity.

Antibody tests usually become positive a week or so after the appearance of the primary lesion: they are virtually always positive in the secondary stage, following which the percentage of positives falls. In neurosyphilis, antibody is more likely to be detected in the cerebrospinal fluid than in the serum.

Following cure, the antibody tests become negative, although the specific treponemal antibodies may persist for some years.

The protective role of specific immunity in syphilis is suggested by the overwhelming infection which sometimes occurs in the immunologically immature fetus. Some of the features of secondary syphilis, including the widespread skin lesions and occurrence of arthralgia and occasionally glomerulonephritis, are suggestive of immune-complex disease. In both congenital and secondary syphilis, lymphocyte depletion in the T-dependent areas of the spleen and lymph nodes, and depressed T-cell function, have been reported.

Other pathogenic spirochaetes

These include the **Borreliae**, which are transmitted by lice and ticks, and cause **relapsing fever** (p. 633) and the **Leptospirae** which infest rodents, etc., and cause febrile illnesses, the best known being Weil's disease (p. 632).

Actinomycosis

This disease is produced by organisms which are normal commensals in the mouth and gut, and only occasionally invade the tissues to produce infection. The actinomyces are branching bacteria which grow in the tissues to produce characteristic radiate colonies, sometimes visible macroscopically. In man, the micro-aerophilic *Actinomyces israelii* is the chief pathogen, but occasionally aerobic organisms—*Nocardia*—are involved, and also other species, which grow more diffusely. In bovines, in which actinomycosis is common, the lesions are localised and are large granulomatous masses which occur especially in and around the jaw. In man, the lesions are of a more suppurative type, and in about 50% of cases are in the region of the mouth or jaws, the parasite gaining entrance commonly from a tooth socket; in 25% the infection is in the appendix or caecal region, from which spread by the blood stream to the liver may occur; in about 15% the initial lesion is in the lung and in 5% it is subcutaneous. The lesion is usually a chronic suppurative one, with formation of multiple abscesses, each containing one or more colonies of the organism—the so-called honeycomb abscess. A fibrous tissue wall forms and

is lined by granulation tissue which characteristically contains many foamy cells—macrophages laden with lipid—which give the lining of each abscess a yellowish colour. In the centre is pus containing actinomyces colonies (Fig. 7.26), which are sometimes visible by

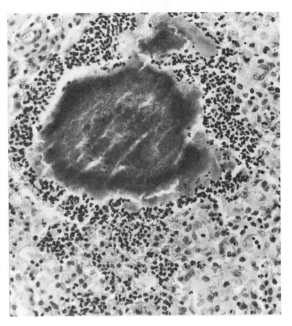

Fig. 7.26 Actinomycosis. A colony of *Actinomyces israelii* in a small abscess, the wall of which consists of granulation tissue heavily infiltrated with lipid-laden (foamy) macrophages. × 190.

naked eye as small yellow or grey, gritty granules. Lesions of the face and neck, originating about the jaw, may produce much granulation tissue in which many small foci of suppuration persist and break down on the surface, resulting in multiple sinuses. The infection spreads directly through the tissues but does not usually involve the regional lymph nodes; if untreated it tends to invade the bloodstream, giving rise to pyaemia with secondary abscesses in the liver, lungs and other organs.

Other Types of Infection

Rickettsial infections

The rickettsiae are micro-organisms of various shapes, which are smaller than bacteria, but

resemble them in their structural and metabolic features, including a cell wall. They are obligatory intracellular parasites and infect many species including arthropods, birds and mammals. Several species of rickettsiae cause disease in man: in most instances they enter the body by the bites of infected ticks or mites, or from infected louse or flea faeces being scratched into the skin. The organisms enter and multiply in the endothelium of the capillaries and other small blood vessels; they are at first localised to the site of infection, but blood dissemination occurs during the incubation period and endothelial involvement then becomes widespread. Capillary obstruction from endothelial swelling or thrombosis occurs, with resultant necrosis in heavily involved tissues, and a mixed cell reaction develops, including polymorphs, macrophages, lymphocytes and plasma cells.

The rickettsial diseases include **endemic (murine) typhus**, caused by *R. mooseri* and transmitted by the rat flea; **epidemic typhus** (*R. prowazekii*) and **trench fever** (*R. quintana*) which are spread by the body louse: the **spotted fever** group (*R. rickettsii*, etc.) transmitted from various animals to man by the bites of infected ticks or mites, and finally **scrub typhus** (*R. tsutsugamuchi*), transmitted from rodents to man by a mite. Epidemic and endemic typhus are of worldwide distribution: the epidemic disease occurs in crowded louse-infested communities, and is common in times of war, earthquakes and other major disasters. Various forms of spotted fever are related to particular localities.

These diseases vary in their severity and pathological detail: in all, the small blood vessels are involved, and lesions tend to result especially in the brain, heart and skin. Infected material is particularly dangerous to laboratory workers, and diagnosis is usually made by demonstrating a rising titre of antibody, either in the patient or in laboratory animals inoculated with the patient's blood, etc. Only *R. quintana* has been cultured successfully in cell-free media.

Q fever is a typhus-like illness caused by the *Coxiella burnetii* which closely resembles the rickettsiae but differs from them in its antigenicity and in being much more resistant to drying, etc: it is a parasite of domesticated animals and man is infected by inhalation of droplets, or by ingestion of animal products. Q fever usually presents as a 'non-bacterial' pneumonia, although lesions may occur in the brain and other organs. *Cox. burnetii* also colonises the valves of the heart, producing a condition closely similar to subacute bacterial endocarditis.

Mycoplasmal infections

Mycoplasmas are very small filamentous or coccobacillary micro-organisms which lack a cell wall but can be grown in cell-free media and are classed as bacteria. They are distributed widely and are pathogenic to many animal and plant species. In man only one species, *Mycoplasma pneumoniae*, has been shown conclusively to be pathogenic, although other mycoplasmas have been isolated from the lesions of various other diseases. A major difficulty arises from their ubiquity and the consequent contamination of culture media; they can pass through bacteria-retaining filters and are also liable to contaminate cell cultures used in virology and for other purposes.

Mycoplasma pneumoniae is the cause of one form of 'non-bacterial' pneumonia, which is endemic in most parts of the world and also occurs as outbreaks, particularly in children. The organism disseminates in the body and may cause a meningo-encephalitis. The immune response includes the production of an antibody which cross-reacts at low temperatures with a human red cell antigen, and is responsible in some cases for acute haemolysis.

Chlamydial infections

The chlamydiae are a group of spherical micro-organisms intermediate in size between the larger viruses and bacteria. They are obligatory intracellular parasites, but otherwise resemble bacteria far more closely than viruses: the vegetative form multiplies by binary fission, and infection is spread by a smaller compact spore-like form (elementary body) which can survive, but not divide, extracellularly.

These organisms are enzootic in certain birds, including the psittacines (parrot family), and also cause infections in sheep, goats and cattle. In man, they are responsible for the sexually transmitted disease **lymphogranuloma inguinale**, for eye infections, the most important being **trachoma**, and for pulmonary infection (**ornithosis**) which results from inhalation of the organism. The initial reaction to chlamydial infection is granulomatous, with accumulation of macrophages and lymphoid cells, necrosis, formation of granulation tissue and scarring. In lymphogranuloma inguinale a small ulcerating primary lesion develops in the genitalia, but the draining lymph nodes become grossly involved and prolonged suppuration and extensive scarring result. Similar lesions occur extragenitally in cat-scratch disease, but the causal agent is uncertain.

Both antibodies and cell-mediated immunity develop in chlamydial infections, the latter probably being the more important in the elimination of the infection. These diseases are considered more fully in the appropriate systematic chapters.

Yeasts and fungi

Yeasts and fungi are primitive forms of plant life which lack the photosynthetic mechanism and obtain energy by breaking down dead organic matter or by parasitism. Only a few of the very many known species are pathogenic to man, and with some exceptions the lesions are superficial and not serious. Good examples of such infection are athlete's foot and tinea (ringworm). In severely ill patients, however, and particularly in those with T-cell deficiency or on immunosuppressive therapy, some of these organisms can cause more extensive or even systemic infections.

Fungi grow typically as filamentous branching hyphae which form an interlacing mycelium; they produce spores, commonly on projecting (aerial) hyphae. Yeasts consist of simple spherical or ovoid cells which multiply by budding, but the distinction from fungi is not sharp, for the so-called dimorphic fungi can assume the form of either hyphae or yeasts, depending on the environmental conditions.

In general, superficial infections with yeasts or fungi promote a mild inflammatory reaction. The reactions to deeper and more extensive infections vary considerably depending on the nature of the parasite and the host responses: they include necrosis, abscess formation, granulation tissue, and aggregation of macrophages, lymphocytes and plasma cells. In some instances, an epithelioid and giant-cell reaction results in appearances similar to those of tuberculosis, and various hypersensitivity reactions may contribute to the pathological changes. Host defence appears to be mediated largely by cell-mediated immunity.

In superficial infections, diagnosis can often be made from the appearance of the lesion, supported by microscopy of skin or mucosal scrapings, but cultivation on suitable media is sometimes necessary.

Some examples of yeast and fungal infections are described briefly below.

Candidiasis. *Candida albicans* is normally present in the mouth and intestine, and on the surface of moist areas of the skin. Superficial invasion and proliferation results in white patches (**thrush**) consisting of yeast forms and elongated cells (pseudohyphae), with mild inflammation of the affected tissue. It occurs in the vagina, particularly in pregnancy, and in the mouth, particularly in infants and in patients on oral antibiotic therapy. More extensive local and systemic infections occur in debilitated, immunodeficient or immunosuppressed patients. *Muco-cutaneous candidiasis*, affecting principally the face, scalp and mouth, is a chronic and extremely disfiguring condition when it affects children with various grades of T-cell deficiency. In some cases, administration of transfer factor (p. 106) has been followed by remarkable and sometimes prolonged remission. Oesophageal thrush (Fig. 18.13, p. 539) is a common finding at necropsy in subjects who have died following a chronic debilitating disease.

Systemic candidiasis is rare; the lesions consist of multiple small abscesses, resembling those of pyaemia, and are usually most numerous in the kidneys.

Aspergillosis. The spores of various species of aspergillus, which are filamentous fungi (Fig. 15.32, p. 427), are present in the atmosphere, and large numbers are inhaled, particularly by agricultural workers: clinical infection is, however, uncommon. It is largely confined to the bronchi and lungs and is usually due to *Aspergillus fumigatus*. In most cases there are predisposing factors, such as steroid therapy or the presence in the lungs of bronchiectatic or old tuberculous cavities in which large aspergillus colonies may develop. The fungus may be more aggressive, and produce suppurating and granulating lesions in the lungs: occasionally it invades blood vessels, causing septic thrombosis, and a pyaemic condition.

The immune response includes antibodies and cell-mediated immunity, and complex hypersensitivity reactions may result. In Northern Sudan, a tumour-like granuloma occurs in the paranasal sinuses and orbit.

Histoplasmosis. This is caused by the dimorphic fungus, *Histoplasma capsulatum*, and occurs in many parts of the world, including some parts of North America and Europe. In Africa, most cases are due to *H. duboisii*. Infection usually results from inhalation of spores, which are present in soil and in the faeces of dogs, cats, rodents, bats and birds. In man, pulmonary lesions are most common; they may be single or multiple and usually heal and become calcified. The hilar lymph nodes are often involved. Progressive lung disease sometimes develops and resembles chronic pulmonary tuberculosis in its effects. The organism multiplies in macrophages, in which it is seen as multiple small yeast-like bodies with a double contour: aggregates of macrophages undergo caseous necrosis. In disseminated infection the macrophages throughout the body are colonised and large lesions occur in the liver, spleen, adrenals, marrow, etc.

In areas of high incidence, skin tests with an extract of *H. capsulatum* elicit a delayed hypersensitivity reaction in most individuals, indicating that a high percentage of the population has developed immunity.

Cryptococcosis is caused by the yeast *Cryptococcus neoformans*, which grows in the droppings of pigeons and other birds. Infection in man occurs sporadically throughout the world. It probably results from inhalation of the organism, and produces a localised granulomatous pulmonary lesion: this may heal or extend, and spread may occur by the bloodstream, resulting in widespread granulomatous lesions mostly in the skin, lymph nodes and bones. A chronic meningitis also occurs, in which masses of yeast are seen macroscopically as gelatinous material.

Sporotrichosis is caused by a dimorphic fungus, *Sporothrix schenckii*, which is saprophytic on plants and is present in soil. Infection in man results from accidental inoculation of wounds or minor trauma. Chronic suppurating lesions develop locally and along the line of the draining lymphatics, but systemic infection is rare.

Protozoal and metazoal parasites

Most of the serious diseases caused by protozoan and metazoan parasites are now largely confined to tropical and sub-tropical countries, where they are responsible for an enormous amount of suffering. Because of the increase in world travel, however, these diseases are now encountered more often in visitors and immigrants to temperate areas, and an awareness of this is of major diagnostic importance.

The nature of the parasites, their life cycles and the features of the diseases they cause, are so varied that few useful generalisations can be made, and accordingly the more important individual diseases are described briefly in later chapters, under the systems in which they produce their major effects.

8

Disturbances of Blood Flow and Body Fluids

Disturbances of the flow of blood are intimately associated with lesions which affect the functioning of the heart and blood vessels: such lesions will be considered systematically in later chapters, but meanwhile it is useful to outline the main features of abnormal changes in total and local blood flow, of thrombosis and clotting of the blood, and of disturbances in composition and volume of the body fluids. Accordingly, this chapter provides a general account of these phenomena.

Changes in Flow and Distribution of the Blood

Increase in total blood flow

This occurs when a sufficient number of arterioles relax to result in significant increase in the rate of passage of blood from the arterial to the venous compartment of the circulation. Physiological examples include the vasodilatation in the skeletal muscles during physical activity and the splanchnic vasodilatation during digestion of a heavy meal. Pathological conditions causing an increase in total blood flow include the following.

(a) Hypoxia, which consists of significant fall in the amount of oxygen carried by the blood and available to the tissues. This occurs in anaemia, i.e. a reduction in the amount of haemoglobin in the blood. In severe anaemia, increased rate of blood flow does not compensate for the reduced oxygen carrying capacity of the blood, and the tissues suffer from **anaemic hypoxia.**

Hypoxia occurs also when, as a result of various abnormalities of pulmonary function, the arterial blood is not fully oxygenated (**hypoxic hypoxia**). In lesions which interfere with pulmonary ventilation, the situation is complicated by increased P_{CO_2} of the blood, which, together with lowered P_{O_2}, is termed **asphyxia**. Congenital abnormalities of the heart or great vessels which result in mixing of venous and arterial blood can also cause hypoxic hypoxia.

Increased cardiac output is a feature of these various conditions, but it does not, of course, occur in heart failure, in which **ischaemic hypoxia** results from diminished perfusion of the tissues due to failing capacity of the heart to maintain the circulation.

(b) Increased metabolic activity. The general body metabolism is increased in hyperthyroidism (thyrotoxicosis), in fever, and convalescence from severe injury. The increased metabolism in these conditions is associated with an increased total blood flow.

(c) Arterio-venous shunts. A single large communication (fistula) between an artery and vein, such as sometimes results from trauma, allows the transfer of part of the cardiac output to the venous side of the circulation, and so reduces the amount of arterial blood available for tissue perfusion. A similar effect is seen in Paget's disease of bone in which vascular connective tissue forms in the marrow spaces: if many bones are involved, this results in considerable blood flow through the vascular tissue, leaving less for the other tissues. Generalised inflammatory skin diseases have a similar effect. Some degree of compensation in these conditions is provided by increased cardiac output.

(d) Liver failure. The cause of increased blood flow in liver failure is uncertain: it may be due to the vasodilator effects of accumulated metabolites, or compounds absorbed from the gut, which are normally removed from the blood by the liver cells.

In these various conditions, increased cardiac output is associated with a lowering of arteriolar tone: the pulse is bounding (of high amplitude) and the skin is warm and pink. The mechanism of these changes is complex and not fully understood: the autonomic nervous system, vasomotor centres, adrenal cortex and medulla, local effects of tissue metabolites, baro- and chemo-receptors, are all involved. If long continued, as in untreated hyperthyroidism, the increased work of the heart is likely to lead to 'high-output' cardiac failure, particularly in older people and especially if the heart is already handicapped by coronary artery disease or other abnormalities.

Locally increased blood flow

The outstanding example of a pathological increase in local blood flow is *acute inflammation*, in which arteriolar dilatation results in active hyperaemia (p. 35) and the characteristic warmth and erythema of the inflamed tissue. Active hyperaemia occurs also following a period of temporary obstruction of the circulation: this is important when the local circulation is arrested to facilitate a surgical operation, e.g. on a limb, for hyperaemia develops gradually, and small vessels which do not bleed immediately after the circulation is restored may subsequently do so.

Reduction in total blood flow

This is a feature of *heart failure*, in which the heart is incapable of maintaining the normal output. The condition may occur acutely, usually as a result of myocardial infarction, or chronic heart failure may result from inadequate function of the myocardium, usually due to coronary artery disease or to increased workload as in valvular lesions or pulmonary or systemic hypertension. Chronic heart failure is often progressive; the heart is incapable initially of supplying the increased output required during physical activity, etc., but eventually it may fail to maintain an adequate circulation even at rest.

Reduced cardiac output is also the major feature of the acute condition of *shock*, in which grossly inadequate tissue perfusion can be fatal (pp. 223–9).

The cardiac output is also reduced in states of *general metabolic depression*, the commonest example being hypothyroidism, but in this instance it simply reflects the reduced requirements for tissue perfusion and is not of pathogenic importance.

The serious effects of heart failure are due very largely to **defective tissue perfusion**, which impairs the functions of all the organs. There are, however, two important structural effects: one is **general venous congestion**, from which the term **congestive heart failure** is derived: it is described below. The other is an increase in extravascular fluid, giving rise to **oedema**, which is described on pp. 216 *et seq.*

Local reduction in blood flow (local ischaemia)

This is of extreme importance since it accounts for a high proportion of cardiac and cerebral disease. Reduction of flow is usually due to *arterial narrowing*, or complete obstruction by thrombosis or embolism. These latter processes are described on pp. 196–207, and local ischaemia on pp. 207–14.

Local ischaemia can result also from *venous obstruction*, when it is accompanied by local venous congestion and commonly by oedema.

Venous congestion

When the heart fails to expel the normal amount of blood, arteriolar tone in general increases and a greater proportion of the blood accumulates in the venous compartment, which is readily distensible. This, together with an increase in blood volume (the mechanism of which is poorly understood) causes the veins to become engorged with blood. Engorgement of the systemic veins (**systemic venous congestion**) is most severe when the failure is predominantly of the right ventricle, as occurs in narrowing (stenosis) of the pulmonary valve orifice and in various diseases of the lungs which interfere with pulmonary blood flow. **Pulmonary venous congestion** develops when there is failure of the left ventricle, as in many cases of coronary artery disease or systemic arterial hypertension: it occurs also when mitral valve stenosis restricts the flow of blood into the left ventricle, and may be present for many years without the development of heart failure. In both conditions, there is a rise in pulmonary arterial pressure due to increased pulmonary arteriolar tone, often leading to right ventricular failure and systemic venous congestion.

Venous congestion may also be localised to parts of the systemic circulation as a result of obstruction to the venous outflow. Such **localised venous congestion** is commonly seen as a result of thrombosis of the leg veins, often extending up to and involving the femoral vein. It occurs in the spleen and gastro-intestinal tract when portal venous flow is obstructed, as in cirrhosis of the liver. Various other veins may be obstructed, either by thrombosis or by pressure or constriction by a tumour or by scar tissue.

Systemic venous congestion

As explained above, this usually results from heart failure and, depending on the nature of the heart lesion, may be acute or chronic. In both instances, the outlook depends on the reversibility or otherwise of the cardiac failure: if this persists for long, the morphological changes of chronic venous congestion are striking, but it must be emphasised that the congestive element is less important than the inadequate tissue perfusion of heart failure.

The systemic veins can dilate to accommodate more blood without an immediate rise of venous pressure, but as the congestion increases, the pressure rises. This may be demonstrated directly by venous catheterisation, but commonly it is apparent from pulsation of the veins in the neck when the patient is sitting or standing. Normally, the neck veins in these postures are partly collapsed and do not pulsate visibly, the pressure in them being slightly below atmospheric. When venous pressure rises, however, the veins in the lower part of the neck are distended, and they pulsate at about the level where the blood is at atmospheric pressure.

Because of the reduced blood flow in heart failure, the degree of oxygen dissociation in the capillaries is greater than normal, and in vascular tissues there may be sufficient reduced

haemoglobin to give the purple-blue colour of **cyanosis**: this is seen, for example, in the lips and buccal mucosa. When there is also systemic venous congestion, the distension of the venules and capillaries, with sluggishly-flowing oxygen-deficient blood, increases the degree of cyanosis. Venous congestion may be present without oedema, but oedema usually accompanies severe congestive heart failure: it is most marked in the lower parts of the body, and chronic hypoxia and the increased venous pressure are probably both contributory factors.

Structural changes of systemic venous congestion. Apart from gravity-dependent oedema (p. 218), the structural changes in systemic venous congestion are most obvious in the abdominal viscera. The **liver** may be moderately enlarged and is often tender and palpable. Microscopically, the centrilobular veins are distended and the central part of each lobule consists of distended sinusoids, the hepatocytes having undergone atrophy and disappeared (Fig. 8.1). Macroscopically, this results in accentuation of the lobular pattern, the dark, congested centrilobular areas contrasting with the paler, some-

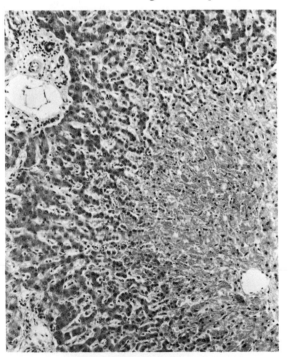

Fig. 8.1 Liver in chronic venous congestion, showing centrilobular atrophy and disappearance of liver cells accompanied by dilatation of sinusoids (rt. side of figure). × 105.

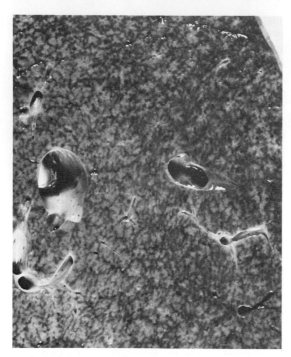

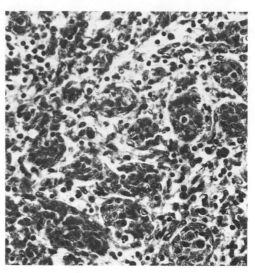

Fig. 8.4 Chronic venous congestion of the spleen. The vascular sinuses are distended with blood, and the intervening medullary cords are relatively inconspicuous. × 250.

Fig. 8.2 The cut surface of the liver in chronic venous congestion. The congested centrilobular zones are dark, and contrast with the pale peripheral-lobular zones, giving the nutmeg-like appearance. × 1·5.

times fatty peripheral lobular cells (Fig. 8.2). Because of its similarity to the surface of a nutmeg cut longitudinally, this appearance has long been described by pathologists as 'nutmeg liver'. In some cases, and particularly when there have been recurrent periods of congestive heart failure, centrilobular fibrosis occurs

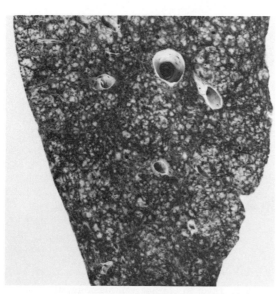

Fig. 8.3 Nodules of hyperplasia in the liver in chronic venous congestion, giving the irregular appearances of so-called cardiac cirrhosis. × 1.

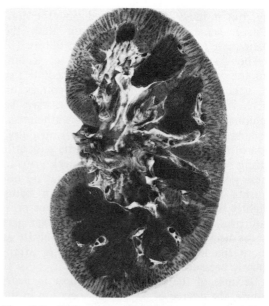

Fig. 8.5 Kidney in chronic venous congestion, showing the intense vascular engorgement. × $\frac{2}{3}$.

and nodules of hyperplastic parenchyma result from compensatory proliferation of surviving hepatocytes. The liver then appears diffusely irregular (Fig. 8.3): although commonly termed *cardiac cirrhosis*, these changes differ from true cirrhosis and do not progress to liver failure.

The **spleen** may be enlarged up to 250 g. It feels firm and maintains its firmness and shape on slicing, little blood escaping from the cut surface. The red pulp is congested and appears almost black: the Malpighian bodies may be visible as contrasting pale spots. Microscopy shows congestion of the venous sinuses in the red pulp, with some thickening of the reticulin framework and atrophy of the medullary cords (Fig. 8.4). More marked congestion of the spleen is seen in portal venous hypertension (p. 509).

The **kidneys** may be slightly enlarged and the medulla is particularly dark and congested; congestion is less obvious in the cortex, and appears as dark radial streaking (Fig. 8.5).

These changes in the abdominal viscera are without serious effects: there may be mild or sub-clinical jaundice, and some red cells and protein in the urine, but the underlying condition of cardiac insufficiency is far more important.

In venous congestion of the **lungs**, the pulmonary venules and alveolar capillaries are engorged with blood (Fig. 8.6) and their walls become thickened. Red cells escape into the alveoli, sometimes resulting in bloodstained sputum, but many of them are broken down by alveolar macrophages, which come to contain large amounts of haemosiderin (p. 239). The macrophages accumulate in the alveoli around respiratory bronchioles (Fig. 9.10, p. 240) and as haemosiderin is gradually released, the reticulin fibres in the alveolar walls become encrusted with it and fibrous thickening occurs. These changes result in increased firmness and give the lung a brown appearance (*brown induration*). They may be associated with attacks of pulmonary oedema and they predispose to pulmonary arterial hypertension with consequent vascular changes. The iron-laden macrophages may be found in the sputum: they have been termed 'heart failure' cells, but are often present in pulmonary venous congestion, e.g. in mitral stenosis, for years before heart failure supervenes. The fine structural changes of pulmonary venous congestion are described on pp. 403–4.

Local venous congestion

As mentioned above, this results from mechanical interference with the venous drainage of blood from an organ, limb, etc. The effects depend on the rapidity, degree and duration of obstruction and also on the local vascular arrangements.

Acute venous obstruction, e.g. by thrombosis or a ligature, would cause complete arrest of blood flow if there were not anastomotic veins to carry the blood away from the drainage area affected. When, rarely, they are absent, the tissue becomes swollen, engorged with blood, and haemorrhagic due to rupture of small vessels. Ischaemic necrosis (venous infarction, p. 211) then develops.

In many sites, acute venous obstruction results in less serious changes, and acute congestion either subsides or becomes chronic. This is illustrated by thrombosis of the deep veins of the leg, which is the commonest example of local venous obstruction, and often extends up to the femoral vein and even beyond. The limb may become cold, cyanosed and oedematous,

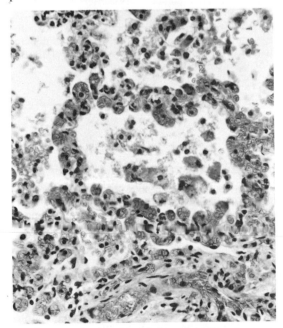

Fig. 8.6 Chronic pulmonary congestion, showing thickening of the alveolar walls, capillary congestion, and free (iron-containing) macrophages in the alveolar spaces. × 210.

but there is nearly always sufficient anastomosis to prevent infarction. The effects tend to subside gradually, partly because the anastomotic channels increase in calibre, and partly because the size of the thrombus is reduced by contraction and by digestion by plasmin. The lumen is thus partially restored, and blood flow increases. Eventually, organisation and recanalisation of residual thrombus may further restore blood flow, but in spite of these changes, deep vein thrombosis, if extensive, sometimes results in chronic venous obstruction and persistent oedema of the limb. Venous valves may be put out of action if they are caught up in an organising thrombus, and this may also be a source of persistent trouble.

Chronic venous obstruction may result from compression or invasion of a vein by tumour, or constriction by fibrous tissue. When obstruction develops gradually, collateral veins enlarge (Fig. 8.7) and drainage is often well maintained.

In chronic portal venous obstruction, which is an important effect of cirrhosis of the liver, the veins connecting the portal venous tributaries with systemic veins become enlarged and help to drain the portal system, but one such group of anastomotic veins, which run longitudinally in the submucosa of the lower oesophagus (Fig. 18.17, p. 544), is liable to rupture, causing serious or fatal haemorrhage.

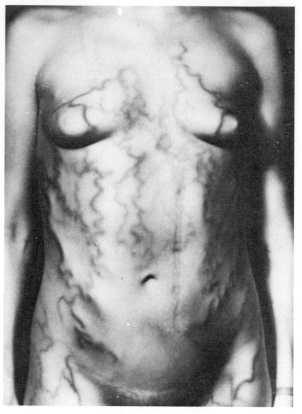

Fig. 8.7 Infra-red photograph showing great enlargement of superficial veins to establish collateral circulation in a patient with obstruction of the inferior vena cava. (Dr. G. Watkinson.)

Haemostasis and Thrombosis

The haemostatic and fibrinolytic mechanisms

The vital importance of keeping the blood fluid within an intact and patent vascular compartment following vascular injury is reflected in the complexity of the mechanisms which exist to this end. Continued blood loss from a leaking vessel is prevented by temporary vasoconstriction and the formation of a haemostatic plug. Initially, the haemostatic plug consists of platelets which rapidly accumulate at the site of vascular injury; the platelet plug is subsequently reinforced by fibrin formation. When the fibrin has served its function, it is removed by the fibrinolytic system, and more permanent repair processes of healing and fibrous tissue replacement then follow.

The haemostatic mechanism can be considered to function at two different levels: (1) in response to an obvious major challenge such as a surgical incision or childbirth to seal off severed blood vessels, and (2) in every-day life to seal off the many tiny injuries to small blood vessels. The 'spontaneous' haemarthroses of patients with a defect in the clotting mechanism, as in severe haemophilia, illustrate the need for effective haemostasis as a continuing physiological mechanism. The opposite effect, inappropriate or pathological thrombosis, is very common, and while there is often some predisposing cause, such as an abnormality of the wall of the blood vessel, or defective blood flow, it is also to be regarded as a disturbance of the haemostatic mechanism.

The normal haemostatic mechanism

There are four components in the haemostatic mechanism: vascular contraction, platelets, the formation of fibrin (blood coagulation), and the fibrinolytic mechanism. Vascular constriction and normal platelet function are themselves not sufficient for physiological haemostasis. When a tooth is extracted from a patient with haemophilia, vascular constriction and the platelet component of haemostasis may prevent bleeding for a few hours after the extraction but unless the platelet haemostatic plug is reinforced by normal deposition of fibrin, haemostasis is only temporarily secured and bleeding, which may be very persistent, then occurs.

Platelet function. In normal blood, platelets circulate as single disc-like fragments of cytoplasm at a concentration of $1·5 - 3 \times 10^5$ per mm³. In addition to providing a factor active in blood coagulation (platelet factor III), the platelets play a vital role in haemostasis. Following injury to the endothelium, they adhere initially, probably to collagen in the connective tissue beneath the damaged endothelium. Contact with collagen provokes complex biochemical and morphological changes in the platelets (see Fig. 8.12). Adenosine diphosphate (ADP) is released from the platelets at the site of injury and causes further aggregation of platelets, leading to progressive occlusion of the vessel by a platelet mass. Simultaneously vascular injury initiates the process of blood coagulation which leads to thrombin production and fibrin formation. Thrombin, in addition to converting fibrinogen to fibrin, causes an explosive release of ADP, 5-hydroxytryptamine and other components from the platelets. These cause further platelet aggregation. The build-up of fibrin around the platelets is an essential step in the formation of an effective haemostatic thrombus.

Platelet function may be studied in various ways, e.g. by assessment of the percentage of platelets in a given sample which adhere to a standard column of glass beads through which the blood is passed, or the aggregation of platelets in plasma following the addition of aggregating substances such as ADP. These techniques have shown that there are a number of syndromes in which, although platelet counts are normal, platelet function is abnormal. Conditions with deficient platelet function include uraemia, the primary thrombocytopathies and hereditary haemorrhagic telangiectasia (p. 503): increased platelet adhesiveness and aggregation have been found in diseases associated with thrombo-embolic phenomena such as ischaemic heart disease, peripheral vascular disease and venous thrombosis. In the puerperium and following surgical operations, platelet adhesiveness is increased, the effect being maximal around the tenth post-operative day. This contributes to the post-operative thrombotic tendency.

Blood coagulation—extrinsic and intrinsic systems. When blood is withdrawn from the body by clean venepuncture and placed in a plain smooth glass test tube it will clot in five to ten minutes. However if the test tube contains an extract of minced tissue, the blood will clot in ten seconds. In this simple experiment the blood *alone* clots under the influence of a system which is derived from the components within the blood itself without any contribution from the tissues. This system is called the *intrinsic* or *blood thromboplastin system*. The more rapid clotting which occurs in the presence of tissue extract is described as clotting under the influence of the *extrinsic* or *tissue thromboplastin system*. The plasma components which contribute to the formation of fibrin by both the intrinsic and extrinsic systems are complex (Table 8.1).

Table 8.1. International classification of the plasma coagulation factors (Roman numerals), together with their commonly-used names. The term 'factor VI', formerly applied to an intermediate product, is no longer used.

Factor I	Fibrinogen
Factor II	Prothrombin
Factor III	Tissue factor
Factor IV	Calcium
Factor V	Proaccelerin
Factor VII	Proconvertin
Factor VIII	Antihaemophilic globulin
Factor IX	Plasma thromboplastin component or Christmas factor
Factor X	Stuart–Prower factor
Factor XI	Plasma thromboplastin antecedent
Factor XII	Hageman factor
Factor XIII	Fibrin stabilising factor (plasma transglutaminase)

The relationships between blood clot, the haemostatic plug and thrombus. When blood is placed in a test tube and allowed to clot, the cellular elements are randomly distributed throughout the fibrin network. However formation of a haemostatic plug or a thrombus takes place in flowing blood, and the cellular elements of the blood are not randomly deposited. In a haemostatic plug an occluding mass of platelets forms at the site of the leakage, and upon this is deposited fibrin which spreads into and reinforces the platelet plug. In a pathological thrombus a similar histological picture is seen with the white 'head' of agglutinated platelets and numerous white cells, followed by a red 'tail' consisting of fibrin and entrapped red cells (see p. 204).

Conversion of fibrinogen to fibrin. The conversion of fibrinogen to fibrin is brought about by the highly specific proteolytic enzyme thrombin, which splits off two small peptides from each fibrinogen molecule, converting it into fibrin monomer. Monomers of fibrin then polymerise to form a network of fibrin. In purified systems fibrin is soluble, but in the body it is converted to an insoluble form by the enzyme transglutaminase (fibrin stabilising factor or factor XIII) which is present in the plasma.

Conversion of prothrombin to thrombin. The ability of the body to keep the blood fluid and free of fibrin formation within the blood vessels is a remarkable phenomenon which suggests that no effective amount of thrombin can be in circulation. Blood coagulation occurs only when the thrombin is elaborated from its inert precursor prothrombin (factor II), under the influence of one or both of the two pathways already mentioned, the intrinsic or blood thromboplastin system and the extrinsic or tissue thromboplastin system.

In both the intrinsic and extrinsic pathways, the components probably do not react together simultaneously to produce their final 'prothrombin converting principle', or thromboplastin; a sequence of reactions probably takes place in stepwise fashion in which one component acts as an enzyme and the other as a substrate. Two essentially similar series of sequential reactions, termed the 'cascade' and 'waterfall' sequences, have been suggested to explain the mechanism of blood coagulation (Fig. 8.8). This hypothesis is likely to be further modified as more information becomes available as the result of purification of known clotting factors. The intrinsic thromboplastin system is activated by contact of blood with a water-wettable surface which activates factor XII (Hageman factor). This reaction presumably occurs in response to relatively minor injuries. (Activated Hageman factor (XIIa) may also have a central role in the functional integration of defence–repair mechanisms, for it triggers the plasmin, complement and kinin systems and also the permeability factor PFdil.) The extrinsic or tissue system is triggered *in vitro* by contact with tissue extract, and presumably operates in more severe injury.

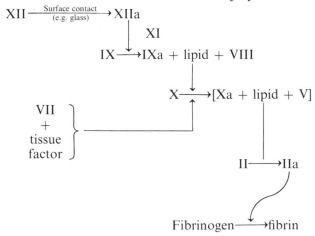

Fig. 8.8 A simplified version of one current concept of the 'cascade' reaction involved in coagulation. A series of reactions is involved in which inactive coagulation factors are converted to active forms, denoted by the letter 'a' after the symbol for the factor.

Normal vascular endothelium appears to have an important role in maintaining the fluidity of the blood within the vascular compartment. In addition, plasma contains natural inhibitors of clotting, and activated clotting factors are removed by cells of the mononuclear phagocyte system. The most important inhibitor of clotting is antithrombin III (heparin cofactor), which inactivates not only thrombin but also factor Xa and probably factors IX and XI; it also has antiplasmin activity. The activity of antithrombin III is much greater against factor Xa than against thrombin. The neutralising effect of the inhibitor is enhanced many times by heparin, which produces a configurational change in antithrombin III and gives better exposure of its binding site. Antithrombin III and other inhibitors are probably of great importance in reducing the risk of inappropriate intravascular fibrin formation when coagulant substances enter the vascular compartment.

The fibrinolytic enzyme system

The fibrinolytic enzyme system has four main components: plasminogen, plasmin, activators and inhibitors. Plasminogen, a β-globulin of the plasma, is converted by activators to plasmin, a proteolytic enzyme which under suitable circumstances digests fibrin to give soluble products (Fig. 8.9). Plasminogen activators are

Plasminogen (inactive plasma globulin)

Activators——→ |

Plasmin (proteolytic enzyme)

Fibrin——→soluble products

Fig. 8.9 The fibrinolytic enzyme system.

widespread throughout the body, being present in almost all the tissues with the exception of liver and placenta. Activity is concentrated around blood vessels, particularly veins and venules. Plasminogen activator is also present in the blood plasma and is responsible for physiological fibrinolytic activity of plasma. It is also present in many body secretions, e.g. milk, tears, saliva, seminal fluid. Normal urine contains urokinase, a physiological plasminogen activator which may represent in part excreted plasma activator and may also be

produced in part in the kidney. In normal plasma, fibrinolytic activity is low, but increased activity is found after exercise or emotional stress, and also following surgical operations and other trauma.

Normal plasma possesses both anti-activator and anti-plasmin activity. Platelets also show anti-plasmin activity.

The fibrinolytic enzyme system is probably in dynamic equilibrium with the blood clotting system, the two acting together to maintain an intact and patent vascular tree. According to this hypothesis the coagulation and fibrinolytic systems may both be continuously active, the former laying down fibrin where needed on the endothelium to seal any deficiencies which may occur, and the latter removing such deposits after they have served their haemostatic function.

Thrombosis

Thrombosis is defined as the formation of a solid or semi-solid mass from the constituents of the blood within the vascular system during life. Coagulation, i.e. deposition of fibrin, is involved in the formation of most thrombi but the composition of thrombus is determined very largely by the rate of flow of the blood from which it forms.

Appearances and composition of thrombi

As a general rule, thrombus forming in rapidly flowing blood, e.g. in an artery, consists mainly of aggregated platelets, with some fibrin; it enlarges slowly and is firm and pale, varying from greyish white to pale red, and is commonly called *pale thrombus*. The proportion of fibrin deposited in pale thrombus depends partly on the rate of blood flow, to which it has an inverse relationship. At the other extreme, thrombus forming in stagnant blood, e.g. adjacent to a complete occlusion of a blood vessel, is indistinguishable from blood which has been allowed to clot *in vitro*: the thrombus is soft, dark *red*, gelatinous and consists of strands of fibrin lying among the elements of whole blood (Fig. 8.10). It may retract from the vessel wall, revealing a smooth, shiny surface. Between these two extremes we have *mixed thrombi* which form in slowly flowing blood, usually in veins, and consist of alternating layers of platelet aggregates and red thrombus.

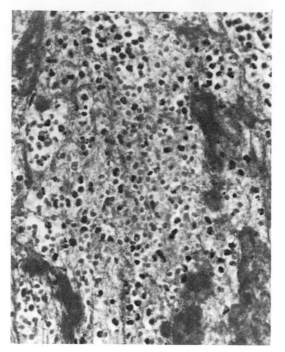

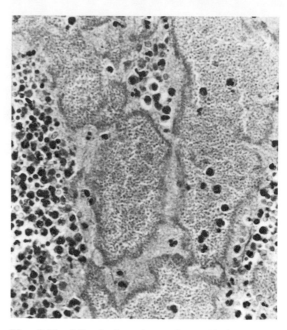

Fig. 8.10 Red thrombus, consisting of strands of fibrin lying among red cells, leucocytes and platelets. In this instance the proportion of entrapped red cells is much lower than in blood clot, suggesting that there has been some movement of blood during thrombosis. × 305.

Fig. 8.11 Mixed thrombus, about 12 hours old, showing dense masses of granular material, composed of fused platelets, with collections of leukocytes between. × 336.

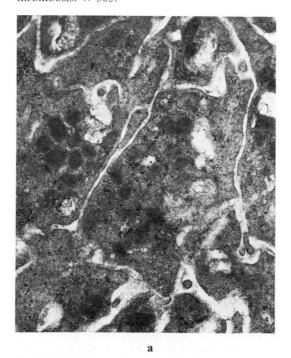

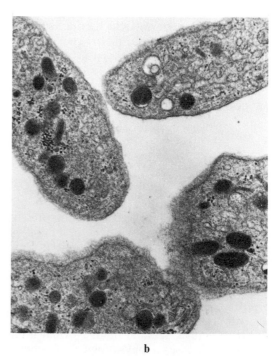

a

b

Fig. 8.12 Electron micrograph of platelet thrombus **a**, compared with free platelets **b**. The platelets forming the thrombus fit closely together and are distorted, but can be readily recognised. × 28 000.

The mixture may be intimate and only recognisable on microscopy: Fig. 8.11 shows such a thrombus in which spaces between masses of aggregated platelets are filled by a fibrin network containing leukocytes and some red cells. In other instances, veins may be filled with columns of red thrombus but with platelet aggregates at points of anastomosis. The formation of such thrombi is explained on p. 204. Except in recently formed thrombi, it is not easy to recognise aggregated platelets, for they soon lose their outlines, presenting microscopically a granular or structureless appearance. Immunofluorescence studies and electron microscopy (Fig. 8.12) have, however, facilitated their recognition.

Factors predisposing to thrombosis

The three major predisposing factors are (a) local abnormalities of the vessel (or heart) wall; (b) slowing or disturbances in the flow of blood, and (c) changes in the composition of the blood. The parts played by these three factors in the formation of thrombi in the heart, arteries and veins are described below.

(a) Cardiac thrombosis. At necropsy, post-

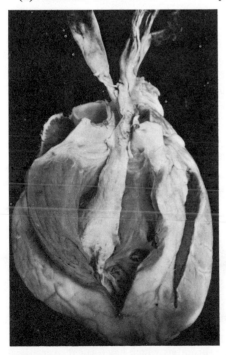

Fig. 8.13 Agonal thrombus in the right ventricle, extending along the pulmonary artery. $\times \frac{1}{2}$.

mortem clots are usually to be found in the chambers of the heart. They are soft and dark red with a glistening surface and are not firmly adherent to the endocardium. Occasionally the red cells settle before coagulation occurs and the upper (usually anterior) part of the clot is then yellow and gelatinous. Thrombi may form rapidly as the circulation is failing immediately before death. They are yellow or pinkish with a glistening surface and have a somewhat stringy appearance (Fig. 8.13). Such agonal thrombi originate at the apex of the ventricle to which they are attached and may extend through the valve orifice. They are composed mainly of fibrin, which separates out from the sluggishly moving blood before death, and may occur in either or both ventricles, although they are commoner in the right side of the heart. Quite apart from these terminal or post-mortem events, thrombi may form in any of the four chambers of the heart. **In the atria**, thrombosis is commonest in the appendices, especially that of the right atrium, in cases of heart failure with atrial dilatation (Fig. 14.25, p. 365). Stagnation of blood is the important causal factor and this is accentuated by atrial fibrillation, which is very commonly complicated by thrombosis. Rarely small flattened globular thrombi form in either the atria or ventricles. They are pale, composed mainly of platelets and may show central softening. In mitral stenosis, a rounded thrombus may develop in the left atrium and lie free. It may exceed 3 cm in diameter and is a rare cause of sudden obstruction of the circulation—the so-called 'ball valve thrombus'. The vegetations which form **on the heart valves** in certain diseases are essentially thrombi. In rheumatic fever the valve cusps are damaged along the line of apposition, and deposition of platelets results in the formation of minute pinkish-grey bead-like vegetations (Fig. 8.14 and Fig. 14.20, p. 361): in bacterial endocarditis the cusps are damaged by bacterial infection and not only platelets are deposited but also fibrin and interspersed leukocytes, and the vegetations are consequently larger, softer and more friable (Fig. 8.15). **In the ventricles**, mural thrombosis commonly occurs on the endocardium overlying an infarct (i.e. a patch of ischaemic necrosis of the heart wall—Fig. 8.16). Depending on the size of the infarct, the thrombus may be large or small. It forms a flat reddish plaque attached to the endocardium. Probably the important factors in its

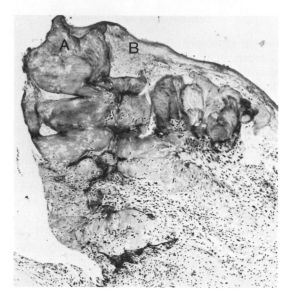

Fig. 8.14 Rheumatic vegetation on a cusp of the mitral valve. The vegetation consists mainly of dense hyaline material (A) composed of fused platelets, and fibrin coagulum (B). × 60.

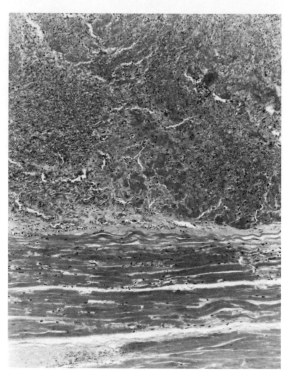

Fig. 8.16 Mural thrombus (*above*) which has formed on the endocardium over a myocardial infarct. Note the necrotic myocardium (*below*). × 120.

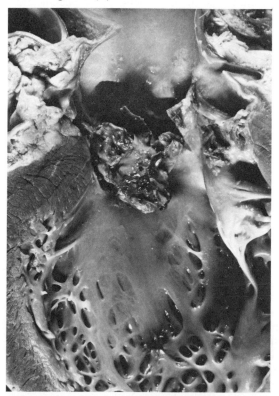

Fig. 8.15 Bacterial endocarditis. The root of the aorta has been cut open and the wall folded back to display the large irregular thrombotic vegetations which have formed on, and are obscuring, the aortic valve cusps.

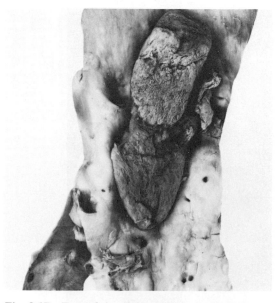

Fig. 8.17 Part of the abdominal aorta opened up to show a large thrombus which has formed over atheromatous patches. The dull, pale, shaggy thrombus consists mostly of fibrin and platelets.

formation are the disturbances in blood flow caused by lack of pulsation in the dead muscle and also diffusion of factor III (tissue thromboplastin) from the dead tissue.

(b) Arterial thrombosis. Probably because of the rapid flow of blood, arterial thrombosis is uncommon in the absence of a local lesion of the vessel wall. In affluent communities, **atheroma** in arteries of various sizes is by far the commonest predisposing local lesion. In the aorta, atheroma is commonly severe and results in gross distortion and unevenness of the wall but, because of the rapid flow of blood, thrombosis is often not superadded. Frequently, however, mural thrombi form over atheromatous plaques which have ulcerated or which have caused a local bulging of the aortic wall (Fig. 8.17). When blood is flowing smoothly in a normal vessel, the particulate elements are separated from the vascular endothelium by a layer of almost pure plasma, but atheromatous plaques, by causing irregularities of the wall, result in turbulent flow, and platelets can then impinge on the wall. This alone probably predisposes to thrombosis, but the ulcerated atheromatous plaque also brings the blood into contact with an abnormal surface on which platelet aggregation occurs. The irregularities also cause local disturbances in the rate of blood flow. Thrombosis also complicates atheroma in medium-sized and smaller arteries, particularly those supplying the heart and brain. Because of their relatively small calibre, which is further reduced by the atheromatous plaques, thrombi readily occlude these vessels completely and ischaemic necrosis commonly results in the deprived tissues. This is described later in the section on infarction and also in the appropriate systematic chapters. When there is gross **localised dilatation (aneurysm)** of the wall of the heart, aorta or other arteries, stagnation and eddying of the blood usually result in some thrombosis. The thrombus may have a laminated appearance and may come to fill the aneurysmal sac (Fig. 8.18). **Inflammatory lesions** in the walls of arteries (p. 327) may also cause thrombosis: contributory factors may be irregularities of the wall, injury to the vascular endothelium, and release of tissue thromboplastin. In **severe arterial hypertension**, necrosis of the walls of small arteries and arterioles is commonly followed by thrombosis.

(c) Venous thrombosis. Because of the

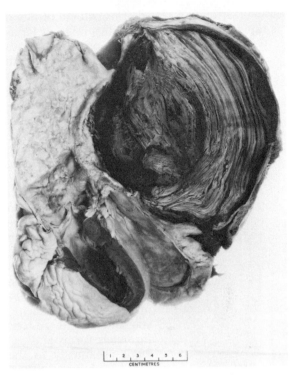

Fig. 8.18 Aneurysm of aorta containing laminated thrombus.

relatively slow flow of venous blood, veins are the commonest site of thrombosis. There may be a local predisposing factor, for example a patch of fibrous thickening in the wall, invasion or compression by tumour, and above all, inflammation of the wall of the vein due either to a phlebitis of unknown cause or to involvement in a pyogenic bacterial infection. Most often, however, there is no demonstrable local predisposing lesion and thrombosis starts by platelet aggregation, usually within a small vein.

The structure of venous thrombi and the factors concerned in their formation are illustrated by thrombosis in the veins of the lower limbs, which is very common in elderly hospital patients, especially following a surgical operation. It is important because it is the usual cause of fatal pulmonary embolism. It starts in the relatively small veins in the calf muscles and may extend proximally as far as the femoral or iliac veins or rarely into the inferior vena cava (Fig. 8.19). The initial thrombus formed in the small calf veins occludes the lumen and for some distance proximal to the occlusion, blood flow is virtually arrested. This column of blood is rapidly converted into red thrombus as far as the next proximal venous tributary. Blood from this tributary continues to flow into the affected vessel and for a time arrests the formation of red thrombus. However, platelets in the moving column of blood coming from the tributary are deposited on the proximal end of the red thrombus, which thus becomes capped with more slowly formed pale platelet thrombus. This may eventually occlude the entrance of the tributary, again producing stagnation, and so red thrombus forms and extends proximally to the next tributary (Fig. 8.20). So the process continues with thrombus extending into larger, more proximal veins. Once a tributary has been occluded, red thrombus also forms in the stagnant blood within it and so the thrombus in the main venous trunks comes to have branches extending into the tributaries. Leg vein thrombosis tends to occur especially in patients lying immobile in the supine position, and impairment of blood flow by pressure on the calves appears to be an important predisposing factor. It is particularly common after an abdominal operation, after childbirth, severe injury, myocardial infarction and in patients with congestive heart failure. Venous return from the lower part of the body is normally aided by muscular movements of the legs and by the pumping action which ensues from use of the abdominal muscles and diaphragm in respiration, and in all the above conditions immobility of the legs interferes with the normal flow. To avoid the pain of abdominal movements, patients who have had an abdominal operation tend to use mainly the

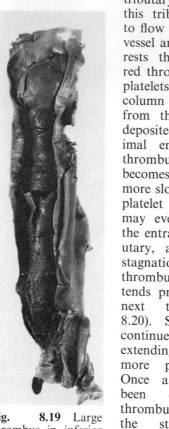

Fig. 8.19 Large thrombus in inferior vena cava, with rounded projection at upper end. × $\frac{2}{5}$.

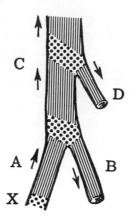

Fig. 8.20 Diagram showing the mode of extension of venous thrombosis. Thrombus occludes a small vein (A) at point X, and red thrombus (lined areas) rapidly extends in the stagnant column of blood up to the entrance of the next tributary (B), where platelet deposition forms a cap of pale thrombus (dotted areas): when this occludes the junction of A and B, red thrombus extends rapidly up to the entrance of the next tributary (C), and so on. Red thrombus also forms in each tributary as its entrance to the major channel is occluded. (Arrows show direction of thrombosis.)

thoracic muscles for respiration, and this is a further factor in impairing venous return from the legs. Thrombosis starts in the small leg veins *during* surgical operations. It extends into the large veins over the next two weeks, when platelet numbers and adhesiveness and prothrombin levels are highest, and as in childbirth and myocardial infarction, pulmonary embolism is commonest around ten days after the event. The main factors predisposing to venous thrombosis in congestive heart failure are venous stagnation and immobility.

Leg vein thrombosis and embolism (see below) of large or small pulmonary arteries is an exceedingly common finding at necropsy on middle-aged and old patients (in our experience over 30%). Recent reports on the prophylactic use of repeated small doses of heparin indicate that this reduces considerably both venous thrombosis and pulmonary embolism, but in surgical cases such therapy is most effective if started at the time of operation. Another common site of thrombosis following operation, etc., is in the veins of the pelvis. This is seen especially after childbirth when the uterine blood flow diminishes considerably, predisposing to thrombosis in the hypertrophied uterine veins. Puerperal sepsis is also a predisposing factor in some cases. Pelvic venous thrombosis may also originate in haemorrhoids. Extension to large veins, including the internal and common iliacs, may complicate pelvic venous thrombosis and fatal pulmonary embolism may follow. It is partly to prevent venous thrombosis that patients are encouraged to leave their beds as soon as practicable after operation, childbirth, etc., and while bedridden to carry out muscular exercises and to practise abdominal respiration.

Venous thrombosis is also a common complication of malnutrition, severe debilitating infections and wasting diseases such as cancer. **Marantic thrombosis** occurs in severe debility in infants and young children. It commonly affects the superior longitudinal sinus (Fig. 8.28). In patients with malignant tumours, and especially carcinoma of the pancreas, repeated episodes of thrombosis may occur in various veins and this may precede other symptoms.

(d) Capillary thrombosis. Thrombosis in capillaries and venules commonly occurs in severe acute inflammatory lesions. It is due partly to endothelial damage and partly to haemoconcentration, the thrombi being composed mainly of packed red cells.

In the Arthus reaction, in which thrombosis of small vessels is often prominent, the endothelial injury is attributable mainly to release of enzymes by neutrophil polymorphs (p. 124).

Fibrin thrombi can be found in the capillaries in some patients dying of disseminated intravascular coagulation (p. 227), although in some cases they are absent, presumably as a result of fibrinolytic activity.

Sequels of thrombosis

Restoration of the vascular channel after thrombotic occlusion may occur by a combination of fibrinolysis and shrinkage of the thrombus. The fibrinolytic mechanism depends on the activation of plasminogen in the plasma and this may become very active when there has been large-scale intravascular coagulation such as may result from the entry of amniotic fluid into the maternal circulation. Unless it is associated with phlebitis, venous thrombus is usually removed, with good restoration of the lumen, within a few weeks, and permanent occlusion only rarely follows. Much of the thrombus is removed by fibrinolysis and the remainder by organisation (p. 79).

Venous thrombi may become infected with pyogenic organisms and undergo suppurative softening; fragments are then liable to be carried away by the bloodstream, giving rise to pyaemia. In some instances, thrombosis is beneficial, for example when it occludes a vessel involved in an ulcerating lesion and thus precludes haemorrhage.

Embolism

By embolism is meant the transference of abnormal material by the bloodstream and its impaction in a vessel. The impacted material is called an **embolus.** In most cases it is a fragment of thrombus, occasionally material from an ulcerated atheromatous patch. A fragment of a tumour growing into a vein may break off and form an embolus, and there may be embolism of the capillaries by fat globules, air bubbles or collections of parenchymal cells. The site of embolism will, of course, depend on the source of the embolus. Thus embolism of the pulmonary arteries and their branches is secondary to thrombosis in the systemic veins or in the right side of the heart. Rarely, where there is a patent foramen ovale, an embolus may pass from the right side of the heart to the left atrium and

thus be carried to the systemic circulation; (*crossed* or *paradoxical embolism*). With this rare exception, emboli occurring in the systemic circulation are derived from thrombi formed in the left side of the heart, from vegetations on the aortic and mitral valves, and occasionally from thrombi or detached portions of atheromatous patches in the aorta or large arteries. Emboli carried from tributaries of the portal vein lodge, of course, in the portal branches in the liver.

Effects of embolism

Systemic emboli. The results are simply those of mechanical plugging and vary according to the site of the embolus, as described in pp. 207 *et seq.*

Pulmonary embolism is a very common and important event: it results from the detachment of a thrombus in a systemic vein, usually in the lower limb. Such thrombi form in conditions which have already been described (p. 204) and in any of them pulmonary embolism may result. It is most common around the tenth day after operation, and may cause sudden death. A large thrombus may become detached *en masse* and be carried to the right side of the heart, causing a sudden blockage of the pulmonary trunk or one of its divisions, death usually occurring at once or after a short period of pulmonary distress. Such fatal emboli are most often derived from the femoral and iliac venous trunk characteristically forming a cylinder about 1 cm in diameter and as much as 30 cm long, which is found at necropsy coiled up like a snake in the pulmonary artery and right ventricle (Fig. 8.21); if smaller, it may be contained within the pulmonary arterial branches. When the patient has lived some time after the em-

bolism, a varying amount of haemorrhagic infarction may be present in the parts supplied by the blocked vessels. Infarction, however, is never co-extensive with the area of distribution, and usually there is none.

Multiple small pulmonary emboli, impacting over a period of time, can rarely cause chronic pulmonary hypertension.

Septic emboli. With the widespread use of antibiotics, septic emboli, containing pyogenic bacteria, have become relatively uncommon. They may give rise to suppuration and this is the usual process by which multiple abscesses are produced by pyaemia. An infective embolus, when arrested in an artery, occasionally weakens the wall and gives rise to an aneurysm—*mycotic aneurysm*. In various septicaemic and pyaemic conditions, capillaries here and there may be plugged by organisms, most frequently pyococci, or by impaction of a small fragment of infected thrombus, the organisms then growing along the capillaries. The number of bacteria seen in necropsy material may have been greatly increased by growth after death.

Embolism from tumours. This is of two kinds. One or a few cells of the tumour may enter the bloodstream and impact in a capillary in some distant organ. In other instances there may be growth of a tumour into a large vein, and a larger fragment may become detached and impact in a vessel, e.g. a branch of the pulmonary artery or of the portal vein. Both of these processes can result in metastatic tumours.

Fat embolism. Entrance of fat into the circulation results from laceration of veins surrounded by adipose tissue. It probably occurs after all fractures with displacement and injury of adipose tissue, in caisson disease (p. 717) and with a fatty liver. In most instances the phenomenon is of no clinical importance but when the amount of fat entering the circulation is large, as in fractures of long bones, the *fat embolus syndrome* may develop within the following 3 days. The syndrome includes mental confusion, fever, dyspnoea, tachycardia, a petechial rash and sometimes cyanosis, haemoptysis, coma and death. It appears to be due largely to hypoxia resulting from pulmonary fat emboli complicated by oedema and haemorrhage. Fat may, however, pass through the lungs into the systemic circulation and cause emboli in the brain, giving rise to multiple small haemorrhages, in the kidneys (Fig. 8.22), and in the skin.

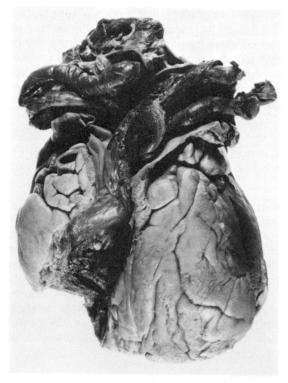

Fig. 8.21 Massive pulmonary embolism. Thrombus from the femoral vein has become detached and impacted in the pulmonary trunk and its right and left branches, causing sudden death.

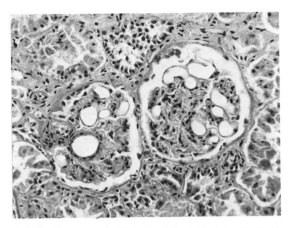

Fig. 8.22 Fat embolism of glomerular capillaries in a case of caisson disease. The globules of fat (dissolved out in processing the tissue) have impacted in glomerular capillaries and caused great distension. × 170. (Professor A. C. Lendrum.)

There may also be thrombocytopenia. In patients who recover, there is usually no residual disability.

Air embolism. This occurs when air is aspirated into a severed vein, especially a large vein near the heart, but air may also enter the circulation in fatal amounts during blood transfusion if positive pressure is used without due care. The frequency and seriousness of the condition have probably been exaggerated. The air may produce effects in two ways. It may become mixed with the blood in the right ventricle, forming a froth which is not readily expelled and interferes with ventricular filling, or the bubbles of air may become arrested in the pulmonary arterioles and lead to the mechanical effects of embolism. When air enters the circulation it is absorbed rapidly, and to produce serious results the sudden entrance of over 100 ml is usually necessary; less than this has provoked alarming symptoms, but recovery has occurred after as much as 300 ml. Injury to the spinal cord and bones can result from formation of bubbles of nitrogen in caisson disease, which develops in divers, etc., from too rapid decompression from a high atmospheric pressure (p. 717).

At necropsy, bubbles of gas may be found in the blood, due to the action of the *Clostridium welchii* after death, and this should not be mistaken for air embolism.

Parenchymal-cell embolism. In certain conditions special types of cells form emboli in the pulmonary vessels, for example the megakaryocytes of the bone marrow in severe infections, the syncytial cells from the placenta, and liver cells after laceration of the liver. Such cellular emboli are without serious effect, the cells in all probability disintegrating. By contrast, the entry of **amniotic fluid** into the maternal circulation during prolonged or obstructed labour may cause serious effects in two ways. Firstly, it may produce extensive and sometimes fatal embolism of the pulmonary circulation by fetal squames, vernix and meconium. Secondly, it may bring about both widespread intravascular fibrin formation and activation of the plasminogen fibrinolytic system, with the result that there is severe hypofibrinogenaemia, and dangerous post-partum haemorrhage commonly results.

Local Ischaemia

Complete arterial occlusion

The term **ischaemic** is applied to tissue in which the blood flow has ceased (complete ischaemia) or is abnormally low (partial ischaemia). Ischaemia localised to an organ, a part of the body, or a patch of tissue, is usually due to obstruction to arterial blood flow.

By far the commonest and most important causes of complete arterial occlusion are thrombosis and embolism; other causes include proliferative changes in the intima of small arteries, and also arterial spasm as in Raynaud's disease or ergot poisoning.

When an artery is obstructed the result depends on the extent of *collateral circulation*, i.e. alternative vascular routes by which blood can reach the deprived tissue. The arterial anastomoses in the limbs are such that blockage of any one artery does not usually result in severe ischaemia provided that the other arteries are not seriously diseased. Similarly, there are effective collateral arteries in the integument and muscles of the trunk. In the internal organs, however, the anatomical arrangement of many of the vessels does not allow a sufficient anastomic supply, and severe ischaemia follows arterial occlusion. When an artery of a limb is suddenly obstructed in a healthy subject, there is an immediate drop in the blood pressure beyond the obstruction, and the circulation is brought almost to a standstill; the arteries then contract and the part contains less blood than normally. Soon, however, the anastomotic arteries dilate and blood thus by-passes the obstruction to enter the vessels of the affected part, through which a flow of blood is gradually established and increased until ultimately it may approach normal. Thus in a healthy subject the femoral artery may be ligated without permanent damage resulting. The limb becomes cold and numb, and some time elapses before the pulse returns at the ankle; and it is much longer before complete muscular power is restored. The collateral vessels remain dilated and maintain the circulation, and in response to the sustained rise in blood flow there occurs a thickening of their walls, with increase of the muscular and elastic tissue corresponding with the enlarged lumen; in other words, the collateral vessels become permanently enlarged or hypertrophied. A good example is provided by the rare congenital localised stenosis (*coarctation*) of the aorta beyond the arch, in which there occurs during development a great enlargement of vessels which link the arteries of the head and neck with those supplying the trunk and legs, the coarctation being thus by-passed.

The development of an efficient collateral circulation often depends on dilatation of healthy anastomotic arteries, and on a healthy heart. If, however, the collateral arteries are diseased, e.g. atheromatous, fibrosed or calcified, they are unlikely to dilate sufficiently to supply the necessary amount of blood to the ischaemic part, and a varying amount of necrosis will follow. In middle-aged or old people blockage of the main artery of a limb, or even of a large branch, may be followed by death of the tissues supplied by the obstructed vessel, the condition of 'senile' gangrene resulting (p. 172). When there are multiple obstructions of limb arteries or spreading thrombosis, as in thromboangiitis obliterans (p. 327), serious results may follow and lead to gangrene even in young adults.

Infarction

Certain arteries of internal organs have imperfect anastomoses and their obstruction is always followed by serious results. Such arteries are called **end arteries**, and they may have no anastomosis, e.g. the splenic artery, or only capillary anastomosis, e.g. the branches of the renal artery, or arterial anastomosis but insufficient to keep the part alive, e.g. the superior mesenteric artery. Obstruction of such vessels leads to ischaemia, usually sufficient to cause tissue necrosis, and sometimes congestion and haemorrhage in the affected tissue. The term **infarct** is applied to the altered area which has lost its blood supply, and use of the term implies that the tissue has undergone ischaemic necrosis. Infarcts are of two main types, *pale* or *anaemic*, and *red* or *haemorrhagic*. Pale infarcts occur in organs where there is little or no anastomosis, e.g. heart and kidneys; while in organs where there is some anastomosis, e.g. the intestine, or a double circulation, e.g. the lungs, red infarcts are found, blood passing from the marginal vessels into the damaged area. Infarction means literally a stuffing-in, and was originally applied to the haemorrhagic type, as the part appeared stuffed with blood. When pale infarcts were found to have a similar cause, the term was applied to them also.

Infarction is usually the result of acute occlusion of an artery by thrombosis or embolism. In the coronary arteries, atheroma with thrombosis is common, and is the usual cause of infarction of the myocardium: in the brain, thrombosis and embolism are both of importance, while in the lungs, kidneys and spleen embolism is a commoner cause than thrombosis.

Features of infarcts in various sites. In the kidneys, spleen and lungs, the vascular arrangements are such that most infarcts are roughly wedge- or cone-shaped, the apex lying most deeply, in the vicinity of the occluded artery, and the infarct enlarging as it extends peripherally, the base being visible as a necrotic area on the surface of the organ (Figs. 8.23 and 8.26). The coronary arteries pass inwards from the epicardium, and accordingly myocardial infarcts involve especially the inner part of the wall, although commonly the whole thickness undergoes infarction.

In the **brain** a reduction in blood flow sufficiently severe to produce infarction is usually due to atheroma of the cerebral arteries or of major arteries in the neck that supply the brain, viz. the internal carotid and vertebral arteries. The artery may be occluded by thrombus formed on an atheromatous plaque but stenosis alone, by severely impairing blood flow through the artery, may cause ischaemic damage in the brain. Indeed cerebral infarction should be equated with a reduced cerebral blood flow rather than actual arterial occlusion as infarction may occur, even when the major neck arteries and the intracranial arteries are normal, as a result of a profound fall in cerebral blood flow due, for example, to cardiac arrest or an episode of severe hypotension. The sites of infarction of the brain depend on the cause of the ischaemia. When a major cerebral artery is blocked, infarction obviously occurs within the territory supplied by it, but blockage of the internal carotid or vertebral arteries, or a hypotensive episode, results in infarction in the so-called *boundary zones* (p. 679) at the margins of the territories supplied by the major cerebral arteries. A not uncommon cause of occlusion of a cerebral artery is embolism. Even when a major cerebral artery is completely occluded, there is considerable variation in the size of the infarct, due partly to the severity and extent of the reduced blood flow and partly to the efficiency of the potential collateral circulation through arteries on the surface of the brain that link the major cerebral arterial territories, and through the circle of Willis. A cerebral infarct may be pale or haemorrhagic (red) depending on whether or not some circulation becomes re-established through it. As the dead tissue soon breaks down and becomes soft, a cerebral infarct is often referred to as a *softening*. Thereafter, over a period of weeks or months, the necrotic tissue is gradually removed by phagocytes. The final result is a cystic shrunken area in the brain (see Figs. 20.23, 20.24, p. 681).

The central artery of the **retina** is an end-artery, and its obstruction causes retinal infarction, with loss of sight in the eye.

In the **heart**, obstruction of a coronary artery or a major branch gives rise to infarction of the ventricular myocardium; it is usually somewhat irregular in form, and is pale but may show congestion and haemorrhage at the margin (Fig. 14.9, p. 352).

Obstruction of even a large branch of a **pulmonary artery** does not always result in infarction. Experimentally-induced pulmonary emboli in otherwise healthy dogs do not usually cause infarction, some additional general impairment of pulmonary blood flow being required for infarction to result from the emboli, e.g. constriction of the pulmonary venous

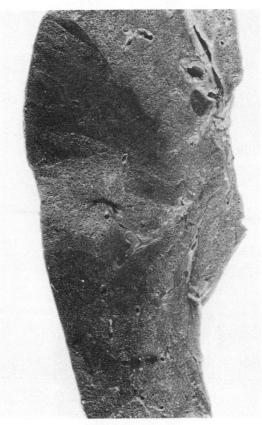

Fig. 8.23 Two haemorrhagic infarcts of lung, seen on section as dark wedge-shaped areas, widening towards the pleural surface (*left*). Note the pulmonary artery occluded by thrombus (beyond the apex of the upper infarct). × 1·3.

drainage. Similarly in man, impaired pulmonary blood flow, due to mitral stenosis, heart failure or lung disease causing obliteration of pulmonary capillaries, predisposes to the development of infarction following pulmonary embolism. The subject is discussed more fully on pp. 405–6.

Pulmonary infarcts are typically wedge-shaped, with the base projecting slightly on the pleural surface (Fig. 8.23). They are firm and

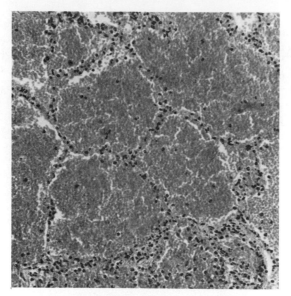

Fig. 8.24 Haemorrhagic infarct of lung, showing alveoli filled with red cells. × 115.

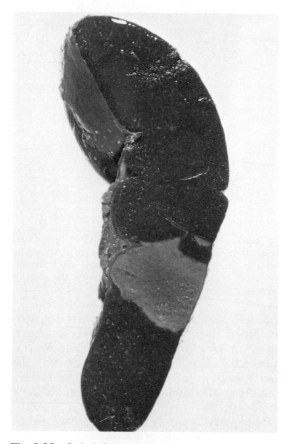

Fig. 8.25 Pale infarct of the spleen.

haemorrhagic (Fig. 8.24). In some instances, pulmonary arterial occlusion results in a wedge-shaped haemorrhagic patch without necrosis, and resolution may then occur, but when there is ischaemic necrosis, i.e. infarction, organisation and scarring follow in patients who survive for more than a few weeks.

Infarcts of the **spleen** are common and result usually from embolism. They are usually pale reddish at first, but soon become yellowish (Fig. 8.25); occasionally they are haemorrhagic. In the **kidneys**, infarcts seen at necropsy are pale, with a deep red periphery due to congestion and haemorrhage. The pale portion involves chiefly the cortex, the affected part in the medulla being usually red and haemorrhagic

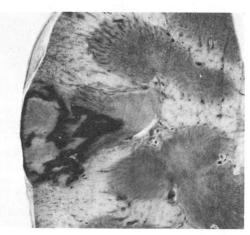

Fig. 8.26 Infarct of kidney, showing pale necrotic centre with haemorrhagic margin. × 1·2.

(Fig. 8.26), but small infarcts may be haemorrhagic throughout. When an arterial branch in a kidney is blocked experimentally, the area supplied becomes at first swollen and red throughout owing to general congestion. Thereafter, the dying kidney cells take up water (p. 6), and their swelling expresses blood from the central part of the infarct, which thus becomes pale. At the periphery and in the medulla the hyperaemia and stasis persist, the ischaemic capillaries rupture, and haemorrhage occurs into the tissues.

Blocking of the superior mesenteric artery produces a haemorrhagic infarct of the **intestine**, (Fig. 18.64, p. 585), which rapidly progresses to gangrene. Death usually results unless the infarcted intestine is removed surgically without undue delay. Obstruction of the in-

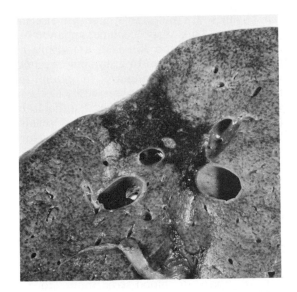

Fig. 8.27 A depressed red patch in the liver due to loss of parenchymal cells and sinusoidal congestion following thrombosis of a portal venous branch (not shown).

ferior mesenteric artery may be without serious effect, but sometimes causes ischaemic colitis.

The sequence of events in the haemorrhagic infarct of the intestine, following obstruction of the superior mesenteric artery, has been studied experimentally in dogs. When this artery is ligated there is at first an arrest of the intestinal blood flow, accompanied by a contraction of the muscular coats of the intestine. The circulation is soon partially restored by blood flowing in from the arterial anastomoses, but without

pulsation being present. The capillaries and small veins become engorged, but the flow through them is inadequate and irregular. Ultimately stasis occurs and there is diffuse haemorrhage into the wall of the intestine and its lumen. Complete deprivation of blood from 5–10 cm of the bowel was found to lead to haemorrhagic infarction. Thus the collateral arterial supply may be able to fill the part with blood, but insufficient to maintain an adequate circulation.

In the **liver**, obstruction of a branch of the portal vein is not followed by infarction, owing to the supply of blood from the hepatic artery. The obstruction does, however, reduce the blood flow sufficiently to cause atrophy and loss of hepatic parenchymal cells, and the sinusoids become dilated, giving a dark red appearance (Fig. 8.27). Obstruction of the hepatic artery or of its branches may result in infarction of the liver (p. 602).

'Venous infarction'. Obstruction of a vein is an uncommon cause of arrest of blood flow through the tissue it drains, partly because in most tissues there is sufficient anastomosis to maintain venous drainage, and partly because thrombosis of veins in internal organs is relatively rare, and emboli do not, of course, impact in veins. When venous infarction does occur the infarct is intensely engorged, oedematous and haemorrhagic. Marantic thrombosis of the superior longitudinal sinus sometimes occurs in severely debilitated children: the engorged cerebral cortical veins may rupture (Fig. 8.28), and there may be patches of

Fig. 8.28 Thrombosis of the superior longitudinal sinus (shown below), resulting in intense engorgement of the cerebral cortical veins and haemorrhage over the frontal lobe.

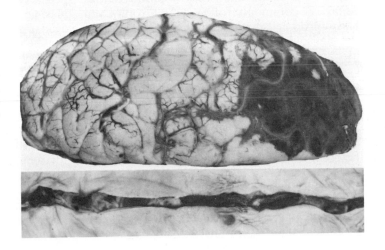

haemorrhagic infarction of the cortex. Thrombosis of the mesenteric veins extending down to the smaller tributaries causes infarction of the intestine, which progresses to gangrene. Venous infarction is also seen occasionally in the liver as a result of extension of hepatic cancer into the hepatic veins. The best examples however are seen in the adrenals, which have several arteries but drain through a single large vein.

The susceptibility of tissues to ischaemia. The extent of infarction is usually less than that of the tissue supplied by the occluded artery, collateral circulation supplying the tissue at the periphery of the area. The extent of infarction may thus vary considerably, depending on whether the collateral arteries are healthy and capable of dilatation. The extent of necrosis is determined also by the capacity of the tissue to withstand ischaemia. As a general rule, the parenchymal cells of the internal organs, which operate at a high metabolic rate, are relatively susceptible to ischaemia, whereas the supporting tissues—connective and fatty tissue and bone, are much less susceptible. The neurones of the central nervous system are perhaps the most susceptible cells of all, and cannot withstand deprivation of blood supply for more than a very few minutes. Glial cells are somewhat less demanding in their requirements, and accordingly at the margin of a brain infarct there is a zone in which partial ischaemia is followed by restoration of the circulation by collaterals; this results in death of the neurones, while the glial cells persist and undergo reactive proliferation. Hepatic parenchymal cells are also highly susceptible to ischaemia and, as described above, thrombosis of a portal venous branch is commonly followed by atrophy and loss of liver cells with survival and dilatation of the sinusoids. The renal tubular epithelium has also a low resistance to ischaemia, and while in the central part of a recent renal infarct all the cells are dead, at the periphery there is a zone in which the glomeruli and intertubular capillaries have survived while the tubular epithelium has died.

Changes following infarction. Following occlusion of an end-artery, some time must elapse before morphological changes take place which allow recognition of tissue death, i.e. before the visible changes of infarction become apparent. The length of this interval depends on the type of tissue undergoing infarction and also upon the method of examination. In general, the changes are detectable first by electron microscopy; later they become apparent on light microscopy, and still later are visible on naked-eye examination. In examining necropsy tissues for the early changes of infarction, the interpretation of changes observed by electron- and light-microscopy is rendered difficult by post-mortem autolysis. The most reliable microscopic change is loss of cell nuclei, which undergo chromatolysis or karyorrhexis (p. 4). In most of the internal organs, infarcts remain solid and coagulative change occurs in the cytoplasm of the dead cells—**coagulative necrosis**: this is the usual sequel to tissue death in the kidneys, liver, myocardium, spleen and lungs. When there has been much exudation from the dying capillaries and venules, or actual escape of blood as in pulmonary infarction, coagulation of fibrin or blood contributes to the solidity and firmness of the infarct. Infarcts of the brain, however, usually undergo **colliquative necrosis** or softening, as described above, and softening occurs occasionally in infarcts of some other organs. For example, a myocardial infarct may undergo autolytic softening (*myomalacia cordis*), and this may be aggravated by the digestive enzymes of neutrophil polymorphs migrating into the dead tissue at the margin of the infarct (see below): rupture of the infarcted tissue may result, with escape of blood into the pericardium and fatal cardiac tamponade (p. 354). Central softening and liquefaction may occur also in a splenic infarct.

Tissue which has undergone coagulative necrosis remains recognisable microscopically for some days or even weeks. Cellular outline persists (Fig. 8.29), although the details of cytoplasmic structure are, of course, lost, and the dead cells have a refractile, homogeneous or hyaline appearance, well seen in myocardial infarction (Fig. 1.4, p. 4): the structural elements of blood vessels and stroma—collagen, reticulin and elastic fibres—persist for longer, and remain demonstrable by appropriate staining techniques.

At an early stage of infarction, products of dead cells at the periphery diffuse into the adjacent tissue and promote a mild **acute inflammatory reaction**, with exudation of fluid from the vessels and migration of neutrophil polymorphs into the peripheral dead tissue. This, together with ischaemia of their walls, accounts for the dilatation of the small vessels

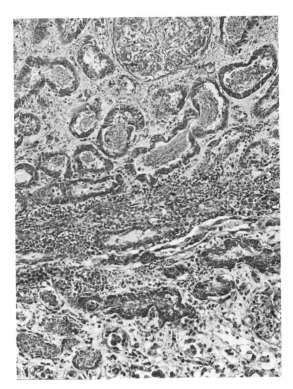

Fig. 8.29 The margin of an infarct of the kidney. The structural appearances of the necrotic tissue are maintained. × 150.

and haemorrhage at the margin of the infarct. The acute reaction soon passes off, and the emigrated polymorphs die. The dead tissue stimulates a reaction similar to that around a foreign body: within a few days a zone of vascular **granulation tissue** forms around the infarct, and ultimately encloses it in a fibrous capsule. The dead tissue is gradually organised; macrophages migrate into and digest it from the periphery inwards, and they are accompanied by new capillary buds and fibroblasts, so that the granulation tissue extends centrally, and as it matures into fibrous tissue the infarct is gradually converted to a **scar**. Extravasated red cells soon lose their outlines, and the pigment is slowly absorbed, although haemorrhagic infarcts, e.g. in the lungs, remain brown for a long time, and macrophages containing haemosiderin may long remain in and around the scar tissue. Loss of parenchymal cells and contraction of the fibrous tissue results in shrinkage; thus an old infarct of the myocardium presents the appearance of fibrosis and thinning of the ventricular wall (Fig. 14.11,

p. 353). In solid organs, old scarred infarcts result in surface depressions, and when they are multiple, e.g. from repeated emboli in the branches of the renal arteries, the surfaces may be puckered and deformed by the scarring.

Septic infarcts. Multiple infarcts due to emboli containing pyogenic bacteria are an essential feature of pyaemia (p. 168) and thus a complication of acute bacterial endocarditis, acute osteomyelitis, carbuncle, etc. The bacteria may extend into, and multiply in, the dead

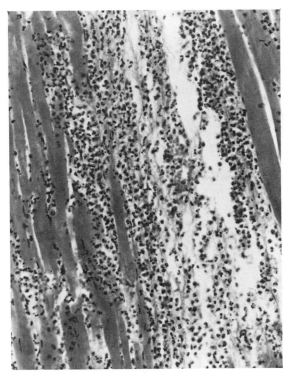

Fig. 8.30 Suppuration at the margin of a septic infarct of the heart. The necrotic myocardium (*right*) is becoming separated from the adjacent living tissue (*left*) by a purulent exudate. × 175.

tissue, and this results in an acute inflammatory reaction in the tissue around the margin of the infarct; thus the central dead tissue becomes surrounded by a ring of suppuration (Fig. 8.30). Occasionally, when putrefactive bacteria are present in the emboli, the infarcts become gangrenous, for example in the lungs as a result of embolism from putrifying thrombi in the pelvic veins in puerperal infection or in the transverse or sigmoid venous sinus in middle-ear infection.

The effects of infarction. The effects of infarction on function depend largely on the location and size of the infarct. In organs such as the kidneys, which have a large functional reserve, extensive or multiple infarctions of both kidneys are necessary to bring about any serious disturbance of function, and serious impairment of liver function also requires very extensive infarction. By contrast, single infarcts of the myocardium are commonly sufficiently large to reduce seriously the functional reserve of the heart, and cause heart failure; infarcts involving the conducting system of the heart may cause heart block, and occlusion of a coronary arterial branch not uncommonly causes death from ventricular fibrillation before infarction has become apparent. Infarcts of the brain are a major cause of serious dysfunction, and even a small one involving the internal capsule is followed by hemiplegia. As already explained, infarction of lung tissue tends to occur especially in association with embarrassment of the pulmonary circulation, and for this reason recent pulmonary infarcts are quite commonly observed at necropsy of patients dying of heart failure.

The effects of infarcts are considered more fully later, in the systematic chapters.

Partial arterial obstruction

Chronic narrowing of the lumen of arteries is very common, and is usually caused by atheroma (p. 313). It brings about the serious effect of ischaemic atrophy of specialised cells with accompanying overgrowth of fibrous tissue, for example in the myocardium and the kidneys. In the brain also, patchy loss of neurones and overgrowth of astrocytes is common, and owing to the prevalence of atheroma in the elderly, is an important cause of senile mental changes. Multiple or extensive atheromatous narrowing of the lumen is common in the arteries of the lower limbs, and the resulting chronic ischaemia brings about various trophic changes, and also limping, and cramp-like ischaemic pain, brought on by walking (*intermittent claudication*). Narrowing of the smallest arteries and arterioles—*arteriolosclerosis*—occurs commonly in the abdominal viscera and central nervous system as an ageing effect, and results particularly from arterial hypertension: it is usually most severe in the afferent arterioles of the glomeruli, where it brings about glomerular sclerosis. These regional changes are, however, more appropriately considered in relation to the various systems and organs.

Disturbances of Water and Salt Balance

Water and salt deficiency

The water content of the average male body, estimated by the deuterium method, is about 62%, and that of the female about 52%, the sex difference being accounted for by the higher fat content in females. A man weighing 70 kg contains about 42 litres and this is distributed as 30 litres of *intracellular* water and 12 litres of *extracellular* water; the latter is subdivided into about 3 litres of *intravascular* fluid, the plasma, and about 9 litres of *interstitial* fluid which is distinguished from the intravascular and intracellular fluids by its very low protein content. The extracellular fluids contain practically all the sodium (except for that associated with collagen and that forming part of bone mineral), balanced chiefly by chloride and bicarbonate ions, whereas the intracellular fluid is almost devoid of sodium and chloride, its proteinate, sulphate and phosphate anions being balanced by potassium and magnesium. It is essential that the interstitial fluid should remain isotonic with the intravascular and intracellular fluids, and it contains a higher concentration of electrolytes which balances the colloid osmotic pressure of their proteins. Reductions in the water and salt content of the body are generally associated, but disproportionate depletion of either water or salt causes disturbances of the normal equilibrium which require different treatment. The continued daily loss by the lungs and by insensible perspiration of about half a litre of water without proportionate loss of salt must always be taken into account. Deficiency of water tends to cause hypertonicity of the extracellular fluids so that water is withdrawn from the cells, which thus share in *primary water depletion*. Conversely, in relative salt depletion the extracellular fluids tend to become hypotonic, but this effect is minimised partly by increased renal excretion of water and partly by diffusion of water from the interstitial fluid into the cells with maintenance of isotonicity. Thus in salt deficiency the extracellular fluids are reduced in volume, but the administration of water or glucose solution without salt is actually harmful as it merely dilutes further the extracellular fluids and increases the diffusion of water into cells. It is curious that whereas the need for water is normally indicated by thirst, in man there appears to be no urgent warning sensation when salt is lacking.

Deficiency in body water may be brought about in various ways and in minor degrees is very common. In hospital patients it is seen most often as a result of insufficient intake owing to physical weakness, coma and pyrexia. The urine is reduced in volume (500 ml) and is highly concentrated, the specific gravity rising to 1·040 or more. The plasma levels of Na^+, Cl^- and urea increase, probably as the result of diminished renal filtration, although the plasma volume is maintained relatively well by withdrawal of intracellular water and by active retention of Na^+ and excretion of K^+ under the influence of the renin–angiotensin–aldosterone system (p. 221) which is stimulated by the diminished blood volume, the so-called reaction of dehydration. More severe water deprivation occurs under exceptional conditions, e.g. in men shipwrecked or lost in the desert, and then the deficiency of body water may ultimately reach over 12% of body weight and amount to nearly 10 litres. Death is thought to be due to rise in the osmotic pressure of the cells. In children the ratio of body surface to weight is higher than in adults so that cutaneous losses of water are proportionately greater; also children cannot produce such a high concentration of urine as can adults. As a result, lack of fluid has a more severe effect in infants and young children than in adults.

Salt depletion is a commoner cause of serious effects than is water depletion, and also is more liable to remain unrecognised. Excessive loss of sodium chloride from the body occurs in various conditions and is commonly only one factor in complex fluid and electrolyte disturbances. Pure loss of salt results from excessive

sweating when water is consumed freely, e.g. in the tropics or when working in a very hot atmosphere. It gives rise to a state of 'heat exhaustion' which necessitates the administration of large amounts of salt as well as of water, the consumption of water alone being liable to produce severe cramps. Clinically, vomiting and diarrhoea are the most important causes of combined water and salt depletion: the former is complicated by alkalosis due to loss of H^+, and the latter by acidosis from loss of the alkaline secretions of the small intestine. If only water is restored the picture of pure salt depletion follows, with lowering of osmotic pressure of the extracellular fluid and so great a reduction in its amount, owing to renal excretion of water and to increased osmotic absorption by the tissue cells, that circulatory collapse (*shock*) soon supervenes. Marriott states that the effects of this *secondary extracellular dehydration* are actually more serious than those of the disturbed acid–base balance which may develop from disproportionate loss of sodium or chloride ions, though the latter condition at one time received more attention. The symptoms of salt depletion when water is consumed freely include lassitude, weakness, giddiness, fainting attacks and cramps; also anorexia, nausea and vomiting occur and tend to aggravate the condition by establishing a vicious circle. Marked loss of weight and mental confusion may occur also. The plasma concentration of sodium, normally about 137–148 mmol/l, falls to 130–120 mmol/l or less. The chloride and bicarbonate concentrations are also reduced *in toto* but their ratio varies with the presence of complicating acidosis or alkalosis. The blood is concentrated, with a rise in haemoglobin, haematocrit value and in plasma protein. The urine contains little or no sodium or chloride except when the salt depletion is due to renal loss, as in Addison's disease or diabetic ketosis. The blood urea rises, often to over 100 mg per 100 ml (17 mmol/l), owing mainly to reduced renal blood flow and diminution in the volume of glomerular filtrate. These are common examples of *pre-renal uraemia* (p. 785).

Combined deficiency of water and salt is more common clinically than of either separately. Vomiting and diarrhoea are probably its most frequent cause. If water is ingested and retained, salt deficiency will predominate, as described above, but without fluid intake water loss exceeds salt loss. In such combined deficiency, the extracellular fluid therefore tends to become hypertonic and consequently fluid is withdrawn from the cells; this leads to thirst and oliguria in addition to the tendency to acute circulatory failure and other symptoms of salt depletion. The rise in blood urea often leads to the erroneous diagnosis of uraemia due to renal failure, but the administration of water and salt in adequate amounts may completely relieve the symptoms.

Regulation of the water content of the blood and urine is normally carried out by the kidneys, which in turn are controlled largely by the neurohypophysis through the action of the antidiuretic hormone on the renal tubular concentrating mechanism. The neurohypophysis is so highly sensitive to the osmotic influence of sodium chloride that an alteration of one per cent in the osmotic pressure of the arterial blood can bring about a tenfold variation in the excretion of water, and the osmotic pressure of the extracellular fluids is thereby regulated so as to maintain a practically constant state. Failure of this mechanism is seen in diabetes insipidus (p. 949), in which intense polyuria approaching maximum water excretion is constantly present. An analogous situation in respect of excessive salt excretion results from failure of the secretion of adequate amounts of aldosterone by the adrenal cortex, e.g. in Addison's disease, in which the cortex is largely destroyed. Uncontrolled sodium loss in the urine leads to fall of the plasma sodium to far below the level at which it normally ceases to be excreted. In consequence serious depletion of the body's store of sodium is brought about and this, if uncorrected, contributes greatly to the severe crises of Addison's disease and the tendency to acute circulatory collapse (p. 977). Other hormones also play minor parts in the regulation of water and salt excretion, e.g. ovarian hormones can cause a distinct retention of water, as is seen in the late phase of the menstrual cycle and in pregnancy.

The pathology of generalised oedema has to be viewed against this background of water and salt balance. Maintenance of osmotic equilibrium is more important for life and is therefore regulated more exactly than the total volume of fluid in the body or within any of its compartments. Most importance was formerly attached to the chloride anion, but it is now recognised that the sodium cation is even more significant in regulating the amount of body fluid in the extracellular compartment of the tissues, and that sodium is intimately concerned in the pathogenesis of oedema.

Water and salt retention: oedema

Oedema is an abnormal increase in the amount of interstitial fluid. It may be localised, e.g. in an organ, limb, etc., or more generalised. In generalised oedema there is usually accumulation of fluid also in the serous cavities (hydrothorax, ascites, etc.). When oedema affects the skin and subcutaneous tissues, swelling may be obvious, and momentary pressure will produce a depression ('pitting') which disappears in a few seconds as the oedema fluid returns to the tissue.

Control of interstitial fluid. The total exchange between the plasma and interstitial fluid is probably of the order of 7000 litres of fluid daily, and fluctuates widely in the varying states of the circulation to different parts. It is generally accepted that the interchange of fluid between the capillaries and venules and the tissue spaces can be explained on a physical basis and that the distribution of fluid within and outside the vessels is regulated mainly by a balance of the two processes of filtration and osmosis. The intracapillary hydrostatic pressure tends to force fluid outwards into the tissue spaces, while the osmotic pressure of the colloids of the plasma tends to attract water and thus to induce its return from the tissue spaces into the capillaries and venules. The permeability of the capillary walls varies in different regions and also under different conditions of physiological activity in any one region, but the filtrate in all situations normally contains at least a small amount of protein, probably not exceeding 0·5% in the more permeable areas such as the liver, and less than 0·1% in the less permeable areas such as the limbs. In the normal exchange of interstitial fluid between vessels and tissue spaces most of the filtrate is returned to the circulation by the veins and only a small amount by the lymphatics, but the latter portion contains practically all the protein, so that the protein content of lymph is higher than that of the filtrate. The protein content of lymph therefore fluctuates widely, depending on the permeability of the capillaries in the area drained: for example, the hepatic lymph is very rich in protein (3–5%).

Water retention. It is important to an understanding of the problems of generalised oedema to realise that, regardless of the cause, this condition is accompanied by retention of water and cannot be regarded as a mere redistribution of the body fluids. There is always an increase in the extracellular fluids of the body and (in an adult) a rise of weight of about 5 kg invariably precedes the appearance of clinically recognisable generalised oedema, a fact utilised in the attention paid to the weight during pregnancy. Indeed generalised oedema can be regarded as a method of disposing of excess fluid, which cannot be discharged by the usual channels, in order to regulate the blood volume. The body appears to tolerate badly an increase in the volume of the intravascular fluid; the excess is shunted into the interstitial spaces where its presence requires the simultaneous retention of a sufficient quantity of electrolytes, chiefly salt, to equalise the osmotic pressure of this fluid with that of the cells and of the plasma. The osmotic effect of the intracellular and plasma proteins is balanced by a higher concentration of electrolytes—chiefly salt—in the interstitial fluid. It is unlikely that increase of capillary permeability to macromolecules plays any major part in the common forms of generalised oedema, for the protein content of oedema fluid is not sufficiently high to support this possibility. Also, there is no gross fall in the blood volume, as might be expected if exudation of protein-rich plasma fluid was an important factor. In rare cases, cyclical oedema has been accompanied by hypovolaemia, and it has been suggested that the oedema of hypothermia may be related to an increase of factors such as bradykinin, which increase capillary permeability.

Local oedema

Active hyperaemia: inflammatory oedema. Active hyperaemia occurs in acute inflammation, in which the exudation of protein-rich fluid from the capillaries and venules gives rise to inflammatory oedema: as indicated in Chapter 2, major factors in the production of inflammatory oedema are increased hydrostatic pressure in the small vessels, capillary and venular dilatation, and increased permeability.

Active hyperaemia of lesser degree occurs also under physiological conditions, for example in the skeletal muscles during exercise, in the gastro-intestinal tract during digestion, and in the skin as an important mechanism of heat loss: the increase in interstitial fluid resulting from such physiological hyperaemia is, however, removed by the lymphatics and oedema does not result.

Oedema is a prominent feature of some types of **hypersensitivity reactions**, for example in hay fever, urticaria, the Arthus and delayed hypersensitivity reactions. These are all described in Chapter 5, and it is sufficient to state here that the oedema is of inflammatory nature, due to active hyperaemia and increased vascular permeability.

Urticaria consists of erythema, itching and wealing (which is sharply localised oedema) of the skin: it is very common, but occurs usually in mild form, with only occasional transient attacks. In some instances, however, attacks are frequent, severe, or more persistent. Although there is often a clear association with eating a particular food or taking a drug (especially aspirin), there is little firm evidence of an immunological hypersensitivity basis in most cases, and the underlying nature of the condition is usually unknown. Histamine antagonists are often beneficial, but in therapeutic dosage these agents have various other effects in addition to anti-histamine activity. Except when it occurs as part of an anaphylactic attack, urticaria is seldom dangerous.

Hereditary angio-oedema. This rare condition is characterised by attacks of acute localised oedema, most often affecting the skin of the face and trunk, but sometimes the larynx: acute abdominal pain, vomiting and diarrhoea can also occur as a result of oedema of a segment of gut, and some patients have undergone several abdominal operations. Death from laryngeal oedema is common in some affected families.

The condition is due to a genetically-determined (autosomal dominant) abnormality of an inhibitor of the activated first component of complement ($C\bar{1}$). In some cases there is insufficient inhibitor, in others it is qualitatively abnormal. The oedema is probably due mainly to a kinin-like fraction of $C\bar{2}$, and transfusion of fresh normal plasma (which contains the inhibitor) has recently been reported to be effective in both prevention and treatment of attacks. Anti-histaminic drugs, adrenaline and steroids are ineffectual. A variety known as Quincke's disease often affects several members of the same family. In this condition the oedema occurs usually in the face or hands but may affect the larynx, and cause death from asphyxia. Oedema of the wall of the bowel with colicky pain has also been described.

Oedema may occur in severe cases of **zoster** (shingles) and is apparently a trophic effect due to inflammatory change in the posterior root ganglia. If the nerve lesion is unilateral, as it usually is, the oedema stops short in the midline of the body.

Local venous congestion and oedema. In a healthy animal, acute venous congestion produced by ligation of a large venous trunk does not usually lead to oedema, although there is an increased filtration of water and electrolytes owing to the heightened capillary pressure, and also an increase in the amount of protein leaving the vessels. Consequently there is increased flow of lymph containing a lowered concentration, but increased amount, of protein, and oedema does not usually develop. If, however, along with the ligation of the vein the vaso-motor nerves supplying the part are cut, the intracapillary pressure is still further increased and localised oedema follows. Similarly, the application of an elastic band to a limb may merely produce venous congestion with increased lymph flow unless the band is tightened sufficiently to prevent the flow of lymph from the part, when oedema will result. These findings indicate that some other factor in addition to acute venous congestion is usually necessary for the production of oedema. In clinical cases, however, local venous congestion often lasts much longer than in the experimental animal, and this may possibly explain the common occurrence of oedema.

In acute venous obstruction there must be sufficient anastomotic drainage of venous blood to permit the circulation to continue; otherwise stasis, thrombosis and haemorrhagic infarction would follow as is seen in mesenteric venous thrombosis. After a time readjustment of the circulation occurs and arterial inflow diminishes. This leads to a reduction in tissue perfusion until, in time, the collateral circulation increases sufficiently to re-establish normal drainage. Until that stage is reached, the combination of venous congestion, tissue hypoxia

and accumulation of metabolites may, by increasing capillary hydrostatic pressure and permeability, result in local oedema.

The oedema of chronic lymphatic obstruction, e.g. that produced by cancer, chronic inflammation, radiotherapy, filariasis, etc. (p. 341), is usually of the non-pitting type, i.e. the swollen tissues do not yield readily to pressure. A characteristic feature of chronic lymphatic oedema is the development of elephantiasis due to overgrowth of the connective tissue in the skin and subcutaneous tissue. Since the plasma protein normally present in the interstitial fluid is returned to the blood by the lymphatics, chronic lymphatic obstruction results in the accumulation of protein in the tissues while most of the water and electrolytes are taken up by the venules as usual. This accumulated protein may, either by providing nutrient or in some unknown way, be responsible for stimulating the connective tissue cells to increased production of collagen.

Lymphatic oedema of the legs also occurs as a primary condition which is sometimes hereditary (Milroy's disease) and is believed to be due to a congenital abnormality of the lymphatics. The legs become permanently thickened.

General oedema

Cardiac oedema is apt to develop at a late stage in cases of right ventricular failure with longstanding systemic venous congestion. It appears first in the most dependent parts of the body and gradually extends upwards. Thus it is usually noticed first round the ankles, and pitting may be elicited by pressure over the lower end of the tibia. When the condition is advanced, the limbs become greatly swollen, while the skin is tense and vesicles may form. Accumulation of fluid may occur also in the serous cavities.

As indicated above, increased transudation from congested, dilated capillaries is not sufficient to produce oedema, because the excess fluid is removed by the lymphatics. When, however, heart failure becomes severe, the diminution in cardiac output adversely affects renal function which depends upon normal renal blood flow. There is evidence that the kidneys can compensate to some extent for reduced blood supply by increasing the proportion of fluid filtered off in the glomeruli; this is probably mediated by increased tone in the efferent arterioles. The volume of urine is reduced and it is highly concentrated, indicating that there is excessive tubular re-absorption of water. The mechanism of this excessive re-absorption is not fully understood, but the reduced renal blood flow may stimulate the juxta-glomerular cells to secrete excess of renin, and this in turn will enhance the secretion of aldosterone by the adrenal cortex, with consequent re-absorption of sodium by the renal tubules. The effect of sodium retention is to stimulate secretion of anti-diuretic hormone by the neurohypophysis, and so more water is re-absorbed in the renal collecting tubules. Direct evidence supporting such a mechanism has been provided in some, but not all cases of cardiac oedema (p. 222). The stimulus to this secondary aldosteronism is not fully understood, as it occurs among different types of heart failure, both in low output and in high output types. The great increase in body weight confirms the enormous amount of fluid retained in the oedematous tissues in some cardiac cases, and the importance of water and salt retention is shown by the effect of diuretics in diminishing the oedema. Reduction in the intake of sodium chloride in the diet has sometimes a markedly diuretic effect, water being eliminated with preservation of the isotonic state of the oedema fluid.

Other factors may play a part in the genesis of cardiac oedema, e.g. the accumulation in the tissues of waste products which by their osmotic action will tend to attract more water from the blood. There is also evidence that chronic hypoxia increases capillary permeability, although this view is not supported by the protein content of the oedema fluid, which is usually about 0·5% or less. We consider, however, that the fundamental cause of cardiac oedema lies in the faulty elimination of fluid consequent upon the deranged renal circulation. The distribution of the retained fluid in the tissues is determined by gravity because, with the reduction in cardiac power, the circulation is unable to absorb the tissue fluid and return it to the right heart against the hydrostatic pressure of the column of venous blood in the dependent parts. The distribution of oedema fluid is influenced also by the degree to which different tissues can be distended without a significant rise in tissue pressure.

In failure of the left ventricle of the heart, venous congestion occurs mainly in the lungs so long as the right ventricle continues to beat forcibly: pulmonary oedema may then develop without generalised oedema.

Renal oedema. Generalised oedema occurs in various diseases which affect the glomeruli including some types of glomerulonephritis, and also in acute renal failure due to injury to the renal tubules. The pathological changes in these conditions are described in Chapter 21. However, an understanding of the factors likely to be involved in the production of the various types of renal oedema depends not so much on a knowledge of the detailed structural changes but rather on the associated functional disturbances. Accordingly, renal diseases which give rise to oedema may be placed within three groups and these are considered below.

(1) Conditions in which all the glomeruli are affected, with reduction in renal blood flow and in glomerular filtration. This group is exemplified by *acute diffuse glomerulonephritis* and *rapidly progressive glomerulonephritis*. There is usually a rise in blood pressure and blood urea level, and production of a diminished amount of concentrated urine containing moderate amounts of protein. The oedema in these conditions is not influenced by gravity to the same extent as is cardiac oedema and is often noticed first in the loose connective tissues, e.g. of the eyelids and face: in ambulant patients, however, gravity is seen to have some effect. The protein content of the oedema fluid is usually less than 0·5% and the oedema therefore cannot be attributed to increased capillary permeability. Also the proteinuria is usually only moderate and the loss does not result in any significant reduction in the levels of the plasma proteins. The blood volume is normal or increased, and the oedema seems likely to be due to excessive re-absorption of salt and water in the renal tubules. The factors responsible for this excessive re-absorption are not, however, clearly defined. The renin–angiotensin–aldosterone system may be implicated, but even this is uncertain.

(2) *The nephrotic syndrome.* In some renal diseases there is persistent and heavy loss of plasma proteins, particularly albumin, in the urine: when this exceeds about 10 g daily, the plasma albumin level falls considerably and this is accompanied by generalised oedema which

often becomes very severe. This condition is known as the nephrotic syndrome. As in other types of renal oedema, the distribution of the tissue fluid is not so dependent on gravity as in cardiac oedema. In patients with nephrotic syndrome, the blood pressure is often not raised and there is commonly no rise in the blood urea, indicating that renal blood flow and glomerular filtration rates are normal. The nephrotic syndrome may arise in a large number of conditions: in some it is regularly present, for example in *glomerulonephritis* of *minimal-change* and *membranous* types (q.v.). It is a common result of amyloid disease involving the glomeruli; it occasionally complicates other types of glomerulonephritis and the glomerular lesions of diabetes mellitus and various other diseases. In all these conditions, its development is dependent on excessive loss of plasma albumin into the glomerular filtrate.

Glomerular leakage of protein exhibits a molecular sieving effect, the amount of plasma albumin which escapes being disproportionately great because of its relatively small molecular size. Also because of its small size and its relatively high concentration in the plasma, albumin is the protein mainly responsible for the osmotic pressure of the plasma, and consequently, in states of severe hypoalbuminaemia, the amount of fluid leaving the capillaries and venules throughout the body greatly exceeds the amount drawn back into them by osmosis. Accordingly, the plasma volume tends to fall and this brings into play the renin–angiotensin–aldosterone mechanism which results in increased re-absorption of sodium and water from the renal tubules: this tends, in turn, to dilute the plasma protein still further and so transudation into the tissues remains excessive; a vicious circle is set up and continues to operate so long as gross albuminuria persists. As would be expected, the oedema fluid in the nephrotic syndrome has a very low protein content, and there is no evidence of general increased capillary permeability for macromolecules.

In experimental studies in which the levels of plasma proteins have been artificially lowered in dogs by plasmapheresis (removal of blood and returning the cells suspended in saline), oedema has not been found to develop unless physiological saline is administered by mouth. Since large amounts of salt and water taken by mouth can cause oedema, even in normal individuals, these findings do not provide strong support for the explanation given above for oedema in the nephrotic syndrome. Nevertheless, the importance of protein loss and hypoalbuminaemia is confirmed by the appearance of similar gross oedema in protein-losing enteropathy (p. 580) in which the kidneys are normal and there is gross loss of plasma protein into the gut. The participation of the renin–angiotensin–aldosterone mechanism is demonstrated by the very high plasma levels of aldosterone found in the nephrotic syndrome.

(3) In *acute tubular necrosis*, the acutely injured tubules lose their capacity for selective re-absorption and concentration of the glomerular filtrate. Consequently, most of the filtrate is re-absorbed and the small amount of urine produced approximates in its composition to a protein-free filtrate of plasma. There is retention of water and electrolytes and a progressive rise in blood urea. Apart from loss by sweating, vomiting, etc., most of the fluid taken by mouth is retained in the body and unless it is seriously restricted, gross oedema develops.

Acute tubular necrosis may result from shock or certain chemical poisons (p. 785). In some cases of acute renal failure following shock, the tubules show no convincing evidence of necrosis in a renal biopsy, and it now appears that hyperactivity of the renin–angiotensin–aldosterone system may be of importance in such cases (p. 788).

In the various forms of renal disease which are complicated by arterial hypertension, cardiac failure is liable to develop with consequent generalised or pulmonary oedema.

Nutritional oedema

Generalised oedema may clearly be caused by malnutrition. Protein insufficiency seems to be the main factor, and the extreme example is termed kwashiorkor (p. 606). Examination of the blood shows a marked fall in glucose, lipids and proteins, the last being sometimes reduced to half the normal. It seems likely that fall in osmotic pressure of the plasma is the most important factor in the production of the oedema, but no strict parallelism has been found, some cases failing to become oedematous in spite of severe depletion of serum albumin, while others show gross oedema with plasma protein levels within normal limits; also the oedema may disappear before there is any significant rise in the colloid osmotic pressure of the plasma. Nutritional oedema is commonly associated with xerophthalmia, a condition in which opacity with ulceration of the cornea occurs, as a result of deficiency in fat-soluble vitamin A; possibly lack of the vitamin B complex is also concerned, and the 'wet' (oedematous) form of beri-beri is perhaps related. A similar form of oedema has been observed in infants when there has been excess of carbohydrates in the diet with marked deficiency in other foodstuffs. In all such examples of nutritional oedema, the problem is a complex one, and the factors which we have mentioned may be concerned in varying proportions.

Oedema may occur in patients with chronic wasting diseases, e.g. cancer, tuberculosis, etc., and is due mainly to cardiac failure, although fall in the plasma proteins is a contributory factor in some cases.

Pulmonary oedema

The osmotic pressure of the plasma (25 mm Hg) is substantially greater than the normal hydrostatic pressure in the pulmonary capillaries (8–10 mm Hg). Consequently, the development of oedema of the lungs usually requires a considerable rise in the hydrostatic pressure. As elsewhere, this occurs, together with increased vascular permeability, in acute inflammatory lesions, and inflammatory oedema is pronounced in severe influenza and lobar pneumonia, etc.

Pulmonary oedema can be produced readily in healthy dogs by interfering with the flow of pulmonary venous blood, for example by compressing the left atrium or ventricle, or constricting the aorta. Similarly, in man, it occurs in left ventricular failure, as in some cases of myocardial infarction and in systemic hypertension. In this latter condition, acute pulmonary oedema comes on especially when the patient is lying down, probably due to improved venous return from the legs, and perhaps also to increase in the blood volume by re-absorption of oedema fluid from the legs when recumbent. The attack is usually relieved by sitting up. Chronic pulmonary congestion, as, for example, in stenosis of the mitral valve, is not alone sufficient to produce pulmonary oedema in man. This is probably because reflex increase in tone of the pulmonary arterioles protects the pulmonary capillary bed from excessive rise in pressure. However, the situation is precarious, and pulmonary oedema is prone to result from physical exertion or other factors which increase the pulmonary blood flow. Chronic pulmonary oedema may occur as part of generalised renal oedema, particularly when there is, in addition, systemic hypertension, as in acute glomerulonephritis. Another important cause is overloading of the circulation by rapid transfusion of blood to patients with severe anaemia. Finally, pulmonary oedema occurs in some cases of increased intracranial pressure, most commonly in head injury or intracranial haemorrhage.

Apart from the above causes, oedema of the posterobasal parts of the lungs is a very common finding at necropsy, particularly in old people and where death is due to a toxic condition or has been preceded by coma. The oedema fluid is very prone to become infected by a mixture of bacteria, usually of low virulence, producing *hypostatic pneumonia* which, if untreated, is likely to be the immediate cause of death.

Depending on the causal factors, pulmonary oedema may be confined within the alveolar walls, i.e. interstitial oedema, or the fluid may pour into the alveolar spaces. The factors concerned are considered on p. 397–401.

The renin–angiotensin–aldosterone system

Renin is an enzyme, stored and probably formed in the renal juxta-glomerular apparatus; it is present in high concentration in the cytoplasmic granules of cells of the wall of the terminal part of the afferent glomerular arterioles. The adjacent macula densa, a plaque of specialised epithelial lining cells in the wall

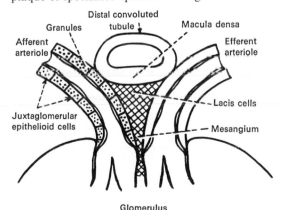

Fig. 8.31 Diagram of the juxta-glomerular apparatus.

of the distal convoluted tubule, is probably a sensory device, regulating the release of renin in response to changes in the composition of the fluid in the tubular lumen (Fig. 8.31).

Renin-substrate (angiotensinogen) is present in the α_2-globulin fraction of plasma and also in renal lymph.

The initial product of the action of renin on its substrate is an inactive decapeptide, angiotensin I. This is converted in the circulation (largely, it now appears, in the lungs) to the active octapeptide, angiotensin II. A much smaller proportion of angiotensin I is converted to angiotensin II within the kidney; nevertheless this is of considerable importance in considering the possible direct renal actions of angiotensin.

Renin is normally present in higher concentration in renal lymph than in renal venous plasma, but because of the much higher rate of renal plasma flow, secretion into the renal vein is greater than that into lymph.

Effects of renin. Renin, by way of angiotensin, has three principal actions:

(a) Aldosterone-stimulating.

(b) Pressor, mediated mainly by peripheral vasoconstriction.

(c) A direct renal effect, modifying urinary output of water and electrolytes.

Other actions, which hitherto have been less fully studied, are the central stimulation of thirst, release of catecholamines and possibly release of kinins.

The relative dominance of the three principal actions mentioned above is much modified by the prevailing sodium status. Sodium deprivation, for example, enhances the aldosterone-stimulating effect, while minimising the pressor action, so that a marked rise in circulating renin, angiotensin II, and aldosterone occurs with little or no increase in arterial blood pressure.

The renal effects of administered angiotensin vary widely according to the dosage, the prevailing sodium status, arterial pressure, and species. At most doses which can safely be given to normal man, angiotensin reduces renal excretion of sodium and water, and this effect is enhanced by severe sodium depletion, as in untreated Addison's disease. By contrast, in hypertension, irrespective of aetiology, and also in hepatic cirrhosis with ascites, angiotensin usually increases water and sodium loss.

Secondary hyperaldosteronism. The renin–angiotensin–aldosterone system is stimulated, and high circulating levels of all three components may be found, in sodium depletion, whether due to dietary sodium restriction, sodium-losing renal disease, diuretics or purgatives: haemorrhage produces a similar response. Because in these situations the increase in aldosterone is thought to be a consequence of a rise in renin, these are regarded as examples of 'secondary' hyperaldosteronism.

Secondary hyperaldosteronism develops in some, but by no means all, cases of untreated congestive heart failure, in hepatic cirrhosis with ascites, and in the nephrotic syndrome. It may seem paradoxical that patients with these oedematous states, with their retention of sodium and water, should react as though sodium-deprived. The explanation lies probably in that the excess sodium is principally extravascular, and thus not capable of recognition by the kidney. The kidney therefore responds as in sodium deprivation; hence plasma renin and angiotensin, and in consequence, aldosterone, are elevated.

Renal artery stenosis is another instance in which the kidney probably receives a stimulus to increased renin release which is inappropriate to the overall requirements of the body. The old belief that renal artery constriction, by leading to increased circulating renin and angiotensin, is simply and directly responsible for hypertension *via* the pressor effect of angiotensin (p. 323) is now known to be a considerable oversimplification. It is clear, however, that in many cases of severe renal artery stenosis with hypertension, both renin and aldosterone are increased. A similar mechanism—possibly multiple intrarenal arterial lesions—may be the cause of the secondary hyperaldosteronism which often accompanies the malignant phase of hypertension, irrespective of aetiology. In advanced chronic renal disease with renal failure, occasionally such severe elevation of renin and aldosterone levels may occur that hypertension cannot be controlled until both diseased kidneys have been excised. This could well be an instance where sufficient angiotensin is circulating to have a direct pressor effect. It is noteworthy that the ability to secrete renin seems to be well maintained even in the terminal stages of chronic renal disease.

A particularly interesting form of secondary hyperaldosteronism is found in the rare condition of renin-secreting renal tumour, which occurs mainly in young patients.

In normal pregnancy, plasma levels of renin, renin-substrate, angiotensin II and aldosterone are all increased. This is an instance of physiological secondary hyperaldosteronism.

Other patterns of variation in circulating renin and aldosterone are readily predictable. Sodium loading, or the administration of sodium-retaining substances such as DOC, fluorocortisone, carbenoxolone or liquorice, depress circulating renin and aldosterone.

Primary hyperaldosteronism. An adrenocortical adenoma secreting an excess of aldosterone will lead to sodium retention, and thus to the combination of renin suppression with elevated aldosterone. This is known as 'primary' hyperaldosteronism (p. 975). The same combination will also be seen in any situation where excess aldosterone secretion is stimulated by mechanisms other than the renin–angiotensin system.

Hypoaldosteronism. In Addison's disease, the sodium deficiency stimulates marked secretion of renin, but aldosterone production remains deficient despite this stimulus, because the diseased adrenal cortex is unable to respond appropriately.

Primary renin deficiency, found mainly in elderly patients, is accompanied by selective aldosterone deficiency, cortisol secretion being normal.

Direct effects of renin and angiotensin on the kidney. The renal actions of angiotensin, although undoubted, are difficult to study in isolation from the pressor and aldosterone-stimulating effects. It has been suggested that phylogenetically, renin and angiotensin may have appeared initially as components of a purely intrarenal sodium-conserving system, and that the peripheral pressor and aldosterone-stimulating actions evolved as subsequent refinements and modifications, perhaps made necessary by a terrestrial, as opposed to an aquatic or semi-aquatic, habitat.

As mentioned earlier, a small proportion of angiotensin I can be converted to angiotensin II within the kidney. The major site of such conversion is, however, the lungs, and it has been suggested that this is an adaptation preventing the accumulation of dangerously high levels of angiotensin II within the kidney. When renal blood flow is impaired, the direct renal effect of angiotensin II may be initially beneficial, preserving glomerular filtration rate, possibly by a tonic action on efferent glomerular arterioles. However, with further elevation of angiotensin II, this beneficial effect is lost, and renal failure with tubular necrosis ensues.

Many years ago Goormaghtigh suggested that a renal effect of renin might be responsible for the reduced renal blood flow and oliguria of acute renal failure (see p. 788); considerable circumstantial evidence now supports the hypothesis that several forms of acute renal failure may be the pathological extreme of the process outlined above. Moreover, very large doses of angiotensin II can produce acute renal failure with tubular necrosis in experimental animals. A wide variety of stimuli causing increases in renin secretion predispose to acute renal failure with or without renal tubular necrosis. These include cardiac failure, sodium depletion, pregnancy, haemorrhage, Addison's disease and renal artery occlusion. Conversely, sodium loading and renal denervation reduce renin levels and are thought to protect against acute renal failure. Moreover, it has recently been shown that very big increases in plasma renin concentration occur after two procedures—the administration of glycerol and the giving of the antibiotic cephaloridine—which each cause severe renal failure and tubular necrosis in experimental animals.

Shock

Definition and nature of shock. Shock is the name given to the complex series of changes which result from an acute fall in cardiac output.

These changes include regulatory mechanisms which are beneficial in that they tend to maintain the circulation, particularly to those organs with the most vital and urgent perfusion requirements—the heart and the central nervous system. Unless the general circulation can be restored without undue delay, the diminished blood flow through most of the tissues results in widespread impairment of cell functions, and this, together with the compensating circulatory changes, is responsible for the clinical features of shock.

Causes and types of shock

The three major causes of shock are:

1. Reduction of blood volume, which induces **hypovolaemic shock**: examples include *severe haemorrhage*, *extensive vascular exudation* as in burns, and conditions such as severe vomiting and diarrhoea, which cause *dehydration*.

2. Acute cardiac failure (cardiogenic shock), due most often to myocardial infarction.

3. Severe infections, usually with bacteraemia or septicaemia, which induce **septic shock**.

Although all three major types have many features in common, they also differ in important ways. It is convenient to give first an account of hypovolaemic shock, and then to describe the special features of the other types. It is also important to emphasise that the longer shock persists, the more complicated it becomes, and in advanced shock all three factors—hypovolaemia, cardiac insufficiency bacterial infection—are often combined.

It is well known that withdrawal of even a few millilitres of blood can induce a *fainting* or *vaso-vagal attack*. This is immediate, can result from all grades of injury, from severe pain, or from psychogenic stimuli such as a fright or witnessing an accident or surgical operation. Fainting is characterised by pallor, sweating, weakness, a slow pulse, marked fall in blood pressure and loss of consciousness; vomiting and convulsions may also occur. These changes last only a few minutes and recovery is rapid. The fainting attack is described here because it used to be known as 'primary shock'. In fact, it is quite distinct from what is now regarded as shock, and should not be confused with it. The nature and features of *anaphylactic shock* and of the shock-like state of *acute immune-complex disease* are described on pp. 118 and 126 respectively.

Hypovolaemic shock

This results most commonly from acute severe haemorrhage, due to trauma, to involvement of blood vessels in disease processes, or to a haemorrhagic disorder. Another important cause is severe burning, in which hypovolaemia results from inflammatory exudation of plasma fluid from the damaged small blood vessels in the vicinity of extensive burns. Thirdly, hypovolaemic shock can develop in severe acute dehydration, for example in cholera or gastroenteritis.

Clinical features

The shocked patient is often restless and confused, has a pale, cold, sweaty skin, often with peripheral cyanosis, a rapid weak pulse, a low blood pressure, increased rate and depth of respiration, and may become drowsy and confused and finally comatose.

Haemorrhagic and traumatic shock

A normal healthy adult can lose 500 ml or so of blood, i.e. about 10% of the blood volume, without any significant disability; the blood volume is almost restored within a few hours, although replacement of plasma proteins takes a day or two, and restoration of red cells takes much longer. Loss of 25% of the blood (about 1250 ml) results in significant hypovolaemia over the next 36 hours, while a rapid loss of about half the blood volume so reduces the circulation that death is likely

unless the blood volume is restored therapeutically.

Early changes. Acute hypovolaemia results in a reduced central (systemic) venous pressure and so a diminished flow of blood into the right atrium. The stroke volume is thus low, and cardiac output and arterial blood pressure fall. These haemodynamic changes trigger off peripheral and central receptors with consequent sympathico-adrenal stimulation, and there is a huge increase in the levels of catecholamines in the plasma, sometimes by over 200 times. As a result of impaired renal perfusion, there is also intense secretion of renin and so greatly increased production of angiotensin II in the plasma (p. 222).

The combined effects of these massive amounts of vasoactive agents result in an increase in the tone of the systemic veins, so that in spite of their reduced content of blood, central venous pressure and right atrial filling are partially restored, the heart rate increases, and cardiac output tends to rise towards normal. The high levels of catecholamines and angiotensin also cause constriction of the arterioles and venules in the skin, splanchnic area, and indeed most of the tissues of the body, so that peripheral resistance is increased, and even without treatment the blood pressure may be partially or fully restored, although tissue perfusion is low. The heart and central nervous system do not suffer to the same extent as the other tissues: their small blood vessels do not contract in response to noradrenaline, etc., but have an inherent property of relaxing when the blood pressure falls and contracting when it rises. In consequence of this autoregulatory mechanism, cerebral and coronary blood flow are maintained close to normal levels at blood pressures down to 50 mm Hg. At this pressure, arteriolar relaxation is maximal and perfusion rapidly falls off at lower pressures.

This, then, is the haemodynamic status in early shock. Compensating changes have tended to keep up the cardiac output and blood pressure, and the brain and heart are preferentially supplied with blood at the expense of diminished perfusion of the other tissues. If less than 25% of the blood has been lost, and if there are no serious complicating factors (see below), the blood volume will rise naturally: vasoconstriction of the arterioles is greater than in the venules, so that the pressure in the capillaries is low and extravascular fluid passes into them (p. 38), and the high levels of angiotensin II stimulate adrenal secretion of aldosterone, which promotes retention of salt and water. The circulation is nevertheless precarious, and further bleeding, major surgery to deal with the causal injury or bleeding vessel, severe pain, or the development of infection, will all tend to increase the circulatory deficit. It is therefore important, in all save the mildest cases, to restore the blood volume by intravenous administration of fluid. The nature of the fluid is not so important as the avoidance of delay: buffered saline or macromolecular solutions (plasma, dextran, etc.) are both effective initially, but macromolecular solutions have the advantage of maintaining the osmotic pressure of the plasma, thus tending to hold fluid in circulation, and are required for losses of around 25% or more of the blood. It is also important to maintain the haematocrit at around 30% in order to minimise tissue hypoxia, and matched blood (or in an urgent situation Group O Rh negative blood) should be administered if haemorrhage has exceeded 25% of the blood volume. Some estimate of the volume of fluids required can be made from the amount of blood lost, the clinical state, and the severity and nature of injury, but account must also be taken of internal haemorrhage, e.g. into the gastro-intestinal tract or around a fracture. The haemoglobin and haematocrit levels are not reliable guides to the degree of hypovolaemia during the first 36 hours. In the absence of cardiac insufficiency, a low blood pressure is an indication of hypovolaemia in early shock, but because of the compensatory mechanisms described above, it may be normal or nearly so in patients with serious hypovolaemia. A low central venous pressure is a useful indication of hypovolaemia, and if possible this should be monitored in all except mild cases of shock.

Although the peripheral vasoconstriction of shock serves a compensatory function, it is also harmful by reducing general tissue perfusion and it may, by increasing peripheral resistance, induce heart failure (see below). In some cases, the blood pressure may rise above normal, and the vasoconstriction may persist in spite of restoration of the blood volume. Drugs which promote vasodilatation (e.g. isoprenaline, thymoxamine) are therefore sometimes beneficial, but only when steps have been taken to restore the blood volume: in the hypovolaemic patient they are liable to cause further circulatory collapse.

The changes of advanced shock. If shock persists, the widespread arteriolar constriction gradually passes off, but venular constriction is more persistent and capillary pressure rises with consequent loss of fluid into the extravascular space and further fall in blood volume. At this late stage of shock, the capillaries are congested with slowly-flowing blood, and *cyanosis* may be apparent. The general reduction in blood supply to the tissues is aggravated by a number of complex factors brought about by changes in the blood itself and by the injury to vascular endothelium and tissue cells resulting from perfusion failure. Some of the changes are as follows:

(a) *Viscosity of the blood* is increased by the haemoconcentration resulting from loss of capillary fluid: This leads to sludging and rouleaux formation (p. 37) and these effects are increased by the rise in plasma fibrinogen which follows haemorrhage.

(b) *Release of thromboplastin* (Factor III) from hypoxic endothelium and tissue cells results in the production of thrombin (p. 197), which promotes aggregation of platelets and occasionally intravascular formation of fibrin. Aggregated platelets release adenosine diphosphate which causes further platelet aggregation.

(c) *Neutrophil polymorphs* adhere to the injured vascular endothelium of small vessels.

(d) *Hypoxic injury* results in release of lysosomal enzymes and secretory products into the blood. Proteolytic enzymes, e.g. trypsin from the pancreas, may activate the kinin system and thus further embarrass the circulation by causing vasodilatation and increased permeability. Production of prostaglandins may also be increased: those of the E group have a kinin-like effect, while the F group may increase the resistance to pulmonary blood flow.

Metabolic disturbances. The hypoxia of shock interferes profoundly with cell metabolism. It prevents the entrance of pyruvic acid into the citric acid cycle and in consequence lactic acid accumulates and glucose passes out of the hypoxic cells, leading to insulin-resistant hyperglycaemia and increased glycogenolysis. These metabolic disturbances, together with high levels of catecholamines, result in rise of fatty acids and amino acids in the plasma. Impaired carbohydrate metabolism results in a fall in production of adenosine triphosphate and so energy is not available for many cell functions, including the sodium pump: potassium leaves the cells and sodium and water enter and cause swelling: these effects, sometimes termed the 'sick cell syndrome' (p. 8) may, by lowering the level of blood sodium, lead to inappropriate administration of salt.

Metabolic acidosis, with rise in blood lactic acid, contributes to the hyperventilation of shock.

Organ function in shock. While all the organs are affected in shock, respiratory and cardiac failure are commonly of fatal importance. Quite apart from cardiogenic shock (see below), **acute heart failure**, first of the left and then of both ventricles, may develop in severe hypovolaemic (and septic) shock, and is particularly common in older patients with pre-existing coronary artery disease. The increased load on the heart resulting from peripheral vasoconstriction and treatment with vasodilator drugs has been considered above. A factor which reduces myocardial contractility (*myocardial depressant factor*) has recently been detected in the plasma of shocked patients who subsequently died of cardiac failure: it is believed to be released from the pancreas. The impaired blood flow of severe shock, together with activation of the clotting mechanism, predispose to coronary thrombosis in patients with coronary artery disease. If operation is necessary, anaesthetic drugs may also impair cardiac function. Monitoring of the central venous and systemic arterial pressures, and particularly of changes in them during intravascular administration of fluid, helps to distinguish between hypovolaemia and cardiac insufficiency in shock. In some cases, drugs such as isoprenaline or digitalis, which increase myocardial contractility, are beneficial.

Failure of gas exchange in the **lungs** is another important complication of shock, and can be assessed by comparing the mixed venous and arterial oxygen tensions. Improvement usually follows restoration of the blood volume, together with intermittent positive-pressure ventilation if necessary, but in some cases pulmonary function continues to deteriorate due to a combination of causes—pulmonary oedema, alveolar collapse, intravascular fibrin formation, embolism, infection, etc., known collectively as **shock lung** (p. 400), and death is then likely to result largely from the additional burden of respiratory failure.

Perfusion of the **kidneys** in shock is directly proportional to the blood pressure. Production of urine ceases at about 50 mm Hg and if the pressure remains low for some hours, focal hypoxic injury to the tubular epithelium may be associated with acute renal failure which persists for days or weeks after recovery from shock (p. 787). Renal damage is particularly common in shock associated with crush injury, childbirth, incompatible blood transfusion or severe infection.

Because of its autoregulatory mechanism, blood flow to the **brain** is relatively well-maintained unless the blood pressure falls below 50 mm Hg. Even a brief period of more severe hypotension can cause severe ischaemic brain damage (p. 212). Ischaemic centrilobular necrosis of liver cells may also occur, although liver failure is seldom prominent.

Other causes of hypovolaemic shock

Burns. In burning or scalding, necrosis of the more superficial tissues is accompanied by a lesser degree of injury to the underlying tissues, the reaction to which is acute inflammation. The small vessels dilate and their permeability increases, so that there is exudation of protein-rich fluid. When the area involved is extensive (10% or more of the skin surface), the loss of fluid is severe enough to induce hypovolaemia and shock. The changes are similar to those following haemorrhage but hypovolaemia develops more slowly, haemoconcentration is more pronounced, with its attendant sludging and rouleaux formation, there is usually a marked leukocytosis, and the state of shock may recur or increase on the second or third days, possibly as a result of infection or absorption of breakdown products from the necrotic tissue. The principles of treatment of burn shock are the same as for haemorrhagic shock, but the loss is of plasma rather than whole blood, so that plasma transfusions are used initially. Some destruction of red cells does, however, occur in the burned area, and in very extensive burning severe anaemia may develop, necessitating blood transfusion. Another important complication of burning is bacterial infection, the dead tissue providing a good culture medium from which bacteria commonly invade the underlying tissue and bloodstream. Streptococci and staphylococci were formerly the most important invaders, but with antibiotic therapy Gram-ve bacilli, and especially *Pseudomonas aeruginosa*, now predominate. The features of septic shock commonly supervene, and sepsis is now the major cause of death from burns.

Dehydration, if severe, causes hypovolaemic shock, although the blood volume is relatively less reduced than the extravascular fluid, and the effects of cellular dehydration are regarded as the usual cause of death (p. 215).

Cardiogenic shock

Acute lesions of the heart may severely reduce cardiac output and the subsequent haemodynamic and other changes are similar to those in hypovolaemic shock. The central venous pressure is, however, raised, and although the clinical features—pallor, weak rapid pulse, sweating, etc.—are the same as in hypo-volaemia, transfusion of plasma, etc., is contra-indicated.

The commonest cause is myocardial infarction, and many patients with this condition develop some degree of shock, which is an important cause of death. Other conditions which can cause cardiogenic shock include rupture of a valve cusp, major arrhythmias, and cardiac tamponade due to haemopericardium (resulting from direct trauma or as a complication of a ruptured myocardial infarct). Although not strictly cardiogenic shock, acute obstruction to blood flow by pulmonary emboli can result in a similar condition. As already indicated, cardiac insufficiency can develop as a complication of haemorrhagic and other types of shock.

Septic shock

Some patients with septicaemia or extensive localised infections, such as general peritonitis, pass into a state of shock which resembles that of hypovolaemia, but is often more prolonged, with a higher incidence of serious complications, and an overall mortality of about 50%.

Septic shock is a common complication of infected burns, and of surgical operations or manipulations (intubation or instrumentation) on the urogenital, gastro-intestinal, biliary or respiratory tracts. It occurs also in patients with immunodeficiency states, such as leukaemia and lymphomas, and as a complication of cytotoxic drugs or immunosuppressive therapy. Many patients are dehydrated, and this is an important predisposing factor.

In a patient with known sepsis, high fever and symptoms and signs of shock, the diagnosis is not difficult, but in many patients, especially the elderly and following surgical procedures, septic shock develops insidiously, often without fever, and there may be an initial 'hyperdynamic' stage in which cardiac output is increased, the blood pressure reduced, peripheral resistance low, and the skin warm: these features may be due to bacteria-mediated release of kinins and other vaso-active agents. More often circulatory changes are similar from the onset to those of hypovolaemia, with pallor, sweating, cold extremities, increased peripheral resistance and reduced cardiac output, etc. Septic shock is particularly difficult to reverse and, as with other forms of shock, the longer it persists the more refractory it becomes. Tissue hypoxia results in widespread derangement of cell function, and features of multi-organ failure often develop. **Respiratory failure** due to 'shock lung' is often combined with **cardiac failure** and arrhythmias. **Acute renal failure** is also very common, although (as in hypovolaemic shock) many of its serious effects develop after recovery from shock.

Disseminated intravascular coagulation (p. 501) is more prone to develop in septic than in hypovolaemic shock. It interferes further with organ perfusion and may greatly aggravate pulmonary failure, or may, by consumption of clotting factors and activation of the plasmin system, progress to a bleeding state with widespread haemorrhage, e.g. from the gastro-intestinal mucosa.

Treatment of septic shock is based on elimination of the causal infection, restoration of the circulation, and correction of metabolic acidosis and electrolyte imbalance. Antibiotic therapy cannot usually await the results of bacteriological culture of the blood etc. and tests for sensitivity, although it may subsequently need to be modified according to the bacteriological findings. The choice and rate of administration of intravascular fluids will depend on the results of monitoring procedures and haematological and biochemical tests. These include monitoring the central venous and systemic arterial pressures, and frequent assay of the blood gases and pH, plasma electrolytes and osmolality, platelet counts and haematocrit. It may also be necessary to assay the status of the coagulation and plasmin systems. Intermittent positive-pressure ventilation, instituted at an early stage, has been shown to decrease the risk of the development of pulmonary failure, and drugs which increase cardiac output and tissue perfusion may be of value. The prognosis depends very much on the availability of experienced staff and facilities.

Aetiology. The microbial factors responsible for septic shock are by no means fully elucidated. With widespread use of antibiotics, the aerobic Gram-ve bacilli have replaced the pyogenic cocci as the major cause of septicaemia and bacteraemia. The organisms most commonly responsible include *Esch. coli*, *Proteus*, *Klebsiella* and in cases of burns *Pseudomonas aeruginosa*. About 50% of patients with blood infection by these bacteria develop septic shock. Bacteroides (the anaerobic non-sporing bacilli which constitute over 99% of the faecal flora) have been recognised quite recently as an important cause of blood infection, and about 30% of cases are complicated by shock. All these Gram-ve bacteria release endotoxins when they die, and there is a widespread belief that endotoxin is a major causal agent of septic shock. Animals injected with endotoxin present many of the features of septic shock, including disseminated intravascular coagulation (the so-called *Schwartzman reaction*), and endotoxin has been detected in the blood of shocked patients with Gram-ve septicaemia by means of the limulus test (in which endotoxin is detected by its property of clotting a lysate of the blood amoebocytes of *Limulus polyphemus*, the horseshoe crab). The limulus test is, however, negative in some cases of undoubted Gram-ve septic shock, and moreover 10% of patients with blood infections with *Staph. aureus* (which does not contain endotoxin) develop septic shock.

Endotoxin may induce the features of septic shock by a combination of its known effects, including activation of complement by the alternate pathway (p. 116), by promoting intravascular clotting, by its cytotoxic effects on neutrophil polymorphs, or possibly by promoting the production of kinins, prostaglandins, etc.

Severe shock sometimes develops in patients with fungal or acute virus infections, and in some instances immune-complex formation may be involved.

Other causes of shock

Some cases of shock do not fall into any of the three major types described above. For example, escape of gastric or duodenal juice into the peritoneal cavity, via a perforated peptic ulcer, causes severe shock, and so does acute haemorrhagic pancreatitis (which is non-bacterial) and, the drinking of many poisons. In these conditions, it is likely that shock is chemically-induced, but there may also be severe pain which, without doubt, aggravates shock.

Severe shock results from transfusion of strongly incompatible blood to which the recipient has iso-antibodies; also in acute circulating immune complex disease (p. 126) and acute generalised anaphylaxis (p. 118).

Pathological changes in shock

The pathological changes in patients dying from shock are often inconspicuous. In spite of the fundamental disturbances of cell function, the parenchymal cells in general usually show only swelling and sometimes fatty change. In addition to the causal changes—injury, haemorrhage, coronary thrombosis, septicaemia, etc., there may be various pulmonary changes, including oedema, congestion, hyaline membrane formation, collapse and bronchopneumonia (p. 401). The kidneys usually show the pallor and cortical swelling of acute tubular injury (p. 786) and there may be centrilobular hepatic necrosis. If the patient has survived sufficiently long for its recognition, there may be acute ischaemic necrosis in the 'boundary' zones of the brain (p. 679). Features of disseminated intravascular coagulation include widespread haemorrhages, and microscopy may reveal fibrin thrombi in the small vessels, especially in the lungs and kidneys. The adrenals show the lipid depletion of the 'stress' reaction (p. 971), but occasionally there is a combination of haemorrhage and necrosis, particularly in septic shock associated with meningococcal septicaemia.

Metabolism after injury

The metabolic disturbances associated with shock (p. 225) include incomplete carbohydrate catabolism, metabolic acidosis, disturbed protein and fat metabolism and a rise in the blood levels of glucose, amino acids and fatty acids. These changes were demonstrated experimentally by Cuthbertson, who termed them the 'ebb phase'. Energy production is consequently depressed, and there is a general disorder of cellular metabolic processes. These changes are liable to develop in the first days following a severe injury, burn or surgical operation. Following the period of shock (or 2–3 days after such injury when shock has been prevented), the metabolism changes to a 'flow phase' in which there is increased energy (and heat) production, due largely to breakdown of depot fat and protein, with consequent loss of weight and a negative nitrogen balance. During this period, which may persist for days or months depending on the severity of the injury, carbohydrate catabolism is complete and there is no metabolic acidosis unless carbohydrate intake is low. The mechanism of the increased metabolic activity, which resembles that in fever, is uncertain, but weight loss can be minimised by a high caloric, high protein diet, and a warm environment.

Blood Groups and Blood Transfusion

Before administering a blood transfusion, it is essential to make sure that the donor's red cells are compatible to the patient, and in particular that the patient's plasma does not contain iso-antibodies reactive with surface antigens on the donor's red cells. The ABO blood group system is of outstanding importance, for iso-antibodies are normally present in the plasma (see Table 8.2) and their reaction with incompatible transfused red cells usually causes a severe haemolytic reaction with fever, shock, often acute renal failure and sometimes death. The rhesus (Rh) blood group system comes next in importance. Unlike the ABO system, Rh iso-antibodies are not usually present in the plasma, but they sometimes develop as a result of an Rh-incompatible blood transfusion or pregnancy.

For blood transfusion, the patient's ABO and Rh types should be determined and blood of the same type should be selected for transfusion. In addition, it is necessary to perform a *compatibility* or *cross-matching* test in which the donor's red cells are incubated in the recipient's serum at 37 °C, and the cells are then examined for agglutination and also by the antiglobulin test (p. 91) to detect non-agglutinating (IgG) antibodies in the recipient's serum. The purpose of this procedure is to detect (1) technical or clerical errors in grouping and in collection and storage of the donor's blood, and (2) the presence of unusual iso-antibodies in the recipient's plasma. Finally, it is good practice for the person administering the transfusion to carry out a simple cross-matching test in which the donor's red cells are mixed with the patient's serum on a microscope slide and examined for agglutination after a few minutes at room temperature. This will detect only major ABO incompatibilities, such as may arise when two patients, or blood from two donors (e.g. with the same surname), are confused.

As a life-saving measure, it may be appropriate to transfuse Group O, Rh−ve blood to a patient of unknown group, but it is usually preferable to administer plasma while grouping procedures are being performed, and in any case the direct matching slide procedure should always be performed.

Incompatibility can also arise when a donor's blood contains high titre antibodies reactive with the patient's red cells. Transfusion reactions from this cause are not usually severe because the donor's plasma (and thus the antibody) is diluted *in vivo* by the recipient's plasma. Screening tests for high titre ABO antibodies are now performed by most transfusion centres, and if donor and recipient are of the same ABO and Rh type the danger is largely excluded.

The ABO groups

Individuals can be classified into four groups by the presence or absence of A and B antigens on their red cells and of anti-A and anti-B antibodies in their plasma (or serum). Table 8.2 shows the features of the four groups.

The Rhesus (Rh) groups

The Rh blood group system was discovered by Landsteiner and Wiener (1940), who were interested in the antigens of human and animal red cells, and noted that guinea-pig or rabbit antisera to the red cells of *Macacus rhesus*

Table 8.2   The four ABO blood groups

Blood group	Red cell antigens	Iso-antibodies in serum	Can accept blood of group	Can donate to patients of group	Incidence in Britain * (%)
AB	AB	nil	all groups	AB	3
A	A	anti-B	A, O	A, AB	42
B	B	anti-A	B, O	B, AB	8
O	O	anti-A + anti-B	O	all groups	47

* The frequencies of the four groups vary greatly between different peoples.

If sera of groups A and B are available one can determine the group to which any individual belongs. If the red cells are agglutinated by both sera the blood belongs to group AB, if agglutinated by group B serum alone the blood belongs to group A, if by group A serum alone to group B, and if by neither serum, it belongs to group O. Since the serum of group AB does not agglutinate the red cells of any of the groups an individual of group AB can receive the red cells of any other group and is thus a 'universal recipient'. The cells of an individual of group O are not agglutinated by the serum of any group; the red cells can be transfused into an individual of any group and such persons are known as 'universal donors'.

The three blood group substances A, B and O are determined by allelic genes, one from each parent, so that there are six genotypes (AA, BB, AB, AO, BO and OO). O substance, however, is for practical purposes non-antigenic, and accordingly grouping is based on the presence or absence of A and B, giving the four phenotypes, which were first detected by Landsteiner. The iso-antibodies are mainly of IgM class, and develop after birth, apparently as a result of exposure to bacterial and other substances antigenically similar to A and B. Group A (or B) individuals are immunologically tolerant to A (or B) and so do not develop the corresponding antibodies.

monkeys agglutinated the red cells of 84% of white Americans; accordingly, these 84% were called Rh-positive, and the 16% of non-reactors, Rh-negative. The human Rh system is, however, more complex, and further elucidation has come from the use of iso-antibodies which, unlike the ABO antibodies, are not routinely present in human serum, but develop in about 50% of Rh−ve subjects transfused with Rh+ve blood, and in about 5% of Rh−ve women as a result of an Rh+pregnancy (p. 122). Once Rh antibodies have developed, a subsequent Rh+ve blood transfusion is likely to cause an acute reaction with immune destruction of the transfused red cells by a cytotoxic antibody (type II) reaction, while an Rh+ve fetus is liable to suffer from haemolytic disease of the newborn (p. 473).

Rhesus iso-antibodies may be of either IgM or IgG class: their demonstration requires incubation with appropriate red cells at 37 °C, and since IgG antibodies sensitise the red cells without agglutinating them, their detection is usually effected by use of the antiglobulin reaction.

Rh sub-groups. In simple terms, Rh blood group antigens are determined by three pairs of allelic genes, one of which codes for antigens C or c, one for D or d and the third for E and e. As the genes are closely linked, they are transmitted as haplotypic 'sets' which may be expressed as CDe, cde, etc., or by a set of symbols (R_1, r, etc.). The frequency of the eight possible haplotypes varies considerably in different peoples: their frequency in this country, together with the alternative symbols, are shown in table 8.3.

Table 8.3 The major Rh haplotypes and their frequency in Britain.

Haplotype	Abbreviation	Frequency*†
CDe	R_1	0·420
cde	r	0·389
cDE	R_2	0·141
cDe	R_0	0·026
cdE	r″	0·012
Cde	r′	0·010
CDE	R_z	very rare
CdE	r_y	very rare

* The frequency varies greatly in different peoples.

† The frequency of any given *genotype* is obtained by multiplying together the frequencies of the two haplotypes as given here: thus CDe/cde occurs in $0.420 \times 0.389 =$ approx. 16% of the population of Britain, and cde/cde in $0.389^2 = 15\%$. Reversing the calculation gives an estimate of gene frequency for known genotype frequencies.

Each individual inherits one of these sets from each parent, and his red cells may thus have from 3 to 6 different Rh antigens. In practice, iso-immunisation develops mainly when an individual of genotype cde/cde receives red cells which are D-positive. Accordingly, individuals whose red cells possess D are termed *Rh-positive* and those without D (i.e. with dd) are termed *Rh-negative*. In Caucasian stock, about 15% of individuals are cde/cde (hence the frequency of cde as calculated in the table is $\sqrt{\frac{15}{100}} = 0.389$). Rh−ve individuals with other genotypes are comparatively rare.

There is also a significant risk of the development of anti-C when C+ cells are transfused to an Rh−ve individual, and it is common practice to use a mixture of anti-C and anti-D for Rh grouping. Iso-immunisation may also result when c+ or e+ blood is transfused to CC or EE individuals respectively, but d+ blood does not iso-immunise DD individuals.

The Rh system is, in fact, much more complex than has been suggested above: a fourth antigen, G, is closely associated with C and D, and further antigens, determined by variants of the common allelic genes or joint products of the genes, also occur.

Other blood group systems

In addition to the ABO and Rh groups many other blood group systems are known, but like the Rh group natural iso-antibodies are absent, and the sera that detect these groups are obtained mostly from persons immunised by transfusion or by pregnancy. These groups only rarely bring about iso-immunisation. Nevertheless the greatly increased use of blood transfusion necessitates their consideration and identification when a cross-matching test reveals an unexpected antibody.

9

Miscellaneous Tissue Degenerations and Deposits

The degenerative changes which result from cellular injury, and the intracellular accumulation of lipids and glycogen resulting from certain disorders of metabolism, have been dealt with in Chapter 1. In the present chapter we describe a group of changes which, although heterogeneous, consist of either the accumulation in the tissues of various substances—amyloid material, mucus, pigmented compounds, calcium deposits and urates—or tissue degenerations which usually affect the stroma of supporting tissues, and are recognised by their microscopic appearances but are ill-defined chemically.

Amyloidosis

Amyloid is a predominantly extracellular fibrillar material composed essentially of protein: it is deposited in various tissues in a number of diseases. Extensive deposits are visible by naked eye, causing enlargement of the involved tissue and giving it a waxy appearance (Fig. 9.1). In sections stained by haematoxylin and eosin amyloid is seen as a homogeneous, pink, refractile material. Electron microscopy shows it to

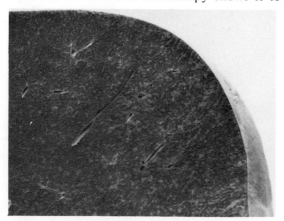

Fig. 9.1 Amyloidosis of liver. The amyloid material renders the organ firm, and gives it a dark, homogeneous appearance. × 1.

consist of filaments of 7·5 nm diameter (Fig. 9.2), which can be dissociated into several protofibrils and are often twisted together in pairs.

Methods of demonstrating amyloid

The wide variety of methods currently used to demonstrate the presence of amyloid is an indication of their lack of specificity. Large deposits of amyloid are usually demonstrable by all the methods. If the amount of amyloid present is small, however, the results with each method vary from case to case and identification is correspondingly difficult; for this reason it is usual to use several methods, the best known of which are as follows.

(1) **Lugol's iodine.** Amyloid has a strong affinity for iodine (hence its name) and this forms the basis for a useful macroscopic test. When Lugol's iodine solution is poured over tissue, the amyloid is stained deep brown in contrast to the normal tissue which is only lightly stained. Congested tissues should first be rinsed free of excess blood as this obscures the test.

(2) **Congo red.** This stain may be used on gross specimens and sections for microscopy. Formerly the rate of disappearance from the serum of an intravenously injected solution of congo red was used as a clinical test for amyloidosis but owing to lack of accuracy it was abandoned. In polarised light amyloid stained by congo red shows a green birefringence.

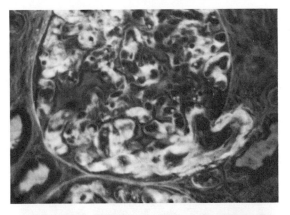

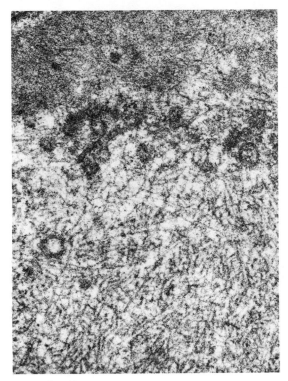

Fig. 9.2 Electron micrograph of kidney showing amyloid deposition. The dense area above is glomerular capillary basement membrane; below, amyloid material is seen as a network of filaments. × 50 000.

(3) Rosaniline dyes. These include gentian violet, methyl violet and crystal violet; they stain amyloid reddish while other tissue elements appear purple. This phenomenon of a dye reacting with a tissue constituent and undergoing a colour change is called *metachromasia*: it is believed that in this instance it is due to selective binding of impurities in the dyes by amyloid fibrils.

(4) Fluorescent dyes. Thioflavine-T binds to amyloid and its presence is demonstrated by fluorescence microscopy (Fig. 9.3).

Classification

Amyloidosis is classified into *primary* and *secondary* types. The primary type occurs apart from any known predisposing cause. The secondary type occurs as a complication of certain diseases. Formerly, chronic infections, and especially chronic pyogenic osteitis, tuberculosis, syphilis and bronchiectasis accounted for most cases. One of the commonest causes today is rheumatoid arthritis in which careful examination of post-mortem tissues reveals

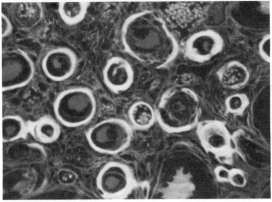

Fig. 9.3 Amyloidosis of kidney, stained by thioflavine-T and photographed by ultraviolet light. Note the bright fluorescence of amyloid in the glomerular capillary and afferent arteriolar walls (*above*) and in the tubular basement membranes (*below*). × 200.

amyloid in approximately 20% of cases. It occurs also in 15% of subjects with multiple myeloma and less commonly in Hodgkin's disease and other malignant tumours. Amyloidosis is also a feature of various hereditary syndromes (see below).

Distribution and effects of amyloid

Organs severely affected by amyloid are enlarged, firm, and of increased specific gravity. The cut surface has a waxy, refractile appearance. In primary amyloidosis the tissues are severely affected in the following order of frequency: heart, alimentary tract, tongue, skin, skeletal muscles, spleen, kidneys, liver and lungs. In secondary amyloidosis the liver, kidney, spleen and gut are most severely affected. In both types, amyloid is deposited in and around the walls of small blood vessels and in relation to epithelial basement membranes. Biopsy of the gum mucosa, or better the rectum, is helpful in diagnosis, but is by no means always positive.

Amyloid produces effects by pressure on adjacent cells and by interfering with the normal transfer of water and solutes across the walls of affected small blood vessels.

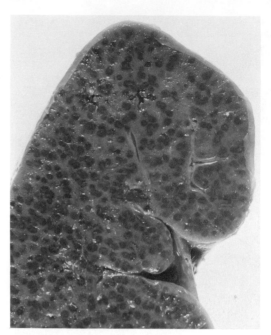

Fig. 9.5 Amyloid spleen of 'sago' type, i.e. affecting the Malpighian bodies.

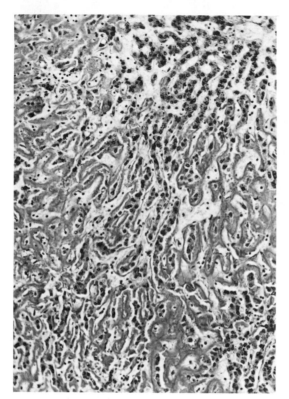

Fig. 9.4 Amyloidosis of the liver. The pale homogeneous amyloid substance occupies the midzone of the lobules. It extends along the walls of the sinusoids, enclosing the liver cells, which are undergoing atrophy. The zone around the central vein (*top right*) is least affected. × 115.

The **liver** is firm and elastic and may be palpable during life. The change usually begins in the sinusoids of the intermediate zones of the lobules: it may become very extensive and produce marked atrophy of the liver cells (Fig. 9.4). Even at an advanced stage, liver function is not usually severely impaired.

The **spleen** shows two distinct patterns of involvement. In one the Malpighian bodies are changed to translucent globules by amyloid

deposition in their reticulum (Fig. 9.5); hence the term 'sago spleen'. In this form splenomegaly is not marked. In the diffuse form, the change affects reticulum of the red pulp, walls of venous sinuses, and many of the small arteries; the spleen may be palpable and weigh up to 1 kg; this variety is rare apart from tertiary syphilis.

Amyloidosis of the **kidneys** is particularly important because of its effect on renal function. Deposition occurs upon the basement membranes of the tubules and in the walls of arterioles and venules (Fig. 9.3), but the most important site is in relation to the glomerular capillary basement membrane (Fig. 21.44, p. 781), which becomes permeable to albumin, etc., with consequent heavy proteinuria and nephrotic syndrome (p. 219).

Eventually many of the glomerular capillaries are obliterated, the kidneys become scarred and shrunken and chronic renal failure develops.

In the **stomach** and **intestines**, amyloid deposits may be widespread and this leads to atrophic changes in the mucosa. Diarrhoea may result from severe involvement of the gut, but even in its absence amyloid material is often demonstrable in rectal biopsy material, providing a useful diagnostic measure. Gingival biopsy is also useful, although less often diagnostic than rectal biopsy.

Deposits of amyloid may also be found in the adrenals, thyroid, lymph nodes and myocardium, especially of the right atrium. The central nervous system is not affected in diffuse amyloidosis, but see p. 710.

Primary amyloidosis tends to occur especially in old age, and involvement of the **myocardium** may lead to heart failure, the cause of which is often obscure during life and is easily missed at necropsy. Careful histological examination reveals minor degrees of unsuspected amyloidosis in a small percentage of old people dying from various causes.

Localised amyloidosis, restricted to one organ or tissue, is relatively common in the larynx where it gives rise to small tumour-like nodules, and is a rare cause of enlargement of the thyroid or other organs. It occurs also in the pancreatic islets in many diabetics, and as a feature of certain tumours, e.g. medullary thyroid cancer.

Genetically-determined amyloidosis. Several familial forms of amyloidosis have been described. The best known are familial mediterranean fever and primary familial amyloidosis.

Familial mediterranean fever is found principally in Mediterranean Jews and Armenians and is inherited as an autosomal recessive factor. In its most typical form, recurrent fever is associated with pain in chest, abdomen, joints and skin; amyloidosis supervenes causing death by renal involvement, but affecting also the spleen, lungs and liver. Variants of the disease are recognised in which the amyloidosis becomes apparent before the other features.

Primary familial amyloidosis. This is least rare in parts of Portugal and is inherited as an autosomal dominant. The disease presents in the 3rd and 4th decades with increasing leg weakness and loss of reflexes. Subsequently sphincteric disturbances and malabsorption from intestinal involvement lead to death within 10 years.

The nature of amyloid

The essential constituent of amyloid is a fibrous protein which forms the amyloid fibrils. In cases which are primary, or secondary to multiple myeloma, this major protein has amino-acid sequences indicating that it consists of the N-terminal parts, and possibly the whole, of immunoglobulin light chains: it is homogeneous in an affected individual, but differs in amino-acid sequences in different cases, and although of low antigenicity has been shown to be of either κ or λ type (p. 88), suggesting production by a plasma cell clone. In hereditary amyloid disease and rheumatoid arthritis, and curiously in amyloidosis secondary to chronic infections in which there is prolonged antigenic stimulation, the major amyloid protein is not recognisable as part of the immunoglobulin molecule: it has been termed 'Protein A' and differs between cases. Protein A is of unknown origin.

Amyloid also contains about 5% of a second ('P') protein, which forms rod-like structures, but is removed from tissues during fixation and processing for electron microscopy: it is apparently present in normal serum. Mucopolysaccharides, including heparitin sulphate and chondroitin sulphate, make up less than 1 per cent, but are readily dissociated from the protein. The properties of amyloid depend on the major protein, which has been shown by x-ray crystallography to have a regular pattern of pleated folding of its peptide chains: this β configuration is biologically unusual.

Amyloid is readily induced in animals by prolonged antigenic stimulation or oral administration of casein, and its deposition is enhanced by thymectomy and by immunosuppressive agents. At present, it seems likely that proteins which assume a β-configuration have the morphological, tinctorial and biological properties of amyloid, including its inertness, muted antigenicity and resistance to proteolytic digestion. Amyloid fibrillar material can be dissociated into components of relatively low molecular weight (5 000–31 000 daltons), and it has been suggested that these result from incomplete digestion, probably by macrophages, of various larger proteins, including immunoglobulins.

There is some evidence that amyloid may be resorbed following effective treatment of the causal disease, but renal amyloid is persistent and steroid therapy has not, in general, proved beneficial.

Hyaline and fibrinoid changes

The term *hyaline* is used to describe material of homogeneous, refractile, eosinophilic appearance seen on light microscopy of stained tissue sections. It is purely descriptive, and many different formed tissue elements, as well as cell cytoplasm, may assume a hyaline appearance. In most instances the chemical basis of hyaline change is not known, although fibrin and amyloid both have a hyaline appearance. The collagen and background material of old dense fibrous tissue and the walls of aged blood vessels are often hyaline and because of its association with age this is often called *hyaline degeneration*. In the kidney and other organs, the walls of arterioles usually become thickened and hyaline in arterial hypertension (Fig. 21.6, p. 750), and glomeruli injured by chronic ischaemia became converted to hyaline balls (Fig. 21.7, p. 750). These changes occur also in diabetic nephropathy, and are believed to be due to accumulation of substances leaking out from the blood (*plasmatic vasculosis*). There are many conditions in which abnormal amounts of plasma proteins leak into the glomerular filtrate; part of the protein is resorbed by the tubular epithelium where it is seen as eosinophil refractile droplets (Fig. 21.23, p. 764) commonly termed *hyaline droplets*. Protein may also coagulate in the tubular lumen and is then secreted in the urine as cylindrical '*hyaline casts*'. In virus hepatitis, damaged liver cells may appear hyaline (Fig. 19.13, p. 612) and '*Mallory's hyaline*' appears in the hepatocyte cytoplasm in alcoholic and certain other forms of liver cell injury. In Cushing's syndrome, hyaline material is seen in the basophil cells of the pituitary (*Crooke's hyaline change*—Fig. 24.4, p. 946). Necrotic tissue, e.g. myocardium (Fig. 1.4) may also appear hyaline, and also fused platelets in thrombi.

These examples serve to show that hyaline material and its pathological associations are widely heterogeneous. It is nevertheless sometimes of diagnostic value, as will be seen from the many examples which crop up in the systematic chapters.

A second term, *fibrinoid change*, has long been used to describe impregnation of tissues with hyaline material which is brightly eosinophilic and has other staining properties similar to those of fibrin. The term became popular in the 1940s when fibrinoid change (incorrectly regarded as diagnostic of hypersensitivity reactions) was noted to be a common feature of the so-called collagen or connective-tissue diseases. More recently, immunofluorescence staining, and to a lesser extent electron microscopy, have provided more specific techniques for identifying fibrin in tissue sections, and have shown fibrin to be present in some, but not all, 'fibrinoid' lesions: in some instances the eosinophilic hyaline is due to ground-substance mucopolysaccharides; in others its nature remains unknown.

Deposition of fibrin in the tissues results from vascular exudation of fibrinogen, which is converted to fibrin by the action of tissue thromboplastin. If the injury causing the exudation is severe, there may also be death of tissue cells, and the changes are then traditionally known as *fibrinoid necrosis*. Examples of this are seen in many acute inflammatory lesions (Figs. 2.3, 2.4, p. 38) including the Arthus reaction, in some infarcts (in which plasma exudes from the ischaemic blood vessels), in the arteriolar lesions of accelerated hypertension (Fig. 13.18, p. 322) and in the necrotic base of peptic ulcers. Fibrin is detectable in some fibrinoid lesions of the connective-tissue diseases, e.g. in some examples of the subcutaneous nodules of rheumatoid arthritis (Fig. 22.55a, p. 857).

Deposited fibrin is usually removed by the action of plasmin or by phagocytic cells. It has, however, been demonstrated in slowly developing, permanent hyaline changes in the walls of arterioles and glomeruli (see plasmatic vasculosis, above) and this supports the view of Lendrum (1969) and others that such hyaline change results from an exudative process (see also p. 750).

Corpora amylacea. Under this term are included a number of rounded or oval hyaline structures, which may stain deeply with iodine, hence the name. They sometimes show concentric lamination and may undergo calcification. Such structures form in various situations and they cannot be regarded as all of the same nature. They are often a prominent feature within the acini of the prostate in the elderly; they occur also in the lungs, in old blood clots, and sometimes in tumours.

In the nervous system they are very common; e.g. in old age, in chronic degenerative lesions, and in the region of old infarcts and haemorrhages. They vary greatly in size, the smallest being spherical and homogeneous, and these usually stain deeply with haematoxylin. They appear to form simply by a deposition of organic material containing acid mucopolysaccharides in globular form in the intercellular spaces, but their exact composition is not known. They are of no importance except as a manifestation of the degenerative condition with which they are associated.

Mucins and myxomatous change

Mucins consist of complexes of proteins with carbohydrates and mucopolysaccharides. They are characterised by their slimy nature and histologically by their affinity for basic dyes and metachromasia with thiazine dyes such as toluidine blue. Most mucins are precipitated by acetic acid.

Mucins are secreted by various glandular epithelia and also by fibroblasts, osteoblasts and chondroblasts as important constituents of the ground substance of the various connective tissues. Both epithelial and connective tissue mucins are mixtures of *glycoproteins*, which are rich in hexose polymers and are stained pink in the PAS method, and *mucoproteins* in which the mucopolysaccharide is rich in hexosamines and which stain metachromatically with toluidine blue at low pH.

Disturbances of epithelial mucin secretion are not of much pathological importance except in *fibrocystic disease of the pancreas* in which an abnormality of mucus secretion occurs in the glands of the intestine, pancreas, bile ducts, bronchi and sweat glands. The thick mucin secreted obstructs gland ducts, with subsequent atrophy and loss of function. The condition is described more fully on p. 657.

Obstruction of the ducts of small mucus-secreting glands, e.g. in the mouth, results in the development of mucous cysts. Chronic irritation of a mucous membrane may result in increase in the number and activity of mucin-secreting cells, as in chronic bronchitis in which there is abundant mucous sputum. Some epithelial tumours secrete mucin, and its detection in relation to tumour cells is sometimes of help in determining the origin of the tumour.

The mucopolysaccharides of **connective tissue mucins** include hyaluronic acid, chondroitin, chondroitin sulphates and other sulphated compounds. They form the ground substances of fibrous tissue, cartilage and bone, and also joint fluid. In the soft tissues, the ground substance is largely in the form of a gel, but in acute inflammatory lesions the mucopolysaccharides are depolymerised, with conversion mainly to a fluid phase, which is more readily permeable to exudate and cells of the inflammatory reaction. Some bacteria also secrete hyaluronidase and other enzymes which may facilitate their spread in the tissues.

Some connective tissue tumours secrete abundant mucin, which appears as a basophilic stroma; they are called *myxomas* (Fig. 12.6, p. 292) and an increase in mucoid ground substance of connective tissue, so that it comes to resemble myxoid tissue of the fetus and umbilical cord, is termed **myxomatous** or **myxoid change**. It occurs in the aortic media in *Erdheim's medial degeneration* (Fig. 13.35, p. 335), and also, together with similar changes in other connective tissues, in *Marfan's syndrome*: in both conditions the inner part of the weakened aortic wall may rupture and blood may track along the media (dissecting aneurysm). Myxomatous change is also seen in the valve cusps of the heart and sometimes results in stretching and incompetence of the valves.

Production of ground substance is influenced by hormones; there is a generalised increase, for example, in *hypothyroidism* giving rise to the term **myxoedema**: the bloated appearance of the face is due to myxomatous change in the dermis, and the croaky voice is due to the same change in the larynx. Curiously, myxomatous change is seen in the pre-tibial region in some cases of thyrotoxicosis (hyperthyroidism).

There are also a number of defects of mucopolysaccharide metabolism—the **mucopolysaccharidoses**—which are inherited as Mendelian recessive characters. Excess mucopolysaccharides accumulate in various types of cell, and are excreted in the urine. The conditions are distinguished by the chemical nature and distribution of the material. The best known example is *Hurler's syndrome* or *gargoylism*, the major features of which include dwarfism, skeletal deformities, a characteristic facies, mental deficiency, corneal opacities and hepatomegaly.

Endogenous pigmentary changes

Pigments are deposited in the tissues in many abnormal states, and may produce changes visible by naked eye or only on microscopy. The two main types of endogenous pigments are melanin and derivatives of haemoglobin.

(1) Melanin pigmentation

The melanins are iron-free sulphur-containing pigments varying in colour from pale yellow to deep brown. They are formed intracellularly from colourless precursors—melanogens—and are very stable substances, resistant to acids and many other reagents, but soluble in strong alkalis; they can be bleached by powerful oxidising agents such as potassium permanganate or hydrogen peroxide. They are related to the aromatic compounds, tyrosine, phenylalanine and tryptophane and may be formed from such substances by oxidation. On treating sections of skin with dihydroxyphenylalanine (dopa), 'dopa-positive' cells in the epidermis oxidise this substance by means of an enzyme like tyrosinase and become blackened in consequence. The only cells in the skin which are 'dopa-positive' *in vivo* are the *dendritic cells*, or *melanocytes*, which lie extended between the basal cells of the epidermis (Fig. 9.6); they are the only melanin-producing cells in the skin and fine granules of melanin in their dendrites are taken up by pinocytosis of the tips of the dendrites, into adjacent epidermal cells and also into certain phagocytic cells (*melanophores*) in the dermis which may thus become heavily laden with coarse pigment granules. Melanin granules possess the capacity to reduce certain silver salts, e.g. ammoniacal silver nitrate, with consequent deposition of metallic silver; melanin can thus be intensified in histological preparations, scanty or light-coloured granules being rendered conspicuous. This property is widely used histochemically. According to Masson, the dendritic cells are of neuro-ectodermal origin, being derived from the cells of the embryonic neural crest, as are also the melanocytes of the squamous mucous membranes, the meninges, choroid and adrenals. This view harmonises well with the evidence about the origin of the naevus cells of pigmented moles from neuro-ectodermal cells and also accords with the ex-

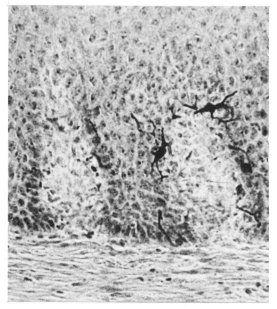

Fig. 9.6 Dendritic cells (melanocytes) in the basal part of the epidermis. (Dopa reaction.) × 220.

perimental work of Billingham and Medawar on the behaviour of melanocytes in skin autotransplants. This work seems to have rendered untenable the alternative view that melanocytes are modified basal epidermal cells. The Langerhans cells of the epidermis are now regarded as macrophages and may play a part in the control of keratinisation. Darkening of the skin on exposure to ultraviolet radiation is brought about first by migration of the melanin granules and subsequent darkening of their colour; later there is increased formation of pigment, apparently by the activity of the dendritic cells, which under further stimulation may increase in number.

In *Addison's disease*, which results from destruction of the adrenal cortex (p. 977), there occurs a general increase in melanin pigmentation of the skin, especially in areas exposed to light and in areas normally pigmented. There may also be pigmentary deposition on the inner surface of the cheeks on a line corresponding to the junction of the teeth, and on the sides of the tongue, the position being apparently determined by irritation. In the skin the pigment is in the form of very fine brownish granules in the deeper layers of the rete Malpighii, and is present also as coarser granules, chiefly within macrophages in the underlying cutis, the appearance and distribution resembling those in the negro skin. The pigmentation in Addison's disease represents an increase of normal pigment, and occurs under the influence of the melanocyte-stimulating hormone of the pituitary (MSH) which is released in excess in the absence of adrenal inhibition (p. 944).

Chloasma is a condition observed principally during pregnancy, and occasionally in association with ovarian disease, in which pigmented patches occur in the skin of the face, and the pigmented parts, e.g. the nipples, may become darker under the influence of oestrogenic and melanocyte-stimulating hormones. A similar condition has been described in women taking oral contraceptives.

Leukoderma (*vitiligo*) denotes patchy depigmentation of skin and this may be accompanied by increase of pigment in the intervening areas. In the affected areas the dendritic cells are of abnormal structure and have lost their capacity to oxidise dopa to form pigment.

Irregular pigmentation of the skin is common in chronic arsenical poisoning and in neurofibromatosis. In haemochromatosis also, the colour of the skin is due partly to deposition of haemosiderin in the cutis, notably around the sweat glands (p. 242), but also to increase in melanin. A striking degree of melanotic pigmentation of the oral and labial mucosa occurs in association with familial multiple polyposis of the small intestine, especially the jejunum (Peutz-Jeghers syndrome): the disorder is transmitted as a Mendelian dominant. The control of pigment metabolism in the skin is obscure, but it is known to be affected by exposure to light, chronic irritation and increased vascularity, activity of endocrine glands including the adrenals, pituitary and ovaries, and nervous influences. Melanin pigment is formed in large amount in the melanotic tumours which arise from pigmented moles and warts of the skin or from the pigmented coats of the eye, and most analyses have been carried out on the pigment from such tumours. The urine of patients suffering from extensive melanotic tumours occasionally contains a melanogen which darkens on exposure to the oxygen of the air.

Melanosis coli. This is a rather uncommon condition characterised by varying degrees of brownish to black pigmentation of the mucosa of the colon, beginning in the caecum and ascending colon, and sometimes extending to the anus. The pigment is contained mainly in macrophages in the lamina propria; it is absent from the epithelial cells. The condition is commonest when there has been intestinal stasis or chronic obstruction, and it is now recognised to be the result of absorption of aromatic products from the gut. This is commonly associated with the prolonged use of anthracene-derived purgatives, e.g. cascara, and the pigment consists of derivatives of anthraquinone combined with products of protein decomposition. The pigment resembles melanin in its reactions, but differs from it in being autofluorescent, weakly PAS-positive, and weakly sudanophilic. The cells containing pigment are dopa-negative.

Ochronosis. In this very rare condition, cartilages, capsules of joints and other soft tissues assume a dark brown or almost black colour, owing to pigment deposition. The pigment resembles melanin in some of its properties but does not reduce silver nitrate. In virtually all cases of ochronosis, alkaptonuria is present, a condition in which homogentisic acid (2,5-hydroxyphenylacetic acid) is excreted by the kidneys and causes the urine to blacken on standing owing to oxidation, especially in an alkaline medium. Homogentisic acid is formed from tyrosine and phenylalanine. Normally it is converted to malylacetoacetic acid by homogentisic acid oxidase in the liver and kidneys, but alcaptonurics lack this enzyme, and consequently homogentisic acid is not metabolised normally, but is oxidised into pigment and deposited in the tissues, producing ochronosis. The metabolic defect in alkaptonuria is inherited as an autosomal recessive character. In the early days of antiseptic surgery ochronosis occasionally followed the use of carbolic dressings for a long time, and the pigment is believed to be formed from the absorbed carbolic acid. This has been called *exogenous ochronosis*.

(2) Pigments derived from haemoglobin

At the end of their life span, red cells are taken up by macrophages in the spleen, marrow, etc. (p. 56): breakdown of haemoglobin (Hb) begins with opening of the porphyrin system of haem, the four pyrrole nuclei and globin now forming a long-chain molecule (choleglobin). The globin and iron are then split off and the residual *biliverdin* pigment, consisting of four pyrrole rings, is reduced to *bilirubin* and passes into the plasma where it is bound to an α-globulin carrier. The bilirubin is taken up by the hepatocytes, dissociated from the protein, and is conjugated with glucuronic acid and excreted as bilirubin glucuronides in the bile. The iron which is split off from haem is stored mainly as *ferritin* and *haemosiderin* and re-used.

Breakdown products of Hb may accumulate in the body in the following circumstances: (*a*) local deposition results from haemorrhage into the tissues; (*b*) more generalised accumulation occurs when there is excessive red cell destruction, i.e. in haemolytic anaemias; (*c*) increase in bilirubin or its glucuronides occurs when there is some defect in the metabolic or excretory pathways by which the iron-free part of haem is delivered into the intestine as bilirubin glucuronide; (*d*) accumulation of iron-containing compounds occurs when the amount of iron entering the body exceeds significantly the small amount which is lost physiologically. The effects of these abnormalities is described below.

Local accumulation of pigments

When haemorrhage into tissues occurs, many of the red cells in the escaped blood undergo lysis; their Hb diffuses away and is taken up and catabolised in macrophages in the draining lymph nodes, spleen, etc. However, some of the red cells are phagocytosed locally by macrophages derived from monocytes which migrate into the lesion and bilirubin and iron com-

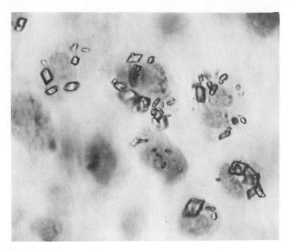

Fig. 9.8 Intracellular formation of bilirubin crystals in macrophages of mouse, 16 days after injection of haemoglobin. × 1200. (From preparations by the late Dr. Janet S. F. Niven.)

pounds are produced as described above: this process is illustrated experimentally in Figs. 9.7 and 9.8: in man it is reflected in the changing colours of a 'black eye' or other superficial bruise. Most of the bilirubin diffuses away and is eventually dealt with by the liver, but some of it may persist locally in crystalline form around an old haemorrhage, particularly in the brain (Fig. 9.9): this may be due to the absence of

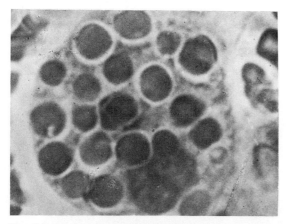

Fig. 9.7 A phagocyte. from subcutaneous tissue of mouse, containing numerous erythrocytes and some haemosiderin granules, 6 days after injection of erythrocytes. × 2000.

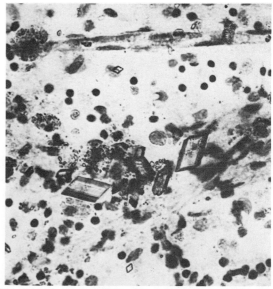

Fig. 9.9 Crystals of bilirubin and granular pigment, some of which is in phagocytes, in the wall of an old cerebral haemorrhage. × 500.

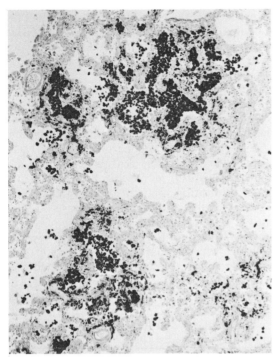

Fig. 9.10 The lung in mitral stenosis. Red cells escaping from the congested pulmonary capillaries are ingested by alveolar macrophages which became engorged with haemosiderin. The macrophages accumulate in the alveoli adjacent to respiratory bronchioles and are thus seen as aggregates. Prussian blue reaction. × 50.

lymphatics in brain tissue. Some of the iron released may also be retained locally as the pigment haemosiderin (see below), either within macrophages or as an incrustation of collagen and other tissue components.

Localised accumulation of haemosiderin may occur in the **lungs** as a result of pulmonary haemorrhages in *mitral stenosis* (Fig. 9.10) and in *idiopathic pulmonary haemosiderosis* where it is accompanied by fibrosis. Haemosiderin deposition also occurs in the **renal tubular epithelium** when haemoglobin leaks into the glomerular filtrate (p. 472).

Generalised increase in haemoglobin-derived pigments

(a) Iron-free pigments

A rise in the level of **bilirubin** in the plasma results from increased breakdown of haemoglobin in haemolytic anaemias or from failure of the liver cells to remove and conjugate it with glucuronic acid. Lesions of the liver or biliary tract which prevent excretion of **bilirubin glucuronide** result in its regurgitation into the plasma. When the levels of either compound exceed 2–3 mg per 100 ml (35–50 μmol/l), **jaundice** develops, i.e. the skin, sclera and various other tissues become distinctly yellow. In adults, jaundice itself causes little disability, but in infants a rise of (unconjugated) bilirubin in the plasma to over 15 mg per 100 ml (250 μmol/l) carries a risk of toxic brain injury. The types of jaundice and their causes and effects are, however, dealt with more fully in Chapter 19.

(b) Iron-containing compounds

Iron metabolism. About 70% of the 3–4 g of iron in the body is incorporated in the haem of haemoglobin: 5% is in myoglobin and small amounts are incorporated in cellular cytochrome, respiratory and metallo-flavo enzymes. The remainder (1–1.5 g) is mostly in storage form in macrophages of the spleen, bone marrow, etc. and in various tissue cells, but particularly hepatocytes. This storage iron is in the form of ferritin and haemosiderin. The **ferritin** molecule consists of a protein shell—**apoferritin**, containing iron as ferric hydrophosphate in micelles. **Haemosiderin** contains a higher concentration of iron in ferric state, and is probably formed from ferritin by degradation of the protein. Normally about 65% of storage iron is in ferritin and 35% in haemosiderin, but with excess iron storage the proportion of haemosiderin increases, and when the stores are diminished, haemosiderin is depleted before ferritin. Haemosiderin is stained by the prussian blue reagent (treatment of tissue with potassium ferrocyanide + HCl converts ferric iron to bright blue ferri-ferrocyanide), and there is normally sufficient in macrophages, e.g. in the bone marrow, to give a faint diffuse staining reaction. Haemosiderin is relatively insoluble, and when present in cells in large amounts it forms irregular granules (Fig. 9.11).

About 4 mg of iron is present in the plasma where it is bound to **transferrin**, a β globulin: this small fraction is very important, because it is the form in which iron distribution occurs between the site of absorption in the gut, the macrophages, the erythropoietic tissue of the marrow, and the various tissue cells. The degree

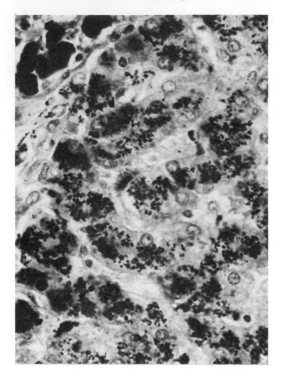

Fig. 9.11 Heavy deposition of haemosiderin in the liver of a patient with haemosiderosis due to multiple blood transfusions. The haemosiderin, which is stained by the prussian blue reaction, is seen as black granules in the hepatocytes and obscures the morphology of macrophages in the portal areas (*upper left*). × 500.

of iron-saturation of transferrin, normally about 30%, may also be of importance in regulating the amount of iron absorbed from the gut (see below).

When released by Hb breakdown in macrophages in the spleen, etc., iron is stored in these cells as described above: its mobilisation involves reduction to ferrous iron which is then bound to transferrin and circulates in the plasma. Contributions to transferrin iron are also made by the gut mucosal epithelium and by hepatocytes. Most of the transferrin iron is used for Hb synthesis by red cell precursors.

Iron balance. Iron loss in the bile, urine and sweat, and by desquamation of cells of the skin and gut lining, totals about 1 mg daily, and there is no physiological means of increasing the loss, except that menstruation accounts for an additional mean daily 0·5 mg and further losses result from pregnancy and lactation. Accordingly, iron balance depends on the amount

absorbed from the gut: this occurs mainly in the duodenum and upper jejunum and is influenced by the amount and form of dietary iron and by the make-up of the diet itself, apart from its iron content. In general, an iron-rich diet increases the *amount* absorbed, although the higher the diet content of iron the smaller is the *percentage* absorbed. Phytates, phosphates and chelating factors in the diet reduce absorption, while gastric juice (and particularly acid) and agents such as ascorbic acid, which reduce ferric to ferrous iron in the gut, increase absorption. Absorption may also be increased in hepatic cirrhosis and in pancreatic insufficiency, but the evidence on this is conflicting. There is, however, no doubt that a fall in total body iron to below the normal range is accompanied by increased absorption, regardless of whether iron-deficiency anaemia has developed. The mechanism controlling this is not understood. One popular view is that the degree of unsaturation of plasma transferrin determines the amount of iron absorbed, the avid uptake of iron by unsaturated transferrin in some way facilitating passage of iron across the gut lining epithelium. It has also been proposed that iron absorption is inversely related to the amount of ferritin in the gut mucosal lining cells. It is known that this is abundant in iron-replete individuals and scanty in states of iron deficiency, and it is probable that the amount of ferritin synthesised by mucosal cells during their development in the mucosal crypts is dependent on the degree of unsaturation of transferrin at the time. When a cell moves up the crypt to its absorbing position on the villus, it is postulated that iron entering it from the lumen would be trapped by the ferritin and progress no further: the cell has a short life span, and when it is shed this trapped iron would be lost. In iron-deficient subjects, with only scanty ferritin in the mucosal cells, iron taken up from the lumen would not be trapped and would traverse the cell and enter the circulation. Thus ferritin, which has been widely regarded as the form in which iron is transported across the mucosa, may actually control iron intake by *inhibiting* absorption.

Disturbances of iron balance. The commonest disturbances are those which result in **iron deficiency**. This results first in depletion of storage iron, secondly in anaemia, and lastly, and less certainly, in fall of the cytochrome content of cells. Most of the important effects of iron deficiency are due to anaemia, and accordingly the subject is dealt with in relation to the blood in Chapter 16.

Iron overload

This may result from prolonged excessive absorption of iron from the gut, as in the disease idiopathic haemochromatosis, excessive oral intake of iron, and in diseases in which there is hyperplasia of the erythropoietic cells in the bone marrow. Overload can result also from administration of iron parenterally, including multiple blood transfusion.

Idiopathic haemochromatosis is characterised by excessive absorption of dietary iron, probably from birth, so that the total iron content of the body gradually increases until, at the age of 40 years or so, it may contain more than 20 g instead of the normal 3–4 g. Occasionally this relatively rare disease, which occurs mostly in men, affects more than one member of a family, and genetic predisposition is suggested also by the demonstration of increased iron absorption and storage in the relatives of patients. Excess storage iron in the form of haemosiderin is widespread. It is seen particularly in the parenchymal cells of the liver and of the pancreas, but also in the myocardium, gastric epithelium and many other organs, and in macrophages in the lymph nodes, marrow and elsewhere. Extracellular deposits of haemosiderin also occur. There is relatively little iron in the spleen and kidneys. In some unknown way, the accumulation of iron in the hepatocytes has a cytotoxic effect and the resultant hepatocyte destruction leads to the scarring and nodularity of cirrhosis, symptoms of which usually appear at about 40 years of age, but sometimes much earlier. Pancreatic scarring also develops, and diabetes mellitus is a common feature. The skin may have a leaden hue due to iron deposition around the sweat glands, but pigmentation due to unexplained excess melanin production is a more striking feature and gives the disease its alternative name of **bronzed diabetes**.

The reason for the excessive iron absorption in haemochromatosis is unknown. The plasma transferrin is not increased, nor apparently qualitatively abnormal, but its percentage saturation is much higher than the normal 30%.

Some patients, but not all, have been found to absorb an unduly high proportion of a test oral dose of ^{59}Fe. In most cases, therapeutic withdrawal of blood to remove iron is followed by increased absorption which gradually decreases towards normal over the next few years. A history of excessive alcohol consumption (which itself predisposes to cirrhosis and chronic pancreatitis) is common, and alcohol is known to increase iron absorption in normal subjects, perhaps by stimulating gastric acid secretion, but in other cases alcohol does not seem to be a relevant factor.

In a minority of patients with other forms of cirrhosis there is excess iron stored as haemosiderin in the liver cells and elsewhere, and in some cases serial biopsy has shown that this *follows* the development of cirrhosis. This contrasts with haemochromatosis in which cirrhosis is the result of prolonged iron overload. Nevertheless in occasional cases of cirrhosis with heavy hepatic siderosis it is difficult to make the distinction.

Dietary iron overload. Over 60% of men of the Bantu race in South Africa have excess of storage iron and in half of these the deposits are very heavy. The incidence of overload is much lower in Bantu women. In most instances haemosiderin is deposited mainly in the macrophages of the liver, spleen and bone marrow, etc., with smaller amounts in the parenchymal cells, and cirrhosis does not develop. This distribution of excess storage iron, with little or no tissue injury, differs from haemochromatosis and is termed **haemosiderosis or siderosis**. In a small proportion of Bantus, however, iron overload has the features of haemochromatosis, but with slight differences in the distribution of iron deposition.

One factor of importance in iron overload in the Bantu race is the high iron content of the food and of Kaffir beer, due to the use of iron cooking utensils and containers. The two patterns of iron overload are, however, unexplained (see below). A condition similar to haemochromatosis is unusually common also in parts of Italy and has been associated with drinking large amounts of iron-rich wine.

Iron overload in anaemia. As mentioned earlier, anaemia is commonly due to iron deficiency. However, it may result also from ineffectual erythropoiesis in 'refractory anaemia' and pernicious anaemia, and from excessive red cell destruction (haemolytic anaemia). In some cases of these conditions, iron storage is excessive and has been shown to be greater than can be accounted for by iron therapy and blood transfusions: it appears that prolonged hyperplasia of the erythropoietic tissue in some way increases iron absorption in the gut.

Patterns of iron deposition. It is apparent from the above account that different patterns of distribution of haemosiderin occur in iron overload. In haemochromatosis there is heavy deposition in the parenchymal cells, with consequent cirrhosis and sometimes diabetes. In haemosiderosis a greater proportion of the haemosiderin is in macrophages, and although there is some redistribution to parenchymal cells (Fig. 9.11), tissue injury does not usually occur. It has been suggested that excessive iron absorption from the gut tends especially to bring about the changes of haemochromatosis, while parenteral iron or excessive red cell destruction produces haemosiderosis. However, this does not explain the distribution pattern in Bantus, and additional factors, at present unknown, must be involved.

Malarial pigmentation

In malaria the parasites within the red cells produce from the haemoglobin a dark brown pigment, haematin, in the form of very minute granules, which accumulates within the parasites. It becomes free when the red cells are broken down, and is taken up by phagocytes and deposited in organs, especially the spleen and liver, where it remains practically unchanged for many years. Malarial pigment is not a melanin; it contains iron, though it reacts negatively in the ordinary prussian blue test. W. H. Brown showed that in its solubilities and spectroscopic properties it is essentially haematin, and it closely resembles the artefact pigment derived from formalin acting on blood. When there is much

blood destruction, especially in severe cases of malaria, haemosiderin may be deposited in the organs in addition to the malarial pigment.

(3) Lipofuscin: age pigment

In the later years of life a fine brownish-yellow pigment tends to appear in the heart muscle, smooth muscle, etc.; and in wasting diseases this accumulation of pigment is more marked. In some cases of malabsorption syndrome, for example due to coeliac disease, it is present in the smooth muscle of the small intestine and oesophagus, and in smaller amounts in that of the stomach and colon: experimental studies suggest that vitamin E deficiency may be responsible.

In the heart muscle the pigment accumulates in the central part of the cells around the poles of the nucleus, and when this is associated with wasting of the muscle, the term *brown atrophy* is applied. Similar pigment may occur in the liver cells, especially in the central parts of the lobules, in the cells of the testis, and in the nerve cells of the cortex of the brain. Heavy deposits of pigment in the cortical neurones is seen in senile dementia and allied conditions. The pigment must be distinguished from that which occurs normally in the pigmented neurons of the locus caeruleus and substantia nigra, which belongs to the melanin group. In brown atrophy the pigment is believed to be chiefly lipid, as it reduces perosmic acid and is usually coloured by the sudan stains. It is often called *lipofuscin*, but differs in its chemical and staining reactions in the various organs, some being fluorescent, doubly refracting or acid-fast in varying degree, e.g. *ceroid*, an acid-fast pigment found in the liver in certain forms of experimental cirrhosis. Electron microscopy suggests that age pigment consists of 'indigestible' residues of lipid metabolism, lying in cytoplasmic vacuoles derived from lysosomes.

Exogenous pigmentation

Inhaled compounds. The most important exogenous pigments are those inhaled as dust particles and entering the body through the respiratory passages. A certain amount of soot, stone dust, etc., enters and accumulates in the

lungs of all individuals living in urban conditions, but the accumulation becomes excessive in those exposed occupationally to an atmosphere rich in dust. The lungs may be infiltrated by foreign particles of various kinds—coal,

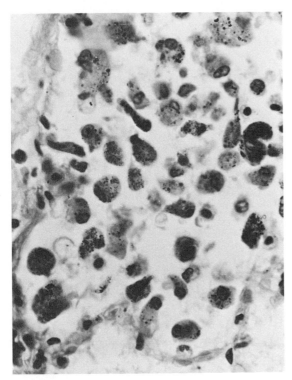

Fig. 9.12 The lung of a coal-miner showing phagocytosis of inhaled particles of coal dust by alveolar macrophages. × 520.

silica, asbestos, iron and other ores and various organic substances. The resulting pathological changes will be described later with the diseases of the lungs.

The entrance of such particles into the lungs is favoured by the presence of chronic bronchitis or other condition in which there is interference with the action of the ciliated epithelium, but even in a healthy animal, dust particles less than 5μm gain access to the pulmonary alveoli if the amount in the inspired air is great. The dust particles are quickly taken up by macrophages in the pulmonary alveoli (Fig. 9.12). Some of the phagocytes with the ingested particles are expelled *via* the bronchi; others enter the interstitial tissue of the lungs, and pass into the lymphatics: others come to lie in the alveoli alongside respiratory bronchioles, and the pigment is eventually incorporated into the respiratory bronchiolar walls. Much of the pigment, however, is carried into the lymphatics; most of it is deposited in the hilar nodes, but some in the pleura. The degree of irritation resulting depends on the nature of the particles. Large collections of carbonaceous particles may provoke little or no overgrowth of connective tissue—*anthracosis*—whereas fibrosis is very marked in the case of silica-containing stone dust, the condition of *silicosis* resulting. The bronchial lymph nodes become pigmented and enlarged, the accumulation within their phagocytic cells being virtually permanent. Some of the pigment which has accumulated in the lungs may be removed by phagocytes which appear in the sputum for a long time after removal of the individual from the dusty atmosphere.

Ingested compounds. Deposition of brownish granules of silver compounds (argyria) was a common result of taking medicines containing silver preparations. The granules are formed by reduction of silver albuminate and are seen especially in the skin (giving a dusky appearance), the gut wall, and the basement membranes of the glomeruli and renal collecting tubules. It is now rare. In *chronic lead-poisoning* an albuminate is produced in a similar way, and around the teeth hydrogen sulphide reacts with it to produce the characteristic blue line on the gums. Melanosis coli (p. 239) is now the least uncommon example of pigmentation resulting from ingestion of chemicals.

Tattooing. In tattooing, fine particles such as india ink, ultramarine, cinnabar (mercuric sulphide), etc., introduced through the epidermis, are taken up by macrophages (p. 55) and lodge in small spaces or clefts in the connective tissue of the cutis. Some particles are carried also by the lymph stream to the regional lymph nodes and then are conveyed by phagocytes into the lymphoid tissue. Both at the site of introduction and in the lymph nodes the pigment persists for life.

Pathological calcification

Pathological calcification of soft tissues occurs most commonly without any general disturbance of calcium metabolism: the level of plasma calcium is normal, and deposition is due to local changes in the affected tissue. This is termed *dystrophic calcification*. Less commonly, pathological calcification is a result of an increase in the level of ionic calcium in the plasma, and occurs in normal soft tissues: this is termed *metastatic calcification*.

In both dystrophic and metastatic calcification the deposits resemble in composition the minerals of bone, but show much greater variations in the proportions of calcium to magnesium and phosphate to carbonate.

Identification of calcium salts in tissues. Calcium salts have an affinity for haematoxylin, forming a lake with it, and the earliest sign of calcification is given by the appearance of hyaline or finely granular material of a deep violet tint. Later the calcium salts form irregular and somewhat refractile masses: they are, of course, readily soluble in weak acids, and small bubbles of carbon dioxide are released from the carbonates. When treated with dilute sulphuric acid, the characteristic crystals of calcium sulphate separate out. This occurs more readily when the sections are in 50% alcohol, in which the solubility of the crystals is low. When calcium salts are treated with silver nitrate, yellow silver phosphate is formed, and this quickly undergoes reduction on exposure to light and turns black (von Kossa's method). Neither the affinity for haematoxylin nor von Kossa's method is specific for calcium. Silver nitrate is reduced by other substances, e.g. iron, and the reaction with haematoxylin is given by a substance formed before the deposition of calcium, and is positive after the tissue is decalcified. The best reagent is alizarin, the staining principle in madder, or its derivatives. Alizarin stains calcium salts red, but the reaction may not be given by very old deposits. When injected *intra vitam*, alizarin colours growing bone (but not fully formed bone) and also pathological deposits of calcium unless they are very old.

Calcification is often accompanied by deposit of iron compounds which give a prussian blue reaction. These may give a diffuse staining or may be granular.

Dystrophic calcification

This consists of the irregular deposition of calcium salts in altered or necrotic tissues and formed elements such as thrombi. Deposition is irregular and may be sufficiently heavy to render the part chalky or even stony hard.

Predisposing changes. The local changes which predispose to dystrophic calcification are as follows.

(1) Hyaline change in fibrous tissue. This occurs as an ageing change in arteries. Increase in calcium in hyalinised artery walls is usual, and

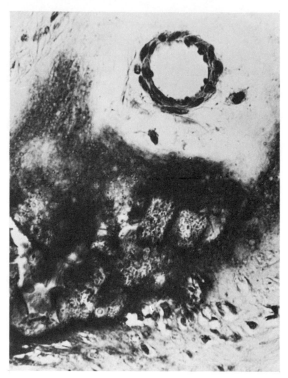

Fig. 9.13 Area of calcification near a blood vessel in a fibroma. Calcified tissue (even after decalcification) is stained by haematoxylin; the earliest change, seen here at the margin, is a fine dark granularity. × 500.

it may be sufficient to convert the vessel to a rigid tube, as in Monckeberg's sclerosis (Fig. 13.19, p. 324). Calcification is also common in dense connective tissues, for example tendons, the dura mater, and the scarred heart valves following rheumatic endocarditis. It occurs in some tumours, for example in fibromas (Fig. 9.13) and in uterine myomas undergoing involution after the menopause. The 'brain-sand' bodies of some meningiomas consist of concentrically arranged cells which undergo hyaline change followed by calcification.

(2) Tissue death, such as caseous patches in tuberculosis, necrotic foci in histoplasmosis, etc., old infarcts and particularly fat necrosis (p. 654) and the lipid-rich debris in atheromatous plaques all tend to become calcified, as do dead parasites (e.g. *Trichinella spiralis* and echinococcal cysts). Calcification of such dead tissue is a slow process, and occurs only when necrotic material persists for a long time without undergoing organisation.

(3) Inspissated pus and *organic material in*

ducts, etc. A large collection of pus, unless discharged, may eventually become inspissated, then calcified, and even ossified. Organic material accumulating in the ducts of salivary glands, or in the appendix, may become calcified, forming 'stones' in these sites. Calcium deposition in the urinary tract, both as discrete stones and as soft, crumbling material, is caused by urinary infections, but stone formation occurs also as a result of increased calcium excretion (see below).

(*4*) *Thrombi.* Calcification occurs very commonly in old thrombi which have not undergone organisation: hard masses are thus formed in veins, e.g. in the legs, and show up on x-ray as *phleboliths*.

The chemical reactions involved in dystrophic calcification are not understood. Factors which may be involved include the following. (*a*) Local changes in pH of hyaline or necrotic tissue, etc.: calcium is deposited more readily from an alkaline medium. (*b*) Breakdown products of cells or tissue elements to provide a nucleus with an affinity for calcium salts. Release of phosphate from nucleoprotein breakdown is a possible example. The strong tendency for calcification of necrotic fatty tissue was formerly explained by the affinity of fatty acids for calcium, forming insoluble calcium soaps. This suggestion lacks supporting evidence, and in particular subcutaneous injection of fatty acids does not lead to calcification. (*c*) Local enzyme changes: the normal process of calcification of growing bone occurs in the presence of high local concentrations of alkaline phosphatase. In experimentally induced lesions, some correlation has been observed between high levels of alkaline phosphatase and deposition of calcium salts, but the correlation is not a very good one, and this is not a convincing factor in dystrophic calcification in man.

Calcinosis circumscripta. This is a condition in which irregular nodular dystrophic calcification occurs in the skin and subcutaneous tissues, especially of the fingers. The overlying skin becomes ulcerated and the chalky material is discharged or may be scraped out. This appears to consist chiefly of calcium carbonate, as shown by solution with effervescence in hydrochloric acid. Microscopically a mild chronic inflammatory reaction with giant cells surrounds the nodules. The causation of the lesion is obscure. The deposits are easily distinguished from gouty tophi by their dense opacity to x-rays and by histochemical tests.

Occasionally calcium deposition is more widespread, involving also muscles and tendons—this is known as **calcinosis universalis**.

Metastatic calcification

This occurs in the following conditions.

(1) Excessive absorption of calcium from the gut. This is seen most commonly in infants with hypervitaminosis D due to over-fortification of infant foods with vitamin D and calcium (p. 827). Similar experimental changes can be produced readily in the rat (Fig. 9.14).

(2) Excessive mobilisation of calcium from the bones. This occurs in patients with widespread bone destruction, as for example in multiple myeloma or metastatic carcinoma. Prolonged immobilisation is also of importance, the bones undergoing disuse atrophy. Excessive mobilisation of bone calcium is also brought about by *primary hyperparathyroidism*, usually due to a parathyroid adenoma (p. 969), and by *secondary hyperparathyroidism* associated with parathyroid hyperplasia and resulting from chronic renal disease with retention of phosphate (p. 970).

Metastatic calcification occurs especially in the walls of arteries, the myocardium of the left side of the heart, the wall of the stomach, the kidneys and lungs. Apart from their arteries, these are otherwise rare sites of calcification, and it may be that the sites of metastatic calcification are determined by a relatively high pH,

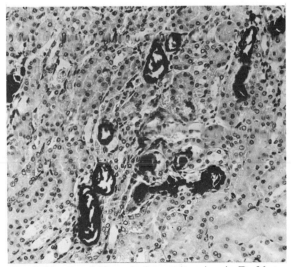

Fig. 9.14 Rat kidney in hypervitaminosis D. Note calcified small vessels. × 120. (From preparation kindly lent by Dr. J. R. M. Innes.)

e.g. around the renal tubules and the acid-secreting gastric glands. Deposition is seen initially on the surface of elastic fibres and other formed elements.

Renal calcinosis, with consequent renal failure, occurs both in hypercalcaemia, and also in renal tubular acidosis, in which the urine is alkaline and contains excess of calcium.

Deposition of uric acid and urates

Uric acid is formed as the final breakdown product of purine bases, and is thus derived from catabolism of nucleic acids. Normal plasma urate levels depend greatly on the assay technique, but levels above 7·2 mg/100 ml (0·43 mmol/l) for men and 5·7 mg/100 ml (0·34 mmol/l) for women are abnormally high. Adults produce 400–700 mg of endogenous uric acid daily and dietary purines contribute 300–600 mg. Most of this uric acid is excreted by the renal distal convoluted tubules, which can normally increase the rate of excretion, as necessary, to maintain homoeostasis.

Hyperuricaemia is not uncommon, particularly in men over 40. It tends to be familial, but sporadic cases occur. The metabolic abnormalities concerned are not clearly understood. In some instances, increased production of uric acid results from a deficiency of the phosphoribosyl-transferase enzyme which is necessary for the re-utilisation of hypoxanthine for purine synthesis. This deficiency results in increased breakdown of hypoxanthine into uric acid. Other enzyme deficiencies with similar effect have been detected in some instances of hyperuricaemia. In others, there is a defect of unknown nature in renal excretion of uric acid. These defects account for at least some cases of *primary hyperuricaemia* in which nucleic acid breakdown is normal. *Secondary hyperuricaemia* results from increased nucleic acid breakdown, as in the myeloproliferative disorders (p. 493).

There is considerable variation in the effects of hyperuricaemia. In most instances, there are no associated pathological changes. In others there is deposition of uric acid or urate in the collecting tubules of the kidneys, seen macroscopically as brown-yellow streaking of the

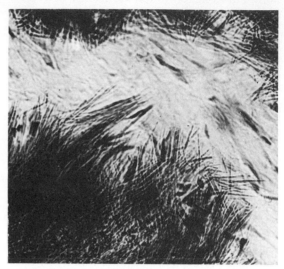

Fig. 9.15 Section through gouty nodule of skin, showing deposit of needle-like crystals of monosodium urate. × 370.

medulla: this may have little or no effect, or may be followed by formation of uric acid stones (p. 805). Uric acid streaking of the medulla is a common necropsy finding, particularly in children, and appears to be associated with a state of dehydration before death. The most important complication of hyperuricaemia is **gout** (p. 861), in which crystals of monosodium urate are deposited in and around the joints, in the skin (Fig. 9.15) and elsewhere. It is always accompanied by hyperuricaemia, and yet the relatives of patients may have equally high levels of plasma uric acid without developing gout. As indicated above for hyperuricaemia in general, a number of individual abnormalities of purine metabolism can result in gout.

10

Tumours

I. General Features, Causation and Host Reactions

Introduction. In previous chapters we have seen examples of cell proliferation and growth of tissues in the process of repair, in response to irritation, and as a hyperplastic process. Such growth is purposeful, and, up to a point, capable of explanation. In a tumour (neoplasm), however, the growth is not only excessive but apparently purposeless, progressing without regard to the surrounding tissues or the requirements of the individual as a whole. While forming a part of the body, a tumour and its cells seem to have become largely unresponsive to the factors which control the proliferation of non-neoplastic cells. Accordingly, tumours exhibit various degrees of uncontrolled growth and in some instances uncontrolled function, e.g. the production of hormones or enzymes. Such behaviour is commonly termed *autonomous*, but a tumour is, of course, dependent on the host for its nutrition, blood supply and supporting stroma, and escape from host control factors is only relative.

Definition. A tumour, or neoplasm, is an abnormal mass of tissue, the growth of which exceeds and is unco-ordinated with that of the normal tissues and continues in the same manner after cessation of the stimuli which have initiated it. This definition covers most tumours, which form discrete lumps, but in the leukaemias, which are tumours of myeloid or lymphoid cells, the tumour cells may extend diffusely through the marrow or lymphoid tissues, and also circulate in the blood.

Origin. Tumours show an extraordinary variety of structure, but the majority retain a resemblance to some normal tissue or cell type; occasionally the resemblance is to some precursor cell or tissue rather than to the fully differentiated adult type. These resemblances are attributable to the origin of all tumours from abnormal and excessive proliferation of a cell derived from the previously normal tissue. (The exact origin of some tumours is unknown or disputed, but this does not affect the general statement.) Tumours arise most often from tissues in which active cell loss and replacement occur normally, and which are exposed to the various noxious agents in the environment (especially the skin and the epithelia of the alimentary and respiratory tracts). Many tumours do, however, originate from highly specialised cells such as those of the liver, thyroid, adrenal, cartilage or fat. The adult neurone is probably the only cell in the body incapable of giving rise to a tumour, and even here tumours derived from the precursor cells—neuroblasts—are not uncommon.

Classification. The cell or tissue origin of a tumour is called its *histogenesis*, and provides the basis of a principal mode of classification. On this basis, nearly all tumours may be classified as *epithelial* or *connective tissue* tumours according to the cell of origin. Tumours are further classified by their naked-eye appearances, their histological features and by the nature of their products. The most important mode of classification is, however, based on behaviour, and divides tumours into **benign** and **malignant** types (see below). So little is known of the precise causal factors of most individual tumours that a classification based on aetiology is not yet widely applicable.

In this book **tumour** or **neoplasm** is used for all lesions of this type, benign or malignant. **Cancer** is used for all malignant tumours, regardless of their origin. **Carcinoma** is used only for malignant tumours of epithelium (see next chapter). Though purists often insist that cancer and carcinoma are the same word, it is quite obvious that 'cancer research' for instance is not limited to epithelial tumours.

Behaviour

Rate of growth. Tumours vary considerably in their behaviour, notably in the following important features. There are all gradations between slow growing tumours which hardly change in size from year to year and those which enlarge so rapidly that differences in size may be detected from week to week. While the rate of tumour cell proliferation largely determines the rate of growth of many tumours, other factors include the rate of tumour cell death, the rate of production of matrix or secretion by some tumours, the induction of vascular stroma by others, vascular engorgement, oedema and infection. Assessment of the *mitotic rate* of a tumour is of assistance in predicting tumour growth, but account must also be taken of the rate of cell loss. Prominent nucleoli, and increased cytoplasmic RNA seen histologically as basophilia, are further pointers to increased cellular proliferative activity. *Nuclear pleomorphism* and *aberrant mitoses* indicate variation from the normal diploid chromosome pattern and are strong evidence of the malignancy of a tumour.

Invasion and spread. The cells of benign tumours remain at the site of origin, forming a single mass. When growing in a solid tissue, they usually become enclosed in a layer of fibrous tissue or **capsule**, formed from the stroma of the compressed surrounding tissue (Fig. 11.8, p. 277). By contrast, the cells of malignant tumours invade locally and also pass via the lymphatics, bloodstream and body cavities to form secondary tumours or metastases, which are remote from the site of origin. Cell motility is probably important in allowing tumour cells to pass through endothelia, basal laminae, etc., and inhibition of such motility by antibodies to the tumour cells or by cytotoxic drugs has therapeutic possibilities.

Differentiation. This is the degree of resemblance of a tumour to its tissue of origin and is applicable to morphology and function of the tumour cells. The naked eye appearances of a well differentiated tumour sometimes reveal its nature: for instance a lipoma is usually recognisable as an encapsulated mass of adipose tissue of essentially normal microscopic appearance. The more undifferentiated a tumour is, the more difficult it is to identify its tissue of origin and the tissue of origin of a poorly differ-

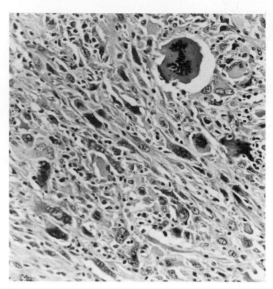

Fig. 10.1 Section of a rapidly growing malignant tumour showing great variation in shape and size of the cells and of their nuclei (pleomorphism). Note also the abnormal mitoses. × 200.

entiated tumour may remain unknown despite naked eye, microscopic and biochemical examination. Partial loss of structural and functional resemblance to parent tissue is called **dysplasia** and total loss is termed **anaplasia**.

There is a general correlation between the above features; malignant tumours are usually rapidly growing, poorly differentiated, and

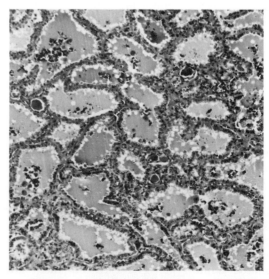

Fig. 10.2 Section of a benign tumour of the thyroid. Note the close resemblance to thyroid tissue. × 75.

have a high mitotic rate with nuclear pleomorphism and aberrant mitoses (Fig. 10.1), while benign tumours are usually slow growing, well differentiated, and show infrequent mitoses and little cytological variation (Fig. 10.2). (See also Figs. 12.2 to 12.15, pp. 290–6.)

Benign tumours seldom kill unless they arise near, and press on, vital structures or secrete excessive amounts of hormone (see below). Most fatal tumours are malignant, and death may result from local invasion, from the effects of metastases, or from a combination of both. The identification of tumours as benign or malignant is therefore crucial and is one of the main functions of the hospital pathologist. Table 10.1 compares the characteristics of benign and malignant tumours. However, the distinction is not absolute and borderline tumours occur. Progression of a benign tumour to malignancy is not common, and most malignant tumours do not arise from a benign

Table 10.1 Contrasting features of benign and malignant tumours

	Benign	Malignant
(a) *Evidence of rapid growth*		
Mitoses	Few and normal	Numerous and often abnormal
Nuclei	Little altered	Enlarged, often irregular (pleomorphic)
Nucleoli	Little altered	Usually large
Cytoplasmic basophilia	Slight	Marked
Haemorrhage and necrosis	Inconspicuous	Often extensive
(b) *Differentiation*		
Naked-eye resemblance to tissue of origin	Often close	Variable: close to none
Microscopic resemblance to tissue of origin	Usually very marked	Usually poor
Function, e.g. secretion	Usually well maintained	May be retained, lost, or abnormal products
(c) *Evidence of transgression of normal boundaries*		
Capsule intact	Frequent	Rare (usually none)
Local invasion	Absent	Very frequent
Metastases	Never	Frequent

tumour. The behaviour of the innumerable different kinds of tumours of different organs varies greatly, and it is necessary to know these variations before one can apply the criteria of the table with safety to the individual case.

Examples of exceptional behaviour. *Rate of growth.* Some benign tumours (especially of the female genitalia, e.g. myomas of the uterus and cystadenomas of the ovary) may grow very rapidly and reach a great size. Some malignant tumours—many rodent ulcers, some breast carcinomas and in particular argentaffinoma and 'latent' carcinoma of the prostate—grow very slowly.

Differentiation. Some benign tumours show a high degree of cellular specialisation and structural arrangement, but do not resemble the parent tissue. Mucinous cystadenoma of the ovary (Fig. 23.35, p. 911) is an example: it is 'well differentiated' but in a different direction from the parent tissue. Some malignant tumours (some squamous carcinomas, for instance, and well differentiated thyroid carcinomas) may closely resemble the parent tissue. Function is not always lost in malignant tumours: indeed, such normal functions as the production of keratin, mucin, melanin, and less often hormones, may be well maintained by malignant tumours arising from the appropriate cell types.

Invasion is perhaps the most nearly reliable criterion of malignancy, but it is often surprisingly difficult to assess in practice, especially where the normal structures are distorted by some other pathological process such as infection, metaplasia or congenital anomaly. A capsule may be absent in some benign tumours, such as papillomas, and present in some malignant tumours, including clear-cell carcinoma of kidney and some thyroid carcinomas.

Metastasis is another generally reliable criterion, but benign tumours and even normal tissue may sometimes become implanted at a distance as a result of trauma or surgical accident. Also some undoubted malignant tumours practically never metastasise: basal cell carcinoma of the epidermis is the best example, but intracranial tumours also fail to metastasise outside the cranio-spinal cavity. The placental trophoblast not only invades the uterus but is often carried to the lungs: and the fetus, incidentally, grows faster than any tumour.

Despite these exceptions, the hallmark of the malignant tumour is its capacity to spread to, and grow progressively in, tissue remote from its site of origin. Spread may occur by lymphatic vessels as tumour cell emboli or a column of tumour cells may grow along the vessel until a lymph node is reached. Invasion of a lymph node may be followed by extension along the efferent lymphatic. Similar invasion and spread by blood vessels is also common. Tumour cells disseminated by the blood stream may involve any organ, but the lungs, liver and bone marrow are specially common sites for the establishment of secondary tumours. It should be noted, however, that by no means all tumour cells which enter the blood stream go on to establish metastases. Circulating tumour cells can be detected in the bloodstream of patients with early cancer and it seems that many such cells are destroyed. Less common but important routes of spread are across body cavities (trans-coelomic spread) and intra-epithelial extension as in Paget's disease of the nipple. The spread of tumours is discussed more fully in Chapter 11.

Effect of tumours

These are various and many of them can be readily understood.

Local effects. The presence of a mass of growing tissue of whatever kind may lead to pressure effects on various important structures, e.g. on blood vessels (especially veins), nerves, tubes and organs, and the usual results will follow. This is true both of benign and of malignant tumours, but in addition the latter infiltrate and destroy such structures, and are especially liable to produce obstructive effects, e.g. stenosis of pylorus, intestine or bronchi.

Extensive replacement of organs by tumour tissue may impair their function: involvement of bones leads to fractures: direct invasion of, or pressure upon, nerves leads to much of the pain associated with malignant disease. Pressure on or infiltration of blood vessels or lymphatics leads to regional congestion, ischaemia and oedema.

General effects. Absorption of bacterial products from infected tumours and of the products of necrosis of tumour tissue contributes to the pyrexia, debility and wasting (*cachexia*) seen in some cancer patients. A further factor in producing cachexia is the competition between tumour and normal tissues for essential nutriments, such as amino acids and vitamins. Actual reduction of food intake is important in patients nauseated from liver secondaries or the effects of cytotoxic drugs, or with dysphagia as a result of involvement of the upper alimentary tract. There is little evidence that tumour cells produce specifically toxic materials.

Anaemia is common in cancer patients; it can result from haemorrhage from, or infection of, an ulcerated tumour, marrow replacement by tumour, or marrow depression by cytotoxic drugs or radiotherapy.

Cancer patients are particularly susceptible to *infections* due to depression of immuno-logical and other defensive mechanisms apparently consequent upon the effects of their tumour. This depression, which may be increased by chemotherapy or radiation, predisposes them to infection with both virulent and opportunistic pathogens.

Occasional effects of cancer include various ill-defined neuropathies and myopathies which interfere respectively with the functioning of the nervous system and skeletal muscles: they are most likely due to humoral products of tumours: also multiple venous thromboses (especially in pancreatic cancer) and various skin rashes. Renal disturbances (usually nephrotic syndrome) occasionally result from deposition of tumour-antigen/antibody complexes in the glomeruli. These and other effects of tumours will be exemplified in the accounts of individual systems and organs.

Hormonal effects. *Syndromes of hormone excess* may result from the production of large quantities of hormone by both benign and, less commonly, malignant tumours of the endocrine organs. These effects may be regarded as appropriate as they reflect 'appropriate' functional differentiation of the tumour cells. Much more surprising is the increasing list of hormones shown to be produced by some tumours arising from tissues with no known relevant hormone secretion. The most commonly encountered examples are production of hormones with ACTH or ADH activity by carcinomas of the bronchi. Syndromes due to such '*inappropriate*' secretion of hormones by tumours of apparently non-endocrine origin occur in relatively few patients with cancer, but a much higher proportion of tumours can be shown to have the enzyme systems necessary for the production of such hormones. The tumours most commonly associated with the inappropriate secretion of hormones are listed in Table 10.2.

The basis of the 'inappropriate' secretion of hormones by non-endocrine tumours remains unclear. The genome of every normal cell contains the whole genetic material of the individual, and during differentiation the genes

Table 10.2 Examples of 'Inappropriate' Hormone Secretion by Tumours

Hormone secreted by tumour	Type of tumour
ACTH	Oat cell carcinoma of bronchus; epithelial thymomas; carcinoid tumours: islet cell tumour of pancreas.
Parathormone	Squamous carcinoma of bronchus; carcinomas of oesophagus, colon, liver, pancreas, kidney.
Antidiuretic hormone (ADH)	Oat cell carcinoma of bronchus; haemangioblastoma of cerebellum.
Insulin	Retroperitoneal fibrosarcoma; mesothelioma; hepatoma; adrenal carcinoma.
Thyroid stimulating hormone	Choriocarcinoma; hydatidiform mole; embryonal carcinoma of testis.
? Haemopoietin (erythrocytosis)	Renal carcinoma; cerebellar haemangioblastoma; hepatoma; phaeochromocytoma.
Gonadotrophin (precocious puberty in males)	Hepatoma.

not required by each particular cell type are suppressed. Apparently the nuclear changes in tumour cells sometimes include re-expression of suppressed genes, but the association between particular types of tumour and hormone production cannot readily be explained by random de-repression. A recent and attractive theory holds that there are widely distributed cells with an endocrine function ('apud' cells) and that tumours arising from such cells ('apudomas') amplify and make detectable their actual or potential hormonal activities (p. 967).

By invading and destroying endocrine glands, tumours can also cause *hormonal deficiencies*.

The causation of tumours

Parodoxically we know many causes for cancer, but not *the* cause of cancer. We know that many things like tar, x-irradiation and (in animals) viruses can produce tumours but we do not know exactly how any of them renders cells neoplastic.

The process of conversion of a normal cell to malignancy is called **carcinogenesis** and agents which cause this are termed **carcinogens**. It seems likely that carcinogenesis is always a complex process involving the interaction of many factors, some of which favour tumour development and others which appear to provide some protection against it. They may be divided into (1) **genetically determined factors**, which in total determine an individual's susceptibility to develop cancer on exposure to (2) the **exogenous influences** encountered in the complex environment in which we live. The complexities of genetic and environmental factors and of their interactions account for many of the difficulties of the epidemiological and experimental investigation of the causes of cancer.

There is great variation in the intensity and length of exposure to individual carcinogens necessary to bring about tumour development. A subthreshold dose of a carcinogen will not produce a tumour, but subthreshold doses of two separate carcinogens given together may be effective (**syncarcinogenesis**). The combinations of certain substances which are not of themselves carcinogenic (**co-carcinogens** or **promoters**) with a subthreshold dose of a carcinogen will also cause tumour development (**co-carcinogenesis**). For example, croton oil, a non-carcinogenic substance, promotes the development of cancer by sub-carcinogenic doses of the chemical carcinogen methylcholanthrene in experimental animals, but only if given simultaneously with, or following methylcholanthrene. Thus the relationship between carcinogens and co-carcinogens requires that initial and persistent carcinogen-mediated changes in the cell must be induced before the promoting substance is effective. The role of co-carcinogens in man is not clear, but the tars of cigarette smoke are active co-carcinogens in experimental animals. It is also possible that there are agents which, when combined with a normally effective dose of a carcinogen, inhibit its action (**anti-carcinogenesis**).

Genetic factors

A few human tumours develop mainly or wholly as a result of a genetic anomaly which makes it virtually certain that affected individuals will develop a particular malignancy. **Familial polyposis coli** is an example in which those affected inevitably develop adenocarcinoma of the colon at an early age. The risk is so high that prophylactic colectomy is essential. **Xeroderma pigmentosum** is another inherited condition, in which exposure to ultraviolet light leads to severe skin damage and the early development of skin cancer. The molecular basis of this condition is the genetically-determined absence of an enzyme which in the normal individual excises pyrimidine bases of DNA which have become irreversibly coupled by ultraviolet rays, allowing their replacement by normal bases. The resulting disturbance of nucleic acid metabolism leads to an increased frequency of mutations, some of which lead to the development of malignancy. It is of interest that an agent as apparently benign as sunlight causes nuclear damage which, if not repaired, gives rise to cancer, and that only the existence of a highly specific enzymic repair mechanism prevents the development of skin cancer in everyone. Other examples of cancers resulting mainly from an inherited abnormality are **retinoblastoma** (p. 743) and less certainly some cases of intestinal polyposis of Peutz–Jegher type and of neurofibromatosis (von Recklinghausen's disease), although sporadic cases of the above conditions may arise as a result of spontaneous mutations.

Certain families have a higher than average incidence of cancer, either of one particular type (e.g. breast cancer or malignant melanoma), which often develops relatively early, or a high frequency of tumours of diverse types. It is difficult to be certain whether this unfortunate tendency is a result of genetic factors or of environmental (e.g. social, dietary and occupational) factors which are shared by family members.

Ethnic factors are also important. A heavily pigmented skin protects against the development of skin cancers and by contrast those whose skins are pale and who show a poor tanning response to sunlight (notably Scots, Welsh or Irish of Celtic stock) are very prone to develop skin cancer if they live in a sunny climate (e.g. immigrants to Australia and S. Africa). Albinos, who lack melanin pigment, are especially vulnerable to solar carcinogenesis, regardless of their ethnic origin. Another possible example of racial predilection to a particular cancer is the high frequency of nasopharyngeal carcinoma in Chinese.

Some assistance in separating heredity and racial susceptibility from environmental factors has been afforded by studies of cancer incidence in immigrant groups. If a cancer is truly hereditary, its high incidence in a racial group would be expected to remain relatively high despite transplantation of that group to a country where the incidence is low. If it is due to environmental factors, the incidence should decline as immigrant peoples modify their traditional dietary and behaviour patterns towards those of their new country.

The transmission of tumour-producing viruses from mother to offspring is a special situation which exists in some animal systems and is at least a theoretical possibility in man. This is discussed in the section on viral carcinogenesis.

Environmental factors

Each individual, with his inherited resistance or predisposition to cancer, encounters an enormous variety of potentially carcinogenic factors during life. The particular pattern depends upon geographical factors, dietary habits based on racial, social, religious and familial practices, socio-economic factors and the nature of occupational and leisure activities.

Geographical factors. The incidence of different cancers varies between countries and even between different areas of the same country. The situation is complicated by regional variations in behaviour patterns, but natural characteristics of different areas are important. These factors include hours of sunlight, the climate as it affects the prevalence of insect vectors of disease and the incidence of parasitic diseases, and the geology of the area with its effect upon the chemical composition of the soil and the background radioactivity of the environment.

Man also modifies geographical characteristics by industrial and domestic pollution of the atmosphere, rivers and seas, and by his use of radioactive materials in industry, power generation and weapons.

Dietary factors. Diets vary widely from area occupations is associated with exposure to specific carcinogens with a consequent high incidence of particular forms of malignancy. The first such association was observed by Percival Pott (also commemorated by Pott's fracture) who in 1775 recorded a high incidence of scrotal cancer in London chimney sweeps (Fig. 10.3). These individuals, who undoubtedly

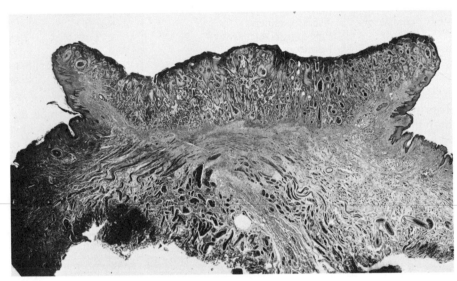

Fig. 10.3 Cancer arising from the epidermis of the scrotum in a chimney sweep. The tumour forms a raised plaque. Numerous small groups of tumour cells are seen invading the dermis. The dark fibres in the deep part of the tissue are cremasteric muscle. × 5.

to area and such variations seem inescapably linked to regional variations in cancer incidence. In addition to the nature and quantity of foods eaten, methods of food preparation and the chemical nature of the cooking vessels may be of importance in determining the presence or absence of carcinogens in the diet. Further possible sources of carcinogens are chemical fertilisers, insecticides, organic and inorganic chemicals fed to livestock, and the materials which are widely used in food preservation. Natural diseases of vegetables, fruits and livestock may be important as evidenced by the induction of liver cancer by aflatoxin, a fungal product found in ground nuts infected by *Aspergillus flavus*. Contamination of stored food is another potential source of trouble and it is likely that some baking flour is contaminated during storage by polyoma virus (a carcinogenic virus of wild mice).

Occupational factors. Employment in certain lacked washing facilities (and perhaps enthusiasm for this activity), retained carcinogenic soot in the rugose scrotal skin. A similar situation was discovered by Volkmann who, in 1874, recorded a high incidence of skin cancer in tar and mineral oil workers. Since that time numerous other examples have been recorded and further examples are given in Table 10.3. Since industry is continually introducing new techniques and using new chemicals, it is of the highest importance that physicians should remain alert to the occurrence of common tumours at an unusually high frequency or in an unusually young group of patients, and to the occurrence of unusual tumours. In fact the earliest warnings of a new carcinogenic hazard have often come from alert general practitioners caring for workers involved in a single factory or industry. In many countries, there are now stringent (although not always totally effective) regulations governing the safety

Table 10.3 Some Examples of Cancer Associated with Occupational Exposure to Carcinogens

Types of tumour	Occupational group	Carcinogen
Skin cancer	(a) Radiologists	(a) 'Soft' x-rays
	(b) Farmers and fishermen	(b) Ultraviolet light
Chronic myeloid leukaemia	Radiologists	'Hard' x-rays
Bladder cancer	Rubber workers	1-hydroxy-
	Aniline dye workers	2-naphthylamine
Lung cancer	(a) Miners	(a) ? Silica
	(b) Uranium miners	(b) γ-radiation
Mesothelioma of pleura or peritoneum	Asbestos miners	Asbestos
	Pipe-laggers, etc.	
Adenocarcinoma of nasopharynx	Furniture makers	Wood-dust
Angiosarcoma of liver	Polymerisation-chamber cleaners	Vinyl chloride monomer

checks necessary before new chemicals can be produced or used in bulk. When a chemical hazard is identified, the dangerous agent is eliminated if an acceptable alternative can be found, or failing this a range of protective measures is devised and enforced.

Bladder cancer was known to occur with relatively high frequency in workers in the aniline dye industry and the compound 2-naphthylamine was suspected from analysis of the occupational histories of affected individuals. Initial studies in a range of laboratory animals suggested that this compound was not carcinogenic. However, feeding it to dogs for 5 years produced bladder tumours and it was found that dogs and men convert the bulk of the non-carcinogenic 2-naphthylamine to carcinogenic 1-hydroxy-2-naphthylamine in the kidney. This compound is excreted in the urine and may induce carcinoma in the transitional epithelium lining the urinary tract, and particularly, because of its relatively large surface area, in the bladder. Most species of animals convert 2-naphthylamine to non-carcinogenic substances such as glucuronides, and this explains the initially negative studies of naphthylamine carcinogenicity. Legislation on the use of 2-naphthylamine followed and urinary-tract cancer was eliminated as a hazard to dye-workers. More recently, however, a high incidence of bladder cancer was observed in workers in rubber tyre factories: this was found to be caused by the contamination of 1-naphthylamine, used as a rubber-curing agent, by 2-naphthylamine.

Another industrial cancer risk, discovered much more recently, occurs in asbestos miners and the industrial users of asbestos (pipe laggers and those involved in insulation) who have an unusually high risk of developing pleural or peritoneal mesotheliomas and bronchial carcinomas as a result of the inhalation or ingestion of asbestos. Since the actual duration of exposure to asbestos may have been short, and the time between exposure and tumour development is many years, a detailed occupational history is vital in tracing the relationship between cancer and exposure to asbestos.

One of the most recent cancer hazards suspected is the development of angiosarcomas of liver (usually an exceedingly rare tumour) in workers involved in the production of the plastic, polyvinylchloride (PVC). PVC is produced by the polymerisation of vinyl chloride monomer (VCM) and it is this latter compound which appears to be carcinogenic. The workers apparently most at risk are those who clean out the polymerisation tanks in which relatively high concentrations of VCM persist. Safety precautions and safe working conditions for these employees are at present receiving urgent consideration.

Progress, however, may not always reduce the hazards or may introduce new dangers. Early radiologists frequently calibrated their machines by exposing their own arms. This cumulative exposure to x-rays was carcinogenic, but as the early x-rays were 'soft' and did not penetrate deeply through the skin, their tumours were accessible squamous carcinomas of the epidermis which could be successfully treated surgically. Later, however, despite the recognition of the hazard and introduction of safe practices, the use of 'harder', more penetrating x-rays led to a raised incidence of deeper tumours, and particularly to the development of chronic myeloid leukaemia originating in the haemopoietic marrow as a result of the capacity of bone matrix to impede and scatter the x-rays. Further developments in safety techniques have now virtually abolished this problem.

Occupation may also have an indirect effect on cancer incidence by influencing personal habits, e.g. cigarette smoking and consumption of alcohol, which are the norm or are acceptable responses to the stresses of the particular employment.

Socio-economic factors. The incidence of different forms of cancer varies between different socio-economic groups, reflecting differences in environment, diet, occupational and leisure activities. Malnutrition is believed to be related to the high incidence of carcinoma of the liver seen in certain areas in Africa. At the other extreme, diseases such as breast carcinoma, malignant melanoma and carcinoma of the colon are undoubtedly becoming more frequent in the affluent, technologically advanced countries of Western Europe and North America. The particular aspects of life in these countries responsible for the observed variations in cancer incidence have not yet been identified.

Chemical carcinogenic agents

In addition to the examples provided above, many chemicals, physical agents and some viruses have been shown experimentally to induce cancer in animals.

In 1917 Yamagiwa and Ichikawa induced carcinomas and tumours resembling human molluscum sebaceum (p. 986) by painting the ears of rabbits with tar. Since that time a very large number of compounds have been tested for carcinogenicity on experimental animals, mainly mice and rats. The experimental design has varied little. Suspected carcinogens are applied by whatever route is appropriate, either alone or combined with co-carcinogens, anticarcinogens or with various manipulations of the animal's hormonal, general metabolic or immunological status. Certain general rules have emerged from such studies.

1. A large number of chemicals have been demonstrated to be carcinogenic.

2. A minimum dose of each chemical—*the threshold dose*—is necessary for carcinogenesis. This is similar for repeated experiments employing the same chemicals and species but varies for different chemicals and between different strains and species. Subthreshold doses of carcinogen will cause tumours only if combined with or followed by either a subthreshold dose of another carcinogenic agent or a co-carcinogen.

3. Once a sufficient dose of carcinogen has been applied, the animal will inevitably develop a tumour, although no morphological, cytological or biochemical abnormalities can usually be detected in the 'target' cells immediately following the period of administration of the carcinogen.

4. There is a *latent period*, which may be prolonged, and is of characteristic length for each chemical/species combination, between carcinogen exposure and tumour development.

5. Tumour development and progression are not dependent upon the continued application of the chemical once the carcinogenic dose has been applied.

6. Some carcinogens act specifically on one organ and this usually implies that the compound is actively metabolised or concentrated in that organ, e.g. the azo-dyes in the liver (see below). Other carcinogens are non-specific in their action and affect sites of maximum exposure, which are often determined by the route of administration of the carcinogen.

7. The physicochemical nature of the carcinogen is important. The effect of a readily soluble material such as urethane, which diffuses widely through the body, is different from that of a relatively insoluble material such as benzpyrene, which remains for some time at the site of application.

Azo-dyes and liver cancer. Carcinogenesis in the liver has been much studied, partly because the liver is a conveniently large organ for biochemical and other investigations, partly because geographical variations in incidence of primary liver cancer in man point strongly to the existence of carcinogens, identification of which might be of great practical value.

There are many liver carcinogens which are relatively non-specific in action. General carcinogens such as acetyl-amino-fluorene can produce liver cancers. Many liver poisons, such as carbon tetrachloride, are not directly carcinogenic, but in certain circumstances cause hepatic cirrhosis, which predisposes to the development of cancer of the liver. There are several with a more specific action, of which *Senecio* alkaloids and *aflatoxin* may prove important (p. 639), but the agents most studied are the *azo-dyes*.

Of these, *o*-amino-azotoluene was the first to be proved active, by Yoshida of Tokyo in 1931; *p*-dimethylamino-azobenzene ('butter yellow') is the most active. Fed to rats in large doses the dyes cause liver necrosis: with smaller doses immediate damage is relatively slight, but if the dosage is continued the liver shows progressive irregular hyperplasia and ultimately cancers develop after 9 months or more.

Dyes of this type are banned from all foodstuffs, and rarely if ever have any opportunity of causing tumours in man: indeed their recognition has probably been valuable in emphasising the need for screening tests on all dyes or similar materials added to food. The lessons which can be drawn from experiments with these dyes are, however, numerous and important.

(1) Cell loss and regeneration. Dye-induced liver damage leads to extensive and continuing loss of liver cells with a consequent high rate of cell regeneration, a cycle which predisposes to the development of cancer. A similar high cell turnover is probably also important in the development of cancers in chronic ulcers.

(2) Progressive change. The transition from normality to malignancy is progressive, probably with several successive stages, each of which seems to blend insensibly into its successor. This applies whether we consider the naked-eye appearance of the liver, the histology or the biochemistry. There is no sudden change from the normal to the malignant state.

(3) Selection of resistant strains of cells. The normal liver cell is damaged by the azo-dye, as shown by measuring oxygen uptake of liver slices exposed to a dilute solution of the dye. If the liver slices are taken from a rat which has been receiving the azo-dye by mouth for a few months, the depression of oxygen uptake produced by the dye *in vitro* is less than with a normal liver. With longer periods of feeding the depression becomes progressively less; when finally a tumour appears its oxygen consumption is found to have returned to normal. The

liver cells appear to become progressively adapted to life in the presence of the azo-dye: very probably this occurs by the selection of resistant strains of cells, just as culture of bacteria in the presence of an antibiotic favours resistant strains of the organism.

(4) Dye-binding. The dye becomes bound to the proteins of normal liver cells. This dye-binding is reduced with time, and little or no binding occurs with tumour cells. We have here an indication of one reason for the selective effect of the dye on the liver, and a possible explanation for the progressive escape of liver cells from the effect of the dye indicated above.

(5) Antigenic changes. In normal liver cells it is possible to demonstrate antigens specific to the liver of the species concerned. Some of these are absent from hepatic cancer cells. There is evidence that the cells of chemically-induced tumours acquire new, tumour-specific antigens (p. 266).

(6) Effect of malnutrition. Production of tumours is much easier in rats on a poor diet. With butter-yellow it has been shown that most of this effect depends on a deficiency of riboflavin, which is required for a detoxification process which involves removal of one of the two terminal methyl groups. Since most geographical areas of high liver-cancer incidence in man are also areas of malnutrition, this may be important; it could well be that in such areas tumours result from exposure to some unrecognised substance which is detoxified, and so rendered harmless, in the well-nourished.

The nature of chemical carcinogens. Thousands of chemicals can produce tumours. The first group of compounds to be identified were the carcinogenic hydrocarbons, discovered by Kennaway, Cook and Heiger in 1931. Important compounds in this group include dibenzanthracene (the first compound identified), benzpyrene (the active compound of soot and tar) and dimethylbenzanthracene. Methylcholanthrene does not occur naturally but is widely used in cancer research. Other compounds used as experimental carcinogens include 2-anthramine, 2-acetyl-aminofluorene and urethane.

A lot has been learned about the structure of chemical carcinogens and their metabolic handling, but few general principles have emerged, and it is usually not possible to predict from its structure how carcinogenic a particular chemical will be. Carcinogenicity also varies considerably with species, and testing for it is a complex and exacting procedure, which is essential if we are to avoid the occurrence of tragedies due to the introduction of carcinogens into drugs, dyes, food, antibiotics, cosmetics and so forth.

The mode of action of chemical carcinogens. This is poorly understood. There are certainly alterations in the chemical composition of the membranes of carcinogen-transformed cells (p. 266) and this suggests that cellular DNA and/or RNA has been altered by exposure to the carcinogen. Some carcinogens probably enter the cell by endocytic vesicles which include that part of the plasma membrane to which the carcinogen is bound. It has been suggested that chemical carcinogens may act by switching on a latent oncogenic virus already present in the cell or by bringing to completion a provirus, that is a virus whose DNA is incorporated in the cell genome but which does not, without an appropriate developing stimulus, affect the host cell.

Physical agents in carcinogenesis

The main physical factor concerned with tumour formation is radiant energy, and much is known of this important form of carcinogenesis. Other predisposing factors, such as mechanical trauma, chronic irritation and the tendency for cancer to develop in scars, are difficult to study and their role in carcinogenesis is poorly understood.

Radiant energy. A detailed account of the effects of radiation on cells is included in Chapter 1. Radiation of diverse kinds, x-rays, α, β and γ rays and ultraviolet light all induce tumours in man and animals. They produce effects by release of energy during their passage through the tissues with resulting alteration of various cellular molecules, including the nucleic acids. The most important long-term consequence of these events is an increased rate of mutation in the irradiated cells. The degree of effect on a tissue depends largely on the total radiation dose, physical characteristics of the radiations (such as their penetrating capacity), and on features of the affected tissues, such as density, mitotic rate, and the nature of their blood supply. Thus short exposure to a high concentration of radiation, as occurred in those exposed to the atomic bomb or to accidents involving nuclear apparatus, and oft-repeated exposure to low doses of radiation, as occurred in the early radiologists, may equally be carcinogenic. Tumours may arise in tissues affected by radiation necrosis (p. 28) and also in those where direct radiation injury appears to have been relatively slight.

The experience of the early **x-ray workers** has been described (p. 256) and indicates clearly the carcinogenic hazards against which workers employing radiant energy must be protected.

The effects of **radio-isotopes** depend on the dosage, and the site of absorption of the radiation produced. Inhaled radioactive dust is likely to produce lung cancers (p. 443). Radio-iodine produces thyroid tumours experimentally because it is concentrated within the gland: external irradiation of the neck with x-rays can produce much the same effect.

The situation with ultraviolet light (UV) is interesting. Long continued exposure to UV, such as occurs in outdoor workers, is associated with the occurrence of basal cell carcinomas, squamous carcinomas, and less often malignant melanomas, all of which arise in those areas of the skin exposed to light. Those most at risk are pale skinned individuals who tan poorly, albinos, and especially those with the genetic predisposition of xeroderma pigmentosum (p. 254). In sunny countries such as Australia, however, the frequency of these skin tumours has reached almost epidemic proportions and affects relatively young people as compared with most other cancers, with some predilection for those of higher socio-economic groups.

Trauma and chronic irritation. Many patients ascribe the onset of a visible (usually skin) tumour to some specific incident of trauma. It is difficult to understand how a gross mechanical injury could cause neoplasia, and it seems likely that, in most cases, an already growing tumour becomes more liable to injury and that this draws the patient's attention to the lesion— *traumatic determinism*. It is possible, however, that mechanical trauma may be important in a few cancers.

Chronic irritation, which could also be regarded as repeated minor trauma, seems important in squamous carcinomas of the mouth associated with ill-fitting dentures and in those cancers which arise in association with longstanding sinuses opening onto the skin. Also, malignant melanoma in African negroes occurs mainly on the soles of the feet of those who go barefoot.

Scars. Tumours do not ordinarily arise in a burn scar or surgical wound scar on a rabbit's skin. But if one paints a carcinogen evenly over an area which includes such a scar, the tumours appear first (and grow largest) in relation to the scar. 'Burn cancers' of man, or 'brand cancers' of animals, occur almost always in areas exposed to excessive sunlight or similar carcinogenic stimulus. Scars thus seem to act as 'co-carcinogens'. The development of cancer in chronic gastric ulcers, but not in the closely similar duodenal ulcers, is explicable on the view that the ulcer scar is acting as a co-carcinogen, but that in the duodenum there is no effective carcinogenic stimulus.

Hormones in the causation of tumours

In general, any induced change of hormone level which causes prolonged hyperplasia of a target organ may cause tumours of the latter, but there are many exceptions. The following are the best known experimental situations.

Oestrogens can undoubtedly cause tumours in susceptible strains of mice; their administration in excess leads to an increased incidence of cancer of the breast in females and the appearance of cancer in males. Reduction of natural oestrogen levels by oophorectomy abolishes cancer of the breast in susceptible females. It might seem that the excessive proliferation of breast ducts induced by oestrogen, carried to excess, has been the actual cause of the cancer. But, as mentioned below, the oestrogens appear to act effectively only in the presence of the mammary tumour virus in mice. In virus-free mice (and in other species) the effect is much harder to demonstrate. In tissues other than the breast the position becomes somewhat anomalous. The most obvious oestrogen target organ, the endometrium, rarely develops tumours in treated animals, though connective-tissue tumours of the uterus are often produced and tumours result also in organs not usually regarded as oestrogen-responsive, for example the kidney in the hamster, and the Leydig cells of the testis in the mouse. These effects appear

to depend only on the oestrogen-activity of the various compounds concerned, and not on their precise structure.

There is controversy over whether oestrogen therapy causes endometrial carcinoma in women. Certainly it produces hyperplasia which can be mistaken for carcinoma. There is also an association between endometrial carcinoma and the oestrogen-secreting granulosa-cell tumours of the ovary.

A good deal has been made of the similarity between the basic ring structure of some of the carcinogenic hydrocarbons—especially methylcholanthrene which has oestrogenic activity in the rat—and the steroid hormones. Various hypothetical transformations of steroid components of bile and sebum have also been based on this resemblance, but there is no solid evidence for any of these attractive speculations.

Disturbances of the pituitary feed-back mechanism. The following three examples, probably the most striking in the endocrine field, all depend on pituitary hormones.

(*a*) *FSH-induced ovarian granulosa-cell tumours.* The ovary is stimulated to various activities, including the secretion of oestrogens, by the follicle-stimulating hormone of the pituitary. A rise of oestrogen level in blood reaching the pituitary reduces the output of FSH, so that the system stabilises. Biskind removed the ovaries of rats and implanted pieces in the spleen. Oestrogen secreted by the grafts in this position passes into the portal blood, and so all of it is carried direct to the liver and is there inactivated by the normal hydroxylation process. Thus very little reaches the pituitary in active form, and FSH rises. This stimulates the grafts both to grow and to secrete oestrogen, but even the excessive oestrogen so produced is prevented from reaching the pituitary. Prolonged over-stimulation of the grafts leads finally to the appearance of granulosa-cell tumours. Although a fascinating experiment, this has no known relation to any situation occurring in man.

(*b*) *Thyroidectomy tumours of the pituitary.* The similar thyroid-pituitary feed-back, with thyroid-stimulating hormone increasing the secretion of thyroid hormone, and a rise of thyroid hormone lowering the secretion of TSH, can lead experimentally to tumours of either organ. If the thyroid is surgically excised or obliterated with radio-iodine, secretion of TSH is raised. In some strains of mice the TSH-secreting cells proliferate so actively under this stimulus that they give rise to malignant tumours of the pituitary. It is a point of special interest about these tumours that they can at first be transplanted only to other mice which have also lost their thyroids, but that after several passages they become resistant to thyroid hormone and can be transplanted to normal mice. Again, there is no evidence of any comparable tumours occurring in man: patients with myxoedema, for instance, do not develop pituitary tumours.

(*c*) *TSH-induced thyroid carcinoma.* If the normal output of thyroid hormones is blocked by thiouracil or other goitrogenic drugs, TSH rises and stimulates thyroid proliferation. In rats, if this is continued for long enough, metastasising thyroid tumours may arise. Even after metastasis to the lungs, such tumours may regress if the goitrogen is stopped. This is a slow and uncertain way of producing thyroid cancers: the combination of a goitrogen with a chemical carcinogen (such as 2-acetyl-amino-fluorene), or with radio-iodine in doses insufficient to cause major damage to the gland, is much more effective than either alone.

This type of experimental tumour is less irrelevant to human cancer than the two preceding. Longstanding TSH-induced goitres, whether due to iodine deficiency or to one of the congenital defects of iodine metabolism, seem to carry a small but significant risk of development of cancer.

Hormone-dependent tumours. The pituitary and thyroid tumours just mentioned both may be 'hormone-dependent' in the sense that they may regress if the hormonal stimulus that invoked them is removed. Related phenomena in man are few, but the following three carcinomas deserve mention. (1) Most **prostatic carcinomas** are sufficiently dependent on a normal male hormonal environment to regress for long periods if oestrogens are given. (2) Some differentiated **thyroid carcinomas** are partially responsive to TSH, and their rate of growth and spread may be reduced or arrested by continued administration of thyroxin which suppresses secretion of TSH by the pituitary. (3) Some **breast carcinomas** regress under a variety of hormonal manipulations—treatment with male hormones or even oestrogens, oophorectomy, adrenalectomy, hypophysectomy. Application of these is largely empirical, and has not so far led to an increased understanding of the tumours concerned. Just as the hormone-dependent pituitary tumours become independent after serial transplantation, the tumours in man practically always ultimately resume growth, though with the thyroid and prostatic carcinomas the period of arrest and partial regression is often very long.

Viruses and tumours

That some human tumours may be caused in part by viruses is an appealing concept, for it raises the possibility of prophylactic vaccination of individuals and populations at risk.

The study of viruses and cancer (viral oncology) is one of the most active areas of current cancer research, but as long ago as 1911 Peyton Rous showed that a sarcoma (i.e. a malignant tumour of connective-tissue origin) of domestic fowls could be transmitted by a cell-free filtrate of the tumour. **Rous sarcoma** virus is an RNA virus related to the myxo-viruses which, in addition to causing the development of sarcomas *in vivo*, can rapidly cause transformation of cells in tissue culture. **Fowl leukosis**, a very variable neoplasm of lymphoid cells, was noted to be transferable by cell free filtrates in 1908, but leukaemia was not recognised as neoplastic at that time and the significance of the finding was not appreciated. Fowl leukosis is caused by an RNA virus which is transmitted to the offspring in the ovum: viral passage in this manner is known as *vertical transmission*, while spread of infection from animal to animal after birth is termed *horizontal transmission*.

Several mammalian tumours were transmitted by cell-free filtrates in the 1930s. Harmless wart-like tumours (**Shope papillomas**) are endemic among the wild cotton-tail rabbits of America and are spread naturally by contact. In the natural host species, tumours develop 21 days after natural contact or the application of a cell-free filtrate of the tumour and rarely if ever become malignant. By contrast, exposure of the domestic rabbit (a separate but related species) to Shope papilloma filtrates induces tumours which are frequently malignant. This was the first example of the important general finding that viruses which do not cause malignant tumours in their natural host species may have this effect in related species in which they are not usually present. Filtrates of the *Shope virus* tumours of *domestic* rabbits are not infective and complete virus cannot be demonstrated in them. However, sophisticated immunological and biochemical tests indicate the presence of at least part of the viral genome integrated into the DNA of the tumour cells.

It may appear that the situations described

above suggest that the viruses are the unique cause of the tumours which develop. However, many factors influence the development of these tumours and not all animals infected with the viruses develop tumours. An excellent example of the complexity of the processes involved is provided by the pathology and epidemiology of breast cancers induced by **Bittner milk factor**. By selective breeding, strains of mice were established in which virtually all the females developed breast cancer late in life, and other strains in which this tumour was rare. This looked like a genetic effect until it was found by Bittner that female neonates of a low-cancer strain suckled by foster mothers of a high-cancer strain frequently developed breast cancer. By contrast, high-cancer strain offspring suckled on low-cancer foster mothers did not develop cancer (Fig. 10.4). Thus the carcino-

genic influence was transmitted by the milk in the post-natal period *and not* by germ cells nor transplacentally by the mother. Investigations with filtrates of 'high-cancer milk', cell-free filtrates of mammary tumour, and electron microscopic studies of milk and tumour tissue, have confirmed that the active principle is a virus, *mouse mammary tumour virus*.

Female neonates which have been infected with the virus are protected from breast cancer by removal of the ovaries, and male neonates infected with the virus only develop breast cancer if given large doses of oestrogens. Thus oestrogenic activity is a necessary co-factor for this virus-induced tumour.

The viruses discussed above all tend to produce a single type of tumour or a restricted range of tumours, usually only in one species of host. **Polyoma virus** is a DNA virus which is endemic in wild mice, and horizontal spread to mature mice causes few, if any, tumours. Infection of neonatal mice, however, induces a wide range of carcinomas and sarcomas which arise in many different organs. This virus will also produce tumours in neonatal rats, rabbits, ferrets and hamsters. In cell cultures, the virus can replicate within cells, causing their destruction (cytopathic effect). It can also transform cells so that they multiply rapidly and acquire other tumour-like features: in cultures, they grow irregularly, piled on top of one another, instead of forming an orderly monolayer (i.e. *loss of contact inhibition*—Fig. 10.5): on injection into suitable host animals, they form tumours. The virus has not replicated in transformed cells and cannot readily be recovered from them. *Polyoma virus* can thus replicate in and destroy a cell or it can transform it: it cannot do both in the same cell. In mouse cell cultures, the virus replicates in and destroys most cells, but a few are transformed. In hamster cells, only transformation occurs. This explains why the virus is transmissible among mice and also causes tumours in neonatal mice, whereas in the hamsters it is not transmissible but can produce tumours from which it is not readily recovered. This is an unusually clear-cut example of viral integration into the host cell genome: it occurs, with variations, in other virus tumours, for instance in the Shope-virus carcinomas in the domestic rabbit (see above). The virus DNA becomes part of the cell and is transmitted by mitosis: it influences cellular activities, but

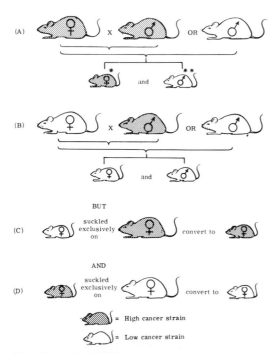

Fig. 10.4 Discovery of the Bittner milk factor. The incidence of breast cancer was high in the daughters of 'high-cancer' strain *mothers* (A), but low in the daughters of 'high-cancer' strain *fathers* (B). The strain of female on which neonates were suckled (C and D) was then found to determine the incidence of cancer, showing the importance of a milk factor, since shown to be a virus. Oophorectomy* reduces the incidence of breast cancer in virus-infected females, and oestrogen** increases the incidence in virus-infected males.

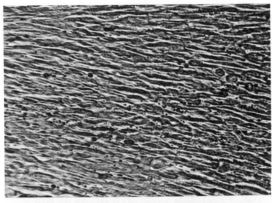

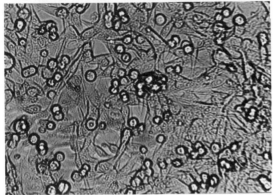

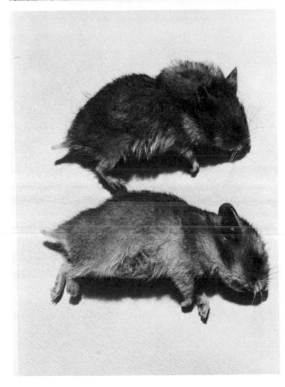

can be detected only by the presence of new cell surface antigens and by the identification of viral nucleic acids or virus-coded enzymes within the cell.

Oncogenic RNA viruses. Rapid and important advances are being made in virus-induced leukaemia in a wide range of species from snakes to higher primates. Proof of a leukaemia-producing virus in man is still lacking, but evidence of it is accumulating rapidly. The *oncogenic RNA viruses* (*Oncornaviruses*) have an RNA core and an envelope which consists partly of the host-cell plasma membrane and which includes components allowing the virus to attach to receptors on host cell surfaces. During some stages of replication the virus particles are visible by electron microscopy and have a characteristic morphology (C-type particles) (Fig. 10.6). In occasional cells, however, the virus does not replicate, but its RNA codes for the synthesis of a remarkable enzyme, termed *DNA polymerase* or *reverse transcriptase*, which promotes the synthesis of specific DNA sequences, using the virus RNA as a template. The DNA thus produced is integrated into the host cell genome and is transmitted to daughter cells as described for polyoma virus. It should be noted that this is a reversal of orthodox nucleic acid production in which DNA is used as a template on which messenger RNA is synthesised. Various methods are now available for identification of the reverse transcriptase, DNA and RNA of oncornaviruses and thus of demonstrating the presence of the integrated virus. Confirmation can be obtained by techniques of viral 'rescue', i.e. activation of integrated viruses (proviruses) by agencies such as x-rays, carcinogens and even by ageing of the host cells.

Huebner and Todaro have postulated that latent, integrated, potentially oncogenic viruses (*oncogenes*) exist in the cells of all humans. They postulate that standard carcinogenic

Fig. 10.5 Cultures of hamster fibroblasts (*above*). The upper culture shows formation of a regular monolayer. The lower culture is infected with polyoma virus and shows cellular pleomorphism and loss of contact inhibition, the cells being piled on top of one another. The upper hamster (*below*) was injected with the polyoma-transformed cells which have grown to form a tumour. The lower hamster was injected with the uninfected cells, and has remained healthy. (Mrs. Joan McNab.)

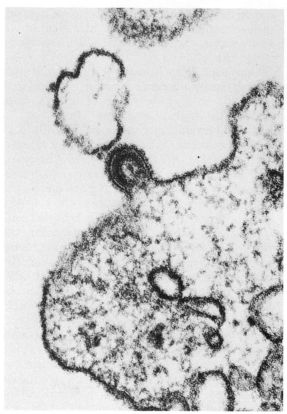

Fig. 10.6 A part of a cell from a cat infected with feline leukaemia virus, showing formation of a virion by budding from the cell surface. Note that the envelope is formed from the plasma membrane, and that the virus particle becomes coated with an outer spiky layer. The section happens to include part of another cell immediately above the virion. × 80 000. (Dr. Helen Laird.)

leukocytes in cats. Spread is usually by horizontal transmission and infected cats excrete large amounts of infectious virus. Infection does not necessarily cause neoplasia and many cats merely develop antibodies against the FeLV antigens. Cats of 'low socio-economic status', which roam freely, are much more likely to be infected with FeLV, and to receive greater dosage, than carefully nurtured housecats. The development of neoplasia appears to be related to the dose of FeLV to which the animal is exposed, probably because in high dosage the virus causes immunodepression. Vertical transmission may also occur and the virus will often remain silent in an integrated form in the host cells for up to ten years after birth. The antibodies to FeLV appear to have a protective effect and animals with tumours have low or undetectable titres of these antibodies. Vaccines containing living attenuated or killed virus have been shown to protect cats against FeLV-induced neoplasia, even when they are administered early in the latent period following infection with the virus.

Viruses and human cancer

The induction of neoplasia by oncogenic viruses has now been demonstrated in several species, and it is therefore likely that viruses are implicated in carcinogenesis in man. However, it must be stated quite unequivocally that, with the exception of the common wart, no human tumour has yet been proved to be caused by a virus. The problem lies not in the demonstration of viruses in association with human tumours, but in proving that they play a causal role and are not merely harmless 'passengers'. In other species, this problem is solved by infecting animals with the suspected virus and observing them for the appearance of tumours. In man, the evidence is necessarily circumstantial.

Leukaemias and lymphomas. It is becoming increasingly apparent, from observations like those in cats, outlined above, that a whole range of leukaemias and lymphomas in various species are caused by oncornaviruses. It would be surprising if man were the exception, and indeed preliminary observations have demonstrated evidence of oncornavirus infection in patients with acute leukaemias. It seems very likely that these and related conditions will be shown to have a viral etiology, in which case

agents activate the oncogenes with the consequent development of a tumour. This interesting idea remains unproved, but it is now known that integrated RNA viruses are ubiquitous in mammalian cells. Not all such viruses are, however, oncogenic.

Oncornavirus was first identified in 1959 by Gross, who injected cell-free extracts of mouse leukaemia cells into neonatal mice: these subsequently developed leukaemia. Many different oncornaviruses have since been identified in a wide range of species. One such agent, the *feline leukaemia virus (FeLV)* has been studied intensively in Glasgow by Jarrett and his colleagues. It has been shown to cause a whole range of neoplastic conditions of the lymphoid cells and prophylactic vaccination may become practicable.

There is recent evidence of a high incidence of **Hodgkin's disease** (a human lymphoma which has no counterpart in oncornavirus-induced neoplasms of cats, etc.) in groups of people known to have had contact with one another: for example, the disease has been shown to have developed in several former classmates of a school in New York State some years after they had been pupils of a teacher who subsequently died of the condition. By analogy with the findings in animals, it is likely that the 'incubation period' of presumptive virus-induced human neoplasia will be long, and that only a minority of those infected will develop neoplasia. Accordingly, epidemiological studies are likely to be extremely complex.

Burkitt's lymphoma (BL). While working in East Africa, Burkitt recognised a rather unusual form of malignant disease—a lymphoma which affected children and young people of either sex, involved the maxillary area or intra-abdominal organs, particularly the ovaries, and had a rather characteristic histology. The tumour occurred only in parts of the region with particular climatic conditions, and this suggested that an insect vector might be involved. A consideration of different areas of the world indicated that similar climatic conditions existed in parts of Nigeria and in New Guinea and investigation of those areas revealed the presence there of a lymphoma similar to that described by Burkitt.

Laboratory studies showed that BL cells released a virus after maintenance in culture for some time. This was identified as a new member of the herpes group of viruses and was called the **Epstein-Barr** (EB) **virus**. Patients with BL all have high titres of antibodies to EB virus-dependent antigens formed within BL cells and on their plasma membranes. The virus can be recovered from most BL cell lines in culture. It replicates in and destroys some of the cells and transforms others by becoming integrated into their DNA. Antibodies to EB virus have also been detected in some patients with nasopharyngeal carcinoma, some forms of Hodgkin's disease and sporadically in various leukaemias; however, the titres of antibodies in these conditions are not as high as in BL.

EB virus is also the cause of the common form of *infectious mononucleosis* (an acute, self-limiting, febrile illness) and community studies have shown that most individuals are infected with EB virus in adolescence or as young adults, and develop antibodies to the virus: infection is followed by a clinical attack of infectious mononucleosis in only a small proportion of those infected. The causal role of EB virus in Burkitt's lymphoma is not proved. If it is the cause, then there must be special factors which determine this outcome: because of the similar geographical distribution of BL and chronic malaria in Africa, the immuno-suppressive effect of malaria has been suggested as a causal factor in BL.

Breast carcinoma. Virus particles similar to those of mouse mammary tumour virus (MuMTV) (p. 262) have been identified in human breast cancer cells and in milk from cancerous breasts. Materials capable of inhibiting MuMTV are present in the serum of breast cancer patients and lymphocytes sensitised to MuMTV antigens have also been reported. Here, then, is evidence of another viral association without proof of its aetiological significance.

Other human tumours. Herpes simplex virus type 2 has been associated with **carcinoma of the cervix uteri** on the basis of raised titres of antibodies to it in groups of women known to be at above average risk of developing the tumour. This includes prostitutes, and sexual intercourse, especially with uncircumcised males, appears to be a predisposing factor: one possible explanation is the carcinogenicity of smegma. It has been suggested that viruses are involved in the aetiology of osteosarcoma, neuroblastoma and possibly other tumours, on the basis of the finding that relatives and close contacts of patients with these tumours possess antibodies and specifically sensitised lymphocytes which react with cells cultured from the tumours of their contacts. A cytopathic effect, suggestive of viral infection, has also been observed in long-term cultures of osteosarcoma cells. More recently, the detection of factors suggestive of integrated RNA viruses (including reverse transcriptase, 70s RNA, and specifically hybridisable DNA and RNA) have been reported in malignant melanoma, leukaemia and various other human neoplasms. It has also been reported that the reverse transcriptase identified is characteristic of an oncogenic virus rather than an integrated non-oncogenic virus.

Immunological aspects of cancer

The natural history of cancer is not determined solely by the qualities of the tumour cells, but also by the host's reaction to them. As indicated below, there is good evidence that protective host mechanisms exist, and that although these are very often unsuccessful in preventing the growth and spread of malignant tumours, and only very rarely bring about their complete destruction, they may nevertheless restrict the rate of tumour growth and spread and contribute to the degree of success achieved by various forms of treatment.

The nature of the host defences is largely unknown, but it has been shown that the cells of human and animal tumours possess surface antigens which are sufficiently foreign to the host to stimulate an immune response. This important property of tumour cells raises the possibility of immunotherapy, and in consequence there is considerable interest in the immunology of cancer, some of the major features of which are summarised below.

Experimental animal studies

Much of the experimental work has involved transplantation experiments, and before the importance of 'transplant' alloantigens was appreciated, rejection of transplanted tumours was frequently observed, but is likely to have been due to histo-incompatibility rather than to a tumour-specific reaction. Since the importance of alloantigens was demonstrated in mice by Gorer, the provision, by close inbreeding, of syngeneic strains of mice and rats has greatly facilitated experimental cancer research, not only by eliminating the 'transplant' antigens as a cause of rejection, but also by excluding other genetically-determined variables and thus allowing the use of smaller numbers of animals.

Protection by specific immunity

Active immunity to tumours has been shown to afford protection against subsequent challenge with the same tumour. Such immunity can be achieved by implanting a tumour into an animal and subsequently excising it, or by inoculating the animal with: (*a*) a number of living tumour cells too small to produce a tumour (the existence of a 'subthreshold' dose is itself evidence of a capacity to deal with small numbers of tumour cells); (*b*) larger numbers of tumour cells made incapable of dividing by irradiation or cytotoxic drugs; (*c*) membrane preparations of tumour cells. Protection against virus-induced tumours can also be provided by administering small amounts of the virus before challenging with the tumour. Only partial protection is provided by these procedures: it varies from tumour to tumour and can be overcome by injecting large numbers of tumour cells.

Tumour-cell antigens. The antigens which render the tumour cell susceptible to immunological attack must be exposed on the tumour-cell surface, and must be foreign to the host. The cells of both human and animal tumours have the surface antigens characteristic of normal cells of the species, and also genetically-determined alloantigens (e.g. H2 antigens in mice and HL-A antigens in man) which are characteristic of the cells of the individual (or inbred strain) in which the tumour originated. Both of these types of antigen may be reduced in frequency on the tumour cell surface. Being present on normal cells, they do not stimulate immunity to the tumour. There are, however, surface antigens which cannot be detected on normal cells. In experimental carcinogenesis, these apparently tumour-specific antigens are in part dependent on the agent which has induced the tumour. All the tumours produced in animals by any one oncogenic virus have been found to have common and relatively strong virus-coded antigens on the surface of the tumour cells. It follows that a vaccine prepared from the cells of a virus-induced tumour will confer immunity against the oncogenic activity of that virus and also against transplants of any tumour induced by it. This has been demonstrated experimentally. By contrast, tumours induced by chemical carcinogens or by physical agents have, at best, only weak common shared antigens: they develop stronger and apparently tumour-specific antigens, but these differ for each tumour, even when multiple tumours are induced in the same animal by the same carcinogen.

In vitro techniques of investigating antibodies

(p. 89) and cell-mediated immunity (p. 94) to tumours have also been used in experimental cancer, and are obviously more readily applicable to man than transplantation experiments. Both antibodies and cell-mediated immunity to tumour cells have been demonstrated to develop in animals bearing tumours. In general, these responses are more readily demonstrable when the tumour is small, and as it enlarges and spreads they tend to diminish or disappear. Both types of response have been observed to be more readily detectable after excision of the tumour, and then to diminish gradually unless the tumour recurs or is re-introduced into the animal.

Both *in-vivo* and *in-vitro* investigations indicate that any protection provided by specific immunity against solid tumours is due mainly to cell-mediated immunity. Antibodies appear to afford little protection, and may indeed enhance the growth of the tumour (see below). By contrast, antibody affords some protection against the neoplastic cells present in the blood in leukaemia and the cells of 'ascites tumours' which grow as a cell suspension in the pleura or peritoneum and induce an inflammatory exudate.

Enhancement and 'blocking' factors. The injection into animals of antibody to the surface antigens of tumour cells has been observed, under certain conditions, to reduce the dose of the tumour cells necessary to cause a tumour, and to enhance the growth of a previously-implanted tumour. This *experimental enhancement* of tumour growth is antigen-specific; it appears to be due to the antibody combining with antigen on the surface of the tumour cells and thus protecting them from attack by specifically primed lymphocytes. In other words, the antibody blocks the delayed hypersensitivity reaction of T lymphocytes with the tumour cells. In animals with large and progressing tumours, *blocking factors* have been detected in the serum; they have been shown to interfere with the killing of tumour cells *in vitro* by specifically-primed lymphocytes. It now seems unlikely that these are antibodies, for they disappear rapidly from the blood after excision of the tumour, at a time when the level of antibody increases. Other possibilities are that the blocking factors are free antigen molecules shed by the tumour cells as part of the normal turnover of plasma membrane constituents, or

such antigens combined with antibody, i.e. immune complexes. Free antigen or immune complexes are capable of combining with the tumour-specific receptors on the surface of T lymphocytes or 'specifically armed' macrophages (p. 130), thus preventing them from reacting with tumour cells: immune complexes might, in addition, bind to the Fc receptor sites of 'K' lymphocytes (p. 123) or macrophages, thus inhibiting their antibody-dependent cytotoxic activity for the tumour cells.

Immunology of cancer in man

Once a cancer has spread beyond the possibility of excision, it usually progresses, and eventually proves fatal. There are, however, considerable variations in the rate of growth, even for tumours of the same type and histological appearances. In patients with carcinoma of the breast, for example, surgical excision is sometimes followed by many years of normal health, but with subsequent re-appearance and relatively rapid growth of tumour in the operation scar or of metastases: this is sometimes observed also with some other cancers. Very rarely, complete spontaneous regression of a cancer occurs. Partial regression is more common, and it is not very unusual for patients with metastatic melanoma to have no obvious primary tumour: examination sometimes reveals an area of skin depigmentation which on histological examination shows evidence of a regressing malignant melanoma.

Observations of the sort outlined above suggest that defence mechanisms against cancer can develop in the host, and that in some instances these are partially or even wholly effective. The nature of host defence in these instances is unknown, but there is circumstantial evidence that specific immune responses may influence the course of some tumours. In the rapidly growing form of breast cancer termed encephaloid cancer, for example, a favourable prognosis following excision has been reported to show some correlation with lymphocytic infiltration of the cancer, and this suggests that a delayed hypersensitivity reaction, or possibly antibody-dependent lymphocyte cytotoxic activity, is involved. Seminoma, a rapidly growing carcinoma originating in the germinal epithelium of the testis, is very commonly infiltrated with large numbers of lymphocytes and may also contain tubercle-like macrophage granulomas, both of which are consistent with a delayed hypersensitivity reaction. This may explain why the cure-rate is unusually high for such a rapidly progressing cancer: even when there is extensive metastasis, radiotherapy is often curative. A third example of a cancer which is often highly susceptible to therapy is choriocarcinoma arising from the placental trophoblast. Although it grows and spreads very rapidly, this rare tumour can often be arrested, and sometimes destroyed, by cytotoxic drug therapy. It is, however, unique among human tumours, for it is a tumour of fetal tissue which grows in the mother; the tumour cells thus have HL-A antigens which are inherited from the father and are foreign to the maternal host, so that allograft rejection is likely to contribute to the success of therapy.

Immune responses. As in animal studies, antibodies and lymphocytes which react specifically with tumour cells have been demonstrated by *in vitro* techniques in patients with various types of cancer. They react with the patient's own tumour cells and with the cells of other tumours of similar type, a finding which is consistent with a viral aetiology: they are most often detectable in patients with early cancer, and tend to diminish as the tumour enlarges and spreads. Blocking factors, similar to those in animals (see above) also appear in the blood, particularly when the cancer is advanced. These observations are based on recent work, and the prognostic significance of fluctuations in the immune responses is not yet known. The antigenic preparations have consisted of whole tumour cells or crude homogenates or extracts, and the apparently tumour-specific cell-surface antigens have not yet been fully characterised.

There is at present considerable interest in the so-called *onco-fetal antigens*. These are products of cancer cells which are also produced by immature cells in the embryo, but only in much smaller amounts by normal mature cells. The two best-known examples are *alpha-feto-protein*, which is present in the serum of some patients with liver-cell cancer, and Gold's carcino-embryonic antigen (CEA). The increased levels of CEA in the serum of patients with cancer of the gut, and in the serum and urine in cancer of the urinary tract, provide useful

evidence of post-operative recurrence of these tumours, but high levels do not necessarily indicate cancer, for they occur also in pregnancy, in heavy smokers, and in various neoplastic and non-neoplastic conditions. These 'onco-fetal' cell products have been termed antigens mainly because antibodies produced in animals are used for their detection and assay. There is no good evidence that they are immunogenic to the host.

Immunodepression and cancer. The induction and growth of tumours in experimental animals are facilitated by procedures such as neonatal thymectomy, which depress the immunity system. In man, there is evidence that the incidence of cancer is increased in individuals with congenital immunodeficiency diseases, and in patients receiving prolonged immunosuppressive therapy to prevent rejection of a renal allograft. These observations support the view of Burnet that one of the functions of the immunity system is to detect and destroy antigenically abnormal cells, including neoplastic or potentially neoplastic cells. Such *immune surveillance* may be responsible for preventing many cancers, and those which appear may do so as a result of the (perhaps *relatively* infrequent) breakdown of the surveillance mechanism. It may be significant that most cancers occur in old age, for there is no doubt that immune responsiveness declines in the elderly, but prolonged exposure to environmental carcinogenic factors and the long latent period of human cancers could also account for the age incidence. Tests for immune responsiveness to various antigens have not, in general, revealed immunodepression in patients with early cancer as compared with age-matched control subjects. Advanced cancer patients commonly show evidence of immunodepression, but this is most obvious in those with tumours which invade and destroy the lymphoid tissues, and is likely to *result* from the cancer.

The prospect of immunotherapy. The possibility of immunotherapy for cancer has been appreciated since the early 1900s. The more recent advances in tumour immunology, outlined above, have strengthened the scientific basis of such treatment, but they have also demonstrated that, in spite of the occurrence of anti-cancer immune responses in many patients, their tumours still progress and cause death. It remains possible, however, that boosting the immune response might have some therapeutic effect. The administration of BCG, which acts as an adjuvant (p. 94) in immune responses, has been attempted in various neoplastic conditions, and has been claimed to have some effect in acute lymphoblastic leukaemia: in other neoplastic conditions, conclusions must await further trials. Various attempts have also been made to stimulate active specific immunity by implanting pieces of tumour which have been excised and treated with x-irradiation to prevent the cells from dividing. Such a procedure is not very hopeful, for if the patient's tumour does not stimulate effective immunity it seems unlikely that the implanted cells will do so, but it remains possible that, by increasing the antigenicity of the implanted cells, e.g. by coupling with haptens, or by using homologous tumour with its 'foreign' transplant antigens, the immune response to the relevant tumour antigens may be augmented. Attempts have also been made to provide passive immunity by transplanting tumour to a volunteer in the hope that therapeutically effective antibody will be produced. On at least one occasion, the volunteer failed to reject the transplanted tumour, which proved to be fatal.

Immunotherapy of cancer patients faces at least three major difficulties. Firstly, excision of an early cancer may effect a cure. It is not possible, at present, to identify those patients who will develop recurrences, and it therefore seems unjustifiable to apply to early cancer patients a form of therapy which is of unknown value. Accordingly, attempts at immunotherapy have mostly been made on patients with advanced cancer, when it is likely to be too late. Secondly, there is no guarantee that active immunisation will induce immune responses which contribute to the destruction of the tumour. There is, in fact, a risk of inducing the production of 'enhancing' antibody (p. 267) and thus increasing the rate of tumour growth. Thirdly, problems in assessing the results of any form of cancer therapy result from the natural individual variations in the rate of growth and spread of cancer.

Attention has also been given to the possibility of vaccines to prevent cancer, and this has been achieved in feline leukaemia (p. 264). If it could be shown that some forms of human cancer are due to particular oncogenic viruses, immunisation against the virus, or against tumours induced by it, should be possible, but it would still be necessary to identify those individuals likely to develop that form of cancer unless one is prepared to immunise whole populations.

What makes the cancer cell multiply?

The preceding review of some of the known causes of cancer leaves us with the crucial questions unanswered. A few tentative conclusions can, however, be put forward.

(a) **A somatic mutation** is involved. This means no more than that a change has occurred in the cells of the tumour which can be transmitted to their descendants. The possible effects of a mutation in a somatic cell are limited. Germ cell mutation can of course give rise to changes in a later generation: and it is probable that somatic mutations in cells of the embryo can give rise to local defects. In the adult the fate of a mutation in a cell will depend on the effect of the mutation on the rate of multiplication of the cell. Unless it produces a clone of cells which multiply faster, or survive longer, than the surrounding cells, its presence will not be noticed. It follows therefore that *a tumour is almost the only kind of somatic mutation recognisable by ordinary methods.*

Such a mutation need not, of course, be a classical single-gene mutation. The same kind of inheritable change may be produced by a chromosomal anomaly, or by the incorporation of viral DNA into the genome (see above), and possibly in other ways.

(b) **Loss of specific features** is probably at least as important as *gain*. Malignancy at first sight seems a positive character, a new acquisition by the cell of the ability to do things (multiply rapidly, invade, metastasise, transplant out of its own pure line) that it could not do before. But some changes—dedifferentiation, loss of antigens, loss of hormone–sensitivity—are clearly negative changes. Even active growth and invasion may be less positive characters than appear at first sight. Most normal cells—probably all that are capable of giving rise to tumours—migrate and multiply actively enough under the right conditions, such as following wounds or in tissue culture. They have the capacity both to grow when stimulated to do so and to stop when further growth is not required, i.e. they have brakes as well as accelerator: it is at least as likely that cancer cells have lost their brakes as that they have too powerful an accelerator.

The behaviour of epithelial cells in tissue culture is particularly significant here. Normal epithelial cells multiply and migrate to form a continuous sheet of one cell thickness. The cells then cease growth as though contact with their neighbour inhibited further growth, which occurs only at the edges. Tumour cells grow at first no more rapidly, but they pile on top of each other indiscriminately without any of this contact inhibition (Fig. 10.5). Part of the same difference is the tendency of normal epithelial cells to adhere closely to each other, whereas tumour cells lose such mutual adhesiveness.

(c) **Multiple stages** are usually involved. In most cases (excluding virus tumours) there is no sudden change, but a whole series of changes from normal to malignant tumour. This is obvious from the microscopic study of human material, but it also appears in such experimental situations as the induction of liver cancer in rats already described, where histological, biochemical and immunological changes all reflect a long process of transition. If a mutation is the basic process, there must be a series of mutations. The steep sixth-power rise in the incidence of many cancers with age has been interpreted mathematically as indicating that it depends on the concurrence of an average of seven independent events—which could be successive mutations.

(d) **'Survival of fittest'.** Many experimental situations are most easily interpreted as the selective proliferation of cells which are more resistant to some noxious agent than are normal cells. From the first partly resistant strain, new and even more resistant strains are further selected, to be superseded in their turn. The explanation of why the selected cells are cancerous might lie as far back in evolution as the protozoa, which multiplies freely whenever environmental conditions are suitable. Such a

basic property may be retained in latent form in metazoan cells, and cancer might simply be the natural result of partial re-expression of this property. Such a theory would explain many of the features of cancer, including the 'purposeless' proliferation, reversion to a more primitive cell type (lack of differentiation), and the increase in motility and loss of mutual cell adhesiveness responsible for invasion and metastasis.

Conclusion. The cancer cell, then, is one with a modification which can be regarded as a somatic mutation: the type of mutation is probably very variable, but whatever its precise nature, the change must have two inescapable characters: (*a*) it must be transmitted to the descendants of the cell, and (*b*) it must give the cells some advantage in rate of growth or length of survival over the normal cells.

Most carcinogens, it must be assumed, increase the frequency of mutations within the tissue concerned, and in addition (either alone or aided by a co-carcinogen) increase the rate of turnover of cells so as to increase the chance of selection of a mutation with the essential features of malignancy. An oncogenic virus, however, short-circuits this process and produces the mutation by inserting its DNA into the host cell genome.

Progress in the prevention and treatment of cancer may be considered at three levels. Firstly, considerable advances are likely to arise from a more complete understanding of the nature of neoplastic cell change. At present, the most hopeful approach seems to be investigations on the effects of small oncogenic DNA viruses, such as polyoma virus, which only have sufficient DNA to code for 6–8 proteins. About half of their total DNA is required to code for the virus coat, leaving a very few viral factors to bring about changes in the host cell. Accordingly, any demonstrable virus-induced cell change has a good chance of being the essential one.

Secondly, advances in experimental carcinogenesis have suggested profitable lines of research on human cancers. The developments in animal leukaemias, including successful prophylactic vaccination, are a good example, and much will depend on the clarification of the role of viruses and of immune defence against cancer.

Thirdly, it seems essential to continue to screen for carcinogenicity the enormous numbers of chemicals and other agents which become available for use in industry, food production and preparation, and therapeutically. It is, of course, equally important to make use of existing knowledge, as exemplified by the 30 000 or so annual deaths from bronchial cancer in Great Britain, most of which are attributable to smoking.

11

Tumours

II. Epithelial Varieties

After the introductory account of tumours in the last chapter, we turn for the next two chapters to the more practical questions of what kinds of tumour occur in man, what they look like and how they behave. There are many aspects of tumours that are best described as part of the pathology of the organs from which they are derived: these chapters are concerned with aspects of more general application, though they will be found to include also descriptions of a number of specialised tumours, sometimes because they illustrate some general principle, and sometimes for no better reason than that they are difficult to fit in elsewhere.

Classification

In the introduction to the previous chapter the distinction between *benign* and *malignant* tumours was discussed in some detail. We must now use the other chief mode of classification, the *histogenetic*, which is based on the tissue of origin. We may conveniently distinguish tumours of:

(*a*) epithelia;
(*b*) connective tissues (including muscle);
(*c*) blood vessels and lymphatics;
(*d*) the nervous system;
(*e*) the lymphoid and haemopoietic tissues;
(*f*) other tissues.

Of these, the epithelial tumours are overwhelmingly the commonest and are responsible for 90% of all cancer deaths in this country. This first chapter will be devoted to them alone.

General features of epithelial tumours

Epithelium has two essential characteristics which are carried over into its tumours.

(*a*) It forms continuous *sheets* or *masses* of cells of similar type, which adhere together without any intervening intercellular structures. This adherence of the cells into larger or smaller groups is retained as an indication of an epithelial origin even in tumours which have lost all the other distinctive features of epithelial cells.

(*b*) It requires a stroma of connective tissue and blood vessels for its support and nourishment. This is equally necessary for tumour epithelium, and all epithelial tumours appear to be able to stimulate the local connective tissues and blood vessels to proliferate and supply a stroma which surrounds and supports the epithelial cell groups. This '**desmoplastic reaction**', as it is called, varies in degree; it is often inadequate, so that much of the tumour dies from ischaemia, but it is sometimes excessive, so that the fibrous stroma becomes more conspicuous than the epithelium (scirrhous tumours, so-called). Far from supporting the tumour cells, such excessive stroma tends to interfere with their nutrition, growth and spread. We know very little about the way in which the tumour cells can influence the development of connective tissue. As so often in cancer studies, the basic problem is a much wider one: the relationship between epithelium and connective tissue is established as a convenient form of organisation in a large part of the animal kingdom, and we know little of its basic mechanism. The cancer cells are simply exploiting a normal process.

The way in which an epithelium is organized naturally affects profoundly the structure of the tumours to which it gives rise, and this is especially marked in the case of the slow growing and well-differentiated benign tumours. Epithelia which cover surfaces generally give rise to **papillomas**; epithelia of exocrine or endocrine glands, and of solid organs like the liver and kidneys, give rise to **adenomas**.

Benign Epithelial Tumours

Papillomas

If one considers what will happen to a sheet of epithelium such as the epidermis when its cells have begun to multiply, it is clear that the first effect will be to thicken the layer. But since this is limited by the extent to which nutriments can diffuse from the underlying blood vessels, the tumour cells must soon spread in other directions. So long as the tumour is benign, they do not spread downwards into the underlying tissue, and so can only continue to spread sideways. To some extent this occurs by displacement of the surrounding normal epithelium, but, in addition and usually to a much greater extent, it occurs by expansion of the epithelium occupying the same spot. If one tries to visualise the epithelium as a sheet of cloth which is pinned down at the edges and then increased in area, it is obvious that it will be thrown into folds. If the increase is in one dimension only, the folds will be regular pleats, but since in a benign epithelial tumour it occurs in two dimensions simple folding cannot occur, and the result is an irregular mass of peaks and hollows. Where the epithelium is raised into peaks, a core of connective tissue is drawn into it (the 'desmoplastic reaction' in effect) and the epithelium covering it remains well nourished and continues to grow. Since each peak is compressed by the other peaks around it, it can only grow upward, producing a higher peak which may finally become a long finger-like process. The resulting mass of '*papillae*' constitutes a papilloma.

If such a papilloma arises in a squamous epithelium the processes are naturally covered by squamous epithelium, thickened but otherwise not grossly abnormal. They are well seen in a papilloma of the skin, the commonest form of which is the virus-induced wart of children. (The name papilloma is derived from the prominence of dermal papillae in such tumours, well seen in Fig. 11.1. This is no longer regarded as an important characteristic, but the name has persisted.)

The transitional epithelium of the urinary tract produces papillomas covered by transitional epithelium, in which the papillary processes are often exceptionally long and

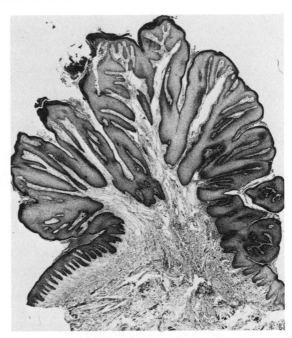

Fig. 11.1   Papilloma of muco-cutaneous junction of lip, showing branching processes of connective tissue covered by stratified epithelium. × 10.

numerous (Figs. 11.2 and 11.3). This is probably not due to any special characteristic of the epithelium, but to the environment provided by the bladder, in which the fronds of the papilloma float like seaweed in a sheltered bay: similar complexity is seen in the rare choroid plexus papillomas which float in the cerebrospinal fluid.

While columnar epithelia can also give rise to papillomas (Fig. 11.4), the relation of these epithelia to glands tends to complicate the picture. Thus at the commonest site for such tumours, the large intestine, a papilloma (the so-called 'villous papilloma') arises from the surface epithelium, and has very much the structure one would expect (Fig. 11.5), but most tumours in this area tend to mimic the glandular structure of the crypts of the mucosa (the *adenomatous polyps* described below).

The papillary structure of papillomas is not usually obvious to the naked eye, though the educated naked eye may recognise it. In most skin papillomas it is hidden by the thick horny layer of keratin which develops on the surface,

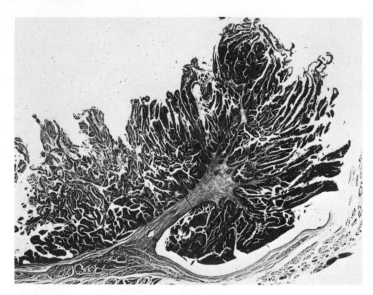

Fig. 11.2 Papilloma of bladder, showing innumerable delicate fronds, which are covered by transitional epithelium. A stalk, as seen in this case, is often absent. It is unusual for a bladder papilloma as large as this to be completely benign. × 4.

filling up the gaps between the fronds and producing a rough dry hard surface in which only an ill-defined cauliflower pattern gives a hint of the underlying structure. The result is a well defined little lump, usually round, always projecting above the surface (except for the plantar wart on the sole of the foot, where pressure flattens it) and at times slightly polypoid—i.e. having a slight neck between it and the skin level. The papillae of excised bladder

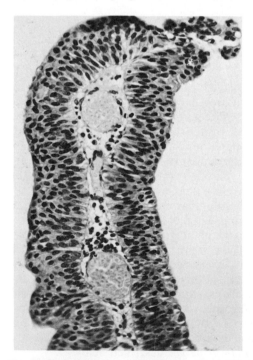

Fig. 11.3 Papilloma of bladder. Section of the tip of a single process, showing a narrow core of connective tissue, including capillaries, covered by transitional epithelium. The epithelium is rather thicker and has rather more cells than normal, but differentiation is still excellent. × 200.

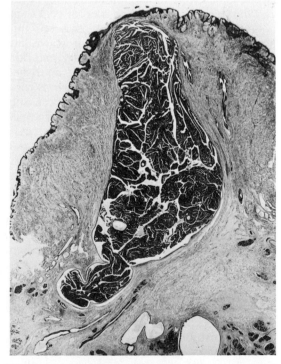

Fig. 11.4 Papilloma of the breast, growing into and distending a duct near the nipple. × 4.

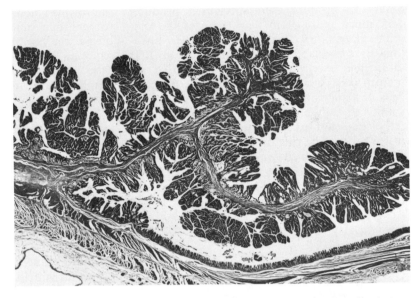

Fig. 11.5 Villous papilloma of rectum. The structure is obviously similar to that of the bladder papilloma, but a higher power would show that the covering epithelium is of columnar type. The majority of papillomas at this site have however a less complicated branching structure, with numerous shorter fronds, arising directly from the mucosa. × 3.

papillomas are thin (often termed *fronds*), and difficult to recognise by naked-eye; unless the excised tumour is submerged in fluid, they collapse against each other and leave nothing but a somewhat velvety surface to indicate their true nature. Seen *in situ* with a cystoscope, or examined with a lens under saline, the fronds will be obvious. The fronds are even harder to see in the soft velvety plaques of a villous papilloma of the rectum, and a dissecting microscope may be necessary.

Adenomas

The simple tumours that arise from acinar glands and ducts vary a great deal in detail, but there is a basic pattern which can usually be recognised through all the variations. As the tumour cells multiply they arrange themselves into rounded packets, into the centre of each of which they usually secrete fluid, thus forming a lumen around which the tumour cells lie in one, or sometimes two, regular layers, each cell assuming a more or less columnar shape. The structure so formed has a fairly obvious resemblance to a gland acinus, and is usually called a tumour acinus. It may resemble quite closely the acini of the original gland from which it has been formed (as in the thyroid, for instance, or to a lesser extent the colon—Fig. 11.6) or it may look very different.

Though each tumour acinus looks like a gland acinus, it has no connection with ducts, so that anything that is secreted by the lining cells can only accumulate in the lumen. The endocrine glands dispose of their secretions directly into the blood, and probably for this reason tumours of endocrine glands retain their

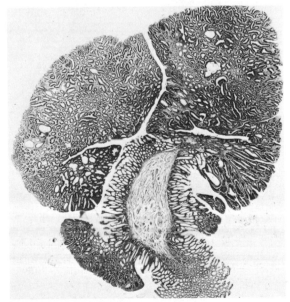

Fig. 11.6 Polypoid adenoma (or adenomatous polyp) of colon. The rounded darker mass of the adenoma is made up of close-packed glands, less regular and more cellular than those of the normal mucosa which is seen below covering the stalk of the polyp. (Unusually, two smaller adenomata arise from the stalk. In this case there were multiple polyps and a carcinoma, seen in Fig. 11.11.) × 8.

ability to produce their specialised products very much more often than those of the exocrine glands, and retain much closer histological resemblance to the parent tissue. It is altogether exceptional to see specialised secretory cells such as gastric parietal or peptic cells or pancreatic acinar cells in tumours: the acinic-cell tumour of the salivary glands is the only significant exception to this rule, and even it is a rarity. The rule does not apply to mucin-secreting cells, which commonly persist in adenomas, and even appear in situations (notably the ovary) where mucin-secreting cells are not found in the normal organ (Fig. 11.7). It will

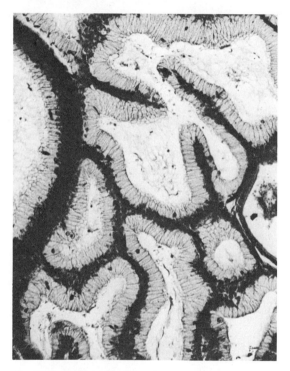

Fig. 11.7 Mucinous cystadenoma (cystic adenoma) of ovary. The cysts (small in this case) are lined by tall mucin-secreting epithelium. The nuclei, lined up at the base of each cell, form a continuous line hardly distinguishable in this picture from those of the next cyst. × 150.

thus be clear that an adenoma of a gland, even though in general it retains a glandular appearance, will often have epithelium that is not easily recognised as derived from the particular gland of origin. Endocrine epithelium, e.g., of the thyroid, may be little altered (Fig. 10.2, p. 250); some mucin-secreting epithelia such as

that of the colonic mucosa may remain readily recognisable; and the same applies to the breast, the normal epithelium of which is not secreting for most of its life. But in most other cases transformation to a relatively nondescript simple or mucus-secreting columnar epithelium occurs.

In addition, the basic pattern of the acini in adenomas may be altered in two main ways:

(*a*) The amount of secretion is usually small, but may be substantial (usually it is then mucous, but there are some special exceptions, chiefly in thyroid and ovary). Since the adenoma has no organised duct system, the acini are distended with secretion, and the epithelium becomes stretched round it. At times the distension is so great that individual acini are large enough not merely to be seen with the naked eye, but to become cysts which may be larger than a football; they are full of secretion and the original epithelium usually persists as a single layer stretched over its surface. Such cyst-containing adenomas, which are quite common in the ovaries, are called **cystadenomas**.

(*b*) The rate of multiplication of the cells may be a more pronounced feature than the production of secretion, the cells tending to pile up round the central lumens, the acini becoming more and more solid: this feature often indicates the onset of malignancy. Sometimes, however, when there is enough secretion to distend the acini, the cells are well enough differentiated to retain the arrangement of a thin sheet, and yet still are multiplying; they behave like a surface epithelium and form papillomas which project into the lumina. Such a tumour is called a **papillary adenoma** or, if the lumens are large, a **papillary cystadenoma**. It might be expected that the pure cystadenomas, in which secretion is abundant and hence differentiation is good, are more benign than the papillary adenomas, in which proliferation is more prominent, and this is generally, although not always, true.

To the naked eye the typical adenoma is a rounded lump, well defined, usually with a thin capsule of fibrous tissue and compressed normal gland. If lumens are small it appears solid when cut across, and is usually paler (because more cellular) and more homogeneous than the normal gland. If secretion is abundant it is obvious on section, and in a cystade-noma the bulk of the tumour consists of a mass of cysts full of mucus or other fluid; it may even sometimes form a single large cyst.

When an adenoma is formed from the glandular parts of a mucous membrane, as in the gut and most commonly the colon, it forms a very characteristic rounded nodule hanging upon a stalk formed by pulled-out normal mucosa, and is called an **adenomatous polyp**. (A 'polyp' is a lump on the end of a stalk, without any commitment as to the nature of the lump.) **Adenomas of solid organs** are not very common, but are seen mostly in the endocrine glands (adrenal, pituitary and parathyroid especially) and occasionally in the liver (Fig. 11.8). They consist of rounded well-defined solid masses of tissue, usually encapsulated and very like that of the tissue of origin: an adrenal cortical adenoma, for instance, is usually a bright yellow lump hardly distinguishable except by its shape and size from the surrounding normal cortex.

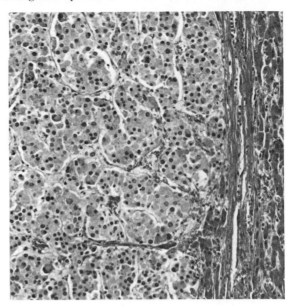

Fig. 11.8 Solid trabecular adenoma of liver. The cells are arranged in irregular columns and are demarcated from the compressed liver cells by a well-defined fibrous capsule. × 150.

Malignant Epithelial Tumours (Carcinomas)

The term **carcinoma** may be applied to any malignant tumour of epithelial origin. It may arise from one of the benign epithelial tumours just described, or arise directly from a non-neoplastic epithelium. In either case, it retains the two features already described as characteristic of epithelium and its tumours—the formation of sheets or masses of contiguous tumour cells, and the ability to excite a stromal reaction between and around the tumour cell masses. In addition, the epithelial element commonly retains some resemblance to the tissue of origin, though in poorly differentiated, and usually more malignant, tumours this may be tenuous.

Naked-eye appearances

While there are many variations, it is possible to describe a typical carcinoma. It forms a firm lump, often irregularly nodular, its edge well defined in places and in others blending into the surrounding tissue (areas of invasion) so that it cannot be dissected out cleanly. On section it is predominantly whitish, as are most dense collections of young cells: there are often red patches of haemorrhage and, especially towards the centre, yellow areas of necrosis. Where the nodule lies on a surface it forms at first an irregularly dome-shaped swelling. The centre of this swelling however has often a poor blood supply and has lost the surface epithelium: it is exposed to trauma, infection and (in the case of lesions in the gut) digestive juices. It therefore often sloughs out, leaving a ragged ulcer. At the edges the tumour has a better blood supply and is partly protected by the surface epithelium, and so survives: the ulcer therefore commonly retains a thick irregular raised edge which is responsible for the highly characteristic appearance of the ulcerated malignant tumour (compare, for instance, Figs. 11.11, 18.31 on p. 554 and 18.32 on p. 556).

Varieties

There are many special types of carcinoma characteristic of particular sites, though the more highly malignant anaplastic ones all tend to look alike. Most malignant epithelial tumours can, however, be included in the two great classes of **squamous carcinoma** and **adenocarcinoma**.

Squamous carcinoma

This is the characteristic malignant tumour of squamous epithelia, both epidermis and squamous mucosae. In addition there are some unexpected sites, where squamous carcinomas arise in organs containing no squamous epithelium: the most important of these is the bronchus, where squamous metaplasia of the bronchial epithelium is the probable explana-

tion; similar metaplasia can account for less common sites such as the urinary tract and the gall bladder. Unstable squamo-columnar junctions such as the uterine cervix are also important sites.

Histologically, most squamous carcinomas are very readily recognisable. In early lesions, the downgrowth of the surface epithelium into the deeper tissues can be detected (Fig. 11.9). At the periphery, small masses and narrow columns of cells burrow into the surrounding tissues. Behind this margin, the invading cell groups have had time to enlarge and differentiate, becoming recognisable as prickle cells and usually forming keratin: the keratin forms rounded concentric nodules in the centre of the cell groups, a very characteristic appearance called 'cell nests' or 'epithelial pearls' (Fig. 11.10). The amount of keratin formed and the proportion of cells recognisable as prickle cells

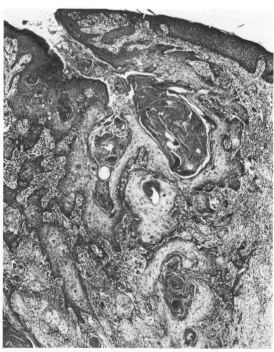

Fig. 11.9 Squamous carcinoma of tongue, showing squamous cell masses with, in places, central keratinisation. These remain in continuity with the overlying epithelium (*above*). Ulceration is beginning (*above left*). There is a well-marked inflammatory infiltrate in the connective tissue, which a little obscures the distinction from the infiltrating tumour. × 38.

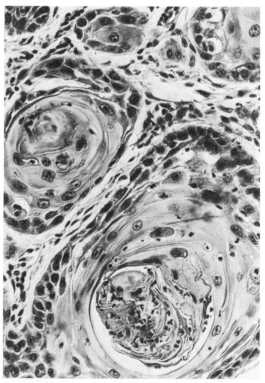

Fig. 11.10 Squamous carcinoma at higher power, showing cell nests. The largest shows central keratin (still with some stratum granulosum granules), then large pale prickle-cells, and a periphery of darker undifferentiated cells. In the smaller cell masses at the top keratinisation has not yet begun: the mass at left centre is at an intermediate stage. × 290.

both vary greatly: they are the best guides to degree of differentiation of the tumour, which, of course, affects its prognosis.

There are some variations from site to site—for instance, a squamous carcinoma of the bronchus or pharynx is usually less well differentiated than one of the lip or the skin. The site also naturally has a profound effect on the signs and symptoms produced by these tumours, and on their accessibility for treatment and hence on their prognosis.

Adenocarcinoma

This second group is a little less homogeneous than the last. Thus a histological section of an adenocarcinoma of the stomach can usually be distinguished from one of the colon with more confidence than a squamous carcinoma of the tongue from one of the bronchus. The grouping of adenocarcinomas together is, however, useful, for most of the malignant tumours of glands have a great deal in common with each other and with those that arise from all the ducts and surfaces lined by columnar epithelium. Important sites of origin include the stomach and colon, the pancreas, gall bladder and its ducts, breast and uterus; also the bronchi, which can produce both squamous and adenocarcinomas.

Histologically, almost everything that has been said of the adenomas applies to adenocarcinomas, with two differences.

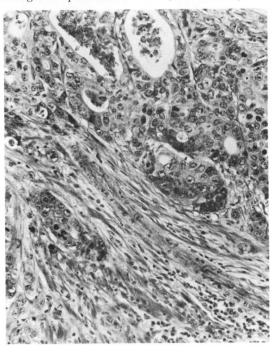

Fig. 11.12 Adenocarcinoma of bowel invading the muscle coat. *Below*, nearly solid strands of tumour are invading smooth muscle on each side of the arteriole which runs up from the bottom right corner. *Above*, the older tumour strands are developing gland-like lumens. × 160.

(*a*) Instead of remaining localised, the tumour cells invade the surrounding tissues (Fig. 11.11).

(*b*) Differentiation is poorer (Fig. 11.12). In

Fig. 11.11 Adenocarcinoma of colon. Ulcerated tumour to left, normal mucosa to right. between them the raised 'rolled margin' formed by a thick layer of tumour still partly protected by the normal mucosa stretched over its upper surface. Invasion of submucosa and muscularis is well seen. × 11.

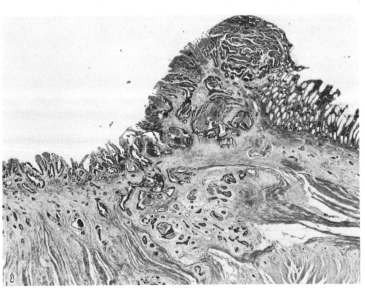

addition to all the general features of malignant tumours listed in the last chapter (p. 251) there is a marked tendency for acini to contain less secretion, to be lined not by one regular layer of epithelial cells but by a thick irregular layer, and in some tumours for most of the cell groups to form solid masses.

Several variations upon the basic pattern are common enough to be worth describing. Mixed and intermediate forms occur, and none of the following should be regarded as completely distinct entities.

(a) Spheroidal-cell carcinoma, (Fig. 11.13) an

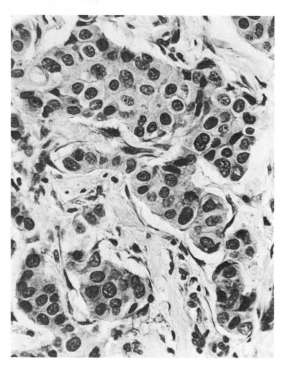

Fig. 11.13 Spheroidal-cell carcinoma of breast infiltrating tissue spaces. The tumour cells are still obviously epithelial, and nuclear changes are not gross, but there is no trace of glandular differentiation. × 300.

adenocarcinoma in which most of the cell masses are solid. This type of tumour is common in the breast, partly because of relatively poor differentiation, and perhaps partly because the gland is in a non-secretory state.

(b) Cystadenocarcinoma, in which cysts lined by columnar or cuboidal cells are prominent. This is common in the ovary and is seen occasionally in the pancreas and kidney.

(c) Papillary adenocarcinoma, in which papillary processes project into cysts. This is seen particularly in the thyroid, ovary and bile ducts.

(d) Mucoid carcinoma. An adenocarcinoma in which mucus secretion is unusually marked. The term should be used only when the whole tumour looks like a mass of jelly, and under the microscope most of the tumour cells float free

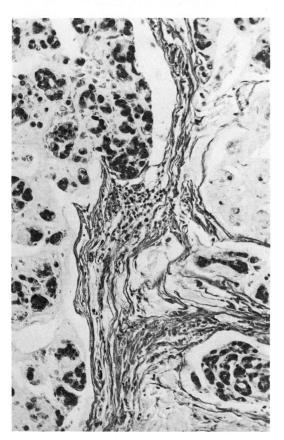

Fig. 11.14 Mucoid carcinoma. The tumour cells, still in this case with some traces of glandular arrangement, lie in large pools of mucin. × 65.

in lakes of mucus (Fig. 11.14). The commonest site of origin is the stomach, but it occurs also fairly often in the colon and breast.

Hard and soft carcinomas

Classification of carcinomas into the two following types depends on features of the stroma and not of the tumour cells. It is thus an essentially different mode of classification. For example both spheroidal-cell carcinoma and

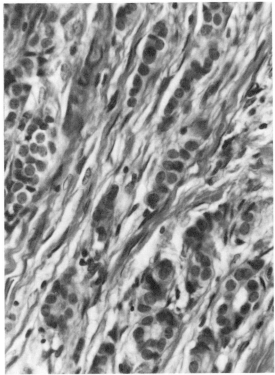

Fig. 11.15 Scirrhous carcinoma of breast, with dense poorly cellular collagen between the tumour cell groups. In this case, in contrast to Fig. 11.13, some of the latter show minimal glandular differentiation. × 240.

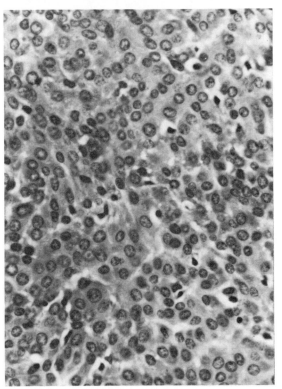

Fig. 11.16 Encephaloid carcinoma of breast, showing cells essentially similar to those of Figs. 11.13 and 11.15, but in larger islands, with very little stroma, the latter being hardly visible here. × 240.

adenocarcinoma can be either scirrhous or encephaloid.

(1) Scirrhous carcinoma (Fig. 11.15) is a carcinoma in which there is an unusually marked fibrous reaction, so that the tumour cells are separated into small groups by dense fibrous tissue. Growth is often slow, but metastasis is not delayed by this reaction. It is common in the breast, and fairly common, in a rather special diffuse form (p. 557), in the stomach.

(2) Encephaloid carcinoma (Fig. 11.16). A carcinoma with minimal stromal reaction, so soft as to be brain-like in consistency, hence the name. The term is rarely used except for the occasional breast carcinoma that contrasts with the more usual scirrhous tumour of that site.

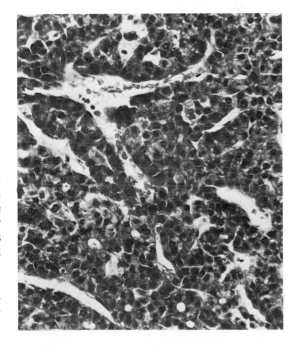

Fig. 11.17 Carcinoma arising from liver cells, showing trabecular arrangement. × 190.

Special types of carcinoma

The names of some carcinomas reflect a striking appearance linked to a distinctive behaviour. Examples include clear-cell carcinoma of the kidney, carcinoma of liver-cell origin (Fig. 11.17), choriocarcinoma of the placenta, and rodent ulcer of the skin; these are highly distinctive lesions with very marked peculiarities of histogenesis as well as appearance and behaviour. They are described in the appropriate systematic chapters.

Spread of carcinoma

Local invasion

Local invasion by a carcinoma depends in part on the sheer expansive pressure of the mass of growing cells, but also on the active migration of motile tumour cells which penetrate the surrounding tissues and then multiply at the new site. Sometimes they appear to migrate as single cells: more often they appear to penetrate as columns of cells which extend by growth at the forward end. We know little about why cancer cells behave thus, but, as indicated in the last chapter, it may be due to increased motility, or to loss of cell adhesiveness or of other normal restraining processes.

Growth is easiest along the planes of loose connective tissue, and may be checked by dense structures such as thick fascia, the walls of large arteries, cartilage and compact bone. Structures such as glands and muscle, once penetrated, are rapidly destroyed, partly by pressure, partly by loss of blood supply. The carcinoma itself tends to outrun its blood supply, and necrosis of the tumour which ensues includes ischaemic destruction of any normal tissues which have been invaded. Unfortunately the growing edge of the tumour is hardly ever included in the necrosis.

Local invasion is important in the establishment of the primary tumour, and may of course result in damage to major structures nearby. Of greater significance from the point of view of the life of the patient in most cases is the appearance of **secondary deposits** or **metastases**— new areas of growth of the tumour at a distance from the primary tumour. These result from spread of tumour cells from the primary growth, usually by the lymphatics or blood vessels, as described below.

Spread by lymphatics

This is one of the most characteristic features of carcinoma and is of prime importance from the surgical point of view. Cancer cells penetrating into the lymphatics may either float free in the lymph and be arrested in the lymph nodes, or they may (probably less often) form columns of proliferating cells filling and growing along the lymphatics (Figs. 11.18, 11.19). Small nodules

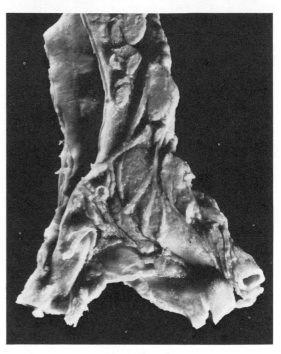

Fig. 11.18 Lymph spread of carcinoma, involving both lymphatics and lymph nodes, around the bifurcation of the aorta. Lymphatics filled with tumour are particularly well seen as they cross the left common iliac artery just below right centre of the specimen. $\times \frac{3}{4}$.

of tumour may be formed along the line of the lymphatics, but the largest nodules are those which form in and replace the lymph nodes. Early lymph node metastases usually lie in the peripheral sinus (Fig. 11.20). While the lymph nodes draining the region of the carcinoma are first and usually most extensively involved, spread may take place in a direction contrary to normal lymph flow (Fig. 11.21) as a sequel to lymphatic obstruction.

Many of the secondary foci in the region of a carcinoma are of only microscopic size, and tissues may be unchanged in appearance though extensively involved. Accordingly it is impossible to assess the degree of secondary invasion by naked-eye examination alone (Fig. 11.22). The presence of these minute collections of cancer cells explains the so-called recurrence

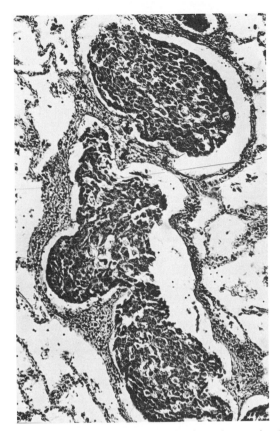

Fig. 11.19 Lymphatic spread of carcinoma in the lung. Two lymphatics (the connective tissue round them indicates that they lie in an interlobular septum) are filled and distended by small dark-staining carcinoma cells. × 45.

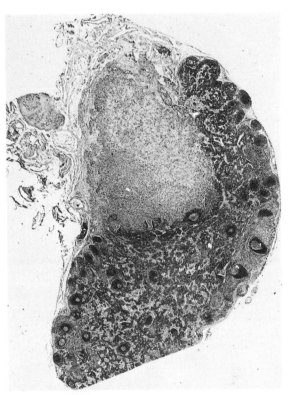

Fig. 11.21 Retrograde invasion of lymph node by carcinoma. The lymphatics at the hilum of the node are filled with cancer cells, which have spread into the node against the normal direction of lymph flow. × 95.

of cancer after surgical removal. '**Recurrence**', in fact, is not usually to be regarded as a fresh start or recrudescence of the disease, but simply the result of growth from cells which have been left behind in the surrounding tissues. Such cells may remain dormant, so that years or even decades may elapse before a recognisable tumour reappears. True recrudescence of growth may, however, occur in an area of premalignant change (p. 287).

Blood spread

With most carcinomas, the effects of blood spread are seen later than those of lymphatic

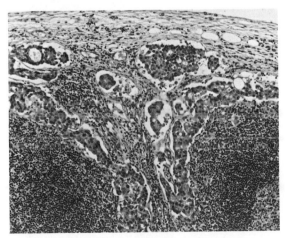

Fig. 11.20 Carcinoma invading lymph node. Carcinoma cells are seen in the lymph vessels in the capsule of the node and in the peripheral lymph sinus, from which they are extending into the medulla. × 66.

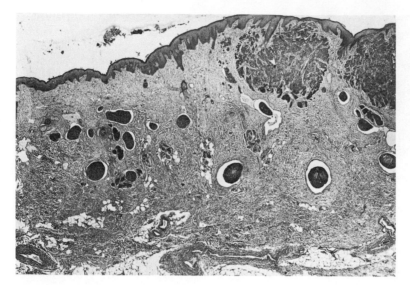

Fig. 11.22 Squamous carcinoma of vulva, showing lymphatic permeation in the dermis beyond the clinically apparent margin. The larger tumour masses (*above right*) would appear to the naked eye to be the edge of the tumour, the bulk of which lies further to the right. Lymphatic permeation can usually only be recognised with certainty in microscopic sections, though when it is as gross as that seen here it may be suspected on careful examination with the naked eye. × 15.

spread, though the wider dissemination makes them usually of more serious consequence to the patient. The small veins in and around the primary tumour are the usual route of entry to the circulation. Tumour cells are then carried away to lodge in the next capillary bed that the blood passes through, e.g. in the liver if the primary tumour is in the portal drainage area (Fig. 11.23), and in the lungs from tumours in most other sites. Thence they may spread further, from the liver to the lungs and from the lungs via the systemic circulation to any part of

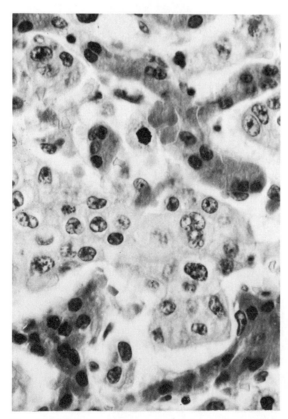

Fig. 11.23 Secondary carcinoma in the liver. Note masses of cancer cells in the sinusoids between the (darker) liver cells, without any formation of stroma. × about 200.

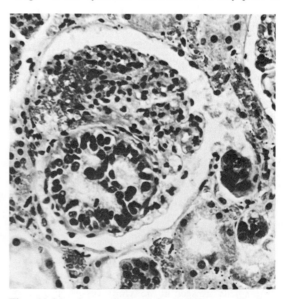

Fig. 11.24 An embolus of carcinoma cells in a glomerulus, with extension into the tubule. × 150.

the body (Fig. 11.24). Blood-spread metastases in a solid organ present a very characteristic picture of multiple rounded nodules, varying in size but with no single nodule conspicuously larger than the rest, and scattered at random through the substance of the organ (Figs. 11.25 and 19.48, p. 640).

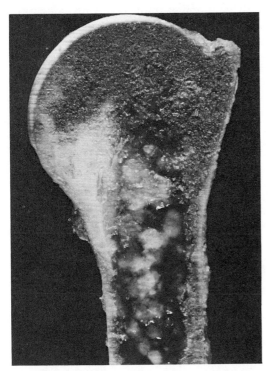

Fig. 11.25 Secondary carcinoma in bone. Multiple rounded white masses in the humerus, in a case of carcinoma of breast. × ¾.

There are in practice many apparent anomalies in the distribution of metastases: some may be due to confusion between blood and lymph spread—there is for instance a strong case for considering the curious predilection of bronchial carcinoma to spread to the adrenals as a consequence of lymph spread rather than (as has been generally believed) blood spread. But even allowing for this, there must be great variations between capacities of different tissues to resist the growth of tumour cells arriving by the bloodstream. It is highly probable that in most cases the great majority of cells leaving the primary tumour by the veins fail to establish themselves.

In a painstaking necropsy study of a large number of cases of carcinoma arising in various sites, R. A. Willis gave the following incidences of metastases in various organs:

liver	36%	brain	6%
lungs	29%	spleen	3%
bones	14%	skeletal muscles	1%
adrenals	9%	skin	1%

These incidences clearly do not correspond with blood flow, and so with the number of tumour cells likely to be arriving in the various organs. The liver and bone marrow are susceptible sites: the spleen and muscles resistant. There is experimental evidence for destruction of tumour cells by the spleen, but the nature of the defence mechanism is not known. The lung, which must receive by far the largest number of tumour cell emboli, provides an environment which is only moderately favourable to their growth. Cases of carcinoma in organs such as the kidney or thyroid often have multiple systemic metastases, for example in bone, with no obvious lung lesions: in such cases it can often be shown that there are minute microscopic foci in the lung where tumour cells have lodged in the pulmonary vessels, and, while failing to grow to any substantial extent at that site, have been able to

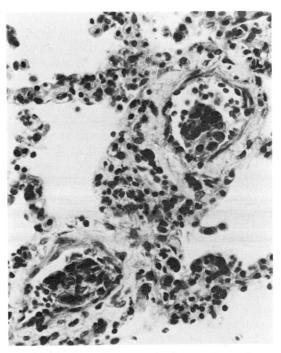

Fig. 11.26 Lung from a case of prostatic carcinoma, showing two pulmonary arterioles containing tumour cells. × 190.

launch further tumour emboli into the systemic circulation (Fig. 11.26).

Retrograde venous spread. One type of anomaly that has a special explanation is the localisation of metastases within the axial skeleton. Carcinoma of the prostate spreads early to the lumbar spine and pelvis, carcinoma of the breast to the thoracic vertebral bodies, and carcinoma of the nasopharynx to the cervical spine and the base of the skull. This is not attributable to direct or lymph spread but to spread by the blood. Yet blood spread in the usual fashion via the lungs should result in all parts of the vertebral column being equally affected, and this is not so. The explanation for the localised involvements of the spine appears to lie in the peculiarities of blood flow in the intra-vertebral venous plexus, in which differences of pressure above and below the diaphragm often lead to reversal of flow: the effect is to draw venous blood at times into the vertebra from neighbouring organs, and this may carry malignant cells, which find a very favourable site for multiplication within the vertebral marrow.

Intracavitary spread

When carcinoma involves a body cavity, cancer cells may be liberated into the space and graft themselves on the surface to form new foci of growth. Any cavity can be involved, and the *subarachnoid space*, for example, is of some importance in the spread of intracranial tumours, but the serous cavities are especially important for carcinoma. Involvement of the *peritoneum* results most often from carcinomas arising in the stomach or the ovary, while the *pleura* and *pericardium* are most commonly invaded by carcinomas of breast or bronchus. In most cases there is an effusion of fluid into the sac concerned, and this may be bloodstained. Malignant cells are often present in such an effusion, but very often it is difficult to distinguish them with certainty from altered serosal cells. A special example of this form of spread is seen in transperitoneal metastasis to the ovary, usually before the menopause and usually from a gastric carcinoma of the 'signet-ring' type (p. 557): the ovaries may become very large, and have the characters first described by Krukenberg, who thought that such tumours originated in the ovaries (see p. 916).

Intra-epithelial and intracellular spread

Cancer cells may invade the epidermis, which is the only extensive epithelium in the body thick enough to withstand such invasion without disruption. Cells may spread for several centimetres in the epidermis without destroying it completely. Paget's disease of the nipple (p. 937) is the only common example involving carcinoma cells (the tumour being derived from the underlying breast): rarely this occurs in the epidermis at other sites, and something similar is seen in malignant melanoma of the skin (p. 1012).

Carcinoma invading skeletal muscle may sometimes be seen under the microscope to be growing within the sarcolemma of muscle cells: this is the only known example of 'intracellular' spread (Fig. 11.27).

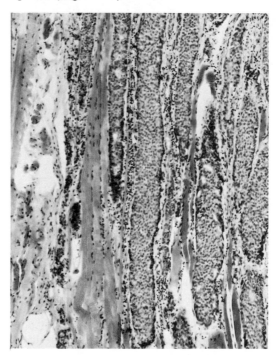

Fig. 11.27   Intracellular invasion. The long sausages of tumour cells have grown within and expanded striped muscle fibres, being still confined by the sarcolemma: compare with unaffected muscle fibres on the left. × 60.

Premalignant lesions

These are conveniently considered here, as most such lesions involve epithelium, and are pre-carcinomatous.

A premalignant condition is one which can be recognised by either clinician or pathologist, and which indicates that the bearer has a substantially greater than the normal risk of developing a malignant tumour. The early stages of premalignant change (which presumably indicate the occurrence of the earlier mutations of a multistage conversion to malignancy) can often be recognised histologically. The signs include nuclear irregularity, increased mitotic activity, and abnormalities of differentiation, often combined with inflammatory infiltrates and stromal changes. The risk of such lesions' becoming malignant can be established only in the light of experience of their behaviour in each particular site in which they occur. The following are examples of premalignant lesions.

(a) Some benign tumours. Probably all benign tumours carry some increased risk of malignancy, but in most it is very little more than that of the normal tissue, while in others it is high. There is little obvious logic about the differences. The villous papilloma of the rectum becomes malignant more often than the adenomatous polyp of the same site: similar tumours of the stomach carry a worse prognosis than either, while the uncommon similar tumours of the small intestine only very rarely become invasive. Comparable anomalies could be quoted at other sites.

(b) Certain chronic diseases. Carcinoma may develop as a more or less common complication of some non-neoplastic diseases, such as cirrhosis of the liver, ulcerative colitis, asbestosis, and a variety of skin diseases.

(c) Carcinoma-in-situ. In the most extreme degrees of premalignant change in an epithelium, all the cytological changes of malignancy are seen in its cells, but the altered cells remain in the intact layer of epithelium and do not invade the underlying tissues. The name carcinoma-in-situ is often given to this lesion: it is not strictly accurate, as no carcinoma is present until invasion begins, but it is a vivid reminder of the need for action. It has been best studied in the cervix uteri, where its detection by the methods of exfoliative cytology is now widely practised in the prevention of invasive carcinoma at that site (p. 904). *Intraduct carcinoma* of the breast (p. 935) is an essentially similar lesion.

The degree of risk of developing malignancy varies greatly with different lesions, and is often hard to determine with any exactness. In a few rare conditions, such as polyposis coli and xeroderma pigmentosa, it is practically 100%. In carcinoma-in-situ of the cervix, extensively studied but still controversial, it may also be high, though a period of twenty years may elapse between appearance of the lesion and the onset of invasive carcinoma. In most other lesions the risk appears to be much lower.

Staging and grading of cancers

A quantitative measure of the factors affecting the prognosis of a particular type of tumour is often required. Sometimes it is used in deciding on the best method of treatment, but it is most useful in statistical studies. If, for instance, a surgeon claims that his new operation is curing more patients than his colleagues (or, to be more precise, raising the proportion of 5-year survivals) it is necessary to be sure that he is not seeing by some accident an exceptionally favourable group of cases—e.g. small, earlier or better differentiated tumours. The production of completely unambiguous criteria is much more difficult than it sounds, and elaborate special systems have been developed for most of the common tumours. All agree, however, in separating two main elements, *grading* and *staging*, and these should not be confused.

Grading. This is a *histological* estimate of the degree of *differentiation*. Exact numerical systems do not work (Broder's system, depending on the percentage of differentiated cells, though still often talked of, has long been abandoned in practice). In general, most tumours are graded for this purpose by the pathologist into well differentiated, average, and poorly differentiated: the system is most useful if the criteria used put about 25% of the tumours into the good group, 50% into the average and 25% into the worst.

Staging. This is a *clinical* estimate of the degree of *spread*. Most systems use four stages, roughly definable as (I) confined to the organ of origin, (II) local spread not interfering with surgical excision, (III) fixation to surrounding structures and (IV) distant spread. A 'Stage O' is sometimes added for tumours of microscopic size.

How this works in practice may be seen from the usual definitions for cancer of the uterine cervix: *Stage I*—confined strictly to the cervix: *Stage II*—local spread, not reaching the pelvic wall or the lower third of the vagina: *Stage III*—fixed to pelvis, or involving lower third of vagina: *Stage IV*— distant metastases, or involvement of bladder or rectum. Stage II is often subdivided, IIa including spread to the uterine body, vaginal fornices and the immediately adjacent connective tissue, IIb everything beyond that. It will be seen that even here the position is not altogether simple. For most other tumours staging is a good deal more complicated and often controversial.

Staging must always be based primarily on the clinical examination, for the assessment at operation often differs from the clinical assessment, and to compare surgical with other forms of treatment, both groups of patients must first be 'staged' in the same way, i.e. clinically. Grading, on the other hand, requires pathological examination of at least a biopsy. The results of the two procedures are not, however, altogether independent: as one might expect, in all series the worse differentiated cases tend to be more numerous in the higher stages.

12

Tumours

III. Other Varieties

There are far more kinds of non-epithelial tissue than epithelial, and equally there are far more kinds of non-epithelial tumour. As already indicated, however, the balance between this chapter and the last reflects the practical circumstance that the carcinomas greatly outweigh all other tumours in clinical importance. Nevertheless, even the tenth of cancer deaths that are due to non-epithelial tumours is a substantial number, and no one can dismiss as unimportant a group that includes the lymphomas, gliomas, melanomas and bone sarcomas. There are moreover some benign tumours, e.g. the myomas, and the tumour-like angiomas, which are very common, although mostly benign and responsible for few deaths.

Though all the main types of non-epithelial tumours will be found mentioned here, detailed description will be given only of those varieties which are of such general distribution as not to be easily included under any one system. Length of description does not therefore always reflect importance.

Tumours of the Connective Tissues

Nomenclature. In this group it is usual to name tumours by adding **-oma** to the appropriate stem for the benign lesion, and **-sarcoma** for the malignant—e.g. fibroma, fibrosarcoma; chondroma, chondrosarcoma.

Benign tumours. These are composed chiefly of fully developed tissues, such as are found in the adult body, e.g. fibrous tissue, cartilage, muscle. They are usually rounded or lobulated and well defined, being generally enclosed within a distinct fibrous capsule. They displace the surrounding tissues and produce atrophy by pressure, but they neither infiltrate tissues nor metastasise. Such benign tumours are sometimes multiple, but then each tumour represents an independent focus of growth. Blood vessels grow in relation to the tumour tissue, and are usually well formed, though the arteries are often deficient in muscle fibres. The well-formed fibrous tissue stroma of epithelial tumours is however altogether absent in most cases, the tumour relying for its support on the matrix produced by its own cells—though exceptions occur, for example in the myomas.

Malignant tumours (sarcomas). In the corresponding malignant tumours, the activity of the cells is mainly proliferative, the tumour is more cellular, and although a certain amount of matrix is formed, this is imperfect and usually scanty. Sarcomas often form large masses, usually soft and with frequent haemorrhage and necrosis (Fig. 12.1). While these malignant tumours may appear to the surgeon to be encapsulated, diffuse destructive infiltration of the surrounding tissue occurs at the margin of most such masses so that wide excision rather than enucleation is required in their treatment. There is an extensive new formation of poorly formed blood vessels. Numerous capillaries, and larger channels composed mainly of a layer of endothelium, are supported by the cells of the tumour, while around the larger channels

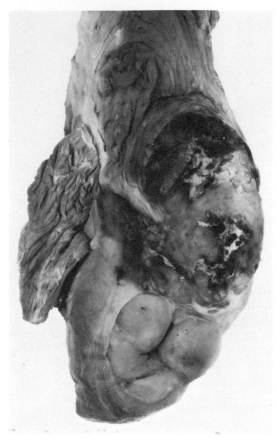

Fig. 12.1 Spindle-cell sarcoma arising in intermuscular fascia of thigh. Above and left there is normal voluntary muscle. The upper half of the ovoid tumour shows extensive necrosis and haemorrhage: the lower half is well-preserved, appearing characteristically greyish-white, soft and slightly lobulated. × 0·6.

there is usually some fibrous tissue. Two results follow—(*a*) the cells of the tumour readily break through the vessel walls and are conveyed in the venous blood until arrested in the smaller vessels of lungs, liver, etc., and thus **metastases** may develop, and (*b*) **haemorrhages** are common. Spread by the lymphatic vessels is unusual, except in the case of synovial sarcoma and lymphoma, and blood-borne metastases in the lungs are the usual cause of death.

Tumours of fibrous tissue

Although it is usual to regard these as the 'typical' connective tissue tumours, they are

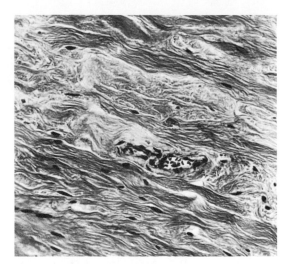

Fig. 12.2 Hard fibroma, showing abundant mature collagen and few cells. Distinction from normal fibrous tissue can be difficult, and depends on careful examination of the whole lesion. × 240.

in fact not very common and wholly typical benign fibromas are rare.

Fibroma. This is the name given to benign tumours of fibrous tissue. The cells of the tumour are fibrocytes; their nuclei are long and narrow and densely staining, the cytoplasm so scanty as to be hard to see, and mitoses are very rare. Bundles of dense collagen separate the cells, and the appearances, in short, may not be very different from that of fibrous tissue as seen in a thick fascia or a scar. A not very important

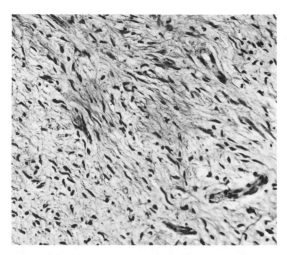

Fig. 12.3 Soft fibroma, showing more numerous cells (which are however mature fibrocytes) and less abundant and looser collagen. × 280.

distinction is sometimes made between hard and soft fibromas on the basis of the amount of collagen present (Figs. 12.2–12.4).

Fibromas are uncommon, but may occur in any type of connective tissue, and may be seen

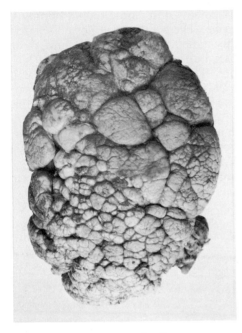

Fig. 12.4 Lobulated soft fibroma removed from buttock. Natural size.

with varying degrees of rarity in most of the internal organs. Special varieties occur in the sheaths of nerves (neurofibroma, p. 733), skin (dermatofibroma, p. 1014) and ovaries (p. 915) which have their own peculiarities of behaviour and which probably do not arise from ordinary fibroblasts.

Fibromatoses. There are a number of fibroma-like lesions which may cause considerable difficulties of diagnosis and which may not be true tumours. They include the following.

(*a*) *Desmoid tumour*, which is a curious lesion seen characteristically in the rectus abdominis muscle of multiparous women. It has the detailed histology of a fibroma, but is not encapsulated and infiltrates the surrounding muscle and destroys the muscle fibres (Fig. 12.5). It often recurs locally after excision, but never metastasises. Desmoids occur also in the thigh and shoulder, where they are difficult to eradicate and tend to recur. Ordinary fibromas are particularly rare in skeletal muscle.

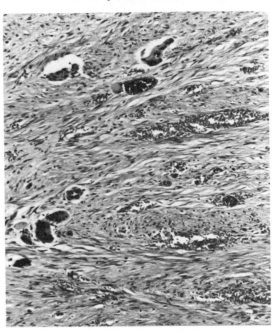

Fig. 12.5 'Desmoid tumour' of rectus sheath. Moderately cellular fibrous tissue forms the bulk of it. The large cells are multinucleate sarcolemmal giant cells, the remains of infiltrated muscle fibres. × 120.

(*b*) *Dupuytren's contracture*. This consists of a fibroma-like lesion, often quite cellular, involving the palmar fascia and producing flexion deformities of the fingers (see p. 867). A similar lesion of the plantar fascia (*plantar fibromatosis*) is often particularly cellular and sarcoma like under the microscope: a similar penile lesion is termed *Peyronie's disease*. Two or even all three of these conditions may occur in one patient, and they are clearly related. Again, none of these ever metastasises.

(*c*) *Keloid*. Some people (negroes more often than others) have a curious tendency to produce excessive masses of poorly cellular fibrous tissue, instead of the normal inconspicuous scars, after injury to the skin. They always cease growth after a time, and are clearly not tumours, but they are sometimes difficult to distinguish from hard fibromas.

Myxoma and mesenchymoma. The rare pure myxomas (Fig. 12.6) are translucent tumours, usually benign, composed of 'myxoid' tissue, a kind of connective tissue with stellate cells widely separated by a ground substance rich in mucopolysaccharide (p. 237). Tumours occur

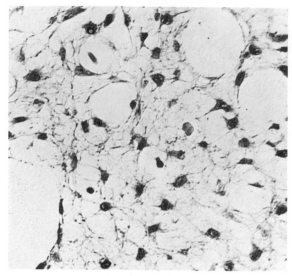

Fig. 12.6 Myxoma. The branching cells lie in a semi-fluid matrix which stains pale lilac with HE but much more deeply with connective tissue mucin stains. The round spaces are included fat cells of the breast, in which this tumour was found. × 300.

also in which similar tissue is mixed with other connective tissue elements (e.g. fat, giving a 'myxolipoma'). Both mixed tumours of this kind and pure myxomas have a greater tendency to recurrence than most benign tumours. There is also a group in which a predominantly

myxomatous tumour contains scattered elements of other mesenchymal tissue types, including muscle and cartilage. The name *mesenchymoma* is usually given to them, reflecting a belief, not necessarily well founded, that they represent a return to the capacity for multipotent differentiation of primitive mesenchyme. These tumours, most often seen in the subcutaneous tissues of the trunk, rarely metastasise but have a high incidence of local recurrence. The '*sarcoma botryoides*' of children (p. 297) also combines myxoid connective tissue with poorly formed muscle cells but has a very different age and anatomical distribution and is much more malignant: it is a rhabdomyosarcoma and must not be confused with the mesenchymoma.

Fibrosarcomas. These tumours arise especially from fascia and subcutaneous tissues, but may occur almost anywhere in the body. Similar tumours arise from nerves, *neurofibrosarcomas* (Fig. 12.7). While most fibro-

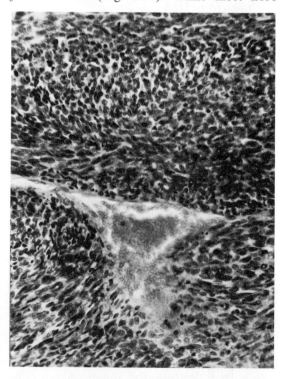

Fig. 12.8 Spindle-cell sarcoma. This is very cellular, but the cells are relatively uniform and still resemble fibroblasts. Special stains would show sparse collagen fibres. The triangular cleft is one of the characteristic poorly formed blood vessels of sarcomas. × 250.

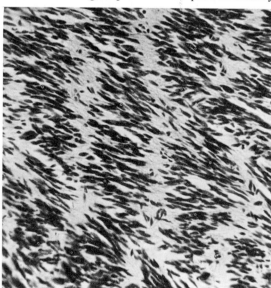

Fig. 12.7 Neurofibrosarcoma arising in recurrent neurofibroma. Note the very pronounced palisading of the nuclei. × 270.

sarcomas are clearly malignant from the start, some progress over a period of many years from an early stage in which they may be difficult to distinguish from a benign fibroma.

Fibrosarcomas differ greatly in their degree of differentiation. *Low grade fibrosarcomas* differ little from cellular fibromas: they are firm and fibrous, produce abundant collagen, and the cells differ little from normal fibroblasts. A moderately high rate of mitosis is often the only real evidence of malignancy. Such tumours are slow growing, are often cured by adequate local excision, and recurrences tend, at least at first, to remain localised. Tumours of intermediate malignancy are often called 'spindle-cell sarcomas' (Fig. 12.8). They are softer, more rapidly growing tumours in which the cells are still recognisably fibroblast-like and regularly arranged, but collagen is relatively inconspicuous: such tumours often metastasise and are usually ultimately fatal. From this type, transitions occur to the *pleomorphic sarcoma* (Fig. 12.9), a

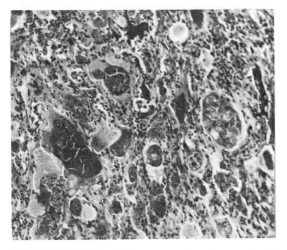

Fig. 12.9 Pleomorphic sarcoma showing great variation in the size of the cells. Note the numerous enormous polyploid nuclei. × 125.

soft, rapidly growing tumour consisting of large irregular cells with large irregular nuclei, with little or no collagen and very little evidence of the tissue of origin; metastasis is usually rapid and prognosis poor. Obviously, in such tumours it may be impossible to identify the cell of origin, and indeed tumours with this kind of histology may arise from dedifferentiation of almost any kind of cell.

Fibrosarcomas, like most other sarcomas, may recur locally or metastasise by the bloodstream, especially to the lungs, but rarely spread by the lymphatics.

The tumour cells of fibrosarcomas, unless very poorly differentiated, form enough collagen to produce an adequate stroma. As noted in the introductory section of this chapter, the blood vessels are often very poorly formed. Where this is very pronounced, the appearance under the microscope may be very striking, leading to their being called 'telangiectatic sarcomas' (Fig. 12.10). Such tumours are

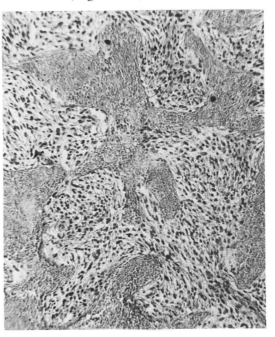

Fig. 12.10 'Telangiectatic sarcoma' showing numerous thin-walled vessels. × 150.

extremely vascular and haemorrhage is especially common. The vascular change is however entirely reactive, and they must not be confused with true angiosarcomas.

Tumours of adipose tissue

Lipoma. This is a benign tumour of adipose tissue. It increases in size by proliferation of fibroblast-like cells which lie around the blood vessels and are typically sparse; subsequently, these cells become ballooned with fat. The common lipoma is a rounded, well-demarcated, subcutaneous mass. It sometimes reaches a considerable size, and may have blunt projections which pass into the tissues around. Multiple tumours may be present and occasionally they are symmetrical. They are commonest over the shoulders and buttocks, and occur also within the abdomen, especially in the perirenal fat, but, like fibromas, they may arise almost anywhere in the body. Should the patient become emaciated, the fat in the tumour is not utilised—a good example of the failure of tumours to respond to the factors controlling the metabolism of normal tissues. In a lipoma there may be areas of fibrous, myxomatous or capillary angiomatous tissue—the tumour being then called a fibrolipoma, myxolipoma or angiolipoma respectively; occasionally there are areas of calcification.

In a rare variant the fat is finely divided in droplets within the cells, which thus closely resemble those of the brown hibernating-fat depots of rodents; this type of lipoma has been called '*hibernoma*' (Fig. 12.11).

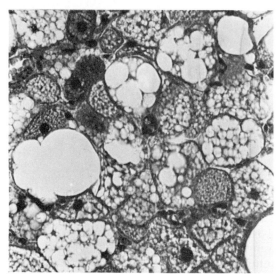

Fig. 12.11 'Hibernoma' showing the characteristic appearances of the fat-laden cells, with central nuclei. × 480.

Liposarcoma. This is rather uncommon. In the less malignant forms the tissue retains some naked-eye resemblance to fat and the microscopic difference from lipoma may not be very striking at first sight. The fat cells vary in size; much more important, the scanty undifferentiated cells from which the benign lipoma arises are augmented to form broad bands of cellular connective tissue, with irregular nuclei, interspersed among the fat-containing cells. These well-differentiated liposarcomas are usually only prone to local recurrence. All transitions occur through myxoid liposarcomas to highly malignant, pleomorphic tumours in some of which gigantic lipoblasts may be seen (Fig. 12.12a). In others, however, the origin in fat

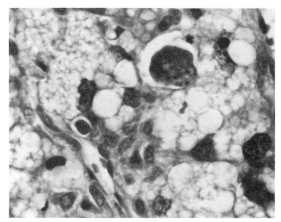

Fig. 12.12a Pleomorphic liposarcoma, consisting of very large cells with very large nuclei, and with much fat in the cytoplasm. × 450.

cells may be hard to establish. Since normal adipose tissue has a lobulated architecture it is not surprising that liposarcomas sometimes show a somewhat lobular or alveolar architecture (Fig. 12.12b) and the cells may rarely be mistaken even for epithelium. Liposarcomas

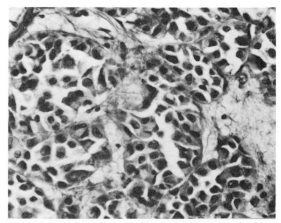

Fig. 12.12b Pseudo-alveolar pattern in a liposarcoma, a rare variant that may be mistaken for carcinoma. × 400.

are commonest about the shoulders, in the peri-renal fatty tissue, and in the intermuscular fasciae of the lower limbs, usually with an admixture of myxomatous tissue.

Alveolar soft tissue sarcoma. This rather uncommon variety of sarcoma arises in the soft tissues, usually of a limb. It is composed of large polygonal or round cells with coarsely granular cytoplasm, and arranged in a curiously alveolar pattern. In paraffin sections the appearances resemble those of liposarcoma or even carcinoma but the granules do not contain lipids, mucin, glycogen or other specifically stainable substance. Its origin and true nature are obscure, but some regard it as a variety of chemodectoma (p. 298).

Tumours arising in cartilage and bone

These are dealt with in detail in Chapter 22. The benign tumours of bone are a perplexingly various group, and their precise histogenesis is often obscure. Most of the masses of cartilage called chondromas and many of those of bone called osteomas are developmental defects or hamartomas (p. 297) and not true tumours. Osteosarcomas and, to a lesser extent, chondrosarcomas are among the commonest sarcomas. Osteosarcoma especially exemplifies many of the most characteristic features of sarcomas generally—a high incidence in childhood, a high mortality and a very low incidence of lymph-spread metastases combined with a high tendency to blood-borne metastases, especially in the lungs.

Fibrosarcomas may arise from bone. Conversely (though very rarely) bone-forming osteosarcomas sometimes arise from connective tissue elsewhere, and sometimes even from such organs as the breast, kidney, etc.

Bone and cartilage are sometimes seen in non-bony tumours. Both are common in teratomas. Cartilage is often seen in the mixed tumours of the parotid and other glands. Bony metaplasia of the stroma of carcinomas is a rare but striking finding, least rare in man in large-bowel cancers, and not uncommon in breast tumours in bitches.

Tumours of muscle

There are two varieties of myoma, the **leiomyoma**, composed of smooth muscle fibres, and the **rhabdomyoma** of striped muscle. The latter is so rare that the term *myoma* without qualification is often used to signify leiomyoma.

The leiomyomas are composed of smooth muscle cells orientated in a more or less parallel manner within bundles, which are arranged in a whorled pattern (Fig. 12.13). A small amount

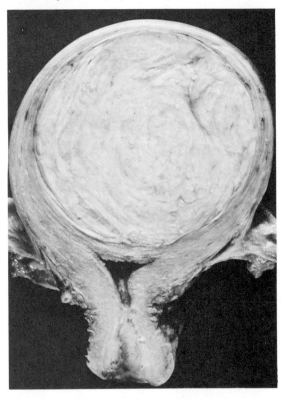

Fig. 12.13 Leiomyoma of uterus. The tumour is paler than the normal muscle because of its higher content of fibrous tissue. The pattern of the cut tumour surface is formed by brownish slightly translucent strands of muscle, here forming an indistinct network but often whorled. Note the distorted uterine lumen. Natural size.

of supporting connective tissue runs among the individual cells, while broader bands separate the bundles. The proportion of fibrous tissue to muscle varies much in different specimens. The tumours are usually firm and rounded, and on section are pinkish with a characteristic whorled appearance due to the arrangement of the fibres (Fig. 12.14).

Leiomyomas of the *uterus* are among the commonest of tumours: their usually high content of fibrous tissue earns them their common

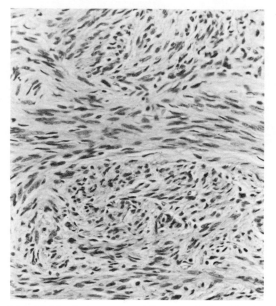

Fig. 12.14   Leiomyoma. The muscle bundles interlace irregularly, and are to be seen cut transversely, longitudinally and obliquely. The cytoplasm of the muscle cells stains somewhat indistinctly but gives a darker shade to the substance of each bundle. Occasional fibrocytes seen between the bundles have smaller darker nuclei apparently devoid of cytoplasm. × 185.

name of 'fibroids', though the muscle is the only true tumorous element and it is incorrect to call them fibromyomas. They are dealt with in more detail in Chapter 23. Of general interest is their tendency to cease growth at the menopause and subsequently regress.

Myomas are probably next most common in the muscular coat of the alimentary canal, though here most are too small to be found without special search and few are large enough to cause trouble. They occur also in the skin, being remarkable here in that some are extremely painful on pressure; they appear rarely in other sites such as ovaries, prostate and bladder.

Leiomyosarcomas occasionally arise from the same sites as leiomyomas, especially the uterus and the stomach. Most appear to be malignant from the start but some may arise by malignant progression in a benign myoma. The histological diagnosis of malignancy is usually easy on general cytological grounds, but the better differentiated tumours can be hard to distinguish from the more cellular benign tumours. It is a useful empirical rule, which cannot be extended to all other tumours, that a smooth muscle tumour in which mitoses can be found easily is liable to metastasise.

Rhabdomyosarcoma. In proportion to their

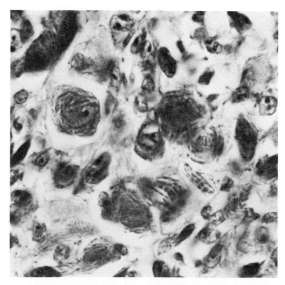

Fig. 12.15a   Rhabdomyosarcoma. Large pleomorphic cells in a slightly myxoid matrix. Special stains and high magnification show coiled myofibrils (best seen in cells just below and to the right of centre).

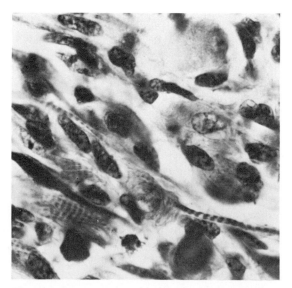

Fig. 12.15b   As 12.15a. The nature of the myofibrils is more obvious when the cells are drawn out into 'strap cells' and the fibrils produce cross striations as seen here, especially below right, but these are usually hard to find.

bulk, the voluntary muscles are one of the rarest of sites for tumours of any kind, both primary and secondary: the reasons for this are not known. The rare tumours in which striped muscle fibres or their precursors are seen are nearly always malignant, and arise mostly in sites where no striped muscle is present normally. They are found most often in the genital tract, characteristically in the cervix or vaginal vault in young girls: probably next least rarely in the soft palate. Usually the tumours have a large myxoid element, and recognisable muscle cells (though very characteristic when found) are often scanty and difficult to find, even with special stains which accentuate their cross striations. Rounded or irregular cells with coiled myofibrils but without cross-striations are usually more readily apparent. (Fig. 12.15). When growing beneath a mucous membrane they often present with numerous blunt translucent processes—hence the name of *sarcoma botryoides* (grapelike sarcoma). These are highly malignant tumours: local recurrence after excision and blood-spread metastases are usual, and (unlike most sarcomas) lymph node metastases are common.

Rhabdomyosarcomas are also seen very rarely in the heart. Benign tumours, perhaps better regarded as hamartomas,* are seen there in children with epiloia (tuberous sclerosis): the lumps consist of swollen muscle cells packed with glycogen and some confusion has in the past existed between these findings and the cardiac lesions of glycogen storage disease (p. 21).

Tumours of Blood Vessels and Lymphatics

Haemangioma. A haemangioma consists of a mass of blood vessels, atypical or irregular in arrangement and size. A corresponding growth, lymphangioma, is composed of lymphatic vessels similarly altered; but, as this is rarer, the term angioma is often used as synonymous with haemangioma.

The majority of the lesions called angiomas are not true tumours, but hamartomas.* They are present at birth, even if not always visible, and their enlargement ceases with the growth of the patient. Most angiomas are well-defined masses of vascular tissue which resemble tumours sufficiently to justify their inclusion here. The two common varieties are as follows.

(*a*) *The capillary angiomas* consist of dense plexiform arrangements of vessels of capillary size (Fig. 12.16). They occur especially in the skin, where they form one of the two common types of *naevus*† or birthmark, but are also seen in the internal organs. Most are small, but larger lesions occur, e.g. the 'port-wine stains' of the face, and these may contain vessels of larger size than capillaries. Capillary angiomas are usually well defined, and deep red or purple. The capillary vessels have a more prominent endothelial lining than normal capillaries. The stroma consists of well-formed collagen. There is no capsule, and outlying groups of capillaries in adjoining tissues often give a false appearance of invasion. The blood supply is usually clearly separated from that of the surrounding tissues, there being generally only one artery of supply.

(*b*) *Cavernous angiomas* are confined to the deeper tissues, being least rare in the liver. They consist of relatively large interconnecting sinuslike vascular spaces (Fig. 12.17). In the liver they form deep-purple well-defined masses, usually polygonal rather than round and not raised above the surface, signs of their lack of expansile growth.

Angiomas are often multiple, and are also an important component of several diseases with a strong hereditary element, e.g. hereditary haemorrhagic telangiectasia (p. 503) (multiple

---

* *Hamartoma* is a convenient term for an ill-defined group of lesions on the borderline of true neoplasia. They are tumour-like lumps present at birth or appearing soon afterwards, growing with the patient and ceasing to grow when general body growth ceases. They can be best understood as a disorder of the relationships of normal tissues in a limited area, leading to a relative over-production of one element but without any tendency to progressive growth characteristic of tumours. Angiomas and pigmented naevi are the common forms, but there are many varieties. With some of them there is a tendency to later development of true tumour.

† A *naevus* (mole or birthmark) is a hamartoma of the skin made conspicuous by some definite colour difference from the surrounding normal area. Angiomas and pigmented naevi (pp. 1007–11) are the two common types.

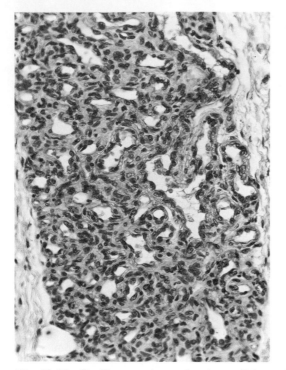

Fig. 12.16 Capillary angioma showing well-formed capillaries with prominent endothelial cells. The solid areas between capillaries include many cells which are believed to be endothelial cells not related to a lumen. × 200.

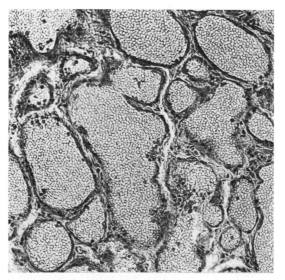

Fig. 12.17 Cavernous angioma of subcutaneous tissue, showing large intercommunicating spaces filled with blood. × 130.

small angiomas in skin and mucosae with a strong tendency to haemorrhage), Lindau's disease (cerebellar and retinal angiomas with cysts of liver and pancreas) and Sturge–Weber syndrome (facial and meningeal angiomas).

A special form of angioma of the skin, the so-called sclerosing angioma, is dealt with later (p. 1014).

Glomangioma (glomus tumour). This uncommon but interesting lesion apparently arises from the glomus bodies, small arteriovenous anastomoses with a coiled arteriole and abundant nerve supply which control blood flow and temperature, particularly in the fingers and toes. In its most characteristic form, the glomangioma is a small bluish nodule, usually near the end of a finger, and extraordinarily tender to even light touch. On microscopic examination the tumour is found to consist of two kinds of tissue variously interblended (Fig. 12.18). The first is angiomatous, with spaces containing blood, lined by endothelium, and separated by connective tissue containing varying amounts of smooth muscle. The other is cellular, with rounded or cuboidal cells called 'myoid', as transitions to smooth muscle fibres can be found. The growth contains numerous medullated and non-medullated nerve fibres and the pain is apparently due to distensile pressures in the blood-containing spaces, though the painfulness is not in proportion to the neural content. A small dermal leiomyoma may likewise be painful and the two forms of growth may be related in origin. Glomangiomas have been described in deeper tissues, including the gut, but the characteristic pain occurs only with those in the limbs.

Chemodectoma. Because of their close anatomical relationship with blood vessels it is convenient to consider here the tumours arising from the chemoreceptor organs, viz. the carotid body, glomus jugulare, organ of Zuckerkandl and no doubt other less clearly defined structures such as the aortic bodies. These tumours have also been called **non-chromaffin paragangliomas**; they do not appear to produce any endocrine effects.

Chemodectomas are usually benign, but their anatomical sites may render complete surgical removal difficult. Thus carotid body tumours, which are the commonest variety, closely embrace the bifurcation of the common carotid artery, and the glomus jugulare tumours involve the middle ear and present as recurrent bleeding aural polyps; they may also present intracranially. Microscopically the architec-

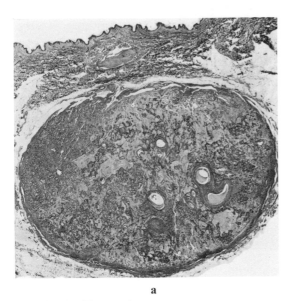
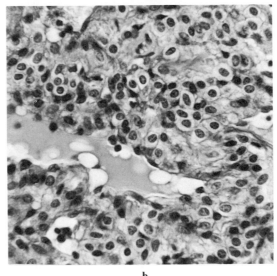

a   b

Fig. 12.18   Glomangioma.
a Small subcutaneous encapsulated growth showing the coiled arteriole. × 8.
b The clear myoid cells surrounding a vascular space. × 350.

tural pattern is similar to the normal structure and consists of many small masses of cells of variable size, sometimes enclosed in a boxlike framework of fine fibrous tissue (Fig. 12.19). The tumour cells are usually polygonal and may be spindle-shaped in places but aberrant types with hyperchromatic nuclei are not uncommon and do not indicate malignancy. The blood supply is very rich and of sinusoidal pattern.

Haemangioendothelioma: haemangiosarcoma. Occasionally tumours with the general histological features of capillary haemangiomas have formed numerous metastases. Fig. 12.20 is an example of this kind which originated in the breast (a not very rare site) and secondary growths developed in the orbit, lungs, liver, etc. Here one finds not only new formation of capillary channels but also active division of the endothelial cells to form solid processes which pass into and blend with the surrounding masses of cells and join with pre-existing capillaries.

Tumours whose origin is traceable to the vascular endothelium and which form both new capillaries and solid masses of cells, the two types being intimately blended, also occur in the intermuscular fascia of the limbs, and may extend much more widely than is clinically apparent. Fig. 12.21 is from such a case; the tumour was in the upper arm and it ramified so extensively in the muscles that ultimately a fore-quarter amputation had to be performed.

Exposure to vinyl chloride may predispose to the

otherwise very rare haemangiosarcoma of the liver (p. 256), but this may yet prove to be of Kupffer cell origin rather than from sinusoidal endothelium.

Kaposi's disease: Idiopathic haemorrhagic sarcoma. This remarkable disorder is rare in Britain. It is more

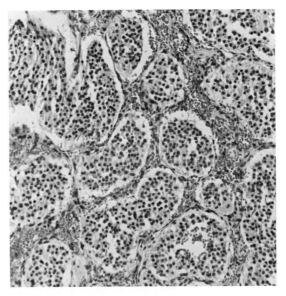

Fig. 12.19   Chemodectoma of the carotid body, showing the characteristic boxlike pattern and highly vascular stroma. × 160.

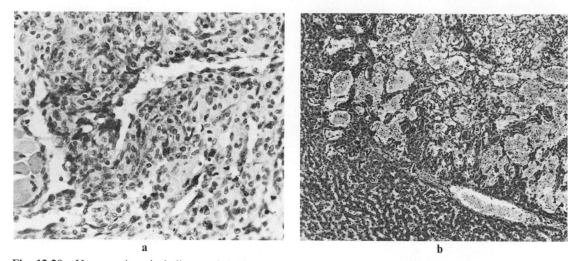

a   b

Fig. 12.20 Haemangioendothelioma of the breast.
a Primary tumour, showing vascular channels and solid masses of endothelial cells. × 270.
b Metastasis in liver, showing wide vascular spaces lined by swollen endothelial cells which invade and replace the sinusoids, becoming continuous with them. × 45.

frequent in some other parts of Europe and Africa, and relatively common in some well-defined areas of Central Africa, where it is much more frequent in males. The condition presents the syndrome of lymphoedema, multiple cutaneous tumours which later ulcerate, lymphadenopathy and ultimately visceral involvement. The skin tumours at first consist of lobulated masses of highly vascular and cellular tissue resembling granulation tissue deep within the corium and separated by fibrous trabeculae (Fig. 12.22). Later there is much haemorrhage in and around the lesions, the spindle cells and vascular sprouts increase progressively, mitoses are abundant, ulceration of superficial lesions occurs and the regional lymph nodes may be replaced by similar highly

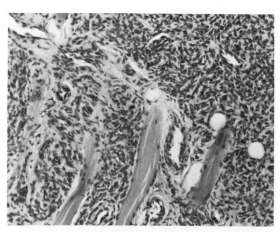

Fig. 12.21 Haemangioendothelioma. The tumour consists of solid cords of endothelial cells and poorly defined capillary channels, invading and destroying skeletal muscle. × 110.

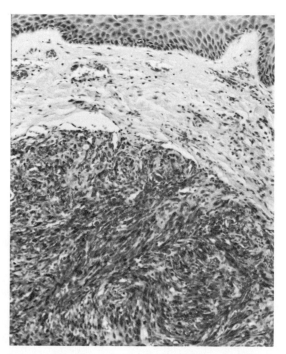

Fig. 12.22 Kaposi's haemorrhagic sarcoma. An early lesion showing the zone of fibrous tissue between the vascular spindle-celled tumour and the epidermis. × 130.

vascular spindle-celled tissue. Despite their tumour-like appearance many lesions ultimately heal, although the disease may progress elsewhere. However, in some cases at least (the proportion is uncertain), the lesions become progressive in internal organs, especially the intestines. This occurs more frequently in Central African cases that in those in South Africa or elsewhere. The superficial lesions respond well to radiotherapy and chemotherapy.

It is uncertain whether this is a true neoplasm but in some cases it certainly behaves like one. Evidence from histochemistry and tissue culture indicates that the spindle cells are not fibroblasts: the lesion may be an angiosarcoma derived from lymphatic endothelium as the cells lack the enzymes characteristic of blood capillary endothelium.

Haemangiopericytoma. This also is a much disputed but probably genuine entity. The tumours are vascular, with uniform sheets of large pale cells around the vessels, the cells being separated from each other by a prominent reticulin network. They are usually malignant. The term should not be confused with 'perithelioma', a term once mistakenly used to describe tumours, usually anaplastic carcinomas, in which the common tendency towards death of cells lying at a distance from blood vessels is exaggerated so that the surviving cells appear to form perivascular sheaths. The true haemangiopericytoma is believed to arise from pericytes, and the perivascular arrangement is not the result of pararterial ischaemic necrosis.

Lymphangioma. This may be composed of numerous lymphatic vessels—the *plexiform* lymphangioma—but more frequently it has a *cavernous* structure. Dilatation and diffuse growth of vessels may give rise to enlargement of a part, e.g. the tongue (*macroglossia*). In such lesions there is even less evidence than in haemangiomas of neoplastic growth, and the more diffuse lesions may be hard to distinguish from the effects of lymphatic obstruction, though in most cases it is clear from the anatomy that no such obstruction can be present, and a congenital malformation (or hamartoma) of the lymphatics is present. It is becoming increasingly common to describe such diffuse leisons as *localised lymphangiectasis* rather than lymphangioma· Lesions, whether diffuse or compact, are commonest in the skin and subcutaneous tissue. Each forms a somewhat ill-defined, doughy, or semi-fluctuant swelling, containing large, intercommunicating lymphatic spaces. The contents are a clear lymph, containing occasional lymphocytes.

Sometimes bleeding into the spaces renders the diagnosis between haemangioma and lymphangioma difficult. Lymphangiomas occur occasionally also in mucous membranes in the wall of the bowel (Fig. 12.23), in the tissues of the orbit and mesentery, and elsewhere.

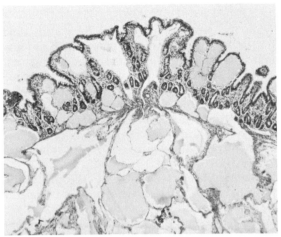

Fig. 12.23 Cavernous lymphangioma of small intestine. It is made up of large intercommunicating spaces filled with clear lymph (which has coagulated then shrunk in processing the tissue). It occupies both mucosa and submucosa, the mucosa being much distorted but otherwise not much damaged.

In rare cases lymphangiomas of neck, retroperitoneum or mesentery undergo great dilatation, forming a multilocular ramifying cystic mass which may reach a large size. Occasionally a single cyst is formed, as in one form of *hygroma* of the neck or axilla. It may be distinguished from other cysts in this region by its endothelial lining.

Lymphangiosarcoma is a very doubtful entity, but has been described as arising in the lymphatics of the arm, following their obstruction by mastectomy and irradiation for mammary cancer. Very similar appearances may result from a slow and rather diffuse permeation of the lymphatics by carcinoma and it remains undecided whether the so-called lymphangiosarcoma secondary to chronic post-operative obstruction is a separate and distinct neoplasm.

'Endothelioma'. This term was once used very freely for tumours of uncertain origin. The angiomas described above could be called vascular endotheliomas, but past misuse has led to the avoidance of this term. Meningiomas, formerly called fibro-endotheliomas, though possibly endothelial in origin, are no longer so described (see p. 729). Tumours of the serosal linings are usually called **mesotheliomas**.

Tumours of Neuro-Ectodermal Origin

From the ectodermal cells of the neural tube and crest are derived the tumours of (*a*) the neuroglia, (*b*) nerve cells and their precursors, (*c*) nerve sheaths, (*d*) peripheral neuro-receptor organs, (*e*) the melanocytes, and possibly also of (*f*) the meninges. These tumours will be discussed in detail in connection with the nervous system and the skin. It will suffice at this stage to mention very briefly a few types and their features.

Glioma. These tumours of the neuroglia occur commonly in the brain, but also rarely in the spinal cord. Because of their anatomical site and the pressure effects they may exercise on vital structures most gliomas in the end are likely to kill the patient, but even those of high cellularity and aberrant cellular structure do not metastasise outside the nervous system. (This absence of distant metastases applies to all intracranial tumours, and appears to be a characteristic of the intracranial site, not of the type of tumour.)

Gliomas may take origin from all types of neuroglia and may be firm, slow-growing, and rich in glial fibrils, but may nevertheless undergo central necrosis. At the other extreme are highly pleomorphic rapidly growing cellular tumours in which necrosis and haemorrhage are conspicuous. A rapidly growing cellular tumour showing little or no pleomorphism occurs in the cerebellum of children—medulloblastoma (p. 727).

Ganglioneuromas are rare tumours composed of mature ganglion cells and nerve fibres. They are found chiefly in relation to the sympathetic chain and adrenal medulla (p. 728). Clinically and histologically they behave as benign tumours except when they contain foci of neuroblasts.

Neuroblastoma or **sympathicoblastoma** is a highly cellular tumour which occurs chiefly in the adrenal medulla or in connection with the sympathetic chain elsewhere, usually arising in children. It consists of small round or oval cells with scanty cytoplasm, in places arranged in ball-like clusters which, on section, appear as rosettes. These tumours are highly malignant and metastasise widely, especially to the skull and other bones (p. 727).

Although strikingly different in appearance, it appears that ganglioneuroma and neuroblastoma are benign and malignant variants of the same tumour. As a rare but remarkable event, neuroblastoma may undergo a form of self-cure by maturing into a ganglioneuroma.

Melanocytic tumours

The cells which form melanin are of neural crest origin and are called melanocytes (p. 1008). The skin and the eye are their chief sites, and in both places they are important sources of tumours.

Skin tumours are dealt with fully in Chapter 25. The so-called **pigmented naevus** is very common. It is a benign lesion, probably better regarded as a hamartoma than a true tumour, formed by a mass of melanocytes ('naevus cells') which accumulate in the dermis as a result of excessive proliferation of melanocytes in their normal site in the basal layer. **Malignant melanomas** are much less common: they arise from epidermal melanocytes, often at the site of a pigmented naevus. They are highly malignant and, unless excised at an early stage, are liable to metastasise extensively, both to lymph nodes and by the blood: since the tumours are often very dark due to melanin production, they can present a striking picture at necropsy.

Ocular melanomas. Malignant melanomas of the eye, though far from common, are the least rare of all intraocular malignant tumours. They are described on page 742.

Melanomas at other sites. Melanocytes spill over all the mucocutaneous junctions into the adjoining mucous membranes to varying distances and in varying numbers, and melanomas occur at the corresponding sites. They are least rare in the nose, but arise also in the mouth, conjunctiva, vagina and anus and even in such deeper sites as oesophagus and rectum. The presence of melanocytes in the meninges is also reflected in the rare occurrence of malignant melanomas, which are remarkable for their inability to metastasise outside the cranial cavity.

Tumours of the Haemopoietic, Lymphoid and Mononuclear Phagocyte Systems

Classification within this group is difficult, and it is only in the last few decades that some of its most important members—the leukaemias and Hodgkin's disease for instance—have become fully accepted as neoplastic. Nomenclature still tends to be anomalous and classification disputed. The principal varieties are described in Chapters 16 and 17 and only a few general points will be made here.

The characteristic cells of these tissues are far more mobile than those of most of the rest of the body. This is obviously true of the blood cells, lymphocytes, macrophages and the like, but applies also to less prominently mobile cells—the blood cell precursors of the marrow, for example, appear in the blood in small numbers in various conditions of stress, and are capable of re-establishing themselves in the spleen and liver. Unlike epithelium, these cells do not adhere to form a compact cell mass; nor are they tethered by the formation of large amounts of extracellular matrix like most connective tissue cells. The tumours accordingly tend not to form a single mass but to spread widely from the start: in most of them the spread is limited to a large extent to the regions which normally contain cells of the same type. This is particularly true of the better-differentiated tumours. For instance, in chronic myeloid leukaemia, a well-differentiated neoplasia of the granulocyte series, very large numbers of tumour cells appear in the blood from the start, but the solid organs most involved are usually the marrow, liver and spleen, i.e. the sites of leukopoiesis in fetal life. The poorly differentiated acute leukaemias on the other hand produce far fewer mobile cells in the blood (and sometimes none at all) and tend to a more destructive infiltration of the marrow and other organs. Similarly the better differentiated lymph node tumours characteristically cause widespread moderate enlargement of multiple lymph nodes and other lymphoid structures but often do not spread very much to non-lymphoid tissues, while the less well differentiated may cause large local masses and less discriminatory spread to other structures.

Any tissue which contains any of the cells belonging to the relevant categories (which means practically any tissue in the body) can give rise to tumours within this group, but the vast majority arise either in the bone marrow (leukaemias and myelomatosis) or the lymph nodes (true lymphomas arising from lymphocytes or their precursors; Hodgkin's disease and 'reticulosarcoma', both of which are of uncertain origin). As will be obvious from what has been said above, a benign tumour in the ordinary sense of the word must be exceptional and may in fact be nonexistent. Localised nodules of abnormal lymphoid tissue are sometimes found, for example in the rectum and skin, and may be called 'benign lymphoma' or 'benign lymphocytoma' but it is doubtful whether these are tumours at all.

The immunological importance of these tissues is naturally reflected in their tumours. Immunological abnormalities are fairly commonly associated with some lymph node tumours, the most striking example being production of immunoglobulin in large amounts by the neoplastic plasma cells of myelomatosis.

The viral aetiology of lymphomas and leukaemias in several animal species is now beyond doubt, and it is very likely that these human tumours are also virus-induced: so far, however, the evidence is inconclusive and relates mainly to acute leukaemia (see p. 264) and to Burkitt's lymphoma.

'Mixed' Tumours

A considerable number of tumours consist of two or more different kinds of tissue. The reasons for this are very diverse: the most important can be classified as follows:

cartilaginous metaplasia of the stroma in mixed-salivary tumours, the bony metaplasia seen in a very few carcinomas of the colon, and the lymphoid stroma of some seminomas all produce

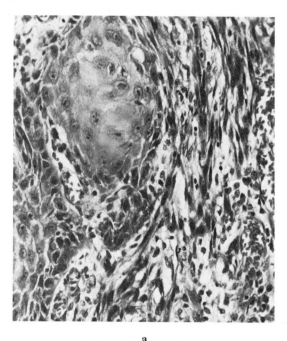
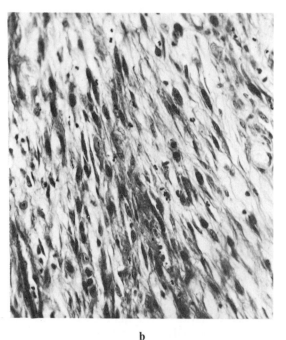

a   b

Fig. 12.24 Squamous carcinoma of tongue, showing so-called carcinosarcoma.
a On the left typical squamous carcinoma, showing continuity with spindle-shaped epithelial cells.
b On the right a purely spindle-cell area containing many mitoses. Transitions from (a) to (b) are readily found. × 200.

(*a*) *'Collision' tumours* result when two different tumours arise close together and intermingle; presumably the juxtaposition may be a chance event, or the result of a single carcinogenic stimulus applied at one point and affecting several tissues.

(*b*) *Stromal changes in epithelial tumours.* The

the *appearance* of a mixed tumour, though only the epithelial element is truly neoplastic.

(*c*) *'Metaplastic' tumours.* Tumours arising from tissues which readily undergo metaplasia from one type to another often reflect this characteristic. Such are the 'adeno-acanthomas', with mixed squamous and glandular elements, which arise especially in uterus and bronchus, and more rarely in the stomach.

(*d*) *Tumours with variable differentiation.* This occurs especially in carcinomas, parts of which are so poorly differentiated as to resemble sarcomas. It is almost certain that most so-called 'carcinosarcomas', both human and experimental, are of this type (Fig. 12.24).

(*e*) *Truly mixed tumours* involving the co-ordinated neoplastic growth of two independent tissues are hard to find. The fibroadenoma of the breast is the only completely acceptable example, though some connective tissue tumours, such as the angiolipoma, may qualify.

(*f*) *'Embryonal' tumours.* There is a group of tumours, mostly highly malignant, which arise usually in infancy and appear to be derived from immature tissue. Most of these (neuroblastoma, medulloblastoma, hepatoblastoma, for example) are not truly mixed, but the partial differentiation of some of the elements, while others continue to resemble primitive embryonal tissue, may give rise to appearances that simulate a mixed tumour.

One of the commonest of these tumours, the renal nephroblastoma (Wilms' tumour), consists of sarcoma-like masses of short spindle cells, among which some elements differentiate to tubules and occasionally glomerulus-like structures (Fig. 12.25). More discordant tissues such as cartilage and striped muscle are occasionally present, possibly representing a derivation of the tumour cells from the myotome at an earlier period in ontogeny.

(*g*) *Teratomas.* These, the most extreme

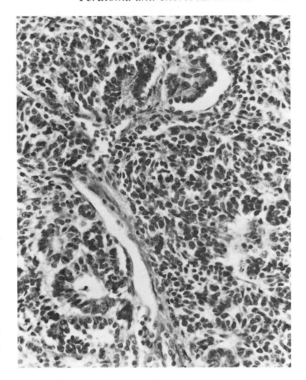

Fig. 12.25 Nephroblastoma (Wilms' tumour), showing cellular sarcoma-like tissue with indistinct differentiation of tubules in several places and a glomerulus-like structure (at *top right*). × 225.

examples of mixed tumours, are dealt with in the following section.

It should be emphasised that the grouping together of these tumours is not intended to indicate any special relation between them: they have, in fact, very little in common except the presence of more than one kind of tissue.

Teratoma and Choriocarcinoma

Teratoma

A teratoma is a tumour composed of various tissues, chaotically arranged and usually of the most diverse types, with no relation to the site of origin. They are not rare and are of practical importance. They are most common in the ovaries and testes, though they occur in other parts, such as the mediastinum, retroperitoneal tissues and pineal. They are usually single but occasionally more than one is present. There is

great variation in naked-eye appearances, and cyst formation may be a notable feature, as in the common ovarian teratoma ('dermoid'). There is endless variety in the tissues and in their arrangement. Cartilage, bone, epidermis, glandular epithelium, hair, teeth, etc., are common components, but other specialised tissues such as liver, kidney, nervous, eye and haemopoietic are also represented (Figs. 12.26, 12.27), and sometimes there are structures resembling early embryos, with trophoblastic

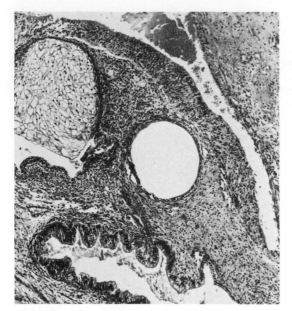

Fig. 12.26 Ovarian cystic teratoma or 'dermoid' (benign). Above there is a cleft lined by squamous epithelium which is part of the main cyst. The cyst on the left is lined partly by columnar, partly by non-keratinising squamous epithelium. The lowest cyst is lined by folded columnar epithelium of alimentary type, and the resemblance to gut is heightened by an incomplete layer of smooth muscle related to it. × 72.

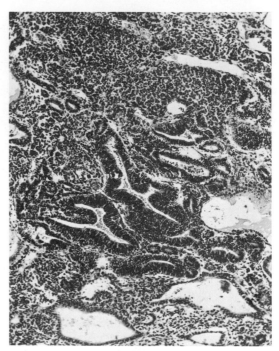

Fig. 12.27 Testicular teratoma (malignant). Because of loss of differentiation the diversity of tissue types is harder to demonstrate, but there is obviously a variety of epithelia present here, the large dark-staining tubules being of primitive neural type. × 62.

epithelium. While a teratoma may be of such a complicated constitution, there is no proper formation of organs, limbs, etc., and a very important fact is that there is no trace of a vertebral column and no metameric segmentation. Germ cells and germinal epithelium are also always absent.

Because of their complicated structure, teratomas were formerly believed to arise from totipotent cells, i.e. from dislocated blastomeres. However, proliferation of a blastomere gives rise to an organised embryo, in contrast to the chaotic mixture of tissues in a teratoma. Another view is that teratomas are derived from the male or female germ cells. The frequency of teratomas in the gonads supports this possibility. Something of the nature of parthenogenetic development would have to be assumed, as is known to occur in amphibian ova under the influence of certain salt solutions. Bosaeus obtained striking results by stimulating frogs' ova to parthenogenetic development and then placing them in the internal tissues: tumour masses developed which he describes as

having the structure of spontaneous teratomas. In cocks the intratesticular injection of solutions of zinc salts during the breeding season or after stimulation by pituitary gonadotrophin has led to the development of highly malignant complex teratomatous tumours closely resembling those in man (Bagg) but similar results do not appear to have been achieved in mammals.

Study of the sex chromatin (p. 884) has provided some evidence in favour of the parthenogenetic origin of teratomas. It has been found that all teratomas in women have female nuclei but about half of those in men have female nuclei, as would be expected if they arose from a cell produced by fusion of two haploid cells in the male gonad. Recent cytogenetic evidence on the occurrence of crossing-over in ovarian teratomas appears to confirm this view.

Many teratomas, especially in the ovary, are benign. Rarely, one element of such a teratoma may become malignant, and if metastases develop they contain only this one type of malignant tissue. Apart from those in the ovary, most teratomas, and especially those in the testis, are malignant from the start, and all of their elements are malignant.

Benign teratomas never contain tissues of extra-fetal origin, such as trophoblast (see below) or yolk sac: whether alone or as part of a teratoma, these always indicate malignancy.

Monstrosities. When identical twins develop from a single fertilised ovum a variable amount of fusion may take place. This may be of limited extent as in so-called Siamese twins, or it may affect a considerable part of the body. Partial fusion of two germinal areas is often invoked. Then there are cases where one fetus is imperfectly represented and fused with the other, growing on it in parasite-like fashion or included within its abdominal cavity—*fetus in fetu*. Many sacral teratomas and epignathi probably belong to this group. All such abnormalities, which are extremely varied, are spoken of as monstrosities. They show wide deviations from the normal, but the formation of parts and the relations of the tissues to one another are well maintained: thus, organs may be doubled, and a limb, though abnormal in size or form, is still a limb. Monstrosities are now generally thought to be of a fundamentally different nature from teratomas and apparent transitions are almost certainly fallacious. A defect in the mechanism of the primary organisers at a very early stage of formation of the embryo may well be responsible for this type of abnormality.

Choriocarcinoma

This is an uncommon and highly malignant tumour which originates from, and retains recognisable features of, trophoblastic epithelium (Fig. 12.28). It also retains the trophoblastic property of invading blood vessels, and so metastases are usually early and widespread. Choriocarcinoma arises occasionally from tro-

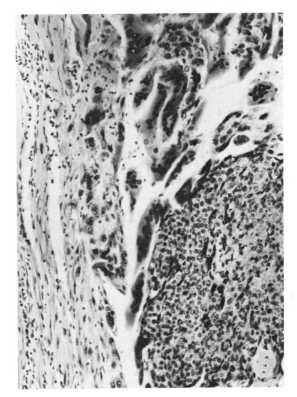

Fig. 12.28 Choriocarcinoma, showing Langhans' cells (cytotrophoblast, *bottom right*) and giant cells (syncytiotrophoblast, *centre*) invading uterine wall (*left*). × 230.

phoblastic differentiation in a teratoma of the testis, mediastinum, etc., but its usual site is in the uterus, where it originates from the placental trophoblast of a pregnancy and is thus a fetal tumour growing in the mother. In spite of this, it grows and extends rapidly, but responds unusually well to chemotherapy, and in some instances removal of the primary tumour has been followed by apparently spontaneous disappearance of metastases. These unusual features, which apply only to the uterine (fetal) choriocarcinomas, are probably due to a homograft reaction.

Cysts

The term 'cyst' properly means a space containing fluid and lined by endothelium or epithelium. Accordingly, cysts are not tumours and are included here only for convenience. Nearly all cysts arise by the abnormal dilatation of pre-existing tubules, ducts or cavities, though such a cyst may lose its cell lining due to inflammatory or other change, and becomes lined by granulation or denser connective tissue. The term is, however, often applied in a somewhat loose way to other abnormal cavities containing fluid. For example, the term 'apoplectic cyst' is applied to a space in the brain containing brownish fluid, which has resulted from haemorrhage. Some tumours, e.g. gliomas, undergo softening in their interior, so that a collection of fluid is formed, and the term 'cystic change' is often used even when no true cyst is formed.

The cysts peculiar to each organ will be described in the later chapters: we shall give here only a classification of their causes. The occurrence of true cysts in tumours—*cystic adenomas and teratomas*—has already been described. Apart from these, cysts fall naturally into two main groups, viz. (1) those due to congenital abnormalities, and (2) acquired cysts, i.e. those produced by lesions in post-natal life.

(1) Congenital cysts. These may also be grouped into two types:

(a). They may arise *within otherwise normal organs or tissues*, as a result of the presence of epithelium of a type not usually present at that site after birth, either as a result of some minor displacement of an embryonal tissue or (more often) the failure to disappear of some embryonic duct or cleft. The commonest site of cysts derived from vestigial ducts is the genitourinary tract, where the disappearance of the mesonephros and its duct in both sexes, and of the Woolffian ducts in females and Mullerian ducts in males, often leaves behind a variety of persistent epithelial remnants: small cysts are very common among these, and larger ones (*parovarian cysts*) are not uncommon in the broad ligaments (p. 910).

Other embryonic ducts which may persist and give rise to cysts include the thyroglossal duct (mid-line of neck, usually near the thyroid, p. 964) and the urachus (usually at the umbilicus). A similar mechanism operates with the branchial clefts; *branchial cysts* are produced at the side of the neck and are lined by squamous epithelium with usually a rim of lymphoid tissue.

A different mechanism produces the *sequestration dermoids* which result from imperfect fusion of embryonal skin flaps. They are lined with squamous epithelium and filled with keratin, and are found mostly in the mid-line of the chest and neck or at the angles of the eye.

The 'pearly tumour' of the meninges (actually a squamous-epithelium-lined cyst, p. 731) is an example of a simple displacement of squamous epithelium into the meninges at the time of neural tube closure.

(b). Cysts arising as *part of a major congenital abnormality of an organ*. Examples are (i) *polycystic disease of the kidneys* (p. 797), in which a major maldevelopment of the renal tubules (of several possible types) results in the formation of cysts in great numbers; (ii) the *meningocele* and other types of cystic swelling that complicate some cases of spina bifida, failure of proper closure of the neural tube being the basic defect (p. 721).

(2) Acquired cysts. These are of several varieties, the three following being the most important:

(*a*) Cysts formed by retention of secretion produced by obstruction to the outflow—*retention cysts*. A single cyst, sometimes large, may be produced by the obstruction of the main duct, e.g. of a salivary gland or of a part of the pancreas. Obstruction of the orifice of a hair follicle gives rise to a cyst-like swelling

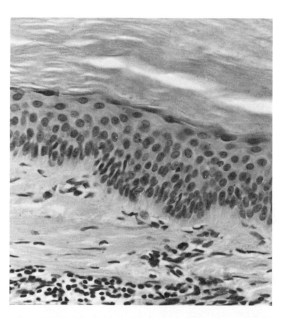

Fig. 12.29 Implantation cyst in subcutaneous tissue, showing lining of stratified squamous epithelium and keratin in the lumen. × 200.

filled chiefly with breaking-down keratin—the so-called sebaceous cyst, seen especially in the scalp. On the other hand, numerous small cysts may result from obstruction of small ducts, an occurrence which is not uncommon in fibrosing lesions of the kidney.

(*b*) Cysts may be formed from natural enclosed spaces, and are then called *distension and exudation cysts*. They occur in the thyroid from dilatation of the acini, and occasionally also in the pituitary: cystic dilatation of Graafian follicles in the ovaries is also common. Distension of spaces lined by mesothelium is also seen; for example, a bursa may enlarge to form a cystic swelling, and there is the common condition of hydrocele due to an accumulation of fluid in the tunica vaginalis.

Occasionally in the adult an *implantation cyst* occurs by the dislocation inwards of a portion of epidermis by injury. The epithelium grows and comes to line a space filled with degenerate epithelial squames (Fig. 12.29); rarely hair follicles are present in the wall. Implantation cysts may result also from wounds of the cornea.

(*c*) *Parasitic cysts*. These are cystic stages in the life cycle of cestode *parasites*. The most striking examples are the 'hydatid' cysts produced by *Taenia echinococcus*, though small cysts may be produced in the brain and other parts by the cysticerci of *Taenia solium*.

13

Blood Vessels and Lymphatics

Arteries

Introduction

Lesions of the arteries are very important because of their frequency and serious consequences. The commonest important disease is **atheroma**, which consists of prolonged, slow, patchy deposition of lipids and fibrosis, in the intima of arteries of various sizes. The patchy thickening results in narrowing of the lumen with consequent chronic ischaemia of the various organs and tissues. Acute ischaemia can result from the occlusion of an artery by local **thrombosis** or **embolism**; these processes have been dealt with in Chapter 8, but it is important to emphasise here that arterial thrombosis is usually the result of disease of the artery wall, and atheroma is the commonest predisposing cause.

Another very common arterial change is termed **arteriosclerosis**. This is a diffuse change in the walls of arteries, in which the muscle and elastic tissue slowly diminish and are replaced by fibrous tissue, with the result that the arteries become more firm and rigid. These changes occur in various degrees with increasing age, but they are aggravated and accelerated by systemic hypertension in which the fibrous replacement is preceded, at least in some instances, by hypertrophy of muscle and elastic tissue. Arteriosclerosis alone is usually without serious consequences, but the accompanying changes in the arterioles—**arteriolosclerosis**—result in ischaemia, particularly of the kidneys. It should be mentioned that some writers apply the term arteriosclerosis to any condition causing increased firmness of the walls of arteries or arterioles: such usage, in which arteriosclerosis would include atheroma, medial calcification (p. 324) and arteriolosclerosis, has led to considerable confusion between these conditions, and we prefer to restrict use of the term to the changes described above.

A very common and important condition which affects the arteries and arterioles is **systemic hypertension**. In most cases, the cause of the rise in blood pressure is not known, but it is likely that, in all instances, the rise is mediated by increased muscle tone in the arterioles. Prolonged hypertension, as mentioned above, leads to severe arteriosclerosis and arteriolosclerosis; it is by far the commonest cause of rupture of the cerebral arteries to produce haemorrhage into the brain, and is an important cause of heart failure.

Diseases of the arteries which bring about severe destruction of the muscle and elastic tissue, particularly of the media, may weaken the wall to such an extent that dilatation results, and if localised this is termed an **aneurysm**; rupture of the vessel wall may occur, with or without preceding dilatation. Severe weakening can result from various forms of **arteritis**, including that due to syphilis, but also from atheroma and from degenerative changes of unknown nature in the media. All three of these conditions can give rise to aortic aneurysm. Aneurysm formation and rupture may result also from developmental defects, as seen in the arteries at the base of the brain. Another effect of the various types of arteritis is to promote thrombosis, although atheroma is a much more important cause of this in certain arteries.

Effects of ageing. Throughout adult life, the walls of arteries of all sizes become gradually less resilient and more rigid; they tend to enlarge both in diameter and in length. These changes constitute **senile arteriosclerosis**: they are well illustrated by the prominence and tortuosity of the temporal arteries in older people, and are due to gradual increase in collagen and ground substance at the expense of smooth muscle and fine elastic fibres. The media is mainly affected, but also the intima which becomes appreciably thickened. Chemical analysis has shown that there is also a gradual increase in calcium salts in the artery walls. Senile arteriosclerosis has little effect on function. Similar changes, but with some thickening of the artery walls, are a feature of chronic hypertension.

Patchy thickening and hyalinisation of the walls of arterioles (**hyaline arteriolosclerosis**) also occurs with increasing age, particularly in the spleen and kidneys, but also in other viscera. When severe, it results in luminal narrowing, and may thus cause ischaemia, e.g. of the renal glomeruli. Hyaline arteriolosclerosis is exaggerated in hypertension and diabetes: it is described more fully on p. 321.

Adaptation and hypertrophy. The muscular and elastic nature of the arterial wall readily permits dilatation to provide an increased blood flow to the part supplied. If the requirement is more than transient, the lumen becomes persistently dilated and there is hypertrophy of the muscular and elastic tissue, e.g. the physiological hypertrophy of the uterine arteries during pregnancy. Similar compensatory hypertrophy is seen in the walls of collateral vessels when a main artery is obstructed.

In persistent hypertension, a state in which the arterial blood pressure is abnormally raised, the tendency for the increased pressure to dilate and lengthen the arteries is partly prevented by compensatory hypertrophy of the circular muscle of the media and the intimal longitudinal muscle fibres which lie next to the internal elastic lamina (Fig. 13.1). The vascular changes in hypertension are described in more detail on pp. 319–22.

Endarteritis obliterans. Intimal thickening of arteries occurs when well-vascularised concentric laminae of cellular connective tissue form in the intima and obliterate or narrow the arterial lumen. New elastic tissue is laid down independently of the internal elastic lamina and may appear as a layer under the endothelium or as a number of small new laminae at various points in the intima. This lesion is called *obliterative*

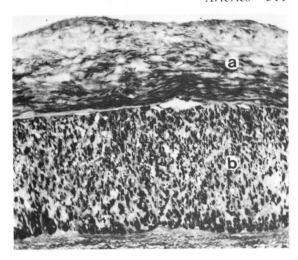

Fig. 13.1 Longitudinal section of the wall of an artery in essential hypertension, showing hypertrophic thickening of the longitudinal muscle in the intima **a** and of the circular muscle in the media **b**. (Myocytes stained black.) × 110.

endarteritis and is found in chronic inflammatory lesions. It is well seen in the base of chronic peptic ulcers (Fig. 13.2) and in the walls of tuberculous cavities, where it is beneficial in tending to prevent haemorrhage. Also in the lesions of syphilis, in tuberculous meningitis (Fig. 20.35, p. 691), silicosis, and in small arteries exposed to radiotherapy. Similar obliterative changes occur in the smaller arteries in severe hypertension and in progressive systemic sclerosis.

When the functional requirements for blood

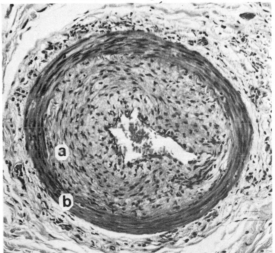

Fig. 13.2 Endarteritis obliterans in the base of a chronic peptic ulcer, **a** = intima, **b** = media.

flow through an artery are greatly reduced, the lumen is narrowed by obliterative endarteritis, which is the physiological mechanism of arterial involution. It occurs, for example, in the umbilical arteries and ductus arteriosus after birth, in the uterine and ovarian arteries after the menopause, and in the arteries supplying an area which is excised (e.g. a limb) or destroyed by disease.

Atheroma

Definition. The lesions of atheroma consist of patches of intimal thickening of the walls of arteries, due mainly to deposition of lipids and formation of fibrous tissue. The alternative term *atherosclerosis* (which literally means hard porridge) is inappropriate, particularly in Scotland, and its use has served merely to confuse the subject.

Naked-eye appearances. The early lesions are visible on the luminal surface of the walls of arteries as yellow patches, scarcely raised above the surface, and sometimes called *fatty streaks* or *patches*: they vary in diameter from 1 mm up to several centimetres in the aorta and larger arteries. They are due to deposition of lipids in the intima (Fig. 13.3), and occur at all ages, even in young children who have died from injury or various other causes..

At this stage, the changes may be reversible, but intimal lipid deposits are found in the coronary arteries in older children, and it seems

certain, from the atheromatous changes observed in the coronary arteries of groups of subjects of increasing age, that these are the forerunners of atheroma. As the condition progresses, the patches enlarge and thicken by further deposition of lipid deep in the intima and by fibrosis more superficially (i.e. adjacent to the lumen): the patches become distinctly raised and when viewed from the intimal surface they may appear yellow or white depending on the amount of white fibrous tissue overlying the yellow lipid deposits. In affluent communities, atheroma is often present in young adults and is virtually always present in some degree in middle-aged and old people. In any one individual, the patches are at various stages of development, indicating progressive formation.

Aorta. Atheroma occurs throughout the length of the aorta, but the abdominal aorta is usually most severely affected and patches often develop first around the origins of the intercostal and lumbar branches (Fig. 13.4): the plaques

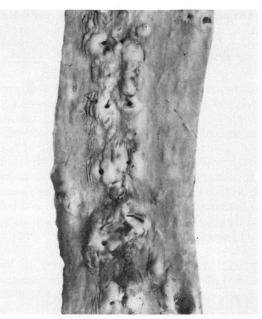

Fig. 13.4 Mild atheroma of the abdominal aorta. The lesions are seen as raised patches and are located mainly around the origins of the arterial branches. × 0·8.

vary in size up to several centimetres diameter and may in places become confluent. If a sizeable plaque is cut across, lipid-rich paste-like material can be expressed from its deeper part, and fibrous thickening is seen as a white layer

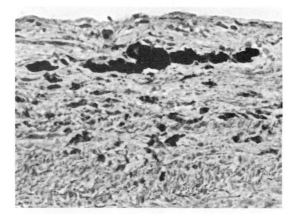

Fig. 13.3 Intimal lipid deposit in the aorta of a child aged 11 years: accidental death. (Frozen section; lipid stained black.) × 200.

Fig. 13.5 Lengths of the abdominal aorta: *left*, minimal atheroma; *middle*, severe atheroma with cracking and early ulceration of patches; *right*, very severe atheroma with ulceration and mural thrombosis. Note also that the two atheromatous aortas have lost their elasticity and stretched: this may be due to atrophy of the media beneath the extensive atheroma, but could also be the result of arteriosclerosis.

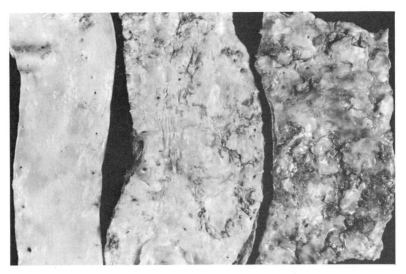

overlying this. The fibrous layer may break down, resulting in *ulceration* of the plaque, and *mural thrombus* is then likely to be deposited on the ulcerated surface; another common change is *deposition of calcium salts* which may convert the plaque to a hard brittle plate. Plaques showing ulceration, calcification or thrombus deposition are commonly referred to as *complicated atheroma*, and may produce great irregularity of the luminal surface of the aorta (Fig. 13.5). Another important feature of aortic plaques is *thinning of the overlying media*, and in some instances extension of the plaque into the adjacent media: the wall is thus weakened and an *aneurysm* may result and even rupture (p. 333).

Other arteries. Atheroma occurs in arteries of all sizes down to approximately 2 mm diameter and is seen occasionally in mild form in even smaller vessels. The features are similar to those seen in the aorta except that the plaques are necessarily smaller, often involve the whole circumference of the intima, and can cause all degrees of *luminal narrowing* down to virtual occlusion (Figs. 13.6, 13.7, 13.8). Atheroma tends to affect especially arteries supplying the heart, brain and abdominal viscera, and also the

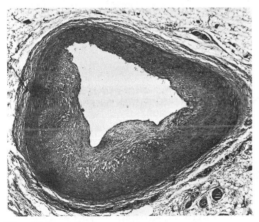

Fig. 13.6 Atheroma of a coronary artery causing moderate narrowing of the lumen. The spaces in the deep part of the plaque represent lipid accumulation. × 10.

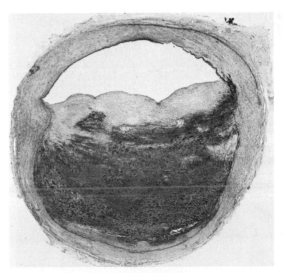

Fig. 13.7 Severe atheroma of the superior mesenteric artery, causing marked reduction of the lumen. Frozen section, stained with Scharlach R, showing the large amount of fatty material in the patch. × 15.

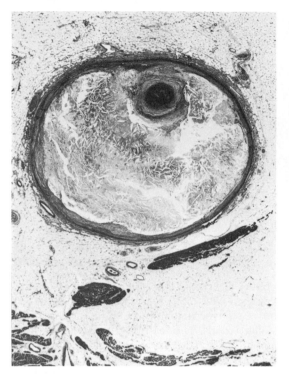

Fig. 13.8 Severe atheroma of the left coronary artery in a patient with myxoedema. The lumen has been greatly reduced by atheroma and occluded by recent superadded thrombosis. × 10.

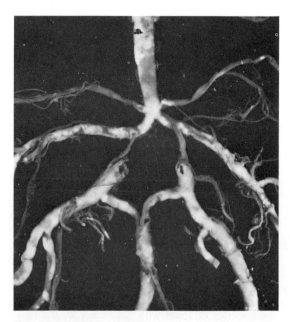

Fig. 13.9 Circle of Willis and branches, showing marked patchy atheroma.

arteries of the lower limbs. There is considerable individual variation in its distribution, in some instances the aorta being mainly affected, in others the arteries at the base of the brain and/or the coronary arteries. The coronary arteries are often severely affected and are more often involved at a relatively early age than any other arteries. The cerebral arteries also are subject to severe atheroma, but this is found chiefly in elderly persons. For unknown reasons, the renal arteries are seldom severely affected except in diabetics, in whom atheroma is often widespread and very severe.

In smaller arteries, e.g. those of the brain, the patches are visible from both inner and outer aspects of the vessels, and their yellow opaque appearance contrasts with the reddish translucency of the normal parts of the vessel wall (Fig. 13.9).

Complications include: (*a*) **haemorrhage into a plaque**, which increases the degree of luminal narrowing (Fig. 14.2, p. 348); (*b*) **rupture or ulceration of a plaque** (Fig. 14.12, p. 354), and (*c*) **occlusive thrombosis** (Fig. 14.6, p. 351) which is a major cause of infarction in the heart, brain and intestine, and of ischaemia of the legs.

Microscopic appearances. The early changes, consisting of fatty streaks or patches, are due to accumulation of lipids in proliferated spindle cells, shown by electron microscopy to be smooth muscle cells, lying in the intima (Fig. 13.10). Lipids also accumulate between cells

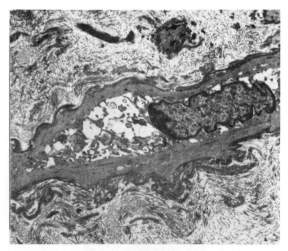

Fig. 13.10 Electron micrograph of part of a smooth muscle cell in an atheromatous plaque. The cytoplasm is made up largely of myofibrils, and contains globules of fat, shown as light spaces. The fine fibres on either side of the cell are collagen. × 7500.

deep in the intima (i.e. close to the media), particularly in relation to elastic fibres and the internal elastic lamina. As the patch develops, thin laminae of connective tissue appear in the more superficial part of the intima and form the fibrous part of the lesion. Lipid-containing cells lie among the collagen fibres in this region. Areas of necrosis then develop, converting the deep part of the patch into a structureless accumulation of lipids, tissue debris (Fig. 13.12) and sometimes altered blood, and the necrosis gradually extends into the overlying fibrous tissue. Calcium deposition may be visible microscopically. Infiltration of neutrophil leukocytes and other inflammatory cells is common, and lipid-laden macrophages—'foamy cells'—may appear around the lipid deposits, which usually contain crystals of cholesterol, represented in paraffin section by the typical elongated clefts (Fig. 13.11). The internal elastic

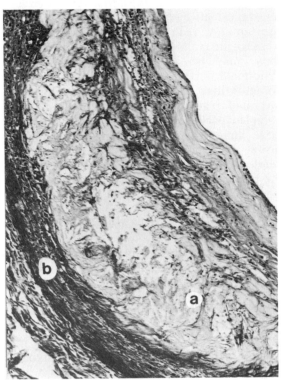

Fig. 13.12 Atheroma of a cerebral artery. The intima is greatly thickened with accumulation of lipid in its deeper part **a** and dense overlying fibrosis. The media **b** shows local atrophy over the patch. × 110.

apart from this, the media deep to the plaque becomes thinned and atrophic (Fig. 13.12).

Small blood vessels grow into the atheromatous patch from the adventitia of the affected vessel and sometimes also from the intimal surface. These may be the source of the haemorrhage which commonly occurs in the patch, although, as already stated, the overlying fibrous patch may be very thin and may rupture, allowing blood to track in from the lumen.

Chemical analysis of the lipids of atheroma have shown that cholesterol esters and unesterified cholesterol, with smaller amounts of triglycerides and phospholipids, make up the bulk of the lipids within the plaques. Their composition closely resembles that of the low density lipoproteins of the plasma except in the most advanced lesions where there is a disproportionate increase in the quantity of unesterified cholesterol.

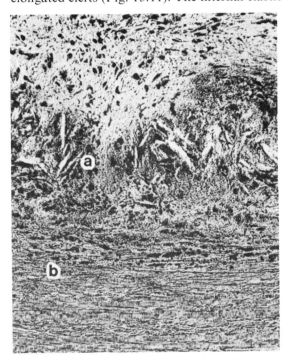

Fig. 13.11 Section showing part of an atheromatous patch of the aorta. In the deep part of the intima there is degenerate lipid-rich material **a**, the spindle-shaped spaces being due to cholesterol crystals. Lipid accumulation stops abruptly at the junction with the media **b**. × 110.

lamina deep to the plaque usually disrupts and lipid deposition, necrosis and fibrosis may then extend into the adjacent media. Quite

Effects

Although the changes of atheroma are essentially the same in all arteries, their effects vary in arteries of different sizes.

Large arteries. Uncomplicated atheroma of large arteries, such as the aorta, very often has no clinical effect because usually it does not substantially reduce the lumen or seriously weaken the wall. In advanced cases, however, there may be aneurysm formation in the abdominal aorta (p. 333) or occasionally in a common iliac artery. Thrombi which form on ulcerated plaques in the aorta seldom cause complete occlusion, probably because the rapid flow limits platelet adhesion. Occasionally, however, thrombus may extend to occlude the whole aortic lumen and when this occurs at the bifurcation it can result in gangrene of the legs unless adequate collateral circulation has developed, in which case there may be merely coldness and weakness of the legs with muscle wasting and sexual impotence but without ischaemic pain or gangrene (Leriche syndrome). Apart from occluding the aorta, thrombi and atheromatous debris from ulcerated plaques may break away and form emboli in the arteries of the lower limbs and abdominal organs such as the kidneys.

Smaller arteries. By far the commonest important effects of atheroma are due to involvement of smaller arteries, the lumen of which may be progressively narrowed by an atheromatous patch, or suddenly occluded by superadded thrombosis (Fig. 13.8). These effects are well seen in the coronary arteries. Atheroma is the chief cause of *ischaemic heart disease*, the largest single cause of death in Europe and North America today (p. 350). *Ischaemic brain damage* is also very common and is usually the result of atheroma of the carotid, vertebral and basilar arteries, vessels of the Circle of Willis and cerebral arteries (p. 679). Atheroma does not cause aneurysms of smaller arteries.

Arteries supplying the legs are often severely atheromatous, with consequent progressive diminution in blood supply. Eventually the collateral circulation becomes inadequate: relative muscle ischaemia can then be induced by the increased metabolic demands of exercise, which produces severe pain in the leg, relieved by rest. This is the clinical syndrome of *intermittent claudication*. In time ischaemia may be so severe as to cause *gangrene*, which usually starts in the toes and spreads proximally. Examination of legs amputed for gangrene usually shows narrowing or obliteration and calcification of the main arteries of the leg. Because atheroma is often widespread, patients with severe involvement of the arteries of the lower limbs frequently suffer also from ischaemic heart disease (p. 314). The arteries of the arms are rarely severely affected by atheroma.

Aetiology

Many factors lead to the development of atheroma. Its patchy nature indicates that local factors are involved, and the siting of the earliest lesions at bends and branching points suggests that local stresses in the arterial wall or turbulence of blood flow are important initially.

A study of atheromatous lesions at different stages shows that the early change is deposition of fatty material in the intima and that the fibrous thickening occurs later, perhaps as a result of irritation due to the lipid.

There are two major theories on the intimal accumulation of lipid.

The filtration theory. The arterial intima has no vasa vasorum and is nourished by diffusion of fluid and solutes across the vascular endothelium. The filtration theory explains the intimal site of the early deposits by assuming that lipids filtered from the lumen are unable to penetrate the internal elastic lamina. If the lipids are not removed as quickly as they accumulate, atheromatous deposits will then occur. This explanation is supported by chemical analysis of the deposited lipids, which resemble those of the plasma lipoproteins.

The thrombogenic theory of Rokitansky (1852) was forgotten until independently suggested by Duguid (1946). It proposes that the lipid accumulation of atheroma is due to repeated formation of mural thrombi in arteries, each thrombus being rapidly covered by growth of endothelium and thus incorporated into the intima, where it results in fibrosis and lipid accumulation in the deeper layers. Some intimal lesions probably do originate in this way. Fibrin and platelet constituents can be demonstrated by immunological methods within atheromatous plaques, findings which suggest that mural thrombosis contributes to their development. However, thrombosis does not readily explain the *gross* accumulations of lipids which are such an important feature of atheroma, and is not widely regarded as a major pathogenic mechanism.

Atheroma may develop in almost any artery but is more common and severe in certain situations; this indicates that local factors determine the site of formation. The distribution of lipid deposits around the origins of arterial branches, e.g. in the aorta (Fig. 13.4, p. 312) and in various smaller vessels which are poorly supported (e.g. the coronary, cerebral and splenic arteries) suggests the importance of local shearing strain, leading to loosening of the sub-endothelial connective tissue. This may explain the tendency for the disease to be most marked in the lowest part of the aorta. The deposition of lipids in the intima of arteries can be induced experimentally in animals by lipid-rich diets, and the lesions are enhanced if, at the same time, the animal is subjected to generalised immune-complex disease (p. 125). This has led to speculation on a possible role for hypersensitivity in human atheroma, but supporting evidence is lacking. It is perhaps worth noting that, like many postulated causal factors, immune-complex disease could be used to support either theory of atherogenesis, for it both increases vascular permeability and enhances thrombosis.

Predisposing factors. While the pathogenesis of atheroma is not fully understood, there are a number of factors which are known to predispose to its development. These are as follows.

Age. Necropsy studies have shown that atheroma increases with advancing age except in extreme old age. This suggests that atheroma is a cumulative effect of causal factors operating usually over long periods. The apparent reduction in old age may be due to earlier deaths among those with advanced atheroma.

Sex. Atheroma is more severe in males than in females of the same age. Women do not usually develop it in severe degree until after the menopause, when it progresses as in men. This is believed to be related to the known effects of oestrogens on lipid metabolism.

Hypertension. Atheroma is commonly found in the systemic arteries in patients with normal blood pressure but is, in general, more intense in patients with hypertension. The effect of hypertension is well shown in cases of coarctation of the aorta; in the segment proximal to the stenosis, the blood pressure is raised and ather-

oma is more severe than in the distal segment where the blood pressure is low. In the pulmonary arteries, atheroma develops only in patients with chronic pulmonary hypertension (e.g. with mitral stenosis).

Blood lipids. Several facts suggest that abnormal lipid metabolism is important in the genesis of atheroma. (1) The earliest recognisable atheromatous lesions are lipid in nature. (2) Atheroma is increased in severity in patients with hyperlipoproteinaemia (e.g. in diabetes mellitus, myxoedema, familial hypercholesterolaemia and xanthomatosis or the nephrotic syndrome). (3) Patients with prolonged wasting diseases are found at necropsy to have, in general, less atheroma than others. (4) Atheroma and its complications are much more prevalent in wealthy societies than in undernourished communities. (5) Lesions closely resembling atheroma can be produced by the administration of large quantities of cholesterol to rabbits (which, being herbivorous, have a low blood cholesterol). Similar lesions are produced in dogs only when thyroid function is simultaneously reduced, as by the use of thiouracil.

High levels of serum cholesterol during life are related to severe atheroma and its complications, confirmed by necropsy. More elaborate physico-chemical investigations of lipid metabolism have been made in people with a history of ischaemic heart disease, which is nearly always due to coronary artery atheroma. There is, however, no test applicable during life by which the severity (or presence) of uncomplicated atheroma can be established, and the 'normal' controls in such studies are likely to have atheroma, even in severe degree; furthermore the commonest presentation of ischaemic heart disease is myocardial infarction, and since this is usually due to atheroma with superadded occlusive thrombosis, any predisposing factors demonstrated may predispose to atheroma, to occlusive thrombosis, or to both.

As explained on p. 15, lipids are carried in the plasma as complexes with proteins; these complexes, or lipoproteins, contain protein, phospholipid, cholesterol (and its esters) and glycerides of fatty acids: they can be differentiated by electrophoresis, molecular size and density, into chylomicrons, which transport glycerides from the gut; pre-β-lipoproteins, which carry endogenously-formed glycerides, and β-lipoproteins, which are rich in cholesterol. In addition, free fatty acids released from the fat depots are transported as complexes with plasma albumin.

In population surveys, it has been shown that elevation of plasma levels of lipid, cholesterol, or any of the complexes mentioned above, is associated with an increased risk of ischaemic heart disease. Classification of hyperlipoproteinaemia (World Health Organisation, 1970) is based on the work of Fredrickson and his co-workers: six types are recognised, partly by the pattern of lipoprotein elevation and partly by aetiology. Three types of hyperlipoproteinaemia are particularly important because they are quite common and are associated with a greatly increased risk of ischaemic heart disease: they are type IIb, in which the β- and pre-β-lipoprotein levels are both raised due to a diet rich in cholesterol and saturated animal fats; type IV, in which excessive dietary carbohydrate results in a raised pre-β-lipoprotein, and type IIa (familial hypercholesterolaemia) in which β-lipoprotein is raised, apparently due to a genetically-determined metabolic peculiarity. The other types are either rare or do not greatly increase the risk of ischaemic heart disease. There is increasing evidence that the high incidence of ischaemic heart disease in patients with those types of hyperlipoproteinaemia susceptible to dietary control (including IIb and IV) can be reduced greatly by a diet low in cholesterol and saturated animal fats and of reasonable total calories. Unsaturated vegetable oils are not atherogenic and may have a positive protective role against the development of atheroma: nor is there evidence that raised levels of the high density α-lipoproteins predispose to atheroma. From these findings, the concept of 'atherogenic' lipoproteins and lipoprotein patterns has arisen, and is supported by the lipoprotein changes which occur in diseases which, like diabetes (see above), predispose to atheroma: further support is provided by the lipoprotein changes which accompany atheroma-like lesions induced experimentally in animals by lipid-rich diets.

Smoking. There is a substantially greater mortality rate from coronary artery disease in cigarette smokers than in individuals who have never smoked or have given up smoking. The death rate correlates well with the number of cigarettes smoked. A factor of this sort may explain the increased death rate from ischaemic heart disease during the present century despite the lack of change in incidence of calcification of the coronary arteries as determined by necropsy.

Physical activity may reduce the incidence of complicated atheroma for it has been shown that people with sedentary occupations generally suffer more from coronary artery disease than those with strenuous jobs.

Psychological factors may be important by their effect on choice of occupation, smoking or eating habits or in some other way.

Prospective population studies have shown that the risk factors act synergistically; for example, a subject with type IIb hyperlipoproteinaemia, hypertension and obesity is *especially* likely to develop serious atheroma: smoking seems to increase the risk particularly in people with raised plasma lipids, and so on.

Systemic hypertension

Definition

Blood pressure usually increases with age, but there is considerable individual variation in the increase, and recordings of the blood pressures in a general adult population show a wide range. Any definition of hypertension must therefore be arbitrary, and there is no general agreement on the level of blood pressure to be regarded as pathological. There is, however, good evidence, for example from insurance companies' statistics, of a general inverse relationship between the height of the blood pressure and the expectation of life.

Classification

In about 85% of cases of hypertension the cause is not apparent and these patients are said to have **primary, essential** or **idiopathic** hypertension. In the remaining 15% hypertension is **secondary** to other disease processes: nearly always diseases of the kidneys are responsible (**'renal hypertension'**) but occasional cases result from certain functioning adrenal tumours or as a feature of Cushing's syndrome (see Table 13.1). Coarctation of the aorta (p. 375) is accompanied by hypertension in the arteries arising proximal to the constriction. It is likely that, as diagnostic techniques improve, further

Table 13.1 Classification of systemic hypertension

I. Essential $\left\{\begin{array}{l}\text{benign}\\\text{malignant}\end{array}\right.$

II. Secondary $\left\{\begin{array}{l}\text{benign}\\\text{malignant}\end{array}\right.$

   (*a*) of renal origin ('renal hypertension'), due to:
      chronic pyelonephritis
      glomerulonephritis
      diabetes
      polycystic disease of the kidneys
      renal amyloidosis
      connective tissue diseases, particularly poly-
        arteritis
      urinary tract obstruction (occasional cases)
      renal artery disease
      radiation nephritis
      some renal tumours
      some congenital diseases of kidney, possibly
        by predisposing to pyelonephritis
   (*b*) adrenal-mediated hypertension.
      Conn's syndrome (primary hyperaldosteron-
        ism)
      Cushing's syndrome
      phaeochromocytoma
   (*c*) coarctation of the aorta.

causes of hypertension will be identified, and the proportion of patients with so-called essential hypertension will thus become smaller. Conn's syndrome (primary hyperaldosteronism, p. 975) is an example of a condition which has recently been distinguished from essential hypertension.

Regardless of the aetiology, hypertension may be divided into **chronic**, so-called **'benign'**, and **accelerated**, so-called **'malignant'** types. In benign hypertension the rise of blood pressure is usually moderate, although sometimes marked. Many patients with benign hypertension lead active lives for many years with few or no symptoms, and may die of some independent disease. Unless the blood pressure is controlled by antihypertensive drugs, however, it frequently causes disability and death from heart failure, and also increases the risk of myocardial infarction and cerebral vascular accidents.

Malignant hypertension is characterised by a very high blood pressure, by eye changes which include retinal haemorrhages and exudates and sometimes, papilloedema, by rapidly progressive renal injury terminating in uraemia, and by hypertensive encephalopathy. The pathological hallmark of this state is fibrinoid necrosis of arterioles (see later). These special features appear to depend on the rapid development of a very high blood pressure. Unless treated, patients with malignant hypertension usually die within six months or so, but frequently the blood pressure can be reduced by antihypertensive drugs, and the outlook is then greatly improved.

Benign and malignant hypertension should not be regarded as independent conditions. Malignant hypertension supervenes in about 10 per cent of cases of benign essential hypertension and is commoner than this in patients with renal hypertension. Hence it is sometimes referred to as the **malignant** or **accelerated phase** of hypertension. However, it can also arise apparently *de novo*, i.e. without evidence of preceding benign hypertension.

Changes in the blood vessels

In addition to left ventricular hypertrophy (p. 347) changes develop in arterial vessels of all sizes as a result of hypertension. In the larger arteries, from the aorta down to vessels of about 1 mm diameter, the changes are widespread, and are termed *hypertensive arteriosclerosis*. Changes in the vessels below this size, i.e. in the smallest arteries and arterioles, tend to affect especially the small vessels of the viscera, and in particular those of the kidneys. The changes occurring in the larger arteries are of the same nature in all types of hypertension, but those in the smaller vessels, particularly the arterioles, are different in benign and malignant types of hypertension, and require separate descriptions.

Large and middle-sized arteries. The vascular changes in hypertension, uncomplicated by the arterial lesions common in the aged, are most readily studied in young patients with high blood pressure secondary to renal disease. **In the early stages** they consist mainly of hypertrophy of smooth muscle and elastic fibres. In the aorta, there is increase in both of these elements in the media. In muscular arteries the increase is mainly in the circular muscle of the media (Fig. 13.14) but also in the longitudinal muscle fibres of the intima; the internal elastic lamina becomes thickened, and very often new laminae are formed towards the intima (Fig. 13.15). **In longstanding hypertension**, which is

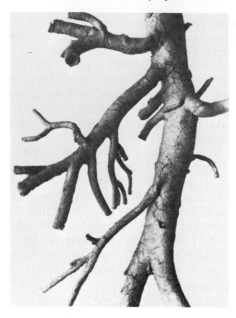

Fig. 13.13 Arteriosclerosis of the aorta and its branches in a patient with hypertension who died aged 36 from chronic renal failure. The walls of the vessels are thickened and rigid: they are also dilated, although this is not readily apparent. × 0·35.

usually of benign essential type, these hypertrophic changes give way to fibrous replacement of muscle and the elastic tissue may break up and undergo partial absorption. The arterial walls are thickened and of increased rigidity, the

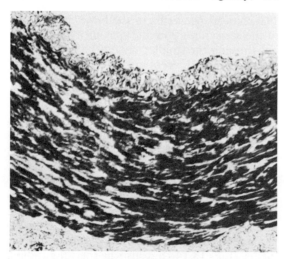

Fig. 13.14 Section of hypertrophied radial artery, from a case of chronic glomerulonephritis in a young subject, showing hypertrophy of the media. (Myocytes stained black.) × 140.

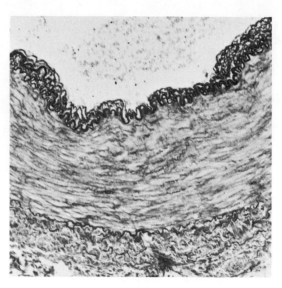

Fig. 13.15 Another section of the same artery as in Fig. 13.14, showing increase of elastic tissue formed by replication of the internal elastic lamina. (Elastic tissue stained black.) × 120.

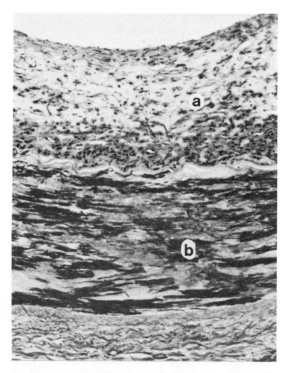

Fig. 13.16 Part of a transverse section of an arteriosclerotic artery. The intima **a** is thickened, while the muscle (stained black) of the media **b** is partly replaced by fibrous tissue. (Compare with Fig. 13.14.) × 200.

lumina are dilated (Fig. 13.13) and the vessels are often elongated and tortuous. In the aorta, there is increase in the elastic and fibrous tissue of the media. In the muscular arteries, the media is thickened and fibrosed with patchy loss of smooth muscle, and there may be fibrous thickening of the intima (Fig. 13.16). These changes are widespread, and vary in degree. They are without important effects, but in the brain they may be associated with formation of multiple micro-aneurysms of deep penetrating arteries, and rupture of these is the usual cause of cerebral haemorrhage (p. 338). Hypertension also increases the risk of rupture of the larger 'berry' aneurysms which develop in the arteries at the base of the brain in some individuals (p. 337) resulting in subarachnoid haemorrhage.

The arteriosclerotic changes described above are similar to those observed in normotensive elderly subjects (*senile arteriosclerosis*) but in the absence of hypertension they are usually less pronounced, and the media, although fibrosed, is often not thickened.

Atheroma tends to be particularly severe in individuals with chronic hypertension, and there is no doubt that prolonged elevation of the blood pressure aggravates this condition.

Hypertension thus results at first in hypertrophy of the arterial walls, with increase in muscle and elastic fibres, followed by arteriosclerosis and a tendency to severe atheroma. The early hypertrophic changes are usually observed only in young hypertensive subjects: in older patients with chronic hypertension, arteriosclerosis and atheroma predominate.

Small arteries and arterioles. In arteries of 1 mm diameter or less, and in the arterioles, the changes differ from those in the larger vessels, and they differ also in benign and malignant hypertension.

(*a*) *Benign hypertension.* The small arteries show the medial thickening seen in the larger vessels, but a more pronounced degree of intimal thickening, due to concentric increase in connective tissue; in the smallest arteries the intimal change predominates, and may result in narrowing of the lumen in contrast to the dilatation seen in the larger arteries.

The *arterioles* undergo *hyaline thickening* of their walls (*hyaline arteriosclerosis*), which consists at first of patchy deposition of hyaline material, often beneath the endothelium, but

sometimes more peripherally: the hyaline change gradually extends to involve the whole circumference, and when severe it replaces the normal structures of the wall apart from the endothelium. This change occurs also apart from hypertension, and is seen especially in old age. In both normotensive and hypertensive subjects it is observed most commonly in arterioles in the spleen, then in the afferent glomerular arterioles of the kidneys (Fig. 13.17),

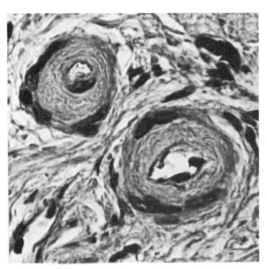

Fig. 13.17 Hyaline arteriolosclerosis of afferent glomerular arteriole in chronic systemic hypertension. The arteriole is not only thickened, but also tortuous, and so has been cut twice in cross-section in the same plane. × 1500.

and in the pancreas, liver and adrenal capsules. In all these sites, the change is appreciably commoner and usually more severe in hypertensives than in normotensive subjects of corresponding ages. Hyaline arteriolosclerosis is uncommon in the arterioles of the brain, gastro-intestinal tract, pituitary, thyroid, heart, skin and skeletal muscles (Smith, 1956). When severe, hyaline arteriolosclerosis results in considerable narrowing of the arteriolar lumen. This has important effects upon individual glomeruli, but does not usually cause renal failure. The nature of the change is not fully understood: initially, the hyaline material resembles fibrin in its staining properties, but later it stains like collagen. It also contains lipid material, and there is evidence that it may result from an exudative process in which plasma seeps into the arteriolar wall (p. 750). Apart from its occurrence as an ageing process and in hypertensive subjects, hyaline arteriolosclerosis is often severe and extensive in diabetes mellitus (pp. 779, 967).

(*b*) *Malignant hypertension*. In this condition, the concentric fibrous thickening of the intima of the small arteries is often of extreme degree, particularly in the interlobular arteries of the kidneys (Fig. 21.10, p. 752). The arterioles are thickened and of hyaline appearance, as in benign hypertension, but the change is relatively acute, and consists of necrosis of the arteriolar wall, accompanied by permeation with plasma and deposition of fibrin (**fibrinoid necrosis**): pyknotic nuclei, neutrophil polymorphs and red cells can often be found in the necrotic wall. The lumen is considerably narrowed, and superadded thrombosis may complete its occlusion. These changes affect especially the viscera, and the arteriolar lesions may result in haemorrhages and in

Course of chronic and of accelerated hypertension

Chronic ('benign') essential hypertension. As already stated, this is much the commonest type of hypertension. The blood pressure rises very gradually over a period of years, in most cases to moderately high levels, e.g. 180/110 mm Hg but occasionally much higher. The increase nearly always starts before the age of 45 years, and individuals with a resting-blood pressure consistently below 140/85 at this age are very unlikely to develop essential hypertension. The diastolic pressure is less subject to physiological variations than the systolic pressure, and a diastolic pressure persistently exceeding 90 mm Hg is generally regarded as abnormal. However, the disease develops very slowly, and it may be some years before the rise in pressure clearly exceeds that which occurs normally with age.

The condition may be symptomless, and

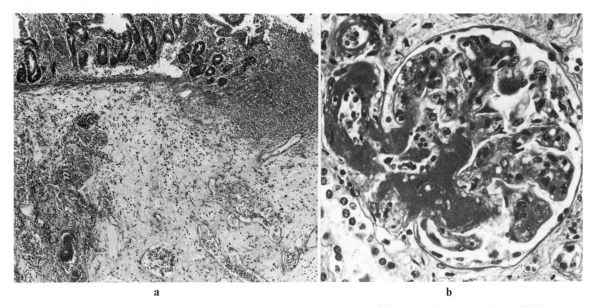

a   b

Fig. 13.18 Arteriolar lesions in malignant hypertension. **a** Ulceration of the colonic mucosa due to fibrinoid necrosis and thrombosis of arterioles: one such vessel is seen (*lower left*) in the submucosa. **b** Fibrinoid necrosis of a glomerular afferent arteriole and part of the tuft.

ischaemic necrosis (Fig. 13.18). Focal fibrinoid necrosis may develop also in the small arteries.

In both benign and malignant hypertension, the changes in the small vessels in the kidneys bring about renal damage, as described on pp. 749–53.

many cases come to light during routine medical examination for insurance or other purposes. Common symptoms include palpitations, audible pulsation in the head, headaches, attacks of dizziness particularly on stooping, and reduced exercise tolerance.

Approximately 60% of deaths in patients

with this so-called 'benign' form of essential hypertension are from left ventricular or total heart failure, and this is due to the increased work load thrown on the left ventricle and the commonly associated severe coronary atheroma. About 30% of patients die from cerebral haemorrhage, and the remainder from various causes unrelated to the hypertension. Although changes occur in the kidneys as a result of the vascular lesions, renal failure is uncommon in benign essential hypertension. When heart failure develops, however, there is usually a moderate rise in the blood urea level. In those patients who progress from chronic to accelerated hypertension renal failure commonly supervenes.

Accelerated ('malignant') essential hypertension. This develops in approximately 10% of cases of chronic essential hypertension. In those cases not preceded by chronic hypertension, the onset is usually between 30 and 45 years. It can result in heart failure or cerebral haemorrhage, but without effective treatment *renal injury* is severe and usually causes death within a few months (p. 751).

Eye changes are another important feature in malignant hypertension: lesions in the small arteries in the retina result in oedema, haemorrhages, infarcts and exudates, and blindness may ensue. Papilloedema, associated with cerebral oedema, is often present. *Hypertensive encephalopathy*, characterised by epileptiform fits and transient paralysis, is not uncommon, and is attributable to cerebral oedema, resulting from arterial spasm and focal cerebral ischaemia. This has been observed directly in rats with experimental hypertension and the fits have been shown to cease when the blood pressure is lowered and cerebral vasoconstriction ceases.

Secondary hypertension. Hypertension is a feature of chronic renal failure, and is more often of malignant type than is the case in essential hypertension. The superadded imposition of further renal injury from hypertensive vascular lesions, whether benign or malignant, aggravates and accelerates renal failure.

Aetiology of hypertension

In all types of hypertension, the raised blood pressure is a result of increased peripheral vascular resistance. In normal circumstances the peripheral resistance is controlled by the muscular tone in the arterioles throughout the body, and the major aetiological problem is the elucidation of the factors which, by increasing arteriolar tone, bring about the various types of hypertension. The possibility that the structural changes of arteriolosclerosis initiate the hypertensive state is extremely unlikely, for such changes are sometimes absent, particularly in early cases, and moreover structural changes do not develop in arterioles which are protected from hypertension by occlusive changes in the larger arteries supplying them. For these reasons, it is widely accepted that the observed structural changes in the arteries and arterioles are the result of hypertension, and not the cause. It is likely, however, that structural changes in the arterioles and small arteries of the kidneys impair renal blood flow, and this may play a part in maintaining hypertension once the vascular changes have become pronounced.

Humoral vasoconstrictive factors. In patients with hypertension due to a phaeochromocytoma, the large amounts of catecholamines released by the tumour into the blood (see p. 981) are very likely to be the cause of the hypertension.

The vasoconstrictor substances renin and angiotensin (p. 221) may contribute to the increase of blood pressure in malignant hypertension secondary to renal disease, as plasma concentrations of these substances are increased in this state. By contrast, the levels of plasma renin in most patients with benign essential hypertension are quite normal, and in patients with Conn's syndrome (primary aldosteronism, p. 975) plasma renin concentration is actually reduced. It cannot be concluded from this that renin and angiotensin do not contribute to the increased blood pressure in these conditions, as sensitivity to the pressor effects of injected angiotensin is known to be increased in hypertensive patients, and thus the normal or subnormal amounts of angiotensin in the blood might conceivably raise the blood pressure to abnormal levels.

Search for other vasoactive substances in the blood of patients with hypertension has failed.

Renal hypertension. A firm experimental basis for renal hypertension was provided in 1934 by Goldblatt and his colleagues, who showed that partial clamping of the renal arteries produced hypertension in dogs. This has been confirmed repeatedly in several species and it has been shown that hypertension can be produced in the rat by partial clamping of the artery to one kidney. Vascular hypertensive changes have been produced by this method, and it is of interest that they do not affect the kidney which is protected by the clamp from hypertension. Experimental hypertension of short duration produced in this manner may be abolished by removing the clamp or excising the clamped kidney, but if the clamp has been left in place for some months, the hypertension persists in spite of these manipulations, because of arteriolar changes produced in the unclamped kidney.

Renal hypertension in man is similar in many ways to the experimental condition. The diseases which cause it are listed in Table 13.1 on p. 319 and are described in Chapter 21: because of their relatively high incidence, *chronic glomerulonephritis* and *chronic pyelonephritis* are the most important ones. Release of excess renin from the abnormal kidney or kidneys may be an important factor in producing hypertension in such diseases. However, high levels have usually been found only in malignant hypertension with underlying renal disease, and even in these the importance of renin is not fully established.

Secondary hyperaldosteronism in hypertension. In some cases of severe hypertension, particularly those with malignant hypertension and/or renal disease, secondary hyperaldosteronism develops. Plasma renin concentration is invariably increased and this leads to stimulation of aldosterone secretion which in turn produces potassium depletion (see p. 222). The condition is recognised usually by a decrease in the concentration of potassium, and often of sodium, in the plasma. It must be distinguished from primary hyperaldosteronism (Conn's syndrome) in which the hypertension and hypokalaemia are associated with *increased* sodium and *decreased* plasma renin concentration (see p. 975).

Neural factors in the pathogenesis of hypertension. The possibility that neural factors may play a role in primary hypertension deserves consideration. There is evidence that in both human and experimental hypertension the threshold of the vascular receptors is elevated, so that abnormally high pressures are necessary to initiate neurogenic anti-pressor reflexes. It may also be that variations in sensitivity to pressor agents, possibly genetically determined, are involved.

Pulmonary hypertension

In contrast to systemic hypertension, a rise in blood pressure in the pulmonary arterial system is usually explicable on the basis of disease of the lungs, heart or major vessels. These causes, and the effects of pulmonary hypertension, are described on pp. 401–5.

Calcification of the media (Mönckeberg's sclerosis)

Definition. This is a degenerative disease of unknown cause characterised by dystrophic calcification (p. 245) in the media, especially common in the major arteries of the lower limbs in elderly people.

Naked-eye appearances. The affected vessels are generally dilated and show transverse bars of medial calcification due to deposition of calcium in the circular medial muscle fibres (Fig. 13.19). At a later stage, lengths of the arteries may be converted into rigid tubes. There may be no noteworthy alteration of the intima though atheroma is sometimes present in addition.

Microscopic examination shows that the earliest change is hyaline degeneration of the muscle fibres and connective tissue, usually starting about the middle of the media (Fig. 13.20). Calcium salts are deposited first as fine granules, and continuous calcification

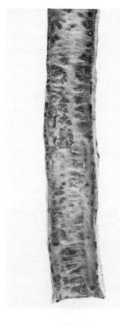

Fig. 13.19 Calcification of media of iliac artery, showing transverse markings caused by confluent calcification. × ⅔.

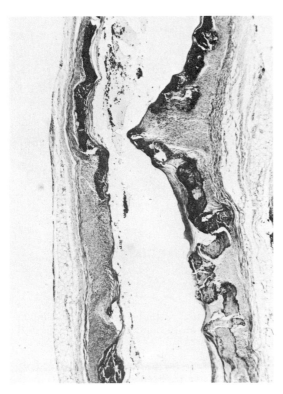

Fig. 13.20 Calcification of media. The calcified tissue is darkly stained. × 16.

follows. There may be little or no cellular re-action. Occasionally true bone may be formed in an area of calcification, and may even contain red marrow.

Aetiology. This is generally regarded as an exaggeration of the natural increase of calcium salts in the arteries with age. It sometimes oc-curs earlier in arteriosclerotic vessels but in man is not intimately related to high blood pressure. A similar lesion has been produced in the aorta of rabbits by injections of adrenaline.

Effects. The radiological appearance is strik-ing but the lumina of the arteries are seldom narrowed. Ischaemic effects, if present, are usually due to co-existing atheroma and its complications.

Syphilitic arteritis

Small arteries

Wherever syphilitic lesions occur there is intimal and adventitial fibrosis of small arteries associated with infiltration of lymphocytes and plasma cells (endarteritis and periarteritis).

These changes are due to the presence of spiro-chaetes in the adventitia. In some cases the change is diffuse and a number of the vessels show general thickening, while in others it is of a patchy or nodular type.

Effects. Reduction of the arterial lumen due to endarteritis may contribute to the necrosis in gummas. The essential change in syphilitic mesaortitis is probably involvement of the small nutrient vasa vasorum of the aortic media. Effects purely attributable to ischaemia are seen in the brain in tertiary syphilis (meningo-vascular syphilis) due to endarteritis obliterans of cortical vessels (Fig. 13.25) and this may be com-plicated by thrombosis leading to cerebral soften-ing at an early age. Widespread obliteration of small pulmonary arteries, resulting in pulmonary hypertension, has been attributed to syphilis.

Syphilitic mesaortitis

This is a common manifestation of tertiary syphi-lis and an important cause of death in this disease. It occurs occasionally in congenital syphilis.

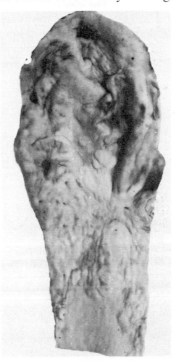

Fig. 13.21 The thoracic aorta in syphilitic aortitis. The arch of the aorta is stretched, with localised bulgings, thickened intimal patches and irregular wrinkling and scarring. The changes stop abruptly below the arch. × ½.

Naked-eye appearances can best be studied in untreated young subjects, in whom the disease occurs in the absence of other vascular lesions. The first visible lesions are greyish-white translucent areas of thickening in the intima, with little tendency to degenerate. Later they extend and fuse, forming areas with wavy or slightly wrinkled surface, while the intima in the parts between appears healthy (Fig. 13.21). In places, contraction of the tissue may occur with formation of stellate scars. Localised depressions which are potential aneurysms may be seen. In older subjects, yellow patches of atheroma, which is often severe, may be associated with the syphilitic lesions. Occasionally, on cutting through the wall of the aorta, gummatous change may be seen extending inwards from the adventitia.

The part of the arch immediately above the aortic valve is usually involved first and the aortic arch is by far the commonest and at times the only part of the aorta with syphilitic lesions. Syphilitic changes are usually limited to the thoracic aorta.

Microscopic appearances. The earliest change is periarteritis and endarteritis of the vasa vasorum in the adventitia (Fig. 13.22). These changes then extend into the aortic media, in which foci of cellular infiltration appear (Fig.

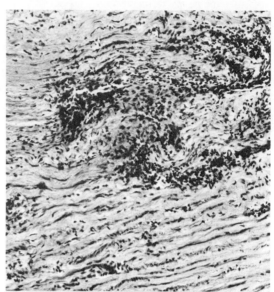

Fig. 13.23 Section of syphilitic aorta, showing cellular accumulations around the small vessels in the media, with destruction of the laminae. × 160.

13.23), with new formation of thin-walled vessels. This leads to breaks or windows in the elastic tissue and muscle of the media, best seen in a section stained to show the elastic fibres (Fig. 13.24). The elastic tissue and muscle are replaced by fibrous tissue, but gummatous necrosis may also occur.

Dense fibrous thickening of the intima occurs over the lesions of the media (Fig. 13.24), and vasa vasorum may extend into these intimal

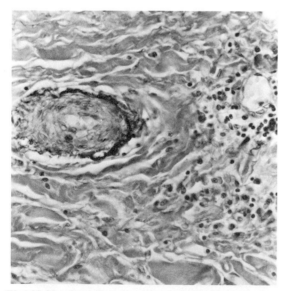

Fig. 13.22 Syphilitic aortitis, showing severe endarteritis of an arteriole in the adventitia of the aorta, and infiltration by plasma cells and lymphocytes around two small vessels (*right*). × 330.

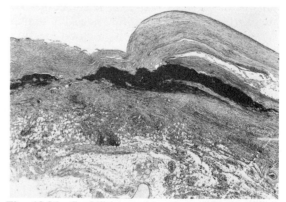

Fig. 13.24 Syphilitic aortitis; elastic tissue stained black. The section shows part of a thickened intimal plaque (*upper right*) and irregularity, thinning and interruptions in the elastic tissue of the media. *Note:* the muscle of the media is also destroyed, leaving a weakened wall. × 10.

patches, which account for the pearly-white raised areas seen by naked eye.

Effects. *Aneurysm formation* is an important complication of syphilitic mesaortitis and is due to weakening of the vessel wall from loss of medial elastic and muscle tissue: the effects of aneurysm are described on p. 334.

Aortic incompetence. The dilatation of syphilitic aortitis may involve the root of the aorta, with consequent incompetence of the aortic valve. The cusps become stretched, thickened and distorted (p. 367).

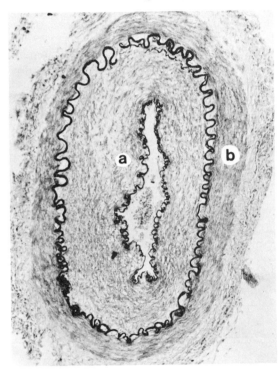

Fig. 13.25 Endarteritis obliterans of a cerebral artery due to meningovascular syphilis. The intima **a** is greatly thickened and a new elastic lamina has formed internal to it. The media **b** appears normal, and there is increase of adventitial fibrous tissue. × 80.

Coronary artery narrowing due to involvement of their orifices by mesaortitis is now a rare cause of myocardial ischaemia.

Idiopathic aortitis in Africans

An inflammatory lesion affecting all parts of the aorta has been described in young Africans. There is infiltration of the adventitia and media with lymphocytes and plasma cells, and destruction of the elastic tissue, ending in dense collagenous fibrosis. The mouths of the renal arteries are often involved, resulting in unilateral or bilateral renal artery stenosis often leading in turn to hypertension. Micro-organisms have not been demonstrated and the aetiology of the lesion is unknown.

Tuberculosis

Marked periarteritis and endarteritis sometimes occur in relation to tuberculous lesions. They are often a prominent feature in tuberculous meningitis, especially with late or inadequate treatment. These changes may lead to complete obstruction of the vessel and cerebral infarction. Occasionally, however, the wall of an artery adjacent to a pulmonary tuberculous cavity may be weakened before obliteration occurs and an aneurysm may form (p. 424).

Thrombo-angiitis obliterans (Buerger's disease)

Definition. Buerger's disease is a painful inflammatory condition of arteries and veins, with thrombosis, organisation and recanalisation of the affected vessels. It occurs almost exclusively in men, and affects mainly the vessels of the lower (but also the upper) limbs, giving rise to pain and progressive ischaemic changes.

Pathological changes. The early changes (which are not often available for histological examination) consist of occlusion of the affected vessel by thrombus which contains foci of intense polymorph infiltration. The whole thickness of the vessel wall is also infiltrated with polymorphs. These acute changes give way to chronic inflammation, and the thrombus is replaced by granulation tissue containing lymphocytes, macrophages and multinucleated giant cells (Figs. 13.26, 13.27). The inflammatory changes eventually subside, and although the original vascular lumen has been obliterated there is often a surprising degree of recanalisation. The inflammation of the vessel wall also progresses to a chronic stage but without the degree of disruption which occurs in polyarteritis nodosa (see below). Fibrosis extends into the adjacent connective tissue, and the

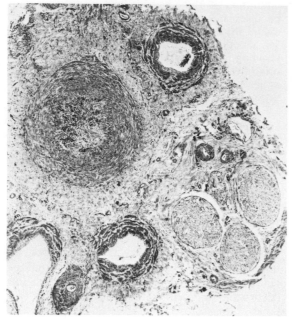

Fig. 13.26 Thrombo-angiitis obliterans. Occlusion of the posterior tibial artery (*upper left*) and surrounding fibrosis extending around the adjacent veins and nerves. × 32.

burned-out lesions thus consist of recanalised vessels with thickened fibrosed walls, enclosed in fibrous tissue which may envelop and compress adjacent nerves (Fig. 13.26).

The lesions affect short lengths of the small and medium sized arteries and veins of the limbs, but seldom the larger vessels. The legs are usually more severely affected than the arms, and in some cases the lesions are confined to the legs. The disease is chronic, acute lesions developing intermittently over a period of years. It may involve mainly arteries or veins, but usually both. The changes of ischaemia, including gangrene of the extremities of the affected limbs, eventually result.

Aetiology. Features which distinguish Buerger's disease from atheroma with superadded thrombosis are its relatively early onset, inflammatory nature, predilection for smaller vessels, involvement of veins as well as arteries and of the upper limbs as well as the lower, and its rarity in women. Suggestions that the lesions are simply a variant of atheroma are almost certainly mistaken, and have probably arisen from the examination of limbs amputated after

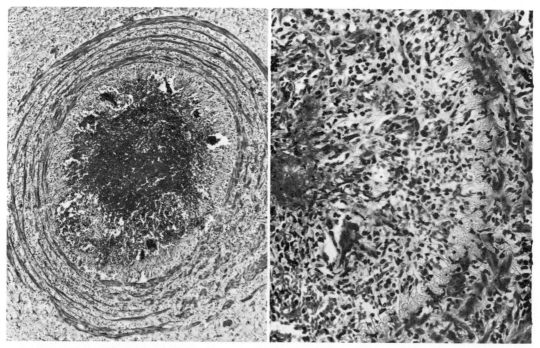

Fig. 13.27 Thrombophlebitis in Buerger's disease. *Left*, a superficial vein, showing inflammation of the wall, thrombosis and early organisation. Several multinucleated giant cells lie in and adjacent to the thrombus. × 60. *Right*, an older lesion with more advanced organisation of the thrombus: note the giant cell (*below centre*) and pleomorphic inflammatory infiltrate. × 250.

prolonged disease, when the lesions are burned-out and there is co-incidental atheroma. It is also a misconception that the disease occurs especially in Jews.

The inflammatory nature of the early lesions suggests a specific causal agent (as was postulated by Buerger) but none has been detected. The single known important predisposing factor is cigarette smoking. The disease is practically confined to heavy smokers, and there is a strong clinical impression that its progress is arrested or diminished by giving up smoking.

Clinical features. The symptoms are varied and depend on the degree of arterial obstruction. The earliest are pain, paraesthesia, and circulatory disturbances—local redness which disappears on elevating the limbs. On walking there is often cramp-like pain and inability to progress—'*intermittent claudication*'; this is a result of ischaemia of the calf muscles and

affected, the condition may stimulate Raynaud's disease in the male.

Polyarteritis nodosa (*Periarteritis nodosa*)

The lesions of this disease consist of multiple foci of necrosis, inflammation and usually thrombosis, followed by healing, in the walls of medium sized and small arteries and arterioles. Vessels in any part of the body may be affected, and there is involvement of many organs and tissues. In its most severe form, with many simultaneous acute lesions, it is rapidly fatal from haemorrhage due to rupture of a weakened artery, or more often from ischaemia of vital organs. Most cases are, however, chronic, with acute lesions developing over years, and usually causing death from ischaemic effects.

Pathological findings. The early lesion consists of a focus of fibrinoid necrosis of the media and intima of a small or medium sized artery (up to about 3 mm

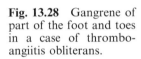

Fig. 13.28 Gangrene of part of the foot and toes in a case of thrombo-angiitis obliterans.

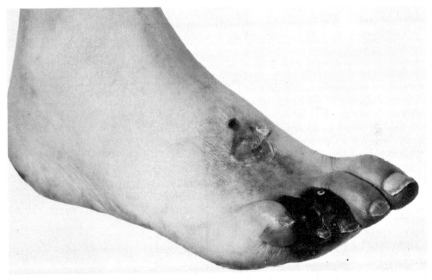

occurs in other forms of arterial disease. Later, more severe trophic changes appear, including intractable ulceration, and gangrene which is apt to spread slowly (Fig. 13.28); amputation, sometimes repeated, is often necessary but the need for surgery may be minimised by therapy which improves the collateral circulation. In view of the widespread involvement of the arteries it has now been recognised that amputation, if required, should be performed at a high level. If the vessels of the arms are severely

diameter) or an arteriole. Necrosis is accompanied by acute inflammation with polymorph infiltration (often including eosinophils) of the whole thickness of the vessel wall and particularly intense in the adventitia and surrounding tissue (Fig. 13.29). Lesions affect the whole circumference of smaller arteries, but often only a segment of the wall of the larger vessels (Fig. 13.30). Occlusive thrombosis is common in the acute stage, but in some cases there is severe haemorrhage. The acute changes progress to more chronic inflammation, with replacement of the necrotic vessel wall by fibrous tissue infiltrated with

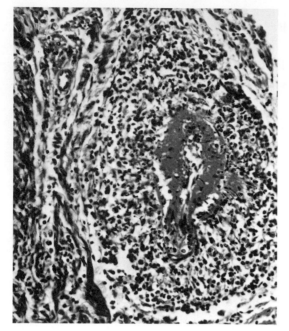

Fig. 13.29   An acute lesion of polyarteritis nodosa in a small artery in the kidney. There is fibrinoid necrosis and an intense inflammatory cellular infiltrate in and around the wall of the artery. × 100.

lymphocytes, plasma cells and macrophages, and the thrombus undergoes organisation. The weakened wall may stretch to form an aneurysm (Fig. 13.31), but even without this the healed lesion may project as a nodular thickening of the vessel wall, and microscopy then shows a sharply-defined zone of fibrous replacement of the artery wall (Fig. 13.30).

The lesions are multiple; they occur in almost any small or medium-sized artery or arteriole, but are commonest in those of the kidneys, heart, gut, liver, pancreas and nervous system, and also in the skeletal muscles. Their effects, apart from haemorrhage, are due to acute or chronic ischaemia, and depend on the distribution of the lesions and arterial anastomoses in particular sites. Infarcts and patches of chronic ischaemic atrophy result in the heart, kidneys, etc.

The disease may be severe and progress rapidly to death, but more often the course extends over some years, with periods of quiescence alternating with the development of new lesions. In most cases, death eventually results from lesions in the kidneys, heart or other vital organs.

Clinical features depend on the number and sites of lesions. In severe cases there is fever, prostration, neutrophil (and sometimes eosinophil) leukocytosis and a very high ESR. In less acute cases the disease fluctuates, with quiescent periods and exacerbations. Lesions in the peripheral nerves result in paraesthesias, etc., and symptoms may arise from ischaemic

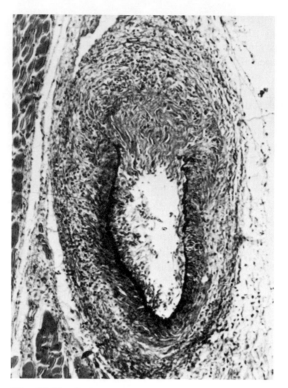

Fig. 13.30   Polyarteritis nodosa involving a coronary artery. The lesion is less acute than in the previous figure. Part of the circumference of the vessel wall (*above*) has been severely damaged, with interruption of the internal elastic lamina (stained black) and replacement of the inner part of the wall by fibrous tissue. There is more diffuse inflammatory cellular infiltrate. × 70. (The late Dr. Janet Niven.)

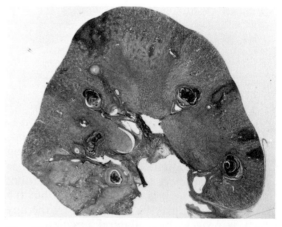

Fig. 13.31   Transverse section of the kidney of a patient who died of acute polyarteritis nodosa. In this instance, the necrotising lesions have resulted in aneurysmal dilatation, together with thrombosis. This has led to multiple infarcts. × 1·4.

injury to virtually any tissue. Angina, cardiac failure, renal failure and hypertension are among the commoner clinical manifestations, but infarction of the gut, etc., can also cause death.

Diagnosis depends on suspecting the disease from the clinical features, blood changes, etc., and confirmatory biopsy. The choice of tissue for biopsy depends on the clinical features, but confirmation is often obtainable from skeletal muscle biopsy, particularly if tissue is removed from a focus of tenderness in a muscle. Inflammatory changes are much more severe than in the necrotising arteriolar lesions of malignant hypertension.

The aetiology of polyarteritis nodosa is unknown. Focal necrotising arteritis of similar appearance can be induced in animals as part of the picture of acute immune-complex disease (p. 125), but only as an acute condition. It is difficult to understand how immune-complex disease can induce acute lesions over a prolonged period, as occurs in polyarteritis nodosa. Nevertheless, a hypersensitivity reaction to microorganisms, drugs, or auto-antigens has often been assumed. Recent reports claim that, in a high proportion of cases, there is serological evidence of infection with B hepatitis virus, electron-microscopic evidence of the virus (Australia) antigen complexed with antibody in the plasma, and antigen in the lesions.

Variants

A **microangiopathic form** of polyarteritis nodosa affects mainly arterioles and very small arteries in the kidneys and elsewhere, and gives rise to haemolysis and uraemia, sometimes without hypertension: the renal lesions include **focal** and **rapidly progressive glomerulonephritis** (p. 771).

Wegener's granulomatosis is a variant in which lesions in vessels in the nasopharynx result in an ulcerating granulomatous lesion, and lesions also tend to occur especially in the lungs and kidneys.

Localised polyarteritis, with lesions indistinguishable from polyarteritis nodosa, occurs in the gallbladder and appendix, and has an excellent prognosis. *Necrotising vasculitis of the skin* is a complex subject (p 996). The lesions of polyarteritis nodosa can remain confined to the skin for some years, but there are other, localised forms of dermal vasculitis which are distinct from polyarteritis nodosa.

Other forms of arteritis

Rheumatic arteritis. Lesions similar to those found in the heart are produced by rheumatism in the walls of large arteries. In the aorta they commence in the adventitia and consist of an infiltration of the tissues with lymphocytes and plasma cells. There may be foci of histiocytes, and typical Aschoff bodies with characteristic cells (p. 362) may form. The cellular infiltration may spread into the media and lead to absorption of elastic tissue, but this rarely extends beyond the outer third of the media. Such lesions do not weaken the wall sufficiently to produce aneurysms.

In the smaller arteries, rheumatic lesions of varying distribution have been found, especially in the visceral branches. They are acute and may be accompanied by necrosis of the media as well as by leukocyte infiltration; they thus resemble the lesions of polyarteritis nodosa but thrombosis and aneurysm have not been found. Further work is required to establish the relation of rheumatism to disease of the smaller arteries. The lesions are clinically silent, but they may form the basis of the subcutaneous lesions which sometimes occur in rheumatic fever and illustrate its systemic nature.

Aortitis in ankylosing spondylitis. Unexplained lesions of the aortic valve and ascending aorta, identical in appearance to syphilitic arteritis but without serological evidence of syphilis, sometimes develop in males with ankylosing spondylitis.

Giant-cell or temporal arteritis. This is a fairly uncommon condition, occurring mostly in old people of both sexes. It affects mainly arteries of the head, but is sometimes much more widespread, and the aortic arch and its major branches are occasionally involved. Diagnosis is often based on clinical examination and biopsy of the temporal artery, which is conveniently superficial and often affected.

The lesion is an inflammation of the whole thickness and whole circumference of the affected arteries, affecting either a continuous length of the vessel or appearing as multiple focal lesions along it. The vessel wall is infiltrated with leukocytes (mainly polymorphs) in the early stages, but the subsequent reaction is granulomatous, with accumulation of lymphocytes, macrophages and multinuclear cells (of both Langhans' and 'foreign-body' types) which sometimes appear to develop in relation to fragments of the disrupted internal elastic lamina. Fibrous thickening of the intima, fibrous replacement of the media, and commonly thrombosis and organisation, result in a severely scarred vessel with a narrowed or obliterated lumen (Fig. 13.32).

Clinically there may be localised reddening of the skin over an affected vessel, which is usually tender or painful and sometimes nodular. Depending on which arteries are involved, there may be headache, visual disturbances and even blindness (from involvement of the retinal arteries), facial pain, and sometimes features resulting from more extensive arteritis. In some instances, the disease occurs in association with polymyalgia rheumatica. It is of entirely unknown aetiology and usually self-limiting.

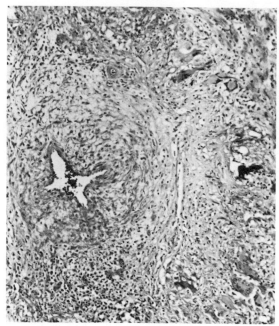

Fig. 13.32 Section of the temporal artery in giant-cell arteritis, showing multinucleated giant cells lying in relation to the internal elastic lamina (now disrupted and seen only as small fragments). There is gross intimal thickening, possibly from organisation of thrombus, and a very narrow lumen. × 120.

Takayashu's disease

This is a rare condition, first reported from Japan, in which the aorta and the large arteries arising from the aortic arch are affected by an arteritis which may resemble syphilitic aortitis, caseating tuberculosis, or temporal arteritis. Intimal thickening, sometimes with superadded thrombosis, severely narrows or occludes the subclavian, carotid and innominate arteries (hence the term *pulseless disease*), with resulting ischaemia of the head and arms. The disease affects mainly young women, and the aetiology is unknown. Occasional cases with vascular occlusions suggestive of Takayashu's arteriopathy are encountered in Britain. The patients are usually older, and may be of either sex. These cases are attributable to severe atheroma or syphilitic arteritis of the major arteries.

Thrombotic microangiopathy (thrombotic thrombocytopenic purpura)

This is characterised by the deposition of homogeneous eosinophilic material, at least some of which is fibrin, in the intima and lumen of visceral arterioles, without an associated inflammatory reaction. It sometimes accompanies, and may belong to, the group of connective tissue diseases. Further details are given on p. 477.

Raynaud's disease

Nomenclature. The name Raynaud's disease has been applied to a variety of conditions in which there is excessive vasomotor response to cold. It is now thought desirable to subdivide these conditions and to use the following arbitrary nomenclature—Raynaud's phenomenon, Raynaud's disease (primary or secondary).

Raynaud's phenomenon affects the extremities, usually the fingers, but occasionally also the ears, tip of the nose and the toes. It is provoked by cold, and consists of attacks of local ischaemia with intense pallor or cyanosis, coldness and disturbance of sensation; the patient suffers from 'dead fingers'. Pallor is due to spasm of all the arteries and arterioles of the affected part. Cyanosis may be accompanied by oedema, and is due to continued arterial contraction, but presumably with, in addition, venular constriction. In Raynaud's phenomenon the circulation through the hands is normal between

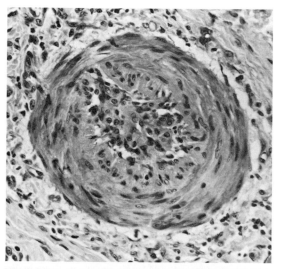

Fig. 13.33 Transverse section of a digital artery in Raynaud's disease. The lumen is obliterated by cellular fibrous tissue which has resulted from organisation of thrombus. × 250.

attacks; these can generally be terminated by warming even after the condition has existed for many years, and the structure of the digital vessels remains normal. There are no trophic changes.

The disorder is familial, predominantly affects women, develops in early adult life, and is an exaggeration of the normal reactions to cold; the prognosis is excellent.

Raynaud's disease consists of attacks resembling Raynaud's phenomenon but progressing to trophic changes or even gangrene. The tips of the digits develop atrophy of the skin with blisters, minor infections and finally progressive necrosis and ulceration of the fingertips, the changes usually being symmetrical. Angio-graphy shows some degree of permanent obstruction of the digital arteries, due either to intimal fibrous thickening or to thrombosis and imperfect recanalisation (Fig. 13.33). *Secondary Raynaud's disease* results from the use of vibrating tools. It occurs also in scleroderma and the other connective tissue diseases (p. 876); in a paralysed limb following poliomyelitis; as a stage in the symptomatology of obliterative arterial disease; in certain forms of paroxysmal haemoglobinuria as a result of cold agglutinins acting on the red cells in the digital circulation; in chronic ergot poisoning. In a few cases no underlying cause is found and these are described as *primary Raynaud's disease.*

Aneurysms

Definition. An aneurysm is a local enlargement of the lumen of an artery.

Classification. A *true* aneurysm is formed by slow dilatation of an artery, the blood being contained by the stretched vessel wall, or, when this is no longer recognisable, the surrounding connective tissue. A *false* aneurysm is produced by rupture of the vessel, the blood being enclosed from the start by the surrounding tissues. After a time the two forms come to be closely similar in structure.

A *diffuse* or *fusiform* aneurysm involves the whole circumference of the wall symmetrically whereas the *saccular* type is an asymmetrical bulge communicating with the artery through an aperture which does not involve the whole circumference. These terms may not be applicable to advanced lesions which are often very irregular in form.

Pathogenesis. The force which expands an aneurysm is the blood pressure, but for an aneurysm to form there must be an arterial lesion which weakens the media locally. Stretching usually results in further weakening, so that once an aneurysm has started it tends to expand and commonly ruptures. Occasionally thrombus forms in thick layers which fill the whole sac.

Dissecting aneurysm. In this, the wall of the artery (usually the aorta) splits, and blood tracks along the media, separating the inner from the outer layers. The essential cause is some lesion in the media.

Other varieties of aneurysm are mentioned briefly on p. 338.

Atheromatous aneurysm

In Europe and N. America, atheroma is now by far the most common cause of aortic aneurysm, due to the decline of syphilis and the concurrent increase in atheroma. Atheromatous aneurysms occur usually after the age of 50, and much more commonly in men than women. They are usually fusiform (Fig. 13.34) and may rupture while still quite small. The aneurysm forms as a result of penetration of the media by ulceration of necrotic atheromatous patches or from calcified plaques impinging on the media and causing pressure atrophy. The microscopic changes seen at the edges are those of atheroma, sometimes with a marked leukocytic reaction around the fatty debris, and there may be some lymphocytic infiltration round the vasa vasorum in the adventitia and media. Atheromatous aneurysms occur mainly in the presence of very severe atheroma and affect especially the abdominal aorta or a common iliac artery. They usually arise below the level of the renal arteries.

Effects. Death is usually due to rupture with retroperitoneal haemorrhage, the clinical features being those of an acute surgical abdominal emergency. In some cases thrombosis of

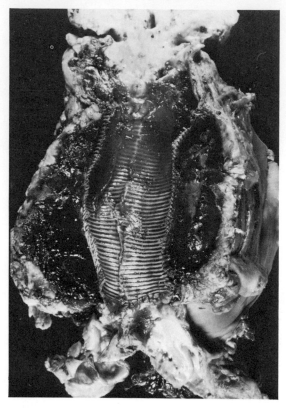

Fig. 13.34 Atheromatous aneurysm of the abdominal aorta arising below the origins of the renal arteries. The aneurysm, which is fusiform, has been repaired by a dacron tube, but death resulted from haemorrhage from rupture at the suture line.

the aorta or its branches takes place, producing ischaemia in legs, kidneys, etc. Pressure effects are not conspicuous.

Syphilitic aneurysm

This usually occurs between the ages of 40–50, when tertiary syphilis is most common and the individual is still able to indulge in strenuous physical activity. Large aortic aneurysms were previously due in most instances to syphilis, but are now rare as a result of successful treatment in the primary and secondary stages of the disease. The commonest site is the aortic arch, because it is the part most frequently affected by syphilitic mesaortitis (p. 325), of which aneurysm is a complication. The focal loss of elastica and muscle in the media results in weakening of the wall, and there may be diffuse

dilatation of the ascending aorta and arch: more localised stretching results in a fusiform or saccular aneurysm, which is often accompanied by smaller aneurysmal bulgings, along with the stellate scars and intimal thickening characteristic of syphilitic mesaortitis. As an aneurysm forms, the elastic tissue and muscle of the artery wall soon degenerate and the sac comes to be composed of layers of fibrous tissue, on which laminated thrombus forms. Blood infiltrates the wall of the aneurysm and may ooze for some distance into the tissues around; accordingly the limits of the aneurysm are badly defined.

Effects. *Pressure* on surrounding structures leads to the syndrome of superior mediastinal compression; the great veins may be displaced and undergo thrombosis, resulting in congestion of the head and neck and the enlargement of collateral channels. Involvement of the oesophagus may cause dysphagia, while pressure on a major bronchus may cause retention pneumonia. Aneurysms of the transverse part of the aortic arch may compress and stretch the left recurrent laryngeal nerve and cause paralysis of the left vocal cord. Rigid structures such as the bodies of vertebrae may be eroded and the bare bone come to form part of the wall of the sac; the intervertebral discs offer greater resistance to absorption and persist longer.

Rupture of an aneurysm may occur into practically any tube or cavity in its neighbourhood, and occasionally takes place externally through the chest wall.

Embolism from thrombus within an aneurysm is uncommon.

Cardiac hypertrophy and dilatation occur only when the syphilitic mesaortitis results in aortic-valve incompetence. Otherwise aortic aneurysms, even very large ones, do not affect the heart as there is no interference with cardiac output.

Dissecting aneurysm

This is much less common than true aneurysm of the aorta. In most cases it results from rupture of the inner part of the wall of the aorta (Fig. 13.36) due to degenerative and cystic changes in the media, the elastica and muscle being replaced by a metachromatic mucoid sub-

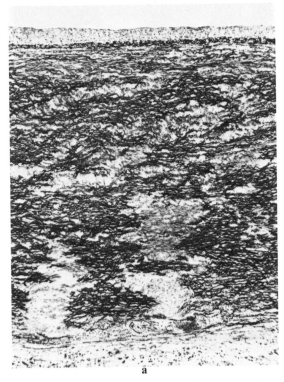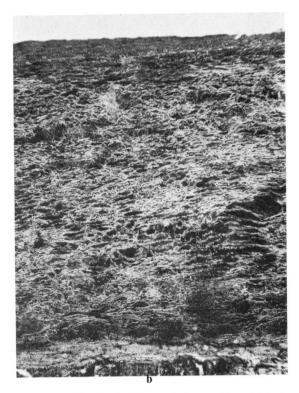

Fig. 13.35 Medial degeneration of the aorta. There are gaps in the elastic tissue of the media, which is stained black in the left (**a**) illustration. In the right (**b**) photomicrograph, myxoid ground substance is stained black and is patchily increased. The patient was a woman of 24 who died of spontaneous rupture of the aorta. × 50.

stance—**Erdheim's medial degeneration**—(Figs. 13.35a and b). Sometimes there are small areas of necrosis with softening (*medionecrosis*) but in our experience this is rare. The cause of these conditions is unknown. Dissecting aneurysm is commonest in old people and high blood pressure with hypertrophy of the heart is present in most cases but they occur also in young people without hypertension.

The commonest site for rupture is shortly above the aortic cusps (Fig. 13.36); next in frequency is a point just distal to the insertion of the ductus arteriosus. The tear is usually transverse and it may extend around almost the entire circumference. Rupture is probably brought about by the frictional tractive effect of blood flow during systole pushing the intima longitudinally; the intima is able to slide to and fro on the media because of the mucoid degeneration and ultimately it ruptures. The outer parts of the media and adventitia are not usually severed, but are widely infiltrated with blood, and dissecting aneurysm is thus produced. In proximal ruptures, blood commonly passes backwards and within a few hours bursts into the pericardial sac and causes death acutely from cardiac tamponade; intra-pericardial rupture may be preceded by signs of coronary occlusion from pressure upon these vessels at their origin. In other cases the blood strips open the media distally between the outer and middle thirds and passes along the wall of the thoracic, and even the abdominal aorta, finally rupturing into the retroperitoneal tissues. Occasionally the blood bursts back into the lumen of the aorta or iliac vessels at a lower level. When this happens the blood may flow through a new channel from the proximal tear to the point of re-entry in the lower abdominal aorta and the patient may survive for some time (Fig. 13.37). Occasionally a dissecting aneurysm remains localised (Fig. 13.38).

Marfan's syndrome. This is a disorder of connective tissue, inherited usually as an autosomal dominant, and characterised by laxity of ligaments, e.g. of joints and of the eye lens, inadequate elastic fibre

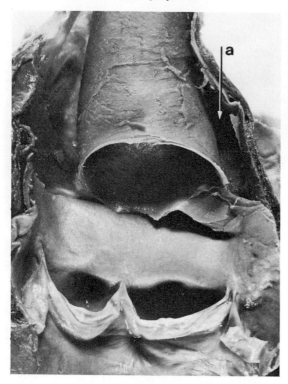

Fig. 13.36 Dissecting aneurysm of the aorta. A rupture of the inner part of the wall, above the aortic valve, extends almost around the circumference, and blood has tracked up between the inner and outer parts of the wall **a**, producing the so-called dissecting aneurysm. × 1.

formation in the aorta, tall slim build, long tapering fingers (*arachnodactily*) and other skeletal abnormalities. Disturbances of vision result from subluxation of the lens, and there may also be deafness. The aortic media lacks elastic fibres, the appearances

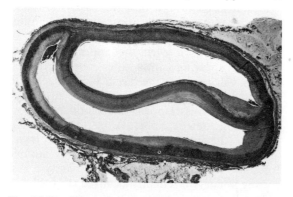

Fig. 13.37 Dissecting aneurysm of the aorta. In this case the blood burst back into the lumen through a second rupture, giving a 'double-barrel' aorta, seen here in cross section. × 2.5.

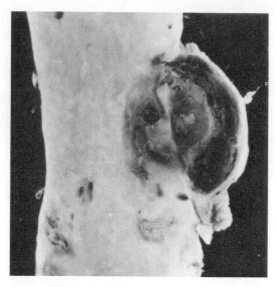

Fig. 13.38 Localised chronic dissecting aneurysm; the space in the media is filled with dense thrombus. × 1.2.

resembling those in Erdheim's medial degeneration. Fusiform aneurysm or dissecting aneurysm may result, and at necropsy there may be multiple healed aortic intimal tears.

Other causes of aortic rupture. Apart from aneurysm, rupture of the aorta may result from damage to its wall from outside, as by the perforation of an impacted fishbone or other sharp foreign body in the oesophagus; also from very severe injury such as crushing of the chest. In children traumatic rupture can occur without fracture of the ribs. Carcinoma of bronchus or oesophagus may invade the aortic wall and cause fatal haemorrhage.

Infective aneurysm (Mycotic aneurysm)

This may occur at the beginning of the aorta as the result of *direct extension* of organisms from vegetations in bacterial endocarditis, mainly the staphylococcal type (Fig. 14.32, p. 370). The organisms settle on the intima, an infective thrombus forms, invasion and weakening of the wall follow, and an *acute aneurysm* is produced, which may rupture; occasionally multiple aneurysms are present. In smaller arteries infective aneurysms result from lodgment of small infected emboli in the vasa vasorum, rather than from the presence of an infected embolus in the lumen of the artery. Inflammatory softening of the arterial wall results. They may occur in a limb or viscus, and the effects are similar to those seen in the *non-infective* aneurysms of polyarteritis nodosa where the vessel is weakened by inflammation due probably to a hypersensitivity reaction. Infected emboli in the lumen of an artery may give rise to acute inflammatory softening with rupture and cerebral haemorrhage, e.g. in staphylococcal pyaemia.

A mycotic aneurysm is sometimes seen in the wall of a tuberculous pulmonary cavity, instead of the usual occlusion of the vessel by endarteritis obliterans or thrombosis.

Cerebral aneurysms

Berry aneurysms of the circle of Willis and its branches occur at all ages and appear to be due mainly to congenital weakness of the arterial wall. Evidence of this is destroyed when the aneurysm forms but a deficiency in the medial muscle, especially in the acute angle between large branches, is demonstrable in other arteries at the base of the brain and similar deficiencies are sometimes found in apparently normal brains. An inherent defect in the elastica has not been demonstrated, but when dilatation starts the elastica probably soon degenerates. These aneurysms are often known as *congenital*, but only the defect is congenital. The aneurysms usually occur singly, but may be multiple: they are usually less than 1 cm diameter, but may be much larger. The commonest site is at the origin of the middle cerebral followed by the anterior communicating artery (Fig. 13.39), but they may arise practically anywhere on the circle of Willis and its major branches. Rupture of these aneurysms is the principal cause of spontaneous subarachnoid haemorrhage, but in some cases the sac is buried in the cortex and they bleed into the brain. Accordingly aneurysm should be suspected in the examination of any cerebral haemorrhage in an unusual situation. Not uncommonly, these aneurysms become partly or completely occluded by thrombus (Fig. 13.40). Occasionally aneurysms of the larger cerebral arteries are due to atheroma.

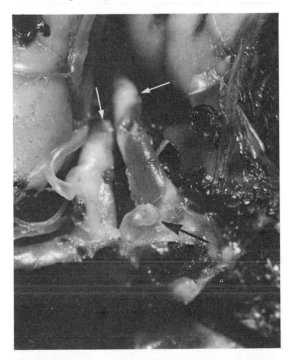

Fig. 13.39 Base of the brain showing subarachnoid haemorrhage which resulted from rupture of a berry aneurysm of the basilar artery (not shown). A second, intact berry aneurysm (black arrow) is seen on the anterior communicating artery. The anterior cerebral arteries are marked by white arrows.

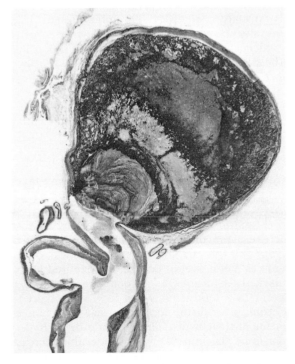

Fig. 13.40 Aneurysm of circle of Willis, almost completely filled with thrombus. × 7.5.

Micro-aneurysms. The occurrence of multiple micro-aneurysms on the small cerebral arterial twigs in hypertensive subjects was described over a century ago, but they are difficult to find without special, techniques, and only recently has their common occurrence been reaffirmed. In a painstaking study, Cole and Yates (1967) using a micro-angiographic necropsy technique reported the occurrence of multiple (usually 15–25) aneurysms of up to 2 mm diameter, occurring mainly on arteries of less than 250 μm diameter. They were detected in over 50 per cent of hypertensives over 50 years of age, and the incidence increased with age: in normotensives, the incidence was low, aneurysms being found in only a few subjects over 65 years old. The aneurysms were most numerous in and around the basal ganglia, and occurred usually at or near branchings of the striate arteries: they were found also in the subcortical white matter and in the mid-brain and cerebellum.

The aneurysms may be saccular or fusiform, and the adjacent artery and wall of the sac show hyaline thickening of the intima, sometimes with fibrinoid change: the internal elastic lamina is usually absent from, or fragmented in, the wall of the sac, and muscle is usually absent. Thrombus, sometimes organised, may fill the sac, and there is often evidence of old or recent leakage of blood into the surrounding tissues.

Cole and Yates detected micro-aneurysms in 18 of 20 hypertensives dying from cerebral haemorrhage, and they provide evidence which suggests strongly that rupture of such aneurysms is the usual cause of cerebral haemorrhage in hypertensive subjects (p. 676).

Other forms of aneurysm

Traumatic aneurysm may be produced by injury to the vessel wall by a stab or bullet wound, or by a spicule of fractured bone. A localised haematoma forms and later a layer of granulation tissue develops around it and matures into a remarkably well-defined wall.

If a vein and adjacent artery are both injured, the arterial blood flows into the vein; if a blood-filled sac develops between artery and vein this is known as an **arterio-venous aneurysm.** Blood flow between a large artery and vein may seriously disturb the circulation and cardiac failure due to increased volume load (p. 345) may quickly follow.

A **cirsoid** or **racemose aneurysm** is a form of arterio-venous fistula which appears as a pulsatile swelling consisting of tortuous and dilated arteries and veins with multiple intercommunications. The commonest site is the scalp, and atrophy of the underlying bone may be produced. The condition is sometimes of congenital origin, but more often is the result of a blow on the head; some of the allegedly congenital cases are probably the result of birth injury. Similarly a carotid-cavernous sinus aneurysm resulting from fracture of the skull base gives rise to great engorgement of the orbital veins and oedema of the orbit and conjunctiva.

Diseases of Veins

Compensatory enlargement of the veins takes place, as in the arterial system, when an increased collateral flow is produced by obstruction in a large vein. As in the case of arteries, the dilatation is followed by hypertrophy of the various elements in the wall of the vessels. Veins are, of course, not exposed to the marked variations of blood pressure which occur in arteries, but when they are subject to chronic over-distension, compensatory changes occur in their walls. There is little or no hyperplasia of the muscle, but considerable increase of the elastic tissue occurs. This later undergoes degeneration, and the fibrous tissue becomes thickened and hyaline. Localised patches of thickening in the intima of veins are not uncommon, but the lipid aggregates which are so prominent a feature of atheroma are rare.

Acute thrombophlebitis

A distinction is sometimes made between *thrombophlebitis*, by which is meant a primary inflammatory condition of the vein, with secondary thrombosis, and *phlebothrombosis* (p. 203), in which a bland thrombosis of the vein occurs with, at most, mild preceding inflammatory change. In many instances, however, the distinction is more theoretical than practical because the presence of thrombus in the lumen of the vein sets up reactive changes so that the distinction between mild thrombophlebitis and phlebothrombosis may no longer be possible. It is, however, of value to distinguish between the relatively rare septic venous thrombosis, due to involvement of a vein in a pyogenic infective lesion and liable to cause pyaemia (p. 168), and milder conditions where the effects are chiefly those of local mechanical occlusion and of bland embolism.

Pyogenic thrombophlebitis was formerly common in the veins of the diploë and dural sinuses in middle-ear disease, in the uterine veins in puerperal sepsis, in the veins of the bone marrow in suppurative osteomyelitis, and occasionally in the pulmonary veins in cases of bronchiectasis. Veins involved in such lesions undergo thrombosis and the thrombus becomes invaded by bacteria, and then by polymorphs, so that it breaks down and disseminates, producing the pyaemia.

In the rare condition known as *pylephlebitis suppurativa* the inflammatory process starts in a small tributary of the portal vein and leads to progressive ascending thrombosis and suppuration, from which multiple abscesses in the liver may result.

Thrombophlebitis may also appear as a complication of conditions in which there is a bacteraemia, notably typhoid fever, and it is presumed that organisms circulating in the blood settle in the intima and produce an acute endophlebitis with secondary thrombosis.

Thrombophlebitis migrans consists of multiple incidents of venous thrombosis. It is a conspicuous feature of many cases of Buerger's disease (p. 327) but it is also seen in association with carcinoma. It is a particularly common complication of carcinoma of the pancreas, but occurs also in association with carcinomas of breast, stomach, bronchi, etc.; it is then usually accompanied by vegetations on the mitral and aortic cusps. Thrombophlebitis migrans may be the presenting sign before the underlying malignancy has been recognised.

Tropical thrombophlebitis. Fisher in Northern Rhodesia described a variety of acute phlebitis occurring in adults, both European and Bantu, accompanied by fever, muscular spasm and pain and tenderness along the course of the veins, the femoral being most frequently affected. The disease runs a self-limited course, but in about 10% of cases proves fatal from involvement of visceral veins. It is probable that this form of *primary tropical phlebitis* is the underlying cause of 'Serenje leg', a fairly common disorder in Africa characterised by chronic oedema. Bacteriological studies failed to demonstrate micro-organisms of any kind. Lendrum described the histological appearances as a peculiar type of inflammatory reaction characterised by gross interruption of the vein wall by new capillaries with many polymorphs and macrophages, some of which contained phloxinophil inclusion bodies of unknown nature. Thrombosis is secondary to the lesion of the vein wall.

Chronic phlebitis

Chronic inflammatory processes may spread to the walls of the veins and lead to reactive thickening; in fact, the minute veins are affected in this way in all chronic inflammatory conditions. Chronic phlebitis is seen in the smaller venous branches, in the primary and later stages of syphilis and in association with syphilitic periarteritis (p. 184). Chronic phlebitis of obscure origin is occasionally observed in the large vessels, for example, in the portal vein, and may lead to thrombosis; after some time it may be impossible to say whether the changes present in the vein wall are primary in nature or secondary to the thrombosis.

Endophlebitis of the hepatic veins is the basis of the veno-occlusive disease of Jamaica and certain other tropical regions (see p. 604) and involvement of the hepatic ostia with thrombosis gives rise to the Budd–Chiari syndrome (p. 603).

Tuberculous invasion of veins most commonly results when a caseous lesion—usually in a pulmonary hilar lymph node—involves and destroys the wall of a vein: huge numbers of tubercle bacilli then enter the bloodstream and cause generalised miliary tuberculosis. Smaller numbers of bacilli may enter the blood, either from lesions in the walls of veins or via the thoracic duct, and settle in various tissues to cause single or multiple metastatic lesions.

Veins are often invaded by **malignant tumours** which may then release cells singly or in groups, with the danger of metastatic growth in the lungs, etc. Cancer may also grow along the lumen of veins, an example being clear-cell carcinoma of the kidney, which commonly extends along the renal vein and even the inferior vena cava. Such invasion is usually accompanied by thrombosis.

Varicose veins

Dilatation and tortuosity of veins is termed *varicosity*. The changes may affect a group of veins diffusely or in the form of saccular dilatation. Varicose veins arise from chronic continuous or recurrent increase in the pressure of the blood within them, and this results mainly either from (*a*) the effects of gravity, e.g. in the leg veins, sometimes aggravated by compression proximally, or (*b*) when a major vein is obstructed, leading to increased pressure in collateral veins.

'Gravitational' varicosity occurs in the saphenous system of the legs, notably the long saphenous vein. The condition is much commoner in women and there is a distinct *hereditary predisposition. Prolonged standing* upright without much muscular movement causes marked rise in pressure and distension of the long saphenous vein. Eventually the veins become permanently stretched, so that the valves are now incompetent, and even muscular activity does not protect them from increased pressure in the upright position; in consequence, stretching tends to progress and the veins become visibly swollen and tortuous, i.e. varicose. Venous stasis in the legs, due to the pressure of the gravid uterus on the iliac veins, often results in the development of varicose veins. Without doubt *pregnancy* is a predisposing cause, perhaps accounting for the higher incidence in women than men, although *obesity* is also a predisposing factor. The increased column of blood, giving greater hydrostatic pressure, further increases the dilatation. The venous valves and the muscle and elastic tissue ultimately atrophy somewhat irregularly so that thinning of the wall and pouchlike dilatations occur; finally the wall comes to be composed chiefly of fibrous tissue. The nutrition of the skin over varicose veins of the legs may be impaired. The skin becomes eczematous and pigmented, and chronic indolent ulceration often follows: haemorrhage from the dilated veins may be severe, but is easily stopped by raising the leg with the patient lying flat. Thrombosis is also apt to follow. Organisation of the thrombus is generally imperfect and calcification may result.

Varicocele is another common example of 'gravitational' varicosity, in the pampiniform plexus of veins around the spermatic cord: it is commoner on the left side than on the right and various ingenious explanations have been suggested for this.

'Obstructive' varicosity. This is exemplified by chronic *obstruction to the portal venous blood flow* (due most commonly to cirrhosis or schistosomiasis of the liver), in which the vessels which form anastomoses between the portal and systemic venous systems become varicose (p. 602): the most important ones are those running longitudinally in the oesophageal and gastric submucosa (Fig. 18.17, p. 544), for they may rupture and bleed profusely. While it is true that haemorrhoids ('piles')—varicosity of the communicating veins between the haemorrhoidal venous plexuses in the rectal wall—are a complication of portal obstruction, they are also extremely common in otherwise healthy individuals. *Obstruction of the inferior vena cava* brings about dilatation of the veins of the abdominal wall, establishing a collateral circulation through the upper thoracic veins (Fig. 8.7, p. 196). *Obstruction of the superior vena cava* may occur in cases of bronchial carcinoma and leads to severe dusky cyanosis of the head, neck and arms, sometimes accompanied by pitting oedema of the hands.

Diseases of Lymphatic Vessels

The lymphatic vessels form a closed system separated by an endothelial layer from the tissue spaces. The walls of the small lymphatics are, however, extremely delicate, consisting mainly of a very thin endothelium and an incomplete basement membrane. Moreover, the junctions between endothelial cells are readily disrupted (p. 47). In consequence organisms, leukocytes and tumour cells readily pass into the lymphatic vessels; also red cells which escape from the capillaries by diapedesis may be present in considerable number in the lymphatics draining an inflamed area. The lymphatic vessels thus afford an easy means of communication between the tissues and lymph nodes. Involvement of the lymph nodes in this way occurs in two main conditions, **infections** and **tumours**, especially carcinoma. In both, the extension may be due to transport of the organism or tumour cell by the lymph stream, i.e. metastasis in the strict sense. There may also be progressive involvement of the lymphatic vessels by the disease. In infections, this may involve either acute or chronic lymphangitis; in tumours, the growth of the cells within the lymphatics leads to lymphatic permeation.

Acute lymphangitis. This is seen in pyogenic infections, and most commonly in erysipelas and infections of the hand, etc., due to haemolytic streptococci. The spread of infection along the lymphatics is sometimes accompanied by visible reddening of the overlying skin, with pain and tenderness and often swelling. Spreading lymphangitis is an important feature in puerperal sepsis and septic abortion and may be followed by suppuration in the loose connective tissue around the uterus. In other cases of bacterial infection, the organisms are carried by the lymphatic vessels without settling in their walls. Inflammation of the axillary lymph nodes may result in this way from an infected wound on the hand, without the occurrence of lymphangitis along the arm. A similar striking example is seen in bubonic plague, where even at the site of infection there is usually no inflammatory reaction, the first lesion appearing in the related lymph nodes.

Chronic lymphangitis occurs in a variety of conditions; it may follow *repeated acute attacks of erysipelas*, and is an important feature in many types of *chronic inflammation*. In various chronic infections the spread of organisms by the lymphatics is of great importance. In *tuberculosis*, a disease which in the early stages may be regarded as essentially one of the lymphatic system, the organisms may be carried to lymph nodes without causing lesions on their way.

They may, however, settle in the walls of the lymphatic vessels and give rise to tubercles which thus come to form rows along the vessels. In tuberculous ulceration of the intestine, small tubercles may be found along the lymphatics passing from the floor of the ulcer (Fig. 18.54, p. 576), and also in the mesenteric lymphatics. The thoracic duct may become involved by spread of bacilli along the lymph stream and ulceration of these lesions may set free a large number of tubercle bacilli into the circulation to set up acute miliary tuberculosis (p. 179).

In *syphilis* also, chronic lymphangitis is a prominent feature in connection with the primary lesion, and induration spreading along the lymphatics leads to the characteristic bubo in the regional lymph nodes. The spirochete has a predilection for perivascular lymphatics, and the serious results caused in the aorta by this mode of spread have already been described (p. 325).

Lymphatic obstruction: lymphoedema. Chronic obstruction of lymphatics may give rise to interstitial accumulation of lymph (lymphoedema). When this is prolonged there is proliferation of connective tissue in the lymphoedematous area, resulting in a firm, non-pitting oedema. The most striking examples are seen in *filariasis*, in which obstruction of major lymphatics, together with recurrent inflammation in the affected region, may lead to gross thickening of the tissues known as **elephantiasis**: the lower limbs and sometimes the male external genitalia may be involved (see below). In this country, lymphatic obstruction was formerly not uncommon as a result of recurrent erysipelas, in which scarring and obstruction of multiple small lymphatics may lead to lymphoedema. Nowadays, extensive carcinomatous permeation of lymphatics is a more common cause, but surgical removal of lymphatics or destruction of lymphatics by radiotherapy can cause lymphoedema. This is sometimes seen following radical mastectomy and radiotherapy for breast cancer, where the ipsilateral arm may be sufficiently deprived of its lymphatic drainage to develop gross lymphoedema without carcinomatous involvement of lymphatics. Several instances of tumour growth resembling lymphangiosarcoma have been observed in the lymphangiomatous arm. It is not clear whether they are true sarcomas, or metastatic breast carcinoma, the appearance of which is modified by the lymphoedematous environment.

Filarial disease. The term *Filaria sanguinis hominis* is applied in a general way to the embryos of at least four species of filaria found in the tissues of the human subject, which are distinguishable by morphological and other characters. Microfilariae may appear only periodically in the blood, for example, at night— *Microfilaria nocturna*, during the day— *Microfilaria diurna*, or at all times—*Microfilaria perstans*. The most important of these filariae is *Wuchereria bancrofti*, the embryo of which is the *Microfilaria nocturna*. A brief account of this parasite is given below.

Wuchereria bancrofti. The parasite is widespread in tropical and sub-tropical countries, and more than a quarter of certain populations may be infested (Manson). The adult worms, male and female, are thin filiform organisms, little thicker than coarse hairs; they are whitish and show wriggling movements. The female is about three inches in length, while the male is shorter, thinner, and has a spirally twisted tail. Within the thoracic duct or in large lymphatic vessels, in the pelvis or groins, several worms often occur together coiled up in a

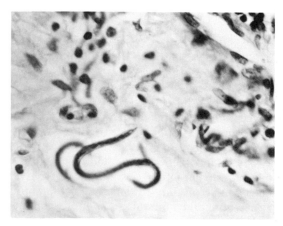

Fig. 13.41 Microfilariae of *Wuchereria bancrofti* in a skin biopsy. × 200.

bunch. The females are viviparous and produce microfilariae, which pass by the lymphatics to the bloodstream, where they are readily found on microscopic examination. The microfilariae, about 0·3 mm in length and about 8 μm in thickness (Fig. 13.41), are each enclosed in a loose sheath within which the young worm may be seen to move backwards and forwards. The microfilariae, which apparently do no harm, appear in the blood in the evening, and they

are readily detected microscopically in a fresh, wet blood film by the agitation their movements produce among the red cells. During the daytime they disappear from the peripheral circulation; some think that they collect in the blood vessels of the lungs, but others believe that they are quickly destroyed, and that their periodicity is due to daily discharge of larvae by female worms in the lymphatics. The intermediate host is a female mosquito, usually of the *Culex* genus, one of the culicines which becomes infected by sucking blood containing the microfilariae. Within the stomach they escape from their sheaths and pass to the muscles, where they undergo further development, and thereafter pass to the labium, where they are in a position to enter human tissues when the insect bites.

In man, the adult worms in the lymphatics cause mechanical obstruction and also low-grade inflammation with gradual injury, scarring and permanent obliteration of the lymphatics. Obstruction of the thoracic duct results in dilatation and varicosity of its tributaries, sometimes forming large masses in the abdominal cavity. The anastomoses with the lymphatics, especially of the abdominal wall, become varicose. Thus the scrotum may become greatly swollen and swellings may form in the groins. These lesions are, however, only the outlying manifestations of the general lymphatic varicosity. The dilated lymphatics contain chyle which is passing along collateral channels, and when rupture occurs a milky fluid escapes, containing fatty globules, red cells in varying number, and sometimes microfilariae. When rupture takes place into the peritoneal cavity *chylous ascites* is produced; when it occurs in the kidneys or bladder *chyluria* results.

Another important result of filarial infection is the production of a form of elephantiasis— *elephantiasis Arabum*—which is of common occurrence in filarial regions. The condition usually starts with an attack of erysipelatoid inflammation and lymphangitis, and is intensified by subsequent attacks. The skin and subcutaneous tissues undergo marked thickening and swelling and become indurated, irregularly folded or nodular. In more than 90% of cases, a lower limb is affected; less commonly the scrotum, breast or an upper limb, are involved. The leg may slowly reach an enormous size, while the enlarged scrotum may exceed 15 kg. According to Manson, elephantiasis occurs when the lymphatic vessels become completely obstructed because the ova of the parasite are set free instead of the living embryos. Since the ova are broader than the living microfilariae, they could more readily cause obstruction and irritation. Thickening of connective tissue results also from attacks of secondary bacterial infection. As a rule microfilariae are not found in the blood in cases of elephantiasis. Manson considered this to be due to complete obstruction of the lymphatics, or to death of the adult parasites.

14

The Heart

Introduction

Disease of the heart now causes more deaths in Western countries than disease of any other organ, amounting to more than a third of all deaths in England and Wales according to the Registrar General's Statistical Review for 1973. Atheroma and thrombosis of the coronary arteries account for most of these deaths by causing ischaemic heart disease in its various forms. The other frequent causes of cardiac disease are congenital abnormality, rheumatic fever and its sequelae, hypertension in the systemic or pulmonary circulations, thyrotoxicosis and anaemia.

The work of the heart. Assuming that at rest the stroke volume of the heart is 66 ml and the rate 72 beats per minute, the left ventricle has a minute volume of about 5 litres, and a daily output of 7200 litres (about $7\frac{1}{2}$ tons). The normal heart has great reserve power, and this can be substantially increased by physical training. During exertion, there is a greater venous return to the heart with consequent increase in diastolic filling and stretching of the muscle fibres; the response is a more vigorous contraction (Starling's law) and the blood pressure is raised. The rate of contraction also increases during exertion and these two factors together can raise the minute volume to about seven times that of the resting state.

This physiological performance can be maintained only if the myocardium is intrinsically healthy, if the valves function efficiently and if the conducting system of the heart co-ordinates contraction of the chambers.

Cardiac Failure

Congestive cardiac failure. Cardiac decompensation.

Definition. Cardiac failure is that state in which the ventricular myocardium fails to maintain a circulation adequate for the needs of the body despite adequate venous filling pressure. Failure of one or both atria is common, but the effect on cardiac function is relatively unimportant unless ventricular function is also deficient.

Causes

Cardiac failure is due to weakness or inefficiency of myocardial contraction, to an abnormal increase of the work required of the myocardium, or to a combination of both. These two basic causes may be further classified as follows.

(1) Intrinsic pump failure. This is most commonly due to *weakness of the ventricular contraction*, the commonest cause of which is myocardial ischaemia resulting from coronary artery disease: other causes of myocardial weakness include acute rheumatic myocarditis, viral myocarditis, severe toxic bacterial infections and congestive cardiomyopathy.

Systolic emptying of the affected ventricle(s) is incomplete, and during diastole the chamber dilates to contain both the residual blood and that received from the atrium. In its defective state, the myocardium cannot respond normally to stretching, i.e. by increasing the force of contraction, and the dilated chamber works at a disadvantage because the force required to provide a given pressure is greater in a large than in a small chamber. Consequently, unless the cause is reversible, dilatation and failure tend to be progressive. Moreover, left or right ventricular dilatation results in stretching and incompetence (functional incompetence) of the mitral or tricuspid valve respectively, and this, as described below, increases the work of the dilated ventricle.

A less common cause of intrinsic pump failure is *impaired compliance of the myocardium*, as in hypertrophic cardiomyopathy and amyloid disease of the heart. In such conditions, the ventricles fail to relax to accommodate the normal amount of blood during diastole, and so the stroke volume is diminished. In addition, the abnormal rigidity may interfere with myocardial contraction. Pericardial haemorrhage or effusion and restrictive pericarditis can produce similar effects.

Disorders of cardiac rhythm, resulting from various conditions, are also included in this group. Although minor irregularities such as sinus arrhythmia and occasional extrasystoles do not significantly impair cardiac function, severe tachycardia so shortens the time for diastolic filling of the ventricles and diastolic flow in the coronary arteries that the efficiency of the heart is substantially decreased; this happens in atrial fibrillation and flutter and the paroxysmal tachycardias. The bradycardia seen in complete heart block (about 30 beats a minute) causes a marked fall in cardiac output.

(2) Increased pressure load results from any condition which increases the resistance to expulsion of blood from the ventricles. The commonest examples are systemic arterial hypertension, and pulmonary arterial hypertension due to mitral stenosis or disease of the lungs: other causes include aortic or pulmonary valve stenosis and coarctation of the aorta.

If the cause is chronic, the affected chamber undergoes hypertrophy, but eventually dilatation and failure develop.

(3) Increased volume load. This arises when a ventricle is required to expel more than the normal volume of blood. It occurs when, owing to incompetence of a heart valve, some of the blood leaks backwards (e.g. through the aortic valve during diastole), and also in conditions in which the general circulation is increased, e.g. anaemia, thyrotoxicosis and hypoxia resulting from lung disease. Other causes include shunts between the left and right sides of the circulation, and arterio-venous shunts.

(4) Coincidence of multiple factors. Each of the above aetiological groups may independently produce cardiac failure, but various factors often operate simultaneously. For example, a patient with mitral stenosis and myocardial fibrosis due to previous rheumatic fever may have only impaired exercise tolerance (i.e. diminished cardiac reserve) without evidence of cardiac failure at rest; with the onset of atrial fibrillation cardiac failure at rest may develop. An individual with systemic hypertension may develop cardiac failure as a result of occlusion of a minor coronary artery which would go virtually unnoticed but for the hypertension, or cardiac failure may be precipitated by an attack of pneumonia in a person with pulmonary hypertension due to chronic lung disease.

Manifestations of cardiac failure

In mild failure, cardiac function is adequate for the needs of the body at rest, and failure becomes apparent as undue breathlessness on exertion; this is attributable to congestion of the lungs, which stimulates respiratory reflexes. In more severe cardiac failure, cardiac output is inadequate even at rest and structural changes in various organs result. The nature of the changes depends on the duration of the cardiac failure, and on which ventricle predominantly fails.

Acute cardiac failure is due to conditions of sudden onset, e.g. coronary artery occlusion, pulmonary embolism, acute infections, the hypertension of acute glomerulonephritis, the development of an arrhythmia, or rupture of a chamber or valve cusp. When cardiac failure is acute and severe (most often due to myocardial infarction) the acute fall in cardiac output, with consequent diminished tissue perfusion, results in a reaction closely similar to that in hypovolaemic shock, with selective vasoconstriction. The term *cardiogenic shock* (p. 227) is appropriate, but the central venous pressure is raised, and the principles of treatment are quite different. Acute heart failure may, however, develop as a result of severe, prolonged hypovolaemic or septic shock (pp. 224–9). If death occurs rapidly the organs behind the failing ventricle show acute venous congestion and no compensatory changes are found in the heart except in cases where there has already been a cardiac lesion.

Chronic cardiac failure may follow acute cardiac failure if death or recovery does not occur rapidly. In cardiac disease of gradual onset, e.g. acquired valvular lesions, chronic failure is particularly common. At death the changes of generalised chronic venous congestion (see p. 193) are found, and the heart, in addition to the features of the causative lesion and the dilatation of failure, shows compensatory enlargement of the chambers. These are described below.

Left ventricular failure causes 60% of deaths in untreated essential hypertension, and is a common cause of death in myocardial infarction, a condition which mainly affects the left ventricle. It is often the cause of death in patients with disease of the aortic valve. The clinical and pathological manifestations are predominantly pulmonary, for in the presence of an efficient right ventricle, congestion is confined to the pulmonary circulation in which an excessive volume of blood accumulates. Severe breathlessness, cyanosis and pulmonary oedema are the outstanding clinical features and there may be no evidence of right ventricular failure, though some congestion of the neck veins is usual. Paroxysmal nocturnal attacks of dyspnoea are common in systemic hypertensive patients and are due to acute left ventricular failure following a rise in pulmonary blood volume, perhaps from resorption of peripheral oedema fluid when the patient is recumbent at night. At necropsy there is dilatation of the left ventricle and functional mitral incompetence: acute or chronic venous congestion of the lungs is found with pulmonary oedema and froth in the bronchi.

Right ventricular failure in its most acute form is found in cases of massive pulmonary embolism. The more chronic forms are found in patients with pulmonary hypertension due to lung disease (e.g. fibrosis or chronic bronchitis and emphysema) and to mitral stenosis. In pure right ventricular failure pulmonary congestion is absent and the findings, besides those of the causal disease and also dilatation of the right ventricle with secondary tricuspid incompetence, distension of the great veins, e.g. in the root of the neck, and acute or chronic venous congestion of the liver, spleen and kidneys. Oedema, ascites and pleural effusions are conspicuous in untreated advanced cases. Right ventricular failure also occurs in mitral stenosis, but in this condition chronic venous congestion with or without pulmonary oedema is found in the lungs owing to the rise in pulmonary venous pressure required to force enough blood through the mitral valve during diastole.

Total heart failure combines the features of left and right ventricular failure and is found not only in diseases which cause diffuse myocardial damage (e.g. extensive infarcts, myocarditis) but also in states requiring a persistently high cardiac output (thyrotoxicosis, etc.). In addition, when there is left ventricular failure the strain imposed on the right side of the heart by the raised pulmonary pressure sooner or later leads to right ventricular failure.

In some cases of heart failure due to lack of ventricular compliance, there may be little or no ventricular dilatation.

Hypoxic phenomena. When left ventricular output falls suddenly and markedly, the cerebral blood supply is so diminished that the patient loses consciousness. This may be momentary, as in a vaso-vagal attack (p. 223), or it may be rapidly fatal when, due to occlusion of a main coronary artery, massive pulmonary embolism or rupture of a cardiac chamber. When the condition is reversible, e.g. during an attack of complete heart block, transient loss of consciousness may occur (*Stokes-Adams attack*); similar attacks occur in patients with incompetence of the aortic valve. In chronic cardiac failure, oxygen deficiency in the tissues is less marked and is seen clinically in the form of cyanosis, sometimes accompanied by mental confusion. Pathologically, the effects of stagnation hypoxia are best seen in tissues such as liver where centrilobular loss of liver cells is usually present in association with venous congestion. A compensatory increase in red cells (polycythaemia) may occur due to hypoxia.

Cardiac oedema is dealt with on pp. 218–19.

Thrombo-embolic phenomena. Patients with cardiac failure are especially prone to develop deep venous thrombosis in the legs as a result of venous stagnation and muscular inactivity associated with lying in bed: in consequence, there is a serious risk of pulmonary embolism. Thrombus is also common in the atria and, in some forms of heart failure, in the ventricles: such cardiac thrombi, depending on their site, can give rise to pulmonary or systemic emboli.

Compensatory enlargement of the heart

When extra work is imposed on the myocardium as a result of a chronic disease (e.g. a valvular lesion or hypertension) compensatory myocardial hypertrophy occurs in the walls of the affected chambers and enables them to deal more effectively with the increased work of maintaining the circulation. As already explained, in conditions of increased volume load, due for example to valvular incompetence, the affected ventricle(s) dilate passively during diastole to contain an increased volume of blood. This occurs before the supervention of heart failure, i.e. when ventricular systolic emptying is normal, and has been termed *compensatory dilatation*. Use of the term 'compensatory' for passive over-dilatation is perhaps not well justified, but it does serve to emphasise the difference from the dilatation of ventricular failure, in which emptying is incomplete. Both hypertrophy and compensatory dilatation cause cardiac enlargement, which is further increased by the dilatation of cardiac failure.

The limiting factors in cardiac hypertrophy are not understood. A likely one is the difficulty in maintaining adequate myocardial perfusion and respiratory exchange when the diameter of the fibres is increased. Because of the vascular arrangements of the coronary supply, ventricular hypertrophy renders the inner part of the myocardium particularly liable to ischaemia in the presence of coronary artery disease (p. 352).

The assessment of cardiac enlargement. In left ventricular hypertrophy, the weight of the heart is increased above the normal 300–350 g, often to over 500 g. Because of its smaller mass, hypertrophy of the right ventricle is only occasionally sufficient to increase markedly the total heart weight. Although hypertrophy of either ventricle is usually obvious at necropsy from the increased thickness of its wall (Fig. 14.1), the degree of hypertrophy is not readily assessed without taking account of the volume of the chambers, i.e. the degree of dilatation. A more reliable method is to separate and weigh the individual ventricles, making allowance for epicardial fatty tissue and any gross fibrous scars, etc.

Increase in size of the hypertrophied heart is often not readily assessed by clinical or radiological measurements unless there is also

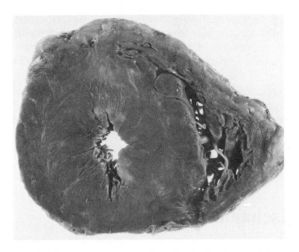

Fig. 14.1 Transverse section through the ventricles of the heart in a case of hypertension, showing obvious hypertrophic thickening of the left ventricle. $\times \frac{1}{2}$.

dilatation, in which case it is difficult to distinguish, from size alone, between the two processes.

Characteristic electrocardiographic changes accompany ventricular hypertrophy, especially when only one ventricle is involved.

Causes of left ventricular hypertrophy. The common causes of marked left ventricular hypertrophy are (1) systemic hypertension (essential, or secondary to renal disease, coarctation of the aorta and certain endocrine tumours), (2) stenosis of the aortic valve, (3) compensatory dilatation of the left ventricle (in aortic or mitral incompetence), (4) persistently high cardiac output (thyrotoxicosis, anaemia, arterio-venous fistula and Paget's disease of bone). Mild and focal left ventricular hypertrophy is found in the absence of hypertension or valvular lesions in certain patients with healed myocardial infarcts, and is presumably compensatory for the loss of muscle. Various cardiomyopathies (p. 365) are a less usual cause of hypertrophy.

Causes of right ventricular hypertrophy. Most examples of right ventricular hypertrophy are found in patients with pulmonary hypertension. The common causes are (1) chronic lung disease, especially bronchitis and widespread pulmonary fibrosis; (2) stenosis and/or incompetence of the mitral valve; (3) congenital heart disease with large shunts of blood from one side of the heart to the other, and also in cases of stenosis of the pulmonary valve; (4) frequently right ventricular hypertrophy without obvious cause occurs in patients with massive left ventricular hypertrophy. This may be due to distortion of the right ventricular lumen by the hypertrophied ventricular septum. Rarer causes of right ventricular failure include multiple small pulmonary emboli and other unusual causes of pulmonary hypertension (p. 401).

Causes of compensatory dilatation. Compensatory dilatation of the left ventricle results from incompetence of the mitral or aortic valve or of both, and right ventricular dilatation from incompetence of the tricuspid and/or pulmonary valves. A lesser degree of compensatory dilatation of both ventricles occurs in patients with persistently high cardiac output, e.g. in thyrotoxicosis or arterio-venous shunts.

Compensatory dilatation is accompanied by hypertrophy of the affected ventricle, the degree of which depends on the increase in its work load.

Ischaemic Heart Disease

Myocardial ischaemia is one of the major causes of disability and death in affluent communities, the outstanding cause being atheroma of the coronary arteries, often complicated by occlusive thrombosis. Practically everybody in such communities has some degree of coronary atheroma by the age of 40, and deaths even earlier than this are increasing in frequency. Severe atheromatous narrowing, particularly of more than one major coronary artery, can give rise to (1) **angina pectoris**, severe chest pain brought on by factors which increase the work of the heart; (2) **myocardial infarction**, usually precipitated by superadded occlusive thrombosis; (3) **sudden death**; (4) **cardiac failure**, and (5) **cardiac arrhythmias**, due to ischaemic injury to the conducting system.

These last three effects may occur either with or without a history of angina pectoris or myocardial infarction.

Angina pectoris

This consists of attacks of severe, sometimes agonising chest pain of sudden onset, due to acute ischaemia of a part of the myocardium with an inadequate blood supply. The pain is brought on by factors which increase the work of the heart and is relieved by rest and by vasodilator drugs such as nitroglycerin. Physical exercise, anger, anxiety, a heavy meal and exposure to cold can all induce an attack.

Aetiology and structural changes. The primary factor in nearly all cases is atheromatous narrowing of the coronary arteries. *Coronary atheroma* shows the usual features of atheroma in other arteries (p. 313). There is patchy fibrous thickening of the intima with accumulation of lipid debris (Fig. 14.2). Calcification is usually present, and confluent calcified patches of atheroma may convert lengths of the vessel into a rigid tube which cannot be cut with a knife; it is then very difficult to examine satisfactorily without decalcification. Atheroma affects all the main branches of the coronary arteries but the earliest and most severe lesions often develop in the first 2–3 cm of the left coronary artery or in its anterior descending branch. Even small distal epicardial branches may be narrowed, although branches that have pene-

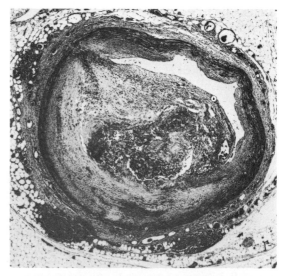

Fig. 14.2 Severe atheromatous narrowing of a coronary artery. In this instance, the lumen has been further reduced by haemorrhage into the soft lipid-rich material, seen as the dark area in the atheromatous patch. × 20.

trated into the myocardium are usually free of atheroma. At necropsy, occlusion of one or more major coronary vessels by organised thrombus can often be demonstrated, with some restoration of blood supply to the distal part of the occluded vessel by enlarged anastomotic arteries (Fig. 14.3). In most cases of angina pectoris, at the time of death there is myocardial scarring or recent myocardial infarction (Fig. 14.4), but myocardial lesions are not invariably present.

Severe atheromatous coronary narrowing may account for the finding of areas in which the myocardium is partly replaced by scar tissue, but in which some myocardial fibres persist (Fig. 14.5), particularly around blood vessels. Old, organised coronary occlusions are, however, commonly present in such cases, and it is often not clear whether the scarring has resulted from chronic ischaemia or myocardial

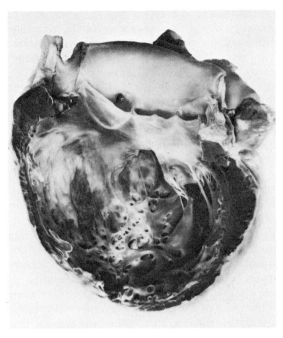

Fig. 14.4 Extensive fibrosis of left ventricle with marked thinning at places; secondary to coronary disease. $\times \frac{1}{2}$.

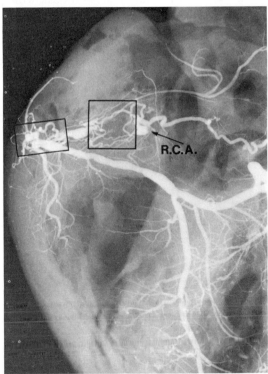

Fig. 14.3 Post-mortem radiograph of part of the right coronary artery in a case of angina. Shortly after its origin (*arrow*), a length of the artery is occluded (*square*) and adjacent vessels have enlarged to provide a collateral route, so that the artery is filled beyond the occlusion. A second occlusion (*oblong*) is present, but is partly obscured by the curving course of the artery. (Dr. M. J. Davies.)

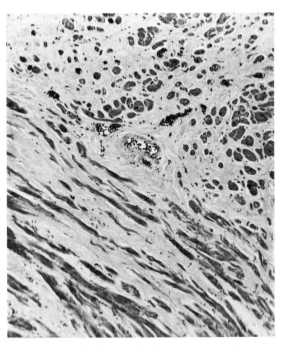

Fig. 14.5 Part of a large zone of myocardial scarring throughout which some myocardial fibres have survived.

infarction. On the basis that the resistance to coronary blood flow is mainly in the arterioles and capillary network, it has been calculated that an atheromatous lesion of a coronary artery must reduce the sectional area by 70% or more to cause a reduction in blood flow. This may be true for resting conditions, but lesser degrees of narrowing, especially if multiple, will inevitably restrict the increased flow which occurs when the arterioles relax, as in physical activity.

In most cases of angina pectoris, there is some degree of left ventricular hypertrophy, usually due to systemic hypertension: by increasing the amount of muscle supplied by the coronary arteries, this aggravates coronary insufficiency and acts as a predisposing cause. Ventricular hypertrophy due to lesions of the cardiac valves or to cardiomyopathy (see later) has a similar effect. Narrowing of the ostia of the coronary arteries by syphilitic aortitis is now a rare cause of angina pectoris.

Clinical Course. In general, chronic coronary insufficiency can be expected to shorten life, although there are wide variations in the clinical course and some patients survive for more than 20 years. Many patients die suddenly and unexpectedly; in some this is due to sudden occlusion of a coronary artery by thrombus, but in about half the cases no recent occlusion can be demonstrated. Death in these cases is assumed to be due to the sudden onset of ventricular fibrillation, and this has been confirmed in patients being monitored by electrocardiography at the time of death.

Myocardial infarction

Myocardial infarction is the commonest cause of death in many parts of the world today. Approximately 33% of males and 25% of females coming to necropsy in this department have evidence of old or recent myocardial infarction and mortality statistics for England and Wales and especially for Scotland suggest that the death rate from this disease is still increasing.

Like infarction in other tissues, it is due to acute ischaemia, usually caused by occlusive thrombosis of a coronary artery over an atheromatous patch.

Clinical course

The onset of myocardial infarction is signalled by the appearance, often abruptly, of severe persistent chest pain. Many patients already suffer from angina pectoris and they often recognise that the pain is different, being continuous for some hours and failing to respond to rest and nitroglycerin. With the onset the patient may experience profound weakness and breathlessness, and there is usually evidence of peripheral circulatory failure with hypotension, cyanosis and a cold clammy skin. Fever, leukocytosis and a raised erythrocyte sedimentation rate are commonly observed within the first 24 hours. Certain tissue enzymes are released by the dead heart muscle, with a consequent rise in blood levels, which is of diagnostic value. The plasma concentration of glutamic oxaloacetic transaminase, for example, rises within 6 to 12 hours, and reaches a peak within 2 or 3 days. Characteristic abnormalities of the electrocardiogram are often demonstrable, but by no means always. The prognosis of myocardial infarction depends on a number of factors including the size of the infarct, its site (e.g. whether it involves the conducting system), the patient's age, and whether or not he has hypertension. Approximately 25% of the patients admitted to hospital die, mostly within the first week, but this excludes a large number who die before they can reach hospital. Death is most commonly caused by ventricular fibrillation, cardiac failure or secondary embolic disease (see below).

Structural changes

The changes found in the heart at necropsy depend on how long the patient has lived since the onset of infarction.

The **coronary arteries** usually show extensive atheroma, but in some cases there will be only one or two patches causing severe narrowing. The occluding thrombus typically overlies an atheromatous patch, but may extend along a considerable length of the vessel. At first, it is usually composed mainly of red thrombus (Fig. 14.6); subsequently it becomes pale and is eventually organised, often with some recanalisation (Fig. 14.7).

Thrombosis of the anterior descending branch of the left coronary artery is particularly

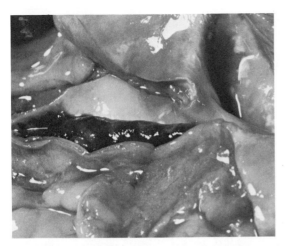

Fig. 14.6 Recent thrombotic occlusion of the right main coronary artery: death resulted 12 hours after the onset of symptoms.

common and usually causes an infarct involving the anterior wall of the left ventricle together with the apex and sometimes extending to the anterior part of the interventricular septum and the adjacent part of the anterior

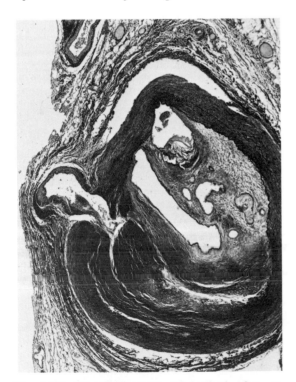

Fig. 14.7 Coronary artery recanalised after occlusion by thrombus. There was extensive healed myocardial infarction. ×25.

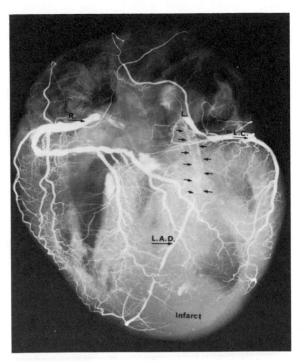

Fig. 14.8 Post-mortem angiograph in a case of recent myocardial infarction. The anterior descending artery (LAD) is occluded proximally (*arrows*), and although there was sufficient collateral supply to fill the artery distally, extensive infarction had occurred over the anterior wall and apical region. Note also the atheromatous narrowings of the right coronary artery. (Dr. M. J. Davies.)

wall of the right ventricle (Fig. 14.8). Occlusion of the right main coronary artery is almost as frequent and is associated with infarction of the posterior wall of the *left* ventricle, sometimes involving also the posterior part of the septum and posterior wall of the right ventricle. Occlusion of the circumflex branch of the left coronary artery can cause infarction of the lateral wall of the left ventricle, but occlusion of the descending and circumflex branches of the right coronary artery are relatively rare causes of infarction. In some instances, recent thrombus is found in two major vessels, and infarction is accordingly extensive.

The extent of infarction varies considerably, depending on the severity of atheromatous narrowing, and the presence or absence of previous thrombosis, in other coronary arteries. There is considerable normal variation in the relative sizes of the left and right arteries, and atheromatous narrowing of a branch may result in enlargement of collateral vessels (Fig. 14.3) so that its final occlusion causes a lesser infarct than usual, or even none at all.

The detection of thrombus in coronary arteries narrowed by atheroma is not always easy. If the arteries are opened lengthwise with scissors, a small thrombus may be displaced and disrupted by the point of the blade without being noticed. A more satisfactory method of examining the vessels is by transverse section at close intervals. The presence of extensive and grossly calcified atheromatous lesions prevents satisfactory naked-eye examination of the affected parts of the vessels at necropsy, and decalcification is first necessary.

The infarct may involve the whole thickness of the myocardium, or it may be confined to the inner part of the wall. Occasionally infarction involves the deeper, subendocardial myocardium throughout most of the circumference of the left ventricle: there is usually severe atheromatous narrowing of the left and right main

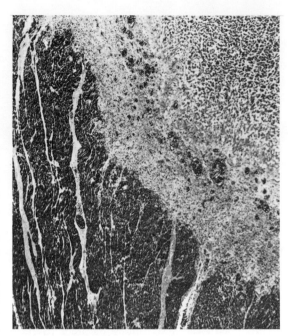

Fig. 14.10 Infarct of myocardium of 12 days' duration. The necrotic heart muscle (*upper right*) is separated from the surviving muscle by a zone of cellular and vascular granulation tissue. × 40.

coronary arteries and the anterior descending branch, but without recent thrombosis. It appears that such extensive arterial narrowing renders especially precarious the blood supply to this part of the myocardium and that subendocardial ischaemic necrosis can occur without superadded occlusive arterial thrombosis (Davies, Robertson and Woolf).

Although ischaemic death of myocardium results within a few minutes of loss of blood supply, the visible changes of infarction in the dead muscle do not appear for 8 hours or so. Accordingly, in patients who die suddenly at the time of coronary occlusion, or within the next few hours, acute changes in the myocardium are not observed by naked-eye or ordinary light microscopy. The first changes noticed by naked eye are blotchy congestion and pallor. Although the muscle undergoes coagulative necrosis, the infarct can usually be felt after a day or so as a patch of softening, and during the next few days its colour changes from brown to yellowish-grey (Fig. 14.9). After a week or so it becomes more sharply defined by the development of a zone of vascular granulation tissue along the margin, and removal of the

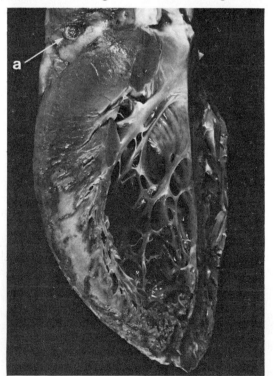

Fig. 14.9 Myocardial infarction of 11 days duration. The anterior descending branch of the left coronary artery (**a**) is occluded by thrombus and there is extensive infarction of the wall of the left ventricle, seen as areas of pallor and surrounding congestion. Note also mural thrombus at the apex.

dead tissue by organisation gradually proceeds. When the infarct extends to the outer surface of the myocardium, the pericardial surface is often covered by a layer of fibrinous exudate with marginal haemorrhages. On the inner aspect, the endocardium and a thin layer of adjacent myocardium remain alive, nourished by blood from the lumen, but in patients surviving for several days this does not prevent thrombosis on the endocardial lining (see below).

Under the microscope the infarcted muscle shows the usual features of necrosis (Fig. 1.4, p. 4). The necrotic muscle is invaded by polymorphonuclear leukocytes and, after a few days, digestion by macrophages and organisation can be seen at the margins (Fig. 14.10). Gradually, the dead muscle is replaced by fibrous tissue, the process taking some weeks or even months, depending on the size of the infarct, and eventually a pale fibrous scar remains (Fig. 14.11).

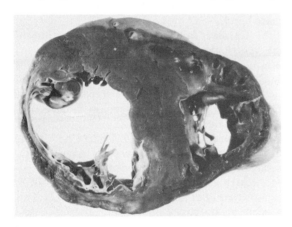

Fig. 14.11 Old infarct represented by replacement of the lateral and posterior wall of the left ventricle by a relatively thin fibrous scar.

As already stated, it is sometimes not possible to determine whether myocardial fibrosis has resulted from infarction or chronic ischaemia.

Aetiology

The important cause of myocardial infarction is atheroma of the coronary arteries with superadded occlusive thrombosis over an atheromatous patch. The aetiology of atheroma, and the factors associated with an increased risk of myocardial infarction, have been discussed on p. 317. These include raised levels of various plasma lipids, obesity, hypertension, cigarette smoking and a sedentary occupation. These factors are all of long duration, and are likely to promote the gradual development and extension of atheroma, but they may also predispose to superadded thrombosis. Enhanced coagulability of the blood has been shown to be common in patients with ischaemic heart disease, and correlates partially with the levels of plasma lipids. It has also been shown that coronary blood flow is affected by cigarette smoking, and this also, by stimulating catecholamine secretion, may predispose to thrombosis.

Patients with severe coronary atheroma are particularly liable to myocardial infarction following a severe injury or major surgical operation. This may occur during a period of shock, but the risk is high for some weeks following the injury, etc. The circulatory disturbances of shock, the effect of anaesthetic agents on the heart, and the increased coagulability of the blood following injury are probably of importance.

Relationship of coronary thrombosis to myocardial infarction. The reported incidence of recent coronary thrombosis in patients dying of acute myocardial infarction varies greatly. In some series, the incidence has been only about 50%, and considerably lower in those patients dying within a few hours of the onset of symptoms. Accordingly, it has been suggested that coronary thrombosis may not be the cause of infarction, and that it occurs *after* the muscle has died. The validity of this view depends upon the care with which the coronary arteries are examined (see above). By careful examination of the coronary arteries by close transverse section, preceded when necessary by decalcification, workers at St. Georges' Hospital, London, have found an occlusive thrombus in the expected artery in virtually all cases of myocardial infarction in patients dying 12 hours or more after the onset of clinical symptoms, and Harland's experience in our own Department has been similar. In patients dying within a few hours of onset, infarction cannot be identified morphologically, and the diagnosis is insecure. These findings relate to regional infarcts occurring mainly within the territory supplied by a major coronary artery. By contrast, circumferential sub-endocardial necrosis of the myocardium (see above) is not usually associated with recent coronary thrombosis, but this lesion accounts for only about 6% of all infarcts (Davies, Robertson and Woolf).

Microscopic examination of recent coronary occlusions shows that the thrombus very often forms over a *ruptured* atheromatous plaque (Fig. 14.12), and this suggests that the rupture

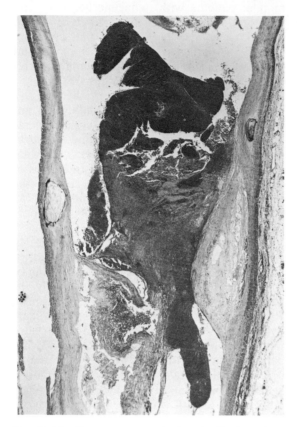

Fig. 14.12 Coronary artery in longitudinal section, showing an ulcerated atheromatous plaque (*left, lower*) with occlusion of lumen by thrombus. × 15.

(and not necrosis of muscle) has promoted thrombosis. It follows that, in such cases, infarction is the *result* of the occlusion. Admittedly, old organised occlusive coronary arterial thrombosis is sometimes found without evidence of previous infarction (i.e. a myocardial scar), but this is probably attributable to enlargement of anastomotic arteries, and thus an increased collateral circulation, before the thrombosis occurred.

Experimental animal studies also support the causal role of thrombosis, for occlusion of a major coronary artery results in infarction,

whereas myocardial necrosis induced by other means is not followed by coronary thrombosis.

Infrequent causes of myocardial infarction. Occlusion of the ostia of the coronary arteries by syphilitic aortitis is nowadays a rare cause of infarction, and so are coronary lesions due to polyarteritis nodosa or Buerger's disease. Occlusion of a coronary artery by embolus is also much less common than thrombosis, but sometimes results from bacterial endocarditis, and also from detachment of thrombus forming in relation to valve prostheses.

Effects and complications

(a) Arrhythmias. Death from myocardial infarction most frequently results from arrhythmias, particularly ventricular fibrillation. Healed infarcts may also be associated with cardiac arrhythmias and are the chief cause of heart block.

(b) Cardiac failure. Extensive infarction of left ventricular muscle can cause acute heart failure, and if severe this results in **cardiogenic shock**, the prognosis of which is poor. Loss of the infarcted muscle also predisposes to chronic heart failure, which may develop at any time after infarction.

(c) Mural thrombosis. Following acute myocardial infarction, release of tissue thromboplastin from the damaged muscle and localised eddying of blood lead to thrombosis in the ventricular chambers (Fig. 8.16, p. 202). This is seen at necropsy in about 30% of cases: in patients who survive, the thrombus is eventually organised. Systemic emboli can result from mural thrombosis, but are not very common.

(d) Venous thrombosis. Presumably because of reduced blood flow, systemic venous thrombosis is an important complication of myocardial infarction and tends to occur especially in the veins of the legs. Detachment of this thrombus is common and consequently pulmonary embolism and infarction are not infrequently a cause of death in this disease.

(e) Rupture of the left ventricle due to myocardial softening (*myomalacia cordis*) causes 10% of all deaths from myocardial infarction. It generally occurs 4 to 14 days after infarction, when autolysis of the infarct is active, and especially when leukocytic invasion is marked but repair just commencing. Rupture leads to sudden death from massive haemopericardium. When the interventricular septum is involved in infarction, it may rupture, leading to sudden onset of severe cardiac failure and a loud heart murmur. Rupture of a papillary muscle in the left ventricle may also occur, leading to incompetence of the mitral valve, with

infarction has occurred, there is likely to be adjacent myocardium which, although not infarcted, is ischaemic (and is presumably the source of the prolonged pain associated with infarction). As anastomotic channels dilate and enlarge, the blood supply to such areas of partial ischaemia will improve. However, in some patients angina pectoris dates from a myocardial infarction, and it is apparent that throm-

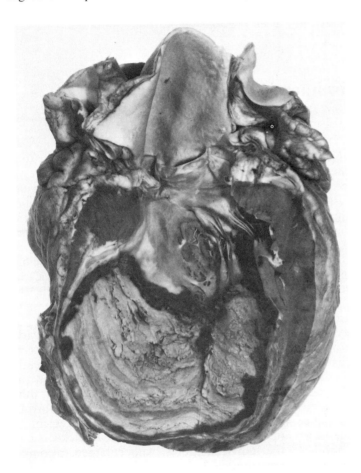

Fig. 14.13 Aneurysm of the left ventricle following ischaemic myocardial fibrosis. Much of the anterior wall (*left*) of the ventricle has been replaced by fibrous tissue, which has stretched to form an aneurysm, now largely filled with laminated thrombus. $\times \frac{2}{3}$.

a loud murmur and intractable pulmonary oedema. Persistence of hypertension and physical activity after infarction predisposes to cardiac rupture.

(f) Cardiac aneurysm. In rare instances the fibrosed wall of a healed infarct of the left ventricle may stretch to form a cardiac aneurysm. As with other aneurysms, laminated thrombus tends to form in the cavity (Fig. 14.13).

(g) Angina pectoris. Whenever myocardial

bosis of a major coronary vessel may render areas of myocardium chronically ischaemic. In some instances, angina is cured by myocardial infarction, presumably because an area of myocardium which was previously clinically ischaemic has been included in the infarct and destroyed.

(h) Recurrence of infarction. Because atheroma is generally extensive, individuals who have had a myocardial infarct are prone to recurrence.

Other effects of ischaemic heart disease

Ischaemic heart disease is the usual cause of **sudden death.** There may be a history of angina, previous infarction, or evidence of chronic heart failure, but sometimes there have been no warning symptoms. At necropsy, there is usually severe coronary atheroma, with or without old organised thrombotic occlusions. In a minority of cases, there is a recent occlusive thrombus which has apparently caused death before there has been time for the morphological changes of infarction to develop. The occasional unexpected deaths which have occurred during ECG recording suggest that ventricular fibrillation is the usual cause.

Ischaemic heart disease is also the most important cause of **chronic heart failure** and of **cardiac arrhythmias**, whether or not there has been previous myocardial infarction.

Non-inflammatory, Non-ischaemic Disorders of the Myocardium

Fatty change of the myocardium (p. 16) is an expression of impaired metabolism of the heart muscle most frequently seen in severe prolonged anaemia. *Adiposity of the heart* is a deposition of fat in the epicardium which extends between cardiac muscle fibres (Fig. 1.18, p. 19). It affects the right ventricle especially and is usually, but not always, associated with general obesity. Very rarely cardiac function is impaired by this deposition of adipose tissue. *Brown atrophy* (p. 29) is not related to the occurrence of cardiac failure. *Primary amyloid disease* (p. 235) commonly affects the heart and is a rare cause of cardiac failure. The clinical picture may be similar to that of restrictive cardiomyopathy, and diagnosis may be difficult both clinically and at necropsy, unless the possibility of amyloidosis is kept in mind. *Segmentation and fragmentation of the myocardium* indicate conditions in which the heart muscle cells either separate from one another at the intercalated discs or show irregular tearing. These changes have been observed in cases of violent death. It is supposed that they result from irregular contraction at the time of death.

Cardiomyopathy

Cardiomyopathy is a convenient term for the classification of a heterogeneous group of chronic myocardial disorders which are not due to ischaemia, hypertension, valve disease or shunts, and appear non-inflammatory. The four main types are as follows.

1. Hypertrophic obstructive cardiomyopathy (asymmetrical septal hypertrophy). In this condition there is asymmetric hypertrophy of the left ventricle, and especially of the septum. Function is effected by (*a*) undue rigidity of the left ventricle, which interferes with diastolic filling, and (*b*) in many, but not all cases, the bulging, hypertrophied septum obstructs the outflow of the left, and less commonly the right, ventricle.

Clinically, the condition presents from early childhood to old age, usually as heart failure or atypical angina: it can also cause sudden death. It is often familial and has been detected (by echo cardiography) in some apparently healthy relatives. Microscopy shows interstitial fibrosis, areas of disordered, whorled arrangement of muscle fibres, and very marked thickening of the individual fibres, with enlarged, pleomorphic nuclei and increased glycogen content. These features are useful in diagnostic biopsy. The nature of the basic abnormality is unknown and current views are largely speculative.

2. Congestive cardiomyopathy. This consists of congestive heart failure which is not due to any of the known causes, and is thus diagnosed by exclusion. At necropsy, the myocardium is pale and unduly flabby, and there is often ventricular mural thrombus and endocardial thickening. Microscopy shows interstitial fibrosis and vacuolation and loss of myofibrils in some fibres: these changes are not diagnostic.

Congestive cardiomyopathy sometimes shows a familial tendency, and may be associated with alcoholism or follow childbirth, but the causation is entirely unknown. Congestive failure is a complication of various other conditions, e.g. dystrophy of the skeletal muscles, Friedreich's ataxia, glycogen disease of the Pompe type, and acromegaly. Such cases are sometimes included as congestive cardiomyopathy but the cause, if known, should be specified.

3. Restrictive cardiomyopathy is also known as **endomyocardial fibro-elastosis.** It is a rare disorder, mainly of infants, characterised by a thick smooth layer of collagenous and elastic tissue between the endocardial and muscular layers. Involvement of the left ventricle, which may be hypertrophied, is most common. Cases have been attributed to fetal endocarditis, to anoxia due to origin of the left coronary artery from the pulmonary trunk, and to hypoplasia of the left ventricle associated with premature closure of the foramen ovale.

Amyloid disease of the heart can cause a restrictive cardiomyopathy in adults.

4. Obliterative cardiomyopathy (endomyocardial fibrosis) is of unknown cause and found mainly in tropical Africa where it is one of the common forms of left or total heart failure. It occurs in many other parts of the world. In the absence of significantly narrowed coronary arteries there is dense fibrosis of the endocardium affecting usually the apex and posterior walls of one or both ventricles. Sometimes the fibrosis partially obliterates the ventricular cavity and, by enveloping the posterior papillary muscles and chordae tendineae, distorts the posterior cusps of the mitral and tricuspid valves with resulting incompetence. Mural thrombus overlying the fibrotic endocardium is common though embolism seldom occurs. The fibrosis is dense and acellular on the surface but more loose with some inflammatory reaction in the deeper layers. Fibrous tissue bands may spread through the inner third of the myocardial wall and there may be atrophy of myocardial fibres with loss of sarcoplasm. Bacterial endocarditis is recorded in about 10% of fatal cases.

Inflammatory Lesions of the Heart

Myocarditis

The term myocarditis is used loosely to cover various lesions of diverse nature. some of which are due to bacterial and viral infections, others to the effects of bacterial toxins. Rheumatic myocarditis appears to be, at least in part, a hypersensitivity reaction to streptococcal antigens. The subject is difficult because of the impossibility of confirming myocarditis in suspected cases which recover, and the poor correlation between pathological lesions in the myocardium and clinical evidence of heart disease. The possibility of serious metabolic disorder with no structural change in the myocardium, and the difficulty of interpreting the results of bacteriological cultures of necropsy material, further complicate the subject.

Toxic myocarditis is a major feature of diphtheria. Similar appearances, presumed to be toxic in origin, may be seen in pneumococcal

pneumonia, typhoid fever, septicaemia and other extensive septic conditions.

Naked-eye appearances. The lesions are not recognisable by naked eye: there may be patches of myocardial pallor and rarely extensive mural thrombus between the columnae carneae of the left ventricle, overlying damaged areas.

Microscopically there is a parenchymatous lesion with numerous small foci of coagulative necrosis in the muscle. The affected fibres appear swollen and glassy, with loss of striations and nuclei, and around them there is infiltration, mostly of mononuclears and lymphocytes, but polymorphs also may be present. The necrotic fibres afterwards undergo absorption, while the supporting cells in the areas of infiltration proliferate, and small fibrous patches ultimately result (Fig. 6.1, p. 148). The nature of the infection cannot be deduced from the appearances of the cardiac lesions. In the toxic

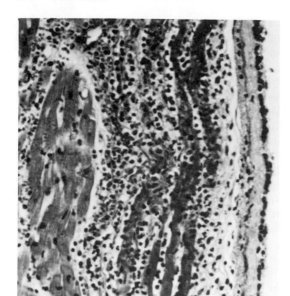

Fig. 14.14 Necrosis of the fibres of the left bundle branch, with an inflammatory reaction, in a fatal case of diphtheria. × 225. (Professor A. C. Lendrum.)

myocarditis of diphtheria, in some cases the conducting system is severely affected (Fig. 14.14), with resultant heart block.

Clinically toxic myocarditis is recognised by the onset of cardiac arrhythmia or acute cardiac failure in a patient with diphtheria, pneumonia or other 'toxic' illness. It may cause sudden death. Peripheral circulatory failure may also be present in severe cases.

Suppurative myocarditis is due to direct extension of pyogenic organisms from an adjacent

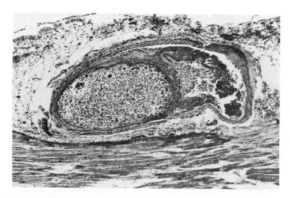

Fig. 14.15 Septic embolus in coronary artery in acute bacterial endocarditis. × 36.

valve in bacterial endocarditis, or to infection by way of the bloodstream. The myocardium is a common site of multiple abscess formation in septicaemia or pyaemia, particularly when due to *Staph. aureus*. In pyaemia, the abscesses have the usual haemorrhagic margin, and their presence is suggested at necropsy by small epicardial haemorrhages, incision of which may reveal underlying abscesses. Septic emboli may be found in coronary branches (Fig. 14.15).

Involvement of the myocardium in acute bacterial endocarditis is described on p. 371.

Virus myocarditis. Coxsackie viruses of Group B cause myocarditis and pericarditis: men are most often affected but outbreaks in infant nurseries have been described. The myocardium shows widespread damage to the muscle fibres with abundant macrophages, lymphocytes, plasma cells and eosinophils in the interstitial tissue (Fig. 14.16).

Isolated myocarditis. Various forms of subacute and chronic myocarditis without concomitant endocarditis or pericarditis have been described, and although the appearances resemble those in Coxsackie infection in the

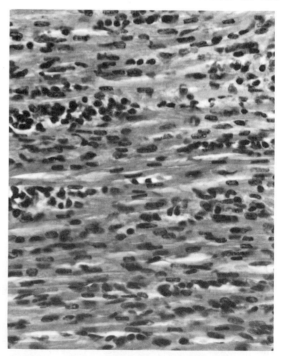

Fig. 14.16 Myocarditis due to Coxsackie B virus from a child of 11 months. The field illustrates the extensive focal infiltration with macrophages, lymphocytes, etc. × 320. (Dr. J. F. Boyd.)

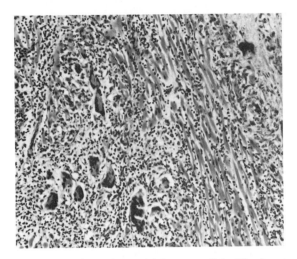

Fig. 14.17   Acute interstitial myocarditis. The heart muscle fibres are replaced by a granulomatous reaction, in which there are many giant cells derived from the muscle fibres. × 85. (Professor T. Symington.)

newborn, nothing is known of their causes or relationships. In one variety, known as *interstitial myocarditis* (*Fiedler's myocarditis*), the heart is dilated and hypertrophied and mural thrombi are common. Yellowish-white foci of necrosis may be visible and microscopically these show conspicuous infiltration of the interstitial tissue around the necrotic muscle fibres with macrophages, lymphocytes, plasma cells, eosinophils and multinucleated giant cells apparently derived from the damaged muscle fibres. Figure 14.17 is from a boy aged 14 who died suddenly after a brief illness.

Clinically the disease presents with cardiac arrhythmias, chest pain and embolic phenomena, progressing in a few weeks or months to cardiac failure without obvious cause.

Sarcoidosis may involve the heart, granulomas developing in the myocardium. The endocardium and pericardium are not usually involved.

Syphilis was formerly a frequent cause of serious heart disease. It may affect the heart in four ways. *Incompetence of the aortic valve* is the commonest form and is due to stretching of the valve ring as a result of its involvement in syphilitic mesaortitis. Because they do not meet,

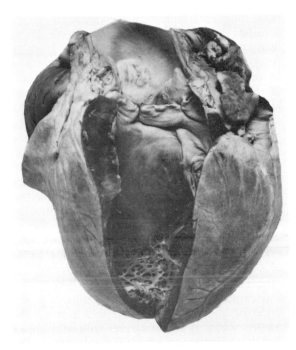

Fig. 14.18   Syphilitic aortitis, affecting the origin of the aorta. Stretching of the aortic ring has resulted in sagging and thickening of the cusps: dilatation and hypertrophy of the left ventricle are secondary to aortic incompetence. × ½.

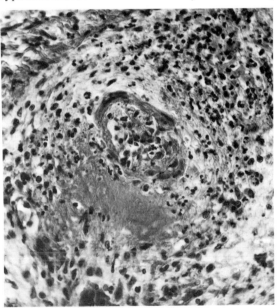

Fig. 14.19   A miliary gumma in the myocardium of a child with congenital syphilis. There is a patch of necrosis adjacent to a small thrombosed artery, and the usual surrounding infiltrate of lymphocytes, plasma cells and macrophages. × 300. (The late Professor J. W. S. Blacklock.)

the cusps become elongated and pendulous (Fig. 14.18). The effects on the chambers of the heart are similar to those resulting from any other variety of aortic incompetence (see p. 367).

Myocardial ischaemia may follow narrowing of the orifices of the coronary arteries by intimal fibrous plaques formed over areas of mesaortitis or by cicatricial contraction of heal-ing lesions. Angina pectoris, myocardial infarction and sudden death are, however, rarely due to syphilis nowadays.

Gumma of the heart is very rare. It may involve the conducting system and cause heart-block. In *congenital syphilis*, there may be miliary gummas (Fig. 14.19) or interstitial fibrosis of the myocardium.

Rheumatic heart disease

Rheumatic fever (Acute rheumatism)

This is an inflammatory disorder of the connective tissues which follows streptococcal pharyngitis. It affects especially the heart and has a marked tendency to recur.

Age incidence. In about 50% of cases the first attack develops during the second decade; of the remainder about one half occur earlier, usually between the fifth and tenth year. The primary attack occurs only rarely after the age of 30 years. Onset in childhood or adolescence is especially likely to result in a severe general involvement of the heart—pancarditis—whereas in adults it tends to progress insidiously to chronic valvular disease.

Aetiology. Most attacks of rheumatic fever occur 2–4 weeks after infection of the throat by β-haemolytic streptococci of Lancefield group A. There is no doubt that such throat infection is a major aetiological factor since prolonged administration of penicillin to patients who have had an attack of rheumatic fever greatly reduces the incidence of further attacks of this notably recurrent disease. Presumably the high incidence of rheumatic fever in the economically poor is due to increased likelihood of streptococcal infection.

It is far from clear how preceding infection of the throat leads to the cardiac and other lesions of rheumatic fever. The 2–4 weeks delay in onset speaks against a direct infection of the heart, etc., or a direct effect of exotoxin. Streptococci have not been demonstrated convincingly in the cardiac lesions, and the failure of antibiotics to prevent the disease when first administered during the interval between the sore throat and the onset of rheumatic fever is not in keeping with simple spread of infection.

There is strong evidence that the disease has an immunological basis. Compared with those who make an uncomplicated recovery from streptococcal sore throat, patients who develop rheumatic fever have unusually high antibody levels against various streptococcal antigens (including antistreptolysin O (ASO) titre, which is widely used as a diagnostic aid). The serum of many patients contains auto-antibody which reacts *in vitro* with myocardial fibres, and becomes fixed to the patient's myocardial fibres *in vivo*. It is of particular interest that Kaplan has shown that certain antigens are shared by some types of group A streptococci and by myocardial fibres. A simple explanation of the pathogenesis of rheumatic myocarditis is that throat infection by streptococci leads, in certain susceptible individuals, to strong immunity against various streptococcal antigens; if, among these, the antibody response is directed towards the antigens shared by streptococcus and myocardium, an immunological cross reaction with myocardium takes place with fixation of antibody and complement and this leads to cytotoxic effects on the myocardial fibres. The real explanation is likely to be more complex since the above does not take into account the occurrence of rheumatic fever following infection by streptococci which do not contain the shared antigen, nor does it explain the typical lesion, the Aschoff body (see below) which does not contain fixed immunoglobulin and is widely regarded as a lesion of connective tissue rather than one centred around myocardial fibres.

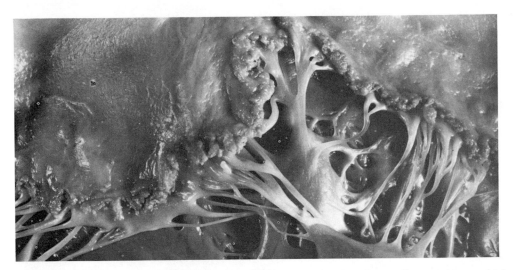

Fig. 14.20 Mitral valve in acute rheumatic endocarditis, showing the small vegetations which form along the line of apposition of the cusps. × 2.

Furthermore some unexplained factor must render the cardiac tissues abnormally permeable to permit the union of antibody and complement with cardiac muscle sarcoplasm *in vivo*.

Naked-eye appearances. Death may occur in the first attack of acute rheumatism or in an early recrudescence and at this stage is due to **myocarditis** and **acute myocardial failure**. This is often precipitated by the onset of **pericarditis** which may further increase the load on the heart, especially if there is much effusion. Aschoff bodies may be just visible as small pale foci in the heart wall, especially behind the posterior mitral cusp.

An **acute endocarditis** usually accompanies the myocarditis, but plays little part in causing death in the acute disease. The endocarditis affects mainly the valves, and small thrombi referred to as **vegetations** are formed, first as minute rounded bodies of greyish or pinkish-grey translucent appearance along the lines of contact of the cusps (Fig. 14.20). In the aortic valve they are found on the ventricular aspect of the cusps a short distance from the free margins, and in the mitral on the atrial aspect. Pressure along the lines of contact between the cusps is obviously a determining factor in the formation of the vegetations. It acts as a slight trauma on the surface endothelium altered by subjacent inflammatory oedema; the resulting lesion leads to the deposition of platelet thrombi. This factor has greater effect on the left side of the heart where the blood pressure is higher, and vegetations predominate on the valves of the left side. The mitral valve is more commonly affected than the aortic, the tricuspid being rarely and the pulmonary valve very

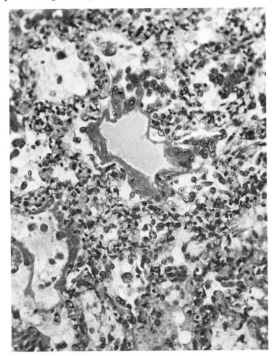

Fig. 14.21 The lung in a case of cardiac failure due to acute rheumatic myocarditis. The lung shows hyaline membranes lining alveolar ducts and mononuclear cells in the alveolar walls and lying free in the alveoli. × 220.

rarely involved. The vegetations later enlarge and may extend on to the mural endocardium; for example, from the mitral valve they may spread over the atrial aspect of the cusps to the atrial endocardium, especially on the posterior aspect. In cases with a history of previous acute rheumatism, patches of endocardial fibrosis may be extensive. In early fatal cases the lungs are congested, sometimes brownish and of firm rubbery consistence, with hyaline membranes in the alveolar ducts (Fig. 14.21). These appearances, previously thought to indicate a specific rheumatic pneumonia, appear to be merely the result of fairly acutely developing left heart failure and are sometimes seen in acute left heart failure from other causes.

Microscopic appearances. The cardiac lesion of acute rheumatism is a **pancarditis**, i.e. lesions occur in myocardium, endocardium and pericardium.

Myocardium. The characteristic lesion of acute rheumatic fever is the **Aschoff body** which, when fully developed, shows hyaline change of collagen bundles surrounded by an infiltrate of lymphocytes, macrophages and occasional polymorphs. It often contains one or more giant cells (Fig. 14.22), though these are

relatively small, with only a few nuclei or a convoluted nucleus. Aschoff bodies are scattered throughout the myocardium (Fig. 14.23) and later become fibrosed. There also occur more diffuse polymorphonuclear and lymphocytic infiltrations along the connective tissue planes, and inflammatory oedema. Bacteria are not demonstrable in these lesions.

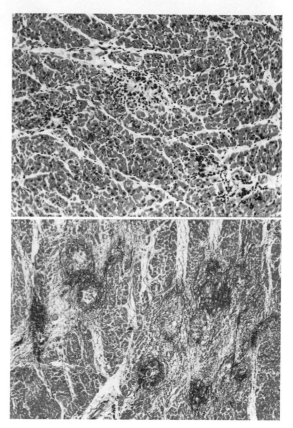

Fig. 14.23 Rheumatic myocarditis. *Above*, the acute stage, showing several Aschoff bodies. × 80. *Below*, later stage, showing fibrosis around the Aschoff bodies (Masson's trichrome stain: collagen appears dark). × 48.

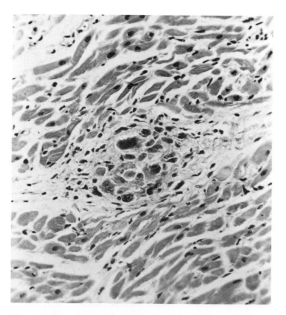

Fig. 14.22 Aschoff body in the myocardium of a child who died of heart failure during an attack of acute rheumatic fever. Central hyaline material is surrounded by macrophages, some with large or multiple nuclei, and by lymphocytes, etc. × 220.

Aschoff bodies are more common in the left side of the heart, both in atrium and ventricle. They are especially abundant beneath the endocardium of the left atrium just above the posterior mitral cusp; in long-standing cases this area becomes thickened, roughened and fibrous. The clinical effects of rheumatic fever indicate extensive myocardial damage, which, as suggested above, may be due to immunological injury (p. 360).

Endocardium. The whole of the endocardium may show innumerable focal lesions and more diffuse inflammatory oedema and cellular infiltration, particularly over the chordae and papillary muscles.

At an early stage the connective tissue of the valves shows inflammatory oedema, most marked in the subendothelial layer, where there may be localised swellings almost like vesicles. The condition is a general valvulitis and where the valve cusps come into contact on closure the additional effect of slight trauma results in ulceration and formation of the thrombotic vegetations (Fig. 14.24). The inflammatory

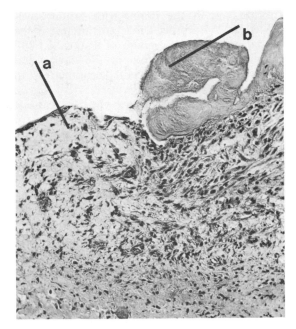

Fig. 14.24 Section of the mitral valve in early acute rheumatic endocarditis. The valve cusp shows inflammatory oedema **a**; where the cusps meet, the oedematous tissue has ulcerated and platelets have been deposited on the ulcerated surface to form the early vegetation **b**. Subsequently, fibrin also is deposited (see Fig. 8.14, p. 202). × 80. (Professor A. C. Lendrum.)

oedema is soon followed by proliferation of fibrocytes and sometimes by the formation of poorly defined Aschoff bodies, especially near the base of the valve cusps, and there is also an ingrowth of capillaries into the valve cusps which normally are avascular in man. The vegetations are composed chiefly of blood platelets and fibrin (Fig. 8.14, p. 202). They tend to glue the valve cusps together at their lines of mutual contact, and later, when organisation occurs, the adherence becomes permanent and results in fibrous thickening, and often calcification, of the valve cusps: these changes can result in serious deformity.

Pericardium. Fibrinous pericarditis is common in rheumatic fever, giving rise to pain and a friction rub, and later undergoing organisation with resulting adhesions.

Clinical features. In children, early evidence of cardiac involvement includes tachycardia, disorders of conduction and dilatation of the heart with the murmurs of secondary valvular incompetence and, at a later stage, signs of pericarditis. The vegetations on the valves have no clinical effect in acute rheumatic fever for they do not impair valvular function or give rise to emboli. Other features which may be seen are *chorea*—a mild encephalitis with degeneration of nerve cells of the basal ganglia which leads to involuntary movements: also various skin rashes of which *erythema marginatum* is most common, and *subcutaneous nodules* consisting of areas of fibrinoid necrosis surrounded by a granulomatous reaction. Salicylates relieve the joint pain and pyrexia of acute rheumatic fever, but do not prevent or arrest the development of heart lesions. Recurrences of rheumatic fever are common. In adults, the joint lesions tend to be more severe, but frequently chronic rheumatic valvular disease presents in adult life in the absence of any history suggestive of rheumatic fever (see below).

Laboratory findings. There is no specific test for rheumatic fever but a raised erythrocyte sedimentation rate, anaemia, slight leukocytosis and high titres of streptococcal antibodies are commonly present. C-reactive protein appears in the serum at an early stage but it is one of the so-called 'acute phase reactants' which are found in many acute illnesses.

Subclinical rheumatic fever. Latent rheumatic fever is important for it may lead to chronic rheumatic carditis. In atrial biopsies from patients operated upon for mitral stenosis (without clinical evidence of active rheumatic disease), the incidence of recent sub-endocardial Aschoff bodies is surprisingly high except in the older patients. Since Aschoff bodies are generally accepted as an indication of active rheumatism, it is clear that the disease can persist in a very chronic smouldering form.

There may be no history of illness suggestive of acute rheumatic fever.

Chronic rheumatic heart disease

Chronic rheumatic heart disease is a common sequel to acute rheumatic fever and is characterised mainly by chronic endocarditis in which overgrowth of connective tissue and its subsequent contraction leads to valvular deformities. Compensatory dilatation and hypertrophy of the chambers are found, depending on the nature of the valvular lesions. In many cases Aschoff bodies are present together with minute foci of myocardial fibrosis representing healed Aschoff bodies. Pericardial adhesions are common but these impede cardiac action only when the fibrous thickening is unusually severe and especially when the pericardium is adherent to other mediastinal structures.

Pathogenesis of lesions. The lesions represent a healing stage of acute rheumatic endocarditis and fibrosis results in all the sites previously inflamed in the acute stage. Thus the valves affected are the mitral, aortic and tricuspid in that order of frequency, and the chordae tendineae are much thickened and shortened. Fusion of the cusps along their contiguous edges by organisation of vegetations and fibrosis leads to permanent *stenosis* of the aperture. The chronic inflammatory process leads to thickening and retraction of the valve cusps which prevents efficient closure; valvular *incompetence* thus results. Both effects are frequently present.

Effects

(1) **Cardiac failure** is common, mainly as a result of the mechanical problems created by stenosed and incompetent valves. These are considered in detail below.

(2) **Thrombi** frequently form in the atrial appendages, especially in patients with mitral or tricuspid stenosis and atrial fibrillation, and may cause emboli in the lungs and systemic arteries, e.g. in the brain, with serious consequences. A rare occurrence of interest is the formation in the left atrium of a so-called ball thrombus which lies free in the cavity and which may reach several centimetres in diameter.

(3) **Angina pectoris** occurs when the cardiac output is so reduced that coronary blood flow to the hypertrophied myocardium is inadequate.

(4) **Cardiac arrhythmias**, especially atrial fibrillation, are a common consequence and may be due to myocardial and subendocardial scar tissue.

(5) **Subacute bacterial endocarditis** is particularly prone to develop on valves even slightly damaged by rheumatic fever.

Deformities of the valves of the heart

Mitral stenosis

This is nearly always due to rheumatic endocarditis. The orifice may be reduced, by fusion of the cusps, to a diameter as small as 5 mm (normal 25–30 mm), the area then being diminished to about one twenty-fifth. The fused cusps may form a thin fibrous diaphragm which is pliable and mobile; closure of the orifice during ventricular systole can then be adequately brought about by the constriction of the annulus fibrosus, approximation of the nodular ridge, and ballooning of the cusps towards the atrium. In such cases of pure stenosis, surgical relief is often successful, but unfortunately recurrence is common. In other cases the cusps are much shortened, thickened and rigid, as well as fused at the commissures, and a dense fibrous diaphragm with a slit-like aperture results (Fig. 14.25). There may be marked thickening and shortening of the chordae tendineae, and also fibrous induration of the apices of the papillary muscles so that the valve comes to form a funnel-shaped structure with a small oval aperture. Calcification of the cusps and valve ring may be present. The endocardium of the left atrium is thickened and opaque in most cases.

Effects. The left ventricle can receive a normal volume in the diastolic interval only if the blood is propelled more forcibly through the narrowed mitral orifice; commonly, it gets less blood than normally, can easily pass it on and

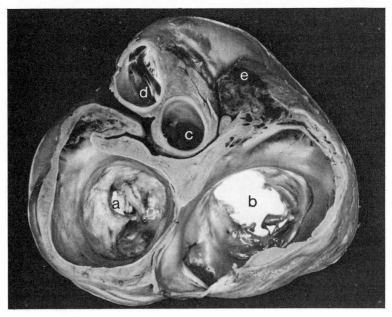

Fig. 14.25 Horizontal section through atria in a case of mitral and tricuspid stenosis, as seen from above. **a**, mitral valve, severely stenosed; **b**, tricuspid valve, moderately stenosed; **c**, aorta; **d**, pulmonary artery; **e**, right atrial appendage containing thrombus. × ⅗.

therefore does not undergo hypertrophy; indeed it is often slightly atrophied. The left atrium hypertrophies and it readily dilates, sometimes to gigantic dimensions (500 ml in place of the normal 30–40 ml). Blood is retained within the pulmonary veins and the intra-pulmonary blood pressure is raised. The work of driving the blood into the pulmonary artery against the raised intrapulmonary pressure falls upon the right ventricle, which undergoes great hyper-

trophy (Fig. 14.26), until the pressure in the pulmonary veins is enough, in conjunction with atrial systole, to fill the left ventricle adequately during diastole. The stroke volume of the left ventricle may thus be normal—or very nearly so—even in quite severe mitral stenosis, and the patient may be very little incapacitated at rest. This is an extremely dangerous position, because if the tricuspid valve is competent then the relatively healthy and powerful right ventricle

Fig. 14.26 Transverse section of the ventricles in a case of mitral stenosis, showing the comparatively small left ventricle and the greatly enlarged and hypertrophied right ventricle (on the right). × ¾.

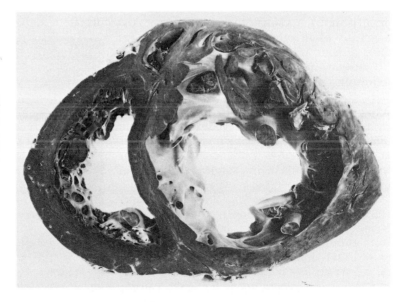

may, in response to physical exercise, raise the pulmonary capillary pressure to levels which produce pulmonary oedema.

In patients with mitral stenosis and tricuspid incompetence, any severe rise of pulmonary artery pressure is prevented by regurgitation into the easily distensible systemic venous system *via* the right side of the heart; this has the effect of decompressing the pulmonary circuit and bringing on right heart failure (p. 346), which is the common mode of death in mitral stenosis.

The venous congestion of the lungs in mitral stenosis cannot be alleviated by any compensatory process. The changes (p. 195) often cause slight haemoptysis, to be distinguished from the more severe haemoptysis which results from pulmonary infarction when the heart is failing. The changes in the pulmonary vessels due to pulmonary hypertension, and the factors involved in pulmonary oedema, are dealt with on pp. 397–405. In mitral stenosis the heart comes to have a quadrangular form, but its weight is not greatly increased. Mitral stenosis usually gives rise to a distinct presystolic murmur over the precordium and sometimes to a palpable thrill during atrial systole.

Mitral incompetence

Competence of the mitral valve depends on a complexity of factors, including the size and flexibility of the annulus and cusps, and the state of the chordae tendineae, papillary muscles and left ventricle. In consequence, the diagnosis of incompetence at necropsy is far more difficult than that of mitral stenosis.

Causes. Mitral incompetence results from the following.

1. Rheumatic endocarditis, where it is due to retraction of the cusps and shortening of the chordae tendineae. Pure incompetence from this cause is now quite rare; combined stenosis and incompetence is more common, and is sometimes a result of the surgical treatment of mitral stenosis.

2. Myocardial ischaemia. Mitral incompetence from this cause is now relatively common. It may develop suddenly and in severe form from rupture of papillary muscles involved in myocardial infarction, or insidiously from ischaemic fibrosis of the papillary muscles.

3. Myxoid degeneration of the cusps, causing

a 'floppy' mitral valve, occurs usually in old people. Disintegration of the collagen of the valve cusps, accompanied by increase in basophilic ground substance (p. 237), results in weakness and stretching of the cusps. Minor degrees are common but without effect: if the changes are severe, the cusps are liable to prolapse during ventricular systole with consequent regurgitation.

Similar changes occur rarely in young people, sometimes as a complication of Marfan's syndrome.

4. Changes in the annulus. Closure of the mitral valve is dependent on the size and shape of the mitral ring during ventricular systole. Regurgitation due to stretching of the ring is a regular feature of the dilatation of the failing left ventricle, and occurs also in some cases of Marfan's syndrome. Senile calcification of the ring can also cause incompetence.

Effects. Mitral incompetence results in compensatory dilatation and hypertrophy of the left ventricle. From the outset, the left atrium is dilated and the pulmonary circulation congested. Increased work is thus thrown on the right ventricle, which also becomes hypertrophied. The subsequent effects are similar to those occurring in mitral stenosis. Mitral incompetence is associated with an apical murmur throughout, or late in, ventricular systole.

Aortic stenosis

Except in countries where rheumatic heart disease is still prevalent, aortic stenosis alone is

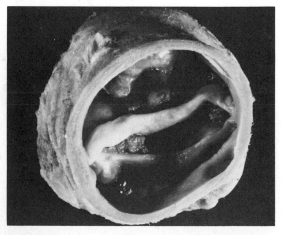

Fig. 14.27 Calcific aortic stenosis arising in a congenitally bicuspid valve. × 1·5.

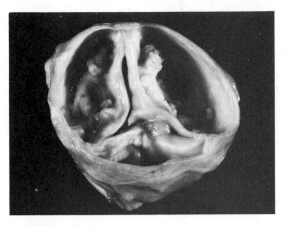

Fig. 14.28 'Senile' calcific stenosis in an aortic valve without obvious predisposing abnormality. × 1·5.

probably as common as isolated mitral stenosis, and most cases are probably non-rheumatic. The commonest form is **calcific aortic stenosis** without evidence of rheumatism, and many cases appear to result from the chronic fibrous thickening and calcification of congenitally bicuspid valves (Fig. 14.27), so that aortic stenosis develops in middle age. The condition occurs also in old age, but usually without the underlying bicuspid abnormality (Fig. 14.28).

Fibrous and calcification occur in the connective tissue of the cusps, which become hard and rigid. Irregular calcified nodules commonly project from the upper surface of the thickened cusps. Stenosis is often very severe and, as with mitral stenosis, it is surprising how small an orifice is compatible with life.

Turbulence of blood flow may account for those cases with a bicuspid aortic valve, but the aetiology in other cases is unknown.

Congenital aortic stenosis usually becomes apparent in infancy. The valve cusps are replaced by a single diaphragm-like membrane with a central hole. Obstruction of the left ventricular outflow by a sub-valvular membrane is a rare congenital abnormality.

Effects. Pure aortic stenosis produces hypertrophy of the left ventricle. When the valve is both stenotic and incompetent, the ventricle dilates and hypertrophies; the cavity becomes lengthened and more pointed. Later, the hypertrophied muscle may fail and then dilatation is the prominent feature. The passage of the blood during systole through the narrow aortic orifice gives rise to a loud ventricular systolic murmur audible over the base of the heart, and a systolic thrill. The pulse pressure is characteristically low, and some patients die suddenly.

Aortic incompetence

This results from dilatation or distortion of the root of the aorta, from contraction or stretching of the cusps, or from a combination of both types of change. In rheumatic aortic incompetence, the cusps are thickened and contracted. In syphilitic aortitis, dilatation of the root of the aorta prevents complete closure of the valve cusps, and the resulting haemodynamic disturbance is the probable cause of the stretching, thickening and distortion of the cusps. Aortic incompetence occurs in some cases of Marfan's syndrome, due to weakness and stretching of the root of the aorta, and rarely to myxoid degeneration of the cusps. In ankylosing spondylitis (another rare cause) the aortic root is distorted and there is also damage to the cusps. Congenitally bicuspid aortic valves may also be incompetent.

Effects. Aortic incompetence is associated, from the outset, with compensatory dilatation of the cavity of the left ventricle, accompanied by hypertrophy of the wall. The internal length of the cavity may reach 12 cm or more (normal 8–9 cm), resulting in twice the normal capacity. This indicates a very gross leakage. Thick white collagenous patches often develop on the mural endocardium beneath the incompetent valve and are known as 'jet lesions', being attributed to forceful reflux of blood during diastole. So long as the mitral valve is competent the effects of the aortic lesion may not extend backwards to the lungs and venous system. But as the enlargement of the left ventricle progresses, and especially as the muscle fails, the muscular ring round the mitral orifice becomes stretched and secondary mitral incompetence results; the effects of the latter lesion then become superadded. Incompetence of the mitral valve from rheumatic endocarditis may be present as a concomitant lesion, and such a combination causes most striking enlargement of the heart—the so-called *cor bovinum*, which may weigh 1 kg or more. The pulse in aortic incompetence is characteristic: there is a large systolic wave owing to the increased output by the left ventricle, and this is followed by a rapid fall. The pulse has a bounding and collapsing character—the so-called 'water-hammer pulse'. A ventricular diastolic murmur, corresponding with the regurgitation, is usually audible over the base of the heart. There is a high risk of sudden death in cases of aortic incompetence.

Tricuspid valve

Tricuspid stenosis is usually due to rheumatic endocarditis, and nearly always accompanied by mitral and aortic valve lesions. It is usually less severe than mitral stenosis (Fig. 14.25).

Tricuspid incompetence, most often secondary to cardiac failure, produces enlargement of both right atrium and right ventricle, while tricuspid stenosis affects mainly the atrium.

Effects of valvular lesions on right side of heart. Tricuspid stenosis restricts right ventricular filling and this diminishes the likelihood of developing pulmonary oedema from the mitral stenosis, which is almost invariably present. **Pulmonary stenosis** causes hypertrophy of the right ventricle. It is very rare, but occurs as a congenital abnormality, or in the carcinoid syndrome (Fig. 14.33, also p. 371).

Infective endocarditis

Classification. Bacterial endocarditis of the heart valves is classified traditionally into *acute* and *subacute bacterial endocarditis*, the latter being a prolonged illness due to organisms of relatively low virulence and the former acute and due to virulent pyogenic bacteria. Because of the differences in the clinical pictures, the distinction between the two conditions is still valid and important, but the pattern has been somewhat altered by the widespread use of antibiotics and of drugs which depress the resistance to infection. Cases now occur which are intermediate between the two conditions, and moreover the use of the latter drugs has resulted in cases of endocarditis due to a wider range of 'opportunistic' micro-organisms, including fungi.

Subacute bacterial endocarditis

Definition. An infection of the endocardium with bacteria of low virulence characterised by the formation of large crumbling vegetations, sometimes on a pre-existing cardiac lesion, by bacteraemia and often multiple embolic episodes over a period of months or years.

Aetiology. Many cases are produced by non-haemolytic streptococci of the type classified as *Streptococcus viridans*; these are by no means uniform in their biological characters. Other causal organisms include *Staphylococcus albus*, *Enterococci*, Gram-negative bacilli, including *Haemophilus influenzae* and *Esch. coli*, and occasionally fungi. Infection results from bacteraemia, usually transient and silent, following dental extraction, tonsillectomy or even firm biting on infected teeth. Operations on the nose, an infected urinary tract, etc., or on the heart itself, may also introduce infection. Abnormal valves, e.g. congenitally malformed or roughened and distorted from any cause, are particularly susceptible to bacterial colonisation. The roughened surface of the abnormal endocardium tends to attract platelet deposition, and bacteria in the bloodstream, like other finely divided particulate matter, become attached to platelets and are deposited with them.

In countries where the incidence of rheumatic fever has declined, the age-incidence of subacute bacterial endocarditis has increased, the peak now being around 50 years: also, it is nowadays more often encountered in the absence of obvious previous valvular lesions. It occurs also in relation to obliterative cardiomyopathy and valvular prostheses, and a similar infective thrombosis can affect a patent ductus arteriosus or foramen ovale, and prosthetic vascular shunts inserted into a limb for chronic haemodialysis.

Naked-eye appearances. *The affected valve*(s) may show evidence of chronic rheumatic endocarditis or other acquired or congenital abnormality. The vegetations are larger, softer and more crumbling than those in rheumatic fever (Fig. 14.29). In post-rheumatic cases the mitral valve alone, or both the mitral and aortic valves, are usually involved: the aortic valve alone is involved in about 10% of cases. The vegetations tend to spread on the endocardial

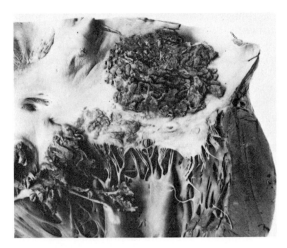

Fig. 14.29 Bacterial endocarditis of the mitral valve. The vegetations on the valve cusps are much larger than those in rheumatic endocarditis (cf. Fig. 14.20). In this instance, vegetations have formed also on the posterior wall of the left atrium. × ⅔.

surface and very frequently develop on the wall of the left atrium just above the posterior mitral cusp, which frequently is the site of previous rheumatic lesions (Fig. 14.29). Pos-

sibly this results from a jet-stream effect of blood against the atrial wall due to mitral incompetence. The lesions are not usually so destructive as in acute bacterial endocarditis (see below), but give rise to emboli, both large and small, and consequently infarcts are common in the internal organs.

Other organs. The skin often has a brownish colour and clubbing of the fingers is usual. Large emboli cause infarction in various organs but the infarcts seldom suppurate, probably owing to the high content of streptococcal antibodies which develop in the blood in the course of the prolonged infection. Petechiae found in the skin, beneath the nails and in the conjunctiva and retina, may be due to embolism (Fig. 14.30). The renal complications are described on p. 771. They include focal glomerulonephritis, which is common in cases of some months duration and is responsible for haematuria; also diffuse glomerulonephritis which may bring about renal failure. As a rule the spleen is enlarged, sometimes markedly so.

Microscopic appearances. The vegetations consist mostly of fibrin and platelets and contain colonies of bacteria (Fig. 14.31). Polymorphs are usually scanty. The underlying cusp

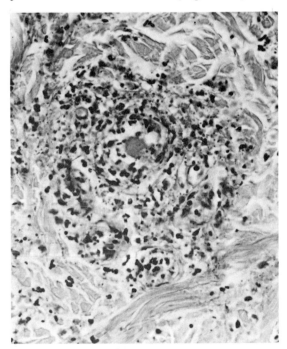

Fig. 14.30 Section through haemorrhagic spot in dermis in subacute bacterial endocarditis. Note small thrombosed and degenerate arteriole surrounded by leukocytes—the result of infective embolism. × 160.

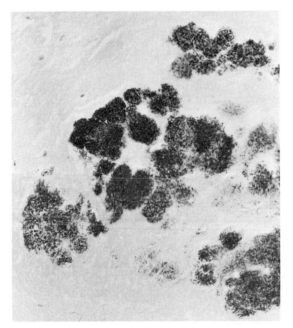

Fig. 14.31 Colonies of *Streptococcus viridans* in a section of a vegetation in subacute bacterial endocarditis. (Eosin, methylene blue.) × 320.

may be vascularised: it is oedematous, often infiltrated with polymorphs and macrophages, and there are usually foci of necrosis.

The myocardium, though grossly normal, often shows microscopic areas of infarction and inflammation.

Clinical features. Subacute bacterial endocarditis is relatively uncommon, but its early diagnosis is very important because antibiotic therapy has reduced the mortality from virtually 100% to about 30%. An irregular fever, with splenomegaly and haematuria (often only microscopic) are usually present. There may be evidence of previous rheumatic or congenital heart disease, and cardiac murmurs which, as the vegetations grow, alter from week to week. Various clinical effects also arise from multiple emboli, including petechial haemorrhages in the skin. Without treatment, the disease is fatal within two years from cardiac or renal failure or the effects of emboli.

Diagnosis depends on the isolation of the causal organism by blood culture. This is often difficult, perhaps because of a high level of serum antibody, and repeated cultures may be necessary. The decision on when to stop searching for bacteria and start therapy on suspicion is often a difficult one.

Healed subacute bacterial endocarditis following antibiotic treatment leaves fibrosis and distortion of the valve cusps, which are sometimes also calcified. The valvular defects often lead to cardiac failure later.

Coxiella burnetii endocarditis complicating Q fever or subclinical *Coxiella* infection is clinically and pathologically closely similar to subacute bacterial endocarditis. It should be suspected when blood cultures are persistently negative and the leucocyte count is normal.

Acute bacterial endocarditis

Definition. An infection of the endocardium by virulent pyogenic bacteria associated with the formation of large crumbling vegetations and severe damage to cardiac valves, septicaemia or pyaemia. Acute and subacute bacterial endocarditis are not, however, clearly demarcated by their morbid anatomy, and a distinction is based chiefly on the clinical course and on the finding of the responsible micro-organism.

Aetiology. The disease is produced most frequently by *Staph. aureus. Strep. pneumoniae* and *Strep. pyogenes* are now less common than formerly, probably due to their susceptibility to antibiotics, and Gram—ve bacilli and fungi are responsible for some cases. Infection of the valves is in most cases secondary to some obvious lesion caused by one of these organisms; it thus occurs in septic conditions of the lungs, urinary tract, etc. Occasionally, however, the path of infection is obscure. Virulent organisms can attack previously healthy valves, as is shown by experimental work, but a pre-existing lesion may sometimes be found.

Pathological appearances. The vegetations are large and tend to break down; and the valve cusps may be largely covered by crumbling masses, which consist of layers of fibrin containing clumps of bacteria, enclosed by a zone of leukocytes, macrophages and granulation tissue. The substance of the cusps may be extensively destroyed by suppuration (Fig. 14.32): rupture, especially of an aortic cusp, may occur, leading to severe incompetence. Aneurysm of a cusp is common, the organisms causing suppuration of one side of the curtain, so that the thin tissue is stretched by the blood pressure and forms an aneurysmal bulging. The vegetations

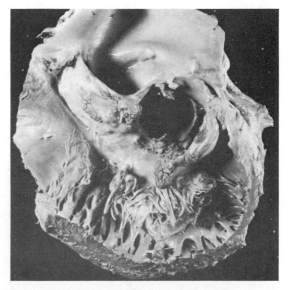

Fig. 14.32 Chronic rheumatic and superimposed acute bacterial endocarditis of aortic valve. The vegetations are large and irregular and there is severe damage to one of the cusps. Involvement of the root of the aorta has resulted in an acute aneurysm. × 0·5.

may spread also to the chordae tendineae, which may rupture. Infection may extend to the intima at the commencement of the aorta and an acute mycotic aneurysm may be formed (Fig. 14.32). The organisms may also pass directly into the adjacent heart wall, and lead to ulceration or to abscess formation. The valves most often affected are those on the left side of the heart. Involvement of the tricuspid is not uncommon, but vegetations on the pulmonary valve are rare.

The lesions are more often localised to one part of a valve or are more irregularly disposed than in the other forms of endocarditis; for example, there may be massive vegetations at the junction of two aortic cusps, the rest of the valve being free.

Embolism is common and the resulting infarcts may undergo suppuration; multiple small abscesses may also be present in organs without gross infarction.

The clinical features of acute bacterial endocarditis are those of septicaemia or pyaemia in the course of which signs of acute cardiac involvement appear. Rupture of a valve cusp may be followed by the development of a very loud coarse murmur and acute heart failure.

Other valvular lesions

Atheroma-like degeneration of mitral valve. Yellowish patches of thickening and degeneration similar in structure to atheroma are fairly common in the mitral valve and may be attended by fibrosis and calcification, especially at the base of the cusps. The chordae tendineae are not affected and there is seldom any effect on cardiac function.

Valvular lesions in carcinoid syndrome. Patients with secondary carcinoid tumours in the liver may develop stenosis of the pulmonary and, less often, the tricuspid valves. The cusps show marked fibrous thickening, have a rolled edge and are adherent along the lines of the commissures. Fibrosis may extend over the adjacent endocardium both in the right ventricle and in the wall of the right atrium (Fig. 14.33). Only trivial lesions are found in the left side of the heart, probably because of the amine oxidase enzymes in the lungs (p. 393).

Libman-Sacks endocarditis occurs in many patients with systemic lupus erythematosus. The vegetations are similar in appearance and consistency to those of acute rheumatism but are larger and are found on unusual sites such as the ventricular aspect of the mitral valves. Embolism and functional impairment of the valve do not occur.

Terminal endocarditis. A few vegetations on the mitral and aortic cusps are sometimes found in cases where death has occurred from wasting diseases, especially carcinoma. The vegetations are usually patchy and soft and consist of fibrin and platelets but no bacteria. There is sometimes an associated peripheral neuritis.

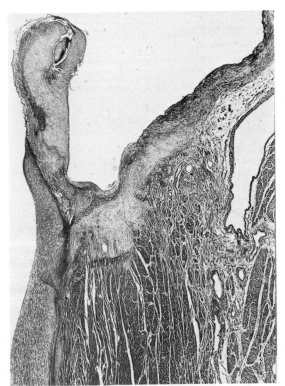

Fig. 14.33 Pulmonary valve in carcinoid syndrome showing great fibrous thickening of the cusp and of the subendocardial connective tissue. × 12.

Disorders of the conducting system

As indicated in preceding sections of this Chapter, disturbances of cardiac rhythm commonly complicate various types of heart disease. Many of them, e.g. extrasystoles, paroxysmal tachycardia and atrial fibrillation, are not usually attributable to changes in the conducting system.

The most vulnerable part of the system is the A–V bundle and its right and left branches: injury may result from the various types of myocarditis (see Fig. 14.14, p. 358), chronic myocardial ischaemia or myocardial infarction, trauma during cardiac surgery, and invasion by metastatic tumours. Bundle branch fibrosis also arises from unknown cause. The various grades of heart block can often be explained by such

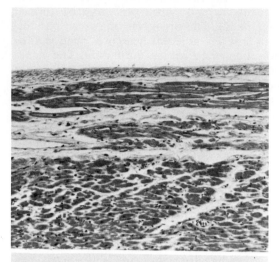

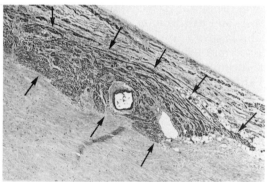

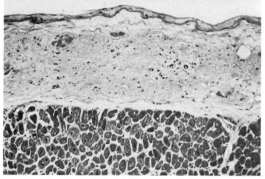

Fig. 14.35 'Idiopathic' bundle branch fibrosis. *Above*, normal left bundle branch from the heart of a young man, consisting of groups of fibres lying between the ventricular myocardium and endocardial surface. *Below*, almost complete loss of left bundle branch in a case of heart block. (Some loss of fibres occurs as a normal feature of ageing.) (Dr. M. J. Davies.)

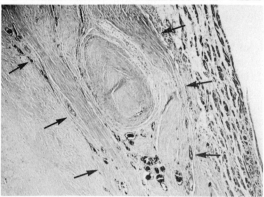

Fig. 14.34 Ischaemic fibrosis of A–V node. *Above*, normal A–V node (outlined by arrows), lying between the endocardium and central fibrous body. *Below*, ischaemic fibrosis of A–V node from a patient with heart block. (Dr. M. J. Davies.)

injuries (Figs. 14.34, 14.35), but in some instances lesions have been sought in vain, while in others the finding of lesions has been associated with normal ECG patterns during life. This lack of close correlation probably reflects the large amount of work involved in thorough histological examination of the conducting system and the difficulties which arise from various artefactual changes.

Congenital Abnormalities

Introduction

Little is known of the causation of congenital abnormalities, but the part played by rubella infection of the mother in the first three months of pregnancy is well established. About 10–20% of the infants show serious abnormalities, of which heart disease constitutes about 50%.

A high proportion of congenital abnormalities of the heart result from defects or variations in the formation of the septa in the primitive heart. For details the student must consult a work on embryology and the classical studies of Maude Abbott and Helen Taussig, but it may be recalled that the heart at an early stage of development consists essentially of three chambers or parts, an atrial, a ventricular and the aortic bulb; division of each of these into two takes place separately. Of special importance in this connection is the relation of the ventricular septum to the division of the distal portion of the bulb into two, which division results in the formation of the beginning of the aorta and of the pulmonary artery. The ventricular septum grows upwards from the apex, with a curved margin resulting from the growing folds on the anterior and posterior walls, until ultimately there is a relatively small aperture at the base. The aortic bulb undergoes division into two nearly equal parts by the formation of longitudinal folds in its wall, which meet, and the two vessels formed undergo a certain amount of rotation in conformity with that of the ventricles. The septum of the bulb ultimately fuses with the up-growing ventricular septum, the last portion to close being represented by the *pars membranacea*. Important abnormalities occur in connection with the growth of these two septa. It is to be borne in mind that the positions of the semilunar valves do not correspond exactly with the junction of the primitive ventricle and the aortic bulb. This is especially the case on the right side, where the lower part of the bulb becomes the upper part of the right ventricle or conus, and, as we shall see, this part is sometimes abnormally narrow.

While some of the anomalies are incompatible with extra-uterine life, in many the circulatory dynamics are such that the patients may survive birth for varying periods of time. With the diagnostic methods of cardiac catheterisation and angiocardiography, successful surgical cure or alleviation of many of the conditions can be effected. It is convenient to divide the anomalies into those which produce *cyanosis* of the patient and those which do not. The cyanosis is produced by admixture of a relatively large amount of reduced haemoglobin, from the systemic venous return, with the oxygenated blood leaving the heart, i.e. a venous-arterial shunt exists.

The resulting unsaturation of the arterial blood leaving the heart leads to an increase in the number and concentration of red cells in the blood, i.e. (there is a *compensatory* or *secondary polycythaemia*). Cyanosis is then prominent. Later, when changes in the lung vessels occur and the heart begins to fail there may be added to this *admixture type of cyanosis* an element of faulty oxygenation of the blood by the lungs.

Cyanotic group

Malformations in connection with the aortic bulb.—Pulmonary and aortic stenosis. The commonest of these result from an unequal division of the bulb, and most frequently the septum is pushed to the right, so that the aorta is abnormally large and arises partly from the right ventricle, there being usually a defect in the ventricular septum at the same time. The result is pulmonary stenosis or obstruction, in the wide sense of the term, but the condition of the pulmonary artery varies. Sometimes the pulmonary artery is small, the division of the bulb being markedly unequal and occasionally the small pulmonary artery is even obliterated or atretic. In other cases the narrowing is mainly at the valve, the cusps sometimes being partly fused to form a thickened diaphragm with an aperture of varying size. A third abnormality occasionally met with is a narrowing of the part of the right ventricle below the valve, that is, the part which is derived from the bulb. All these abnormalities interfere with the flow of blood into the pulmonary artery, and lead to a varying degree of hypertrophy of the right ventricle. Part of the blood from the right ventricle passes through the aperture in the interventricular septum and then into the aorta, and after birth the ductus arteriosus usually remains open and the lungs receive part of their blood supply through it. The foramen ovale also remains open and may be of considerable size.

The commonest anomaly of this group and one which is amenable to surgery is the *tetrad of Fallot*. In this there is obstruction in the outflow tract of the right ventricle, usually from stenosis of the pulmonary valve but the obstruction may be in the infundibular portion of the right ventricle. This results in right ventricular hypertrophy and the pressure in this chamber is raised so that some of the reduced blood in the chamber is shunted through a high interventricular septal defect into the aorta, which, in addition to receiving the oxygenated blood from the left ventricle, partially overrides the septal defect and is thus in communication with the cavity of the right ventricle. In other words the aorta is dextraposed. All degrees of severity exist in the stenosis of the right ventricular outflow, the size of the septal defect and the dextraposition of the aortic root. In extreme cases the pulmonary orifice and artery may be atretic and blood reaches the lungs from the aorta through a patent ductus arteriosus. Obviously such cases will die when the ductus closes.

In about 25% of cases of Fallot's tetrad, there is a right aortic arch.

Eisenmenger's complex. In this there is a strong resemblance in the gross morphology of the heart to that just described but there is no obstruction to the outflow from the right ventricle. The pressure gradients across the high interventricular septal defect are such that little right-to-left shunting of blood, and hence little cyanosis, occurs at first. Later, with the onset of pulmonary hypertension and changes in the pulmonary vessels, overt cyanosis occurs, partly from admixture cyanosis and partly from faulty oxygenation of the blood by the lungs.

Transposition of the great vessels. A curious anomaly results from failure of the septum which divides the aortic bulb longitudinally to develop with the normal spiral twist necessary for the establishment of its correct relationship to the interventricular septum. In consequence, the origins of the great vessels are anomalous, the aorta arising from the right ventricle and the pulmonary artery from the left. While such a condition alone is incompatible with extra-uterine life, it may sometimes be compensated, for a time, by persistence of the ductus arteriosus, patent foramen ovale or a defect of the interatrial or interventricular septum; often these defects are present in combination. In this condition, the chief difficulty is not the volume of blood reaching the lungs but how effective is the mechanism allowing oxygenated blood to reach the systemic circulation. Hence the greater the volume of the shunt, the better the admixture of arterial blood to venous blood and the less marked is the cyanosis.

Truncus arteriosus. In this the arrangement of the heart and emergent arteries resembles that met with in elasmobranch fishes in that the aorta and the pulmonary arteries arise from a common stem vessel. The pulmonary arteries may be replaced by enlarged bronchials. The truncus arises from both ventricles, overriding a ventricular septal defect. Sometimes the septum may be missing so that a single ventricular cavity exists. Defects of the interatrial septum are also common.

Single ventricle with a rudimentary outlet chamber. This latter lies in the position of the normal conus of the right ventricle, and communicates with the main ventricular cavity which receives blood from both atria. One or both great vessels may arise from the rudimentary chamber; most often the pulmonary artery arises thus, with the aorta coming off the single ventricle. The interatrial septum may or may not develop normally, resulting in cor binatrium triloculare or cor biloculare respectively.

Tricuspid atresia. This is associated with defective development of the right ventricle which in extreme cases is virtually absent. Blood passes from the right to the left atrium through a defect in the septum between these two cavities. The pulmonary artery is small, arising from the underdeveloped right ventricle. In some cases the vessel is atretic or occupies an abnormal position. Usually blood reaches the lungs from the aorta by a patent ductus arteriosus.

Aortic atresia. In this rare condition the aortic orifice is hypoplastic, the ascending aorta hypoplastic or atretic and the left ventricle poorly developed or absent. Circulation of blood is maintained by shunting of oxygenated blood from the left atrium into the right atrium and thence to the right ventricle and pulmonary artery. From this the aorta is filled *via* a patent ductus arteriosus.

Pure pulmonary stenosis. Here the course of the circulation is essentially normal except for possible patency of the interatrial septum. The lesion is either a stenosis of the pulmonary valve or of the infundibulum of the right ventricle. The right ventricular myocardium is hypertrophied in order to force the blood to the lungs past the obstruction. If the interatrial septum is intact, cyanosis need not be present; if there is interatrial communication a right-to-left shunt may be established and cyanosis will then result.

Anomalies of the venous return. These may involve the systemic or the pulmonary veins. In the former the superior vena cava and/or the inferior cava may open into the left atrium, thus shunting reduced systemic venous blood into the arterial side of the systemic circulation. If, on the other hand, some of the pulmonary veins open into the right atrium the result will be merely that an excessive amount of oxygenated blood is pumped around the pulmonary circulation and cyanosis will not occur.

Acyanotic group

Aortic valve stenosis and subaortic stenosis. Apart from these localised abnormalities, the heart is normal. Another isolated abnormality here is bicuspid aortic valve, which may later become the site of bacterial endocarditis or calcific stenosis.

Patent ductus arteriosus. While it will be appreciated from the foregoing description that this may coexist with many other anomalies, patency of the ductus may be the only abnormality present and closure by surgery restores the patient to complete normality. Failure to close the ductus leads eventually to heart failure or the development of bacterial 'endocarditis' (endarteritis) at the site of the ductus. In a few cases there is associated pulmonary hypertension and in some the direction of blood flow in the ductus may be reversed so that unoxygenated blood passes from the pulmonary artery into the ductus and aorta distal to the ductus, usually immediately beyond the origin of the left subclavian artery. Such a patient may thus have a cyanotic tinge in the nailbeds of the toes but not in those of the hands.

Interatrial septal defect. This is one of the commonest congenital malformations of the heart. Such defects, even when of considerable degree, appear to have little effect on the circulation. They may occasionally be the means of allowing a portion of thrombus from a vein to pass from the right atrium into the left, in which case *crossed* or *paradoxical embolism* results. While probe patency of the foramen ovale is not uncommon in normal hearts (25% approximately), the important malformations are of three main types, persistent ostium primum, ostium secundum and persistent atrio-ventricularis communis. In this latter condition, there is often fusion of the tricuspid and mitral valves to form a common atrio-ventricular valve. Lutembacher's disease consists of an interatrial septal defect with mitral stenosis.

Interventricular septal defect. A high septal defect is frequently part of another congenital anomaly, e.g. tetrad of Fallot, but an isolated high interventricular septal defect is not uncommon. Maladie de Roger is the name sometimes applied to an isolated perforation of the interventricular septum; the size and location of the aperture varies.

Anomalies of the aortic arch. As shown by Blalock, these are common in association with tetrad of Fallot, but as isolated anomalies they rarely cause symptoms. When, however, a vascular ring is formed around the trachea and oesophagus by a right aortic arch and left descending aorta together with a persistent ductus arteriosus or ligamentum arteriosum or from an anomalous left subclavian artery, pressure effects mainly on the trachea may result. A double aortic arch may give similar symptoms.

Coarctation (stenosis) of the aorta. Slight narrowing of the aorta between the left subclavian artery and the orifice of the ductus arteriosus, i.e. in the interval where the two main streams of the fetal circulation cross, is not very uncommon. The stenosis is rarely marked, but it may be severe and all degrees of narrowing up to complete atresia of the aorta at this point have been recorded. In such a condition an extensive collateral system from the carotids and subclavians links the aorta above and below the narrowed segment. The pulses in the lower limbs are poor as compared with those of the upper. Hypertension develops and death is likely to ensue from cardiac failure, cerebral haemorrhage or less commonly from local complications associated with the coarcted site, e.g. aneurysm or rupture of the aorta. Coarctation of the aorta may be associated with other congenital abnormalities, but frequently it is the only abnormality present and, moreover, it is one that can be cured by surgery. The condition is distinctly commoner in the male sex.

Ebstein's disease. In this condition there is downward displacement of the tricuspid valve so that the upper part of the right ventricle comes to be a functional part of the right atrium. The course of the circulation is normal.

Other abnormalities of the valves. Sometimes there is excess or deficiency in the number of the segments of the semilunar valves; occasionally there are four segments, usually somewhat unequal in size, but, as a rule, there is no interference with the efficiency of the valve. Occasionally, on the other hand, only two segments are present, and this abnormality is more frequently met with at the aortic valve. One segment is, as a rule, somewhat larger than the other and often shows evidence of fusion of two segments; the competence of the valve may not be interfered with. Such valves have a tendency to develop calcific aortic stenosis (p. 367) and also bacterial endocarditis. Very rarely cases have been recorded in which two mitral valves have been present.

Diseases of the Pericardium

Pericarditis

Inflammation of the pericardium can be caused by bacterial and viral infections: it is also a complication of myocardial infarction, and a feature of acute rheumatic fever and of uraemia.

Classification. Pericarditis may be classified according to its cause and may be acute or chronic. Acute cases are usually fibrinous and are divided into those with effusion (which may be serous, haemorrhagic or purulent), and those without. Some chronic cases are classified according to their effects on cardiac function (e.g. chronic constrictive pericarditis).

Aetiology. *Pyogenic infection.* Acute pericarditis may be the result of invasion by organisms from a lesion in the vicinity, e.g. empyema, suppuration in the mediastinum, or from some ulcerating tumour, e.g. of the oesophagus. In some cases, however, infection is by the bloodstream in the course of septicaemias. The suppurative type is produced chiefly by pneumococci, streptococci and staphylococci; and infection by the last may be secondary to small abscesses in the heart wall.

Tuberculosis. The pericardium and heart are relatively immune in cases of acute miliary tuberculosis; but tuberculous pericarditis is not uncommon, due to spread of infection along lymphatics from caseous upper mediastinal lymph nodes.

Non-infective types. A sterile pericarditis commonly occurs in the later stages of an acute attack of rheumatic fever and may gravely impair the heart's action. In uraemia, pericarditis is a common terminal event, and appears to be due to metabolic disturbances rather than infection. Acute fibrinous pericarditis usually accompanies myocardial infarction and is often more extensive than the infarct. Pericarditis is a feature of polyserositis (Pick's disease, Concato's disease, p. 598), in which great thickening of the subserous fibrous tissue occurs.

Naked-eye appearances. *Fibrinous pericarditis* is found in rheumatism, uraemia, myocardial infarcts and some infective cases. The exudate usually appears first posteriorly round the large vessels at the base of the heart as an opaque, dull and roughened layer, and when it becomes abundant it forms a rough covering to the heart with irregular projections (Fig. 2.15, p. 50), giving the so-called 'bread and butter' appearance. *Pericardial effusion* up to or over a litre is usually accompanied by fibrinous pericarditis. The effusion may be serous in rheumatic fever or myocardial infection, haemorrhagic in tuberculosis, uraemia, myocardial infarction and metastatic tumours, and purulent following invasion by pyogenic bacteria. Pericarditis due to *Coxsackie B virus*, sometimes accompanied by myocarditis, occurs as outbreaks among infants and also affects adults.

Chronic pericarditis. The ordinary sequel to pericarditis is organisation of the deposited fibrin, and adhesions ultimately form with partial or complete obliteration of the pericardial sac. Sometimes, especially in rheumatic cases, there may be repeated attacks, and great thickening of the pericardium may result. Adherent pericardium may contribute to the development of cardiac hypertrophy.

Slightly thickened patches of opaque and whitish appearance in the epicardium are known as 'milk spots'. They occur especially over the anterior surface of the right ventricle and the apex of the left ventricle, and occasionally a large area of opacity is present. They are common in hypertrophied hearts and occasionally fibrous adhesions are present over an area of thickening. Milk spots are of no clinical significance.

Tuberculous pericarditis. At an early stage the disease may appear like an ordinary fibrinous pericarditis and its real nature may be discovered only on microscopic examination. In other cases the pleura may contain caseous material and this is usually followed by much thickening of the layers of the pericardium, and sometimes by calcification. In some cases at an early stage there is an abundant exudate, both fibrinous and fluid, and it may be heavily blood-stained. Ultimately the sac may be enormously distended. Tubercle bacilli are sometimes present in very large numbers in the exudate.

Chronic constrictive pericarditis is a rare condition of dense fibrous adhesions around the heart, usually commencing in childhood with a febrile illness and pericarditis clinically resembling rheumatism. Pericardial effusion is often followed by pleural effusion and later by absorption and healing with very dense fibrous tissue and sometimes calcification. The effect is to constrict the chambers of the heart and vena caval openings, which interferes with diastolic filling; a marked rise of venous pressure occurs and so the effects resemble those of cardiac failure. Most cases are either of tuberculous or unknown origin. Surgical resection of the visceral and parietal layers of the pericardium gives relief of symptoms in about one-third of the cases.

Effects of pericarditis. Many examples of pericarditis are not recognised during life. In acute pericarditis there may be pain in the chest or neck, and pericardial friction. Signs of pericardial effusion include enlargement of the 'heart' on percussion and radiologically with a feeble apex beat in the normal position. Chronic constrictive pericarditis may be associated with systolic retraction of the chest wall and with increased venous pressure and ascites due to interference with filling of the heart; the pulse pressure is low and decreases on inspiration (pulsus paradoxus).

Pericardial haemorrhage

Haemorrhage into the pericardial sac, giving rise to *haemopericardium*, may be due to rupture of the heart itself following infarction, to rupture of an aortic aneurysm, to rupture of the aorta (p. 336) caused by an acute dissecting aneurysm which strips open the aortic wall to the base of the heart, or to a stab wound involving the heart or a large vessel. When the bleeding takes place rapidly, the pressure of the accumulated blood interferes with the diastolic filling of the chambers. The output of blood from the left ventricle is greatly diminished, the blood pressure rapidly falls and death from heart failure results—this is known as **cardiac tamponade.**

Multiple minute haemorrhages occur into the layers of the pericardium in the various purpuric conditions. They are sometimes a prominent feature also in cases of death by suffocation.

Tumours of the Heart and Pericardium

Primary tumours of the heart are rare. *Fibroma, myxoma, lipoma, haemangioma* and *lymphangioma* are occasionally encountered, especially in the left atrium, the commonest being a myxomatous mass of considerable size, the so-called **cardiac myxoma**, projecting into the cavity from the margin of the foramen ovale: the commonly-associated mitral valve lesions may be due to haemodynamic or traumatic effects of the tumour. Cardiac myxoma sometimes has various unexplained effects, including weight loss, anaemia, a high ESR, serum protein disturbances, Raynaud's phenomenon and arthralgia. *Rhabdomyoma* of congenital origin occurs especially in the ventricles as multiple rounded nodules of pale and somewhat translucent tissue. It consists of large branching cells in which striped fibrils are found; the cells have a somewhat vacuolated appearance and contain much glycogen. In a number of cases, the tumour has been associated with multiple discrete gliomatous growths in the cerebral hemispheres—*tuberous sclerosis* (p. 722); in some cases there have been also malformations of the kidneys and liver, and adenoma sebaceum on the face (Bourneville's disease).

Metastatic tumours in the heart and pericardium are less uncommon than is generally realised, occurring in about 10% of all fatal malignancies, secondary melanotic tumours being disproportionately numerous in relation to their total incidence. Primary carcinoma of the bronchi spreads to involve the heart more frequently than any other neoplasm (31% of cases); no doubt the proximity of the primary growth is a factor in this high incidence, as direct extension readily occurs to the base of the heart and pericardium. There is, of course, an element of selection in the cases studied at necropsy, as those with bronchial carcinoma more commonly die in hospital.

Neoplastic invasion of the pericardium often causes a haemorrhagic inflammatory exudate. Spread of tumour into the wall of the right atrium is liable to cause arrhythmias.

15

Respiratory System

Introduction

The primary function of the respiratory system —oxygenation of the blood and removal of carbon dioxide—requires that air be brought into close approximation with blood. Accordingly, the respiratory tract is particularly exposed to infection, both by microbes in the inspired air and by spread downwards of the bacteria which commonly colonise the nose and throat. Another important hazard is presented by inhalation of pollutants contributed to the air we breathe in the form of dusts, smokes and fumes, a particularly important example being cigarette smoke. Thirdly, the lungs are the only organs, apart from the heart, through which all the blood passes during each circulation: accordingly, cardiovascular diseases which disturb pulmonary haemodynamics are likely to have serious secondary effects on the lungs, such as pulmonary oedema, and conversely diseases of the lungs which interfere with pulmonary blood flow have important effects on the heart and systemic circulation. In short, normal cardiac and pulmonary function are closely interdependent.

Apart from infections, injury due to inhaled pollutants and the effects of cardiovascular disease, the respiratory tract is remarkably trouble-free, and most of this chapter will be devoted to the effects of these three hazards.

Although the respiratory tract, like other systems, is best considered on a regional basis, the continuity of the mucous membranes from nose to alveolus, and the microbial contamination of inspired air, allow ready spread of infection, and accordingly it seems appropriate to give a brief general account of the main factors concerned in respiratory tract infections before proceeding on a regional basis.

Respiratory infections

The defences of the respiratory tract against infection have been described in Chapter 6: they include upward flow of the surface film of mucus which coats the air passages and is impelled by ciliated epithelium; the cough reflex; the secretion of IgA antibodies; and the phagocytic activity of alveolar macrophages.

Bacterial infections of the respiratory tract may be primary (i.e. occur in healthy individuals), or secondary to a large number of conditions which depress resistance. *Primary infections* are now relatively rare in many parts of the world: they include laryngeal or nasal diphtheria, bacterial pneumonia due usually to *Strep. pneumoniae*, and pulmonary tuberculosis. Other examples include pneumonic plague and anthrax pneumonia. Primary pneumonia due to various pyogenic bacteria is, however, relatively common in infants and old people. *Secondary bacterial infections* occur especially when the local resistance of the respiratory mucosa is lowered by various infections, e.g. the common cold, influenza and measles: in these conditions, bacteria growing in the nose and throat extend downwards, usually giving a mixed infection, but in hospitals and other institutions, outbreaks of respiratory virus infections may be complicated by spread of virulent pathogenic bacteria from patient to patient. Chronic liability to bacterial infections also results from persistent abnormalities of the bronchi, especially chronic bronchitis and bronchiectasis, from various debilitating and wasting diseases, and from congenital and acquired immunodeficiencies.

Virus infections. Most acute respiratory disease seen in general medical practice every winter is caused by viruses. Over 150 different viruses have been isolated and antibody

Table 15.1 The respiratory viruses (after Hobson)

Group	Virus
MYXOVIRUSES	Influenza virus Parainfluenza viruses Respiratory syncytial virus
PICORNAVIRUSES	Rhinoviruses Echoviruses Coxsackieviruses
CORONAVIRUSES and ADENOVIRUSES	
VIRUS PNEUMONIA AGENTS (not true viruses)	*Mycoplasma pneumoniae* *Chlamydiae* (Psittacosis-ornithosis agents) *Coxiella burnetii* (Q fever)

acquired against one virus rarely gives any cross-protection against any of the others. Many virus infections of the respiratory tract such as 'viral sore throat' and the common cold are frequent and comparatively trivial. Others, like bronchiolitis in infants due to the respiratory syncytial virus, may be fatal.

Most of the respiratory virus pathogens fall into a few well-defined major groups which replicate readily in tissue culture (Table 15.1).

The clinical syndromes due to acute respiratory virus infections depend to some extent on the age of the patient and the depth to which the respiratory tract is invaded. These syndromes are not sharply defined and may be produced by many different viruses. Nevertheless, recognisable clinical syndromes produced by viruses in the respiratory tract are the common cold (coryza), viral sore-throat, influenza and febrile catarrh, infantile croup, infantile acute bronchiolitis and 'atypical pneumonia'.

The **common cold** occurs throughout the world, including tropical countries, and exposure to low temperature does not appear to be a predisposing factor. The main cause is the group of *rhinoviruses* composed of about ninety serologically distinct picornaviruses (pico = small, RNA viruses). There is no cross immunity so that repeated infections are common. Other viruses causing common colds are the parainfluenza, respiratory syncytial, Coxsackie and Echo viruses.

Adenoviruses give rise to ill-defined syndromes of 'viral sore-throat' in which pharyngitis and conjunctivitis are prominent. They

may cause epidemics of acute respiratory disease or endemic pharyngitis and follicular conjunctivitis. There are about thirty serological types of these DNA viruses.

The *parainfluenza viruses* cause a febrile catarrh that is intermediate in severity between the common cold and influenza. They are the

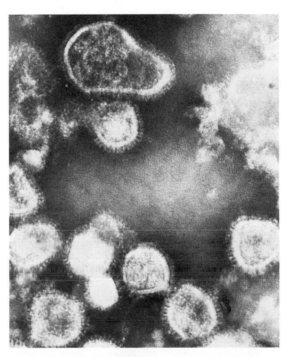

Fig. 15.1 Individual virus particles of the influenza A2/Hong Kong strain showing spikes of haemagglutinin by which the particle attaches itself to susceptible cells in the respiratory mucosa. Electron micrograph. × 128 000. (Dr. D. Hobson.)

major cause of acute laryngo-tracheo-bronchitis (succinctly termed 'croup') in young children. There are four serological types of these large RNA viruses.

Respiratory syncytial viruses are widespread in adults, giving rise to trivial signs and symptoms because they are usually re-infections in the presence of partial immunity. However, they are highly virulent for children under two years of age and account for most of the young children admitted to hospital each winter with acute bronchiolitis and pneumonia.

The most serious disease of the upper respiratory tract caused by a virus is **influenza**. This is an acute febrile illness attended by malaise, often followed by lassitude and depression. In a minority of cases this may progress to influenzal pneumonia, which is commonly fatal. From time to time new antigenic strains arise and cause world-wide pandemics in the population having no immunity to the new strain. Three major types of this RNA myxovirus exist, called A, B and C in decreasing order of virulence (Fig. 15.1). The first influenza A virus, AO, was isolated in 1933. Strain A1 emerged in 1947 and A2, causing 'Asian flu', appeared ten years later. When a new virus variant appears, as in 1918 or 1937, rapidly fatal virus pneumonia with extreme cyanosis may occur in previously fit young people but in most epidemics bacterial complications are the chief cause of pneumonia. During influenza epidemics it is important to protect those who are at special risk, such as chronic bronchitics. The pathology of influenza and viral pneumonias is considered later in this chapter. **Measles**, and in lesser degree the other viral exanthemata of childhood, cause an acute tracheo-bronchitis, which is commonly complicated by bacterial infection sometimes progressing to pneumonia.

Nose, Nasal Sinuses and Nasopharynx

Inflammatory conditions

Acute rhinitis is the common inflammatory disorder of the nasal mucosa. The familiar clinical form, the common cold (acute coryza), is caused by any one of a group of rhinoviruses or sometimes by parainfluenza virus and may be followed closely by secondary bacterial infection. The specific infectious fevers, such as measles, are often preceded by acute rhinitis. Nasal diphtheria is another cause but is now a rarity in many countries.

Another common clinical disorder is hay fever, or acute allergic or *atopic rhinitis*, which occurs as a result of sensitisation to certain pollens, such as the pollen of Timothy grass, or to house dust, animal dandruff, feathers or other specific allergens (p. 118). Atopic hypersensitivity is also a factor in some cases of nasal polyposis.

Acute sinusitis is generally a complication of acute infection of the nose, less commonly of dental sepsis. Gram +ve cocci such as *Streptococcus pyogenes*, *Streptococcus pneumoniae* or *Staphylococcus aureus* are the usual causal organisms.

Acute nasopharyngitis usually accompanies either acute rhinitis or acute tonsillitis in which *Streptococcus pyogenes* is the common pathogen.

The histopathology of acute inflammation of the nose, sinuses and nasopharynx is similar. There is hyperaemia and oedema of the mucosa, and the mucosal glands are hyperactive. In virus infections, neutrophil polymorphs are generally sparse in both the mucosa and the exudate until secondary bacterial infection supervenes, but thereafter increasing numbers of neutrophils migrate through the mucosa and the exudate becomes mucopurulent in character. There is a variable degree of loss of the superficial ciliated epithelium. In atopic inflammation, oedema of the submucosa is a prominent feature, giving rise to polypoid thickening of the mucosa. The mucosal glands are often enlarged and distended and the oedematous stroma is characteristically infiltrated by numerous eosinophil polymorphs.

Chronic rhinitis, sinusitis and nasopharyngitis may follow an acute inflammatory episode which has failed to resolve. Inadequate drainage of the sinuses, nasal obstruction due to polypi, or enlargement of the nasopharyngeal lymphoid tissue (adenoids), may be underlying factors.

Nasal polypi. Chronic inflammation of the

nose may lead to polypoid thickening of the mucosa. Polyps are rounded or elongated masses commonly arising from the region of the middle turbinate. They are often bilateral, a point of distinction from nasal tumours. Nasal polypi are usually gelatinous in consistency with a smooth, shiny surface. Their microscopic structure consists of a core of loose oedematous connective tissue containing occasional mucous glands and covered by normal ciliated respir-

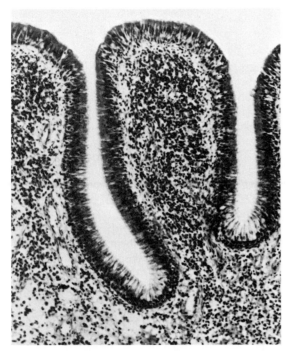

Fig. 15.2 Section through the margin of a nasal polyp, showing the respiratory epithelial lining and the loose oedematous stroma infiltrated with chronic inflammatory cells. × 100.

atory type of epithelium (Fig. 15.2). Lymphocytes, plasma cells and eosinophils infiltrate the submucosa to a variable degree. Polypi in which eosinophils predominate in the inflammatory infiltrate are considered to have an atopic basis.

Chronic granulomatous rhinitis. In contrast to acute infection, specific forms of chronic infection of the nose are rare in most communities. Chronic granulomas may be due to tuberculosis, tertiary syphilis, leprosy, scleroma or fungal infections such as aspergillosis or rhinosporidiosis.

Two rare forms of necrotising granuloma of uncertain nature occur in the upper respiratory tract. In one form, **Wegener's granuloma**, a necrotising lesion with giant cells develops usually in the nose or the maxillary sinus, followed by necrotic lesions in the lung and associated with disseminated lesions of polyarteritis, particularly in the lungs and kidneys. The other, so-called **malignant granuloma of the nose**, presents as an ulcerated lesion which spreads progressively to erode the soft tissues and bones around the nose. Histologically the lesion consists of proliferating lymphocytes and macrophages: some authorities consider it to be a lymphoid neoplasm.

Tumours

Benign tumours. The common benign lesions of the nose are haemangioma of the septum and *squamous papilloma* of the vestibule. A much less common tumour is the *juvenile angiofibroma* which usually occurs in the nasopharynx. It appears in childhood, almost exclusively in boys and tends to become quiescent by the end of the second decade. It is an enlarging vascular tumour which may cause bone erosion and destruction by pressure atrophy. The histological structure consists of numerous small vascular spaces set in poorly cellular fibrous tissue. The histogenesis of the lesion is uncertain and, like haemangiomas, it may be a hamartoma of the nasal erectile tissue rather than a true neoplasm. Angioma may also occasionally present as a nasal polypoid lesion, but in this form does not show the same predilection for adolescent males.

Malignant tumours. *Transitional-cell epithelial tumours* are common in the nasal passages. Some of these do not recur, and may be termed transitional cell papillomas: some recur in the same form, and some show a rapid change to squamous carcinoma. The fact that transitional cell tumours are found mainly in the nasal cavity itself, most tumours in the maxillary sinuses being squamous carcinomas, is usually attributed to transitional cell papillomas being difficult to diagnose in the sinuses, so that they remain undiscovered until they become frank squamous carcinomas. *Squamous carcinomas* are common in the nose and nasal sinuses, but anaplastic carcinoma and adenocarcinoma also occur. The so-called lympho-epithelioma of the nasopharynx is now generally accepted as a highly anaplastic carcinoma invading the normal non-neoplastic lymphoid tissue of the region.

Nasopharyngeal carcinoma, usually squamous, often poorly differentiated or of lympho-epitheliomatous type, is particularly common in China, Malaysia, Indonesia and East Africa, where there is some evidence that the anaplastic forms of this tumour are associated with the same (EB) virus as Burkitt's lymphoma (p. 265). *Adenocarcinoma of the nose and nasal sinuses*, especially in the ethmoid, has been found to be unduly frequent in wood-workers in the furniture industry in Southern England. It arises after a very long latent period, sometimes of 40 years or more.

Larynx and Trachea

Inflammatory conditions

Acute inflammation

Mild *acute laryngitis and tracheitis* are commonplace in the conditions of modern urban life with its atmospheric pollution with cigarette smoke, car exhaust fumes, industrial and domestic smoke, etc. While these factors in themselves are rarely the cause of significant clinical laryngeal disease, they may be of importance in predisposing to viral and bacterial infections. The viruses concerned have been considered above. The bacteria commonly involved are *Streptococcus pneumoniae*, *Streptococcus pyogenes* and *Neisseria catarrhalis*. Once secondary bacterial invasion occurs it may progress to bronchitis. Acute laryngo-tracheitis commonly complicates acute febrile states such as measles, influenza and typhoid. It usually subsides but it may pass into the chronic stage.

Pseudomembranous inflammation may be due to diphtheria (see below) or may be associated with secondary infection by *Streptococcus pyogenes*, *Staphylococcus aureus* or *Streptococcus pneumoniae* following infection with parainfluenza virus. Frequently such infections spread to involve the bronchial tree as laryngo-tracheo-bronchitis. In this condition there is necrosis of epithelium and the formation of an extensive fibrinous membrane in the trachea and main bronchi. There may be pronounced oedema of the subglottic area, resulting in stridor. In a minority of cases *Haemophilus influenzae* is the secondary invader, with severe sore throat, fever, tender lymph nodes and swelling of the epiglottis. In most cases of laryngo-tracheo-bronchitis the danger of laryngeal obstruction is greater than that of toxaemia or lung infection but bronchopneumonia and lung abscess are recognised complications. Pseudomembranous inflammation may result also from the action of corrosive substances or from the inhalation of irritating gases, notably ammonia.

Diphtheria is an acute pseudomembranous inflammation which is now very rare in countries where prophylactic immunisation is carried out. It affects more frequently the fauces, soft palate and tonsils but it may also involve the nose, larynx, trachea and bronchi. The local lesions are characterised by the formation on the affected surface of a false membrane composed of fibrin, neutrophil polymorphs and necrotic epithelium and containing clumps of *Corynebacterium diphtheriae*. In the larynx and trachea the epithelium is columnar and the coagulated exudate rests on the basement membrane from which it separates easily and is coughed up. Over the vocal cords, where the mucosa consists of squamous epithelium, the membrane is firmly adherent. When it is coughed up from the trachea, it may remain attached to the vocal cords and may then impact in the larynx and cause death from suffocation. In nasal diphtheria the infection is often unilateral and the child may appear to have a cold with discharge from one nostril. This type may be overlooked until the appearance of such toxic manifestations as palatal paralysis or myocardial failure.

Acute epiglottitis. This condition, which is caused by *Haemophilus influenzae* type B, is a disease of early childhood which may lead to death within a few hours of onset. Histological examination shows swelling of the tissues due to acute inflammatory oedema and infiltration by neutrophil polymorphs. There is no mucosal ulceration.

In typhoid fever there may be laryngitis and bronchitis. Typhoid bacilli may be recovered from such lesions but more commonly the inflammatory reaction is produced by infection by other bacteria. Occasionally ulceration involves the perichondrium of the laryngeal cartilage, sometimes followed by necrosis and suppuration.

In smallpox, in addition to catarrhal or membranous inflammation, nodular inflammatory foci, similar to those in the skin, may form in the larynx and especially in the trachea. They are accompanied by intense congestion and haemorrhage but have less tendency to necrosis than those in the skin. Sometimes, however, they break down and form ulcers.

Endotracheal intubation. Sore throat, hoarseness, subglottic oedema and non-specific arytenoid granuloma may follow brief endotracheal intubation during general anaesthesia for a surgical operation. Endotracheal intubation exceeding 48 hours, using a tube with an inflatable cuff, may lead to excoriation of the trachea with production of large ulcers which expose the underlying cartilaginous rings. Such ulcers, which may be oval or linear transverse lesions, are often located on the antero-lateral surface of the trachea: they may become infected by organisms such as *Pseudomonas aeruginosa* and *Candida albicans* and may be covered by a pseudomembrane. Occasionally, prolonged intubation is complicated by the development of tracheo-oesophageal fistula or tracheal stenosis. A rare and dramatic complication of prolonged endotracheal intubation is haemorrhage due to erosion of the tube through the tracheal wall into the adjacent pulsating innominate artery. The prevention of tracheal injury is a matter of concern in intensive treatment units. Recent studies have implicated excessive balloon pressures associated with non-compliant cuffs leading to ischaemic necrosis of the mucosa. The piston-like motion of the endotracheal tube induced by intermittent positive pressure ventilation may lead to shearing forces between the inflated cuff and partially fixed trachea.

Oedema of the glottis. This is an acute inflammatory oedema of the loose tissue of the upper part of the larynx and not of the vocal cords. The aryepiglottic folds and the tissues around the epiglottis become greatly swollen and tense. The false cords also are affected. This is an important lesion as the swelling may lead to obstruction and death by suffocation. It should be noted that after death the tissues become less swollen and tense than they were during life. Oedema of the loose tissues mentioned may occur in cardiac and renal diseases but rarely to such an extent as to cause serious results. The severe type occurs as a complication of other lesions of the larynx such as diphtheria or the deep-seated ulceration and perichondritis seen in tuberculosis and syphilis and sometimes in typhoid. It may result also from erysipelas or from the spread of inflammation from tonsillitis and suppurative conditions in the neighbourhood, and from agranulocytic angina. Oedema of the glottis is also caused by the trauma following impaction of a foreign body in the larynx and may be produced by irritating gases or scalding fluids. It occurs in angio-oedema (p. 217) and in some cases this form has proved fatal.

Chronic laryngitis

Chronic catarrhal inflammation of the larynx and trachea is frequently associated with excessive smoking. The mucous glands are swollen and give the surface a granular aspect. Heavy smoking also leads to extension of the normal distribution of squamous epithelium in the larynx.

The normal adult larynx is lined by squamous epithelium over the true cords, posterior glottis and a variable rim at the lateral margins and tip of the epiglottis on its posterior surface, and by respiratory epithelium over the central parts of the posterior surface of the epiglottis, the false cords, the ventricles and the subglottis. Staining of the whole larynx by methods which allow naked-eye distinction between squamous and respiratory epithelium have shown that squamous metaplasia is a common occurrence among city dwellers, chronic bronchitics and smokers. Watt has shown that among heavy smokers, the entire larynx, including the subglottis and upper trachea, may be lined by squamous epithelium, thus interfering with clearance of mucus. Extensive squamous metaplasia is almost invariably present in association with carcinoma of the larynx.

Both tuberculosis and syphilis may give rise to a chronic inflammation of the larynx but in most countries these conditions have become much less common.

Tuberculous laryngitis occurs secondary to

pulmonary disease, the tubercle bacilli being carried directly to the larynx in the sputum: they enter the mucosa and give rise to tubercles which caseate and form small ulcers which tend to spread. Any part of the larynx, or less commonly the trachea, may be affected but the disease usually starts first, and is most pronounced, in the arytenoid region and on the vocal cords. Occasionally small papilliferous outgrowths form at the margins of the tuberculous ulcers, and epithelial hyperplasia in biopsy material may be mistaken for carcinoma. Tuberculosis may spread deeply and involve the perichondrium of the arytenoid cartilages, there being chronic thickening with caseation and ulceration from which portions of dead cartilage may be separated and discharged. These various changes are often accompanied by great pain and considerable inflammatory swelling. Sometimes oedema of the glottis is superadded.

Syphilis. In the secondary stage there may be a catarrhal laryngitis, white 'mucous' patches or superficial erosions (p. 184). The most important effects, however, are in the tertiary stage: the lesions usually start in the submucosa of the larynx or trachea, or in the perichondrium as a diffuse but irregular thickening and stiffening which often leads to immobility of the cartilage. Gummatous change follows. The epiglottis and affected cartilages may be extensively ulcerated and the latter may become necrotic and separated. There is a pronounced tendency to extensive scarring, with stenosis and deformity of the larynx. The upper part of the trachea may also be involved and narrowed, but the commonest site in the trachea is at the bifurcation, where ulceration with secondary scarring can cause stenosis of a main bronchus.

Tumours

Benign tumours. Small inflammatory polyps are common and may contain amyloid or show myxoid degeneration. They may simulate neoplasms. The *squamous papilloma* is the commonest benign tumour of the larynx. It occurs usually on the vocal cords and especially at the commissure. In adults, it is generally single, but in children less than five years old it may be multiple and arise anywhere within the larynx. Papillomas in children are mostly of viral origin

and they regress spontaneously at puberty, sometimes with great rapidity. In the adult, a papilloma may recur after removal, but seldom undergoes malignant change. The *laryngeal fibroma* is less common. It is usually small, rounded, and sometimes pedunculated. Like the papilloma, it is common on the vocal cords, and both are apt to occur in singers and others who use their voices a lot. Angioma, myxoma and lipoma are all very rare.

Granular cell myoblastoma (p. 532) sometimes arises in the larynx.

Malignant tumours. *Carcinoma* is the commonest malignant tumour of the larynx, is usually squamous, and occurs most often in men over 50 years old. An association with pipe smoking has been postulated. When the tumour is on the true or false vocal cords, it is usually less invasive and has a better prognosis, after removal, than when it arises in the upper part of the larynx or in the subglottic region. Carcinoma of a vocal cord appears first as a small indurated patch, sometimes with a papillary surface, and subsequently ulcerates (Fig. 15.3).

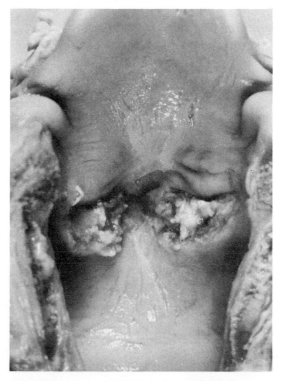

Fig. 15.3 Carcinoma of the larynx, causing extensive ulceration of the vocal cords. The false cords are intact. × 2. (Dr. J. Watt.)

In the latter case, diagnosis will be unsatisfactory if only a superficial part is removed for microscopic examination. A carcinoma of the larynx infiltrates and destroys the surrounding parts by ulceration. This may be accompanied by septic infection from which the discharge passes down the bronchi into the lungs and causes aspiration pneumonia.

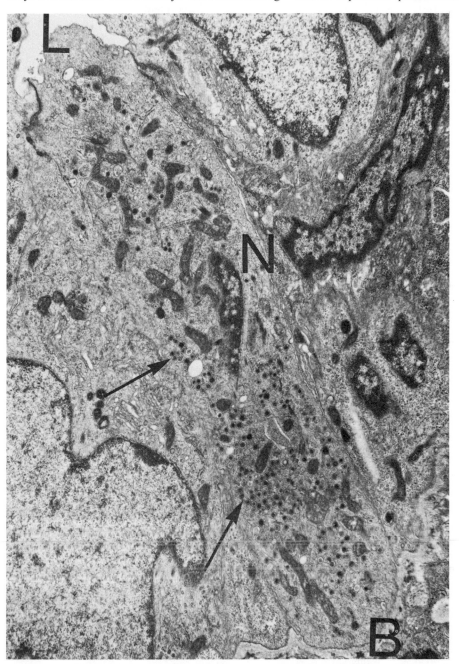

Fig. 15.4 Feyrter cell. Electron micrograph of bronchial epithelium from a neonatal rat showing a Feyrter cell lying on the basement membrane (B) with its tip exposed to the lumen of the bronchus (L). The cell contains characteristic round osmiophilic bodies (arrows) and elongated mitochondria. Only part of the nucleus (N) is shown in the figure. × 12 500.

The Bronchi

The cells of the bronchial epithelium in health and disease

As explained in Chapter 6, the ciliated and mucus-secreting cells of the bronchial epithelium are intimately concerned in the defence of the airways and lungs against microbes and foreign material. Certain viruses may damage the ciliary mechanism of the respiratory epithelium, thus facilitating invasion of the deeper reaches of the bronchial tree and lung by bacteria. Chronic irritation of the bronchi by polluted air and particularly by cigarette smoke may lead to the hyperplasia and hypertrophy of goblet cells and mucous glands which is an important feature in chronic bronchitis. Other, less familiar cells are present in the bronchial epithelium and subserve functions which are not yet well understood. An appreciation of the role of these cells in pulmonary pathology awaits detailed investigation but we may briefly consider them here in anticipation of a fuller understanding of them in the near future.

Within the bronchial epithelium there are argyrophilic cells, termed *Feyrter cells* (Fig. 15.4), which have the cytological and ultrastructural features of the chief cells of the carotid body. They appear to belong to the group of 'apud' cells, many of which are associated with the secretion of polypeptide hormones (p. 589). Feyrter cells may possibly have an endocrine function and may be responsible for the hormonal effects of some types of bronchial carcinoma. On exposure to chronic hypoxia, these bronchial argyrophilic cells show the same ultrastructural changes in their intracytoplasmic vesicles as those shown in the chief cells of the carotid body. They may act as airway chemoreceptors. It has been postulated that bronchial argyrophilic cells may produce histamine and catecholamines which may be of importance in dilating the pulmonary arterial musculature of the fetus, thus aiding adaptation to neonatal life.

Scattered among the ciliated respiratory epithelial cells in the bronchi and especially in the respiratory bronchioles are the non-ciliated *Clara cells* (Fig. 15.5). These have all the features of apocrine secretory cells; the secretory product accumulates within smooth cisternae at the apex of the cell, and the apical region is then extruded into the bronchiolar lumen. Adminstration of chlorphentermine to rats will induce a hyperplasia of Clara cells with accumulations of phospholipid within them and in the alveolar spaces. On evidence of this sort, it is possible that these cells may be one source of pulmonary surfactant.

Brush cells are also found in the epithelium of the conducting airways. They resemble alveolar brush cells, or type III pneumocytes. Their most striking feature is the large regular microvilli which cover their relatively small free surface. Their function is as yet unknown but they may be some type of receptor because their ultrastructural features are similar to those of the chemoreceptor cell in taste buds.

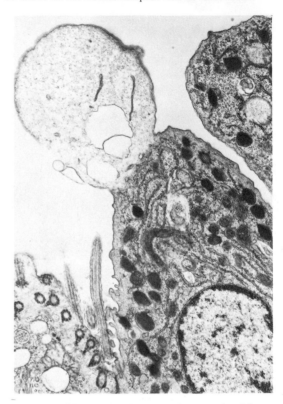

Fig. 15.5 Clara cell. Electron micrograph of bronchiolar epithelium from a neonatal rat showing the apex of the cell caught in the process of extrusion into the bronchiolar lumen. It contains little smooth endoplasmic reticulum. The main body of the cell contains rough endoplasmic reticulum and mitochondria. × 12 500.

Acute bronchitis

A distinction must be made between acute inflammation of the larger bronchi which lie outside the lung lobules (*acute bronchitis*) and of the small, intralobular bronchi and bronchioles (*acute bronchiolitis*). These different anatomical sites influence the likely consequences and hence seriousness of the inflammatory reaction. The common acute bronchitis of the adult affects the large and medium-sized bronchi. It is usually mild but may be the cause of much disability when it aggravates an established chronic bronchitis, especially in aged or debilitated subjects. Except as a complication of influenza, acute bronchiolitis is rare in healthy adults, because bacteria do not readily spread so far down the bronchial tree. It does, however, occur in children, old people and in states of debilitation: it is a serious condition owing to the liability of the organisms to spread to the adjacent acini and cause bronchopneumonia. Accordingly, acute bronchiolitis is dealt with in relation to pneumonia on pp. 413, 416.

The larger bronchi have mucous glands in their walls so that their involvement in acute inflammation is characterised by excessive production of mucus. Acute bronchitis may be catarrhal, membranous or putrid.

Catarrhal bronchitis is characterised, as the name suggests, by an excessive secretion of mucus. As in the acute inflammatory response anywhere in the body there is vasodilatation and exudation of oedema fluid, some of which escapes into the lumen and is added to the bronchial secretion. Should the inflammatory stimulus remain, a cellular response follows so that neutrophil polymorphs appear and the sputum changes from a mucoid secretion to yellow muco-pus. Finally, in very severe cases the superficial part of the bronchial wall may be shed with exposure of deeper tissues—the so-called *ulcerative bronchitis*. Much acute bronchitis is probably initiated by viruses or mycoplasma which impair local defence mechanisms and allow secondary bacterial invasion by the more pathogenic bacteria present in the upper respiratory tract at the time. Of these, *Haemophilus influenzae* and *Streptococcus pneumoniae* are the commonest, being found in the upper respiratory tract in half the adult population and in an even higher proportion of children. *Staphylococcus aureus* and *Streptococcus pyogenes* can produce a severe purulent bronchitis in infants. Sometimes catarrhal bronchitis is an early symptom of typhoid. A much rarer cause of acute bronchitis is the inhalation of smoke or irritant gases such as sulphur dioxide or chlorine.

Pseudo-membranous bronchitis sometimes occurs in diphtheria, which has been described above. Rarely it may be produced by severe infections due to *Staphylococcus aureus* and the croup virus.

Putrid bronchitis commonly occurs in dilated bronchi or bronchiectatic cavities as a result of decomposition of stagnating bronchial secretions by putrefactive bacteria, such as *Borrelia vincenti* and anaerobic streptococci. It is also associated with aspiration pneumonia following inhalation of infected fluids during narcosis or coma, and is a common result of ulceration of malignant tumours growing into the trachea or bronchi.

The bronchi become covered with necrotic debris consisting of fibrin, dead tissue and the bacteria concerned, and the sputum is abundant and foul-smelling.

Chronic bronchitis

In spite of its name, chronic bronchitis is not primarily an inflammatory disease but consists of metaplastic and other changes resulting from chronic irritation of the bronchial epithelium. The two main irritants responsible are cigarette smoke and atmospheric pollution, aggravated by dampness and fog. Accordingly, it is exceptionally common in heavy smokers and in industrialised areas. It is especially prone to occur in middle-aged men and is a major cause of absenteeism from work, of great economic and sociological importance. Under certain atmospheric conditions, sulphur dioxide and other pollutants accumulate in the air and give rise to the lethal aerosol called smog which will kill sufferers from the disease. One serious aspect of chronic bronchitis is that it frequently becomes associated with the condition of pulmonary emphysema, which is described later (p. 407).

The chronic irritation of the bronchial epithelium leads to a pronounced hypertrophy and hyperplasia of mucous glands within the bronchial wall and an increase in the number and proportion of goblet cells, at the expense of ciliated cells, in the lining epithelium. Goblet cells appear also in the terminal bronchioles, where they are normally absent. The hypertrophy and hyperplasia of mucous glands can be detected and assessed by quantitative histological techniques, such as point counting, or less accurately by comparing the thickness of the mucous gland layer, which is in fact very irregular, with that of the bronchial wall. These changes are persistent and lead to an excessive production of mucus, which is the hallmark of both the histological and the clinical pictures. In fact chronic bronchitis has been defined by the British Medical Research Council as a clinical entity characterised by a cough productive of sputum, in the absence of cardiac or other pulmonary disease: to fulfil the definition sputum must be produced on most days for a period of at least three months of the year, during at least two consecutive years.

Excessive production of mucus, combined with the loss of ciliated epithelium, results in accumulation of mucus which penetrates even into the alveolar spaces. There is a tendency for colonisation of the retained secretion by bacteria, although they are of little importance in the primary causation of the disease. The bacteria usually found are *Haemophilus influenzae* and *Streptococcus pneumoniae*. Thus in chronic bronchitis the lower respiratory tract, which is normally sterile, is very liable to be infected, and an episode of virus infection or of irritation by atmospheric pollution, fog or cigarette smoke could be sufficient to precipitate an acute exacerbation, with more extensive invasion of tissues by bacteria already present in the bronchial tree.

When such secondary pyogenic infection occurs, the sputum changes in character from a glairy mucus to a frankly yellow pus. Bouts of acute infection of this type may occur several times during the course of a year, especially during winter.

It is important to distinguish between chronic bronchitis, which is based on a chronic irritation of the bronchial tree, and emphysema, which is a destructive disease of the lung substance. The two conditions commonly exist together but they are quite distinct. Chronic bronchitis must also be distinguished from bronchial asthma. Clinicians and respiratory physiologists are inclined to refer to chronic bronchitis and emphysema together as 'chronic obstructive airways disease' but this is not a pathological diagnosis. Organic obstruction to airways may, in fact, occur in cases of chronic bronchitis without emphysema. The episodes of mucopurulent inflammation may give rise to ulceration, scarring and destruction of the walls of bronchioles and this may lead to multiple stenoses and airway obstruction. This should be contrasted with the much rarer condition of *bronchiolitis obliterans* where bronchiolar epithelium may be destroyed by irritant gases such as ammonia or by a severe infection, and replaced by polypoid masses of granulation tissue.

Bronchial asthma

In bronchial asthma there is widespread bronchial obstruction due to muscular spasm and plugging by thick mucus.

Aetiology and types. Bronchial asthma may be classified into extrinsic and intrinsic types. *Extrinsic asthma* usually starts in childhood or early adult life and may be preceded by infantile eczema or hypersensitivity to foodstuffs in childhood. It is due mainly to atopic (type I) hypersensitivity (p. 117) to one or more extrinsic antigenic substances ('allergens') and inhalation of the offending allergen brings on an attack within a few minutes. As already explained, such hypersensitivity occurs in individuals who have a genetically-determined predisposition to develop reaginic antibodies of IgE class, and skin tests or provocative inhalation tests with the allergen(s) responsible typically produce an immediate (type I) reaction. The allergens commonly responsible include various pollens, animal dandruff, house dust and various fungi.

The most important allergen in house dust is provided by house mites and particularly *Dermatophagoides pteronyssinus* (Fig. 15.6) which infests mattresses and lives on human squames. This mite is commonly found in house dust, and inhaled excreta or fragments of the mite produce an asthmatic reaction in sensitised individuals. The prognosis in extrinsic asthma is good, although deaths may result from overmedication or from sudden withdrawal of corticosteroids.

Intrinsic asthma usually develops later in adult life in subjects without an individual or family history of previous atopic diseases. In contrast to extrinsic asthma, skin tests or provocative inhalation tests fail to reveal a responsible allergen. Nasal polypi are common, and microscopic examination of them shows infiltration with eosinophils. The prognosis is less good than in extrinsic asthma. Patients tend to develop drug hypersensitivities, particularly to aspirin and penicillin, and administration of these drugs may then be followed by a generalised atopic reaction which is sometimes fatal.

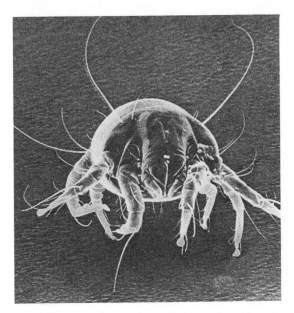

Fig. 15.6 The house mite, *Dermatophagoides pteronyssinus.* × 300. (By courtesy of Bencard.)

Intrinsic asthma is commonly associated with chronic bronchitis, and atopic hypersensitivity to allergens provided by bacteria in the infected bronchi has been suggested, although this has seldom been established.

Psychological factors are of importance in asthma and in many patients the attacks are more likely to occur during periods of anxiety or emotional disturbance.

Clinical features. Asthmatic patients usually suffer from acute attacks characterised by a feeling of tightness in the chest, difficulty in breathing, and particularly in exhaling, which is accompanied by loud wheezing, and often coughing which, during the attack, tends to be non-productive. As the attack subsides, thick viscid sputum, which contains eosinophils, is coughed up. An attack may last from a few minutes to days and may vary in severity from mild dyspnoea to wheezing with severe respiratory distress. Attacks may occur in an unremitting manner, the so-called *status asthmaticus*. Recently there was a striking increase in mortality in Britain associated with the use of pressurised aerosols of sympathomimetic drugs. This declined following the issue of warnings against excessive use of such aerosols.

During attacks the lungs become overdistended with air, but such distension should not be confused with pulmonary emphysema (p. 407), which is only likely to complicate bronchial asthma when there is associated chronic bronchitis. Right ventricular hypertrophy does not result from uncomplicated bronchial asthma.

Pathology. When death has occurred during an acute attack, at necropsy the lungs appear overdistended with air and fail to collapse. Their cut surfaces show occlusion of many segmental bronchi by plugs of tough mucoid

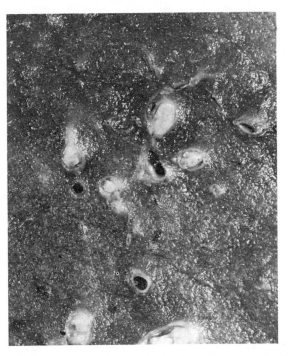

Fig. 15.7 The cut surface of a lung from a patient who died during an acute attack of bronchial asthma. The bronchi are distended by plugs of tough white mucoid material. × 2. (Dr. P. S. Hasleton.)

material (Fig. 15.7). Occasional areas of bronchiectasis may be seen but there is a notable absence of emphysema. The outstanding histological feature in sections of asthmatic lung during an attack is the plugging of the bronchial lumen by mucinous material containing eosinophils and normal or degenerate columnar respiratory epithelial cells. The cellular elements tend to form twisted strips, known as Curschmann's spirals, which are sometimes found in asthmatic sputum. The bronchial epithelium is shed into the lumen, exposing the basal layer of cells overlying the basement membrane which shows a characteristic hyaline thickening. The submucosa shows vascular congestion, oedema and infiltration by eosinophils from which Charcot's crystals are derived. There have been claims that the number of mast cells is increased. There is hypertrophy of the smooth muscle of the small bronchi, clearly associated with the repeated spasm of these air-

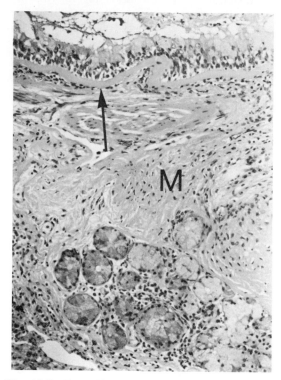

Fig. 15.8 Bronchial asthma. The bronchial lumen (top) contains mucinous material and is lined by intact respiratory epithelium. The basement membrane shows a characteristic hyaline thickening (arrow). The layer of bronchial smooth muscle (M) is hypertrophied and there is a proliferation of mucous glands (bottom). × 130.

ways (Fig. 15.8). Eventually the changes of chronic bronchitis may supervene, i.e. hypertrophy and hyperplasia of the mucous glands in the bronchial walls and extensive replacement of ciliated epithelium by goblet cells.

Bronchiectasis

Definition and classification. Bronchiectasis means an abnormal and irreversible dilatation of the bronchi, which may be generalised or localised, and may result in the formation of multiple large spaces or cavities. It is said to be *cylindrical* when the bronchi are affected over most of their length; this is most pronounced in the lower lobes. In the *saccular* form the dilatation is more localised and severe. *Congenital bronchiectasis* results from agenesis of pulmonary alveolar tissue and failure of large portions of a lobe or lobes to expand at birth (atelectasis): the affected lobe is small and shrunken and dilated bronchi form cyst-like spaces which extend almost to the pleural surface, there being virtually no trace of lung substance between them.

Structural changes. In chronic bronchitis the transverse markings of the bronchial lining are often increased and depressions are present between the ridges; from this condition all degrees of generalised dilatation are seen up to fully established cylindrical bronchiectasis. Saccular bronchiectasis (Fig. 15.9) is usually due to

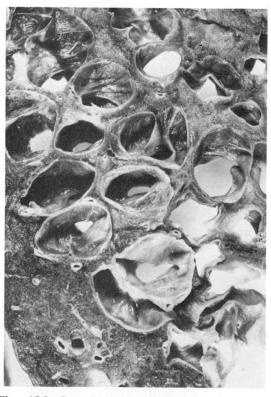

Fig. 15.9 Bronchiectasis. There is pronounced dilatation of bronchi which appear crowded together with obliteration of intervening lung substance. The dilated bronchi have thick white fibrous walls and their lumens are tortuous and lined by congested mucosa.

fibrosis of the surrounding lung tissue with obliteration and destruction of the smaller bronchi and bronchioles. The dilated sacs so clearly displayed in a bronchogram appear to be the expanded terminations of the first few branches of the segmental bronchi. The lining of the bronchiectatic spaces resembles an irregularly swollen and vascular bronchial mucosa and is often congested. For a time the cavities are almost dry, but later secretion accumulates, becomes purulent, and ulceration of the wall occurs. Bilateral saccular bronchiectasis is seen in the upper lobes in the more fibrotic varieties of chronic tuberculosis, where the true nature of the lesion may be difficult to prove; such cases are now becoming rare in countries where tuberculosis has declined. Apart from tuberculous infection, saccular bronchiectasis is usually unilateral and is commonest in the lower lobes of the lung, especially in the left posterior basal segment.

On microscopic examination of the bronchiectatic cavities an epithelial lining may be present to a varying extent, the cells being columnar, rounded or flattened. They may occur in single or several layers; sometimes there is squamous metaplasia. In specimens removed surgically at an early stage, the walls of the larger affected bronchi often show surprisingly good preservation of their structural elements, the chief change being dilatation of the lumen, with collapse and obliteration of their terminal divisions and fibrosis of the lung tissue. In the later stages the epithelium disappears, the surface being formed by a thinned basement membrane beneath which there is granulation tissue. Deeper ulceration also may be present. The various structures of the bronchial wall such as muscle, elastic tissue and glands become atrophied and may disappear. This is the usual state found in necropsy specimens.

Effects. Ultimately an abundant purulent secretion accumulates within the bronchiectatic cavities and this tends to stagnate and undergo decomposition. Accordingly, patients suffering from bronchiectasis often have halitosis and abundant foul-smelling sputum. Organisms may extend from the bronchiectatic cavities to the alveolar tissue, either by the air passages or by direct ulceration, and cause pneumonia or a lung abscess. In such conditions the wall of a vein may become involved, with the formation of septic emboli and the development of secondary abscesses, particularly in the brain. The abundant putrid secretion from the bronchi may lead to infection of the nasal sinuses.

In chronic bronchiectasis pulmonary haemodynamic changes may occur. There is usually considerable enlargement of the bronchial arteries with the development of bronchopulmonary anastomoses so that the bronchial blood flow is substantially increased. This may be a factor in raising pulmonary arterial pressure and increasing the degree of right ventricular hypertrophy that results. Left ventricular hypertrophy may also occur.

Aetiology. In the production of bronchiectasis three main factors may be concerned:

(a) loss of aerated lung substance so that the force of inspiratory expansion of the chest falls, in the affected part of the lung, on the bronchial walls alone, **(b)** weakening of the supporting tissue of the bronchial wall caused by inflammatory changes, and **(c)** contraction of fibrous bands connecting the bronchial wall with the fibrosed and adherent pleura.

In long-established cases these factors are variously combined and usually all three are present, but it is important to ascertain which is of primary importance in the pathogenesis of the condition.

Bronchiectasis is usually a sequel of bronchiolitis and bronchopneumonia in childhood with partial collapse and imperfect resolution; it may also follow congenital atelectasis of a portion of the lung. In children the bronchopneumonia may be primary or it may complicate whooping cough or measles. In adults, influenza may have similar effects. In some early examples of bronchiectasis obtained from children by lobectomy, Macfarlane and Sommerville have shown the bronchi to be ensheathed in hyperplastic lymphoid tissue, which causes narrowing of the lumen (Fig. 15.10). The condition closely resembles that seen in certain virus infections of the lung in cattle ('cuffing pneumonia'), and in most of these cases evidence of the presence of one of the adenoviruses has been obtained, either by isolation of the virus or by means of serological tests. Infection by adenoviruses may prove to be important in the aetiology of this variety of bronchiectasis in children, to which the name *follicular bronchiectasis* has been applied.

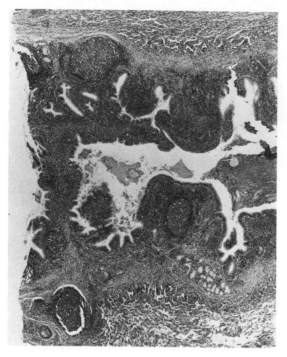

Fig. 15.10 Juvenile bronchiectasis associated with adenovirus infection. A bronchus showing the massive lymphoid infiltration of the submucosa and pronounced irregularity and narrowing of the lumen. × 21. (Dr. Peter Macfarlane.)

There has been much uncertainty about the relative parts played by infection with consequent weakening of the bronchial walls and by collapse of lung tissue with subsequent fibrosis. Radiological investigations clearly indicate that any major degree of pulmonary collapse with negative intrapleural pressure is followed almost at once by dilatation of the bronchi supplying the collapsed zone; this dilatation may subsequently disappear when the lung becomes re-expanded. Permanent collapse is, however, followed by fibrosis and the bronchi remain dilated. Radiographic examination indicates that this state is commoner than had been supposed and that it may exist for long periods without the clinical symptomatology associated with bronchiectasis. The dilated bronchi are relatively dry, and if lobectomy is performed at this stage, remarkably little structural change in the larger bronchial walls may be seen. Infection, with destruction of the specialised elements and consequent weakening of the wall cannot, therefore, be the

primary change in these cases, and it is probable that pulmonary collapse is the all-important initial causal lesion. No doubt bronchial dilatation is hastened by the forced inspiration which follows the act of coughing. A vicious circle is thus set up, the effects of which become more severe when the accumulation of infected secretions has produced inflammatory damage to the bronchial walls with the loss of the cartilage, muscle and elastic tissue.

Undoubtedly the bronchopneumonias of childhood are the most important antecedent to bronchiectasis, but any extensive pulmonary fibrosis may have this effect. In chronic pulmonary tuberculosis with fibrotic change, saccular bronchiectatic cavities are common in association with tuberculous cavities, and they also occur in silicosis and fibrotic conditions generally. In infants a few months old suffering from fibrocystic disease of the pancreas, the trachea and bronchi are lined by tough mucoid secretion which soon becomes purulent; bronchopneumonia follows, and if the infant survives, bronchiectasis is a common sequel.

Bronchial obstruction

Various degrees of obstruction may occur up to complete occlusion and either large or small bronchi may be affected, the causation being different in the two cases. Progressive obstruction of a **large bronchus** is most frequently produced by a primary carcinoma infiltrating the wall and growing into the lumen, or by pressure of massively enlarged lymph nodes. A rare cause of progressive bronchial obstruction is pressure on a main bronchus by an aneurysm of the aortic arch. Sudden obstruction may be produced by a foreign body lodging in a large bronchus. This may obstruct the bronchus completely, whereupon the air in the related part of the lung is absorbed rapidly and pulmonary collapse follows. Usually, however, obstruction is partial at first, resulting in the accumulation of oedema fluid and secretions with some degree of bronchial dilatation. Bacterial infection in the part beyond the obstruction follows, leading to a purulent bronchitis which by further extension may bring about suppurative bronchopneumonia. This is the usual sequence of events when a major bronchus is invaded by a neoplasm or is otherwise progressively obstructed.

Obstruction of individual **small bronchi** does not lead to collapse of the segment of lung supplied, because collateral ventilation from adjacent lobules through the pores of Kohn and canals of Lambert, connecting bronchioles to distal air passages, supplies enough air to expand the obstructed segment. It is more likely to become distended.

Obstruction of **bronchioles** is usually produced by inflammatory exudate, such as purulent plugs of bronchopneumonia, or by fibrinous exudate. In bronchial asthma the obstruction is due to the spasmodic contraction of the walls of the bronchioles, aided by the presence of tough secretion. If the obstruction is such that air can be sucked in and cannot be expelled, as may occur in bronchiolitis and in asthma, then hyperinflation may occur in the area supplied by the obstructed bronchioles. Such hyperinflation is at first reversible when the obstruction is removed. When the bronchiolitis is repeated, destruction of the wall of the respiratory bronchiole may occur, leading to centrilobular emphysema.

The Lungs

Functions

The essential function of respiration is to provide oxygen to the cells of the body and to remove excess carbon dioxide from them. In large animals such as man, respiration in its broader physiological context involves four processes. The first act of respiration is *ventilation* which is the exchange of gases between the alveolar spaces and external atmosphere. Then in the lungs the blood gases exchange with alveolar air by *diffusion* across the alveolar walls. Finally the blood circulatory system is used to *transport* gases to and from the tissues, while *exchange* between blood and tissue cells occurs in the systemic capillaries. Respiration in its clinical sense is generally restricted to those aspects which concern the major airways and lungs. The primary function of the lungs is, therefore, to oxygenate mixed venous blood. This involves the controlled absorption of oxygen and the elimination of carbon dioxide so that the blood gas tensions are maintained within normal limits.

Although primarily involved in gas exchange, the lungs also have important non-respiratory functions: they act as a filter for the blood passing through them and are also concerned in the metabolism of certain vasoactive substances. Their anatomical situation is ideal for these roles for, apart from the heart, the lungs are the only organs through which all the blood passes in a single circulation. The pulmonary capillary bed is a huge network, the average diameter of the capillaries being about 8 μm.

Particles ranging in diameter from 10 to 75 μm tend to be delayed in passing through the pulmonary circulation. Small emboli such as fibrinous clots, bone marrow, fat, placental tissue and particulate matter contaminating intravenous infusions, are trapped in the lungs and may be cleared by the action of proteolytic enzymes and phagocytosis. The lung, therefore, plays an important role as a sieve in protecting organs such as the brain and kidney.

The lungs also have the ability to clear certain vasoactive substances from the blood and to synthesise or activate others. Thus significant proportions of the 5-hydroxytryptamine, bradykinin and noradrenaline present in the blood are removed during its passage through the lungs. The lung is probably the main site for the conversion of the relatively inactive decapeptide angiotensin I to the potent systemic vasoconstrictive octapeptide angiotensin II. The enzyme mechanisms responsible for the clearing and activation of these vasoactive substances are probably localised in the endothelial cells lining the pulmonary arteries, capillaries and veins.

Respiratory failure

The primary function of the lungs is to maintain the blood gas tensions at normal levels. Respiratory failure exists when a patient is unable to maintain his blood gas tensions within normal limits and it is usually said to be present when the systemic arterial oxygen tension

(Pa_{O_2}) falls below 60 mm Hg or when the carbon dioxide tension (Pa_{CO_2}) exceeds 50 mm Hg, while the patient is breathing air. Figures such as these imply that the patient's respiratory function is impaired, but it should be emphasised that many people are able to live comparatively unrestricted lives with blood gas tensions at least as abnormal as these.

The maintenance of normal blood gas tensions depends on the following factors.

1. Adequate ventilation of the alveolar spaces.
2. Unimpaired diffusion across the alveolar-capillary wall.
3. An even distribution of ventilation to the alveoli relative to the pulmonary capillary blood flow (perfusion).

The causes of respiratory failure may, therefore, be divided into 3 groups: *hypoventilation, impaired diffusion* and *uneven ventilation and perfusion.*

Hypoventilation

Ventilation of the lung is the volume of gas inspired in unit time and is 7 litres per minute in a normal adult breathing a tidal volume of 500 ml at a respiratory rate of 14 breaths per minute. This quantity of gas does not reach the alveoli because part of each breath merely fills the large conducting airways and takes no part in gaseous exchange. This is the *anatomical dead space* which amounts to about 150 ml. *Alveolar ventilation* in a normal adult, therefore, amounts to $(500 - 150) \times 14 = 4900$ ml per minute. Alveolar ventilation is achieved not only by the mass movement of gases caused by the rhythmic expansion and deflation of the lungs, but also by diffusion of gas molecules within the airways. The total cross sectional area of the airways at the level of alveolar ducts and spaces is many times greater than that at the levels of the bronchi and bronchioles. This means that the mass flow of gas which is the major transport mechanism in the relatively narrow bronchi and bronchioles suddenly drops to zero as the airways abruptly widen into the alveolar ducts and spaces. Thus, transport of gas over the few millimetres between the respiratory bronchioles and alveolar-capillary wall is achieved by molecular diffusion. An important adverse effect of airways obstruction is to impede the mass transport of

gases and consequently increase the distance over which molecular diffusion has to take place, so giving rise to a state of alveolar hypoventilation.

Causes of alveolar hypoventilation. In its broadest sense the term alveolar hypoventilation means that the volume of gas reaching the alveolar gas-exchanging interface is inadequate to maintain the normal systemic arterial tensions of oxygen and carbon dioxide. However, alveolar hypoventilation in the clinical sense is usually applied to those patients with evidence of respiratory failure without underlying disease of the lungs. Ventilation is a complex process which requires intact airways and involves the co-ordinated action of the respiratory centre, peripheral nerves, respiratory muscles and thoracic cage. Hypoventilation may, therefore, be caused by depression of the respiratory centre, neurological disease, muscular disorders and disorders of the chest wall and pleura.

Respiratory centre depression. Alveolar hypoventilation, leading to cyanosis and carbon dioxide retention, is a common complication of overdosage or poisoning with narcotic drugs such as the barbiturates and morphine. The action of the medullary respiratory centre may also be impaired by the direct or indirect effects of cerebral infarcts, cerebral haemorrhage and intracranial neoplasms.

Neurological disease. Conditions such as poliomyelitis, acute polyneuritis and spinal cord lesions at or above the origin of the phrenic nerve (C3, 4, 5) may cause hypoventilation due to paralysis of the respiratory muscles. Tetanus, botulism and neuromuscular block produced by curare or by ganglion-blocking agents may produce a similar effect.

Muscular disorders. These include conditions such as myasthenia gravis, dermatomyositis and muscular dystrophy which may affect the intercostal muscles and diaphragm.

Chest wall disorders. Multiple fractures of the ribs may produce a 'flail chest' in which the affected part of the chest wall collapses inwards on inspiration, so reducing effective ventilation of the alveoli. Severe kyphoscoliosis can interfere with the respiratory excursions of the thoracic cage and produce hypoventilation.

Pleural disease. Large pleural effusions and pneumothorax induce hypoventilation by causing compression collapse of the adjacent lung.

Excessive obesity (Pickwickian syndrome).

Some excessively obese people develop hypoventilation although objective tests of pulmonary function are normal. They are liable to episodes of somnolence and develop cyanosis with secondary polycythaemia, hypercapnia and often pulmonary hypertension leading to right ventricular failure. Numerous factors have been suggested to account for the ventilatory disorders in these subjects, including mechanical impairment of respiration due to fatty infiltration of the respiratory muscles, excessive elevation of the diaphragm in the supine posture, and decreased compliance of the thoracic cage.

Effects of hypoventilation. Alveolar gas differs from the inspired air because carbon dioxide is being continually added to it, and oxygen removed from it, by the blood perfusing the alveolar capillaries. Its composition depends on a balance between ventilation and blood flow. Hypoventilation causes a fall in alveolar oxygen tension and an increase in the carbon dioxide tension. This is accompanied by an elevation in the systemic arterial carbon dioxide tension (*hypercapnia*) and an arithmetically equivalent depression of the oxygen tension. The main effects of hypoventilation are attributable to hypercapnia. Oxygen desaturation with cyanosis are late events. The symptoms and signs of hypercapnia are a rapid bounding pulse, moist warm hands, small pupils and elevation of the systemic blood pressure. Dyspnoea is often absent. Severe carbon dioxide retention leads to confusion, drowsiness, coarse tremors and eventual coma. The tendon reflexes are depressed and the plantar response is extensor. An important feature of hypoventilation as a cause of respiratory failure is that the lung is normal and the prognosis is excellent, if the precipitating cause can be removed.

Impaired diffusion

In the normal lung, alveolar gas is separated from capillary blood by the alveolar-capillary membrane which is 0.2 μm wide at its thinnest points and is composed of three distinct anatomical layers: alveolar epithelium; a narrow interstitial zone; and capillary endothelium (Fig. 15.11). The exchange of respiratory gases

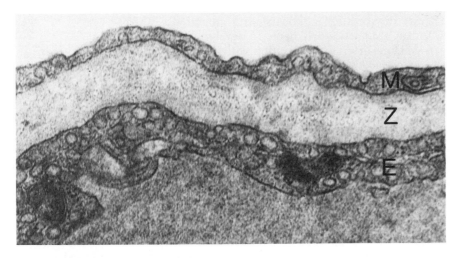

Fig. 15.11 Alveolar-capillary wall in normal human lung. The capillary endothelial cell (E) is separated from the membranous pneumocyte (M) by an amorphous granular zone (Z) consisting of their fused basal laminae. Electron micrograph. × 50 000.

between the alveolar space and capillaries is by diffusion, the gases flowing from a region of high partial pressure to one of low partial pressure. Blood entering the alveolar capillaries is mixed venous blood having a relatively high carbon dioxide tension and a low oxygen tension. It gives off carbon dioxide and takes up oxygen from the alveolar gas. In a healthy individual at rest, equilibration between alveolar gas and capillary blood is virtually complete. Lung disease may impede the diffusion of gases if the thickness of the alveolar-capillary membrane is increased, or if there is a decrease of the anatomical surface area available for diffusion due to resection of lung tissue or its destruction by disease such as emphysema. There are conditions such as diffuse fibrosing alveolitis, sarcoidosis, asbestosis and alveolar cell carcinoma where microscopically the alveolar-capillary wall appears to be thickened and it is probable that some of the systemic arterial hypoxaemia in these conditions is caused by defective diffusion. The term 'alveolar-capillary block' was coined for this condition but it should be used with caution because the diffusion of oxygen through tissues is very rapid and calculations have suggested that the observed degree of thickening of the alveolar-capillary wall is insufficient to impair oxygen diffusion seriously. The hypoxaemia in such patients is now known to be due mainly to a disturbed ratio of ventilation/perfusion (see below) rather than to impaired diffusion.

The functional effect of impaired alveolar-capillary gas exchange is interference with oxygen uptake and the development of systemic arterial desaturation. Patients with impaired diffusion are particularly liable to develop sudden systemic arterial desaturation with cyanosis on exercise or if alveolar hypoxia occurs. The effect of exercise is to reduce the time spent by the blood in the pulmonary capillaries and thus reduce the time available for diffusion and equilibration. In alveolar hypoxia the difference between the oxygen tension of alveolar gas and mixed venous blood is reduced, so decreasing the diffusion gradient across the alveolar-capillary wall and slowing the rate of diffusion of oxygen. Carbon dioxide is much more soluble than oxygen and diffuses twenty times more readily through the tissues, so that thickening of the alveolar-capillary wall has no effect on the exchange of carbon dioxide between alveolar gas and capillary blood.

Uneven ventilation and perfusion

A factor of fundamental importance in gas exchange in the lungs is the ventilation/perfusion ratio, usually signified by the formula $\dot{V}A/\dot{Q}$. That is, the distribution of alveolar ventilation $(\dot{V}A)$ relative to the pulmonary capillary blood flow $(\dot{Q})$. The dots indicate that the volumes are expressed in unit time, e.g. ml per min. When the lung is considered as a whole, under normal circumstances the overall $\dot{V}A/\dot{Q}$ ratio approximates to unity:

$$\frac{\dot{V}A}{\dot{Q}} = \frac{\text{Alveolar ventilation}}{\text{Pulmonary capillary blood flow}}$$
$$= \frac{4900 \text{ ml per min}}{5000 \text{ ml per min}}$$

The situation in an 'ideal' lung is shown diagrammatically in simplified form in Fig. 15.12. In each of the two alveolar units, ventilation is closely matched by perfusion. In practice, the

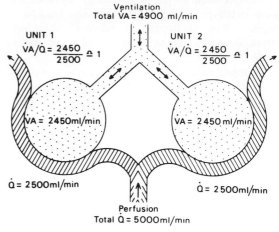

Fig. 15.12 The ideal distribution of ventilation $(\dot{V}A)$ and perfusion $(\dot{Q})$ in a lung composed of 2 alveolar units. Both ventilation and perfusion are evenly distributed to all parts of the lung. Ventilation and perfusion are almost precisely matched to give a $\dot{V}A/\dot{Q}$ ratio of approximately one.

situation is more complicated because gravity affects the distribution of ventilation and perfusion. In a normal healthy individual who is upright, the alveoli at the apex of the lung have almost no blood flow and a moderate ventilation, while at the base the blood flow is much larger, but the ventilation only slightly increased. The result is that the ventilation/perfusion ratio decreases down the lung.

The anatomical organisation and physiological regulation of the lungs, which are composed of three hundred million functioning alveolar units, allow a large volume of gas and blood to be brought into close proximity over an enormous area (about 70 m²). The efficiency of gas exchange is largely dependent upon the precision with which appropriate proportions of the total ventilation and total pulmonary blood flow are conveyed to each alveolus. Uneven distribution of ventilation and perfusion is the most common cause of respiratory failure. It may arise either because ventilation is uneven but perfusion is normally distributed, as in acute bronchial asthma, or because perfusion is uneven but ventilation is normally distributed, as in multiple pulmonary emboli. More commonly, both ventilation and perfusion are irregularly and unevenly distributed as in chronic bronchitis and diffuse fibrosing alveolitis. The effects of irregular and uneven distribution of ventilation and perfusion are illustrated diagrammatically in Fig. 15.13, from

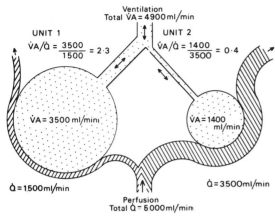

Fig. 15.13 Uneven ventilation ($\dot{V}A$) and perfusion ($\dot{Q}$). Unit 1 is excessively ventilated but underperfused ($\dot{V}A/\dot{Q} = 2\cdot3$). Unit 2 is underventilated and overperfused ($\dot{V}A/\dot{Q} = 0\cdot4$). The blood leaving unit 1 has a normal oxygen tension. The blood leaving unit 2 has a reduced oxygen tension due to hypoventilation. Thus, although the overall ventilation and perfusion of the lung are the same as in the ideal lung (Fig. 15.12), the effect of unevenness is to reduce the systemic arterial oxygen tension.

which the following three points should be noted:

1. The excessive ventilation of unit 1 cannot materially increase the oxygen tension of the blood perfusing that alveolus. This excessive ventilation which is superfluous to the respiratory capacity of the perfusing blood is wasted. The *physiological dead-space* is wasted alveolar ventilation added to the anatomical dead space.
2. The mixed venous blood reaching unit 2 is unable to be fully saturated with oxygen because of the hypoventilation. The blood flow which is superfluous to the ventilatory capacity is wasted.
3. Although the overall blood flow and ventila-

tion of the lung is the same as in the ideal lung (Fig. 15.12), the effect of the uneven distribution of ventilation and perfusion is to produce a decrease in the oxygen tension of arterial blood.

Although inequalities of both ventilation and perfusion commonly occur together in the same patient, it is easier to consider the pathological causes of each separately.

Uneven distribution of ventilation. This may be caused by narrowings and dilatations of airways, by variations in the distensibility of airways, and by the presence of oedema fluid and exudate.

Narrowing of airways. This occurs in acute bronchial asthma, chronic bronchitis and acute bronchiolitis.

Dilatation of terminal airways. If the terminal airways such as the respiratory bronchioles are dilated, as occurs in bronchiolar emphysema, ventilation of the alveoli diminishes because part of every inspired breath is used to fill these abnormal airspaces. The distance over which gas molecules have to travel by diffusion is increased.

Variation in distensibility of different airways leads to uneven ventilation because those with stiff, inelastic walls expand to a smaller extent for a given intrathoracic pressure change than those which are compliant and easily distensible. This type of uneven ventilation is probably the major cause of impaired gaseous exchange in patients with diffuse pulmonary fibrosing diseases.

Alveolar exudates. In pneumonia, the alveolar capillaries are perfused but the alveolar gas is replaced by inflammatory exudate.

Uneven distribution of perfusion. This may be due to conditions leading to obstruction of the pulmonary vascular bed such as multiple pulmonary emboli, fibrous obliteration secondary to pneumoconiosis or diffuse fibrosing alveolitis, the occlusive lesions of severe hypertensive pulmonary vascular disease, and pulmonary vasoconstriction resulting from hypoxia. This last mechanism may have a compensatory effect by reducing perfusion of poorly ventilated alveoli and thus improving the ventilation/perfusion ratio.

Pulmonary oedema

This condition may be defined as an excessive extravascular accumulation of fluid within the lung. It can result from (1) an *imbalance of hydrodynamic forces* across the alveolar-capillary wall which causes more fluid to leave the capillaries than can be removed from the tissues, and (2) *toxic agents* which damage the alveolar-capillary wall, increasing its permeability to water, electrolytes and protein.

Previous conventional teaching based on light microscopy has described pulmonary oedema in terms of an extravasation of plasma filtrate from the pulmonary capillaries directly across a simple membrane into the alveolar spaces. However, ultrastructural studies have revealed that the barrier between pulmonary capillary blood and alveolar gas is more complicated than the histologists suspected, and that alveolar oedema is a late and not invariable manifestation of the excessive accumulation of fluid in the lung. The ultrastructural appearance of the alveolar septum is shown in Figure 15.11. Capillary blood is separated from alveolar air by 3 distinct anatomical layers: capillary endothelium; a narrow interstitial zone; and alveolar epithelium. The alveolar capillaries are lined by the thin cytoplasmic extensions of endothelial cells which contain few organelles apart from numerous small pinocytotic vesicles. Normal alveolar capillary endothelial cells are not fenestrated. They are joined by 'tight junctions' containing *zonulae occludentes* (p. 39). Sandwiched between the capillary endothelium and alveolar epithelium is an interstitial zone of variable width. Over the convexities of the capillaries protruding into the alveoli, there is no true interstitial space because the contact surface between the endothelium and epithelium is formed exclusively by the fused basement membranes of these two cell layers. In other regions, the epithelial and endothelial basement membranes are separated by an interstitial space containing fine elastic fibres, bundles of collagen fibrils, fibroblasts and macrophages. The alveolar septa are devoid of lymphatics, which first appear in the interstitial space surrounding terminal bronchioles, small arteries and veins. Over 95% of the area of the alveolar walls is lined by the thin, extensive membranous pneumocytes. The cytoplasm of these epithelial cells closely resembles that of the subjacent endothelial cells. The margins of adjacent membranous or granular pneumocytes (p. 428) abut bluntly or overlap with the formation of narrow clefts. However,

unlike the endothelial cell junctions, which allow exchange of fluid between intravascular and extravascular spaces, the clefts between adjacent epithelial cells are actually obliterated by fusion of opposing cell membranes. Escape of fluid through the inter-endothelial junctions is dependent, as elsewhere, on capillary intraluminal pressure: a rise in intravascular pressure results in an increase in the amount of fluid entering the interstitial space of the alveolar septum. It is the alveolar epithelium rather than capillary endothelium which is the critical barrier to the entry of fluid into the alveolar spaces.

The distribution of interstitial oedema fluid in the alveolar septum appears to depend on whether pulmonary oedema is produced by haemodynamic changes or by the action of toxic agents on the alveolar-capillary wall. In haemodynamic pulmonary oedema, such as may occur in patients with mitral stenosis or left ventricular failure, the fluid is restricted to the collagen-containing portions of the alveolar wall. It does not accumulate in the thinnest portions of the blood-air pathway over the convexities of the alveolar capillaries, where there is fusion of the basement membranes of membranous pneumocytes and subjacent endothelial cells. In 'toxic' pulmonary oedema such as may follow the aspiration of acid gastric contents, there may be degeneration of both membranous pneumocytes and capillary endothelial cells. Fluid accumulates in the thinnest convex portion of the alveolar-capillary wall leading to detachment of the endothelial cell from the basement membrane. This causes the formation of endothelial blebs or vesicles which protrude into the capillary lumen and partially occlude it (Fig. 15.14).

In the early phases of haemodynamic pulmonary oedema, fluid first accumulates in the collagen-containing portions of the alveolar septum. This stage of interstitial oedema is undetectable by light microscopy. The earliest histological evidence of pulmonary oedema is seen in the connective tissue surrounding small bronchioles and blood vessels and at this stage excess water is rapidly transferred from the alveolar septa to the lymphatic channels surrounding small blood vessels and bronchioles. The classical histological picture of eosinophilic coagulum in the alveolar spaces is a late sequel to excess water accumulation in the lungs.

Pulmonary oedema may occur in patients

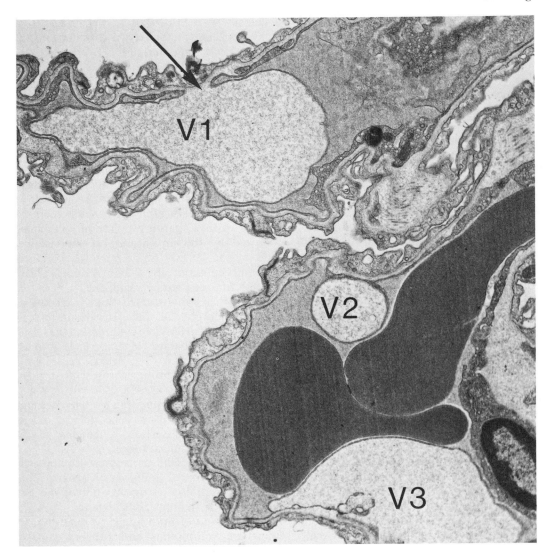

Fig. 15.14 Electron micrograph of two pulmonary capillaries from a rat showing the features of early pulmonary oedema, in this instance brought about by exposure to simulated high altitude corresponding to the summit of Mount Everest. The lower capillary contains two erythrocytes appearing as large dark masses. Three endothelial vesicles, V1, V2 and V3, are seen. The upper has been cut in longitudinal section and assumes the shape of the capillary into which it projects. Its pedicle is indicated by an arrow. The middle vesicle, V2, has been cut in transverse section and gives the spurious appearance of lying free in the capillary. × 12 500.

with left ventricular failure or mitral stenosis due to elevation of the pulmonary venous pressure. The lung oedema which follows overloading of the circulation with intravenous infusions is probably also due to failure of the left ventricle. The acute pulmonary oedema which may follow sudden withdrawal of a pleural effusion is generally attributed to a sudden increase in the negative intrathoracic pressure. Pulmonary oedema may occasionally occur in patients with raised intracranial pressure resulting from head injuries, neurosurgical operations, intracerebral haemorrhage and neoplasms. The mechanism of production of this oedema is not clear. High altitude pulmonary oedema is a rare complication following ascent to altitudes over 3000 metres. It is unusual in that it occurs in otherwise healthy individuals, such as mountain climbers and military personnel. The mechanism of its production is unknown. Rats subjected to a simulated high altitude show endothelial vesicles within the pulmonary capillaries. Susceptibility to high altitude pulmonary oedema is not limited to men from low altitude, for if a high-altitude dweller spends a few weeks at sea level, he may develop pulmonary oedema soon after returning to his usual altitude of residence. Toxic gases and fumes such as nitrogen dioxide, chlorine and phosgene may damage the alveolar wall and produce pulmonary oedema.

Hyaline membrane disease. The respiratory distress syndrome is a serious disorder of newborn infants with a mortality rate of between 20 and 40%. It is most common in premature infants and 10–15% of those with a birth weight of 2500 g or less develop the syndrome. Infants born by Caesarian section and those born of mothers with diabetes mellitus are also particularly susceptible. The disorder is characterised by increasing respiratory difficulty which starts a few minutes to a few hours after birth. There is hypoxaemia and cyanosis despite high concentrations of inspired oxygen. Physiologically, the babies have large functional right-to-left shunts and very low lung compliance. At necropsy the lungs are collapsed, firm, and resemble liver in appearance and consistency. Microscopically, the alveoli are collapsed while the terminal and respiratory bronchioles are distended and lined by thick, eosinophilic 'hyaline membranes' of variable composition: they may contain fibrin, necrotic epithelial cell debris, and keratinised cells presumably derived from inhaled amniotic fluid. If the infants survive the first few days, they seem to recover completely, although pulmonary fibrosis may ensue in a small minority.

The aetiology of this disorder remains obscure. Important factors seem to be high pulmonary vascular resistance, impaired or deficient surfactant activity, increased permeability of the alveolar capillaries, and inhalation of amniotic fluid. Continued breathing for some time is essential for the formation of the hyaline membranes, which are generally thought to be an effect of the disease rather than its cause. The lungs of infants dying at the height of the disease invariably have a deficiency of pulmonary surfactant, which normally lowers the surface tension of the alveoli. Although this deficiency is regarded as a crucial factor by some workers, whether it is a cause or effect of the disease remains unsettled. It has also been suggested that some component of the fibrinolytic system may be defective, so that once fibrin is formed in the airways of the lung, it is not removed.

Massive pulmonary haemorrhage in the newborn. Sometimes infants thought clinically to have died from hyaline membrane disease are found at necropsy to have massive haemorrhage involving two or more lobes of the lungs. The condition may arise from about half an hour to two weeks after birth. First there are periods of slow, gasping breathing or apnoea, followed by the appearance of bloodstained fluid in the larynx. Sometimes the condition becomes apparent in a baby already being treated for respiratory insufficiency in a respirator, when bloodstained fluid is discovered in the endotracheal tube. Evidence of disseminated intravascular coagulation has been found in some babies. Haemorrhage into the subarachnoid space or cerebral ventricles is sometimes also found at necropsy. At present, it is impossible to ascribe a single common cause for massive pulmonary haemorrhage. Some believe that it may be due to oxygen toxicity or to the insertion of catheters too far down the endotracheal tubes.

Uraemic lung. This term is used to describe a chronic form of pulmonary oedema long known to radiologists on account of the butterfly-shaped shadow that extends outwards from the hilum of both lungs. At necropsy, the lungs are voluminous and rubbery and, on squeezing, a frothy fluid exudes from the cut surface. Microscopically the reluctance of the oedema fluid to drain out of the cut surface is seen to be due to a fine fibrin network in the alveoli, and hyaline membranes may be formed. In longstanding cases organisation of the exudate may take place in some areas.

Shock lung. It has been known for some years that respiratory failure is the cause of death in many patients who have suffered major trauma, haemorrhage or other catastrophe. With improved techniques of resuscitation and blood transfusion, the syndrome of post-traumatic pulmonary insufficiency or 'shock-lung' has emerged as one of the most frequent and life-threatening complications to occur in both civilian and military casualties. Shock lung occurs within one or two days of the traumatic episode, following the initial resuscitation procedures. The patient gradually becomes hypoxic with acidosis despite oxygen therapy, and frequently dies. Initially, the chest radiograph shows patchy opacities attributed to pulmonary oedema and collapse, which progress to almost totally opaque lung fields in the severely affected patient. At necropsy, the lungs are heavy, beefy and oedematous. Microscopically, in early cases there is intra-alveolar oedema with extravasation of erythrocytes. Fibrinous exudate and hyaline membranes which line the alveolar walls develop later. In longstanding cases, pulmonary fibrosis ensues, and the alveolar walls become lined by metaplastic cuboidal epithelium.

There are many possible explanations for shock lung, including fat embolism, over-transfusion, pulmonary oedema, aspiration of gastric contents, oxygen toxicity and pulmonary micro-embolism. It is probably not a single entity, but has several causes. It has been suggested that micro-emboli originating in damaged tissue, in transfused whole blood or reconstituted dried plasma, may be responsible for the pulmonary changes. Disseminated intravascular coagulation and endotoxaemia have been recognised in some cases.

Pulmonary vascular disease

Diseases of the heart affect the lungs and diseases of the lungs affect the heart. The anatomical pathway through which this inter-relationship is effected is the pulmonary vasculature. Normally the blood pressure in the pulmonary arterial tree is only one sixth of that in the systemic. This is reflected in the fact that the right ventricle is thinner than the left. The pulmonary arteries are also thinner than the systemic and consist of a layer of circularly orientated smooth muscle sandwiched between elastic laminae. The pulmonary arterioles, unlike their counterparts in the systemic circulation, do not have a muscular media but instead have a wall composed of a single elastic lamina. Normal pulmonary arterioles are thus incapable of exerting significant resistance to the flow of blood through the lungs. The main way in which diseases of the heart and lung affect each other is through the production of pulmonary arterial hypertension and associated hypertensive pulmonary vascular disease.

Pulmonary hypertension

There are many diseases which will cause pulmonary arterial hypertension and associated pulmonary vascular disease (Table 15.2). Pul-

Table 15.2 The causes of pulmonary arterial hypertension and hypertensive pulmonary vascular disease

Disease group	Examples
Pre-tricuspid congenital cardiac septal shunts.	Atrial septal defect.
Post-tricuspid congenital cardiac septal shunts.	Ventricular septal defect. Patent ductus arteriosus.
Elevation of left atrial pressure.	Mitral stenosis. Chronic left ventricular failure. Left atrial myxoma.
Massive pulmonary fibrosis.	Silicosis.
Fibrosing alveolitis.	Rheumatoid disease. Scleroderma. Berylliosis.
Chronic hypoxia.	Normal subjects living at high altitude. Chronic bronchitis and emphysema. Kyphoscoliosis. Pickwickian syndrome.
Liver disease.	Cirrhosis. Portal vein thrombosis.
Pulmonary thrombo-embolism.	Secondary to thrombosis in deep veins of limbs.
Primary pulmonary hypertension.	Classical variety. Pulmonary veno-occlusive disease.
Diet.	Crotalaria alkaloids. Some anorexigens suspected.

monary hypertension may be arbitrarily defined as a systolic blood pressure in the pulmonary circulation exceeding 30 mm Hg. There are various forms of hypertensive pulmonary vascular disease, and one cannot predict what vascular lesions are present from a knowledge of the level of the pulmonary arterial pressure. Rather the form of the hypertensive pulmonary vascular disease depends upon the nature of the underlying disease process. This is of considerable practical importance, since the different forms of pulmonary vascular disease are reflected in different levels of pressure, flow and resistance in the pulmonary circulation, which, in turn, have an important effect on the clinical picture and course. The causes of pulmonary hypertension and the various forms of hypertensive pulmonary vascular disease that they are associated with are as follows:

Congenital cardiac shunts. A large congenital cardiac defect between the right and left ventricles or between the aorta and the pulmonary trunk will lead to pulmonary arterial hypertension from birth, due to direct transmission of systemic arterial pressure and flow into the pulmonary circulation. Examples of such *post-tricuspid shunts* are ventricular septal defect, patent ductus arteriosus, persistent truncus arteriosus and aorto-pulmonary septal defect. *Pre-tricuspid shunts*, such as atrial septal defects, produce pulmonary hypertension in adolescence or adult life as a result of the effect of a prolonged excessive blood flow on the pulmonary vasculature.

Provided the defect is large enough, a characteristic form of pulmonary vascular disease occurs in association with the raised pulmonary arterial pressure. The form of disease produced by pre- and post-tricuspid congenital cardiac shunts is identical. Initially there is increased thickness of the medial coat of the small pulmonary arteries. The pulmonary arterioles develop a distinct muscular media and resemble systemic arterioles. This is followed by intimal thickening of the pulmonary arteries and arterioles, at first cellular, then fibrous, and finally fibro-elastic. These intimal changes lead to *organic occlusion* of pulmonary arteries. This is followed by dilatation of the pulmonary vasculature which may be generalised or localised. Localised 'dilatation lesions' develop. These are clusters of thin-walled branches of small pulmonary arteries arising proximal to the sites of occlusion. They form a collateral circulation

to maintain a flow of blood to the pulmonary capillary bed, and may be termed '*angiomatoid lesions*'. Sometimes a characteristic proliferation of endothelial cells takes place within them in a plexiform pattern to give the structure its name of

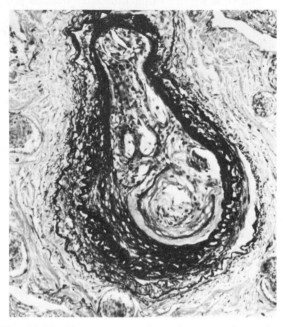

Fig. 15.15 Transverse section of a muscular pulmonary artery from a young woman with severe pulmonary hypertension secondary to a large ventricular septal defect. Internal to the hypertrophied media is a thick zone of elastic tissue (stained black). The lumen of the parent artery contains a proliferation of endothelium which extends into the branch (above). This is a plexiform lesion. (Elastica and Van Gieson stain.) × 150.

'plexiform lesion' (Fig. 15.15). These thin-walled branches rupture to give rise to *pulmonary haemosiderosis*. Finally, *fibrinoid necrosis* of the small pulmonary arteries may occur if the pulmonary arterial pressure rises rapidly or severely.

This form of pulmonary vascular disease offers a good example of how pathological changes in the pulmonary circulation may exert a profound effect on the clinical picture and course. It illustrates too how these effects may change according to the stage of the pulmonary vascular disease. Thus the early stages of medial hypertrophy and intimal fibrosis are associated with pulmonary arterial hypertension with a high pulmonary flow, and a moderate increase in pulmonary vascular resistance which is largely reversible. The later dilatation lesions and necrotising arteritis are associated with severe pulmonary hypertension, a reduced pulmonary blood flow, and a severely and irreversibly increased pulmonary vascular resistance. Hence, the early phase of the clinical picture of a large congenital cardiac shunt is dominated by signs of left ventricular hypertrophy, increased pulmonary blood flow, and left-to-right shunting of blood with no cyanosis. The later phase, however, is dominated by clinical signs of right ventricular hypertrophy, diminished pulmonary blood flow, and right-to-left shunting of blood with cyanosis. In the early stages of hypertensive pulmonary vascular disease, surgical correction of septal defects is usually followed by the reversal of the associated pulmonary hypertension. In the later stages, however, the pulmonary hypertension is irreversible and this is considered by some to contraindicate attempts at corrective surgical treatment.

This florid form of hypertensive pulmonary vascular disease is characteristic of **congenital cardiac septal defects** but is not exclusively produced by them. It can also complicate an **acquired ventricular septal defect** such as septal rupture following infarction, or the rare cases of cirrhosis of the liver associated with pulmonary hypertension. It is also found in **primary pulmonary hypertension** which is a rare disease occurring in young women with no underlying disease of the heart or lungs.

Hypoxia. Any state of chronic hypoxia will induce pulmonary arterial hypertension and associated changes in the pulmonary arteries. Thus pulmonary hypertension occurs in anyone living at high altitude and is consistent with a healthy and active life. It also complicates chronic bronchitis and emphysema when there is associated chronic hypoxia. Kyphoscoliosis, Monge's disease (so-called 'chronic mountain sickness') and the Pickwickian syndrome are all likely to become complicated by hypoxic hypertensive pulmonary vascular disease, which occurs also in occasional subjects with enlarged adenoids.

The hallmark of this variety is muscularisation of the terminal portions of the pulmonary vascular tree, which increases pulmonary vascular resistance. There is insignificant intimal fibrosis and the important functional implication of this is that the pulmonary hypertension and associated pulmonary vascular

disease of chronic hypoxia are largely and rapidly reversible. This may be readily confirmed by subjecting rats to a diminished barometric pressure in a vacuum chamber, when they develop muscularisation of their pulmonary arterioles. After removing them from the chamber to ambient room air for a month or so, both the pulmonary hypertension and muscularisation regress virtually completely. Another effect of hypoxia is the development of longitudinal muscle in the intima of pulmonary arteries and arterioles, usually ascribed to longitudinal stretching of these vessels.

Elevation of left atrial pressure. Any disease that brings about a sustained significant elevation of blood pressure in the left atrium is complicated by pulmonary hypertension and associated hypertensive pulmonary vascular disease. This is characterised in its early stages by medial hypertrophy and intimal fibrosis of pulmonary arteries and muscularisation of pulmonary arterioles. Rarely in the later stages there is fibrinoid necrosis of pulmonary arteries. Plexiform and other dilatation lesions do not occur in this group. The pulmonary hypertension associated with the early vascular changes is reversible whereas that associated with fibrinoid necrosis is not. Diseases which lead to chronic left atrial hypertension include mitral stenosis and incompetence (acquired or congenital), myxoma of the left atrium and any cause of chronic left ventricular failure. The interesting association of pulmonary capillary hypertension and normal left atrial blood pressure occurs in pulmonary veno-occlusive disease which is a rare form of primary pulmonary hypertension.

Pulmonary venous hypertension produces a collection of pathological effects which have been traditionally referred to as *chronic venous congestion of the lung*. As the blood pressure rises in the pulmonary venules and capillaries, they become congested with blood. This may become associated with pulmonary oedema in which, in addition to the presence of oedema fluid in the alveolar spaces, there may be collections of fluid in the interlobular septa of the lung and in the distended peri-arterial and peri-bronchial lymphatics. Such collections of oedema fluid may present radiographically as *basal horizontal lines* (Kerley B lines), which indicate that the pulmonary venous blood pressure exceeds a mean level of 25 mm Hg.

Persistent pulmonary congestion and oedema are associated with a hyperplasia of granular pneumocytes (p. 428) and the development of interstitial fibrosis of the lung. Red blood cells may be extruded from the distended pulmonary capillaries into the alveolar walls and spaces (Fig. 15.16). Their phagocytosis and destruc-

pulmonary arteries and veins where it may provoke a giant cell reaction. The combination of rusty discolouration of the lung due to this deposition of ferric salts, and firmness of the pulmonary parenchyma due to increase in fibrous tissue in the alveolar walls, accounts for the classical term of *brown induration*.

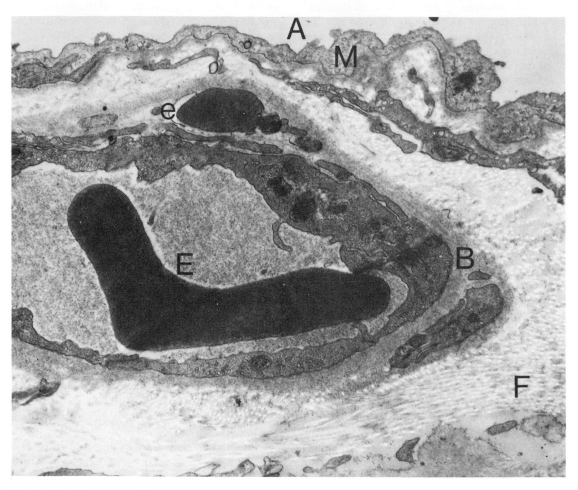

Fig. 15.16   Alveolar wall in mitral stenosis. The alveolar capillary contains an erythrocyte (E) and is surrounded by dense fibrous tissue (F) which displaces it inwards from its normal superficial position beneath the membranous pneumocyte (M) lining the alveolar space (A). The capillary basement membrane (B) is thickened and contains a disintegrating extravasated erythrocyte (e). Electron micrograph. × 16 500.

tion in macrophages results in collections of haemosiderin-laden macrophages within the alveoli, giving rise to the condition of pulmonary haemosiderosis (Fig. 9.10, p. 240) which may present to the radiologist as a 'snow storm effect' on chest radiographs. The liberated ferric iron salts may also be deposited on reticulin and elastic fibres in the walls of alveoli and in

Other mineral deposits may occur in states associated with chronic pulmonary venous hypertension. They include nodules of osseous metaplasia which present a characteristic radiological picture. A much rarer manifestation is the deposition in the alveolar spaces of myriads of microliths composed of laminated concretions of calcium phosphate bound within an organic envelope containing ferric salts. This condition, which may transform the lung into a rock-hard mass that may require sawing for dissection, is called *microlithiasis alveolaris pulmonum*.

The pulmonary veins themselves show the effects of increased pressure within them by the formation of a distinct muscular media so that they may resemble small muscular pulmonary arteries. They also show intimal fibrosis.

Pulmonary fibrosis. Both massive and interstitial pulmonary fibrosis may become complicated by pulmonary hypertension and pulmonary vascular changes which are initially muscular in type and reversible. Later there is obliterative fibrosis of pulmonary arteries and arterioles with an irreversible increase in pulmonary vascular resistance.

'Cor pulmonale'. The term 'cor pulmonale' has been used in a general sense to mean involvement of the heart secondary to lung disease. Unfortunately it is used equally to describe either hypertrophy or failure of the right ventricle, brought about by involvement of the pulmonary circulation by lung disease. Since this term has no precise meaning its use is best avoided.

Pulmonary hypotension

Diminished pulmonary arterial pressure is usually associated with reduction of pulmonary blood flow. This may occur in pulmonary stenosis, which may be isolated or associated with cardiac septal defects as in Fallot's tetrad. In patients with pulmonary stenosis and reversed flow (from right to left) through a congenital cardiac septal defect there is pronounced cyanosis. This leads to compensatory polycythaemia. The net result is the circulation of viscous blood at diminished pressure and flow through the pulmonary vessels. This leads to atrophy of the media of the pulmonary arteries with thrombosis, subsequent organisation, and recanalisation of these vessels. The media of the pulmonary trunk shows atrophy with clumping of its elastic tissue. This is in contrast to states of pulmonary arterial hypertension where there is thickening of the media even to the extent of the pulmonary trunk becoming as thick as the aorta. In states of pulmonary hypotension with an inadequate flow of blood to the pulmonary capillary bed, there is compensatory enlargement of the bronchial arteries.

Pulmonary embolism

Thrombo-embolism

By far the commonest sites of origin of thrombi leading to pulmonary embolism are the deep veins of the legs, especially in the calf. *In vivo* studies using intravenous injections of fibrinogen labelled with ^{131}I have confirmed this. Pulmonary thrombo-embolism is very rare in children but opinion is divided as to whether age or sex affects its incidence in adults. Predisposing factors are described on p. 204. They include also some blood dyscrasias, e.g. polycythaemia vera, and possibly the use of contraceptive pills.

There is no doubt that pulmonary thrombo-embolism is very common indeed. In one study, carried out in hospitals in Oxford, its incidence, as determined by examination of the left lung in a routine necropsy service, was 12%. A detailed histological examination of the right lung from the same cases revealed an incidence of 52%. Morrell and Dunnill believe that pulmonary thrombo-embolism is even commoner than indicated by their results and that it is almost ubiquitous in hospital patients coming to necropsy.

The lungs have an astonishing capacity to dispose of thrombo-emboli. Even large fresh thrombi are absorbed by the lungs in dogs in six weeks and small ones much more rapidly. Two main groups of processes are involved, chemical and cellular. Chemical disposal is by fibrinolysis and predominates in the disposal of small thrombi. Lung tissue has a high content of fibrinolysins, which have been shown to be present in the intima of both pulmonary and systemic arteries. Cellular processes of organisation and recanalisation seem to be more important in the disposal of larger thrombo-emboli. In a few days fibroblasts and capillaries grow into the emboli, which are gradually reduced to patches of intimal fibrosis.

The clinical effects of pulmonary thrombo-emboli depend upon the size of the pulmonary artery involved and on the speed with which the occlusion occurs. Sudden blocking of the pulmonary trunk or a large pulmonary artery may be rapidly fatal owing to the inability of the right ventricle to maintain the circulation. Under certain conditions, blockage of smaller pulmonary arteries will give rise to pulmonary infarction. In the third and rarest groups of patients, multiple small thrombo-emboli lodge in the smaller branches of the pulmonary arterial tree over a period of time and give rise to severe pulmonary hypertension.

Massive pulmonary thrombo-embolism. Massive pulmonary embolism is a classical clinical emergency brought about by sudden occlusion of the pulmonary trunk (Fig. 8.21, p. 206) or one of its main branches by a large embolus (Fig. 15.17). In the normal human lung, rather more

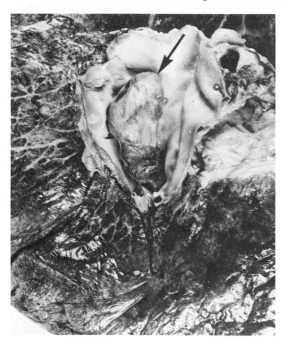

Fig. 15.17 Pulmonary thrombo-embolism. The main pulmonary artery at the hilum of the lung has been opened to reveal a pale thrombo-embolus (arrow) lying free in its lumen.

than half the pulmonary arterial bed has to be occluded before the clinical syndrome of acute massive embolism will appear. In the presence of pre-existing pulmonary hypertension, however, occlusion of one primary branch of the pulmonary trunk has important haemodynamic effects. The increased pulmonary vascular resistance which occurs in pulmonary embolism in man is more likely a mechanical effect of blockage of pulmonary arteries rather than due to

the effect of serotonin liberated from pulmonary emboli: the latter has a greater effect on the pulmonary circulation of dogs and cats than on that of man.

Pulmonary infarction. The pathogenesis of pulmonary infarction is something of an enigma, for pulmonary arterial occlusion alone fails to produce it. An additional important requirement appears to be an increased pulmonary venous pressure and infarction is therefore common in patients with mitral stenosis. In experimental studies, the presence or absence of the bronchial arterial supply seems to make no difference to the development of infarction. Pulmonary infarction occurs more often in the lower lobes, where the pulmonary venous pressure is likely to be higher. In addition, the lung bases are more prone to be affected by bronchial occlusion, pleural effusion, and infection, all factors shown experimentally to favour infarction. The appearances of pulmonary infarcts are described on pp. 209–10.

Recurrent pulmonary embolism. In this condition there is a gradual occlusion of the pulmonary arterial bed over a period of time which may extend to several years. Infarction is not a feature but there is a progressive increase in the pulmonary vascular resistance, leading to severe pulmonary hypertension, right ventricular hypertrophy and failure. The muscular pulmonary arteries show medial hypertrophy and excentric nodular fibro-elastic thickening of the intima due to organisation of the thrombo-emboli. The larger elastic pulmonary arteries may show lattices, due to recanalisation of thrombo-emboli. Smooth muscle develops in the walls of pulmonary arterioles.

In many patients with recurrent pulmonary thrombo-embolism the source of venous thrombi is not found. As already explained, the recurrent impaction of small thrombo-emboli in the pulmonary circulation is a normal phenomenon. Hence it may well be that chronic pulmonary thrombo-embolism is not caused by the production of an excessive number of thrombo-emboli, but by the intrinsic inability of the pulmonary circulation to deal with them. So far, no evidence has been found of inadequate fibrinolytic activity in the blood of these patients. The abnormality may lie in the pulmonary vascular endothelium.

Non-thrombotic pulmonary embolism

The pulmonary capillary bed is a most effective filter of particulate matter in the blood and all manner of fragments may be found impacted in it. The commonest and most important clinical form is pulmonary thrombo-embolism, but fragments of various materials other than thrombus can cause pulmonary embolism, as described below.

Bone marrow embolism may follow accidents with bone fractures, thoracic operations involving cleavage of the sternum, rib fractures due to external cardiac massage, or spontaneous fracture due to tumour metastases in bones. Masses of megakaryocytes may be found impacted in the pulmonary capillaries, especially after surgical operations and in cases of pulmonary thrombo-embolism. *Fat embolism* commonly occurs after accidents involving fractures of bones or contusion of adipose tissue (p. 206). It is detected as oily patches in the blood and can be readily demonstrated by the usual stains for fat. Fat embolism to the lungs is very common but a rare cause of significant symptoms, but when very extensive it can cause death. *Amniotic fluid embolism* to the lung is a clinical and pathological entity which may occur in women during or shortly after childbirth. It causes a sudden onset of dyspnoea, cyanosis and shock, and may be fatal. It is also possible that non-fatal amniotic fluid embolism is a cause of primary pulmonary hypertension. By contrast, small fragments of trophoblast are frequently found in the lungs of pregnant women dying from various causes, but rarely give rise to symptoms. *Cancer cells* get trapped in the pulmonary capillary bed like other particulate matter. They degenerate or grow to form metastases. Recurrent emboli from the right atrium in cases of cardiac myxoma may lead to pulmonary hypertension. *Air embolism* to the lung may arise from many causes, including various surgical and diagnostic procedures such as intravenous injections and infusions, abortions, and the induction of a pneumothorax. The air turns into a frothy mass inside the pulmonary artery but will not easily pass the capillary bed. At necropsy, the pulmonary trunk must be opened under water to reveal air embolism. Other materials entering the pulmonary circulation include cotton wool fibres and materials injected by drug addicts.

Pulmonary emphysema

Pulmonary emphysema is a permanent enlargement of the respiratory passages or air spaces distal to the terminal bronchiole. By using this anatomical definition it is possible to avoid the use of words such as 'destructive' or 'distensive emphysema' which depend on the assumption of mechanisms of causation the evidence for which is by no means clear. Under certain circumstances air may escape into the interstitial connective tissues of the lung. This condition is called *interstitial emphysema* and should not be confused with pulmonary emphysema as defined above. It will be considered briefly later.

Bronchi and bronchioles. To understand emphysema it is necessary to be familiar with the micro-anatomy of the terminal air passages. Large bronchi have complete rings of cartilage in their walls. They divide into small bronchi with cartilage in the form of plates which do not completely surround the lumen of the bronchus. With further division, the airways increase in number and decrease in size, and the point at which the cartilage disappears is taken as the dividing line between the small bronchus and the bronchiole. Small bronchi still have a few mucous glands left in their wall, whereas in the bronchioles the only mucin-secreting cells are goblet cells in the lining epithelium. The terminal bronchiole is the last small air passage not to bear alveoli and the respiratory bronchiole is the first in which they appear.

The cut surface of distended lung shows hexagonal areas of parenchyma, some 1 or 2 cm across, delineated by fibrous septa (Fig. 15.18). Each hexagonal area is a section of a **secondary lung lobule**; it contains the lung tissue supplied by the 3 to 5 terminal bronchioles, which radiate from the centre, accompanied by muscular pulmonary arteries. This is the unit referred to subsequently in this account as '*the lobule*'.

The respiratory acinus. The structure of the respiratory acinus is central to our understanding of the pathology of pulmonary emphysema. The acinus (previously termed a 'primary lobule') is that portion of lung tissue formed by the branching from a single terminal bronchiole (Fig. 15.19a). Hence one lung lobule (see above) consists of 3–5 respiratory acini. The respiratory bronchioles may branch three or as many as five times. The first order of respiratory

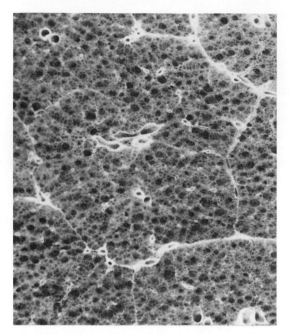

Fig. 15.18 Normal adult lung. Note the hexagonal lobule in the centre of the field with the terminal bronchioles in its centre. (Barium sulphate impregnation.) × 4. (Dr. W. R. Lee.)

bronchioles have only a few alveoli but they increase in number with each division. The walls of the alveolar ducts are lined entirely by alveoli, the dividing walls between the spaces ending in small knots of smooth muscle.

The varieties of pulmonary emphysema. There are complicated and detailed classifications of all the possible localised and generalised forms of pulmonary emphysema but a simple classification of the generalised form, which may cause death from respiratory or cardiac failure, follows from the micro-anatomy of the lung that we have just considered. The respiratory acinus consists of respiratory bronchioles, alveolar ducts and alveoli (Fig. 15.19a). There are two main forms of pulmonary emphysema. One is characterised by permanent dilatation of the respiratory bronchioles, the other by permanent dilatation of the alveolar ducts or alveoli.

In **bronchiolar emphysema** the enlarged terminal air spaces are respiratory bronchioles (Fig. 15.19b). In the early stages of the disease the alveolar ducts and alveoli distal to the dilated bronchioles are normal. The disease is readily recognised by naked-eye examination of slices of fixed distended or inflated lungs, as the enlarged airspaces are seen in clusters, at the centres of the secondary lung lobules, surrounded by normal lung tissue (Fig. 15.20). In histological sections, the emphysematous spaces appear to be derived from respiratory bronchioles, but it may be difficult to be certain of this unless many lesions or serial sections of a single lesion are examined. There is a great contrast between the greatly enlarged respiratory bronchioles and the normal alveolar ducts and alveoli distal to the emphysematous spaces.

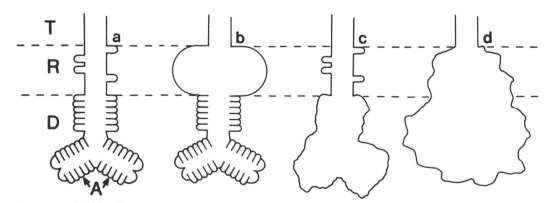

Fig. 15.19 Models of the normal respiratory acinus and the changes of emphysema. The normal acinus (**a**) consists of a terminal bronchiole (T), leading into respiratory bronchioles (R) and alveolar ducts (D) from both of which alveoli (A) arise. (For clarity, only one respiratory bronchiole is shown arising from the terminal bronchiole.) Dilatation of air spaces is confined initially to the respiratory bronchioles in centrilobular and focal duct emphysema (**b**), and to the alveolar ducts and spaces in alveolar duct emphysema (**c**). In panacinar emphysema (**d**) dilatation of the alveolar ducts and spaces extends to the respiratory bronchioles.

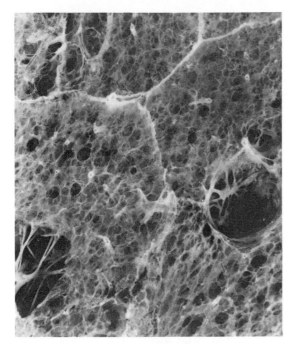

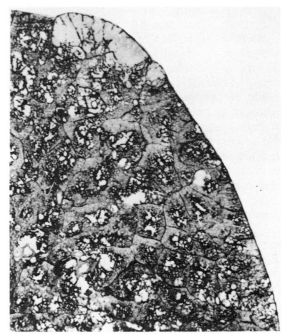

Fig. 15.20 Section of lung impregnated with barium sulphate, showing centrilobular emphysema. Note the punched out centrilobular spaces containing fibrous strands and blood vessels and the relatively normal parenchyma at the periphery of the lobules. × 7. (Dr. W. R. Lee.)

Fig. 15.21 Focal dust emphysema in coal-worker's pneumoconiosis. × 1.

There are two varieties of bronchiolar emphysema. The first is **focal dust emphysema** which is virtually confined to coal workers (Fig. 15.21). (A minor form, which has been termed 'soot emphysema', occurs in the general population.) The second, more serious and commoner form, is found in the general population and is called **centrilobular emphysema** (Fig. 15.20). (Because the respiratory bronchioles lie centrally in the lobule, the dilated spaces are, in fact, centrilobular in both focal dust and centrilobular emphysema.)

The distinction between focal dust emphysema and centrilobular emphysema depends to some extent on the occupational history but there are also micro-anatomical differences. In the focal variety, there is a fusiform dilatation of all orders of respiratory bronchioles and they are surrounded by coal dust. In centrilobular emphysema, the distal orders of respiratory bronchioles are first affected and there is little surrounding dust but evidence of chronic bronchiolitis. Right ventricular failure is common in centrilobular but not in focal dust emphysema,

which is discussed in the later section on pneumoconioses.

In **alveolar emphysema** there is permanent enlargement initially of alveolar ducts and alveoli and subsequently of respiratory bronchioles (Fig. 15.19c). The first stage is called **alveolar duct emphysema**, although it has also been called the *vesicular* variety. In slices of distended or inflated lung it may be recognised as diffuse areas of abnormally large air spaces. Histological sections show enlarged alveolar ducts and alveoli, the latter becoming wider at their mouths and shallower in depth. The respiratory bronchioles are normal. In the second stage of alveolar emphysema, the enlargement of air spaces extends from the alveolar ducts proximally in the respiratory acinus to involve the respiratory bronchioles and so the entire acinus (Fig. 15.19d). This is called **panacinar emphysema**: in lung slices it is readily recognised by areas of grossly abnormal air spaces scattered irregularly throughout the lung. Macroscopically the lungs appear voluminous; the anterior surface of the heart is covered and the diaphragm pressed downwards. The edges of the emphysematous lung are raised above the surface, rounding off the sharp edges. The emphysematous tissue is paler than the rest of the lung as less carbon pigment is present: it contains little blood and pits on pressure owing to lack of elasticity. Emphysema is most pronounced at the apices of the lungs and along the margins, especially the anterior borders, but in extreme cases practically the whole of the lung substance may be affected, although the condition is usually slight on the posterior aspect. When the disease is severe, the involved areas frequently merge with one another so that there is little or no intervening normal lung tissue. Some of the enlarged abnormal air spaces in the lung may become cystic and project from the pleural surface; these are called *bullae*. In histological sections the alveoli are few and greatly enlarged. In some cases of centrilobular emphysema the dilatation of the respiratory bronchioles may be so pronounced that it becomes impossible to distinguish them from cases of panacinar emphysema.

The demonstration of emphysema at necropsy. Adequate fixation is very important for the demonstration of emphysema. The usual practice of cutting lungs at necropsy results in collapse and could hardly be better designed to obscure the appearances of the air spaces. Careful examination or 'point-counting', as described below, requires that the whole lungs should be distended with formol-saline until the pleural surfaces are smooth and then left for two to three days before cutting. Impregnation of slices of fixed lung with barium sulphate will allow the relationship of the abnormal air spaces and their connections to be assessed in three dimensions with the dissecting microscope (Fig. 15.20). Sections of an adequately fixed lung can be used for 'point-counting' to estimate the distribution and severity of emphysema. This may be carried out by placing over the slice of lung a perspex sheet divided into equilateral triangles with 1 cm sides, at the corners of which are small punched-out points. This enables one to determine the percentage of emphysema present by counting the number of points lying over air spaces. Such quantitative studies have not revealed any simple relation between the amount of lung destroyed by pulmonary emphysema and the weight of the right ventricle (see below). Another technique for the demonstration of emphysema is the preparation of sections, approximately 300 μm thick, of gelatin-embedded lungs. Such sections may be

mounted on paper and preserved as dry specimens. If morphometric studies on histological sections are to be carried out, the lung should be inflated with formalin vapour in a vacuum chamber.

Clinicopathological correlations. There are two main clinical syndromes associated with what physicians call '*chronic obstructive airways disease*', the pathology of which is chronic bronchitis and emphysema. The 'type A' patient is characterised by obvious radiological evidence of emphysema, reduced diffusing capacity; Pa_{O_2} and Pa_{CO_2} are both normal at rest, and there is little tendency to develop congestive cardiac failure. This patient is the 'pink puffer' and his main disability is breathlessness. He has emphysema without significant hypoxia and the emphysema is commonly but not invariably of the panacinar type. The 'type B' patient does not have much radiological evidence of emphysema; diffusing capacity is normal; at rest, Pa_{O_2} is low and Pa_{CO_2} raised. This is the 'blue bloater' who has significant hypoxia and is likely to die in congestive (right ventricular) cardiac failure. The emphysema is commonly of bronchiolar type with associated bronchiolitis. Chronic hypoxia causes pulmonary hypertension and the hypoxic form of pulmonary hypertensive vascular disease (p. 403).

Morphometry in emphysema. Quantitative methods have proved useful in the study of pulmonary emphysema. It is quite inadequate now to talk of 'severe' or 'moderately severe' emphysema. The application of histological morphometric techniques derived from principles used by geologists for a century in the study of rocks enables one to establish fairly easily the internal surface area of the lung and the number of surviving alveolar spaces. In one study the normal internal surface of both lungs together was 70 m². The corresponding area in centrilobular emphysema was reduced to 61 m² and in alveolar emphysema to 46 m². The total number of alveolar spaces in the normal left and right lungs together was 273×10^6, while in centrilobular emphysema it was 215×10^6, and in panacinar emphysema 63×10^6. There is no relation between the reduction in internal surface area in pulmonary emphysema and the weight of the right ventricle, suggesting that the classical concept that right ventricular hypertrophy in emphysema is due to loss of pulmonary capillary bed is incorrect. In fact, right ventricular hypertrophy appears to be commoner in centrilobular emphysema in which the reduction in internal surface area, and so presumably in capillary bed, is smaller.

The pathogenesis of emphysema. There is evidence to suggest that certain proteolytic enzymes can cause emphysema. It can be induced in animals by aerosols of papain, a proteolytic enzyme which attacks elastin. Emphysema can also be produced in dogs by aerosol homogenates of human leucocytes which are thought to contain an elastase capable of damaging the lung. Alpha$_1$-antitrypsin, which is an inhibitor of such enzymes, is synthesised in the liver and is a normal constituent of the α_1-globulin fraction of the plasma proteins. Some people have an inherited deficiency of this inhibitor in their blood. In the rare homozygous state, the deficiency is severe and there is a high frequency of emphysema. It is not generally accepted that heterozygotes are more prone to emphysema, but deterioration in lung function in cigarette smokers, and the loss of elastic recoil with increasing age, proceed more rapidly in heterozygotes than in the normal population. It is now possible to measure the serum trypsin inhibitory capacity. The emphysema associated with α_1-antitrypsin deficiency in man is panacinar in type and is mainly basal in situation. This has been attributed to the fact that in the upright posture basal perfusion exceeds that of the apex and that the proteolytic enzyme presumed to be the causative agent is blood-borne.

By contrast, the known air-borne factors predisposing to emphysema, including cigarette smoke and coal dust, tend to induce centrilobular or focal dust emphysema, most severe in the apices of the lung. Such apical predominance may relate to the lung apex being subject to greater inflationary stresses and having a higher ratio of ventilation to perfusion than the base. Centrilobular emphysema is associated with chronic bronchitis leading to postinflammatory weakening and dilatation of the respiratory bronchioles. In focal dust emphysema the accumulation of dust in and around the walls of respiratory bronchioles leads to rigidity and loss of the smooth muscle, so that the affected segments are progressively dilated under the pressure of inspired air.

Once the initial damage to the lung tissue has occurred, the force which expands the damaged portions into emphysematous spaces is the atmospheric pressure of the inspired air. The force required to distend an elastic sphere is inversely proportional to the radius and therefore becomes progressively less as the sphere enlarges. A vicious circle is initiated as soon as a weakness develops in the air passages, and continuing dilatation and destruction is inevitable, particularly if the emphysematous lung is subject to the powerful inspiratory effort of the coughing which is associated with chronic bronchitis.

'Compensatory emphysema' is a term sometimes used to describe the overdistension of alveoli which may occur around areas of collapsed lung tissue and during acute attacks of bronchial asthma.

With increasing age there is a concomitant increase in the size of the alveolar spaces and a decrease in the internal surface area of the lungs. In some elderly subjects these changes are of sufficient magnitude to suggest to some pathologists that they constitute **'senile emphysema'**.

'Interstitial emphysema'. This condition follows laceration of the lung substance. It may be produced by overdistension of the alveolar spaces as may occur with severe coughing or in dyspnoea with forced inspiration. It may also follow traumatic laceration of the lung tissue by a fractured rib or by a perforating wound. Interstitial emphysema due to rupture of alveolar walls from over-distension is much commoner in children than adults and occurs in such conditions as whooping cough, bronchiolitis, and in diphtheria of the larynx and trachea. The alveolar walls rupture as the result of over-expansion during forced inspiration, and air, in the form of small bead-like collections or blebs, extends along the lines of junction of the interlobular septa with the pleura, thus producing a reticulated appearance on the pleural surface. When the air is abundant, it passes by the lymphatics to the rest of the lungs, and in exceptional cases it may extend even to the tissues at the root of the neck and give rise to subcutaneous emphysema.

Collapse of lung tissue

Atelectasis and collapse. There is a distinction to be made between these two conditions. The term atelectasis is derived from the Greek for 'imperfect expansion' and it should be restricted to denote failure of the lungs to expand properly at birth. *Atelectasis*, which is thus congenital, should be distinguished from acquired *collapse* of a previously expanded lung. A lung may collapse because something presses on it from without; this is *pressure collapse*, or because there is obstruction of a bronchus with resulting absorption of air in the corresponding area of lung tissue; this is *absorption collapse*.

Pressure collapse. The lung may be compressed from without by a pleural effusion, haemothorax, empyema or pneumothorax. Spencer points out that the pulmonary changes which follow this type of collapse differ from those which follow absorption collapse because the absence of bronchial obstruction leaves the secretions from lung and bronchi free to drain in the normal fashion up the bronchial tree. Thus the changes that eventually occur within the lung parenchyma do not result from infection, but from the haemodynamic alterations and associated vascular changes. Collapse due to pyothorax may be considerable so that the lung becomes very small and lies posteriorly against the side of the vertebral column. When the exudate on the pleural surface becomes organised, pleural thickening results and prevents re-expansion of the lung even when the infection is overcome. Accordingly it is important to drain the pleural cavity and obtain re-expansion of the lung before this happens. In pressure collapse, the reduction in lung volume may be pronounced.

Absorption collapse. This is a commoner condition than pressure collapse and follows *acute and complete obstruction* of a large bronchus. Following such obstruction, collateral air ventilation may for a time keep the obstructed segment of lung filled with air provided the surrounding lung is free from pulmonary oedema, haemorrhage or pneumonia. However, as the air gradually disappears it is largely replaced by secretion and oedema fluid so that the lung does not change very much in size. Acute absorption collapse follows inhaled foreign bodies and collections of mucus occurring in terminal illnesses, after tracheostomy, anaesthetics or in lung infections. *Chronic bronchial obstruction* may be caused by tumours growing in the wall of the affected bronchus or pressing on it from without. Other lesions which may press on bronchi and obstruct them are aneurysms and enlarged lymph nodes. In absorption collapse, bronchial secretions beyond the obstruction are very likely to become infected and suppuration may extend through the collapsed segment of lung tissue.

In collapse of the lung the pleural surfaces are wrinkled and the cut surface is airless. Portions of the collapsed tissue sink in water. As explained above, the reduction in volume is often much greater in pressure than in absorption collapse. The alveolar walls are pushed together. There is no respiratory movement of air in the bronchial tree in the collapsed area of lung so that the haemoglobin in its dilated alveolar capillaries is largely in a reduced state. As a result the affected lung appears purple. When the collapse has lasted for some time, there is a proliferation of granular pneumocytes, associated with progressive pulmonary fibrosis. This permanently prevents re-expansion and a return to normal. In the early stages there is a constriction of the pulmonary arteries but later they show intimal fibroelastosis.

Massive collapse, affecting most of one or both lungs, is rare and is usually caused by wounds or injuries of the chest wall. It may also follow the use of lipiodol for bronchography, and may complicate laryngeal paralysis in diphtheria.

Atelectasis. Incomplete expansion of the neonatal lung may be caused by failure of the respiratory centre or because the lung is insufficiently developed owing to the child being born prematurely. It may follow hyaline membrane disease (p. 400), or may result from laryngeal dysfunction and obstruction of the air passages. Finally, congenital lung disease may prevent expansion of the lung. All these causes are, however, responsible for only a small proportion of atelectatic neonatal lungs. In many infants with severe atelectasis, no cause can be demonstrated at necropsy.

Acute bacterial infections

The most common acute inflammatory disorders of the lung are the various types of **pneumonia**, which is defined as an inflammatory disorder of the lung characterised by consolidation due to the presence of exudate in the alveolar spaces. The term **pneumonitis** is sometimes used to denote an inflammatory condition of the pulmonary interstitial tissues without consolidation of the alveolar spaces.

The pneumonias may be classified anatomically into lobar pneumonia and bronchopneumonia. In **lobar pneumonia**, the causative bacteria lead to the production of a watery inflammatory exudate in the alveoli. This flows directly into bronchioles and related alveoli, filling them and spilling over into adjacent lobules and segments of the lung. Damage to the bronchiolar walls, although present, is relatively unimportant. The exudate and bacteria spread through the lumen rather than the walls of the terminal airways. The consolidation is sharply confined to the affected lobe, which is diffusely affected. In **bronchopneumonia**, the inflammation occurs primarily in the terminal and respiratory bronchioles. The walls are damaged so that exudate spreads into the surrounding peribronchiolar alveoli and into the acinus supplied by the affected terminal bronchiole (Fig. 15.22).

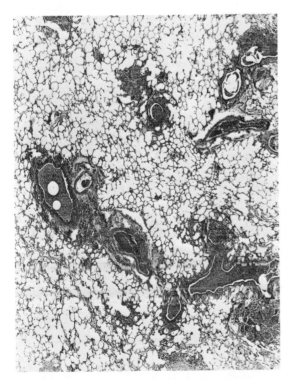

Fig. 15.22 Acute bronchiolitis and early bronchopneumonia. The bronchioles are filled with exudate which is extending into the associated respiratory acini and peribronchiolar alveoli. × 10.

The resulting pneumonia consists of numerous discrete foci of consolidation centred around inflamed terminal bronchioles.

The anatomical type of pneumonia (lobar or bronchopneumonia) and the subsequent liability to develop complications depend on the aetiological agent responsible. Hence the older anatomical classification is being superseded by a classification based on the causative agent.

Pneumococcal lobar pneumonia

Since the widespread use of antibiotics the fully-developed picture of classical lobar pneumonia is not often seen in Britain. However, fatal untreated cases may still be encountered in those who lie neglected at home, in those who decline medical aid, in vagrants and in alcoholics who become exposed to cold. Classical lobar pneumonia is still a common disease in many areas of the world where medical services are poorly developed. Thus it is still very frequent and an important cause of death in many parts of Africa. The disease predominates in males and occurs at all ages, although it is uncommon below the age of one year. It is still most commonly seen between the ages of 30 and 50 years.

The causative agent is *Streptococcus pneumoniae*, a Gram + ve diplococcus which can be serologically typed according to the antigenic properties of its polysaccharide capsule. About 90% of cases are caused by the following types in descending order of frequency: I, III, II, V, VII, VIII and IV. The first three types are responsible for 70% of cases. Types I and II cause pneumonia mainly in younger persons who were previously healthy, and type III mainly in patients over the age of 50 suffering from some other form of chronic disease. Type III has always been known as a particularly lethal strain and it is still likely to cause high mortality in spite of the use of antibiotics and modern supportive measures. Type III pneumococci have an abundant capsular mucopolysaccharide which imparts a slimy quality to the exudate and thus to the cut surface of the lung at necropsy. Pneumococcal pneumonia with abscess formation is most likely to be caused by this organism.

Structural changes. Infection is acquired by inhalation of pneumococci. If the organisms are virulent and the resistance of the patient low, a disease process commences which, if untreated, runs a fairly well-defined course, usually terminating in resolution. It has been customary to recognise the following four stages in the progress of untreated pneumococcal lobar pneumonia: acute congestion; red hepatisation; grey hepatisation; and resolution. It must be emphasised that these stages occur in untreated cases in adults. The use of sulphonamides and antibiotics profoundly alters the classical clinical and pathological picture.

Acute congestion. This initial phase, which lasts for one or two days, is one of acute congestion and oedema. Macroscopically the affected lobe is heavy, dark red and firm: abundant frothy red fluid can be squeezed from it. Large numbers of pneumococci are seen in stained smears made from the cut surface. Microscopically the alveolar capillaries are engorged with erythrocytes. There is venular margination of neutrophil polymorphs which can be seen to be migrating into the alveolar spaces. These are filled with eosinophilic oedema fluid which contains many Gram + ve diplococci.

Red hepatisation. This phase lasts from the second to the fourth days of the disease. The pleural surface of the affected lobe is covered by greyish-white friable tags of fibrin. The cut surface appears dry, firm, red and granular and has the consistency of liver (Fig. 15.23). Affected lung tissue is airless and sinks in water. Histologically, the capillary engorgement persists, but the exudate occupying the alveolar spaces now contains a fine network of fibrin (Fig. 2.4, p. 38), large numbers of extravasated red cells and increasing numbers of emigrated neutrophil polymorphs.

Grey hepatisation. In this stage of late consolidation (4 to 8 days) the affected lung may weigh as much as 1500 g. Fibrinous pleurisy is present and the cut surface is dry, granular and grey. The affected lobe still has the consistency of liver and slices of it retain straight, sharp edges. Histologically, the alveolar spaces are distended and consolidated by a denser network of inspissated fibrin containing neutrophil polymorphs, many dead and disintegrating, and occasional degenerating erythrocytes (Fig. 15.24). During this stage, antibodies to pneumococci appear in the blood, pneumococci are eliminated, and the fever subsides by crisis.

Resolution occurs on the eighth day with the

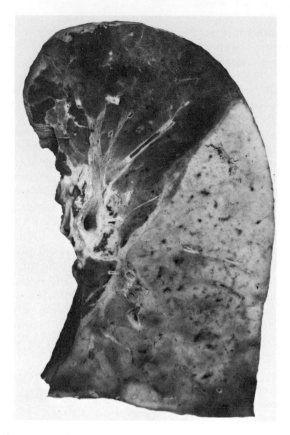

Fig. 15.23 Acute lobar pneumonia with grey hepatisation in lower lobe and red hepatisation in part of upper lobe. × 1/3.

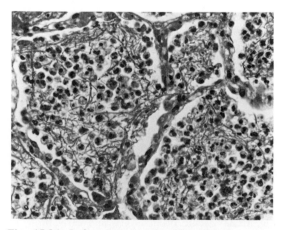

Fig. 15.24. Lobar pneumonia. The alveolar spaces are filled with exudate containing a fibrin network and many neutrophil polymorphs. × 235.

migration of macrophages from the alveolar septa into the exudate, which is gradually liquefied by fibrinolytic enzymes and absorbed or coughed up. The cut surface of the affected lung is at first friable and mottled red and grey in colour. Complete resolution and re-aeration take from one to three weeks. Since there is virtually no tissue destruction in lobar pneumonia, the lung parenchyma returns to normal, but the pleural exudate is commonly organised with the formation of fibrous adhesions between the two surfaces.

As already mentioned, the above account refers to cases not receiving antibacterial therapy. Sulphonamide or antibiotic therapy rapidly eliminates the pneumococci and resolution follows.

Clinical features. The onset is sudden and the patient has a fever with rigors and sharp pleuritic pain on respiration. When a lower lobe is involved, diaphragmatic pleural pain may be referred to the tip of the shoulder. Partly because of the pain, breathing is shallow and rapid, and there is usually a cough productive of brown or blood-stained sputum. There is a well marked neutrophil polymorphonuclear leucocytosis from an early stage. Bacteraemia is common, blood cultures being positive in about 65% of cases. Usually the systemic arterial oxygen saturation is only slightly reduced. As in acute inflammation in general, blood flow through the consolidated lobe(s) is at first rapid, but soon slows down, and becomes very low, although the total pulmonary blood flow is increased, as in any infective fever.

Complications. The principal complications of pneumococcal lobar pneumonia are as follows:

Organisation of exudate. In about 3% of cases resolution does not occur and the fibrinous exudate occupying the alveoli becomes organised (Fig. 15.25). The fibrin is slowly digested by macrophages, while fibroblasts grow in from the alveolar septa, and the tissue becomes fibrosed, tough, airless, leathery and grey. There is an impression that the incidence of organising pneumonia has increased since the introduction of antibiotics. Possibly these drugs cut down the inflammatory response and reduce the numbers of emigrating polymorphs, which are important in digestion of the fibrin.

Pleural effusion occurs in about 5% of treated cases.

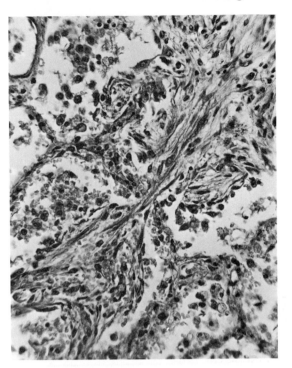

Fig. 15.25 Organisation of alveolar exudate in the lung. The inflammatory exudate has been replaced by cellular fibrous tissue which can be seen passing from one alveolus to another through the pore of Kohn in the centre of the picture. × 390.

Empyema occurs in less than 1% of treated cases.

Lung abscess is a complication which has practically disappeared since the introduction of antibiotics.

Cardiac complications include suppurative pericarditis, acute bacterial endocarditis and various degrees of acute failure from toxic myocarditis.

Bacteraemic complications include bacterial endocarditis, suppurative meningitis, acute otitis media and arthritis.

Bronchopneumonia

Bronchopneumonia is an inflammatory condition of the lung that occurs when micro-organisms colonise the bronchioles and extend into the surrounding alveoli, leading to numerous discrete foci of consolidation (Fig. 15.22). Many types of bacteria can cause it, including *Strep. pneumoniae, Staph. aureus, Strep. pyogenes, Klebsiella* and *Haemophilus influenzae.* It occurs most commonly in infancy, in old age, and in patients with some debilitating condition such as cancer, uraemia or a stroke. Acute respiratory virus infections, and chronic diseases such as chronic bronchitis, bronchiectasis and cystic fibrosis predispose to bronchopneumonia. It may develop in patients with congestive cardiac failure and after surgical operations under general anaesthesia, due to the adverse effect of narcotic drugs on respiration and ciliary activity.

At necropsy, bronchopneumonia is commonly found in the lower lobes of the lungs, where it appears as focal dark red or grey areas of about 1 cm diameter, which are firmer than the surrounding lung, and appear to be centred around a bronchiole from which a bead of pale yellow pus can be expressed. If progressive, the focal areas of consolidation become larger and eventually coalesce to simulate lobar pneumonia. The microscopic lesions of bronchopneumonia are an acute bronchiolitis with filling of the surrounding peribronchiolar alveoli with inflammatory exudate rich in neutrophil polymorphs.

Complete resolution is uncommon in bronchopneumonia because, except in mild cases, there is usually a variable amount of damage to, and destruction of, the walls of bronchioles. In consequence, the lesions usually result in the development of small foci of fibrosis. If fibrosis of the lung is extensive, bronchiectasis may develop.

Staphylococcal pneumonia. *Staphylococcus aureus* rarely causes pneumonia as a primary event; it is usually encountered as a secondary infection in patients debilitated by chronic lung disease, such as cystic fibrosis, where antibiotics have been used for long periods. Its incidence rises sharply during epidemics of influenza, measles and pertussis, when it may be responsible for an acute, short-lived, lethal pneumonia in children and adults. In acute cases, staphylococci invade the lungs about 36 hours after the onset of influenza. At necropsy, the lungs appear purple and are heavy due to haemorrhagic pulmonary oedema. The bronchi are filled with blood-stained fluid which drains away to reveal an inflamed mucosa, sometimes covered by a grey membrane of fibrin. There is no pleural reaction. Microscopically there is an acute ulcerative bronchitis and bronchiolitis: the alveolar spaces are filled with oedema fluid containing fibrin coagulum, much extravasated

blood, scanty neutrophil polymorphs and abundant clusters of Gram + ve cocci.

In older children and adults who survive this acute phase, multiple foci of greyish-white consolidation develop which break down to form abscess cavities containing sticky yellow pus. There is much lung destruction and the pleura at this stage is thickly coated with fibrinous or fibrino-purulent exudate. Empyema and pneumothorax may occur from rupture of pulmonary abscesses into the pleural cavity. In children, a valvular obstruction may occur at the junction of an abscess cavity and bronchus to produce a rapidly-expanding air-filled *tension cyst* or *pneumatocele*. Such lesions rarely occur in tuberculosis treated with drugs but are otherwise a complication peculiar to staphylococcal pneumonia in children. The cyst, which can be several centimetres in diameter, may rupture into the pleural cavity to produce a *tension pneumothorax*. Usually the air is absorbed after the infection is overcome.

Klebsiellar pneumonia. *Klebsiella pneumoniae* (Friedlander's bacillus) is a Gram − ve bacillus with an abundant mucoid capsule. It is an infrequent cause of pneumonia but important because the infection is destructive, with a mortality rate of about 40% and a high incidence of sequelae. The organism is a commensal in the upper respiratory tract in about 5% of normal individuals, but more frequently in people with advanced dental caries and periodontal disease. Klebsiellar pneumonia tends to occur especially in men over the age of 50 who are chronic alcoholics, diabetics or have oral sepsis. It is about thirty times commoner in men than women. About 75% of infections commence in the right lung, usually in the posterior segment of the upper lobe. Clinically, the onset is acute with severe prostration and a cough with blood-stained gelatinous sputum resembling red currant jelly. Pathologically, red-grey areas of consolidation become confluent, leading to involvement of the entire right upper lobe. The cut surface of the affected lung is mucoid. Destruction of lung tissue leads to the formation of a large apical abscess in about 80% of cases, and this may be mistakenly diagnosed as tuberculosis. The infection may become chronic with severe progressive destruction of lung tissue so that the patient becomes a permanent respiratory cripple.

Streptococcal pneumonia. Cases of pneumonia due to *Strep. pyogenes* are rare and usually secondary to influenza or measles. Death occurs within 36 to 72 hours and at necropsy the lungs appear purple with a fibrinous pleurisy. In cases dying after a week, yellow areas of consolidation are present in the lungs. These consolidated foci may cavitate, with the formation of abscesses leading to empyema and bronchopleural fistulas.

Pseudomonas pneumonia. Following the introduction and combined use of antibiotic and corticosteroid drugs, Gram − ve organisms in general, and *Pseudomonas aeruginosa* in particular, have become of greater importance as causes of bacterial pneumonia. Another factor is the increased use of tracheostomy and mechanical ventilation. Both the tracheostomy wounds and ventilation apparatus commonly become colonised by *Pseudomonas aeruginosa*, which spreads rapidly to infect neighbouring patients. It is most important to sterilise respiratory equipment properly after use to prevent the spread of infection. Unfortunately, *Pseudomonas aeruginosa* may survive and proliferate in water, soap solution, stored blood, infusion fluids and in some antiseptics. In pseudomonas pneumonia, the air spaces in the affected lung are filled with blood, oedema fluid, scanty neutrophil polymorphs and innumerable causative organisms which can be demonstrated by appropriate staining methods. A characteristic feature of pseudomonas pneumonia is bacterial invasion of pulmonary arteries, leading to necrosis of the vessel with subsequent haemorrhage or thrombosis and then pulmonary infarction.

Aspiration pneumonia results from the inhalation of food, gastric contents, or infected material from the oropharyngeal region. It may follow anaesthesia administered on a full stomach because of an obstetric or other emergency. It may complicate pyloric stenosis, hiatus hernia, oesophageal obstruction and any condition associated with persistent vomiting. The likelihood of food or gastric contents being inhaled is increased in unconscious patients, drunkenness, epilepsy and neurological disorders affecting swallowing.

Massive inhalation of gastric contents may lead to rapid death from asphyxia. The aspiration of smaller amounts of sterile acid gastric contents produces pulmonary oedema due to chemical irritation of the alveolar walls: a few

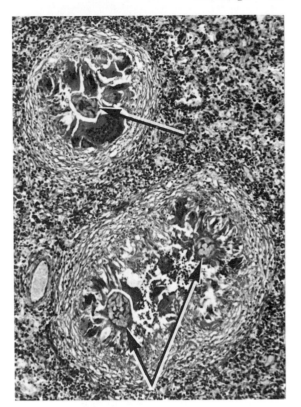

Fig. 15.26 Aspiration bronchopneumonia showing inhaled lentil-starch grains (arrows) with granulomatous foreign-body giant cell reaction. × 72.

hours after aspiration the patient dramatically develops cyanosis, dyspnoea and shock, with bloodstained sputum. If the acute episode is survived, secondary bacterial infection is likely to follow. Non-sterile aspirate rapidly causes widespread bronchopneumonia, which becomes confluent with multiple areas of necrosis. The microscopic picture is of a suppurative bronchopneumonia with destruction of alveolar walls and abscess formation. Foreign-body giant cells may be seen surrounding vegetable matter from food, giving rise to a granulomatous reaction (Fig. 15.26).

Aspiration pneumonia with suppuration may also result from partial drowning, particularly in dirty water.

Lung abscess

Lung abscess presents clinical and radiological features which must be distinguished from those of necrosis in a malignant tumour or cavitation due to tuberculosis; these two diagnoses must be automatically considered whenever there is a clinical suspicion of lung abscess.

The commonest cause of a lung abscess is inhalation of infected material during unconsciousness and sleep. Such material may be food, gastric contents, decaying teeth or necrotic tissue derived from lesions in the mouth, upper respiratory tract and nasopharynx. An abscess may form beyond an obstructed bronchus and this may be the first sign of a bronchial carcinoma or impacted foreign body. Pyogenic infection of bronchiectatic or tuberculous cavities results in abscess formation, and another important group of lung abscesses is that arising as a complication of bacterial pneumonia. The organisms most likely to be concerned are the type III *Strep. pneumoniae*, *Klebsiella pneumoniae*, *Staph. aureus* and *Strep. pyogenes*. Less common causes of lung abscess include infection of a pulmonary infarct, septic emboli in the lung as in pyaemia due to acute osteomyelitis or bacterial endocarditis, amoebic 'abscesses' due to *Entamoeba histolytica*, trauma to the lung, or direct extension from a suppurating focus in the oesophagus, mediastinum, subphrenic area or vertebral column.

Abscesses due to inhalation of infected foreign material are likely to be located in the inferior portion of the right upper lobe or at the apex of the right lower lobe. The right bronchus is more in line with the trachea than the left and is thus more receptive to aspirated foreign material. An abscess resulting from inhalation of a large foreign body will develop beyond where the body is impacted. Small foreign particles are able to travel further into the lung and may evoke inflammation in the alveoli to produce an abscess just beneath the pleura. An abscess arising as a result of bronchiectasis tends to be centred around the affected bronchus, while an abscess complicating pneumonia has no primary relationship to a major bronchus. Pyaemic abscesses, which are usually staphylococcal or streptococcal in nature, are scattered widely throughout the lungs, although they are likely to be small and mainly subpleural.

It is possible for a small lung abscess to heal completely, leaving a fibrous scar with a small central sterile cavity. An abscess located near the pleura induces a fibrinous or purulent pleurisy which may progress to empyema. An abscess communicating with a bronchus may rupture into the pleural cavity to give a bronchopleural fistula and pyopneumothorax. Serious haemorrhage may occur if an abscess erodes a pulmonary or bronchial artery. A distant complication of lung abscess is dissemination of infection to the brain which occurs in 5 to 10% of cases, with the development of meningitis or cerebral abscess. Abscess formation in staphylococcal pneumonia may result in *tension cysts* or *pneumatoceles* (p. 416).

Gangrene of the lung

The term gangrene cannot be accurately used with reference to the lung, because massive necrosis followed by putrefaction does not occur in this organ. The aspiration of non-sterile gastric contents may produce a widespread bronchopneumonia which becomes confluent, with the development of rapidly progressive multiple abscesses in which anaerobic organisms such as bacterioides, streptococci, clostridia and fusiform bacteria, in addition to aerobic organisms, play an active role. These abscesses are not walled-off and lung destruction is very extensive. There are irregular cavities containing foul-smelling pus surrounded by soft, friable, moist, green or black tissue.

Virus pneumonia

In viral respiratory infections there may be proliferation of bronchial, bronchiolar and alveolar epithelium, which may form multinucleated giant cells, followed by necrosis. The bronchial, bronchiolar and alveolar walls are infiltrated by lymphocytes and mononuclear cells. There is an almost total absence of neutrophil polymorphs from the inflammatory cell infiltrate, which is mainly interstitial. Inclusion bodies are unusual in pulmonary viral infections, and unless specific tests are performed, the viral nature can often only be inferred from the above histological features. Moreover, as previously implied, many viral infections of the lung predispose the respiratory tissues to secondary bacterial invasion and when this occurs the distinctive histological appearances of viral pneumonia are lost. Much of the mortality attributed to viral pneumonia is, in fact, due to secondary bacterial infection.

The nature of a viral pneumonia can be confirmed by identifying the infecting organism, using complex methods for the culture and isolation of the virus, or by demonstrating a rising or high titre of specific antibodies in the patient's serum. In spite of their varied pathogenesis, viral pneumonias mostly present a broadly similar clinical picture which is commonly referred to as **atypical pneumonia**.

Influenza

Influenza occurs endemically in most countries, but about every three years it causes an epidemic. Every forty years or so a major epidemic or worldwide pandemic appears, as in 1918 when a large percentage of the world's population was affected. Infection is probably spread by droplets of infected secretions reaching the respiratory tract of susceptible subjects.

Influenza virus produces its effects within the epithelial cells lining the respiratory tract. It has been suggested that the susceptibility to influenza of patients with chronic heart failure is due to the proliferation of granular pneumocytes in the alveoli in this condition, thus providing more cells suitable for virus growth. The whole respiratory tract is commonly invaded. The trachea and large bronchi usually show signs of intense inflammation, which may be accompanied by haemorrhage and occasionally, in very severe cases, also by some superficial necrosis of the mucosa and fibrinous exudate. There is leukopenia, and neutrophil polymorphs are absent from the lesions. In most cases the disease progresses no further, but during epidemics, when the virulence of the virus may have become enhanced, extension of the disease to involve the bronchioles and lung parenchyma (Fig. 15.27) is much more common, although it also occurs in severe endemic cases.

In *primary influenzal pneumonia* the alveoli are filled with a mixture of oedema fluid, fibrin, red blood cells and mononuclear cells. These changes are accompanied by an interstitial mononuclear cell infiltrate in half the cases. In the most severely affected parts of the lung there may be focal necrosis of the alveolar walls, which are lined by hyaline membranes.

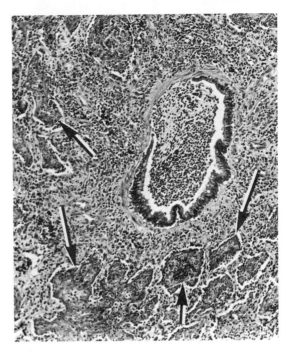

Fig. 15.27 Influenzal bronchopneumonia. There is acute inflammatory exudate in the bronchiole and in the surrounding alveolar spaces (arrows): the exudate in the alveoli is rich in fibrin and appears dark. × 60.

At necropsy, the lungs are heavy, bulky and purple-red. The cut surfaces exude bloodstained frothy fluid from the bronchi and lung parenchyma: the latter shows extensive dark areas of haemorrhage, particularly in the lower lobes.

The lowering of the resistance of the respiratory tract to secondary bacterial infection is a striking and characteristic feature of influenza. The development of *bacterial pneumonia* is usually due to *Haemophilus influenzae*, *Streptococcus pneumoniae*, *Streptococcus pyogenes* or *Staphylococcus aureus*.

Other viral pneumonias

Giant-cell pneumonia. In cases of measles dying early in the disease, the epithelium of the bronchioles may be hyperplastic and contain intracytoplasmic inclusion bodies (Fig. 15.28). The alveoli may show many giant cells derived from the lining epithelium by fusion, and they, too, contain inclusion bodies. There is good evidence that this form of giant-cell pneumonia is due to the measles virus and that it represents an altered immune response to the virus, in which the titre of serum antibody remains low or

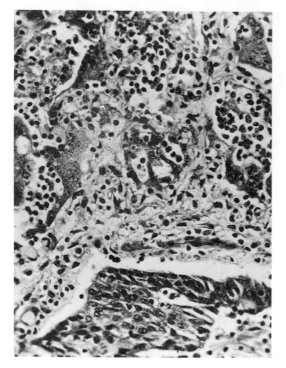

Fig. 15.28 Giant cell pneumonia in measles. There is hyperplasia of the bronchiolar epithelium and numerous giant cells in the alveolar spaces. × 240.

nil. In cases developing a secondary bacterial pneumonia the characteristic changes are lost.

Cytomegalovirus lung disease. Cytomegalovirus causes opportunistic infections in man, notably in the fetus, in premature infants, and in subjects with immunodeficiency diseases or whose immunity is depressed by corticosteroid therapy, immunosuppressive drugs, irradiation or cytotoxic drugs. In the adult form of disease, the lungs are usually involved as part of a serious widespread infection, the salivary glands and kidneys being affected more frequently than the lungs. The changes occur in both bronchiolar and alveolar epithelium. Cells enlarge so that they are five to six times the size of their uninvolved neighbours (Fig. 21.60, p. 796). *Pneumocystis carinii* is often present in addition (see below).

Other types of pneumonia

Psittacosis and ornithosis. Infection with various species of *Chlamydiae* (p. 188) is very common in birds. Infection in man is acquired by inhalation of virus particles derived from the excreta of infected birds. Cross infection from human patients to healthy attendants may occur by droplet spread. The infection should be suspected in any patient who presents with atypical pneumonia where there is a history of contact with birds, especially parrots, budgerigars and pigeons. If the disease is acquired from parrots and budgerigars, it is termed *psittacosis*, while *ornithosis* is used to describe the disease acquired from other birds. Infection produces a haemorrhagic consolidation of the lungs.

Q fever. This condition is caused by *Coxiella burnetii* which primarily infects cattle, sheep and goats. Cases of human disease usually originate from the handling of carcasses of infected cattle and sheep, the inhalation of dust from infected barns and straw, or from the drinking of raw milk containing the organisms. Stockyard workers, farmers, shepherds and medical laboratory staff may be exposed to infection during the course of their work. The disease most commonly presents as an atypical pneumonia, with headache and muscle pains as prominent symptoms. The course of the illness is usually short (up to 8 days) and benign, but chronic infection can occur. Endocarditis is a rare complication and is frequently fatal. It occurs particularly in patients with pre-existing valvular disease. Great care should be taken when necropsy is performed in cases of atypical pneumonia, for small outbreaks of Q fever have occurred in those performing or attending necropsies on patients dying with coxiellar pneumonia.

Mycoplasma pneumonia. This is caused by *Mycoplasma pneumoniae* (p. 188). The lesions consist of a low-grade inflammation of focal character centred on the bronchioles, the walls of which are thickened by interstitial mononuclear cell infiltration, while the lumina contain mucopurulent material. In some alveoli there is fibrinous exudate tending to undergo organisation, in others oedema and haemorrhage. The onset is usually gradual and the mortality is low but resolution is often somewhat delayed.

Pneumocystis pneumonia. This usually occurs as an opportunistic infection in premature and debilitated babies, in older children with hypogammaglobulinaemia, and in patients with immunological deficiency due to lymphoid neoplasms or to the administration of cytotoxic or immunosuppressive drugs. Microscopically, the alveoli are filled with a foamy, pale eosinophilic substance containing innumerable minute haematoxylinophilic dots, 1 μm in diameter, representing the trophozoites of the protozoal parasite *Pneumocystis carinii*. Cystic forms, 8–12 μm in diameter, may also be present and are best demonstrated by methenamine silver staining. The alveolar septa are distended with an infiltrate of plasma cells, lymphocytes and mononuclear cells, but in cases of hypogammaglobulinaemia plasma cells may be absent and so the term *interstitial plasma cell pneumonia* is unsatisfactory. Pneumocystis pneumonia is sometimes accompanied by cytomegalovirus disease.

Unusual causes of pulmonary consolidation

Lymphoid interstitial pneumonia is characterised by a chronic cough, dyspnoea and pyrexia, together with enlargement of the spleen and liver. Radiologically, nodular and patchy opacities with some linear markings are present in the lower lobes of the lungs. Many patients have hypergammaglobulinaemia. The disease, which is of unknown cause, affects persons of all ages, including infants. It is a slowly progressive condition and the diagnosis is usually made following lung biopsy. Histologically, the alveolar septa are distended with masses of mature lymphocytes intermingled with large pale macrophages and plasma cells. Large lymphoid follicles may be present. Differentiation from a malignant lymphoma may be difficult.

'Desquamative interstitial pneumonia' is now regarded as a cellular form of diffuse fibrosing alveolitis and is discussed in the section on pulmonary fibrosis (p. 430).

Pulmonary alveolar proteinosis. This is a rare chronic disease of unknown cause, which can affect persons of all ages from infancy to old age. It is manifested clinically by dyspnoea, a cough often productive of yellow sputum, increasing fatigue and loss of weight. Some patients recover spontaneously but the disease is fatal in about one third of cases. At necropsy, confluent grey areas of consolidation are found in the lungs. A little milky or pale yellow fluid may be squeezed from the cut surface. Histologically, the alveolar spaces are distended by a granular eosinophilic substance, and lined by prominent granular pneumocytes. The granular eosinophilic intraalveolar material contains lipid and protein and is apparently derived from the cytoplasm of granular pneumocytes which have degenerated, become necrotic and detached from the alveolar walls. The alveolar septa are devoid of inflammatory cells and fibrosis is usually absent. The nature of pulmonary alveolar proteinosis is obscure. It may represent a stereotyped reaction of the lung to different types of injury, rather than being a single disease entity. Some fatal cases show evidence of pneumocystis infection or nocardiosis. An identical condition can be produced in rats by exposure to quartz, aluminium and siliceous dusts.

Lipid pneumonia The inhalation of oily material into the lungs may cause a lipid pneumonia. This is associated with the long-term use of oily drops or sprays taken for rhinitis. Mineral oil (liquid paraffin) taken regularly at bedtime is readily aspirated during sleep in small amounts which fail to excite the cough reflex. There is a danger of aspiration when oily vitamin preparations are given to reluctant young children or debilitated elderly persons. Occasionally, radio-opaque contrast medium used for bronchography may be retained in the lungs with a resulting lipid pneumonia. Olive oil and neutral vegetable oils are the least irritant. They stimulate slight fibrosis but are slowly absorbed. Mineral oil, although chemically inert, is much more irritant and evokes a granulomatous reaction with considerable fibrosis.

Lipid pneumonia tends to be symptomless and is usually revealed by chance during radiographic examination or at necropsy. The lesions are commonly located in the middle or lower lobes of the right lung or in the left lower lobe. There may be diffuse fibrosis of the affected lung or the formation of a well-circumscribed *oleogranuloma*. This latter firm tumour-like mass may be mistakenly diagnosed as carcinoma in a chest radiograph or during thoracotomy. The histological picture of lipid pneumonia is the presence of oil, either free or in foamy macrophages, and multinucleate giant cells with accompanying lymphocytic infiltration and fibrosis.

Chronic bacterial and fungal infections

Tuberculosis

The general features of tuberculosis have already been discussed (p. 173). The causative organism, *Mycobacterium tuberculosis*, is a slender, straight or slightly curved rod, 1 to 4 μm long, which is stained red by the Ziehl-Neelsen method. In most communities, the lungs are more commonly affected by tuberculosis than any other organ, partly because inhalation is now the commonest mode of infection, but also because lung tissue provides a favourable environment for the growth of the organism. Certain diseases and occupations predispose to the development of tuberculosis. Thus it occurs with increased frequency in chronic alcoholics and in workers with silicosis. It is an occupational hazard for all hospital personnel, particularly those who work in pathology laboratories and necropsy rooms. Corticosteroid therapy, diabetes mellitus and partial gastrectomy are associated with an increased liability to develop the disease. In all developed countries where treatment and prevention of tuberculosis is actively undertaken, there has been a tendency for the incidence of the disease and its mortality to decline steeply among the younger age groups of both sexes during the past twenty years. However, this decline in incidence and mortality has been much less pronounced among the elderly, particularly men. Thus, in countries with a low case rate, tuberculosis now tends to be a disease of older people.

Pulmonary tuberculous lesions vary widely in appearance and behaviour. In communities with a high infection rate, tuberculosis is usually contracted during infancy and childhood, and the resulting *primary* lesions may either heal or prove fatal. During this primary infection, a state of cell-mediated immunity to tuberculoprotein develops. Subsequent infection may occur in adult life, giving rise to *re-infection* or *post-primary* tuberculosis, which

1 to 2 cm in diameter, and situated just beneath the pleura, usually in the mid-zone of either lung. Microscopic examination of the early Ghon focus shows central caseation and peripheral tubercles; the lesion enlarges by spread of mycobacteria, which are taken up and carried by macrophages, so that tubercles form in the adjacent lung tissue, replacing alveolar walls and filling air spaces, and as they enlarge these peripheral tubercles become incorporated in the central caseous area.

Lymphatic spread of *Myco. tuberculosis* takes place in the primary infection; tubercles are frequently seen along the line of the lymphatics between the Ghon focus and the hilar lymph nodes, and both the tracheobronchial and adjacent mediastinal nodes often become extensively involved (Fig. 15.29). Tubercles are

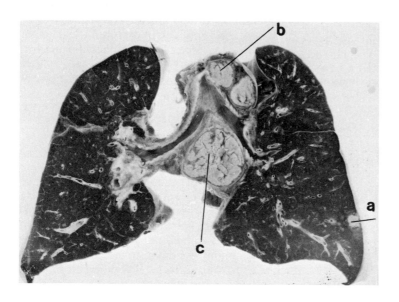

Fig. 15.29 Primary pulmonary tuberculous complex. Lung of child with primary lesion (a) in right lower lobe and enlarged tracheobronchial lymph nodes (b and c).

may either heal or produce chronic pulmonary disease. In communities with a low rate of tuberculous infection, primary lesions may occur in adult life. Thus it is no longer appropriate to refer to primary and re-infection tuberculosis as the childhood and adult types respectively. The basic features of delayed hypersensitivity reactions, which are necessary for the full understanding of this account, have been given in pp. 127–30.

Primary pulmonary tuberculosis. In patients who have not previously had tuberculosis, inhalation of tubercle bacilli and subsequent infection gives rise to a primary lesion, also termed the *Ghon focus*. This is usually single,

found in large numbers in these nodes, which undergo caseation and coalesce, finally converting the nodes into large caseous masses with marginal tubercle follicles. The combination of the Ghon focus and tuberculous lymphadenitis is termed the *primary complex*. In children, the affected hilar and tracheobronchial lymph nodes form a caseous mass which is much larger than the peripheral Ghon focus. In some adults, the reverse is the case.

In most instances, the Ghon focus undergoes healing: if small, it may be replaced completely by fibrous tissue but, if larger, the caseous centre usually persists and is converted into a hard calcified nodule, often partly ossified and enclosed in fibrous tissue: such a healed lesion is readily visible in chest radiographs. The affected hilar and tracheobronchial lymph nodes usually heal and may become heavily calcified but rarely ossified.

Progressive primary pulmonary tuberculosis. Healing of the primary tuberculous complex with a favourable outcome is usual but not invariable. Sometimes infection may spread from the Ghon focus to the pleural cavity causing *pleural effusion* or even occasionally *tuberculous empyema.** Hilar lymphadenopathy may cause bronchial obstruction by pressure and lead to segmental or lobar *consolidation or collapse*. Spread of the disease along the submucosal lymphatics of the bronchi produces a series of tubercles and sometimes ulceration of the bronchial mucosa. Involvement of the bronchial blood vessels has been said to impair the blood supply to the bronchial walls, resulting in destructive changes and subsequently *bronchiectasis*. The disease may progress to *tuberculous bronchopneumonia* or to *blood-borne* spread which gives rise to innumerable disseminated lesions in various organs (*generalised miliary tuberculosis*), to smaller numbers of disseminated foci, or to one or two metastatic foci.

Acute tuberculous bronchopneumonia can develop from the primary infection by aspiration of infected caseous material throughout the bronchial tree, either from the Ghon focus or, more commonly, from caseous lymph nodes at the hilum or in the mediastinum. In the former case, the Ghon focus continues to enlarge until eventually it incorporates a bronchus in the caseous process. Caseous material is then discharged into the lumen, from where it may be aspirated through adjacent and more distant parts of the bronchial tree. Bronchial dissemination results similarly when a caseating lesion in the hilar or mediastinal lymph nodes ulcerates into a major bronchus. The resulting tuberculous bronchopneumonia is relatively acute, and usually affects both lungs, although one is often involved more extensively than the other. The lung tissue is studded with numerous small pneumonic patches, which are arranged in groups or clusters around the terminal bronchi. The tubercle bacilli, after reaching a bronchiole, produce bronchopneumonic consolidation followed by caseation. The histological features of this condition are described on p. 177.

There may be considerable fibrinous exudate in and around the lesions, which advance too rapidly for tubercle formation or the development of granulation or fibrous tissue. As the condition progresses, the lesions may become confluent in the lower parts of the lungs, where they are most numerous. The enlarging caseous patches may also soften and discharge into bronchi, with dissemination of more mycobacteria and aggravation of the condition. The cavities resulting from discharge of caseous material have ragged caseating walls without surrounding fibrosis, and in these respects they contrast with the smooth fibrous walls of chronic tuberculous cavities. Tuberculous pleurisy usually develops in tuberculous bronchopneumonia. A small cavity opening into a bronchus may rupture also into the pleura, resulting in pneumothorax. Extensive tuberculous bronchopneumonia is associated with fever, severe debility and rapid weight loss. Unless treated early and effectively it is rapidly fatal. As stated below, acute tuberculous bronchopneumonia can occur also in patients with re-infection pulmonary tuberculosis.

Re-infection (post-primary) tuberculosis. During the primary tuberculous infection, the patient develops cell-mediated immunity to antigens of the tubercle bacillus: this is demonstrable by a positive tuberculin skin test (a delayed hypersensitivity reaction to tuberculoprotein) which is associated with increased resistance to subsequent infection.

Post-primary infection can be endogenous, resulting from re-activation of a dormant primary or post-primary lesion, or it may be exogenous, i.e. caused by organisms inhaled from the external environment. The causes of re-activation of a dormant primary lesion include malnutrition, the development of other severe illness, intercurrent lung infection, and systemic corticosteroid therapy, but in many instances, none of these factors is responsible.

The common sites for post-primary pulmonary tuberculosis are the posterior segment of the upper lobe and the apical segment of the lower lobe. The anatomical location of the lesion is attributed to the good ventilation but relatively low blood flow in these areas. The

---

* Unless there is superadded pyogenic bacterial infection, tuberculous lesions do not usually suppurate, but tuberculous lesions of the kidney, bones and pleura sometimes produce pus.

re-infection lesion results from proliferation of *Myco. tuberculosis* in the wall of a bronchiole or of an alveolus. The usual reaction takes place, with formation of tubercle follicles, and the lesion enlarges by formation of new tubercles at the margin and in the adjacent lung tissue. The infection spreads by the lymphatics, but, as it induces a delayed hypersensitivity reaction from the onset, lymphatic spread is not usually extensive, and the hilar lymph nodes are not usually affected. The developing re-infection lesion thus comes to consist of a cluster of follicles which, as they enlarge and caseate, tend to become confluent, producing one or more larger lesions. Because of the partial state of immunity which exists, progress of the lesions is slow, the tubercles are well developed and there is conspicuous formation of fibrous tissue at their periphery. The caseous material is yellowish or sometimes greyish due to inclusion of carbon pigment, which is often abundant in the fibrous tissue. If healing does not now occur, some of the nodules will spread to involve the wall of a bronchus in caseous necrosis and blockage of the lumen follows. The lesion may become encapsulated by fibrous tissue or the caseous material may be gradually discharged along the bronchus leaving a small cavity. Bronchial spread to the upper parts of other lobes and to the other lung may occur, and chronic pulmonary tuberculosis is frequently bilateral.

The cavities may coalesce and can become very large (Fig. 15.30). Even with cavitation, enlargement of the tuberculous lesions is usually slow: there is considerable overgrowth of fibrous tissue, not only around the cavities, but also in a diffusely spreading manner. In this way the lung shrinks and bronchiectasis may be superadded. Ultimately a cavity may become very large and occupy a considerable portion of the upper lobe. The walls of the chronic cavities are somewhat irregular and contain raised bands, which represent obliterated blood vessels and other structures with more resistance than the rest of the tissue. In very chronic cases the lining of the cavities may be comparatively smooth, but there is usually adherent caseous material, or there may be debris with sometimes an admixture of blood. The contents of the cavities do not usually have a putrid odour, and the organisms present along with the tubercle bacilli are chiefly pyogenic cocci. Pulmonary

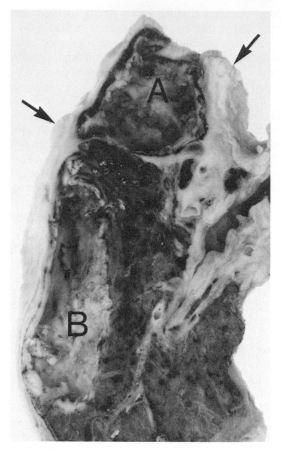

Fig. 15.30 Cavitating post-primary tuberculosis. The upper lobe of the left lung is shrunken and almost completely occupied by a tuberculous cavity with an irregular white wall (A). A similar oval cavity is situated just beneath the pleura at the apex of the lower lobe (B). There is considerable fibrous thickening of the pleura overlying the cavities (arrows).

and bronchial blood vessels involved in the wall of a cavity usually become occluded by endarteritis obliterans (p. 311). Sometimes, however, the wall of an artery may be weakened and rupture when the vessel still contains blood; this may be preceded by aneurysm formation. Serious and sometimes fatal haemorrhage results. This is to be distinguished from the coughing up of bloodstained sputum, or the slight bleeding which commonly occurs from small vessels in the wall of a cavity.

If at any time there should occur a rapid diffusion of large numbers of bacilli by the air passages, as may happen when a caseous focus suddenly discharges into a bronchus, the patient's resistance may be overcome and acute rapidly spreading tuberculous broncho-pneumonia supervenes. It is not uncommon to find the latter in the lower parts of the lungs, while chronic cavity formation is present in the upper lobes. This is likely to occur if the patient is debilitated by intercurrent disease such as influenza or diabetes, or by overwork, malnutrition and unfavourable environmental conditions.

In patients dying from chronic pulmonary tuberculosis, and particularly when there has been breakdown of resistance and extensive bronchopneumonia, blood dissemination with acute miliary tuberculosis may occur, but this is much less common than in primary tuberculosis in young children.

Tuberculous ulcers may develop in the intestine from infection by bacilli in swallowed sputum (p. 575). Tuberculosis of the larynx (p. 383), likewise produced by direct infection from the sputum, is a serious complication.

Secondary amyloidosis is a common complication of chronic tuberculosis.

The effects of specific chemotherapy. The above account refers essentially to the disease unmodified by chemotherapy. The general changes produced in tuberculous lesions by streptomycin alone and in combination with ethambutol and isoniazid have been discussed on p. 180. In pulmonary tuberculosis, combined therapy is imperative in order to render the patient non-infective and to reduce quickly the risk of producing antibiotic-resistant strains. If adequately carried out in the early stages of the apical lesion, chemotherapy leads to rapid healing with minimal fibrosis. In excavated lesions, the caseous lining disappears and is replaced by a layer of vascular granulation tissue which, in turn, is converted to a thin smooth fibrous layer, over which an epithelial lining may eventually grow, leaving a persistent cavity which may or may not communicate with a bronchus. The epithelial lining is rarely complete except in very small lesions. If small, fibrocaseous lesions may be almost completely absorbed; if larger, they may become hyalinised and acellular with a thin fibrous capsule. In favourable cases even actively caseating bronchopneumonia may cease to progress, the caseous material becoming liquefied and absorbed or discharged. The cavities become walled off by granulation tissue, which eventually becomes fibrosed and re-lined to some extent by epithelium. A notable feature is the lack of the dense fibrosis which characterises healing under natural conditions. Large open cavities may become epithelialised and inactive, but since there is always a danger of subsequent aspergillosis, secondary pyogenic infection and re-activation, surgical removal is frequently performed. Patches of active disease may persist for long periods and tubercle bacilli may be isolated from such resected cavities despite long-continued chemotherapy, so that it is advisable to regard the disease process as arrested, rather than cured, by specific therapy. The naked-eye appearance of the treated lesions is an unreliable guide to the bacteriological state. Infection also commonly persists in lesions healing naturally, i.e. without chemotherapy.

Generalised miliary tuberculosis. The pulmonary lesions in this condition are part of an acute

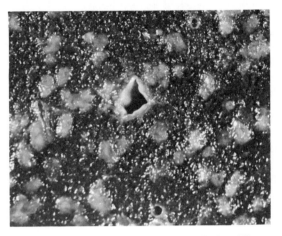

Fig. 15.31 Acute miliary tuberculosis. The cut surface of the lung shows numerous discrete grey tubercles. × 5.

generalised tuberculosis, which occurs when a considerable number of mycobacteria gain entrance to the bloodstream. The ways by which this is brought about have already been considered (p. 179). In miliary tuberculosis, lesions are usually more numerous in the lungs than in any other organ. They consist of grey tubercles which may be too small to be visible by the naked eye or up to 3 mm in diameter (Fig. 15.31). Commonly, they are more numerous and rather larger in the upper lobes than in the lower.

Microscopically the early tubercles are seen to be in the peribronchial connective tissue, fibrous septa, and in the alveolar walls but they enlarge by consolidation of the surrounding alveoli. Necrosis then occurs in the centre of the tubercle. In very acute cases the tubercle follicles are poorly formed and giant cells are virtually absent. In miliary tuberculosis there is no cavitation of the lesions, and *Myco. tuberculosis* is rarely found in the sputum.

The pleura in pulmonary tuberculosis. At a very early stage of localised lung disease, tubercles may form in the visceral pleura, and this may be followed by an extensive effusion into the affected pleural sac. Tuberculosis is a frequent cause of the apparently idiopathic pleurisy of young adults. The fluid is usually clear and the cells in it are scanty and mainly lymphocytes. A large proportion of desquamated mesothelial cells, as is seen in the centrifuged deposit of the serous transudate of cardiac failure, strongly contra-indicates tuberculosis. In many cases tubercle bacilli cannot be found. Sometimes the exudate is serofibrinous and there may be some admixture of blood. The lesion usually resolves and the fluid is absorbed, leaving only scanty adhesions to mark its previous existence. In chronic tuberculous lung lesions there is fibrous thickening and adhesion of the overlying pleural layers, and in long-standing cases this may be pronounced. Owing to such adhesions, perforation of an underlying cavity into the pleural sac is uncommon. As mentioned on p. 423, pulmonary tuberculosis sometimes causes empyema, and secondary pyogenic infection cannot always be incriminated.

Sarcoidosis

Sarcoidosis is a systemic disease of unknown aetiology in which non-caseating epithelioid cell follicles are scattered throughout several organs. The general features of the condition are described on pp. 182–3.

The lungs are involved more frequently than any other organ. In Europe the commonest presentation of the disease is an abnormal routine chest radiograph. The four following patterns of radiological abnormality can be distinguished. (1) Hilar node enlargement with normal lung fields (38%). (2) Hilar node enlargement with pulmonary infiltration (50%). (3) Pulmonary infiltration without hilar node enlargement (7%). (4) Pulmonary fibrosis with honeycomb lung (5%).

In most cases the patients have no physical disability and the radiological changes regress within two to three years. About 13% of patients develop chronic progressive pulmonary sarcoidosis, which is frequently associated with crippling dyspnoea, respiratory failure and pulmonary hypertension. Right ventricular failure may also ensue. About half the patients with chronic progressive pulmonary sarcoidosis die within ten to fifteen years of the disease being recognised.

Pathological examination of the lungs at an early stage of the disease reveals typical non-caseating epithelioid cell granulomas in the alveolar walls and fibrous septa. These lesions usually heal with minimal fibrosis. If the disease becomes progressive with extensive involvement of the lung, an interstitial fibrosis develops which leads eventually to honeycomb change (p. 431): in this late stage, no trace of the original sarcoid granulomas can usually be found.

Syphilis

Pulmonary syphilis occurs in congenital and acquired forms, both of which are extremely rare in most medically advanced countries. The majority of infants with *congenital* pulmonary syphilitic lesions are stillborn. The lungs are enlarged, pale and firm due to diffuse fibrosis of the alveolar septa and peribronchial and perivascular tissue. The interstitial fibrous tissue is diffusely infiltrated by lymphocytes and plasma cells and contains abundant *Treponema pallidum* which can be demonstrated by silver impregnation methods such as Levaditi's stain. In *acquired* syphilis, gummas may rarely develop in the lung.

Actinomycosis and nocardiosis

Actinomycosis is caused by *Actinomyces israelii* (p. 187) which produces a chronic granulomatous reaction with pus formation. About 20% of actinomycotic infections involve the lungs and thorax. Pulmonary actinomycosis may be primary or secondary, the latter usually resulting from the spread of disease from below the diaphragm, particularly from the liver. About 75% of pulmonary cases are primary and the disease commonly occurs in the lower lobes, where it forms a dense fibrotic lesion honeycombed with small abscess cavities. The pus contains 'sulphur granules' which are colonies of *Actinomyces israelii*.

Nocardia asteroides is an aerobic, branching filamentous organism similar in some respects to *Actinomyces israelii*. The lungs are involved in about 60% of cases of nocardiosis. The incidence of infection appears to be increasing, and to be associated with diseases or therapy that impair the patient's immune mechanisms. At necropsy the lungs show a suppurative pneumonia that may be lobular in distribution. The organism does not form colonies, but occurs as branching filaments which are not stained with haematoxylin and eosin. It is Gram +ve and appears black using the silver methenamine stain.

Fungal infections

Most pulmonary fungal infections are *opportunistic*, arising as a result of breakdown in cellular and humoral defence mechanisms (p. 140), and from the sustained use of antibiotics, which may so alter the normal human bacterial flora that fungi which are normally non-pathogenic may grow and invade the tissues. Until recent years, many of the pulmonary fungal diseases (mycoses) were little known and constituted an unimportant group of conditions. However, since the introduction of the therapeutic immunosuppressive agents and antibiotics, the importance of fungal diseases has changed dramatically

The pulmonary mycoses usually encountered in Britain are aspergillosis, candidiasis and cryptococcosis, but increasing foreign travel has also brought occasional cases of histoplasmosis, coccidioidomycosis and blastomycosis from overseas

Aspergillosis. This is the commonest pulmonary mycosis in the British Isles and it is usually due to infection by *Aspergillus fumigatus*. The hyphae are 3–4 μm in diameter, show frequent transverse septa, and exhibit dichotomous branching at acute angles (Fig. 15.32). It may give rise to four types of lung disease in man. Firstly, atopic subjects may develop reaginic antibodies to antigenic constituents of *Aspergillus*, and as a result suffer from attacks of *bronchial asthma* following heavy exposure to the spores. Secondly, some patients develop precipitating antibodies, and on further exposure to the spores may have attacks of *extrinsic allergic alveolitis* (p. 440). Thirdly, *Aspergillus* can colonise tuberculous or bronchiectatic cavities in the lung producing a rounded mass of fungus (*mycetoma*) with a characteristic

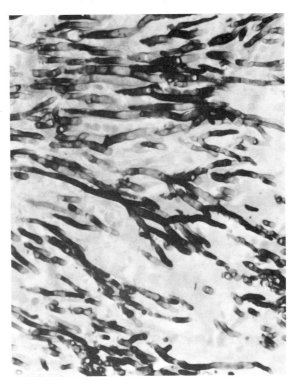

Fig. 15.32 Invasive pulmonary aspergillosis. The hyphae of *Aspergillus fumigatus* show frequent transverse septa and exhibit dichotomous branching at acute angles. From a patient who received cytotoxic therapy for Hodgkin's disease. Silver methenamine stain. × 375.

radiographic appearance. The chest radiograph shows an opaque spherical mass which almost completely fills the cavity, leaving a crescentic 'halo' of air between the mycelial mass and cavity wall. Fourthly, in immunosuppressed patients, and in patients with Hodgkin's disease or leukaemia, aspergillus infection may produce nodules of *haemorrhagic consolidation and necrosis* scattered throughout the lungs. Such consolidated areas contain ramifying hyphae of *Aspergillus fumigatus* which may invade pulmonary arteries and veins leading to thrombosis and metastatic foci in other organs.

Candidiasis. *Candida albicans* (p. 189) is a normal commensal in the pharynx, where it can give rise to the lesion of *thrush*. Bronchopulmonary infection with *Candida* is rare, occurring as a result of severe underlying disease, immunological deficiency, or because of long-term treatment with antibiotic or corticosteroid drugs. Sometimes the trachea and bronchi are lined by a mass of fungus and sections show hyphae growing down through the mucosa. The lungs may show pneumonic consolidation with areas of necrosis and infiltration by neutrophil polymorphs.

Cryptococcosis (torulosis). *Cryptococcus neoformans* (p. 190) tends to cause disease in patients whose resistance to infection is diminished by leukaemia, Hodgkin's disease or by systemic corticosteroid therapy. Although rare, the incidence of infection is increasing. The most usual presentation is a meningo-encephalitis, but respiratory tract infection can occur with the production of an atypical pneumonia. At necropsy, the lungs contain firm rubbery areas of consolidation which are devoid of necrosis but show a mucoid cut surface.

Pulmonary fibrosis

Pulmonary fibrosis is a result or complication of many of the diseases described in this chapter. Localised fibrosis, for example, may result from organisation of acute pneumonias, from tuberculosis, and inhalation of silica. More diffuse fibrosis may result from chronic interstitial oedema and haemorrhage secondary to pulmonary hypertension complicating mitral stenosis or chronic left ventricular failure. Chronic diffuse pulmonary fibrosis may be caused by inhalation of toxic dusts or fumes, by certain connective tissue diseases, ionising radiation, sarcoidosis and as an adverse reaction to certain drugs.

This section includes accounts of diffuse alveolar fibrosis, so-called honeycomb lung, and the effects of various drugs and chemicals which cause pulmonary changes, including fibrosis.

Before proceeding, however, it seems appropriate to give a brief account of the major features of the alveolar lining cells, or pneumocytes. Although the elucidation of the functions of these cells is still at an early stage, sufficient is known to indicate that they are of importance in the reaction of lungs to various forms of injury, including those which result in fibrosis.

Alveolar lining cells (pneumocytes)

The alveolar walls consist of a meshwork of capillaries covered in the main by the ultrathin cytoplasmic extensions of **membranous (type I) pneumocytes**. These extensions have a large area but possess few organelles so that they are probably metabolically dependent upon the central perinuclear portion of the cells which lie in the corners and angles of alveoli. This may explain why membranous pneumocytes are vulnerable to a variety of injuries. They appear to be involved in one of two ways in pathological processes. First, they may be destroyed by toxic substances such as paraquat. This herbicide will cause membranous pneumocytes to develop a grossly cystic, oedematous cytoplasm which bulges into the alveolar space. Second, they may show intracytoplasmic micropinocytotic vesicles due to haemodynamic disturbances in the lung, e.g. in mitral stenosis or high-altitude pulmonary oedema.

In striking contrast to the relatively quiescent membranous pneumocytes are the **granular (type II) pneumocytes**, which undergo pronounced hyperplasia and shedding into the alveolar spaces in various conditions. They are interposed between the flat membranous pneumocytes and unlike them do not have squamous extensions. The basal portion of the cell is attached to the underlying basement membrane of the blood–air barrier while the free convex surface of the cell projects into the alveolar space (Fig. 15.33). This free, curved surface of the granular pneumocyte is covered by microvilli which are short, straight and fairly regular. Within the abundant cytoplasm are prominent lamellar bodies which are considered by some to be the source of pulmonary surfactant (Fig. 15.33), although others would at present attribute part or all of this substance to the bronchiolar Clara cell (p. 386). Granular pneumocytes have a much greater capacity for division and a shorter turnover time than membranous pneumocytes and probably represent the reserve cells of the alveolar lining epithelium. They proliferate and replace mem-

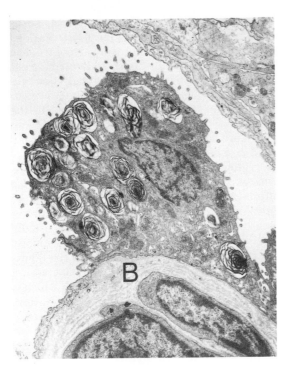

Fig. 15.33 Granular pneumocyte. The cell rests on the basement membrane (B) and projects into the alveolar space. Its surface is covered by microvilli and within its cytoplasm are lamellar bodies, considered by many to be the source of pulmonary surfactant. Electron micrograph. × 7500.

branous pneumocytes when the latter are destroyed. Thus, hyperplasia of granular pneumocytes can occur in a wide variety of circumstances and appears to be a basic mechanism of repair. Hyperplasia of granular pneumocytes assumes importance in the primary cellular and desquamative stage of fibrosing alveolitis, which subsequently proceeds to the mural stage of interstitial pulmonary fibrosis. This is considered in greater detail below.

Brush cells are common in the bronchial tree and may be demonstrated elegantly by scanning electron microscopy. They also occur rarely in the alveolar walls, where they are sometimes called **type III pneumocytes**. They are shaped like a truncated pyramid, the base being situated on the basement membrane and the tip protruding above the surrounding epithelial surface. The lateral aspects are covered by adjacent membranous or granular pneumocytes. Their most striking feature is the large regular microvilli which clothe their

relatively small free surface. These thick microvilli contain fine filaments which extend down into the cell body to the basement membrane. The ultrastructural features of the alveolar brush cell are similar to those of the chemoreceptor cell in taste buds.

Diffuse fibrosing alveolitis

This term describes a group of diseases characterised by inflammatory changes in the lung parenchyma beyond the terminal bronchioles, with two main histological features.

1. Cellular fibrous thickening of the alveolar walls.
2. Proliferation in the alveolar spaces of large cells, the nature of which is discussed below.

The relative predominance of each of these two features varies from case to case but a study of lung biopsy specimens has revealed that there appears to be an inverse relationship between the degree of alveolar wall fibrosis and

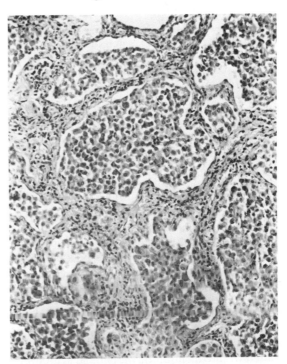

Fig. 15.34 'Desquamative interstitial pneumonia', regarded by most as an early cellular stage of fibrosing alveolitis. The alveolar spaces are filled with a mixture of macrophages and granular pneumocytes. There is only slight fibrous thickening of the alveolar walls. × 130. (From a section kindly donated by Professor D. B. Brewer.)

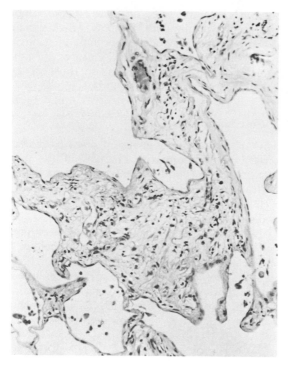

Fig. 15.35 Mural stage of fibrosing alveolitis in which the alveolar walls are greatly thickened by fibrous tissue. There are no cells in the alveolar spaces. × 130.

the number of proliferated intra-alveolar cells. Thus there is a histological spectrum ranging between a *desquamative pattern* with masses of large cells filling the alveolar spaces, accompanied by only scanty alveolar wall fibrosis (Fig. 15.34), and a *mural pattern* characterised by pronounced fibrous thickening of the alveolar walls combined with only occasional cells in the alveolar spaces (Fig. 15.35). The condition **desquamative interstitial pneumonia** is now believed by most workers to be identical to the cellular desquamative phase of diffuse fibrosing alveolitis. Electron microscopy has revealed that the proliferated alveolar cells consist mainly of granular (type II) pneumocytes, together with some macrophages. The histological pattern observed at lung biopsy seems to be unrelated to the duration of the clinical symptoms.

Diffuse fibrosing alveolitis may be associated with several types of extrapulmonary disease. Thus about one eighth of cases also have rheumatoid arthritis. Some patients with progressive systemic sclerosis develop an indolent fibrosing alveolitis of mural pattern. The prolonged administration of busulphan, hexamethonium, bleomycin or high concentrations of oxygen may induce a fibrosing alveolitis. The inhalation of cadmium fumes and excessive exposure of the lungs to ionising radiation are among other causes of this condition. However, in more than half the cases conforming to the description of diffuse fibrosing alveolitis, no cause can be found and these are commonly called *cryptogenic fibrosing alveolitis*.

Cryptogenic fibrosing alveolitis. This condition, which used to be known as *idiopathic diffuse interstitial pulmonary fibrosis* or the *Hamman-Rich syndrome*, is an uncommon disease that affects both sexes equally, usually after middle age, although it occasionally occurs in young people. The onset of the illness is usually insidious with gradually increasing dyspnoea on exertion. There is a cough which is dry or productive of scanty mucoid sputum, although occasionally there is slight haemoptysis. Clubbing of the fingers may occur. Cyanosis increased by exertion is characteristic of advanced disease. The course of the disease is variable. There is a rare subacute form which presents abruptly with fever and dyspnoea and progresses to death within a few months. In a recent published series of over 50 cases, the mean survival from the onset of the first symptom to death was four years. In most cases, the cause of death is right ventricular failure or respiratory failure precipitated by a superimposed respiratory tract infection. Recently it has become apparent that patients with fibrosing alveolitis have an increased tendency to develop bronchial carcinoma.

The aetiology of cryptogenic fibrosing alveolitis is, by definition, unknown. About one third of patients have antinuclear factor in the serum and about one third have rheumatoid factor, although only a few have both. The titres are usually low. These serum changes and the association of fibrosing alveolitis with connective tissue diseases like rheumatoid arthritis and progressive systemic sclerosis led to speculation that the pulmonary lesions have an autoimmune basis. It has been suggested that the lung disease may depend on the combination of circulating auto-antibodies and an external provoking agent, such as inhaled dust particles, or viral or bacterial infection. Since some drugs may induce fibrosing alveolitis, the possibility must be borne in mind that ingested substances, as yet unidentified, may be concerned in the causation of some cases at present classified as cryptogenic. Very rarely cryptogenic fibrosing alveolitis affects more than one member of the same family, suggesting that there can be an inherited predisposition to the disease.

Honeycomb lung describes the naked-eye appearance of an acquired condition in which a large number of small cystic spaces develop in fibrotic lungs. Honeycomb lung is the non-specific final end-stage of many disease processes of diverse aetiology including asbestosis, beryllium and cadmium intoxication, extrinsic allergic alveolitis, cryptogenic diffuse fibrosing alveolitis, sarcoidosis, rheumatoid disease, progressive systemic sclerosis and Hand-Schüller-Christian disease. The cysts are up to 1 or 2 cm in diameter, have smooth grey-white walls, and the surrounding lung is pale, firm and fibrous. The cystic change is usually most pronounced in the sub-pleural regions on the anterior borders of the upper and lower lobes (Fig. 15.36). The presence of cysts

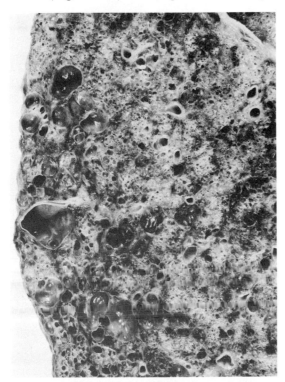

Fig. 15.36 Slice of lung showing a subpleural band of honeycomb change brought about by dilatation of terminal bronchioles. The condition is quite distinct from pulmonary emphysema.

beneath the visceral pleura gives the external surface of the lungs a nodular appearance which simulates that of the liver in macronodular cirrhosis. The essential change in honeycomb lung is obliteration by fibrosis or granuloma of some of the bronchioles and alveolar spaces with compensatory dilatation of unaffected neighbouring bronchioles. Thus the cysts are lined by columnar or cuboidal epithelium which may be ciliated or mucin-secreting. The interstitial and pericystic tissue is composed of young fibroblasts and collagen infiltrated by scanty lymphocytes, plasma cells and histiocytes. There may be an interstitial hyperplasia of smooth muscle cells probably derived from obliterated bronchioles and pulmonary blood vessels. Right ventricular hypertrophy is present in more than half the cases at necropsy. Pulmonary hypertension in honeycomb lung is attributed to a combination of chronic hypoxia, fibrous obliteration of the pulmonary vascular bed, and the development of bronchopulmonary anastomoses.

The causes of impaired gas exchange in pulmonary fibrosis are discussed in the section on respiratory failure on p. 396.

The effects of drugs and toxic compounds on the lung

A wide range of drugs and toxic compounds may give rise to clinical signs and symptoms which may resemble those of naturally occurring disease. Thus bronchial asthma may result from hypersensitivity to a wide variety of drugs, including aspirin. Some drugs, herbal substances and poisons, however, may give rise to other organic diseases in the lungs and we shall consider a few of them now.

Paraquat. This is the widely used weed-killer, 1,1-dimethyl-4, 4-bipyridylium chloride. When ingested, it may produce ulceration of the mouth within two days. Acute renal failure may result from tubular injury, but renal function usually returns, sometimes with the help of haemodialysis. The most serious effect of paraquat, however, is on the lung. Within hours of ingestion there is an initial destructive effect on the alveolar epithelium. The membranous pneumocytes become swollen and vacuolated and project into the alveolar spaces. The granular pneumocytes also show vacuolation of their lamellar bodies and disruption of their endoplasmic reticulum. Two days after administration of paraquat, many alveolar walls are denuded of their epithelial lining and there is commonly pulmonary oedema and the formation of hyaline membranes. This destructive phase is followed by a proliferative phase.

Three days after a single injection of paraquat into rats, mononuclear cells are found in the alveolar spaces. They resemble macrophages, but mature into fibroblasts (Fig. 15.37)

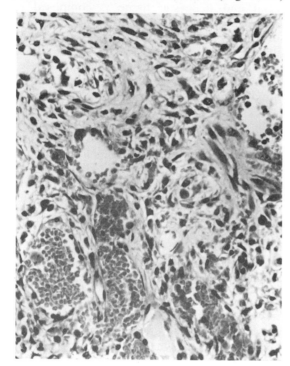

Fig. 15.37 Lung of a rat ten days after an intraperitoneal injection of paraquat. The lung architecture is obliterated by a dense mass of fibroblasts and small quantities of collagen. × 330.

and accordingly may be termed profibroblasts. They form collagen in the alveolar spaces and thus paraquat produces intra-alveolar rather than interstitial fibrosis. There may be some associated dilatation of respiratory bronchioles. Paraquat appears to kill plants by entering the chloroplasts and then taking part in an oxidation-reduction cycle in which hydrogen peroxide is liberated. A similar type of catalytic activity may occur in animal tissue, in which a small concentration of paraquat can lead to the synthesis of a high concentration of toxic by-products.

Busulphan. This drug is widely used in the treatment of chronic myeloid leukaemia. It can cause damage to the lung parenchyma which, unlike the intra-alveolar fibrosis following ingestion of paraquat, progresses to true interstitial fibrosis. Patients receiving up to 1 g of the drug over a period of up to two years may become dyspnoeic and develop crepitations in the lungs. Chest radiographs show peri-hilar infiltrates and subsequently diffuse mottling throughout both lungs. Lung function tests often show considerable impairment of oxygen diffusion. At necropsy there is a striking proliferation of granular pneumocytes, many of which disintegrate to produce intra-alveolar debris. There is associated interstitial pulmonary fibrosis. Electron microscopy confirms that the desquamated alveolar cells are granular pneumocytes with characteristic lamellar bodies which break down to form phospholipid myelin figures and lattices (Fig. 15.38). Busulphan

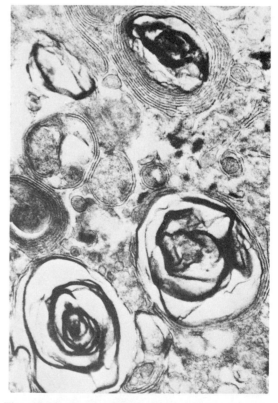

Fig. 15.38 Electron micrograph of intra-alveolar debris from a case of busulphan lung occurring in a man of 61 years who received a prolonged course of the drug for chronic myeloid leukaemia. The apparently amorphous debris is seen to consist of lamellar bodies and myelin figures. × 28 000.

causes pulmonary fibrosis in only a minority of patients receiving it, usually those on a heavy and prolonged dosage. It is a valuable drug in the palliation of chronic myeloid leukaemia and there is no case for withholding its use because it may give rise to pulmonary fibrosis. Pulmonary fibrosis may also occur as a result of administration of bleomycin, salazopyrin, hexamethonium and methotrexate.

Pyrrolizidine alkaloids and anorexigens. Addition of the seeds or foliage of certain plant species of *Crotalaria* or *Senecio* to the diet of rats, causes pulmonary hypertension and associated vascular disease of the lungs, and death from right ventricular failure in one to two months. The plants in question are *Crotalaria spectabilis*, a cover crop grown in the United States, *Crotalaria fulva*, used to prepare bush-tea in Jamaica and a cause of veno-occlusive disease of the liver, and *Senecio jacobaea*, the common 'ragwort' of British hedgerows. The effects of these plants are due to the pyrrolizidine alkaloids they contain.

A recent epidemic of primary pulmonary hypertension in Germany, Switzerland and Austria has been ascribed to the anorexigen, aminorex fumarate. There is as yet no proof of the association, as hypertensive pulmonary vascular disease has not been produced in laboratory animals fed on the drug. An anorexigen available in Britain, chlorphentermine hydrochloride, induces the accumulation of large numbers of prominent foamy macrophages in the alveolar spaces of rats. After prolonged administration of the drug to this species the pulmonary histiocytosis does not progress to interstitial fibrosis but ends in disintegration of the cells to produce a picture mimicking alveolar proteinosis. The alveoli become packed with lamellar bodies and phospholipid lattices.

Pulmonary oxygen toxicity. One of the commonest therapeutic agents used in intensive treatment units is oxygen. The prolonged use of high concentrations of inspired oxygen can cause lung damage which may be irreversible and is potentially fatal. There is controversy as to the concentration of oxygen and the length of administration necessary to produce lung injury. Examples of pulmonary damage have been described in patients who breathed 40% oxygen at atmospheric pressure for several days. There are conflicting views on the possible protective effect of pre-existing cyanosis with hypoxia on the lungs of patients receiving oxygen. The initial damage in pulmonary oxygen poisoning seems to be an increased permeability, followed by disintegration, of capillary endothelial cells and alveolar epithelium. The alveoli become filled with oedema fluid, fibrinous exudate and extravasated blood. Hyaline membranes line the alveolar walls. If the patient survives, there may be replacement of the intra-alveolar exudate by fibroblastic tissue which becomes incorporated into the alveolar walls. The thickened alveolar walls become lined by proliferated granular pneumocytes. It is of interest to note that some of the changes induced in the lung by oxygen toxicity are similar to those produced by the weed-killer, paraquat.

Pneumoconiosis and industrial lung diseases

Pneumoconiosis is a comprehensive term covering a group of lung diseases resulting from the inhalation of dust. This group of conditions grows continuously as fresh industrial hazards are created. The type of lung disease varies according to the nature of the inhaled dust. Some dusts are apparently inert and cause little or no damage, whereas others may cause widespread lung destruction and fibrosis. Certain dusts are antigenic and cause damage through immunological reactions, while others may predispose to tuberculosis or to neoplasia. The factors which determine the extent of damage caused by an inhaled dust include its physical state, its chemical composition, its concentration, the duration of exposure, and the co-existence of other lung diseases.

The size of the inhaled dust particles is of great importance as it is this factor which largely determines whether particles will reach the alveoli and whether they will adhere to the alveolar wall. Particle size is also important in determining whether dust will penetrate the thin alveolar epithelium or remain within the alveolar lumen. Practically all inhaled non-filamentous particles of more than 10 μm diameter are trapped in the nasopharynx, trachea and major bronchi, from where they are swept upwards, entangled in mucus, by the action of cilia. Many inhaled particles of 5 μm diameter gain access to the alveolar spaces, where they tend to collect in the lower halves of the upper lobes, the upper halves of the lower lobes, and the right middle lobe.

When particles measuring from 0·5 to 5 μm reach the alveolar walls, they adhere to the surface film of fluid and within minutes are ingested by macrophages. Ultra-fine particles, less than 0·02 μm in diameter, rapidly penetrate the alveolar epithelium. Coarse filamentous particles 30–60 μm in length, such as asbestos fibres, can reach the alveoli, but they tend to slip down and lodge in the larger bronchi and the resulting lesions are found mainly in the lower lobes of the lungs.

The pneumoconioses may be classified according to whether the dusts inhaled are inorganic or organic.

Inorganic dusts

The principal varieties are anthracosis, coal worker's pneumoconiosis, silicosis and asbestosis.

Anthracosis

This is a pneumoconiosis caused by the inhalation of atmospheric soot particles: it is found to a greater or lesser extent in all adults, and is more marked in those who live in the highly polluted atmosphere of large industrial cities. Most of the inhaled carbon particles are dealt with by the normal pulmonary mechanisms for ridding the lungs of dust and are expectorated, but some are engulfed by macrophages and retained within the relatively immobile alveoli adjacent to bronchioles, blood vessels, fibrous septa, beneath the pleura and at the edges of lung scars. Some soot particles reach the lymphatic channels of the lung and are carried to the hilar lymph nodes. Thus anthracosis is the innocuous, well-known blackening seen in virtually every adult lung at necropsy.

Coal-worker's pneumoconiosis

This condition is due to the inhalation of coal dust and occurs in persons who handle soft bituminous coal, either in mines or by shovelling it in large quantities, as in the holds of ships. It occurs in two forms or stages: *simple coal worker's pneumoconiosis* in which the lungs become impregnated with dust, leading to a minor degree of fibrosis and causing few if any symptoms; and *progressive massive fibrosis (complicated pneumoconiosis)* which develops in a small proportion of patients with simple pneumoconiosis.

Simple coal worker's pneumoconiosis. This is due to the inhalation of coal dust particles measuring less than 5 μm in diameter. Silicosis is not involved. The inhaled dust is fairly evenly distributed within the lungs but maximal changes occur in the upper two thirds of each lung. The particles are ingested by macrophages which are then carried to the alveolar spaces surrounding the respiratory bronchioles. These dust-laden macrophages tend to be retained and adhere to the relatively immobile walls of the peribronchiolar alveoli in the centres of the lobules. Thus the respiratory bronchioles become surrounded by a sleeve of alveoli which are consolidated due to the accumulation of dust-laden phagocytes. The phagocytes eventually die and a network of fine collagen fibres develops in between the liberated dust particles; the aggregates also become covered by alveolar epithelial cells and thus incorporated into the alveolar walls. The upper two thirds of an affected lung contain numerous black, firm, spidery nodules and streaks measuring a few millimetres in diameter which produce a radiographic appearance known as *dust reticulation*. After several years there is fibrous obliteration of the peribronchiolar alveoli and atrophy of bronchiolar smooth muscle. The collagenous tissue then shrinks but the lung as a whole is not reduced in size, because the respiratory bronchioles dilate to produce *focal dust emphysema*, characterised by abnormal clusters of dust-blackened centrilobular airspaces (Figs. 15.39 and 15.21, p. 409).

Simple pneumoconiosis may be seen in the chest radiographs of coal workers who are free from symptoms. It appears to have no adverse effect on pulmonary function and does not significantly alter life expectancy. Coincidental chronic bronchitis in such patients may, however, cause great concern in men who are aware that their chest radiograph is abnormal.

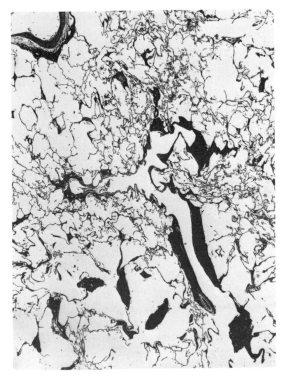

Fig. 15.39 Simple coal worker's pneumoconiosis. Focal dust emphysema showing the localisation of dust accumulation in the walls of the second order of respiratory bronchioles. × 7.

Progressive massive fibrosis. After 10 to 20 years at the coal face a small proportion of workers with simple pneumoconiosis may develop massive confluent areas of fibrosis in one or both upper lobes, which may ultimately involve an entire lobe. Irregular masses of jet-black rubbery fibrous tissue with well-defined margins are present in the affected lobe, which is commonly adherent to the chest wall (Fig. 15.40). Sometimes the fibrous tissue contains cavities filled with black fluid resembling India ink. These cavities result either from tuberculous infection or ischaemic necrosis consequent upon fibrous obliteration of branches of the pulmonary artery in the affected lobe. Histological examination shows that the fibrous lesions are composed almost entirely of dense collagenous tissue arranged in bundles. Between the bundles are collections of coal dust

and scattered lymphocytes. There has been considerable debate about the nature of progressive massive fibrosis and the factors which promote its development in a small proportion of cases of simple pneumoconiosis. Concomitant silicosis does not appear to be a factor. Careful examination of the lungs at necropsy, including culture and guinea-pig innoculation, yields evidence of tuberculous infection in about 40%

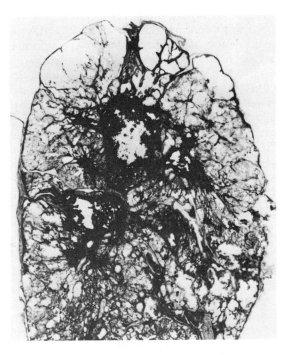

Fig. 15.40 Thick section of the lung of a coalminer, showing very severe emphysema and two foci of progressive massive fibrosis, seen as solid black areas with, in this instance, central cavitation. × 0·5.

of cases, and many people accept that concomitant tuberculosis leads to the development of massive fibrosis in workers with simple pneumoconiosis. Progressive massive fibrosis is a serious and incapacitating disease. It may develop after exposure to coal dust has ended, and nothing can be done to halt its course once it is established; eventually death results from respiratory failure, tuberculosis or right ventricular failure secondary to pulmonary hypertension. The pulmonary hypertension is probably due to a combination of chronic hypoxia and fibrous obliteration of a significant proportion of the pulmonary vascular bed.

Caplan's syndrome (rheumatoid pneumoconiosis)

This is characterised by rounded nodules, up to 5 cm in diameter, scattered fairly evenly throughout the lungs of workers who are exposed to inhaled dusts, including coal dust, silica and asbestos. Rheumatoid arthritis is usually present but occasionally the nodules develop several years before the arthritic manifestations. Rheumatoid factor is present in the blood. Cavitation and calcification of the nodules is common and clinically they may be mistaken for tuberculosis, bronchial carcinoma and secondary carcinoma. Not all patients with rheumatoid disease and pneumoconiosis develop Caplan's syndrome. The central parts of the nodules show concentric black and pale yellow rings, the pale zones frequently being liquefied. Histologically, the lesions are modified rheumatoid nodules with a central zone of dust-laden fibrinoid necrosis, separated by a cleft from an outer layer of palisaded fibroblasts and mononuclear cells.

Silicosis

The changes of silicosis are seen in the lungs of workers who inhale fine particles of silica (SiO_2) for many years. Silica and silicosis have a world-wide distribution. Wherever rock is cut, as in granite, sandstone and slate quarries or in the mining of coal, gold, tin or copper, silica dust is likely to fill the air. In the case of coal, it is the hard anthracite variety which is accompanied by significant quantities of silica. Other workers also face the hazard, particularly stonemasons, sandblasters, boiler scalers and those involved in glass and pottery manufacture. Inhaled particles of less than 5 μm in diameter are liable to cause silicosis: they reach the alveoli, where they are phagocytosed by macrophages which tend to congregate in the relatively immobile alveolar spaces adjacent to respiratory bronchioles, blood vessels, fibrous interlobular septa, and beneath the pleura. The characteristic lesions therefore develop in these sites. Silica induces production of relatively acellular collagenous fibrous tissue which is often hyaline and arranged in a concentric laminated fashion (Fig. 15.41). These silicotic nodules measure up to 5 mm in diameter and are pathognomonic of the disease. The fine silica particles are birefringent and are readily

detected within the fibrous nodules on examination by polarising microscopy. The fibrosis obliterates the lumen of bronchioles and pulmonary blood vessels. As nodules increase in size beneath the pleura, adhesions form and in advanced cases the pleural cavity may be

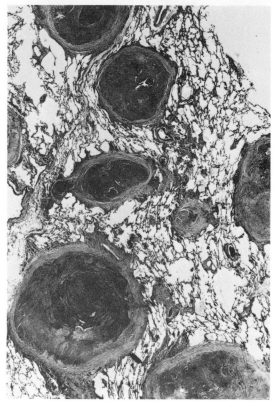

Fig. 15.41 Silicosis. The lung contains multiple nodules consisting of laminated fibrous tissue. There is no inflammatory cellular infiltrate. × 7.

obliterated. At necropsy the pleura is thickened and adherent and the lungs feel gritty on cutting and palpation due to the presence of innumerable discrete fibrous nodules. Some of these may coalesce to form large confluent masses of fibrous tissue. In a severe case the lungs may be largely solid. The silicotic nodules are well circumscribed and greyish-black in colour. Silica dust is carried to the hilar lymph nodes, which become enlarged, fibrous and nodular.

The cause of lung fibrosis in silicosis is uncertain. The solubility theory postulated that silica particles slowly dissolve to form silicic acid, which in turn stimulates fibrogenesis: this has become unacceptable because there is no relation between the severity of fibrosis and the solubility of different forms of silica. Two alternative but unproven biological theories are that silica is antigenic and provokes fibrosis through an immunological mechanism, and that collagen formation is stimulated by the release of phospholipid from dead silica-laden macrophages.

Silicosis leads to progressive respiratory impairment, although twenty years exposure may have occurred before symptoms appear. Death may be due to respiratory failure. Progressive fibrous obliteration of the pulmonary vasculature, together with chronic hypoxia, may induce pulmonary hypertension with the development of right ventricular hypertrophy and eventual failure. There appears to be a synergism between silica and tuberculosis and the reported incidence of tuberculosis in patients with silicosis varies between 10 and 75%. Tuberculosis tends to progress rapidly in silicotic patients and may terminate in tuberculous bronchopneumonia and miliary tuberculosis. It may also lead to the development of progressive massive fibrosis.

The effects of asbestos

Asbestos is a general term embracing a number of complicated fibrous silicates of magnesium of differing chemical composition and morphology. It is imported into Britain mainly from mines in South Africa and Canada. The three types of asbestos which are most important commercially are *chrysotile* (white asbestos), *crocidolite* (blue asbestos) and *amosite* (brown asbestos) which is rich in iron. Chrysotile consists of soft, curly pliable fibres which tend to split progressively into finer fibrils. Amosite and crocidolite fibres are in general rigid and harsh even when fine. The physical properties of the fibres determine the industrial use of various types of asbestos, and to some extent the depth to which they travel along the airways during inspiration and thus perhaps their differing pathological effects. The behaviour of inhaled particles is determined by their aerodynamic properties as well as their size. Chrysotile fibres are apparently more likely to be retained higher up the small airways, particularly at bifurcations, while the rigid fibres of crocidolite and amosite travel

readily in the airstream and so reach the periphery of the lung. It has been suggested that these properties may explain why chrysotile has rarely been associated with pleural mesothelioma (see below) though often with asbestosis. All forms of asbestos are fire-resistant and are good acoustic and thermal insulators. Chrysotile can be spun into yarn and incorporated into textiles. Crocidolite and amosite are noted for their resistance to acids and alkalis. Large amounts of asbestos (mostly chrysotile) are used in asbestos-cement products for corrugated roofing, pipes, gutters, chimneys and tiles. Chrysotile is also used in the manufacture of floor tiles, brake linings, clutch facings, plastics, paint, and in asbestos-paper products including engine gaskets, roofing felts and wall coverings. Both crocidolite and chrysotile have been used for pipe and boiler lagging and as a spray with synthetic resins for thermal and acoustic insulation of buildings and ships.

Occupational exposure to asbestos occurs to a small extent in miners who obtain the mineral but is potentially high in the crushing and extraction processes which follow. Bagging of the fibre used to be a dusty process and before the introduction of modern methods and leak-proof bags, dockers and warehouse personnel were exposed to hazard. The asbestos textile and insulation industries have produced the highest incidence of asbestosis. There is little risk associated with cutting, sawing and trimming asbestos-cement products because the fibres are trapped within the cement matrix. In Britain, rigorous standards came into force in May 1970. The most stringent rules apply to crocidolite because of its association with mesothelioma; the use of this fibre has latterly been discouraged and much reduced in many countries.

Exposure to asbestos dust may be associated with the development of the following lesions: *pleural fibrous plaques, asbestosis* and *mesothelioma of the pleura or peritoneum*. Mesothelioma is considered on p. 447.

Pleural fibrous plaques. These are distinct from the fibrous thickening of the visceral pleura which accompanies asbestosis, in that they are located in the parietal pleura on the posterolateral aspects of the lower chest wall, mainly over the ribs, and on the diaphragm. They are bilateral, well-circumscribed, irregularly-shaped areas of hyaline fibrosis. The surface may be nodular, or smooth and polished resembling articular cartilage. Histologically the plaques consist of hyaline acellular collagenous lamellae. Extensive foci of calcification may be present. Asbestos bodies (see below) are not found in the plaques but may be detected in the lungs. Calcified parietal pleural plaques may be visible in chest radiographs but they do not produce symptoms and are free from complications. At present there is no evidence that pleural plaque formation is a precursor of malignant mesothelioma.

Asbestosis. This term means fibrosis of the lungs due to inhaled asbestos dust (Fig. 15.42).

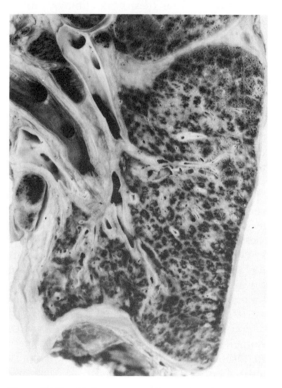

Fig. 15.42 Pulmonary asbestosis showing pronounced fibrosis and shrinkage of the lower lobe and gross pleural thickening. × 3/4.

It is specific and excludes pleural fibrous plaques and mesothelioma. Chrysotile, crocidolite and amosite are all capable of producing pulmonary fibrosis, though of differing degrees of severity, probably due to differences in their penetration and retention in the lungs as a result of their aerodynamic and physical properties. The most important factors in the development of asbestosis are the concentra-

tion of dust to which an individual is exposed and the duration of exposure. Heavy exposure for a few years and exposure to fairly low concentrations over many years are equally likely to result in asbestosis. As will be seen later, this contrasts with the exposure levels associated with the development of malignant mesothelioma. The chief symptom of asbestosis is dyspnoea on effort and this usually takes more than ten years to develop. Occasionally the onset of symptoms may be delayed up to even forty years after exposure.

Inhaled asbestos fibres (50 μm long and 0·5 μm in diameter) are mostly retained in the respiratory bronchioles of the lower lobes. In time a number of them pass into the alveolar ducts and spaces. Experimental evidence suggests that short fibres or fragments less than 10 μm long are engulfed by macrophages, whereas larger fibres cannot be properly ingested but become surrounded by macrophages. In time, the asbestos fibres become coated with endogenous iron and mucopolysaccharide to produce the characteristic **asbestos body** (Fig. 15.43). When well formed, these are long (50 μm), golden-yellow or brown structures consisting of an asbestos fibre coated with layers of iron-containing protein which gives the prussian blue reaction for ferric iron (p. 241). The proteinaceous coat is usually segmented along the length of the fibre and bulbous at its ends, producing a 'dumb-bell' or 'drumstick' appearance. It should be emphasised that the finding of asbestos bodies in the sputum or lung is only an indication of past exposure to asbestos and is *not* proof of the presence of disease due to asbestos. Asbestos bodies have been found in the lungs of 20 to 60% of otherwise normal urban dwellers with no known industrial exposure to asbestos. There is a tendency for these bodies to fragment. The mechanism by which asbestos causes pulmonary fibrosis is not understood. It has been suggested that macrophages which have ingested asbestos may release a fibrogenic substance. Immunological factors may play a part: this is suggested by the finding of a high prevalence of circulating antinuclear antibody (25%) and rheumatoid factor (23%) in cases of asbestosis. Fibrosis is first evident around respiratory bronchioles and then spreads to involve alveolar ducts, atria and alveolar walls. There is progressive obliteration of alveolar

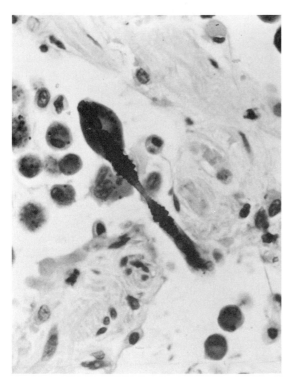

Fig. 15.43 Asbestos body. The proteinaceous coat is segmented along the length of the fibre. Its upper extremity appears to lie within the cytoplasm of an alveolar macrophage. The adjacent alveolar walls are thickened. × 600.

spaces with compensatory dilatation of unaffected bronchioles which may progress to honeycomb lung. Asbestos bodies are found free in alveolar spaces and also enmeshed in fibrous tissue. The disease commences in the sub-pleural region of the lower lobes and then progresses inwards and upwards so that eventually the middle lobe and lower parts of the upper lobes may be affected.

Patients with asbestosis may develop respiratory failure and also secondary pulmonary hypertension, which may in turn lead to right ventricular hypertrophy and failure. Asbestosis does not predispose to pulmonary tuberculosis.

Asbestosis is the only form of pneumoconiosis with a high risk of bronchial carcinoma. Approximately half of British male asbestos workers with asbestosis die of bronchial carcinoma, which arises in the vicinity of the fibrosis and is, therefore, most commonly found in the lower lobe. The neoplasm may be of any cell type but it is usually an adenocarcinoma. There is no evidence that an excess of bronchial carcinoma is related to asbestos exposure in the absence of asbestosis.

Other inorganic dust diseases

Pulmonary siderosis. This occurs in silver polishers (who use rouge containing iron oxide), arc-welders and haematite miners. Iron oxide itself appears to be almost innocuous, and does not cause fibrosis or chest symptoms, but frequently in the case of haematite miners a quantity of silica accompanies it. The result is a modified silicosis. The haematite lung is rusty brown and may be extensively fibrosed. Macroscopically, free haematite pigment is brownish-yellow and does not give a prussian blue reaction: after ingestion by macrophages, however, it reacts positively.

Berylliosis. This affects workers who extract beryllium from ores or who handle it in industry, as in the making of alloys. Heavy concentrations of dust produce an acute chemical pneumonitis. Prolonged exposure, such as formerly occurred in the fluorescent lighting industry, induces a chronic granulomatous reaction histologically similar to sarcoidosis, and sometimes with similar lesions in the liver and other organs. The pulmonary lesions progress to generalised fibrosis and sometimes honeycomb lung.

Cadmium fumes, in high concentration, cause an acute pneumonitis with hyaline membranes and a proliferation of alveolar cells. This condition may progress to pulmonary fibrosis and honeycomb lung. Pulmonary emphysema has been described in the lungs of workers chronically exposed to cadmium fumes. The risk from cadmium arises during the manufacture of alloys for use in the electrical industry and nuclear reactors, and in the cutting of scrap metal by welders.

Aluminium is a rare cause of pulmonary fibrosis among workers in the fireworks industry.

Tin causes a simple pneumoconiosis (stannosis) without fibrosis or functional disability.

Other metals encountered in industry may be very harmful and, when inhaled as fine dust or fumes, may cause an acute chemical pneumonitis. These include manganese, osmium, vanadium and zinc.

Organic dusts

Inhaled organic dusts may affect the bronchi, as in the case of byssinosis, or produce an *extrinsic allergic alveolitis*.

Byssinosis. This is an occupational disease of

extrinsic allergic alveolitis. Their symptoms and pathological manifestations are similar but their origins diverse. The individual diseases are generally recognised by names descriptive of their occupational or antigenic origin (Table 15.3). The inhaled organic material may be

Table 15.3 Examples of extrinsic allergic alveolitis

Disease	Occupation	Dust Exposure	Circulating Precipitating Antibodies Against
Farmer's lung	Dairy farmers, cattle breeders	Mouldy hay	Thermophilic actinomycetes, usually *Micropolyspora faeni*
Bagassosis	Manufacture of paper and cardboard from sugar-cane bagasse	Mouldy sugar-cane bagasse	Thermophilic actinomycetes, usually *Micropolyspora faeni*
Mushroom worker's lung	Cultivation of mushrooms	Mushroom compost dust	Mushroom spores and/or *Micropolyspora faeni*
Maple-bark stripper's disease	Maple-bark stripping	Mouldy maple bark	*Cryptostroma corticale*
Suberosis	Cork workers	Mouldy oak-bark and cork dust	Mouldy cork dust
Malt worker's lung	Distillery or brewery workers	Mouldy barley, malt dust	*Aspergillus fumigatus*
Bird fancier's lung	Pigeon breeders, parrot and budgerigar fanciers, chicken farmers	Pigeon, parrot, budgerigar and hen droppings	Serum proteins and droppings
Pituitary snuff-taker's lung	Patients with diabetes insipidus	Porcine and bovine pituitary powder	Serum proteins and pituitary antigens

the cotton, flax and hemp industries. The illness comes on after many years of exposure. The early stage is the typical syndrome of 'Monday Fever': following the weekend break, the worker returns to the dusty atmosphere and after a few hours develops a characteristic tightness of the chest with a cough productive of scanty sputum. The symptoms persist during the day but regress for the remainder of the week. As time goes by, the symptoms persist for longer and finally progress to permanent dyspnoea with cough and sputum, and there may be severe disability. Respiratory failure, pulmonary hypertension and right ventricular failure occur in the late stages of the disease. The pathogenesis is uncertain. Byssinosis is *not* associated with pulmonary fibrosis and at necropsy the lungs show the features of chronic bronchitis.

Extrinsic allergic alveolitis. In addition to their causal role in asthma, inhaled organic dusts can induce in the alveoli an Arthus (type III) reaction (p. 123) in which circulating precipitating antibodies react with inhaled antigen. The clinical syndromes produced by this latter reaction are known collectively as

antigenic moulds, bird droppings, fungus in dead wood or heterologous pituitary powder. The clinical features consist of acute episodes of fever, headache and malaise with cough, dyspnoea and basal pulmonary crepitations, arising 4 or 5 hours after exposure to dust and persisting for 24 hours. There is seldom opportunity to examine the lung tissue during the acute stage of the Arthus reaction, with polymorphonuclear infiltration, acute exudation, etc. Subsequently, the alveolar walls are thickened by an infiltrate of lymphocytes, plasma cells and mononuclear cells and by sarcoid-like granulomas. Repeated exposure, as commonly occurs with bird fanciers, is associated with chronic ill health, weight loss, etc, rather than acute episodes, and leads to the development of a diffuse interstitial fibrosis which may progress to honeycomb lung. Of all the forms of extrinsic allergic alveolitis so far known, the most acute and severe is *farmer's lung* (which also occurs in cows). However, new sources of environmental contamination are constantly being found, and consequently new types of the disease emerge every year.

The Pleura

Pleural effusions

The passage of fluid in and out of capillaries is mainly dependent upon a balance between the colloid osmotic pressure exerted by the plasma proteins and the hydrostatic pressure within the capillary lumen (p. 38). In the systemic circulation the averages of these two forces in capillaries and venules are normally approximately equal. In the pulmonary circulation, however, the intracapillary hydrostatic pressure is only about one-third of that in the systemic capillaries, so that it is normally exceeded by the colloid osmotic pressure. The pleural surface is an interface between the pulmonary and systemic circulations. There is a pressure gradient from the interstitial tissue beneath the parietal pleura to the pulmonary interstitial tissue beneath the visceral pleura, producing a net absorptive force of about 13 mm Hg into the visceral pleura. The continuous removal of fluid from the pleural cavity into the visceral pleura creates a sucking force which normally maintains the two pleural surfaces in apposition.

Causes. Pleural effusions can be caused by diseases which interfere with the mechanisms that maintain the normal balance of entry and removal of water, electrolytes and protein into and out of the pleural cavity. The following are the more important causes.

Increased intracapillary pressure may cause a pleural effusion in patients with either left or right ventricular heart failure or an increased blood volume.

Increased capillary permeability is responsible for effusions complicating pleural inflammation which may be due to pneumonia, pulmonary tuberculosis, pulmonary infarction, connective tissue diseases, bronchial carcinoma, mesothelioma, subphrenic abscess and acute pancreatitis.

Hypoproteinaemia may cause pleural effusions in patients with the nephrotic syndrome or cirrhosis of the liver.

Impaired lymphatic drainage of the lung may occur in lymphangitic carcinomatosis and in neoplasms involving the hilum of the lung.

As with oedema fluid in general, pleural effusions may be rich in plasma proteins when they are due to increased capillary permeability, i.e. **inflammatory exudates**, or of low protein content when due to haemodynamic or osmotic disturbances or lymphatic obstruction, i.e. **transudates**. As elsewhere, inflammatory exudates may be serous, serofibrinous, purulent or haemorrhagic. A haemorrhagic exudate should always raise the suspicion of tuberculosis, neoplastic infiltration or pulmonary infarction.

Empyema or pyothorax is a collection of purulent exudate or pus in a pleural cavity. It may be due to infection of the pleura from the lung or occasionally from penetrating injuries of the chest wall. Less commonly infection of the pleura may arise from the bloodstream or through the diaphragm from abdominal disease such as a subphrenic abscess. In lung abscess, bronchiectasis and bronchial cancer, infection of the lung may extend into the pleural cavity and cause empyema. A post-pneumonic lung abscess may discharge both into a bronchus and into the pleural cavity, resulting in a broncho-pleural fistula and **pyopneumothorax**. Empyema may also result from perforation of the oesophagus and mediastinitis, and may arise as a complication of thoracic surgery. A large empyema compresses the lung, which becomes collapsed against the side of the vertebral column: a layer of granulation tissue then forms on the pleural surfaces and matures to dense fibrous tissue. This is followed by fibrosis in the collapsed lung. These changes prevent the proper expansion of the lung and hence it is of great importance that pus in the pleural cavity should be evacuated without undue delay. If the empyema is small, its contents may be absorbed or changed into inspissated material. Great pleural thickening, sometimes followed by calcification, is apt to occur.

Haemothorax is a collection of blood in a pleural cavity. It may be due to trauma to the chest wall and lung, or result from rupture of an aortic aneurysm. The pleural cavity may be distended with fluid and clotted blood, with associated compression-collapse of the ipsilateral lung.

Chylothorax is the accumulation of an opalescent creamy fluid in the pleural cavity due to obstruction of, or injury to, the thoracic duct. Obstruction is commonly due to pressure exerted by enlarged mediastinal lymph nodes, while trauma may be accidental or a complication of thoracic surgery. The fluid is an emulsion of fat globules which separate into an upper fatty layer on standing. It is odourless and alkaline, can be cleared by adding fat solvents, and stained with dyes such as sudan III.

Pleural fibrosis

This condition, often with pleural adhesions, and sometimes with obliteration of the cavity, may follow acute pleurisy, or may be the result of chronic pulmonary lesions such as silicosis and tuberculosis, as already described. The presence of some pleural adhesions is common after middle adult life. Hyaline fibrous plaques may develop on the diaphragmatic and posterior costal portions of the parietal pleura in persons exposed to asbestos.

Pneumothorax

Pneumothorax is the presence of air in a pleural cavity. It causes the lung on that side to collapse to an extent depending on the volume of air admitted. Pneumothorax may be therapeutic or traumatic, or it may arise spontaneously due to the escape of air from the lung through a hole in the visceral pleura. Traumatic pneumothorax may be due to a penetrating injury of the chest wall or it may occur accidentally during the withdrawal of pleural fluid.

Primary spontaneous pneumothorax occurs in the absence of any clinical evidence of underlying disease, most commonly in young males between the ages of 20 and 40 years. In some cases it is recurrent and rarely bilateral. Occasionally thoracotomy has revealed a tear in the visceral pleura at the site of attachment of a fibrous adhesion. The association of spontaneous pneumothorax with the Ehlers-Danlos syndrome and Marfan's syndrome (p. 335) is attributed to the rupture of gas-filled cystic spaces beneath the visceral pleura, formed as a result of the inherited defect of connective tissue.

Secondary spontaneous pneumothorax occurs in patients who have evidence of underlying lung disease—most commonly emphysema or active pulmonary tuberculosis. Other causes include sarcoidosis, honeycomb lung, pneumoconiosis, bronchial asthma, lung abscess, bronchiectasis and bronchial carcinoma.

Once rupture of the lung surface has occurred, air continues to escape into the pleural cavity until the pressure gradient reaches zero or until the aperture is sealed by collapsing lung tissue. Occasionally, a valve-like mechanism occurs so that air enters the pleural cavity during inspiration but cannot escape during expiration: the pressure within the affected pleural cavity then steadily increases to produce a *tension pneumothorax* leading to mediastinal shift and compression also of the opposite lung. In uncomplicated cases, air in the pleural cavity is gradually absorbed, a 50% pneumothorax taking about six weeks to re-expand fully. Possible complications include pleural effusion, haemorrhage and infection.

Tumours of the Bronchi, Lungs and Pleura

Benign tumours

The so-called *chondroma* or *adenochondroma* of the lung forms an ovoid mass largely composed of cartilage. It usually presents as a chance finding on radiological examination as a discrete rounded shadow which requires surgical intervention to exclude a bronchial carcinoma. These tumours consist almost entirely of mature cartilage with clefts lined by flattened or respiratory type epithelium and with collections of adipose and fibrous tissue (Fig. 15.44). They are best regarded as hamartomas. The so-called *bronchial adenomas* are described in the following section on malignant tumours.

Fibromas and *lipomas* occur in the lung but they are very rare.

Malignant tumours

Bronchial carcinoma

This is the commonest primary tumour of the lung. At the turn of the century it was seen

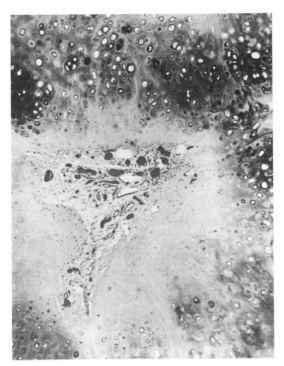

Fig. 15.44 Section of a cartilaginous hamartoma ('adenochondroma') of lung. The bulk of the lesion consists of cartilage but small epithelium lined spaces are present. × 50.

infrequently but since that time it has become a major health problem in most parts of the world. The reports of the Registrar-General for England and Wales show a rise in the number of deaths registered as due to cancer of the lung from 6500 in 1944 to over 30 000 in 1969. Bronchial carcinoma is considerably commoner in men than women. Like other carcinomas, the incidence increases with age, but it is now not exceptional for it to cause the death of young men in their thirties.

Aetiology. There is now little doubt that the most important factor in this dramatic rise in the incidence of bronchial carcinoma is the habit of **smoking, particularly cigarettes**. There is good statistical evidence that the risk increases proportionately to the consumption of cigarettes and inversely to the length of the cigarette stub left. The smoking of cigars appears to be safer and the smoking of pipes safer still, although here the risk of carcinoma of the tongue is apparently increased. In spite of reports from the World Health Organisation and the Royal College of Physicians on the relationship between cigarette smoking and bronchial carcinoma, this lethal habit still maintains a grip on modern society. The risks have been clearly indicated by retrospective statistical studies and confirmed in a prospective study of the causes of death of medical practitioners. In this country, the habitual smoking of 25 cigarettes or more a day over a period of years is associated with a 12% risk of dying from bronchial carcinoma. The mode of action of cigarette smoke is uncertain. There is about 1 μg of 3:4 benzpyrene in the smoke of 100 cigarettes. This is not much (see below) and it is by no means certain that benzpyrene is the only carcinogen involved; it may be more important that the tar from cigarette smoke has been found to be a powerful co-carcinogen. Accordingly, the relationship of bronchial carcinoma with smoking may represent the summation of the effects of a number of different substances, including carcinogens and co-carcinogens.

Another important source of smoke, apart from tobacco, is **atmospheric pollution**. Statistical evidence shows that bronchial carcinoma is commoner in towns than in rural districts and that its incidence is closely correlated with the degree of atmospheric pollution. It is commonest in large towns with an atmosphere heavily polluted by industrial and domestic smoke and by the fumes from internal combustion engines. The carcinogenic agents liberated in the combustion of coal include benzpyrene and arsenic and the concentration of the former in the air of large towns, up to 5 μg per 100 cubic metres of air, is such that under normal weather conditions about 0·5 μg may be inhaled in 12 hours. The amount is greater in winter than in summer and may be increased almost tenfold in foggy weather.

There are much rarer but established causes of bronchial carcinoma. Thus workers in the chromate industry have an abnormally high death rate from bronchial carcinoma. Other industrial workers at risk are those engaged in nickel refining, workers with asbestos and haematite miners. A much quoted example of industrial lung cancer, now of little practical importance, is that of the workers in the Schneeberg cobalt mines in Saxony. It is almost certain that radioactive substances were concerned. In these miners, as in cigarette smokers, the tumours were largely of oat-cell and squamous type.

Naked-eye appearances. Bronchial carcinoma presents a variety of appearances depending upon the site of origin, the extent of local spread, and the degree of bronchial obstruction produced.

Hilar type. Usually the tumour forms a mass surrounding the main bronchus to the lung or

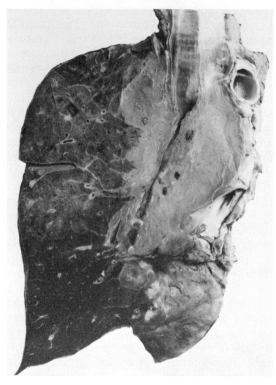

Fig. 15.45 Bronchial carcinoma showing pronounced obstruction of the bronchus from which it has arisen. There is pneumonic consolidation and abscess formation in the lower lobe resulting from the retention of secretions. × 2/5.

to one lobe (Fig. 15.45). The bronchial mucosa may be ulcerated or may be merely roughened and nodular. Lymphatic spread often produces further nodules in the mucosa towards the bifurcation of the trachea. The carcinoma narrows the lumen of the affected bronchus, causing obstruction. Retention of secretions then occurs and is followed by infection with consequent bronchopneumonia and abscess formation. The tumour soon spreads by the lymphatics, giving rise to massive metastases in the mediastinal nodes, which are often so incorporated with the bronchial mass as to be indis-

tinguishable separately. Extension upwards into the lymph nodes of the neck is often seen. Retrograde spread also occurs along the peribronchial and perivascular lymphatics so that even the smaller bronchi and vessels may be ensheathed by whitish collars of tumour. Permeation of lymphatics just beneath the visceral pleura produces a delicate white lacework pattern, visible on the external surface of the lung (*'lymphangitic carcinomatosis'*). Invasion of the pericardial sac occurs by direct extension along the lymphatics around the walls of the pulmonary veins and the carcinoma may compress and occlude the superior vena cava, causing marked cyanosis. Infiltration of the heart is sometimes obvious on gross examination, and on careful histological examination of necropsy material it is found to be frequent.

Peripheral type. Less frequently the tumour originates from a peripheral bronchus and sometimes apparently arises in such a small bronchus that the exact site of origin is uncertain. Some workers claim to recognise a form

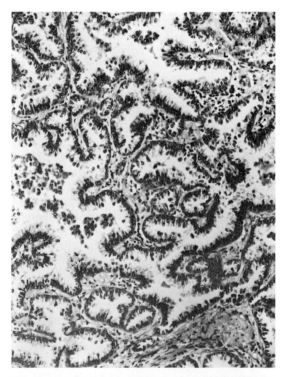

Fig. 15.46 Pulmonary adenomatosis. The alveolar walls are lined by tall columnar neoplastic cells. × 125. (From a section kindly loaned by Dr. F. Whitwell.)

arising in the pulmonary alveoli. However, the histological appearances are deceptive and both carcinomas of unequivocally bronchial origin and metastatic tumours may use the alveolar walls as a convenient stroma and thus simulate an alveolar origin. Tumours behaving thus are usually, but not invariably, mucus-secreting adenocarcinomas and they may produce consolidation of large areas of the lung resembling pneumonia, the cut surface presenting a greyish, mucoid appearance. A variant of this neoplasm appears to arise in the respiratory bronchioles and may spread by way of the air passages producing a characteristic type of pulmonary invasion to which the name *pulmonary alveolar adenomatosis* has been applied (Fig. 15.46).

The spread of lung cancer. The early and widespread invasion of the lymphatics has been emphasised and this may involve the pleura, forming a thick ensheathment of the surfaces or taking the form of multiple discrete nodules. Pleurisy with effusion, often haemorrhagic in character, is common. When the tumour is at the apex of the lung, extension to the adjacent thoracic cage may involve the lower cords of the brachial plexus and the sympathetic chain, so that pain and sensory disturbances occur. This is the so-called *'Pancoast's syndrome'*. Owing to the peripheral situation of the lung cancer, symptoms and signs referable to the lung may appear only late in the disease.

Metastases. Metastases are widespread and may involve virtually any organ in the body. Spread may occur to the lymph nodes of the neck, axilla or groin, before the primary tumour presents localising signs. Ipsilateral spread to the adrenals is common and this favours the lymphatics rather than the bloodstream as the route of spread. The kidneys, with a much larger arterial supply, are less often involved by metastases. Ipsilateral spread also tends to predominate in the liver and kidneys.

There is a special tendency to the formation of secondary tumours in the brain, which may overshadow the primary bronchial tumour clinically. Surgical exploration for a cerebral neoplasm should always be preceded by a careful survey of the lungs to exclude primary bronchial carcinoma. Metastases in the bones are common, the thoracic vertebrae being especially frequently involved, possibly by the retrograde venous route. It should be kept in mind that widespread metastasis may have occurred from a small and clinically silent bronchial carcinoma. Even at necropsy the primary tumour of lung may be very difficult to find.

Associated clinical phenomena. Bronchial carcinoma is sometimes associated with neuropathy and myopathy mediated by humoral factors of the tumour. Cushing's syndrome with adrenal cortical hyperplasia is due to secretion of ACTH by the tumour, which is almost always of the oat cell type. Other rare systemic effects of bronchial carcinoma are the carcinoid syndrome, hypercalcaemia, hyponatraemia, encephalopathies, neuropathies, hypertrophic osteoarthropathy and gynaecomastia. Migrating phlebitis and gross lymphoedema may also occur and may cause the initial symptoms.

Histological types. There are four main histological types of bronchial carcinoma. They are the squamous cell carcinoma, oat cell carcinoma, adenocarcinoma and undifferentiated carcinoma. The structure may be mixed. Thus there may be gland-like structures in the oat cell type and some degree of squamous metaplasia in the adenocarcinoma. Squamous cell, oat cell,

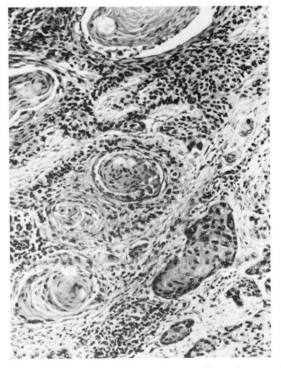

Fig. 15.47 Keratinising squamous cell carcinoma of bronchus with well-developed cell nests. × 130. (From a section kindly loaned by Dr. F. Whitwell.)

and anaplastic carcinomas comprise over 90% of bronchial cancers in countries where the incidence is high, and are the histological forms related to the smoking of cigarettes. Their increased frequency accounts for the striking male predominance of bronchial carcinoma.

Squamous cell carcinoma is the most common form of bronchial cancer (Fig. 15.47), and presents macroscopically as a dense whitish hilar mass, often with a flaky surface. It arises from bronchial epithelium which has undergone squamous metaplasia, areas of which are frequently seen in the bronchial mucosa of cigarette smokers and patients with chronic bronchitis.

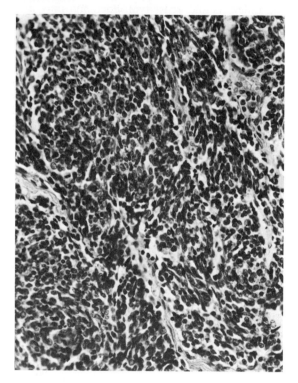

Fig. 15.48 Oat cell carcinoma of bronchus. This neoplasm is composed of small, uniform, darkly-staining ovoid cells, with scanty supporting stroma. × 115.

Oat cell carcinoma. (Fig. 15.48) commonly arises near the hilum of the lung. The cells are very short darkly-staining spindle cells and may appear oval or round, depending upon the plane of section. They are usually arranged in solid masses or anastomosing trabeculae. These tumours were formerly confused with lympho-

sarcoma but are now recognised as being of epithelial origin. On electron microscopy the tumour cells are found to contain neurosecretory granules and it has been postulated that oat cell carcinomas are derived from argyrophilic cells ('apud' cells—p. 967) in the bronchial mucosa. Perhaps this is why most endocrine syndromes caused by lung cancer are associated with the oat cell variety.

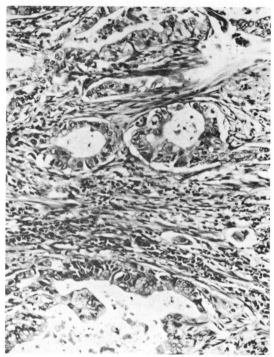

Fig. 15.49 Adenocarcinoma of bronchus. The neoplasm is composed of columnar cells which form acini situated in a dense fibrous stroma. × 130. (From a section kindly loaned by Dr. F. Whitwell.)

Adenocarcinoma. (Fig. 15.49) is the least common of the four main types and is composed of cubical or columnar cells which are usually mucus-secreting in places. Sometimes the tumour has a distinctly papillary structure or it may be more scirrhous. Adenocarcinomas account for 5–10% of primary lung cancers and more than half arise in the more peripheral intrapulmonary sites. It is not possible to distinguish an adenocarcinoma from the other types merely by its site and naked-eye appearance. In striking contrast to the other types, adenocarcinoma occurs with equal frequency in the two sexes.

'Bronchial adenoma'

This term should mean a benign glandular proliferation of bronchial epithelium. However, in practice it is used to designate a group of slowly growing malignant tumours which not uncommonly metastasise to regional lymph nodes and other organs such as the liver. A disturbing feature is that it is not possible to predict their prognosis on the basis of their histological appearance. 'Bronchial adenomas' form some 3 to 10% of surgically excised tumours of the lung and they occur most commonly in people under the age of 40 years and with equal frequency in the sexes. Macroscopically the tumour forms a 'dumb-bell' lesion, intraluminal growth being connected by a relatively narrow neck to invasive growth in the adjacent lung tissue. Endoscopic resection is therefore not practicable. The tumour usually causes partial bronchial obstruction, with bronchiectasis and sometimes haemoptysis. Histologically, most 'bronchial adenomas' resemble the carcinoid tumours of the alimentary canal. They rarely show the argentaffin reaction but occasionally give rise to the carcinoid syndrome (p. 590) and excretion of 5-hydroxy-indole-acetic acid in the urine. On electron microscopy, they show characteristic intracytoplasmic secretory vesicles (Fig. 15.50). The remaining adenomas show a glandular histological pattern rather like tumours of the salivary glands: this suggests that they arise from the bronchial submucosal glands. These glandular variants are designated cribriform (adenoid cystic) and muco-epidermoid carcinomas.

Secondary tumours in the lung

The lung is the great filter of the bloodstream so it is not surprising that a wide variety of tumours may give rise to pulmonary metastases. Sarcomas of all types show frequent metastasis to the lung by the bloodstream. Spread of carcinoma to the lungs is also common both by the lymphatics and by the bloodstream. **Spread by lymphatics** is common in breast carcinoma, the tumour cells of which may spread to the pleural lymphatics and thence to the lungs. Abdominal carcinomas may spread to hilar lymph nodes and thus extend into the lung. When the lymphatics of the lung are involved, lymphangitis

carcinomatosa may be visible to the naked eye (p. 382). Lymphosarcoma may involve the bronchial lymph nodes, primarily or secondarily, and show a tendency to extend along peribronchial lymphatics, forming an encasing sheath to the bronchi. Some **blood-borne metastases** may be very large. Such is the case with the 'cannon-ball' metastases which may originate from a renal carcinoma or from testicular tumours.

Pleural mesothelioma

Until recently this neoplasm was considered to be very rare. In 1960 a relation was noted between mesothelioma and occupational and environmental exposure to asbestos in South Africa. Since then the number of recorded pleural and peritoneal mesotheliomas has been steadily increasing in many countries. Only about 10 to 15% of the cases recorded in Britain appear to be unrelated to asbestos. On the other hand the incidence of the tumour in people with industrial exposure to asbestos is very low. In cases of pleural mesothelioma, the amount of asbestos inhaled has usually been low and the duration of exposure short, amounting to 1 or 2 months. The latent period which elapses between exposure to asbestos and the development of mesothelioma is very long, usually more than 20 years and sometimes more than 40. Because of this long delay an increasing number of mesotheliomas can be expected to occur until well into the twenty-first century. The fibre type which has been most associated with mesothelioma is crocidolite. The source of exposure has usually been occupational but cases have occurred in people exposed to air pollution in the vicinity of asbestos mines and factories. The tumour affects both the visceral and parietal layers of the pleura, leading to the formation of a scabbard-like mass of grey-white tissue 0·5 to 3 cm in thickness, which obliterates the pleural cavity, ensheaths and compresses the lung, and extends into the interlobar fissures. Areas of necrosis within the tumour give rise to large cystic spaces containing mucinous fluid. The histological picture presents a variable pattern with either carcinomatous or sarcomatous features or a mixture of the two. The carcinomatous pattern usually consists of tubular and papillary structures in a loose stroma. The sarcomatous pattern consists of spindle

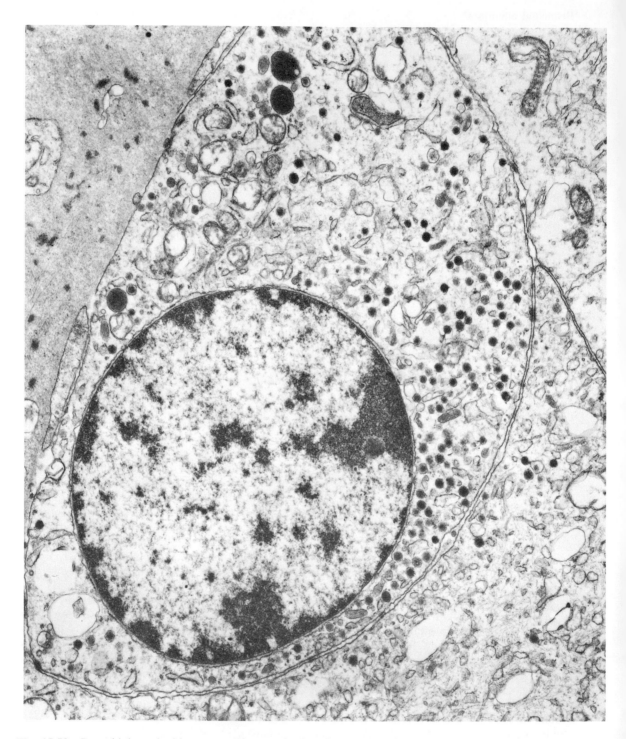

Fig. 15.50 Bronchial carcinoid tumour. The neoplastic cell contains a large round nucleus and numerous small electron-dense neurosecretory granules. × 18 750. (Dr. W. Taylor.)

cells. Asbestos bodies are seen in the lungs but not in the mesothelioma tumour tissue. The neoplasm is thought to be derived from the mesothelial lining of the pleura. Metastasis to hilar and abdominal lymph nodes is fairly common. A few years ago it was believed that distant metastasis did not occur: recent studies have, however, shown that secondary deposits can arise in the contralateral lung, liver, thyroid, adrenals, bone, skeletal muscle and brain.

Congenital anomalies

Unilateral **agenesis** of a lung does not in itself endanger life but other serious malformations often accompany it. Sometimes one lobe or an entire lung may be **hypoplastic**. It is not uncommon to find an excessive or diminished number of lobes in a lung and this rarely has an effect on pulmonary function. A **sequestered pulmonary segment** is one which is totally or partially separated from the normal lung. It is usually intralobar but an extralobar variety also occurs. Intralobar sequestration is observed in young adults in whom a large mass is found, usually in the lower lobe of the left lung. The sequestrated lobe does not communicate with the bronchial tree and is supplied with blood from an artery which arises from the aorta above or below the diaphragm. In extralobar sequestration, which is usually encountered in infancy, the lesion is usually basal and on the left side either in the pleural cavity or within the substance of the diaphragm. It is covered by its own pleura and does not communicate with the bronchial tree. Its arterial blood supply is derived from the aorta and its veins drain into the azygos system. Rarely, a sequestration of either variety is served by a bronchus growing directly out of the oesophagus or gastric fundus.

Congenital cysts occur and may or may not communicate with the bronchial tree. In older children and adults, congenital pulmonary cysts may be so altered by inflammation and fibrosis that distinction from acquired bronchiectasis and honeycomb lung may be difficult. Cysts arising near the hilum of the lung may be bronchial or derived from the foregut. The former are lined by bronchial epithelium and their walls contain cartilage, smooth muscle and bronchial glands. Some bronchial cysts may arise near to or within the wall of the oesophagus. Enterogenous cysts derived from the foregut are lined by gastric or intestinal epithelium. Multiple small cysts in the periphery of the lung may be congenital anomalies of the distal bronchi or may be derivatives of the visceral pleura. Multiple lung cysts may be present in patients with Marfan's syndrome.

Congenital cystic adenomatoid malformation is a rare form of diffuse hamartoma usually found in the lungs of premature or stillborn infants. The lesion is generally confined to one lobe which is greatly enlarged to form a firm, white fibrous mass containing small cysts. There is commonly mediastinal displacement to the opposite side and compression of normal lung. Microscopically, the hamartoma consists of an intercommunicating mass of tubules and spaces resembling fetal bronchioles and alveoli. Mucous glands and cartilage may be present.

16

The Blood and Bone Marrow

Introduction

This chapter is concerned with abnormalities of the red cells, leukocytes and platelets of the blood. All of these cellular elements are produced in the haemopoietic bone marrow, and very commonly changes in the blood reflect abnormalities of cell production in the bone marrow. It is also important to appreciate that, while the cells of the blood and their precursors are subject to their own, apparently intrinsic abnormalities, more often than not quantitative and qualitative abnormalities of the cells of the blood and marrow are the result of pathological changes elsewhere. An obvious example is the leukocytosis accompanying pyogenic infection, but the connection between the primary disease and the blood changes may sometimes be so obscure that the haematological abnormality may be mistakenly regarded as the primary pathology. Severe anaemia is, for instance, observed in some forms of renal failure, while the opposite condition, polycythaemia, may sometimes result from a renal tumour or cyst.

Disorders of lymphocytes are considered mainly in the following chapter on the lymphoid tissues, and in Chapter 5, but lymphoid leukaemia is included with other forms of leukaemia in this chapter. Similarly, abnormalities of the plasma and its constituents are dealt with in the appropriate chapters, but tumour-like proliferations of plasma cells, which involve especially the bone marrow and often result in a very high level of plasma immunoglobulins, are described in this chapter.

Development of the cells of the blood

Haemopoietic stem cells appear first in the embryonic yolk sac and subsequently in the primitive blood and fetal liver; in the adult, this stem cell population is maintained in the haemopoietic marrow, and from it the supply of red cells, granulocytes and platelets is provided by proliferation and differentiation. Also, stem cells pass into the blood and supply the thymus and probably other lymphoid tissues, where they differentiate into lymphoid cells. The primitive stem cell is pluripotent in being capable of giving rise to unipotent precursors of red cells, granulocytes,* and platelets. These cells are in a sense end products; they are incapable of further multiplication in the blood-stream, although both erythrocytes and leukocytes undergo some maturation after having entered the circulation.

The evidence for a pluripotential stem cell is based largely on experiments in which mice exposed to a dose of whole-body x-irradiation sufficient to destroy their own haemopoietic cells are then injected with relatively small numbers of normal haemopoietic cells from a donor mouse. Some of the donor cells settle in the spleen and marrow and produce clones in the form of discrete colonies, each of which consists initially of cells which differentiate in one direction, i.e. towards production of red cells, granulocytes or platelets. If the cells obtained from a single colony (i.e. the descendants of one stem cell) are injected into a second irradiated mouse, colonies of all three types are formed from stem cells in the donor colony. These findings have been interpreted as indicating that the mouse haemopoietic stem cell is pluripotent and that the direction in which it differentiates is influenced by the micro-environment provided by the tissue in which it settles. The effect of the micro-environmental factors is to produce progenitor cells of restricted potential.

The case for a single totipotential stem cell in man is supported by the finding of the abnormal 22 Philadelphia chromosome in the red cell and megakaryocyte series as well as in the leukaemic cells of chronic myeloid leukaemia.

---

* There is, however, evidence that the granulocyte precursor can also produce monocytes (p. 155).

These stem cells are known as *haemocytoblasts*. Normally, differentiation proceeds so rapidly that such indeterminate cells appear scanty in marrow samples and the great majority of the early progenitor cells present are recognisable as belonging to either the red or white cell series; only in abnormal conditions, when differentiation is for some reason slowed down, or the intermediate cells are being rapidly destroyed, are such primitive undifferentiated cells readily found. Since granulocytes have a much shorter lifespan in the circulation than erythrocytes, their precursors outnumber erythroblasts in the marrow in a ratio of about 3 : 1.

Erythrocyte production. The developing erythrocyte passes through successive changes

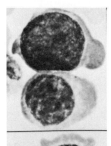
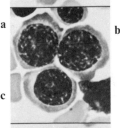
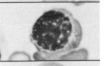
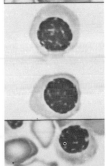

Haemocytoblast with finely dispersed chromatin and basophil cytoplasm.

Pronormoblast: basophil cytoplasm, early condensation of nuclear chromatin.

Early normoblast with basophil cytoplasm and coarse well-marked condensation of the nuclear chromatin.

A slightly later normoblast with commencing haemoglobinisation.

Three early normoblasts: **a** and **b**, polychromatophilic cells; **c**, a well-haemoglobinised normoblast at a later stage.

Late normoblast showing marked nuclear condensation.

Late normoblasts showing early pyknosis and more haemoglobinisation.

Late normoblasts—the lower showing complete pyknosis. The cytoplasm in a Leishman-stained film would still be polychromatophilic.

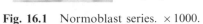
Fig. 16.1 Normoblast series. × 1000.

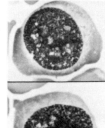
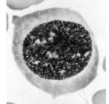
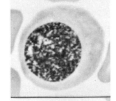
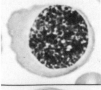
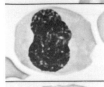
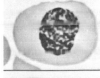
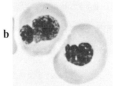

Haemocytoblast: note the basophil cytoplasm and evenly dispersed nuclear chromatin containing several nucleoli.

Promegaloblast: nucleoli persist, nuclear chromatin shows commencing fine reticular condensation, cytoplasm basophilic. Note contrast to the coarse aggregation of nuclear chromatin in the normoblast series.

Early megaloblast: nuclear chromatin is finely reticulate, cytoplasm shows diminished basophilia and early haemoglobinisation.

Polychromatophilic megaloblast with haemoglobinisation in advance of nuclear maturation.

Later polychromatophilic megaloblast.

Late megaloblast with some nuclear condensation.

Two late megaloblasts, one showing nuclear pyknosis (**a**) and the other nuclear fragmentation (**b**).

Fig. 16.2 Megaloblast series. × 1000.

which involve (1) progressive diminution in cell size; (2) progressive reduction of nuclear size with condensation of the chromatin, culminating in pyknosis and ultimate disintegration or extrusion of the nuclear remnant; (3) progressive loss of the basophil substance (RNA) of the cytoplasm and concurrent development of haemoglobin. This process of development must be seen as a continuum, although it is convenient to characterise the stages of maturation as in Fig. 16.1. This process of differentiation and proliferation appears to be under the control of *erythropoietin*, a hormone produced by the juxtaglomerular apparatus of the kidney: when erythropoietin production is acutely stimulated by hypoxia of any type, including anaemia and haemorrhage, there is a resultant increase in red cell production. Normally, only late reticulocytes and mature erythrocytes appear in the peripheral blood, but in states of erythropoietin-induced stimulation early reticulocytes and even normoblasts may enter the circulation. Megaloblasts, produced by an abnormal form of erythropoiesis, are shown in Fig. 16.2 for ease of comparison with the normal red cell precursors. Their significance will be explained later.

After release from the marrow, the normal red cell survives for about 120 days; at the end of this time the cell is phagocytosed by macrophages, and haemoglobin release and breakdown occur (p. 239). About 1% of the total red cells are destroyed and replaced each day as shown in Table 16.1.

Table 16.1 Circulating mass and turnover of red cells and iron compounds

	Circulating mass	Daily turnover
Red cells	2000 g	17 g
Haemoglobin	680 g	5·7 g
Porphyrin pigment	23 g	200 mg
Iron	2·3 g	19 mg

(Values for a normal 70 kg man)

Fig. 16.3　Megakaryocytes and platelets.

a Young megakaryocytes with commencing granulation. × 900.

b More advanced cell showing early platelet formation. × 600.

c Mature megakaryocyte with fully formed platelets. × 600.

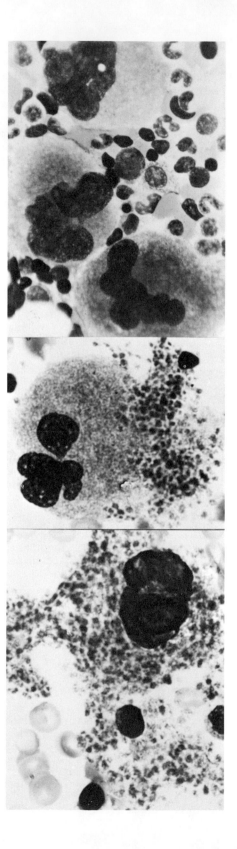

Granulocyte production. The development of granulocytes in the bone marrow has been described on p. 153, in relation to leukocytosis.

Platelet production. Platelets are produced by mature megakaryocytes in the bone marrow (Fig. 16.3) and released into the blood. The megakaryocyte arises from the haemopoietic stem cell by an unknown number of cell divisions, followed by repeated divisions of its nucleus in a common cytoplasm. Thereafter the cytoplasm fragments into platelets. There is approximately one megakaryocyte per 500 nucleated red cells in the bone marrow. It is probable that platelet production is regulated by a humoral factor, rather as erythropoiesis is regulated by erythropoietin.

Extramedullary haemopoiesis. If the bone marrow has been replaced by tumour, fibrous transformation or osteosclerosis (p. 510), blood cell formation may reappear in the primitive fetal sites. There may be extensive formation of marrow in the liver, lymph nodes and spleen, and enormous splenomegaly may result. Extramedullary haemopoiesis is often associated with the presence of primitive red and white cells in the peripheral blood (*leuko-erythroblastic reaction*) possibly indicating that in extramedullary sites there is imperfect control over the entry of immature cells into the circulation.

The blood as a whole

Blood volume. The volume of circulating blood in a normal adult male is about 5 litres; slightly lower values are found in females. There is a relationship between the blood volume and body weight, but a closer correlation is found with lean body mass. Blood volume can also be estimated from height³/body weight. Centrifuging a venous blood sample will show that about 44% of the blood consists of cellular elements (*packed cell volume* or *haematocrit value*), and the remaining 56% of plasma; this gives a rough estimate of the proportion of cells to plasma in the blood as a whole. A rise in the haematocrit value will result equally from an increase in red cell volume (*polycythaemia*) or from a decrease in plasma volume (*haemoconcentration*). Conversely, a fall in the haematocrit value may result from a reduction in red cell mass (*anaemia*) or a rise in plasma volume (*haemodilution*). Other haematological measurements dependent on concentration (e.g. red cell count, haemoglobin level) will vary in a similar way.

Specific gravity and viscosity. These are both dependent largely on the concentration of red cells and the protein content of the plasma. Important increases in specific gravity and viscosity may thus occur in polycythaemia and in conditions such as myeloma where there is a high concentration of globulin in the plasma; similar increases may be associated with very high leukocyte counts in leukaemia. This increased viscosity may slow the circulation and contribute to the thrombotic episodes sometimes found in these conditions.

Erythrocyte sedimentation rate. This is determined by placing the blood, to which anticoagulant has been added, in an upright calibrated tube and observing the rate of sedimentation of the red cells, as indicated by the length of the column of plasma after a given period of time. The range of normality depends on the details of technique, and is greater for women than men. Abnormal variations are chiefly in the direction of increased rapidity of sedimentation and are associated with increased concentrations of fibrinogen and various globulins in the plasma. The test has no specific value but has been found useful as an aid to detection of organic disease in the absence of physical signs, and notably as a prognostic aid in a particular condition, e.g. in tuberculosis or rheumatoid arthritis in which approximation of the rate to normal is taken as a favourable sign.

The Red Cell

Examination of the blood is essential in any disease affecting the haemopoietic tissues; this should include haemoglobin estimation, packed red cell volume by centrifugation in a haematocrit tube, and red cell count. From these may be derived the **absolute values** described below. Since the advent of automatic cell counters, the red cell count and also the mean red cell volume can be estimated directly, and calculations based on these measurements are now more dependable than formerly.

Haemoglobin concentration. This is usually

expressed in g/100 ml of whole blood (males 13·5–18·0; females 11·5–16·5). Various standards are available for haemoglobinometry, e.g. British Standard 3985 (1965), which defines a solution of cyanmethaemoglobin.

Packed cell volume or haematocrit. This represents the proportion of red cells as a percentage in a measured volume of whole blood. The normal range is 40–54% in men and 35–47% in women.

The absolute values

The mean corpuscular volume (MCV) (normal 76–96 fl,* average 86 fl) is given by the formula:

$$\frac{\text{volume of red cells in ml/l}}{\text{no. of red cells in millions}/\mu l}$$

As already mentioned, the MCV can now be measured directly in a cell counter.

The mean corpuscular haemoglobin (MCH) (normal 27–32 pg/cell) is given in picograms by the formula:

$$\frac{\text{grams of Hb/100 ml} \times 10}{\text{no. of millions of red cells}/\mu l\dagger}$$

This indicates the average amount of haemoglobin per red cell.

The mean corpuscular haemoglobin concentration (MCHC) (normal 32–36) gives precise information on the degree of saturation of the red cells with haemoglobin and a low result is valuable in confirming that inadequate formation of haemoglobin is a factor in the development of an anaemia. It is given by the formula:

$$\frac{\text{grams of Hb/100 ml} \times 100}{\text{packed cell volume \%}}$$

and is thus expressed as a percentage.

The main purpose in determining the absolute values is to classify states of anaemia (i.e. reductions in the haemoglobin concentration of the blood) according to the average size of the red cells and their degree of haemoglobin saturation. The terms used in such classification depend upon the appearances of the red cells in a stained blood film and the three main groups are as follows:

* The SI unit femtolitre ($= 10^{-15}$ litre).

Type of anaemia	Absolute values		
	MCV	MCHC	MCH
normochromic/normocytic	normal	normal	normal
hypochromic/microcytic	low	low	low
normochromic/macrocytic	high	normal	high

The absolute values are more reliable than the microscopic appearances of the red cells in making this classification, on which diagnosis and therapy usually depend.

Morphological changes in red cells

Changes in size and shape. Anaemia is frequently associated with variations in the size of the erythrocytes—*anisocytosis*—and irregularities in form—*poikilocytosis*. Abnormally large red cells, termed *megalocytes* or *macrocytes* (see p. 452), are numerous in pernicious anaemia and some related anaemias; in air-dried films they may measure 10–12 μm in diameter (p. 478). Although undersized cells also are present in pernicious anaemia, the *average size* of the red cells is usually greater than the normal, and the anaemia is thus termed *macrocytic*. The typical macrocytes in pernicious anaemia appear well coloured, as the MCHC is normal. Abnormally small red cells, or *microcytes*, occur in all forms of anaemia, but in certain types they preponderate so that the average size of the cells is diminished; the anaemia is then called *microcytic*.

Erythrocytes of irregular shape and usually small, known as *poikilocytes*, may occur in any severe anaemia (Fig. 16.25, p. 478). While their presence is of no absolute diagnostic importance, they are usually a striking feature in pernicious anaemia and may appear even before the anaemia is pronounced. In certain disorders of small blood vessels, e.g. micro-angiopathic haemolytic anaemia (Fig. 16.24, p. 477), triangular helmet-shaped or *burr cells* may be numerous in the circulation; these irregularly contracted cells result from mechanical damage in the abnormal vessels, and are frequently found along with obvious red cell fragments (*schistocytes*).

Another pathological variation is that the erythrocytes may be thicker than normal while their diameter is reduced and their volume is unchanged. They thus tend towards a globular

† 4·5–6·5 × $10^6/\mu l$ depending on age and sex.

shape and the term *spherocytosis* is applied. Characteristically this is associated with red cell membrane damage and haemolysis (p. 467). Other morphological abnormalities are associated with inborn abnormalities of haemoglobin structure, e.g. (*a*) the sickle form assumed by de-oxygenated cells containing Hb-S (p. 469), (*b*) the abnormally thin cells which sometimes have a central area of thickening (*target cells*) found in thalassaemia and other haemoglobinopathies (p. 470). In *hereditary elliptocytosis* the majority of the erythrocytes are oval, but in most instances this is a harmless trait; occasionally a mild haemolytic anaemia is present. The genes for the trait appear to be carried on the same chromosome pair as those for the Rh blood group. (Non-hereditary elliptocytosis occasionally occurs in association with myelofibrosis.)

Variations in haemoglobin content. Reduction in the amount of circulating haemoglobin may be the result either of diminution in the numbers of circulating red cells or of the amount of haemoglobin within them or of both. For example, in pernicious anaemia, reduction in the numbers of red cells is the cause of the anaemia; the increase in size of the individual cells does not compensate for this. In the hypochromic anaemias of iron-deficiency states, on the other hand, the number of red cells may not be much below normal, and the anaemia is due chiefly to reduction in the haemoglobin content of the cells, as a result both of lowered concentration and reduced size of cells: accordingly the MCHC is lowered, e.g. to 25% or less, and the MCH is also low. When the MCHC is greatly reduced, the cells in films show red staining only at the periphery, giving the so-called ring-staining, but there are so many artefacts that this feature, unless gross, is quite unreliable and should not be used as an indication of the haemoglobin content of the cells.

Polychromasia and reticulocytes. If a film of normal blood is stained with a Romanowsky stain, practically all the erythrocytes are purely eosinophilic. In certain conditions, however, in addition to the eosinophilia, a proportion of the erythrocytes show a slight bluish-violet basophilia and the term *polychromasia* is applied to this double staining. These are young cells which have recently lost their nuclei but still retain some of the basophilic RNA which is abundant in the early erythroblast and is con-

cerned in haemoglobin synthesis: as they mature in the circulation, the polychromasia gradually disappears and they become normochromic. The young erythrocytes tend, on the whole, to be slightly larger than those thoroughly mature.

By supravital staining with certain dyes, cresyl blue being most frequently used, any basophil substance remaining in the erythrocytes is precipitated or condensed within the cells as a sharply-stained skein or reticulum, and such corpuscles are called **reticulocytes.** The reticulum has nothing to do with the remains of the nucleus, and it is not visible within the cells by dark-ground or phase-contrast illumination until it has been precipitated by a supravital

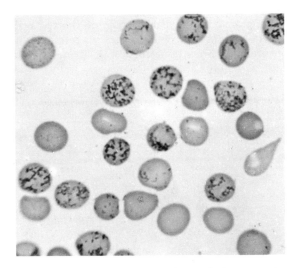

Fig. 16.4 Blood smear in haemolytic anaemia, showing numerous reticulocytes containing various amounts of reticulum. Supravital staining with cresyl blue. × 1100.

basic dye (Fig. 16.4). Reticulocytes are normally present in a proportion of less than 1% in males, but may rise to 2% in females after menstrual loss.

Polychromatic cells and reticulocytes become increased when there is stimulated output from the bone marrow, e.g. after haemorrhage or in haemolytic states. In addition, they may rise during response to specific therapy in a deficiency anaemia, e.g. after injection of vitamin B_{12} in pernicious anaemia.

Red cell inclusions. Various inclusions may occur in erythrocytes, either as vestiges of cell maturation, or as part of a pathological process. A normal function of the spleen is to remove such inclusions from the erythrocytes without destroying the cells themselves; this is achieved in the red pulp and is known as the 'pitting' function of the spleen. If the spleen has been removed, is atrophied or is congenitally absent, cells with such inclusions may be present in large numbers in the circulation without necessarily indicating any blood disorder.

Pappenheimer bodies are small, deeply basophilic granules, usually solitary and less than 1 μm in diameter, which give a positive prussian blue reaction for ferric iron. Red cells containing them appear most abundantly in the peripheral blood of adults after splenectomy, but are present in some erythroblasts in normal marrow (*sideroblasts*).

In *punctate basophilia*, some of the red cells contain clumps of RNA, seen as minute blue granules in smears stained with Romanowsky

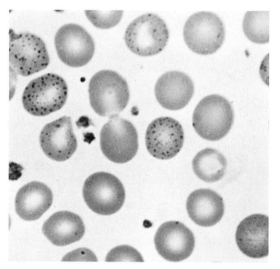

Fig. 16.5 Blood smear showing punctate basophilia. × 1250.

dyes (Fig. 16.5). This is seen in chronic lead poisoning and red cell injury by haemolytic chemicals, but can also occur in other types of anaemia.

Howell–Jolly bodies are granules of nuclear chromatin, 1–2 μm or more in diameter (Fig. 16.26), but which, if very small, resemble Pappenheimer bodies; they are, however, *iron-negative*. They are most common in the red cells in macrocytic anaemias but are found also in a variety of other blood diseases or following splenectomy in normal individuals.

Heinz bodies appear in wet unstained preparations as irregularly shaped, highly refractile granules, which often aggregate or coalesce under the red cell membrane. Not visible in Romanowsky-stained films, they are readily demonstrated in supravital methyl violet preparations (Fig. 16.15, p. 469) or when stained by brilliant cresyl blue. They consist of granules of denatured globin, and are numerous in many forms of chemical haemolytic anaemia, especially those induced by oxidant drugs (p. 476). Evidence of oxidative change to the iron in the haem moiety (methaemoglobin) often co-exists.

The red cell inclusions of *malaria* are described on p. 475.

Presence of erythroblasts. The term *erythroblast* is used throughout to mean nucleated red blood cells of all types; normally in the adult they are present only in the marrow, but they appear in the blood in a variety of conditions.

Normoblasts are about the size of an ordinary red cell or a little larger, and have a single spherical nucleus which is condensed and thus stains very deeply. The nucleus shows a coarse network of deeply staining chromatin, or it may appear very dense and practically homogeneous in the pyknotic nuclei of the more mature erythroblasts (Fig. 16.1). A few normoblasts appear in the blood in various types of anaemia, especially in those characterised by extramedullary haemopoiesis; the rapid appearance of a large number usually indicates a specially active marrow response to demands for new red cells.

Megaloblasts, as their name indicates, are larger; the nucleus is fairly large, is usually of less mature appearance, stains less deeply than the nucleus of a normoblast, and shows a somewhat granular or reticular structure (Fig. 16.26, p. 478); in later forms it may be fragmented or pyknotic. The cytoplasm of megaloblasts often gives a polychromatophilic reaction of varying depth, and may show punctate basophilia; Howell–Jolly bodies are frequently present. Megaloblastic change is due to abnormal erythropoiesis and is seen at all stages of maturation of red cell precursors in the marrow (Fig. 16.2). In megaloblastic anaemia of any cause, the presence of circulating megaloblasts is an important feature, and at least a few are to be found, as a rule, in smears of the buffy coat. They are particularly frequent in megaloblastic anaemias in childhood.

Fragility of the erythrocytes

Osmotic fragility. When red cells are placed in a hypotonic salt solution they become swollen and finally rupture, the haemoglobin diffusing out. With normal blood, the first trace of lysis is usually seen in a concentration of 0·42–0·46% NaCl; initial lysis occurring below 0·4 or above 0·5% may be taken as abnormal, indicating diminished or increased

fragility respectively; in some cases the abnormality may be detected only by careful quantitative methods. There is a close parallel between the thickness/diameter ratio of red cells and their osmotic fragility; increase of the ratio, as in the globular cells of hereditary spherocytosis, conferring increased fragility and conversely the reduced ratio of the thin cells in thalassaemia and other haemoglobinopathies conferring reduced fragility.

Mechanical fragility of erythrocytes (susceptibility to trauma) is much increased in certain states associated with cold agglutinins, and sometimes in lead poisoning.

The Leukocytes

Introduction

The three classes of leukocytes in the blood—polymorphs (granulocytes), monocytes and lymphocytes—differ in their precursor cells, their morphology, and in their function. The three types of **polymorphs**—neutrophil, eosinophil and basophil—originate in the bone marrow (p. 154). The neutrophil polymorphs, as already explained in Chapter 2, are concerned in inflammatory reactions, and their chief function is the phagocytosis and digestion of microorganisms and other foreign materials, damaged tissue elements and dead cells. The **monocytes** of the blood are also phagocytic; they belong to the mononuclear phagocyte system (p. 53) and provide most of the macrophages in inflammatory lesions. They originate in the haemopoietic marrow. Disturbance of the functions of neutrophil polymorphs and monocytes, with consequent tissue injury, is a feature of certain types of hypersensitivity reaction (Chapter 5). The eosinophil polymorphs increase in the blood, and appear in the lesions, of patients with atopic hypersensitivity (p. 121) although their physiological role, like that of the basophil polymorphs, is largely unknown. The origins of **lymphocytes**, and their essential functions in immune responses, have been considered in Chapter 4.

Increase or decrease in the numbers of the leukocytes in disease can affect any or all of the different types; increase in the total number of leukocytes above 11 000 per μl is termed *leukocytosis*, while diminution below 4000 per

μl is termed *leukopenia*: to determine the *absolute numbers* of different types of leukocytes, it is necessary to determine the total number and also the proportion of different types by performing a *differential count* on a stained film. The normal range of numbers of the leukocytes in adults is given in Table 16.2.

Table 16.2 The Normal Number of Leukocytes

	No. per μl blood
Polymorphs	
neutrophil	2500–7500
eosinophil	40–440
basophil	0–100
Lymphocytes	1500–3500
Monocytes	200–800
Total	4000–11 000

Changes in the leukocytes in disease states

Neutrophil polymorphs

Neutrophil leukocytosis. An account of neutrophil leukocytosis, and the accompanying myeloid hyperplasia of the haemopoietic marrow, is given on pp. 152–6. The commonest cause is bacterial infection, which should always be suspected, particularly in a neutrophil leukocytosis of over 20 000 per μl, and may cause an increase to 50 000 per μl. Moderate rises may accompany tissue necrosis without infection, such as myocardial infarction, and occur in burns and crush injuries: leukocytosis also occurs within a few hours after a large haemorrhage, passing off within a day or two; acute haemolysis is also accompanied by a neutrophil leukocytosis, and drug reactions, e.g. to steroids, sometimes promote a leukocytosis.

Increased production of neutrophil polymorphs in the circumstances given above is a controlled response to a stimulus, and may be regarded as a physiological reaction on the part of the myelopoietic (i.e. granulopoietic) marrow. By contrast, the neutrophil leukocytosis which occurs in myeloid leukaemia (p. 491) is not a controlled response to a known stimulus, but is of neoplastic nature.

In any acute neutrophil leukocytosis, the proportion of young neutrophils in the blood

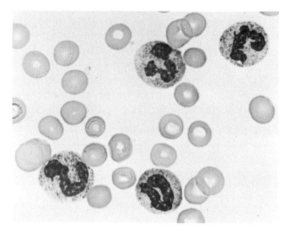

Fig. 16.6   Blood smear in neutrophil leukocytosis. × 850. (Dr. I. Evans.)

increases (Fig. 16.6), and some myelocytes or metamyelocytes may be found. Another change is a moderate increase in neutrophil alkaline phosphatase.

In severe infections and toxic states the young polymorphs entering the circulation may show morphological evidence of damage; their cytoplasm contains deeply-staining granules showing abnormal variations in size, and giving a poor oxidase reaction ('*toxic granulation*'), and their nuclei fail to undergo the normal degree of segmentation. Cell injury of greater degree results in failure of production of polymorphs, and leukopenia is thus a grave sign when associated with severe infection by pyogenic bacteria.

Neutrophil Leukopenia (neutropenia).   The term leukopenia means diminution of circulating leukocytes below the normal limit of 4000 per μl; as the neutrophil polymorphs constitute so high a proportion of the leukocytes, it is for practical purposes synonymous with neutropenia. It occurs both as an isolated haematological feature and also as part of a reduction of all cell types in the blood (pancytopenia). Severe diminution or total absence of circulating neutrophils is termed **agranulocytosis.**

Neutropenia can result either from failure of the marrow to produce adequate numbers of neutrophils, or from excessive peripheral destruction or consumption of these cells. Examples of the former include bone marrow aplasia (p. 486), bone marrow replacement with secondary tumour, leukaemia or myeloma, or severe megaloblastic anaemia (p. 479). Marrow production may also be severely depressed in overwhelming infections such as septicaemias and disseminated tuberculosis, and neutropenia in such conditions is of gráve prognostic significance. A large number of different drugs has been incriminated in cases of agranulocytosis, the most important being phenylbutazone, chlorpromazine and other phenothiazines, sulphonamides and related compounds, e.g. co-trimoxazole and sulphasalazine, frusemide and anti-thyroid drugs. In large doses, many compounds may depress the marrow, but neutropenia is more often the result of the development of an idiosyncrasy towards a particular compound, subsequent administration of even a small dose being capable of inducing the condition. Indeed, it now seems improbable that severe neutropenia arises as a primary spontaneous disease, and in every case the possibility that it is drug-induced must be thoroughly investigated.

The mechanisms underlying idiosyncrasy towards a particular drug are not completely understood. In all probability an immunological mechanism of one kind or another is involved in most instances. Possibly a drug, in binding to the leukocyte surface, acts as a hapten to form an antigenic complex, the resulting antibodies being capable of destroying or damaging the circulating leukocytes and their more mature precursors in the marrow, on re-exposure to the drug (analogous to Sedormid purpura, p. 122). In other instances, leukocytes may be damaged when drug-induced antigen–

antibody complexes bind to their plasma membrane. In any event, with so many new synthetic drugs being introduced into therapeutics, the dangers of sensitisation of this kind must always be kept in mind, since the haemopoietic system and in particular its granulocytic component, is often the first to exhibit signs of unwelcome toxicity.

Immune reactions may also be involved in the neutropenia of primary atypical pneumonia, glandular fever, disseminated lupus erythematosus, and cyclical agranulocytosis. In anaphylactic shock (p. 118), marked leukopenia may develop very rapidly, due apparently to aggregation of leukocytes in the capillaries of the lungs and other internal organs, and endotoxic shock (p. 228) may also be accompanied by leukopenia. The syndrome of hypersplenism, in which leukocytes, erythrocytes and platelets all undergo excessive sequestration in an enlarged spleen, is another example of neutropenia on the basis of 'peripheral' mechanisms.

Severe neutropenia has a high mortality, especially where the absolute neutrophil count falls below 500 per μl. Not only is there an increased likelihood of major infection by pathogenic organisms, but opportunistic infection with organisms normally of commensal type (e.g. gut coliforms, fungi) may become a major factor. There is often a severe inflammation of fauces and gums, which can progress to local gangrene—**agranulocytic angina.**

Defects of neutrophil function. An abnormal susceptibility to infection can be produced not only by a reduction in circulating neutrophils, but also by defective neutrophil function, even when their number is normal. The capacity of the neutrophil to combat infection by pathogenic micro-organisms is dependent upon its ability to respond to chemotactic stimuli, to phagocytose the offending micro-organisms, and to bring about their subsequent destruction intracellularly (p. 150). Defects in all three of these components of neutrophil function have been described and in some of these the abnormality appears to be intrinsic. Perhaps the most important of these is *chronic granulomatous disease of childhood*, in which the neutrophils have an undefined enzyme defect, and as a result lack the capacity to destroy phagocytosed

bacteria, especially staphylococci, Gram −ve species and certain fungi. The disease is transmitted by a gene defect on the X chromosome and so, like haemophilia, affects males; female carriers can be shown to have an admixture of normal and defective neutrophils in their blood, which supports the Lyon hypothesis.* From early childhood, affected males suffer from protracted infections, with extensive suppuration and granulation tissue formation, even from bacteria of low pathogenicity. The enzyme defect can be demonstrated *in vitro* by the failure of neutrophils and monocytes to reduce the yellow dye nitroblue tetrazolium (NBT) to an insoluble precipitate of blue-black formazan. The NBT test may also be useful in other contexts. It has been claimed that in the neutrophilia associated with bacterial infection the neutrophils acquire an increased capacity to reduce the dye, whereas this is not usually seen in the neutrophilia related to other conditions, such as tissue necrosis. Reports on the value of the test in the diagnosis of bacterial infection are, however, conflicting.

Another example is the *Chediak–Higashi syndrome*, a rare condition in which there is a lysosomal abnormality affecting many cell types. The neutrophils possess characteristically large cytoplasmic granules, which are of lysosomal origin and fail to disrupt following the phagocytosis of bacteria: as a result there is an impaired capacity to destroy bacteria intracellularly. The condition, transmitted as an autosomal recessive character, thus gives rise to recurrent infections. Other variable features include leukopenia, defective skin pigmentation, neuropathies, lymph-node enlargement and hepatosplenomegaly: malignant lymphoma commonly supervenes. Of the other neutrophil function defects, which are more common than was previously thought, mention should be made of the *lazy leukocyte syndrome*, in which there is a defect of neutrophil motility. There are also conditions of impaired chemotactic response and phagocytic capacity secondary to an absence of plasma factors, especially components of complement.

Pelger anomaly. This is a genetically-determined morphological curiosity of the nuclei of the granulocytes, which fail to become fully segmented as they mature, two lobes being the maximum. The

---

* This postulates that the inactive X chromosome represented by the sex-chromatin of females' cells (p. 884) can be *either* of the X chromosomes, selection being random in each individual cell.

abnormality is transmitted as a Mendelian dominant factor, and the heterozygous condition has an incidence of the order of 1 in 10 000: it is apparently not associated with susceptibility to infections or other harmful effects. A similar abnormality occurs in rabbits and dogs, where the homozygous condition is accompanied by skeletal and other deformities incompatible with life. The homozygous condition is unknown in man.

The presence of myelocytes. The appearance of these cells in the blood has an important clinical significance. In addition to myeloid leukaemia, where their presence in large numbers along with myeloblasts is a prominent feature, they are found occasionally in pernicious anaemia in small numbers. In the leuko-erythroblastic anaemia accompanying secondary carcinoma of the bone marrow and in myelofibrosis, myelocytes may be found in relatively large numbers, as may also nucleated red cells (p. 453), and the term leukoerythroblastosis is then applied. A few myelocytes may be found also in some very severe infections, particularly if there is a marked neutrophilia.

Eosinophil leukocytes

These differ from neutrophil polymorphs in having larger, brightly eosinophilic cytoplasmic granules, which often appear closely packed. Also, the nucleus usually has only two lobes (Fig. 16.7).

Eosinophil leukocytosis. Just as neutrophil leukocytosis occurs in pyogenic infections, so eosinophil leukocytosis is observed in those conditions which are characterised by infiltration of the tissues with eosinophils. The factors responsible for this local and general increase in eosinophils are not understood, but there is experimental evidence that, in hypersensitivity reactions, they are dependent on a T-lymphocyte response. Eosinophilia occurs in the following conditions.

(*a*) *Parasitic infestation* by various kinds of worm, e.g. *Trichinella spiralis*, ankylostomes and schistosomes. The eosinophil level sometimes exceeds $3000/\mu$l.

(*b*) *Hypersensitivity reactions.* In atopic hypersensitivity reactions (p. 117) such as asthma and hay fever, eosinophilia is usually present, and is related to the local emigration of eosinophils in the tissues. Eosinophilia may also be found in angio-oedema, food sensitivity, and in hypersensitivity reactions to certain drugs. An increase in eosinophils may occur in polyarteritis nodosa. The functions of eosinophil leukocytes and the part they play in the conditions noted above are unknown, in spite of much experimental investigation. There is, however, some evidence suggesting that they may antagonise the effects of histamine.

(*c*) *Chronic skin diseases*, such as dermatitis herpetiformis, psoriasis, etc. In some generalised skin conditions, a hypersensitivity mechanism may be present, e.g. in eczema or urticaria. Eosinophilia also occurs early in scarlet fever.

(*d*) *Malignant tumours.* The eosinophil count rises in some patients with cancer involving the bone marrow. In chronic myeloid leukaemia eosinophils may be increased along with the other granulocyte cells. In certain forms of Hodgkin's disease, the lymph glands are infiltrated with eosinophils, and about 10% of cases show an eosinophilia in the blood.

Eosinophil leukopenia. Diminution in the eosinophils is a practically constant response to increased secretion or therapeutic administration of adrenocorticotrophic hormone and of adrenal glucocorticoids.

Basophil leukocytes

The granules of these cells usually give a purplish metachromatic reaction, and the cells have been known as '*mast cells*' but this term should no longer be applied because the true mast cells in the tissues are of a different nature. The rôle

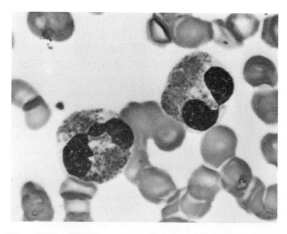

Fig. 16.7 Blood smear showing two eosinophil polymorphs. × 1250. (Dr. J. Browning.)

of the mast cell in atopic hypersensitivity (p. 119) has already been discussed. In chronic myeloid leukaemia, basophils sometimes take part in the leukocyte increase and basophil myelocytes may also appear. In various chronic wasting diseases an increase of basophils in the blood may be present occasionally, but there is no condition known which regularly induces a basophil leukocytosis.

Lymphocytes

Recent advances in our understanding of the life cycle and immunological functions of the lymphocyte have been described in Chapter 4. The picture is far from complete, but it is apparent that the lymphocytes in the blood represent at least two functionally different populations, each being concerned, however, with immune responses and reactions; other functions of the lymphocytes, if they exist, are unknown.

Lymphocytosis. Normally the proportion of lymphocytes in the child is higher than in the adult, perhaps in relation to the relative size of the thymus (p. 528). The number is highest shortly after birth and gradually falls in subsequent years; allowance for age must accordingly be made in interpreting lymphocyte counts. In most patients with leukopenia the fall in total count is attributable to granulocytopenia, and there is thus an increase in the proportion of lymphocytes; a *true lymphocytosis*, that is an increase in the number of lymphocytes per μl, is less common. It usually accompanies specific infective fevers and is a useful diagnostic feature in mild cases of whooping cough, in which it occasionally rises to 100 000/μl. Lymphocytosis also occurs in glandular fever, many of the cells being large and of abnormal appearance. It is usually a marked feature in smallpox, especially in moderately severe cases, both the small and large lymphocytes being increased along with the monocytes. Other infections in which lymphocytosis may be seen include typhoid and paratyphoid fever, brucellosis, influenza and secondary syphilis. High lymphocyte counts are also seen in the acute infective lymphocytosis of young children. The outstanding increase of lymphocytes however is in chronic lymphocytic leukaemia (p. 493), and an increased proportion of lymphocytes may sometimes be observed by a differential count to precede the actual rise in the leukocyte count.

Lymphopenia occurs irregularly in various miscellaneous conditions. In infancy, it is a cardinal feature of some immunological deficiency syndromes (p. 141), in which the near absence of lymphocytes from the blood and lymphoid tissues is associated with a fatal deficiency of the immunological mechanism. Severe lymphopenia results also from x-irradiation and use of cytotoxic drugs for immunosuppressive therapy or treatment of neoplasia.

Monocytes

The monocytes (Fig. 16.8) are circulating cells of the mononuclear phagocyte system (p. 57). When stimulated they enlarge, increase in motility and metabolic activity, becoming macrophages. The release of lymphokines

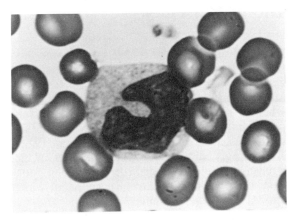

Fig. 16.8 Monocyte in a blood smear. × 1250. (Dr. I. Evans.)

which influence monocytes and macrophages in delayed hypersensitivity reactions is discussed on p. 129.

Like the neutrophil polymorphs, monocytes migrate into inflammatory foci and phagocytose bacteria, damaged tissue elements, dead cells, etc., but they aggregate later than the polymorphs, and are seen in increasing numbers in the late stages of pyogenic infections in the outer part of the wall of persistent abscesses (Fig. 7.26, p. 187), and in chronic inflammations of various types and causes. **Monocytosis** is commonly present in subacute bacterial endocarditis, in undulant fever, and sometimes in systemic lupus erythematosus. In tuberculosis, serial studies on individual cases have shown that the numbers of lymphocytes and monocytes in the blood tend to be inversely proportional to one another, and there is some evidence that a high ratio accompanies healing and that a low ratio is associated with extension of the lesions. The monocytes are increased also in typhus and some other rickettsial diseases, and in certain protozoal infections, e.g. malaria, trypanosomiasis, and kala-azar, in which diseases there is no increase of the neutrophils. In chronic malaria, the presence of numerous monocytes is often a striking feature, and some of them may contain small granules of pigment (Fig. 16.23, p. 475).

The abnormal cells which appear in the blood in large numbers in some cases of *infec-tious mononucleosis* (glandular fever) resemble monocytes, but are really T lymphoblasts (p. 515). In *tetrachlorethane poisoning* there is sometimes a progressive increase in the mono-cytes up to 3–4000 per μl.

The most remarkable example of monocy-tosis in relation to bacterial infection is attribut-able to a micro-organism known as *Listeria monocytogenes* recovered from an epizootic among rabbits. On experimental inoculation of rabbits these cells numbered, in extreme examples, fully 6000 per μl.

Monocytic leukaemia must always be con-sidered in patients with monocytosis (p. 491).

Blood Platelets

Platelets are capable of releasing some his-tamine and 5-hydroxytryptamine, and are weakly phagocytic, but their major functions are in aggregating to form a haemostatic plug when a small blood vessel is severed, and in promoting clotting of fibrinogen by taking part in the cascade reaction described on pp. 197–9. Accordingly, diminution in the number of cir-culating platelets, or disordered platelet func-tion, can result in a state of *purpura*, in which spontaneous haemorrhages occur.

The number of platelets in the blood is nor-mally between 150 000–400 000 per μl. An abnormal but temporary increase in platelets occurs after injury, haemorrhage and par-ticularly after removal of the spleen, which is the major site of normal platelet destruction. The increase in numbers (*thrombocytosis*) in these conditions is also accompanied by an increase in adhesiveness and a tendency to thrombosis. Thrombocytosis also accompanies a prolonged neutrophil leukocytosis, and is commonly seen in the early stages of chronic myeloid leukaemia. There is also a very rare disease—*haemorrhagic thrombocythaemia*—in which there is a tendency to spontaneous bleed-ing in spite of a thrombocytosis which some-times reaches 3 million platelets per μl.

Reduction in the number of platelets (*throm-bocytopenia*) commonly accompanies leuko-penia, e.g. in pernicious anaemia and aplastic or hypoplastic anaemias. It occurs also in acute leukaemias, where consequent haemorrhage may be an early feature.

The most important and commonest primary disease causing serious thrombocytopenia is *idiopathic thrombocytopenic purpura* which, in spite of its name, is due to an auto-antibody which causes excessive platelet destruction in the spleen. Excessive destruction in the spleen also occurs in *hypersplenism*, in which it is ac-companied by abnormal destruction of red cells and leukocytes. Rarely, thrombocytopenia alone, i.e. without reduction of red or white cells, results from marrow failure.

More attention will be paid to these and other platelet abnormalities in the section on abnormal haemorrhagic states (pp. 500–4).

Anaemia

Definition and types of anaemia

Anaemia is defined as a reduction in the con-centration of haemoglobin in the blood below the normal level, and is usually but not invar-iably accompanied by reduction in the number of red cells. Anaemia develops when the rate of red cell production by the bone marrow fails to keep pace with destruction of red cells or with any losses from haemorrhage. Accordingly the anaemias can be classified simply as follows:

(1) Excessive loss or destruction of red cells
   (*a*) haemorrhage—*post-haemorrhagic anaemia*
   (*b*) destruction—*haemolytic anaemia.*
(2) Failure of production of red cells
   (*a*) diminished production with marrow hyperplasia—*dyshaemopoietic anaemia*
   (*b*) diminished production with marrow hypoplasia or aplasia—*hypoplastic* or *aplastic anaemia.*

These categories are not watertight, since more than one mechanism may be involved in the production of the anaemia; for example in pernicious anaemia, which is due to lack of vitamin B_{12}, there is not only insufficient output of red cells by the marrow, but those cells which are produced wear out too quickly, i.e. excessive destruction is also implicated.

Effects of anaemia

The essential feature of anaemia is brought about by a reduction in the level of circulating haemoglobin. There is thus a reduction in the oxygen-carrying capacity of the blood, with resulting **tissue hypoxia.** The patient may complain of tiredness, dizziness, paraesthesia of the extremities, anginal chest pain and breathlessness on exertion.

Certain **compensatory adjustments** to the anaemia come about; there is a reduction in arteriolar tone, the stroke volume of the heart and to a lesser extent the heart rate increase; cardiac output thus rises, circulation time falls, and tissue perfusion is increased. These changes may be reflected clinically in a bounding pulse with a high pulse pressure, palpitations, cardiac enlargement and haemic murmurs; if the condition continues or the anaemia worsens, *cardiac failure* is a serious risk, especially if the load on the heart is increased by injudicious blood transfusion. These effects do not depend only on the severity of the anaemia; if anaemia develops rapidly the symptoms are correspondingly severe, whereas remarkable tolerance is often seen when the haemoglobin has fallen slowly. Co-existing vascular disease, as in the elderly, will also exacerbate the effects of anaemia. Pallor, mild pyrexia and slight splenomegaly may be attributable to anaemia *per se.*

Tissue hypoxia resulting from anaemia will stimulate the production of erythropoietin, which will in turn lead to *marrow hyperplasia*; the yellow fatty marrow of the long bones becomes progressively replaced by dark red cellular marrow, and in extreme cases resorption of bone trabeculae may occur. In haemolytic and post-haemorrhage anaemias, this will lead to a useful output of new red cells from the marrow (*effective erythropoiesis*); in the dyshaemopoietic states, however, although marrow hyperplasia will occur, disordered haemopoiesis usually prevents a useful output of new red cells (*ineffective erythropoiesis*). In an aplastic marrow, compensatory hyperplasia cannot occur despite erythropoietin stimulation.

Fatty change, especially in the liver and heart, is the most constant pathological change in patients dying of anaemia (p. 17).

Post-haemorrhagic anaemia

The restoration of the fluid part of the blood after haemorrhage (p. 224) leads, of course, to dilution of the blood with accompanying fall in the number of erythrocytes per μl. The first evidence of regeneration of red cells after a large haemorrhage is a progressive increase in the number of reticulocytes, and the degree of increase is an indication of haemopoietic activity. They show a varying degree of polychromasia in ordinary stained films. Along with them are often a few normoblasts, which, if there are repeated haemorrhages, may become fairly abundant. As regeneration becomes complete the reticulocytes gradually return to their normal level and normoblasts disappear. These changes are the results of proliferation of erythroblasts in the bone marrow, in which they form a larger proportion of the cells than normally (Fig. 16.9). A polymorphonuclear leukocytosis and thrombocytosis, both of

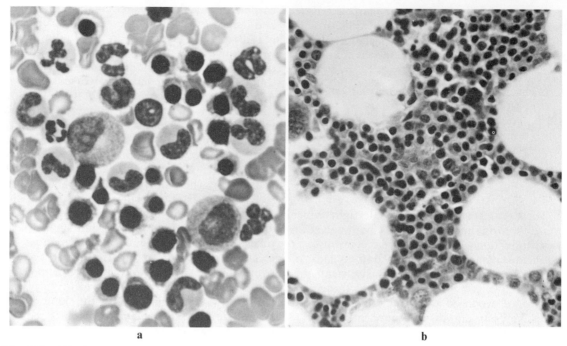

a   b

Fig. 16.9   The haemopoietic marrow, showing an erythroblastic reaction following haemorrhage. **a** Marrow smear: there is an increased proportion of normoblasts, at various stages of maturity, as compared with myelocytes. × 850. **b** Marrow section: the cellular haemopoietic tissue has increased at the expense of the fat cells. × 500.

moderate degree, appear within a few hours after haemorrhage; they pass off in two or three days, unless the haemorrhage is repeated.

Chronic loss of small amounts of blood does not produce anaemia by loss of circulating red cells since the amounts involved are insufficient to alter significantly the red cell mass. However, significant amounts of iron can be lost in this way, and chronic haemorrhage is the most important cause of iron deficiency anaemia, a dyshaemopoietic state (p. 484). In such states the circulating platelets also rise.

Haemolytic anaemias

General features

The haemolytic disorders comprise a group of conditions characterised by an increase in the rate of red cell destruction, and thus a reduction in the normal lifespan of the erythrocyte (100–120 days). There is a compensatory increase in the rate of red cell production, and anaemia will develop only when the rate of destruction exceeds that of production. These processes are common to all haemolytic disorders, irrespective of cause, and these general features will be described more fully before considering the various types of haemolytic anaemia.

Sites of red cell destruction. Red cells may undergo premature destruction either by phagocytosis by macrophages, or by intravascular lysis. In most haemolytic conditions, red cell destruction occurs in macrophages of the spleen, liver and bone marrow. These cells are capable of destroying as much as 20% of the total red cell mass each day. The spleen has a particular capacity for the recognition of mild and moderate damage to red cells, and in such cases the role of spleen in red cell destruction is dominant. More severely damaged cells, however, undergo phagocytosis in all tissues containing vascular channels lined by macrophages (notably the liver, spleen and bone marrow).

Intravascular destruction is relatively uncommon (see below) and complicates blackwater fever, arsine poisoning and severe red cell membrane damage from complement-fixing antigen-antibody reactions as in ABO-incompatible blood transfusions.

Changes resulting from increased destruction of red cells. Following phagocytosis of red cells by macrophages, haemoglobin is broken down to iron and globin, both of which undergo re-utilisation, and the haem is degraded to bilirubin (see p. 239). In haemolytic disease, the production of bilirubin may exceed the capacity of the liver to remove it, and plasma levels rise; clinical jaundice results when the level exceeds about 3 mg/100 ml (50 μmol/litre). The bilirubin is bound to plasma albumin and does not pass into the urine (*acholuric jaundice*). The increased excretion of conjugated bilirubin by the liver leads to excessive formation of stercobilinogen in the gut, so that the faeces are dark. There is increased absorption of urobilinogen which often cannot all be dealt with by the overworked liver and so appears in the urine; measurement of faecal stercobilinogen and urinary urobilinogen are useful confirmatory tests of haemolysis, although time-consuming and not very accurate. The high bilirubin content of the bile may predispose to the formation of pigment stones in chronic haemolytic anaemias, and the high levels of bilirubin found in haemolytic disease of the newborn may cause toxic damage to the brain (p. 662).

Intravascular lysis leads to the appearance of free haemoglobin in the plasma; a proportion of this is bound at once to plasma haptoglobin and the haemoglobin/haptoglobin complex is phagocytosed by the macrophages. If the haemolysis is severe, this mechanism is easily overcome; some free haemoglobin is then converted to methaemalbumin, and the remainder is excreted free in the urine. This form of erythrocyte destruction can be recognised by haemoglobinaemia, haemoglobinuria, by spectroscopic tests for methaemalbumin in the plasma, and by disappearance of plasma haptoglobin levels.

Changes associated with compensatory erythropoiesis. In haemolytic states, erythropoietin stimulation of the marrow induces compensatory hyperplasia of red cell precursors; kinetic studies show that the marrow is capable of increasing red cell production to a maximum of 8–10 times normal. There is thus an increased number of young red cells in the blood; in a Leishman-stained film, many of the erythrocytes show polychromasia, and there may be both early and late normoblasts. Reticulocytes are always increased, often exceeding 20% (Fig. 16.4). In any untreated case of anaemia, such a reticulocytosis is strong evidence of a haemolytic process provided blood loss can be excluded. The anaemia is usually of normochromic and normocytic type; a mildly macrocytic blood picture, may, however, result from macronormoblastic change in the hyperplastic erythropoietic marrow.

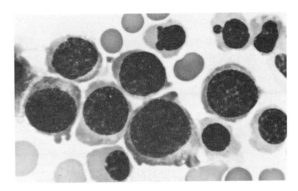

Fig. 16.10 Marrow smear in haemolytic anaemia due to hereditary spherocytosis, illustrating normoblastic hyperplasia: the cluster of erythroblasts includes all stages from early basophilic cells to late normoblasts. × 1100.

The marrow shows erythroblastic hyperplasia (Fig. 16.10), the proportion of erythroblasts is increased, and the fat cells are partly or even completely replaced by haemopoietic tissue, which may also extend down the shafts of the long bones, eventually the medullary cavity may become widened with loss of bony trabeculae and thinning of the cortical bone. In extreme cases of long duration, extramedullary haemopoiesis occurs in spleen and other extraosseous sites.

Measurement of red cell lifespan. Using radiochromium (^{51}Cr), the patient's red cells can be tagged *in vitro* and returned to the circulation. Their fate can be closely followed and the chief sites of destruction found. The rate of disappearance of radioactivity from the circulation can be estimated by serial blood samples, and is proportional to the rate of red cell destruction. Provided loss of blood can be excluded, the red cell lifespan can be estimated from these data. In addition, by placing an external scintillation counter over the liver, spleen and bone marrow, information on sites of red cell sequestration and destruction can be obtained.

Types of haemolytic anaemia

Although recent advances in our understanding of the metabolism of glucose by red cells has

16.11). Such methods are not usually required for routine hospital diagnosis as the various forms of the disease present other distinctive characteristics. However, the availability of radioactive chromium (^{51}Cr) as a means of labelling red cells has brought the red cell survival time into general use as a diagnostic measure. For descriptive purposes, the following subdivisions may be made:

CLASSIFICATION OF HAEMOLYTIC ANAEMIA

(I) Intrinsic defects in the red cells

A. Genetically determined defects

  (1) Hereditary spherocytosis (familial acholuric jaundice).

I. Intrinsic red cell defects

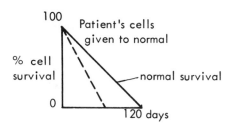
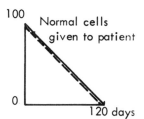

II. Extrinsic haemolytic mechanisms

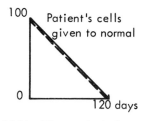
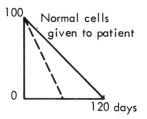

Fig. 16.11 The survival of red cells in cross-transfusion experiments in haemolytic anaemia. The continuous lines indicate the rate of disappearance of transfused red cells from normal donors to normal recipients. The interrupted lines show the rates of disappearance of transfused red cells in the stated circumstances.

helped to clarify the modes of red cell destruction, the causation of the different types of haemolytic anaemia is by no means fully understood, and classification is therefore tentative. Reduced red cell survival time is the essential feature of haemolytic anaemia; it may be the result either of an intrinsic abnormality in the red cells, or of an extrinsic haemolytic mechanism. The distinction is based on red cell survival times in cross transfusion experiments (Fig.

  (2) Hereditary elliptocytosis.
  (3) Red cell enzyme defects
    (*a*) Pyruvate kinase deficiency
    (*b*) Glucose-6-phosphate dehydrogenase deficiency.
  (4) The haemoglobinopathies.

B. Acquired defects

  (1) Paroxysmal nocturnal haemoglobinuria.
  (2) Dyshaemopoietic anaemias.

(II) Abnormal extra-erythrocytic haemolytic mechanisms.

A. Auto-immune haemolytic anaemia
(1) 'Warm antibody' type.
(2) 'Cold antibody' type.

B. Iso-antibodies to red cells
(1) Erythroblastosis fetalis.
(2) Transfusion reactions.

C. Parasitic invasion of red cells
(1) Malaria.
(2) Oroya fever.

D. Haemolytic toxins and chemicals
(1) Bacterial toxins, e.g. *Cl. welchii*, *Strep. pyogenes*.
(2) Chemicals, e.g. phenacetin, phenylhydrazine, potassium chlorate, arseniuretted hydrogen, lead.
(3) Vegetable poisons, e.g. favism.

E. Mechanical damage to red cells
(1) March haemoglobinuria.
(2) Microangiopathic haemolytic anaemia.

NOTE: The groups and types of haemolytic anaemia listed above are not entirely independent. For example, subjects with glucose-6-phosphate dehydrogenase deficiency are abnormally susceptible to haemolysis by various chemicals.

I.A. Genetically determined red cell defects

(1) Hereditary spherocytosis. This common type of chronic haemolytic anaemia, occurring in most parts of the world, is caused by a red cell membrane defect of uncertain nature and inherited as an autosomal dominant trait with incomplete penetrance. In about 25% of patients, however, there is no family history, and the defect presumably arises as a spontaneous genetic mutation in such cases. The membrane defect results in excessive permeability to sodium ions, and red cell integrity can only be maintained by increased glycolytic activity, required to 'pump' sodium ions out of the cell. This metabolic activity is associated with an increased turnover of membrane lipid, some of which is inevitably lost. Membrane loss is responsible for the tendency of the red cells to assume the microspherocytic form, a process which is greatly accelerated in the red pulp of the spleen where the ratio of plasma to red cells is greatly reduced and the availability of glucose diminished (p. 464). Microspherocytes formed in the red pulp become trapped and subsequently lysed, since they lack the pliability necessary to enable them to pass through the clefts between the endothelial cells in the venous sinusoids and return to the circulation. The spleen thus occupies a critical rôle in the disease process, and following splenectomy the survival of the red cells returns to normal.

Clinically the disease is characterised by acholuric jaundice, often mild and fluctuating, and usually dating from early childhood. Anaemia may be mild and even absent although episodes of severe anaemia ('crises') are sometimes experienced. These crises are due either to an increase in red cell destruction, sometimes related to infections or pregnancy and associated with deepening jaundice, fever and leucocytosis, or to reduction in erythropoietic activity in the marrow, when increasing anaemia is accompanied by a fall in the reticulocyte count (hypoplastic crisis). Splenomegaly is invariable, and some patients develop chronic leg ulceration. The diagnosis is suspected when signs of haemolysis, such as persistent reticulocytosis and urobilinogenuria, are associated with the presence in the peripheral blood of microspherocytes, which are small, intensely stained spheroidal red cells (Fig. 16.12). Demonstration of increased osmotic fragility of the red cells (p. 457) confirms the diagnosis. The haemolytic state is cured by removal of the spleen, which is always found to be enlarged, usually weighing about 500 g but sometimes up to 1400 g.

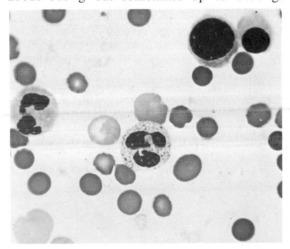

Fig. 16.12 Blood film in hereditary spherocytosis. Note the small, densely staining spherocytes. × 780.

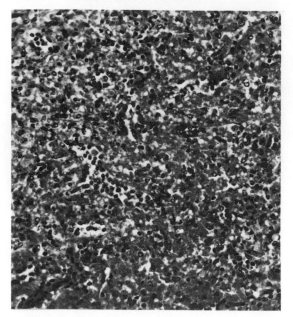

Fig. 16.13 Spleen in hereditary spherocytosis. The pulp is intensely congested and the sinuses are inconspicuous. × 230.

Histologically, the red pulp is distended with red cells, while the venous sinusoids are compressed (Fig. 16.13). Although splenectomy relieves the haemolysis, microspherocytosis and increased osmotic fragility of the red cells persist.

(2) Hereditary elliptocytosis causes a much less pronounced sequestration of cells in the spleen pulp and the anaemia is usually mild. This defect exhibits genetic linkage with the Rh blood group genes.

(3) Red cell enzyme defects. Normal red cell survival is dependent upon the integrity of the two enzyme systems concerned in glucose metabolism, namely the Embden–Meyerhof pathway and the hexose monophosphate shunt (Fig. 16.14). Enzyme deficiencies in either system are usually genetically determined and can lead directly or indirectly to haemolytic anaemia. It is notable that microspherocytosis is not a feature of red-cell enzyme defects, which are usually implicated in the group of conditions described as hereditary non-spherocytic haemolytic anaemia (HNSHA).

(*a*) *Pyruvate Kinase deficiency*, although rare, is the commonest defect in the Embden–Meyerhof pathway. It is inherited as an autosomal recessive trait and produces a mild haemolytic state in individuals homozygous for the abnormal gene. The red cells show minimal morphological abnormality, despite the paradoxically high reticulocyte counts which have been recorded. Trapping of red cells in the spleen is not a prominent feature, and splenectomy confers only minimal benefit.

(*b*) *Glucose-6-phosphate dehydrogenase deficiency* is by far the most common defect in the hexose monophosphate shunt and is, moreover, one of the commonest of all genetic defects, affecting as many as 50% of individuals of negro or Mediterranean ancestry in some parts of the world. Several allotypes of the enzyme (isoenzymes) are known, and the effects of deficiency vary accordingly. Inheritance of the defect is sex-linked, and so males are most often affected. The principal effect of deficiency is a decrease in reduced glutathione: in consequence, the haemoglobin is readily oxidised and ultimately masses of denatured haemoglobin (Heinz bodies) are deposited on the cell membranes (Fig. 16:15). Spontaneous haemolysis has only been described in the rare Caucasian form of the disease, which presents as a form of HNSHA in neonates. Much more often haemolysis only develops following exposure to chemical agents with oxidative potential. In Mediterranean people, even the mild oxidant found

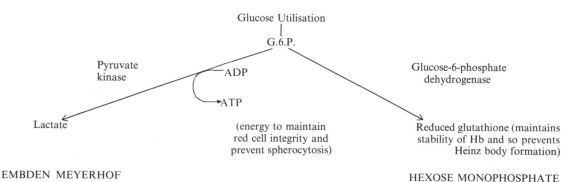

Fig. 16.14 Two enzyme systems of importance in determining the lifespan of the red cells.

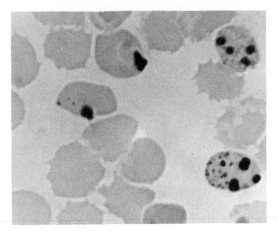

Fig. 16.15 Blood film in sodium chlorate poisoning, stained with methyl violet to show Heinz bodies. × 1400.

in beans, or bean pollen, is sufficient to produce haemolysis—*favism* (p. 477). In negroes, however, oxidative drugs such as phenacetin or the antimalarial primaquine are required to expose the enzyme defect, although the subsequent haemolysis may be severe. The diagnosis is established by enzyme assay techniques or more simply by observing the number of Heinz bodies produced by exposing the red cells to phenylhydrazine *in vitro*.

(4) Haemoglobinopathies. Haemoglobin is a globular protein of molecular weight 68 000, consisting of two pairs of coiled polypeptide chains, a single prosthetic haem group being attached to each of the four chains. The type of haemoglobin is determined by the amino-acid sequence in the polypeptide chains. Four different chains occur normally in adults, termed α, β, γ and δ. The normal haemoglobins consist of a pair of alpha chains combined with a pair of one of the other three chains, as illustrated in Fig. 16.16. Haemoglobins differ in their electrophoretic mobility, solubility and resistance to alkali denaturation; these features, together with chromatography, are used in their identification. Replacement of Hb-F

by Hb-A starts before birth, and Hb-A and Hb-A$_2$ account for over 99% of the haemoglobin normally present by one year of age. In the adult, less than 0·4% is Hb-F. Haemoglobinopathies result from abnormalities in the synthesis of the globin fraction, due to gene mutation, the haem groups being normal. These mutations are of two varieties. The first causes an abnormality in the amino-acid sequence of the polypeptide chain so that an abnormal haemoglobin is produced. By 1970 over one hundred such abnormal haemoglobins had been recognised, the best known being S, C, D and E, in each of which the β chains contain an abnormal amino-acid sequence. In the thalassemias however, the genetic disturbance leads to a reduction in the *rate* of synthesis of one of the *normal* polypeptide chains, most commonly the α or β chain, and abnormal chains are not formed. In α-thalassemia, reduced α-chain synthesis leads in fetal life to an excess of γ chains, which tend to form tetrameric haemoglobin molecules (**Hb Barts**), and in adult life an excess of β chains which combine to form the unstable tetramer known as Hb-H (Fig. 16.17). In β-thalassemia, however, there is no abnormal haemoglobin since although impaired β-chain synthesis leads to an excess of α chains, the latter are incapable of forming tetramers. The effect of a haemoglobinopathy, however caused, is to impair the synthesis of haemoglobin so that anaemia results; the red cells also have a reduced survival time in the circulation, and the anaemia is therefore partly dyshaemopoietic, partly haemolytic. These defects in haemoglobin formation are especially marked in the homozygote.

Sickle-cell or haemoglobin-S disease occurs in individuals homozygous for a gene determining an abnormal form of haemoglobin, Hb-S. It is found in negroes and is often fatal in childhood. Hb-S ($\alpha_2\beta_2^{6val}$) differs chemically from Hb-A in the substitution of valine for glutamic acid in the sixth position of the amino-acid sequence of the β chain. When the β chains move apart on giving up oxygen, the amino-acid substitution results in locking of the adjacent ends of the α chains with the abnormal β chains, and the haemoglobin molecules become stacked in rows.

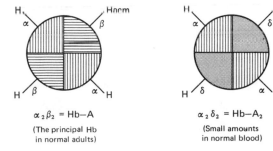
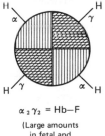

Fig. 16.16 The structure of the normal haemoglobins.

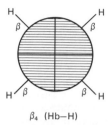
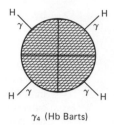
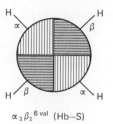

β₄ (Hb—H)   γ₄ (Hb Barts)   α₂β₂⁶ ᵛᵃˡ (Hb—S)

Fig. 16.17   The structure of some abnormal haemoglobins.

This causes distortion of the red cells in the deoxygenated state: *in vitro*, sickling is demonstrable by adding a reducing agent to the blood (Fig. 16.18). Clinically, there is a chronic haemolytic anaemia, painful sickling crises, leg ulceration, recurrent respiratory infection and a cardiomyopathy. The crises affect especially the abdomen, bones and joints: they are due to blocking of small vessels by sickled cells, and infarcts of the spleen, bones, etc. commonly result.

The *sickle-cell trait*, due to the heterozygous state, occurs in negroes (12–20%) and those with negro ancestry. Symptoms are usually absent or mild, but *in vitro* sickling is demonstrable (see above). Hb-S appears to increase the resistance to malaria, and this may account for persistence of the responsible gene—an example of *balanced polymorphism*. The combination of Hb-S and Hb-C causes a mild anaemia with prominence of target cells.

Unstable haemoglobin disease. Certain haemoglobin variants are highly unstable, since the causative amino-acid substitutions affect the attachment site of the haem plate. Even individuals heterozygous for such abnormal haemoglobins, of which **Hb Koln** is

the commonest example, suffer from a spontaneous hereditary non-spherocytic haemolytic anaemia. Since unstable haemoglobins readily become denatured, Heinz body formation is a typical feature and this can readily be demonstrated when the cells are incubated *in vitro*. Heinz bodies are not observed *in vivo* unless splenectomy has been carried out, for the spleen is capable of removing them from circulating red cells (p. 506).

Thalassaemia major and minor. This hereditary anaemia is due primarily to defective globin synthesis but the abnormal cells also have a reduced life span. **Thalassaemia major** occurs in homozygotes: severe anaemia is apparent within a few weeks of birth and splenomegaly is prominent. There is a reticulocytosis and many nucleated red cells are present together with a leukocytosis and occasional myelocytes. Target cells (p. 455) are numerous (Fig. 16.19) and the blood shows increased osmotic resistance owing to the flattened shape of the cells (leptocytes). Many

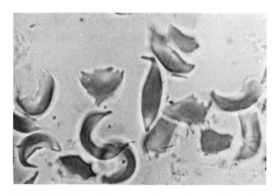

Fig. 16.18   Blood from a subject with sickle cell trait showing the characteristic distorted shapes taken up when the red cells are subjected to a low oxygen tension. × 1000.

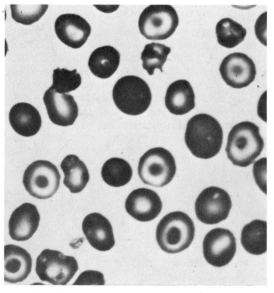

Fig. 16.19   Target cells in a case of thalassaemia minor. × 1000.

such cases die in infancy or early childhood and show widespread haemosiderosis: in cases of long survival hepatic cirrhosis tends to develop. Prolonged active hyperplasia of the marrow causes bone changes, e.g. thickening of the calvarium and great increase in the diploë sometimes giving a rather mongoloid appearance. Haemopoiesis is present in the spleen and other organs. **Thalassaemia minor** (target cell anaemia) occurs in the heterozygote; it is much less serious and presents in adult life merely as a mild anaemia of hypochromic microcytic type highly resistant to treatment with iron. Sometimes, owing to the variable penetrance of the gene, the condition may be symptomless.

The defect in haemoglobin synthesis may affect either the α or β polypeptide chains of the globin molecule (see p. 469). In the classical form the β chains are affected. In consequence, production of Hb-A $(\alpha_2\beta_2)$ is reduced while Hb-A$_2$ $(\alpha_2\delta_2)$ and Hb-F $(\alpha_2\gamma_2)$ are 'compensatorily' increased; no abnormal haemoglobin is formed. In α-chain thalassaemia all three normal haemoglobins are affected since they all contain α chains and so low A, A$_2$ and F values are present but excess β, γ and probably δ units are produced. Although these β, γ and δ chains are normal, their abnormal combination, e.g. as tetramers, results in the appearance of the abnormal haemoglobins, as explained above.

Thus the two biochemical forms of thalassaemia contrast:

α-chain—low A^2 and F, Barts or H present.

β-chain—High A$_2$ and usually high F also. No abnormal haemoglobin present (see Fig. 16.20).

The disease most frequently affects inhabitants of the Mediterranean littoral (hence 'thalassaemia') but is seen also in parts of the world where other haemoglobinopathies occur. When a mixed heterozygous state is encountered, as in thalassaemia—Hb-C or E disease, a clinical picture similar to thalassaemia major results.

I.B. Acquired red cell defects

(1) Paroxysmal nocturnal haemoglobinuria (PNH) is a rare chronic haemolytic disease of insidious onset, most common in early middle life and characterised by haemoglobinuria, weakness, fever, slight jaundice and moderate splenomegaly. *Intravascular haemolysis* occurs mostly during sleep and is attributable to a remarkable sensitivity of some of the red cells, but not all, to slight lowering of the pH; this is the basis of *Ham's test* for haemolysis with acidified serum. The urine passed at night or on rising contains haemoglobin whereas the daytime urine contains less or even none. Lysis is now attributed to an abnormal sensitivity of the red cells to complement. There is also a tendency to venous thrombosis, the cause of which is not clear. Transfusion is dangerous owing to the risk of a haemolytic crisis. Repeated haemolytic episodes cause a marked degree of anaemia with reticulocytosis, marrow hyperplasia and siderosis of the organs, especially the kidneys (Fig. 16.21); granules

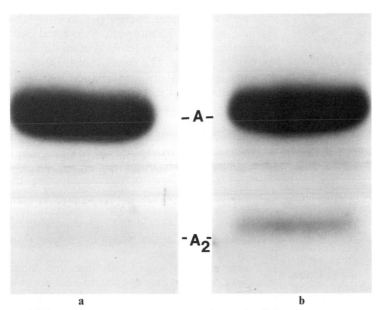

Fig. 16.20 Starch-gel electrophoresis of haemoglobins. **a** Normal. **b** Thalassaemia minor, showing increase in Hb-A$_2$.

of haemosiderin are abundant in the urine both day and night. After a few years death results from thrombosis in the portal or cerebral veins, but milder forms occur and spontaneous permanent remissions have been observed. The essential abnormality in the red cells has not yet been clearly defined but pits in the red cell surface have been detected by electron microscopy and the stromal lipoproteins are abnormal. Occasional patients present with hypoplastic anaemia, the marrow being hypocellular, and it may

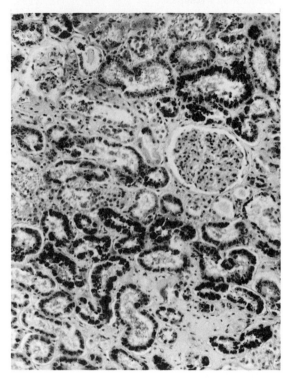

Fig. 16.21 The kidney in paroxysmal nocturnal haemoglobinuria, stained by the prussian blue reaction, showing accumulation of haemosiderin in the convoluted tubules due to prolonged haemoglobinuria. × 100.

be that PNH arises as an acquired red cell abnormality following an aplastic episode.

(2) Dyshaemopoietic anaemias. In many anaemias due primarily to underproduction of red cells, there is also a haemolytic element, the average life span of the red cells being shortened. This occurs in the macrocytic anaemias, iron-deficiency anaemia, in some cases of aplastic anaemia, and in leukaemia. Apart from the macrocytic anaemias, in which the mechanical injury to abnormally large cells during their passage through capillaries may be a factor (p. 478), the nature of the defect in the red cells in the above conditions is unknown.

II. Abnormal extra-erythrocytic haemolytic mechanisms

There are several conditions in which excessive blood destruction results from the presence of an abnormal antibody, which combines with the red cells, rendering them susceptible either to phagocytosis by macrophages, or to the lytic action of complement.

II.A. Auto-immune haemolytic anaemia

One of the commonest causes of acquired haemolytic anaemia is the development of an auto-antibody capable of binding to and damaging the individual's own red cells (cytotoxic antibody, or type II, hypersensitivity, p. 121). Red cells coated with **antibodies of IgG class**, which generally react at 37 °C ('*warm antibodies*'), commonly become microspherocytic and undergo phagocytosis following sequestration in the spleen, liver or bone marrow, i.e. extravascular haemolysis. The clinical picture thus closely resembles hereditary spherocytosis. **IgM antibodies** react at temperatures below 37 °C ('*cold antibodies*') and produce their effects in different ways. Firstly, they may lead to red cell auto-agglutination which produces microvascular occlusion and *Raynaud's phenomenon* (p. 332). Secondly, complement-binding, with consequent haemolysis, is a notable feature and the phenomena associated with *intravascular haemolysis* (p. 465) often dominate the clinical picture. The severity of these effects depends upon the thermal amplitude of the antibody; the higher the temperature at which it can react, the more severe is the disease likely to be.

The mechanism of auto-antibody formation is uncertain. In most instances, however, it seems likely that suppressor T-lymphocyte function has become defective, allowing the development of reactive clones of lymphocytes (p. 135). In other cases, exogenous agents, such as drugs or micro-organisms, may stimulate the formation of antibodies which cross-react with red cell surface antigens.

'Warm antibody' type. Although this condition can develop at any age and in both sexes, it is commonest in women of over forty. Almost half of all cases are primary, while the remainder complicate other diseases, especially systemic lupus erythematosus, rheumatoid arthritis and other putative auto-immune disorders, and malignant lymphomas such as chronic lymphatic leukaemia. Some cases are attributable to drug therapy, α-methyldopa being the most common offender. The clinical picture is that of a chronic, usually fluctuating haemolytic state. Splenomegaly is common. The red cells may show microspherocytosis and increased osmotic fragility, particularly during severe exacerbations. The presence of antibody attached to the red cell surface is the diagnostic feature. The antibody is 'incomplete', i.e., does not agglutinate red cells in saline suspension, and is detected by the direct antiglobulin test (p. 91). Antibody is sometimes present in the serum, and it can be eluted from the red cells. Occasionally it has been found to react with antigens of the Rh system, usually antigen e (p. 230). This might be important in the selection of blood for transfusion. In most cases, the haemolytic process can be controlled by corticosteroid therapy although splenectomy may be beneficial in cases where the spleen is specifically sequestering antibody-coated red cells (p. 121). The excised spleen shows marked engorgement of the red pulp and erythrophagocytosis can sometimes be detected.

'Cold antibody' type. In this group of conditions, the auto-antibodies are usually of IgM class and react only at temperatures below 37 °C. They are often present in the serum in high titre, of the order of 1 in 1000, and give rise to two fairly distinct clinical syndromes. Firstly, *paroxysmal cold haemoglobinuria*, which consists of attacks of haemolysis following exposure to cold, due to union of the antibody with the red cells, and subsequent fixation of complement, causing intravascular haemolysis. Secondly, *cold haemagglutinin disease*, in which the antibody causes also strong haemagglutination, resulting in attacks of cyanosis and Raynaud's phenomenon on exposure to cold, and also chronic haemolytic anaemia in cold weather, due to complement fixation and also to increased mechanical fragility of the agglutinated red cells.

Paroxysmal cold haemoglobinuria. The classical type of this condition occurs in association with syphilis, particularly congenital syphilis. The cold antibody is unusual in being of IgG class; it reacts with antigens of the P system, present in the red cells of nearly all individuals and is capable of strong complement fixation and causes *intravascular haemolysis*. The mechanism of haemolysis was elucidated by Donath and Landsteiner, who demonstrated haemolysis *in vitro* by first chilling the blood to allow the cold antibody to react with the red cells, followed by warming to allow complement activity. This was the first demonstration of an auto-immune disease mechanism, and the test is still used, although paroxysmal cold haemoglobinuria must now be extremely rare as a complication of syphilis, at least in this country. Indeed, most cases of paroxysmal cold haemoglobinuria encountered nowadays are not associated with syphilis, although a false-positive Wassermann reaction is not uncommon.

Cold haemagglutinin disease. This tends to affect middle-aged or older individuals, and while it is sometimes idiopathic, more commonly it is secondary to various diseases, especially lymphomas, connective tissue diseases, or following certain infections, especially *primary atypical pneumonia* due to infection with *Mycoplasma pneumoniae*. The antibody is of IgM class and commonly reacts with the antigen I, which is present in the red cells of nearly all individuals. The thermal amplitude of antibodies of this type varies, and the disease occurs only in those subjects with antibody reacting at temperatures up to about 30 °C. The direct antiglobulin test is usually positive using anti-IgM or antibody to complement, but negative with anti-IgG. The haemagglutinin titre of the serum is usually 2000–64 000 when tested at 2 °C. When the condition follows primary atypical pneumonia it is self-limiting, the antibody disappearing within a few months.

II.B. Iso-antibodies to red cells

(1) Haemolytic disease of the newborn (HDN). Fetal red cells commonly enter the maternal circulation during labour and sometimes they provoke the formation of antibodies to blood group antigens foreign to the mother. Such immune iso-antibodies tend to belong to the IgG class and are thus capable of crossing the placental barrier in subsequent pregnancies, with the result that the fetal red cells will be damaged should they possess the appropriate antigen (Fig. 5.5, p. 122). Since at least twenty common blood group systems are known to exist, some degree of fetal maternal incompatibility is inevitable, but in practice the Rh system (p. 230), and in particular the antigen D, is responsible for most of the severe cases of HDN. The disease only occurs in a small proportion of those at risk (i.e. of those with an Rh −ve mother and an Rh +ve father). This is because: (*a*) the first born child, for reasons already given, is not affected unless the mother has been previously immunised by a blood transfusion or previous abortion; (*b*) the father is sometimes heterozygous (Dd), in which case the fetus has a 50% chance of being Rh −ve; (*c*) ABO incompatibility between mother and fetus often prevents immunisation of the mother with fetal (e.g. D) antigen. Incompatible fetal red cells (say Group A) entering the maternal circulation are destroyed by maternal natural (anti-A) iso-antibody before they can stimulate production of Rh antibodies. ABO incompatibility itself rarely causes severe HDN because the antibodies are usually of the IgM class and incapable of crossing the placenta, although occasionally IgG antibody is present and causes a relatively mild form of the disease.

HDN varies considerably in severity. In milder forms there may only be transient jaundice and anaemia—**congenital haemolytic anaemia**—and treatment is often unnecessary, or simple blood transfusion alone is sufficient. A more dangerous form, known as **icterus gravis neonatorum**, is of extreme importance, for urgent treatment is required and is often successful. In this condition jaundice develops shortly after birth, and if the level of unconjugated serum bilirubin is allowed to exceed 15 mg per ml (250 μmol per litre) there is a serious danger of permanent brain damage—*kernicterus* (p. 662). The infant is usually anaemic, with reticulocytosis and many normoblasts and primitive erythroblasts in the blood. Marked hepatosplenomegaly is usual and in fatal cases there is widespread liver cell necrosis, together with extensive extramedullary haemopoiesis in the spleen, liver, kidneys and adrenals. The only effective treatment of this condition is exchange transfusion, that is the removal of red cells from the fetus and their replacement by compatible red cells (e.g. lacking D antigen). When very severe, HDN causes intrauterine death due to marked anaemia and congestive cardiac failure—**hydrops fetalis.**

The possibility of HDN should become known from blood grouping early in pregnancy, if necessary also on the husband. When Rh incompatibility exists, the mother's serum should be examined during pregnancy for Rh incomplete antibody. Confirmation of HDN can be obtained by detecting a raised level of bilirubin in samples of aspirated amniotic fluid. Early delivery may save some infants, but with others intrauterine fetal transfusion with Rh −ve blood is indicated. Once the infant is born, the diagnosis and treatment are based on the detection of IgG antibody on its red cells by the direct antiglobulin test (p. 91), and assessment of the blood changes and clinical features outlined above.

There have been most significant advances in the prevention of HDN. Trials initiated by Clarke (1963) demonstrated conclusively that intravenous injection of Rh antibody (anti-D) of IgG class into the mother, shortly after delivery, greatly reduces the chance of her developing anti-D antibody herself and lessens the risk of HDN in subsequent pregnancies. Such prophylactic injections are now widely used. It is, of course, most important to avoid Rh-incompatible blood transfusions, which were formerly an important cause of iso-immunisation.

(2) Transfusion reactions. When incompatible blood is transfused into a recipient in whose circulation the appropriate antibodies are already present, a haemolytic transfusion reaction results and the transfused cells are rapidly destroyed. The results of an incompatible transfusion depend to some extent on the speed of destruction of the transfused red cells and this is likely to be greater when abundant iso-antibody is present, e.g. in ABO incompatibility, especially transfusion of Group A blood into a Group O recipient, or of Rh positive blood into an Rh negative *immunised* recipient. These are not the only incompatibilities encountered, but are so much the most common that stringent precautions must be taken to avoid them. The patient is likely to suffer a rigor, pain in the back and pyrexia; shortly thereafter haemoglobinuria appears, followed by jaundice. In a severe reaction death from shock may occur within a few minutes. If the patient survives, haemostatic failure may develop. Later the urinary output may diminish and death may result from acute renal failure (p. 785).

Similar clinical effects may result from the transfusion of blood that is too old, or contaminated by Gram −ve organisms, some of which grow freely at refrigerator temperature (cryophilic bacteria).

II.C. Parasitic invasion of red cells

In malaria and oroya fever the parasites invade and destroy large numbers of red cells, thus producing an anaemia.

(1) Malaria. There are three types of malarial fever caused by four different parasites. These are (*a*) the tertian, with paroxysms of fever every other day, caused by *Plasmodium vivax* and by *Plasmodium ovale,* (*b*) the quartan, with paroxysms at 72 hr intervals, caused by the *Plasmodium malariae* and (*c*) the subtertian or malignant malaria caused by *Plasmodium falciparum*, in which the fever is without a regular cycle. These parasites belong to the *Haemosporidia*, a sub-class of the *Sporozoa*. The first three are closely allied, being of the same genus, and the gametocytes or sexual cells are of spherical form; in the fourth the gametocytes are crescentic. Each parasite passes through two cycles of development—an asexual one or *schizogony* in the human subject, and a sexual one of *sporogony* in the mosquito. In the former cycle, the gametocytes are formed, but undergo no further development in man, while in the latter, conjugation of the gametes formed from the gametocytes takes place in the mosquito. Several species of mosquito of the genus *Anopheles* have been found to be capable of carrying infection. The onset of a febrile attack of malaria coincides with the setting free of a new brood of young parasites (merozoites) by the asexual division of the adult forms within the red cells, and the period of the fever depends on the time taken for the full development from the young to the adult form. Multiple infection occurs when parasites are introduced by mosquitoes on more than one occasion, so that parasites at different stages of development are present. Sometimes also mixed infection occurs, e.g. by the tertian and subtertian parasites.

Cycle of development in man. When man is bitten by infected mosquitoes, sporozoites are injected and are carried to the liver, where they undergo a stage of development within the hepatic cells (Fig. 16.22). Schizogony takes place and culminates after 6–9 days in the liberation of merozoites in large numbers into the blood, where they enter the red cells. This preerythrocytic development constitutes the incubation period of the disease of about 6–9 days. Within the red cells the parasites go through further cycles of asexual proliferation which cause the paroxysms of fever. It is highly probable that in benign tertian malaria there are persistent exoerythrocytic forms of the *P. vivax*, from which the relapses so characteristic of the disease are derived.

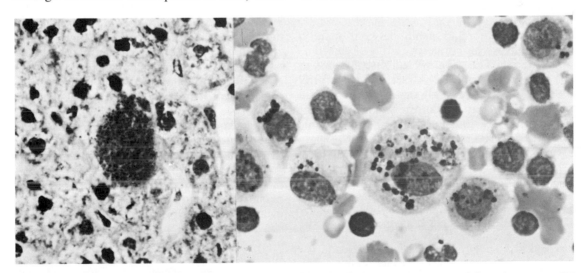

Fig. 16.22 Development of malaria parasites within a liver cell. × 600. (Preparation kindly lent by Professor P. C. C. Garnham.)

Fig. 16.23 Malaria; monocytes containing pigment. × 680

Malarial anaemia. With each bout of fever a large number of red cells are destroyed by the parasites, and the dark brown pigment formed from the haemoglobin is taken up by monocytes and by macrophages in the spleen, liver, etc. It is accordingly not surprising that in chronic malaria anaemia may be severe. *Blackwater fever*, due to intravascular haemolysis, will of course greatly intensify the anaemia. Malarial anaemia is generally of the normochromic or mildly hypochromic type and there is an early reticulocytosis, but in chronic cases deficient formation of red cells may be present. A few normoblasts may sometimes be found. When severe, malarial anaemia may become macrocytic, especially in falciparum infections. This may, in some cases at least, be due to excessive demands for folic acid. There is usually a mild leukopenia, but with an increase in monocytes, some of which may contain malarial pigment (Fig. 16.23).

Blackwater fever is an acute attack of intravascular haemolysis, occurring usually in Europeans who have or have had malaria. There is haemoglobinaemia and methaemalbuminaemia and the urine is dark from the presence of haemoglobin and methaemoglobin. It is accompanied by fever, vomiting, shock, and sometimes convulsions and coma, and is often fatal. Acute renal failure with anuria is common. The haemolytic mechanism is not known: in some cases quinine may precipitate an attack.

The possible relationship between malaria and Burkitt's lymphoma (p. 265) is of considerable interest. The geographical distributions of the two conditions in Africa coincide fairly closely, and it seems likely that either malaria in childhood, or an infective oncogenic agent transmitted by insects, plays a carcinogenic role.

(2) Oroya fever. This is caused by infection with a small gram-negative bacillus—*Bartonella bacilliformis*—which colonises the red cells and macrophages. Infection is transmitted by certain species of sandfly (*Phlebotomus*) and is limited to the slopes of the Andes. The infected red cells show increased mechanical fragility and become sequestered in the liver and spleen, haemolytic anaemia resulting. The organisms can be seen in Romanowsky-stained blood films. Fever, joint and muscle pains, and enlarged lymph nodes are followed by a papular skin eruption.

II.D. Haemolytic toxins and chemicals

(1) Bacterial toxins. Extensive infections with bacteria which secrete haemolytic toxins can result in acute haemolysis. Examples are *Cl. welchii* and *Strep. pyogenes*.

(2) Haemolytic chemicals are numerous. Phenylhydrazine, lead, arseniuretted hydrogen, saponin, potassium chlorate are a few examples which have been extensively investigated. In *chronic lead poisoning* the effect of lead is upon the red cell surface, rendering the cells brittle and increasing the mechanical but diminishing the osmotic fragility: they are short-lived, and anaemia results. Lead also interferes with haemoglobin synthesis and the utilisation of iron; and so the red cells tend to be hypochromic although iron is plentiful in the marrow. Iron accumulates in the nucleated red cell precursors which are then called sideroblasts (Fig. 1.12, p. 11). Lead also precipitates the RNA of young polychromatophilic erythrocytes in the form of punctate basophilia. The anaemia is rarely severe, and the diagnostic feature is the presence of punctate basophil (stippled) cells which are most easily detected in smears from the lower part of the buffy coat. The detection of punctate basophilia is now seldom used in the diagnosis of lead poisoning, which can be achieved earlier and with more certainty by the more specific method of estimating the concentration of lead in the blood. The disorder in haemoglobin synthesis induced by lead is reflected in the high levels of erythrocyte protoporphyrin, urinary coproporphyrin and aminolaevulinic acid, the estimation of which can be valuable in diagnosis.

(3) Drugs. These are an important cause of haemolysis, and can produce this by a variety of mechanisms. Most common is the *Heinz body type* of haemolytic anaemia, in which there is oxidative denaturation of the haemoglobin molecule (p. 456) sometimes preceded by methaemoglobinaemia. Many drugs with oxidative potential have been incriminated, including phenacetin, sulphonamides, salazopyrin, dapsone, primaquine, etc. Individuals with a defective hexose monophosphate shunt mechanism, usually as a result of glucose-6-phosphate dehydrogenase deficiency (p. 468), are particularly susceptible, although if drugs of this kind are taken in large enough amounts even normal individuals are affected. Haemolysis is usually only moderate and tends to be self-limiting since reticulocytes are more resistant to this kind of drug-induced damage. Withdrawal of the drug is curative. Occasionally drugs produce haemolysis by an *antibody-mediated mechanism*. Some drugs, e.g. penicillin, quinidine, phenacetin, may act as haptens which bind to red cells and stimulate the formation of antibodies. The anti-hypertensive drug α-methyldopa, however, appears to induce the production of auto-antibodies, and in about 20% of patients taking this drug the red cells can be shown by the direct antiglobulin test to be coated with antibody (p. 122). Only rarely, however, does a frank haemolytic state supervene: it is indistinguishable from auto-immune haemolytic anaemia of warm-antibody type.

(4) **Vegetable poisons.** The term 'alimentary haemolysis' is used to describe haemolytic states arising as a result of the ingestion of various fruits and vegetables. Usually this only happens in individuals affected by the more severe Mediterranean type of glucose-6-phosphate dehydrogenase deficiency. The best-known example is *favism*, caused by the ingestion of broad beans (*Vicia faba*). The chemical component in beans responsible for haemolysis is uncertain, although it is known to induce oxidative denaturation of haemoglobin with the formation of Heinz bodies (p. 456). Similar haemolysis can result from inhalation of certain pollens.

II.E. Mechanical damage to red cells

(1) **March haemoglobinuria.** This consists of acute haemoglobinuria, usually mild, resulting from long marches. The haemolysis is now believed to be due to mechanical injury to the red cells sustained in the circulation through the soft tissues of the plantar aspect of the feet and brought on by the prolonged mild trauma of long walks, particularly on hard surfaces and carrying heavy loads.

(2) **Microangiopathic haemolytic anaemia** is a haemolytic state of varying severity, associated

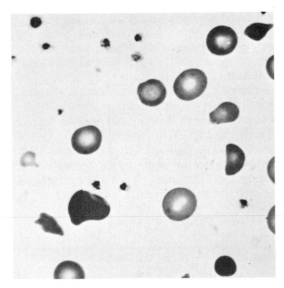

Fig. 16.24 Fragmentation of red cells in micro-angiopathic haemolytic anaemia. × 1000.

with red-cell fragmentation (Fig. 16.24) and thrombocytopenia; it is observed in a variety of clinical situations, including obstetric complications such as ante-partum haemorrhage and pre-eclampsia, malignant hypertension, thrombotic thrombocytopenic purpura (Moschcowitz syndrome), the 'haemolytic-uraemic' syndrome of childhood (p. 789), carcinomatosis, especially if the tumour is of mucin-secreting type, and endotoxic shock (p. 227). A common factor in all these conditions is the presence of widespread fibrin deposition in small arteries, due either to intravascular activation of the blood-clotting mechanism or to vascular damage (microangiopathy). It is thought that the red cells are fragmented when they become enmeshed in fibrin strands, as shown experimentally by Brain and Dacie. A similar form of red-cell fragmentation has also been observed in patients with artificial heart valves, which invariably produce some degree of red cell damage, occasionally resulting in overt intravascular haemolysis with haemosiderinuria and even iron deficiency.

Dyshaemopoietic anaemias

The essential feature of this type of anaemia is the failure to deliver to the blood sufficient numbers of normal red cells despite the presence of adequate precursors in the marrow. Indeed, under the influence of erythropoietin, there is often grossly increased marrow cellularity in dyshaemopoietic anaemias, which contrasts strikingly with the paucity of red cells in the circulating blood. This implies that most red cells produced in the marrow reach an insufficient degree of maturation to be released into the circulation and these may actually undergo destruction within the marrow itself. Much of the erythropoietic activity can thus be regarded as ineffective (p. 463). Anaemias of this type are usually due to failure of the marrow to obtain substrates which it requires for normal red cell maturation. The most important examples are the megaloblastic anaemias and iron-deficiency anaemia.

Megaloblastic anaemia

This form of anaemia is characterised by the presence in the bone marrow of a distinct abnormality of haemopoiesis known as *megaloblastic change*. This affects granulocytes and platelets as well as red cells, but the alteration in erythropoiesis is most conspicuous. By far the commonest cause of megaloblastic haemopoiesis is **deficiency of either vitamin B$_{12}$ or folic acid** although, much less often, similar changes occur in cytotoxic drug therapy, rare inherited enzyme defects, and in the uncommon neoplastic condition of erythraemic myelosis (di Guglielmo's disease). In the peripheral blood, megaloblastic anaemia is typified by an increase in the mean corpuscular volume (MCV) of the red cells and is the commonest cause of 'macrocytic' anaemia. It must be emphasised, however, that other forms of anaemia can be macrocytic in the absence of megaloblastic marrow change. This is especially

true of the anaemia of chronic liver disease, but anaemia following severe haemorrhage, haemolysis or marrow replacement (p. 453) is occasionally macrocytic, presumably because of a high reticulocyte count, although some forms of aplastic or refractory anaemia also show this change.

The effects of vitamin B$_{12}$ and folic acid deficiencies

Of the many tissues affected by deficiency of these two substances, those in which there is a high rate of cell replacement or nucleic acid synthesis are particularly susceptible. This explains the predominant involvement of the haemopoietic system, and the haemopoietic changes are identical in vitamin B$_{12}$ and folic acid deficiency. In some other tissues, however, the effects differ; neurological changes, for example, are only obvious in B$_{12}$ deficiency.

(1) Peripheral Blood. In established cases the red cells, granulocytes and platelets are all reduced in number, i.e. there is a **pancytopenia**. The red cells invariably show an increase in MCV and since the MCHC is normal, the MCH rises in direct proportion to the MCV. These changes may all be evident before anaemia becomes apparent. As anaemia develops, the red cells show increasing variation in size (anisocytosis) with many small cells or cell fragments as well as macrocytes over 10 μm in diameter. Grossly abnormal red cell shapes also become prominent (poikilocytosis), in advanced cases (Fig. 16.25). Nucleated red cells, often with megaloblastic features (see below), can almost always be detected in severe cases (Fig. 16.26), especially in smears prepared from

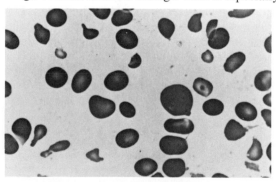

Fig. 16.25 Red cells in pernicious anaemia, prepared from below the buffy coat, showing gross anisopoikilocytosis. × 650.

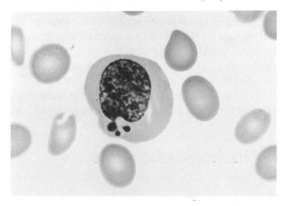

Fig. 16.26 Blood in pernicious anaemia showing a megaloblast with Howell–Jolly bodies. × 1300.

the red cell buffy coat layer in centrifuged whole blood. This technique may be diagnostically useful should marrow examination prove to be impracticable. The reticulocyte count is usually less than 2%, although sometimes there is a slight increase, possibly reflecting a mild haemolytic element in the anaemia, which is suggested also by a slight increase in serum bilirubin. This latter may, however, result from breakdown of red cell precursors in the marrow (see below). There is usually significant neutropenia, associated with the presence of large hypersegmented neutrophils with six or more lobes (macropolycytes), often detectable at an early stage of the disease. Conversely, occasional myelocytes are seen in severe cases. The reduction in platelets is usually moderate, but is sometimes less than 50 000 per μl, and purpura may result (p. 503).

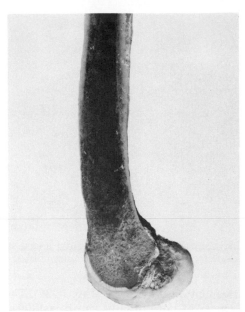

Fig. 16.28 Section of femur in pernicious anaemia, showing the dark red marrow throughout the shaft. × ½.

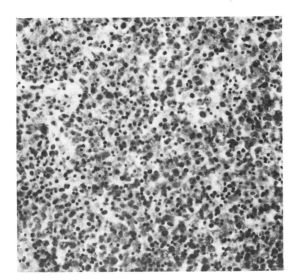

Fig. 16.27 Bone marrow from femoral shaft in pernicious anaemia, showing an extreme degree of megaloblastic hyperplasia with complete loss of fat and absorption of the bony trabeculae. × 250.

(2) Bone marrow. Diagnostic changes are observed in marrow aspirated from sites in the axial skeleton, such as the sternum or iliac crest. The cellularity in such aspirates is maximal, with complete loss of the fat spaces (Fig. 16.27), even when anaemia is minimal. Necropsy studies further reveal the marked expansion in haemopoietic tissue, which may ultimately extend throughout the entire length of the long bones (Fig. 16.28). Cytologically all the

haemopoietic elements are affected to some extent. Erythropoiesis undergoes a profound alteration, described as **megaloblastic change** nearly 100 years ago by Ehrlich, who noted its resemblance to the form of erythropoiesis predominating in fetal life. The essential feature of this change is a delay in nuclear maturation, with the accumulation of many cells in an early stage of development (Fig. 16.29). This phenomenon is described as **'maturation arrest'**, although it is likely that many immature cells die in the marrow without ever delivering functional red cells to the peripheral blood. This is called '*ineffective erythropoiesis*' and is the hallmark of a dyshaemopoietic anaemia. Morphologically, nuclear immaturity is expressed by an increase in nuclear size with a characteristically stippled chromatin pattern. A variety of other 'dyserythropoietic' abnormalities, including polyploidy and nuclear fragmentation with Howell–Jolly body formation, can also be demonstrated. Haemoglobinisation of the cytoplasm of developing erythroblasts is much less seriously affected, and the asynchrony between nuclear and cytoplasmic maturation leads to the appearance of the most distinctive manifestation of megaloblastic erythropoiesis in the marrow, the '**haemoglobinised megaloblast**', a cell which although fully haemoglobinised,

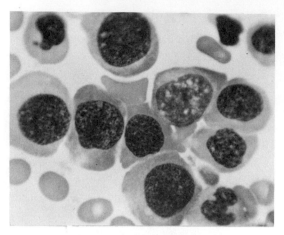

Fig. 16.29. Smear of bone marrow from a case of pernicious anaemia, showing large megaloblasts. × 1100.

possesses an immature nucleus (Fig. 16.30). The various stages of normoblastic and megaloblastic erythropoiesis are compared in Figs. 16.1 and 16.2 (p. 451). Interference with granulocytic development is most readily identified by the presence of abnormality at the metamyelocyte stage. This cell is greatly enlarged, and possesses a large horseshoe-shaped unsegmented nucleus (the giant metamyelocyte). Megakaryocytes are often quite difficult to find, possibly as a result of a defect in the maturation of precursor forms.

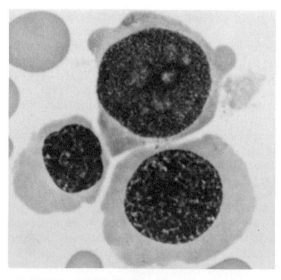

Fig. 16.30 Smear of bone marrow in pernicious anaemia, showing a haemocytoblast (*above*) and two typical haemoglobinised megaloblasts. × 1700.

(3) Neurological changes. These are only conspicuous in B_{12} deficiency, and it is important to note that they may be present when anaemia is mild or even absent. The principal lesion is referred to as **subacute combined degeneration** of the spinal cord, characterised by a discontinuous demyelination of the long pyramidal tracts and posterior columns in the midthoracic region. There is in addition a **peripheral neuropathy**, and foci of demyelination are sometimes found in the cerebral hemispheres. These changes are fully described on p. 715. Early clinical recognition of subacute combined degeneration is extremely important because, although it can be arrested by treatment, it is disabling and not completely reversible. Further, the administration of folic acid alone can exacerbate the condition. Should urgent treatment of a megaloblastic anaemia be required before the cause can be established, it is essential to give both B_{12} and folic acid.

(4) Other tissue effects. Epithelial changes can be detected in both B_{12} and folic acid deficiency. Atrophy of the epithelium of the tongue, sometimes associated with glossitis and focal ulceration, is a common feature of B_{12} deficiency, and megalocytic epithelial cells have also been detected in smears from the cervix uteri. Mild villous atrophy in the small intestine has also been reported (p. 582). Megalocytic changes have been described in the crypts of Lieberkuhn in the small bowel in folic acid deficiency, although villous atrophy has only been observed experimentally. Sterility, presumably due to disturbed maturation of germ cells in the gonads, has been described both in males and females suffering from B_{12} deficiency and can be reversed by specific therapy. Marked haemosiderin deposition in the renal tubules is observed in untreated cases of megaloblastic anaemia, probably a result of the haemolytic element mentioned above. Slight to moderate splenic enlargement, due to increased red cell destruction or to extramedullary haemopoiesis, is often present.

Causes of vitamin B_{12} deficiency

Although existing in several forms, B_{12} is basically a cobalamin which consists of a cobalt-containing porphyrin linked to a ribonucleoside. It is derived mainly from animal sources, such as glandular meats, muscle and eggs, although produced commercially from bacteria and moulds. The minimal daily requirement is approximately 1 μg and the normal serum level as assayed by microbiological techniques is between 160 and 1000 ng/litre (=pg/ml). Normally the liver stores sufficient vitamin to provide the total needs for 6 to 10 years. Absorption from the gut is dependent on the binding of dietary B_{12} to a gastric mucoprotein known as **intrinsic factor (IF)** in deference to Castle who initially demonstrated its existence in 1929. In man, IF is produced by the parietal cells of the gastric fundus and the IF-B_{12} complex formed in the stomach traverses the greater part of the small bowel before the vitamin is absorbed in the terminal ileum. The causes of B_{12} deficiency are as follows.

(1) Dietary deficiency. Diets deficient in B_{12} are quite common in, and largely restricted to, underdeveloped parts of the world. Strict vegetarians would theoretically be expected to develop B_{12} deficiency, but this is observed only occasionally.

(2) Intrinsic factor (IF) deficiency. This is by far the commonest cause of B_{12} deficiency. The classical example is **pernicious anaemia**, recognition of which is usually attributed to Addison in 1855. This disease, described in detail below, is basically a diffuse atrophic gastritis, in which there is almost complete destruction of the specialised fundal cells, including the all important parietal cells, by an inflammatory process now thought to be auto-immune in origin.* Total gastrectomy also eliminates IF secretion, but overt signs of B_{12} deficiency may be delayed as long as 10 years if the liver stores are normal. A small proportion of patients also develops B_{12} deficiency following partial gastrectomy, usually due to chronic gastritis in the remaining portion of the stomach. Rarely, B_{12} deficiency is due to a congenital failure of IF secretion, although the stomach is morphologically normal.

(3) The 'blind-loop' syndrome. There are several conditions in which the IF-B_{12} complex formed normally in the stomach fails to reach its absorptive site in the distal ileum. Uptake of B_{12} by bacteria proliferating abnormally in the more proximal parts of the small bowel is the usual cause. Almost any form of intestinal stasis, if sufficiently prolonged, can cause such

colonisation, although surgical blind loops, jejunal diverticula and chronic obstruction are most often responsible, and co-existent malabsorption of fat can usually be demonstrated (p. 583). Stasis in the afferent jejunal loop might be involved in some cases following partial gastrectomy of the Polya type. In Scandinavia a comparable deviation of B_{12} from its absorptive site can be caused by fish tapeworms in the upper small bowel, although frank B_{12} deficiency usually only develops in those individuals who already have a co-existent defect of IF formation (i.e. atrophic gastritis).

(4) Malabsorption. Extensive disease of the distal ileum interferes with the final stage of B_{12} absorption. This occurs invariably in tropical sprue (p. 582) but in only 30% of cases of adult coeliac disease, in which the mucosal lesions tend to be mild or even absent in the distal ileum (p. 582). In Crohn's disease (p. 562) in which the terminal ileum is frequently involved, B_{12} deficiency is a recognised complication, and of course surgical resection of the ileum inevitably eliminates B_{12} absorption. A rare congenital condition in which there is an isolated defect of B_{12} absorption in the ileum has also been described.

Pernicious anaemia

This disease was the first cause of B_{12} deficiency to be described and is still the most important. It is particularly prevalent in individuals of North European stock and is predominantly a disease of the elderly, being uncommon under the age of 40 years. There is a strong familial tendency, relatives of patients being at much greater risk of developing B_{12} deficiency than the general population. Relatives also have a high incidence of auto-immune thyroiditis, and there is convincing evidence that pernicious anaemia belongs to the group of organ-specific auto-immune disturbances (p. 133). The basic lesion is a diffuse atrophic gastritis (p. 546), involving the fundal portion of the stomach and leading ultimately to histamine-fast achlorhydria and grossly impaired IF secretion. Antibodies to parietal cells are found in the serum in 90% of cases, and in 60% antibodies to IF itself can also be demonstrated. Perhaps more significantly, IF antibodies have been found in the

---

* It is a curious coincidence that both of Addison's diseases should have turned out to be in the organ-specific auto-immune group (p. 133).

gastric juice in about 50% of cases and in the majority the antibodies block the binding site for B_{12} on the IF molecule. Such antibodies have the effect of nullifying the activity of the IF, already severely reduced by chronic gastritis. In the few young patients with pernicious anaemia, IF antibody is more frequently found and there are often associated auto-immune disturbances such as adrenal insufficiency, hypoparathyroidism and malabsorption ('juvenile pernicious anaemia'). The present view of pernicious anaemia is that it is caused by a genetic predisposition to develop auto-immune reactions to gastric antigens; this leads to diffuse atrophic gastritis and reduced IF secretion, the final event ensuring frank B_{12} deficiency in many cases being the appearance of IF antibodies in the gastric juice. Symptoms directly referable to the stomach are seldom evident, and the effects of B_{12} deficiency, especially anaemia and neurological disturbance, dominate the clinical picture. There is, however, an increased risk of gastric carcinoma in patients surviving for long periods on treatment. The anaemia is usually insidious and many patients are severely anaemic before they seek medical advice.

The diagnosis of vitamin B_{12} deficiency states. Once evidence of a megaloblastic anaemia has been obtained, usually by marrow examination, B_{12} deficiency is established by the demonstration of a reduced level of the vitamin in the serum, which is assayed most often by a microbiological technique using *Euglena gracilis* or *Lactobacillus leichmannii* as the test organism. Confirmation is provided by the observation of a distinct reticulocyte response between 5 and 10 days after the parenteral administration of B_{12}, although the marrow reverts to normoblastic erythropoiesis within 24 hours. It is now standard practice to identify the cause of B_{12} deficiency by the use of radio-isotopic techniques, especially the *Schilling test*. In this test, a small dose of B_{12} labelled with ^{58}Co is administered orally, followed by a parenteral loading dose of 1 mg of unlabelled vitamin to prevent cellular uptake of any of the labelled B_{12} absorbed from the gut. The degree of absorption is assessed by measuring either the urinary excretion of labelled vitamin over a 48-hour period, or the serum level after 36 hours. If dietary deficiency is responsible, absorption is normal, whereas in IF deficiency,

as in pernicious anaemia, there is subnormal absorption which is usually rectified by the oral administration of IF with a second dose of labelled B_{12}. In the blind loop syndrome, IF does not improve absorption, although broad-spectrum antibiotics usually do so. More specific therapy is, however, required to improve B_{12} absorption in malabsorptive states, e.g. the gluten-free diet in coeliac disease (p. 582). Although the demonstration of IF deficiency is necessary for certain diagnosis of pernicious anaemia, the demonstration of histamine-fast achlorhydria or of antibody to IF each establishes the diagnosis beyond reasonable doubt. Antibody to parietal cells is not so helpful, for it is common in people with less severe gastritis, without pernicious anaemia.

Causes of folic acid deficiency

The chemical name for folic acid is pteroylglutamic acid and it consists of pteridine and para-aminobenzoic acid coupled to a single glutamic acid molecule, although in nature it usually exists in a polyglutamate form. The main dietary sources are fresh green vegetables, e.g. spinach and lettuce, cereals, meat, fish and eggs. The estimated minimum daily requirement is 50 μg, but much more is needed in pregnancy and in some pathological states (see below). The storage capacity of the body is much less than that for B_{12} and is only sufficient for about 80–100 days. Absorption of folic acid takes place predominantly in the upper small bowel. The causes of folic acid deficiency are as follows.

(1) Dietary deficiency. This is a common contributory factor in many folic acid deficiency states, and is of particular importance in the elderly, who often have suboptimal diets, and in infancy when weaning is delayed; dried milk is also a poor source of folic acid. Any condition in which there is anorexia and poor dietary intake, e.g. alcoholism or chronic gastro-intestinal disease, predisposes to folic acid deficiency.

(2) Malabsorption. Only two conditions are known with certainty to cause malabsorption of folic acid, namely coeliac disease (p. 582) in which folic acid deficiency is invariable, and tropical sprue (p. 582). In both these diseases there are extensive pathological changes in the upper small bowel. Few other intestinal diseases produce chronic lesions of comparable extent, and folic acid deficiency arising in conditions such as Crohn's disease (p. 562) or following partial gastrectomy, are more likely to be due to impaired dietary intake. There is, however, a rare condition known as *congenital malabsorption of folate*, which is thought to be due to an inherited defect in the intestinal mucosal transport system for folic acid.

(3) Increased requirements. The most important condition in which the requirement for folic acid is increased is pregnancy, the haematological complications of which are discussed below. Diseases in which there is greatly increased haemopoietic activity, such as haemolytic states, myelosclerosis (p. 487) or leukaemia, or rapid proliferation (usually neoplastic) of other tissues, can similarly predispose to folic acid deficiency.

(4) Drugs. It cannot be over-emphasised that therapeutic agents can produce an astonishing variety of haematological disturbances, and one of the most notable examples of this is the megaloblastic anaemia associated with anticonvulsant drugs such as phenytoin. The mechanism involved is uncertain, but these drugs probably interfere with folic acid absorption. It is also suspected that oral contraceptives can lead to folate deficiency. Some cytotoxic drugs, such as methotrexate, are folic acid antagonists and are given deliberately to induce folate deficiency in dividing tumour cells; some degree of megaloblastic change in the marrow is thus inevitable.

Anaemias of pregnancy

It is well recognised that the haemoglobin level tends to fall during normal pregnancy. This so-called 'physiological anaemia' is probably due to an expansion of plasma volume rather than to any fall in the total haemoglobin content of the blood. Nevertheless, true anaemia due to haematinic deficiency is common, mainly because of the demands of the developing fetus, particularly for iron and folic acid. These demands are greatest during the later months of pregnancy. An adequate diet will normally meet the increasing requirements imposed on the mother, but haematinic deficiency is especially liable to develop when a woman is in negative haematinic balance at the onset of pregnancy.

Iron deficiency is common enough in non-pregnant women of reproductive age (p. 484) and not surprisingly is the commonest cause of anaemia during pregnancy: although debilitating, it is seldom severe. *Megaloblastic anaemia*, often severe, is not uncommon in the last third of pregnancy. It is due to deficiency of folic acid and so the traditional term 'pernicious anaemia of pregnancy' is not appropriate and should be discarded. Since it is potentially dangerous for a woman to begin labour in an anaemic state, supplementation of the diet with both iron and folic acid is now a routine part of ante-natal care, and it is recommended that the daily intake of folic acid should be not less than 200 μg during pregnancy. Rarely other forms of anaemia, such as aplastic anaemia, arise during pregnancy, although almost any form of blood disorder can complicate pregnancy as a fortuitous event.

The diagnosis of folic acid deficiency

The presence of megaloblastic haemopoiesis in the absence of evidence of B_{12} deficiency strongly suggests deficiency of folic acid. The microbiological assay of the serum folate level, using *Lactobacillus casei* as the test organism, has some diagnostic value if the result is less than 3μg/litre, although the more time-consuming assay of the red cell folate content is more accurate, especially in deficiency of some duration. It must be noted, however, that a low red-cell folate, less than 100 μg/litre, is also found in B_{12} deficiency. The haematological response to a small oral dose of folic acid therefore remains the most convincing evidence of deficiency.

The biological actions of vitamin B_{12} and folic acid

These two substances are obviously of importance for normal cell function, and in particular for normal cell division. Their activities are clearly interrelated, although the nature of this relationship has yet to be fully clarified. Certainly both act as co-enzymes in a number of biochemical reactions. The main function of folic acid co-enzyme is the transfer of single carbon units in such reactions as the breakdown of histidine, the synthesis of methionine and, of particular relevance to the pathogenesis of megaloblastic haemopoiesis, the synthesis of

DNA and RNA. It now seems likely that folic acid is only active biologically in the polyglutamate form, and that B_{12} is required for the intracellular conversion of the transport form of folic acid, 5-methyl-tetrahydrofolate, to the polyglutamate form. This would explain why B_{12} deficiency leads to megaloblastic haemopoiesis, which is largely due to a failure of DNA synthesis, and to neurological disturbance, thought to be a result of impaired RNA synthesis in nerve cells (Chanarin, 1974). It would also account for the observation that biochemical tests of folic acid deficiency, such as the urinary excretion of formimino-glutamic acid (FIGLU) following a loading oral dose of histidine, are often positive in B_{12} deficiency. Co-enzyme B_{12}, however, has other functions, including a critical part in the catabolism of methyl-malonic acid, an intermediate product of valine and propionic acid metabolism: B_{12} deficiency thus leads to the appearance of this metabolite in the urine following a loading dose of valine, a test of potential diagnostic value.

Iron-deficiency anaemia

Since there is no excretory mechanism for iron, body iron content is controlled entirely by absorption from the gut. The mechanism of control of absorption, and the distribution, control and forms of storage of iron are discussed on p. 241 *et seq.*

Less than 1 mg of iron is lost passively from the body every day, and this is easily balanced by absorption of a similar amount of iron from food. In menstruating females, however, the average daily losses are increased to around 1·6 mg daily, and in the second and third trimesters of pregnancy to around 3·0 mg daily; iron balance is thus more precarious in menstruating women in the child-bearing era, and it is not surprising that the majority of patients with iron-deficiency anaemia are women in the reproductive period of life.

Negative iron balance will occur either when there are excessive losses of iron from the body, or when there is impaired intake or absorption of iron relative to demands; co-existence of both processes often occurs in the individual patient. Negative iron balance is compensated for a time by mobilisation of the iron stores and by enhanced absorption from the gut, allowing the haemoglobin to be maintained at normal levels. Eventually, however, the stores become depleted and the characteristic changes of iron deficiency begin to appear in the blood.

Causes of iron deficiency

(1) Dietary failure. Poor intake of iron makes an important contribution to iron deficiency, especially in underdeveloped countries, and in infants before the onset of mixed feeding. Dietary deficiency of iron is, however, rarely the sole cause of anaemia.

(2) Chronic blood loss. Essentially this is the only way by which significant amounts of iron can be lost from the body. Heavy menstrual bleeding is commonest, but any source of chronic or recurrent blood loss will have the same effect. Of particular importance diagnostically is occult bleeding from unsuspected gastro-intestinal tract pathology, especially an ulcerated tumour, since iron-deficiency anaemia may be the only indication of such underlying conditions. Infestation with hookworm (ankylostomiasis), which causes considerable gastro-intestinal bleeding, is probably the most common cause of iron deficiency in the world, and an important cause of chronic morbidity in tropical areas.

(3) Malabsorption of iron. Iron is absorbed mainly in the duodenum and diseases affecting it may cause iron deficiency, e.g. coeliac disease. An intact stomach is also important for iron absorption, and gastrectomy or achlorhydria predispose to iron deficiency.

(4) Increased requirement. The expanding red cell volume of pregnant women, and of actively growing infants and adolescents, may lead to a relative negative iron balance; iron deficiency is particularly common at such periods of life.

The blood picture

The anaemia is of the *microcytic hypochromic type*, the cells being of smaller diameter than

normal and of reduced volume, e.g. 50–70 fl
(μm^3). They are inadequately filled with
haemoglobin so that the MCH is reduced to 27
pg or less; many of the red cells may show ring-
staining owing to deficiency in haemoglobin
(Fig. 16.32), but this is not a reliable diagnostic
feature, and can appear as an artefact in smears
of normal blood. A more useful feature is the
presence of poikilocytes, including rod-shaped

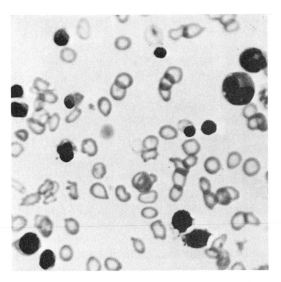

Fig. 16.32 Sternal marrow in hypochromic
microcytic anaemia, illustrating the increased
proportion of erythroblasts, many of which are
poorly haemoglobinised normoblasts. In severe iron
deficiency, as here, ring-staining of erythrocytes may
be conspicuous. × 1000.

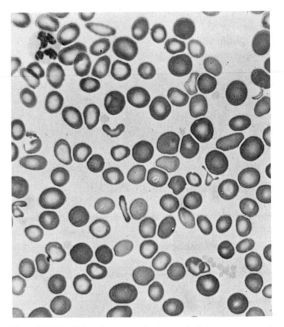

Fig. 16.31 Blood smear in iron-deficiency anaemia,
showing some variation in the size of red cells and
some rod cells: note that ring-staining is not conspicuous and certainly not diagnostic. × 800.

cells (Fig. 16.31). The fall in the number of red
cells is usually slight or moderate, and erythroblasts are rarely found. The leucocyte count
is usually normal. The platelet count is also
normal but in long-standing cases it may be
increased. The concentration of serum bilirubin
is usually normal, although there is sometimes
mild haemolysis, but if blood loss is an important factor there may be a reticulocytosis. The
serum iron is low and the total iron-binding
capacity is increased. **The marrow** is hyperplastic
due to erythropoietin stimulation, but because
of lack of iron, production of haemoglobin, and
therefore of red cells, is inadequate: cytologically there is an increased number of early
forms and of small, poorly haemoglobinised pyk-

notic normoblasts (Fig. 16.32). Sections of marrow stained by the prussian blue reaction show
an absence of stainable iron in the macrophages, confirming that all storage iron has
been used up.

Associated conditions

In iron deficiency, the haematological effects
are the most obvious, but other signs of tissue
iron depletion may be found. The nails become
striated and brittle and may eventually become
spoon-shaped (*koilonychia*). Atrophic glossitis
and angular cheilosis with fissuring of the
angles of the mouth also occur. A minority of
patients suffer from dysphagia, which may be
purely functional. In some patients it is associated with the formation of post cricoid webs
(p. 541). The association of anaemia, glossitis and
dysphagia was first recorded by Brown-Kelly and
Patterson in 1919, but is more usually known as
the Plummer–Vinson syndrome; it may predispose to the later development of post-cricoid
carcinoma of the oesophagus. A high proportion of iron-deficient patients have achlorhydria
and there may be various degrees of gastric
mucosal change ranging from superficial

gastritis to gastric atrophy as severe as that found in pernicious anaemia. In most patients, however, it is possible that the achlorhydria is the result of iron deficiency, analogous to the other tissue changes: only in a minority does it appear to precede the anaemia and play a role in the development of iron deficiency through malabsorption. Once achlorhydria has developed, it will nevertheless tend to aggravate the iron deficiency. The oral and nail changes usually respond to iron, but achlorhydria may be permanent.

Iron deficiency is much the commonest cause of hypochromic anaemia, but any condition characterised by failure of haemoglobin synthesis will have the same effect. In some patients the fault may lie in globin synthesis (p. 470) and in others a failure to synthesise adequate amounts of haem.

Anaemia from disturbances of iron metabolism

Iron deficiency is a disorder of iron balance, but other anaemias are characterised by abnormalities in internal iron exchange. Iron derived from haemoglobin catabolism by macrophages is usually bound to plasma transferrin and returned to the bone marrow for haemoglobin synthesis; such iron is donated to the developing normoblasts by transferrin, and is later inserted into protoporphyrin to form haem. This pathway may be compromised in two situations:

(a) Secondary anaemia of chronic infection and inflammation. Here there is a block in the release of iron by macrophages, with consequent fall in plasma iron and failure of iron supply to the normoblast. This may contribute to the production of a hypochromic red cell. The mechanism of such anaemias is, however, more complex and toxic marrow depression and mild shortening of red cell survival may also play a part.

(b) Sideroblastic anaemia. This is a heterogenous group of disorders which have in common the presence of prussian blue +ve staining granules in the normoblast, usually arranged around the nucleus in a ring fashion. These granules are iron-laden mitochondria (Fig. 1.12, p. 11), and result from impairment of iron utilisation within the cell; since iron is not being inserted into the porphyrin precursors, haem cannot be formed and there is thus poor haemoglobinisation of the red cells. Sideroblastic anaemia may occur in a familial form, or be secondary to a wide variety of differing conditions including carcinomas, leukaemia and exposure to certain drugs and toxins, notably lead and certain anti-tuberculous drugs. Some sideroblastic anaemias may respond to pyridoxine therapy.

Hypoplastic and aplastic anaemias

Anaemia due to diminution in the volume of haemopoietic marrow is termed *aplastic* when little or no cellular marrow exists, and *hypoplastic* when the marrow is merely of reduced cellularity, as is more commonly the case. Aplasia restricted to red cell precursors is rare and it is more usual for all the haemopoietic cell lines to be affected, resulting in pancytopenia in the peripheral blood; the blood picture is thus attributable to marrow failure to produce cellular elements in sufficient numbers to replace natural wastage from ageing or destruction. Pure red cell aplasia and pancytopenia may each occur in a congenital or acquired form:

(a) Pure red cell aplasia

Congenital—Blackfan–Diamond anaemia ('erythrogenesis imperfecta').

Acquired—usually in adults, often associated with thymic tumours.

(b) Pancytopenia

Congenital—Fanconi anaemia, usually associated with other mesenchymal, e.g. skeletal, abnormalities.

Acquired—see below.

All these forms are rare apart from acquired pancytopenia and this will be considered in greater detail below.

Aplastic anaemia with pancytopenia

The characteristic blood findings are normochromic, normocytic anaemia, granulocytopenia and thrombocytopenia; this produces anaemic manifestations which may be severe, increased liability to infection which is often fatal, and thrombocytopenic bleeding. The bone marrow is often difficult to aspirate and contains a reduced number of cells. It is either fatty (Fig. 16.33) or consists of gelatinous connective tissue containing few haemopoietic cells but often some plasma cells.

Aplastic anaemia may be apparently spontaneous or may result from the administration of agents toxic to the bone marrow. Cytotoxic drugs or x-rays used in the treatment of malignant disease regularly produce marrow depression in proportion to the dosage given; usually it is possible to avoid severe damage by careful attention to dosage. In some patients, however, marrow aplasia may result from an *idiosyncratic reaction* to certain drugs, particularly chloramphenicol, sulphonamides, phenylbutazone and other antirheumatic agents, and antithyroid drugs; such drug reactions are now a major problem and are not infrequently fatal. On occasion, the marrow may be found to be hypercellular, e.g. in benzene poisoning, but this group of conditions is poorly understood; the anaemia in such cases is attributed to failure of red cell maturation and release from the bone marrow, rather than diminished precursors.

It is important to distinguish pancytopenia attributable to aplastic anaemia from the other pancytopenias which can occur in marrow replacement (e.g. leukaemia), megaloblastic anaemia, and hypersplenism. Such distinction must usually be based on marrow biopsy.

Agranulocytosis and thrombocytopenia, due to failure of marrow production, may each occur in pure form and are considered respectively on pages 458 and 503.

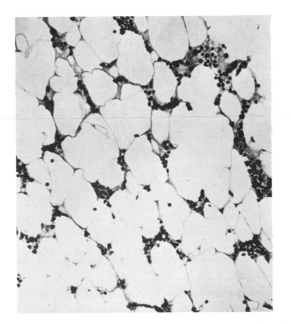

Fig. 16.33 Sternal marrow biopsy in aplastic anaemia due to chloramphenicol. There is great reduction in the numbers of all the cellular elements. × 250.

Myeloproliferative Disorders

All precursor cells of the erythroid, leucocyte and megakaryocyte series may undergo physiological proliferation in response to appropriate stimuli. However, each cell type may also undergo purposeless proliferation; such conditions can be regarded as haematological neoplasia, e.g. red cell proliferation may lead to **polycythaemia vera**, white cell proliferation to **myeloid leukaemia**, megakaryocyte proliferation to **haemorrhagic thrombocythaemia**, and fibrous proliferation to **myelofibrosis** or **myelosclerosis.** These conditions are known as the myeloproliferative disorders. They occur most frequently in a chronic form in which the cell type is well differentiated, but they may also take a more acute or aggressive course when poorly differentiated or primitive cells are involved.

There is some evidence for an interrelationship between these disorders. Firstly, transitions from one to another may occur in the course of the disease; for example, polycythaemia after some years may convert to typical myelofibrosis or terminate in acute myeloid leukaemia. Secondly, features of more than one proliferative condition may be present from the outset; thrombocytosis is for instance, a common early feature of chronic myeloid leukaemia, and polycythaemia vera is usually associated with evidence of increased myeloid cell and platelet production. It is attractive to assume that such inter-relationships between myeloproliferative disorders could have a basis in the common origin of each cell type in the primitive haemopoietic stem cell (p. 450); the final form of the disease in each individual would then be determined by differentiation favouring only one cell type or several types.

It would be a mistake, however, to infer too close a relationship or assume an aetiological connection that is as yet unproven. Fundamental differences do exist between some of these conditions, e.g. the neutrophils in polycythaemia vera are rich in alkaline phosphatase whereas in chronic myeloid leukaemia the enzyme is reduced; the Philadelphia chromosome characteristic of chronic myeloid leukaemia (p. 450) is not found in the formative cells of polycythaemia or myelofibrosis. There is, moreover, no evidence that the haemopoietic stem cell can give rise to fibroblasts, and myelofibrosis and myelosclerosis in some respects resemble reactive more closely than neoplastic changes.

The term myeloproliferative disorder is thus a useful descriptive term but there is a danger that it may be used uncritically to cover a variety of conditions of essentially distinctive nature.

Myelofibrosis

This is an uncommon myeloproliferative disorder occurring in old people. It is characterised by replacement of the bone marrow with fibrous tissue (Fig. 16.34) of both collagen and elastic type. Bone marrow aspiration is usually impossible ('dry tap'), and open trephine biopsy is needed for diagnosis. There is conspicuous extramedullary haemopoiesis, and enormous enlargement of the spleen and liver may occur. The blood picture is leuko-erythroblastic (p. 453). The anaemia is mainly attributable to inadequate red cell production, but a haemolytic element due to hypersplenism may contribute.

The leukaemias

These diseases are caused by neoplastic proliferation of the leukocyte-forming tissues, especially in the bone marrow; this is usually reflected by an overflow of neoplastic cells into the blood and a rise in circulating leukocytes, but sometimes this does not occur (*aleukaemic leukaemia*). In addition the neoplastic cells can infiltrate almost any other tissue, and produce general organ enlargement or tumour masses. Most of the clinical effects of leukaemia can be attributed to tissue infiltration or to interference with normal marrow function by the proliferation of neoplastic leukocytes. Precursors of each of the three main types of leukocyte— granulocytes, lymphocytes and monocytes— can become leukaemic, and each type of leukaemia may be either acute or chronic. The acute forms are characterised by a rapid clinical course and the predominance of primitive cells (myeloblasts, lymphoblasts or monoblasts), both in the marrow and the blood, whereas the chronic forms run a more protracted course and the neoplastic cells are mostly well differentiated. Monocytic leukaemia, the least common of the three major types, almost always presents as an acute or subacute form of leukaemia. Certain rare forms of marrow neoplasia closely resemble acute leukaemia clinically; these include megakaryocytic leukaemia and erythraemic myelosis (di Guglielmo's disease) which are probably both variants of acute myeloid

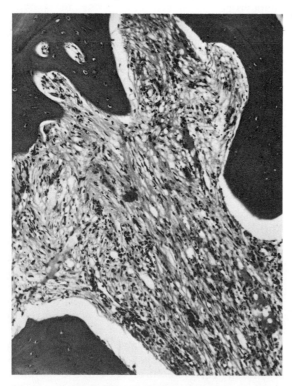

Fig. 16.34 Myelofibrosis. Section of bone showing replacement of the haemopoietic marrow by fibrous tissue.

leukaemia, and plasma cell leukaemia which is a rare feature of myelomatosis (p. 498).

Acute leukaemia

Leukaemia occurring in childhood or adolescence is most often one of the acute types. Acute lymphoblastic leukaemia tends to occur most frequently in the young, whereas acute myeloblastic leukaemia predominates in adults. The clinical features of acute leukaemia are attributable mainly to bone marrow failure, with the characteristic triad of anaemia, infection and thrombocytopenic bleeding. The disease appears abruptly with fever, weakness, pallor, bleeding from the gums and petechial haemorrhages in the skin. Intercurrent infections are very common and the whole course from onset to death may occupy only a few weeks. In adults the disease may be more insidious, but the clinical features are similar.

Blood picture. The peripheral blood usually shows a moderate increase in the total white cell count, 20 000 to 50 000 per μl being common; most of these cells are primitive, with nucleoli and a high nuclear/cytoplasmic ratio (Figs. 16.35, 16.37, 16.38). In over one-third of cases,

however, the total white cell count is normal or even reduced—so-called *aleukaemic leukaemia* —although primitive cells can almost always be demonstrated. The clinical presentation in these cases is that of acute marrow failure.

Bone marrow. In marrow aspirates, a marked increase in cellularity is usual and most of the cells are primitive 'blasts' (Fig. 16.36). Sections

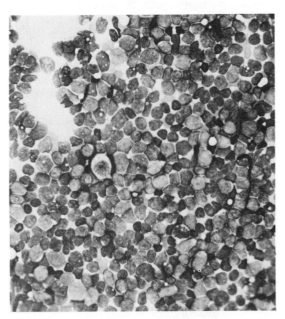

Fig. 16.36 Smear of sternal marrow in acute leukaemia. Nearly all the cells are primitive 'blasts', with a large nucleus. Further details cannot be discerned at this magnification. × 400.

of the marrow show replacement of the fat spaces by the primitive leukaemic cells. Normal haemopoietic elements, especially neutrophils and megakaryocytes, are sparse. At autopsy in untreated cases, there is variable degree of extension of haemopoietic marrow along the shafts of the long bones. It often has a reddish-grey or green hue and a firm consistency.

Other organs. Splenic enlargement is common, but is seldom gross. Lymphadenopathy is unusual in the myeloblastic type but can sometimes be detected in the lymphoblastic type. Of particular interest in the observation that a mediastinal tumour mass histologically of lymphoblastic appearance (p. 526) may precede the onset of acute lymphoblastic leukaemia in childhood. Similarly the onset of frank acute myeloid leukaemia, especially in

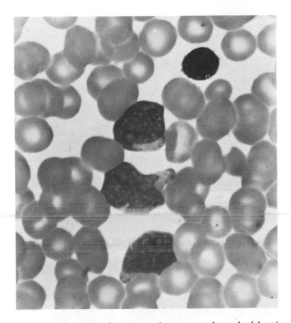

Fig. 16.35 Blood smear in acute lymphoblastic leukaemia, showing three large, primitive leukaemic cells with dispersed chromatin and basophilic cytoplasm. The cell at upper right is a mature lymphocyte. × 1000.

childhood, is occasionally preceded by the discovery of a tumour mass, usually arising under the periosteum of the facial bones; this kind of tumour is called a *chloroma*, since it develops a curious green colour on exposure to air. Histologically it consists of proliferating myeloblasts. More diffuse tissue infiltration occurs during the course of acute leukaemia and almost any organ can be affected. Meningeal infiltration occurs most frequently in acute lymphoblastic leukaemia under treatment; leukaemic cells in the subarachnoid space evade destruction by intravenous cytotoxic agents which fail to cross the blood–brain barrier and provide a nidus of malignant cells from which relapse may develop.

The effects on blood viscosity of high leukocyte counts has already been referred to (p. 453) and occlusion of small blood vessels in the brain by leukocyte thrombi may cause extensive haemorrhagic infarctions.

Identification of cell type. Before effective treatment became available, identification of the cell type involved in acute leukaemia was mainly of academic interest. Nowadays, although sometimes difficult, such identification is critically important from the therapeutic viewpoint and must always be attempted. It is helpful if the primitive blast cells show some degree of differentiation into later forms; thus the association of blast cells with promyelocytes suggests acute myeloid leukaemia, whereas the presence of mature lymphocytes in appreciable

numbers would favour acute lymphoblastic leukaemia. The blast cells themselves occasionally show distinctive features; thus myeloblasts tend to have more nucleoli (2–5) than lymphoblasts and sometimes contain crystalline structures known as Auer rods (Fig. 16.37). Certain cytochemical tests have also proved useful. The Sudan Black B or peroxidase stains can detect the early phases of granulation in myeloblasts, whereas lymphoblasts never show much staining. The periodic acid–Schiff (PAS) reaction for glycogen can demonstrate a distinctive pattern in different blast cells; lymphoblasts commonly show coarse cytoplasmic clumps of PAS +ve material under the cell membrane, whereas myeloblasts are usually negative. It has been shown that high serum or urine levels of lysozyme (muramidase) are characteristic of acute myeloid or myelomonocytic types of leukaemia (see below). In most cases the cells of acute lymphoblastic leukaemia do not have the distinctive features of either T or B lymphocytes (p. 107). In some

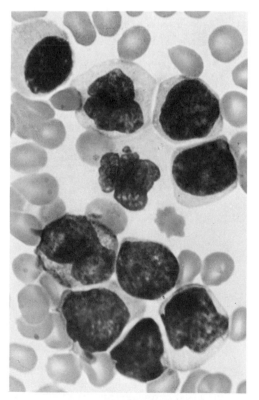

Fig. 16.38 Acute monocytic leukaemia (Schilling type). × 1000.

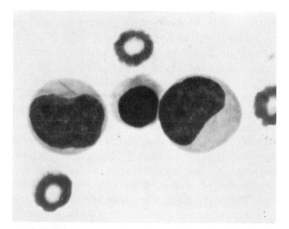

Fig. 16.37 Blood in acute myeloid leukaemia, showing two large myeloblasts; the one on the left contains an Auer rod. The cell in the centre is a lymphocyte. × 1000.

cases, however, they appear to be of T-cell nature. Only rare cases are of B-cell origin and the leukaemic cells closely resemble those of Burkitt's lymphoma (p. 265).

Monocytic leukaemia

This relatively uncommon variety of leukaemia is usually acute or subacute and thus presents clinically with increasing anaemia, pyrexia associated with infective mucocutaneous lesions, and thrombocytopenic purpura. Bleeding, swollen gums and nodular infiltrative skin lesions are characteristic. The total white cell count is not usually very high but in occasional patients may reach 250 000/μl. Most of these cells are monocytes or monoblasts (Fig. 16.38), which may exhibit pseudopodial cytoplasmic projections, a fine peripheral cytoplasmic PAS +ve granularity and lysozyme production (see above). In addition to this purely monocytic form of leukaemia (*Schilling type*), an acute myelomonocytic form of leukaemia in which there is

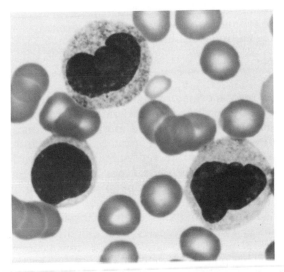

Fig. 16.39 Blood smear in monocytic leukaemia of Naegeli type, showing a myelocyte (*above*) and a promonocyte (*lower right*). The third cell is a lymphocyte. × 1300.

an admixture of myeloid cells and monoblasts (Fig. 16.39) is known as the *Naegeli type*: presumably the leukaemic cells, like the normal myeloid progenitor cell (p. 155), retain the capacity to differentiate into either type of cell line.

Chronic myeloid leukaemia

While commonest in middle-aged and elderly people this disease can occur at any age from birth onwards. The clinical picture is dominated by evidence of organ involvement, particularly of the spleen and liver which become grossly enlarged. Signs of impaired marrow function such as anaemia and thrombocytopenia are usually inconspicuous until late in the course of the disease. After a variable period, usually of some years, transformation commonly occurs to a more aggressive form of leukaemia resembling the acute myeloid type both clinically and pathologically.

Blood picture. The outstanding feature is the very large number of circulating leukocytes which may exceed 300 000 per μl. Most of the cells are mature neutrophil polymorphs (Fig. 16.40) although metamyelocytes and myelocytes are almost always present and in more rapidly advancing cases myelocytes may predominate (Fig. 16.41). Occasionally eosinophils are numerous and a significant increase in basophils is a useful diagnostic feature in the blood film. A substantial increase in promyelocytes and myeloblasts suggests that the disease is undergoing transformation to an acute terminal phase, as mentioned above (*myeloblastic transformation*). While the disease remains chronic, however, anaemia is only moderate and indeed a polycythaemic state has been observed initially in some cases.

Diagnosis is usually easy but rarely a pronounced reactive neutrophilia associated particularly with infections, especially haematogenous tuberculosis, can produce a blood picture closely resembling that of chronic myeloid leukaemia, myelocytes and even less mature cells being observed. Features which help to confirm the diagnosis of chronic myeloid leukaemia include (1) an unusually high proportion of myelocytes, (2) the presence of an absolute basophilia, (3) the almost invariable presence of the Philadelphia chromosome in proliferating marrow cells (p. 450), (4) the markedly reduced level of alkaline phosphatase in leukaemic neutrophils in contrast to the elevated levels observed in reactive leukocytosis, and (5) elevation of the serum vitamin B_{12} thought to be due to an increase in vitamin B_{12}-binding protein.

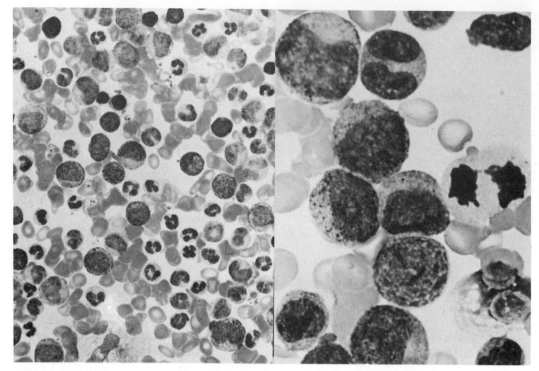

Fig. 16.40   Blood in chronic myeloid leukaemia, showing myelocytes, polymorphonuclear leukocytes and intermediate forms; two erythroblasts are seen above centre of field. × 500.

Fig. 16.41   Blood in chronic myeloid leukaemia, showing finely granular myelocytes and polymorphonuclear leukocytes. One cell is in mitosis. × 1000.

Bone marrow. The medullary cavity of the bones becomes filled with pale, pinkish-grey or slightly greenish cellular tissue (Fig. 16.42). This replaces the red marrow in its normal sites and also the fatty marrow of the shafts and distal ends of the long bones. The marrow cavities are also conspicuously increased by reabsorption of bone trabeculae, and the soft marrow can be cut out in large portions, although at necropsy it is sometimes almost fluid and may even resemble pus. Microscopically there is seen to be a massive increase in the marrow cells; various granulocyte precursors predominate, myelocytes being most numerous except in the acute terminal stage. In some cases megakaryocytes are also conspicuous, while in others there may be a pronounced increase in red cell precursors, the appearances resembling those of polycythaemia vera (p. 496). It is of interest that the Philadelphia chromosome is present not only in the myeloid cells but also in the red cell precursors and megakaryocytes.

Other organs. The spleen is usually massively enlarged and may exceed 3 kg; it often causes great discomfort. It is moderately firm and the cut surface has a pale red mottled appearance, often with even paler patches of infarction. Microscopically the red pulp is packed with leukocytes of the same types as those in the blood; this being partly due to sequestration of circulating cells, but probably also to extra-medullary haemopoiesis, for erythroid precursors and megakaryocytes, in addition to granulocyte precursors, are usually conspicuous. The Malphighian bodies are largely obscured by the massive cellular infiltration of the red pulp. In cases in which the disease advances rapidly, splenic enlargement is usually not so great. **The liver** is usually markedly enlarged and microscopy shows diffuse infiltration with myeloid cells. Diffuse infiltration is usually present in most other organs but varies in degree. In some cases it causes gross enlargement of the kidneys, pancreas, adrenals, etc. The central nervous system may also be involved. In consequence of this extensive infiltration of

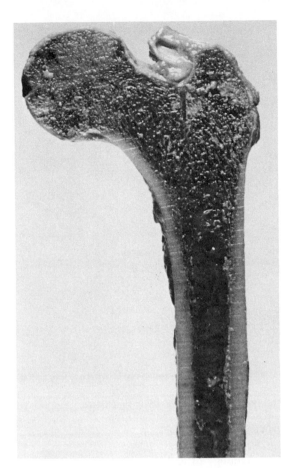

Fig. 16.42 Upper end of the femur in chronic myeloid leukaemia. Pale cellular marrow occupied the whole shaft. There is also resorption of bone trabeculae.

organs and tissues symptomatology varies greatly.

Other features include fatty change of the organs due to anaemia, widespread capillary haemorrhages due mainly to thrombocytopenia, occasionally more extensive haemorrhage, especially in the brain, due to diffuse microvascular occlusion by leukocyte thrombi, and haemorrhagic infarcts in various organs. There is usually a rise in the level of serum uric acid derived from the breakdown of nucleic acids from large numbers of leukaemic cells, especially during cytotoxic drug therapy. Unless prevented by appropriate treatment, for example xanthine oxidase inhibitors, the large uric acid load may lead to formation of urate crystals in the renal tubules and impairment of kidney function.

Chronic lymphocytic leukaemia

This is a disease of middle and old age. It may cause little disability for several or even many years, death commonly resulting from anaemia and infections.

Blood picture. The outstanding feature is a marked increase in leukocytes commonly to around 100 000 per μl and nearly all of these are lymphocytes, mainly with the appearance of

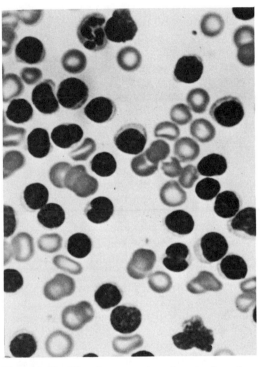

Fig. 16.43 Blood smear in chronic lymphocytic leukaemia. Most of the leukaemic cells have the appearances of normal small lymphocytes, a narrow ring of pale cytoplasm enclosing a round, dense nucleus of about the diameter of a red cell. $\times$ 750.

normal mature small lymphocytes (Fig. 16.43), but with a small proportion of larger, more primitive cells. This disease originates in the lymphoid tissues and extensive replacement of the haemopoietic marrow occurs late. Accordingly, anaemia, granulocytopenia and thrombocytopenia due to marrow replacement are late features. Auto-immune haemolytic anaemia and mild thrombocytopenia, possibly also of auto-immune nature, are complications which sometimes occur quite early in the course of the disease. Extensive involvement of the lymphoid tissues occurs relatively early and may result in a reduction in the normal plasma immunoglobulins and decreased resistance to bacterial infections. Occasionally there is monoclonal gammopathy (p. 498). In most cases the leukaemic lymphocytes can be shown to possess readily demonstrable surface immunoglobulin and sometimes other surface markers characteristic of B cells. Occasional cases however appear to be of T-lymphocyte type.

Bone marrow. In early cases the marrow may appear relatively normal. As the disease advances, however, there is a progressive infiltration of the haemopoietic marrow with leukaemic lymphocytes and as this occurs the fatty marrow is replaced until eventually the shafts of the long bones may be filled with pale leukaemic marrow, resembling that in chronic myeloid leukaemia but usually appearing firmer at necropsy.

Other organs. Generalised enlargement of the lymph nodes is a conspicuous feature and commonly the presenting sign of the disease. The nodes are soft and rubbery and appear homogeneous and pinkish-grey on cutting. Large nodes may cause clinical effects by compressing important structures such as the common bile duct. Microscopically, the enlarged nodes have lost their normal architecture and are occupied by huge numbers of small lymphocytes presenting a monotonous appearance. The spleen is greatly enlarged though not often as massive as in chronic myeloid leukaemia. It usually weighs between 1 and 2 kg and microscopy shows extensive infiltration by mature lymphocytes which fill the red pulp and obscure the Malpighian bodies.

Involvement of the other organs is usually extensive, although it tends to be more patchy than in myeloid leukaemia. The liver is usually enlarged due to infiltration of the portal and periportal areas by leukaemic cells (Fig. 16.44). The kidneys are also usually enlarged, either diffusely or with nodules of leukaemic infiltration. As with chronic myeloid leukaemia the extent of infiltration of the various other organs varies greatly. The risk of renal damage by urate crystals is not as great as in chronic myeloid leukaemia.

Other features include fatty change due to the anaemia, which develops late in the disease, and bacterial infection, especially bronchopneumonia, which is often the immediate cause of death.

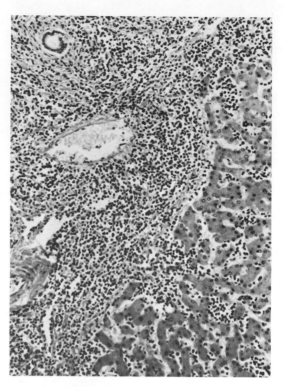

Fig. 16.44 Section of liver in chronic lymphocytic leukaemia, showing infiltration of lymphocytes around the portal tracts. × 60.

The aetiology of leukaemia

The cause of leukaemia in man is still unknown but much has been learned recently about factors that may be involved. The mortality in England and Wales attributed to leukaemia increased from 17 per million in 1931 to 54 per million in 1957. Subsequently, this rate of increase has not been maintained and this provides support for the belief that the increase was due, at least partly, to improved diagnosis.

X-irradiation. There is an undoubted association with ionising radiation; some of the evidence is as follows: (*a*) there is an increased liability to chronic myeloid leukaemia in patients given deep x-ray therapy over the spine for ankylosing spondylitis; (*b*) the incidence of chronic myeloid leukaemia is eight times greater in radiologists than in physicians; (*c*) the incidence of myeloid leukaemia has been high among survivors of the atomic explosions at Hiroshima and Nagasaki. The incubation period between exposure to irradiation and the appearance of the disease is from 6 to over 20 years, and it has been shown that any considerable exposure to x-irradiation produces recognisable chromosome damage which may persist for many years. In all these examples there is a strong indication that the leukaemogenic effect is proportional to the total dose of irradiation.

Less certain are the suggestions that exposure of the fetus *in utero* to diagnostic x-ray examination in the late stages of pregnancy increases the risk of leukaemia in childhood, or that treatment of patients with polycythaemia with radioactive phosphorus increases the incidence of myeloid leukaemia.

Chemical induction. There is considerable evidence that prolonged exposure to benzene may be associated with the later development of acute myeloid leukaemia. The leukaemia is characteristically preceded by bone marrow aplasia which may last for many years if the patient is kept alive by transfusions. Certain drugs known to cause marrow aplasia have similarly been suspected of inducing acute leukaemia, e.g. phenylbutazone and chloramphenicol, although this has not been proved; it has also been suggested that the cytotoxic agent phenylalanine mustard (Melphalan), used in the treatment of multiple myeloma, has been responsible for inducing acute myeloid leukaemia.

The role of viruses. Leukaemia occurs widely in the animal kingdom, and it has long been known that the disease in mice and fowls could be transmitted to unaffected animals of the same strain by the inoculation of cell-free filtrates from leukaemic animals. Mouse leukaemia is also transmissible 'vertically' from mother to fetus, although the latter may not develop leukaemia until it reaches adult life. These features suggest a virus aetiology, and recent work describing the role of viruses in leukaemogenesis in cats, etc., is confirmatory (p. 264). Of particular interest is the integration into the host genome of DNA produced through the action of virus-derived reverse transcriptase on a template of viral RNA.

It has proved much more difficult to obtain firm evidence for a viral role in human leukaemia, although such proof may now be emerging. Many virus particles have been isolated from human leukaemic cells in culture, but their aetiological importance has not been clear, since they may simply be 'passengers'. There is no proof that transmission of leukaemia between humans can occur; in addition, of several hundred reports of pregnant women with leukaemia, the child developed the disease in only two cases. Feline leukaemia virus is widespread in domestic cats, and one study has suggested that the relative risk of leukaemia in children exposed to sick cats was more than doubled, but this is disputed by other investigators; in any case it is improbable that more than a small proportion of childhood cases could be explained on the basis of such contacts.

Genetic factors. There is no good evidence of an increase in the incidence of leukaemia among the relatives of affected patients; a high rate of concordance for leukaemia has, however, been reported for monozygotic twins. Certain genetic diseases appear to predispose to leukaemia, e.g. Fanconi anaemia, and mongolism, and these are associated with a high frequency of chromosomal abnormalities. The abnormal 22 (Philadelphia) chromosome in chronic myeloid leukaemia has already been discussed on p. 450.

In the leukaemias, it seems probable that chromosomal abnormality with the consequent disturbance of the genetic material of the cell is the means by which all these diverse aetiological factors bring about the uncontrolled cellular proliferation which characterises the disease.

Polycythaemia

A true increase in circulating red cell mass is known as *polycythaemia* or erythrocytosis. It may be secondary to various conditions or occur primarily as one of the myeloproliferative disorders.

Secondary polycythaemia is usually the result of stimulation of the bone marrow by erythropoietin. Hypoxia of any type, especially associated with chronic respiratory insufficiency, congenital heart disease with right to left shunts, or living at high altitudes, is the most frequent cause of *secondary polycythaemia*, but inappropriate renal production of erythropoietin from conditions such as hypernephroma, hydronephrosis, or local ischaemic lesions of the kidney may also cause an increase in red cell volume. Tumours elsewhere in the body may rarely produce erythropoietin-like polypeptides, and the resulting polycythaemia may initially be the only evidence of underlying disease. In all such secondary polycythaemias, splenomegaly almost never occurs. The leukocytes and platelets are not usually increased.

Polycythaemia rubra vera (primary polycythaemia) can be regarded as one of the primary chronic myeloproliferative disorders in which an apparently autonomous bone marrow proliferation produces excessive and inappropriate numbers of red cells; this is not a physiological response and indeed renal erythropoietin production is usually suppressed. The disease occurs most commonly in middle or later life. The clinical features include a florid appearance, thrombotic and haemorrhagic episodes and hypertension resulting from the increased blood viscosity. Gout may follow from the grossly increased turnover of nucleoprotein and uric acid production, and splenomegaly is the rule. There is an increased incidence of peptic ulcer. Transformation to myelofibrosis occurs in a proportion of patients, and acute myeloid leukaemia may supervene. Untreated patients survive for around 3 years but the prognosis is improved by efficient therapy.

The blood picture. The circulating blood volume is increased and this is attributable mostly to the often very large increase in circulating red cell mass. The packed cell volume may reach 70–80% in extreme cases, and the red cell count is usually in excess of 7×10^6 per μl. Hypochromia of the red cells is frequent because available iron is insufficient to supply adequate haemoglobin for all the red cells. Unlike secondary polycythaemia, the white cell and platelet counts are often increased, and the latter may contribute to the thrombotic manifestations seen in polycythaemia vera. The marrow usually shows maximal hypertrophy, not solely of red cell precursors, but also of white cell precursors and megakaryocytes.

Plasma cell tumours

Plasma cells are derived from B lymphocytes (p. 101) and are responsible for the synthesis and secretion of antibodies. It is therefore not surprising that those lymphomas which show plasma-cell differentiation commonly produce large amounts of immunoglobulin. Analysis of these so-called *myeloma* or '*M*' *proteins* has shown molecular homogeneity for each tumour, and this has important implications relating both to the nature of tumours and also to the basis of antibody production and specificity (see below).

The most important and best defined of the plasma-cell neoplasms is *myelomatosis*, which differs from other lymphomas in affecting predominantly the bone marrow. Other members of the group are rare: they include *Waldenström's macroglobulinaemia* and *heavy-chain disease*, the morphological and other features of which are intermediate between myelomatosis and the other lymphomas.

Multiple myeloma (myelomatosis)

As stated above, this is a neoplastic proliferation of plasma cells or their precursors, usually confined to the bone marrow, and occurring in elderly subjects, more commonly in men than women. Death results within 2–3 years, mainly from anaemia, infection, renal failure or skeletal lesions. Plasma cells are normally present in the bone marrow and may be increased in chronic infections, connective tissue diseases, etc. The proportion in such reactive states, however, rarely exceeds 10%.

Although not a common disease, multiple myeloma is of considerable interest because investigation of the immunoglobulins ('*myeloma proteins*') produced by the neoplastic cells has contributed significantly to our understanding of both antibody production and neoplasia.

Pathological changes. The neoplastic tissue occurs usually in the form of numerous reddish nodules throughout the bones which normally contain red marrow (Fig. 16.45), but also throughout the long bones. The nodules exert an osteolytic effect so that absorption and rarefaction of the affected bones take place and spontaneous fractures are common, especially in the ribs (Fig. 16.46). The lesions are seen radiologically as sharply punched-out defects in the bone, for example in the calvarium. Less often, widespread plasma cell proliferation in the marrow produces a diffuse osteoporosis without the formation of discrete nodules, and vertebral collapse may occur. Rarely a *solitary plasmacytoma* may develop, usually in a long bone, but in most cases multiple myeloma develops sooner or later. Amputation is there-

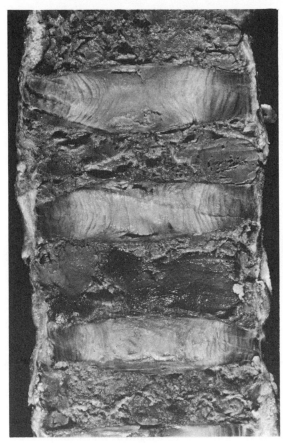

Fig. 16.45 Multiple nodules of myeloma in vertebral column. The vertebral bodies show compression collapse.

fore unlikely to effect cure, though a few successful cases have been recorded. A solitary plasmacytoma may occur in various other tissues, e.g. the nasopharynx, or stomach, and its relation to the true myeloma is uncertain.

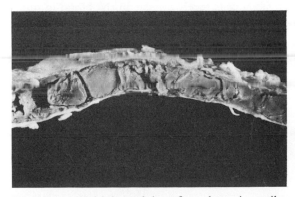

Fig. 16.46 Multiple nodules of myeloma in a rib; numerous spontaneous fractures were present.

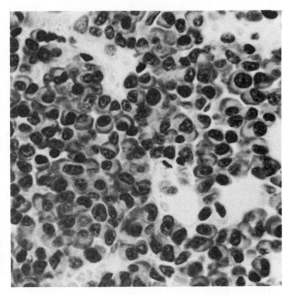

Fig. 16.47 Section of sternal marrow aspirate in myelomatosis: clumps of plasma cells with eccentric nuclei and basophil cytoplasm, showing a marked perinuclear halo. × 600.

Microscopic appearances. The nodules or diffuse infiltrates of myelomatosis are highly cellular and vascular. The appearance of the cells is variable, but most commonly many of them are recognisable as plasma cells (Figs. 16.47, 16.48), having the typical eccentric cartwheel nucleus, and cytoplasm of various grades of basophilia and pyroninophilia due to their content of RNA. There may be a crescentic area of

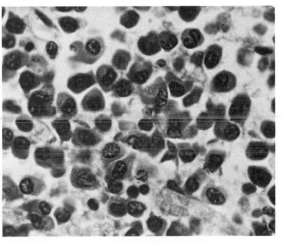

Fig. 16.48 Smear of sternal marrow aspirate showing almost total replacement of the haemopoietic elements by plasma cells. × 600.

pale-staining cytoplasm adjacent to the nucleus, and bi- and tri-nucleate cells are often seen. More primitive cells—plasmablasts—are also present in varying proportions. Cells of intermediate appearance between small lymphocytes and plasma cells may occasionally predominate. There is usually little or no fibrous stroma.

Myeloma proteins. In most cases the myeloma cells, like normal plasma cells, synthesise and secrete immunoglobulin, but when this has been tested for immunological reactivity, it has only rarely been shown to react strongly and specifically, i.e. like an antibody, with any one of a large number of antigens; nor is there any other evidence to indicate that myeloma cells have proliferated as a result of an antigenic stimulus. In most cases, the level of serum immunoglobulins is raised, in some instances exceeding 100 g/litre.

A remarkable feature is the homogeneity of the myeloma protein in each particular case: it is entirely of one or other immunoglobulin class, usually IgG, less commonly IgA, rarely IgD and almost never IgE.* Invariably, its light chains are of one type, either kappa or lambda (p. 88). Its uniformity is most readily shown by electrophoresis, when it appears as a narrow dense 'M' band, contrasting with the broader less well-defined bands of normal serum immunoglobulins. Moreover, evidence from chemical analysis suggests that the individual molecules are identical in the amino-acid sequences of their polypeptide chains. These findings indicate that, in any one case, most or all of the secreting myeloma cells are producing identical molecules of immunoglobulin and this in turn suggests that they have all originated from a single plasma cell or plasma-cell precursor—hence the term **monoclonal gammopathy**. This conclusion supports the view that neoplasms arise from single cells, and also provides strong evidence for Burnet's clonal selection theory of antibody production (p. 104). Comparison of myeloma immunoglobulins of the same class (e.g. IgG) from a number of cases shows that, in contrast to the homogeneity of the protein in each case, the proteins from different cases all differ from one another in their amino-acid sequences.

Another feature of myeloma cells is that they may produce an excess of immunoglobulin light chains in addition to whole molecules, and in 50% of cases light chains in the form of monomers and dimers, of molecular weights 22 000 and 44 000 respectively, are demonstrable in the urine, where they are known after their discoverer as **Bence–Jones proteins**. Adjustment of the pH of the urine to 4–6 and heating results in precipitation of the light chain molecules at about 50 °C, and they re-dissolve at about 80 °C. This test is useful in diagnosis, and especially so in 15% of cases in which only light chains are produced—*light chain myeloma*.

Production of myeloma proteins is often accompanied by a fall in the plasma level of normal immunoglobulins, and it has been suggested that myeloma cells produce a factor which suppresses normal plasma cell function.

Associated changes. *Skeleton.* Myelomatosis causes pronounced bone resorption with focal or generalised osteoporosis, *hypercalcaemia*, and increased excretion of calcium and phosphorus in the urine; the serum alkaline phosphatase, however, is usually not much raised.

Blood. The increased level of immunoglobulin in the plasma results in a tendency to unusually strong *rouleaux formation* and a *high ESR*, while the increase of protein may cause background staining in blood films. *Anaemia* results from extensive infiltration of the marrow by myeloma cells, and is usually of normochromic normocytic type, although blood loss from a haemorrhagic tendency may bring about an iron-deficiency anaemia. A tendency to *haemorrhage* may be due to formation of complexes between myeloma immunoglobulin and several of the clotting factors, but there may also be thrombocytopenia. The neoplastic plasma cells rarely appear in the blood in numbers which warrant the term *plasma cell leukaemia*. Infiltration of various organs may also occur.

Renal changes are common, and result from precipitation of Bence–Jones protein in the lumen of the renal tubules to form dense hyaline casts: these cause tubular obstruction and also stimulate a foreign-body giant-cell reaction, and consequent tubular destruction may bring about renal failure. Nephrocalcinosis resulting from hypercalciuria may also be a contributory factor.

---

* The frequencies of these Ig classes of myeloma proteins correlate with the levels of the classes of Ig in normal serum, and so presumably with the numbers of plasma cells normally producing each class.

Immunological deficiency results from the variable reduction of normal immunoglobulins mentioned above. There is an increased susceptibility to infections and death often results from bronchopneumonia.

Amyloid deposition is a common complication of myelomatosis, and usually presents the pattern of 'primary' amyloidosis (p. 233); it occurs particularly in the light-chain and IgA varieties of the disease and only rarely in IgG myelomas.

Waldenström's macroglobulinaemia

This uncommon condition occurs in individuals over 50 years of age, more often in men than women. The primary form of the disease, which is described below, runs a prolonged course; it is basically a monoclonal gammopathy of IgM class, and may be regarded as a low-grade neoplasm of lymphoid cells. In some cases, however, the syndrome is associated with a frankly malignant lymphoid neoplasm, and the outlook is then poor.

The clinical features include weakness and tiredness; spontaneous haemorrhage from the respiratory, urinary or alimentary tracts and in the periphery of the retinae; susceptibility to bacterial infections, and a variable degree of enlargement of the liver, spleen and lymph nodes. The plasma protein level is usually raised to 80 g/litre or more, and the increase is due to the presence of immunoglobulin of IgM class with a molecular weight of approximately 900 000, and detectable as an M band on serum electrophoresis. It is insoluble in water, and precipitates when the plasma is diluted with water (Sia test).

Of particular importance is the increase in plasma viscosity due to the high level of IgM: this produces extensive microcirculatory stasis with varied symptoms, including blurring of vision, neurological disturbances and haemorrhagic phenomena. This last may also result from the IgM coating the platelets, and preventing release of platelet factor III, but the macroglobulin also interferes with the polymerisation of fibrin.

The macroglobulin also commonly behaves as a cryoglobulin (see above), so that exposure of the patient to cold may result in ischaemia, and even gangrene, of the extremities. The red cells often show a strong tendency to aggregate *in vitro* which renders cell counting difficult, and the ESR is raised.

All these effects are rapidly reversed by the removal of the protein from the patient's circulation by plasmapheresis. The peripheral blood usually shows some degree of anaemia, leukopenia and thrombocytopenia as a result of impaired marrow function, although there is a lymphocytosis in some cases.

Histological changes. There is a diffuse pleomorphic infiltrate of the marrow by small lymphocytes, plasma cells and mast cells, although the most characteristic cell has a morphology intermediate between the lymphocyte and the plasma cell ('*plasmacytoid lymphocyte*') and may have PAS +ve intranuclear inclusions. There are, however, no focal lesions in the bones, which are either normal radiologically or show diffuse osteoporosis. The **lymph nodes** are moderately enlarged and are overrun by the pleomorphic lymphoid infiltrate, although the architecture is not usually destroyed. Similar infiltration is also noted in the portal tracts of the **liver** and the Malpighian bodies of the **spleen**, and has even been observed in the brain—Bing-Neel syndrome. The overall picture closely resembles chronic lymphocytic leukaemia and represents a link between the plasma cell tumours and the malignant lymphomas (p. 526).

Heavy-chain disease

This term is used to describe a group of rare neoplastic conditions in which infiltration of the tissues by lymphoid cells is associated with the presence in the serum of a protein identifiable as the Fc fragment of the immunoglobulin heavy chains (see p. 88). In the most remarkable member of the group, the heavy chain is derived from IgA and lymphoid infiltration with the same pleomorphic character as that noted in Waldenström's disease is largely confined to the mucosa of the small intestine. This unusual type of lymphoma, known as **'alpha-chain disease'**, is mainly found in young adults of eastern Mediterranean origin.

Secondary tumours of bone marrow

Metastatic deposits, both of carcinoma and sarcoma, are fairly common in the bone marrow;

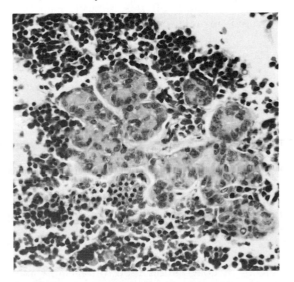

Fig. 16.49 Section of sternal marrow aspirate showing metastatic breast carcinoma. × 250.

and in malignant melanoma and carcinoma of certain organs, especially the breast, bronchus, prostate and thyroid, the nodules may be very numerous and widespread. They occur especially in the red marrow and their presence and nature are sometimes established by histological section of marrow aspirates (Fig. 16.49). When the marrow of the short bones is extensively invaded, there is often a compensatory hyperplasia of red marrow in the long bones. Leuko-erythroblastic anaemia (p. 453) may result, particularly where metastases are numerous and widespread, or when they stimulate an osteosclerotic reaction, a common feature of prostatic cancer metastases.

Haemorrhagic states

Under this heading we have grouped together a number of conditions of different aetiology, which have in common the liability to haemorrhage into the tissues and from mucous membranes. They fall into two broad classes, the **purpuras** and the **coagulation defects**. In purpura, the bleeding is chiefly in the skin and from the surface of mucous membranes and is spontaneous. In coagulation defects, haemorrhage is usually initiated by trauma and is characterised by its persistence rather than by its severity.

Before reading the following account of haemorrhagic disorders, it is essential to have a basic understanding of the physiological mechanisms and the various factors involved in haemostasis and coagulation of the blood. A brief account of this subject has been provided in relation to thrombosis on pp. 196–9.

Defects of coagulation

Coagulation defects may be genetically determined or acquired. The only common examples of the former are haemophilia (deficiency of factor VIII or anti-haemophilic globulin) and Christmas disease (deficiency of factor IX). Genetically-determined defects are due to failure of an individual gene controlling the production of the corresponding clotting factor; thus only single defects occur, affecting one coagulation factor. By contrast, acquired defects of coagulation more often show multiple deficiencies affecting several factors, most frequently II, VII, IX and X.

Congenital defects

Haemophilia. This disease is characterised by a congenital deficiency of factor VIII; this interferes with the intrinsic system of blood coagulation and results in poor formation of thromboplastin. The severity varies widely, but is likely to be the same in affected members, and in different generations, of the same family. The coagulation time of whole blood is greatly prolonged, although it may approach normal after a major haemorrhage. The bleeding time, estimated from a small prick wound, is usually normal, since capillary haemostasis is largely dependent on vasoconstriction and the formation of a platelet plug; for the same reason, venepuncture is usually safe in haemophilic patients.

Excessive bleeding on minimal injury has usually declared itself by the first year of life. Operations such as circumcision, tonsillectomy or dental extractions may cause very severe or fatal bleedings. Recurrent haemorrhage into joints is characteristic; blood in this site is intensely irritant and leads to erosion of cartilage, fibrous adhesions resulting in ankylosis, and eventual crippling. Bleeding can, however, occur from any site, including the nose, gastrointestinal and urinary tracts; haemorrhages into the tissues around the floor of the mouth may cause respiratory obstruction and death by suffocation. Skin petechiae characteristic of the purpuric diseases do not occur.

Haemophilia is restricted to the male sex. It is clearly genetically determined, half of the sons being affected and half of the daughters being carriers. Haemophilia results from a defect in a gene carried by the X chromosome and controlling the development of Factor VIII, the anti-haemophilic globulin normally present in the plasma. The abnormal chromosome (X′) does not cause haemophilia in females (X′X) because the normal X is sufficient to prevent the bleeding tendency; such a heterozygous female does, however, have an abnormally low plasma level of Factor VIII, a feature which is explicable on the Lyon hypothesis (p. 459). Also, half her sons will be haemophiliacs (see below) and half her daughters will be carriers (Fig. 16.50).

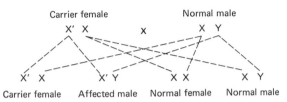

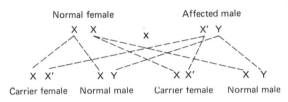

Fig. 16.50 The genetic transmission of the abnormal X chromosome (X′) responsible for haemophilia.

The Y chromosome does not compensate for the X′ chromosome, and so X′Y males are haemophiliacs: their sons will not inherit the defect, but all their daughters will be carriers (Fig. 16.50). Theoretically, half of the daughters of a carrier (XX′) mother and a haemophiliac (X′Y) father would be X′X′ female haemophiliacs, but this must be very rare.

The deficiency can be corrected temporarily by the transfusion of fresh blood or fresh plasma, or more efficiently by the intravenous administration of factor VIII concentrates. After repeated infusions, a refractory state occasionally develops, possibly indicating immunisation of the recipient against anti-haemophilic globulin.

Christmas Disease is due to congenital deficiency of factor IX, which leads to deficient formation of thromboplastin from the intrinsic system. It shows a similar sex-linked inheritance to classical haemophilia, and the clinical pattern of bleeding is identical. Treatment is by the administration of factor IX concentrates.

Von Willebrand's Disease. This condition is acquired by an autosomal dominant inherit-

ance. There is not only marked deficiency of factor VIII, but also capillary fragility; this leads to abnormal bleeding which more closely resembles that of the purpuric diseases than the coagulation defects.

Acquired defects

Combined deficiency of factors II, VII, IX and X in various combinations is seen most commonly in patients on anticoagulant therapy, but occurs also in the following conditions.

(1) *Haemorrhagic disease of the newborn.* This condition, characterised by spontaneous haemorrhages from the umbilicus and mucous membranes, often causes severe melaena; it occurs in about 0·3% of neonates and may be due to inadequate supplies of vitamin K before the intestinal bacterial flora is established: administration of vitamin K to the infant rapidly restores the coagulation time to normal and bleeding ceases. Lack of vitamin K results in the combined deficiency of factors II, VII, IX and X. Administration of 5 mg of the vitamin to the mother in the 24 hours before labour raises the plasma prothrombin of the infant above the danger level. However, if given direct to a premature infant, the dose must be carefully regulated because it may increase haemolysis and thus raise the load of bilirubin which the immature liver cannot conjugate and excrete: the risk of kernicterus is thus increased.

(2) *Malabsorption.* In prolonged obstructive jaundice, or malabsorption from other causes, impairment of absorption of vitamin K may be sufficiently severe to result in combined deficiency of clotting factors; tests for impaired coagulation are therefore of importance before surgical procedures in these conditions.

(3) *Liver failure.* The liver is responsible for production of factor II and other clotting factors. Severe liver insufficiency may thus result in a combined defect, and also in deficiency of fibrinogen (factor I). Needle biopsy of the liver may, in the circumstances, result in severe and even fatal haemorrhage.

Hyperplasminaemic states and the defibrination syndrome. Excessively rapid activation of plasminogen (p. 199) may result in the appearance of free plasmin in the circulation with digestion of plasma proteins, including fibrinogen and coagulation factors. The breakdown products of digested fibrinogen interfere with haemostasis by inhibiting polymerisation of fibrinogen, and there is also accelerated lysis by plasmin of any fibrin which may form. Hyperplasminaemia may occur as a *primary* event when tissues rich in plasminogen activator are traumatised, but is also encountered as a *secon-*

dary phenomenon in response to disseminated intravascular coagulation. Release of thromboplastic substances producing intravascular coagulation may occur as a complication of endotoxic shock (p. 227), surgical operations, certain tumours and obstetric accidents. Treatment of a low fibrinogen level depends on identification of the cause; where primary fibrinolysis is responsible, a fibrinolytic inhibitor (e.g. ϵ-aminocaproic acid) may be used, but if the primary problem is intravascular fibrin formation then either conservative measures, or in some circumstances a heparin infusion, may be indicated.

Afibrinogenaemia occurs also as a rare congenital abnormality; the condition is inherited as a recessive character, and the blood is virtually incoagulable. In severe **liver failure**, production of fibrinogen by the liver may be reduced sufficiently to interfere with coagulation, and afibrinogenaemia may occur also in the cachexia accompanying widespread carcinoma.

Purpura

This term is applied to various conditions in which small haemorrhages occur from *capillaries* throughout the body, resulting in haemorrhagic spots (petechiae) in the skin, mucous membranes and serous surfaces, while more gross bleeding may occur from the mucous membranes of the alimentary, respiratory and genito-urinary tracts; the pattern of bleeding differs from that of coagulation defects, in that haemorrhage from larger blood vessels into tissue spaces is uncommon. In many cases of purpura the bleeding is due to direct damage to the capillaries by an underlying systemic disorder, and the platelets are normal—**non-thrombocytopenic purpura**. Platelets themselves, however, contribute to the integrity of small vessel walls, possibly by continually forming plugs at sites of minimal injury; reduced numbers of circulating platelets may therefore cause abnormal capillary fragility, leading in turn to purpuric bleeding—**thrombocytopenic purpura**. Accordingly it is customary to classify purpura into non-thrombocytopenic and thrombocytopenic types; in each case however the characteristic bleeding occurs from abnormally fragile or permeable capillaries.

Non-thrombocytopenic purpura

(a) Toxic damage to the capillaries may occur in septicaemias, haemorrhagic smallpox and severe scarlet fever. The purpura found in acute meningococcal septicaemia (Fig. 20.25, p. 683) and subacute bacterial endocarditis may be caused by septic micro-emboli or by toxaemia.

(b) Drugs. Many severe cutaneous drug reactions are purpuric, in particular those due to antibiotics and sulphonamides; such vascular reactions must be distinguished from those due to drug-induced thrombocytopenia.

(c) Poor supporting tissues. The common senile or cachectic purpura is probably attributable to poor capillary support from collagen, as is the purpura associated with corticosteroid therapy and Cushing's syndrome. Ascorbic acid is concerned with the synthesis of collagen by promoting the polymerisation of mucopolysaccharide, in conjunction with the phosphatase of fibroblasts, and may also have a role in the formation of intercellular cement substance; thus capillary haemorrhage, most characteristically from the gums around carious teeth, and under the periosteum, but also from other sites as well, is common in **scurvy**. The anaemia of scurvy usually results from haemorrhage but has a mild haemolytic component; since ascorbic acid is concerned also in the conversion of folic acid to active folinic acid, megaloblastic anaemia occasionally results (p. 478). Important changes in the bones also occur (p. 822).

(d) Anaphylactoid (Henoch–Schonlein) purpura. Damage to capillaries may have an *allergic* basis, especially in children. The purpuric rash may develop explosively 2 to 3 weeks after a streptococcal respiratory infection, but the high titres of anti-streptolysin O found in rheumatic fever are not present. Common accompaniments are acute polyarthritis similar to that of rheumatic fever, colic, haemorrhage and serosanguineous effusion into the gut, and an acute haemorrhagic glomerulonephritis (p. 771), which sometimes progresses to renal failure. The preceding streptococcal infection and the lesions resembling rheumatic fever and glomerulonephritis all suggest that this type of purpura is the result of hypersensitivity. Common articles of food, e.g. chocolate, may similarly be responsible for sensitisation.

(e) Congenital abnormalities. Although itself rare, the commonest of these is *hereditary* *haemorrhagic telangiectasia*. This disease is transmitted as a simple dominant in both sexes. Symptoms vary greatly in severity and time of onset, but epistaxis is usually a prominent feature. Multiple small telangiectatic spots, which are, in fact, arteriolar-venular anastomoses, occur in the skin and mucous membranes, and from them repeated haemorrhages occur so that severe anaemia may result. In the lungs similar lesions may give rise to profuse haemoptysis.

Thrombocytopenic purpura

Thrombocytopenia may be said to occur when the platelet count is less than 150 000 μl. It is unusual for there to be abnormal bleeding when the count is greater than 60 000/μl however, and spontaneous haemorrhage does not usually occur until the count has fallen to less than 20 000/μl. Thrombocytopenia may result from impaired marrow production of platelets, as in aplastic anaemias (p. 486), marrow replacement syndromes of all types, and in megaloblastic anaemias (p. 478). Thrombocytopenia may also be caused by damage to platelets in the circulation or by their consumption or trapping in excessive numbers. Such damage may have an immunological basis as in idiopathic thrombocytopenic purpura, the thrombocytopenia of systemic lupus erythematosus, in some cases of chronic lymphatic leukaemia, and in certain drug reactions; excessive consumption or trapping may occur in disseminated intravascular coagulation, in micro-angiopathic haemolytic anaemia (p. 477) or in hypersplenism. In cases where the thrombocytopenia is due to excessive consumption or destruction of platelets in the circulation, normal or increased numbers of megakaryocytes are present in the bone marrow (Fig. 16.51); this is an important point of distinction from thrombocytopenias due to impaired marrow function.

Idiopathic thrombocytopenic purpura. This condition occurs chiefly in children and young adults; it is often a self-limiting disease which disappears spontaneously within 3 months of onset and does not recur, but chronic relapsing cases also occur. In some cases of acute onset, the condition appears to follow an upper respiratory infection, and fulminating cases may occur during pregnancy. The clinical pattern of bleeding may vary from mild cutaneous pur-

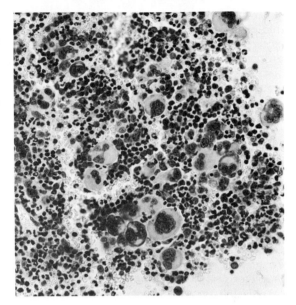

Fig. 16.51 Marrow biopsy in thrombocytopenic purpura showing increased numbers of megakaryocytes, many of which are immature. × 205.

pura to gross uterine, renal or gastro-intestinal haemorrhage. In severe cases, intracerebral bleeding is a particular danger. As in other cases of thrombocytopenic bleeding, the whole-blood clotting time is normal, but the bleeding time is prolonged and clot retraction impaired.

The evidence for an immunological causation for the disease rests on the following: (*a*) the presence of transient thrombocytopenia in neonates born to mothers suffering from the disease, probably due to the transplacental transfer of a maternal antibody; (*b*) the production of the disease in a normal individual following the transfusion of plasma from an affected patient; (*c*) the response of many patients to corticosteroids or ACTH; (*d*) the recent demonstration of specific anti-platelet autoantibodies in many cases; and (*e*) the strong resemblance clinically to the thrombocytopenia complicating systemic lupus erythematosus (SLE). These patients may present only with idiopathic thrombocytopenic purpura, and only some time later manifest the fully developed SLE syndrome.

Many patients respond to corticosteroids, but if these fail, splenectomy may be beneficial; this operation presumably does not affect the degree of platelet sensitisation by antibody, but simply removes the site of their destruction.

Following splenectomy there may be a remarkable overswing in the platelet count which can exceed 1 000 000/μl or more; there is thus a temporary danger of thrombosis, but in such cases the platelet count usually falls to normal again in a week or two.

Immunological drug purpura. Although drugs may produce non-thrombocytopenic purpura by direct capillary damage, and may also cause thrombocytopenia by bone marrow toxicity, some thrombocytopenic drug purpuras are due to immune damage to platelets, the drug acting as a hapten and rendering the platelets antigenic. The best-known example is Sedormid (p. 122), but others include quinine and quinidine.

Other thrombocytopenic states due to excessive platelet consumption or destruction. In states characterised by disseminated intravascular coagulation or **micro-angiopathic haemolytic anaemia** (p. 477), platelet trapping by widespread fibrin deposition in arterioles may induce thrombocytopenia, with the paradoxical result of abnormal bleeding and excessive coagulation co-existing in the same patient. Excessive platelet sequestration or destruction can occur in conditions associated with splenomegaly of any type, e.g. portal hypertension, tropical splenomegaly, myelofibrosis, and this may respond to splenectomy (**hypersplenism**, p. 509). Thrombocytopenia may also result from massive blood transfusion, since stored blood is itself poor in platelets.

Qualitative platelet abnormalities

In certain rare conditions, the platelets may be present in normal numbers but are qualitatively abnormal, resulting in haemorrhage. An example of this is *Glanzmann's disease*, in which the characteristic features of thrombocytopenic bleeding are present although the platelet count is normal. Poor platelet function may also occur in the thrombocytoses associated with some myeloproliferative disorders (e.g. polycythaemia vera).

17

The Lympho-Reticular Tissues

The lymphoid tissues subserve two major functions. Firstly, they are responsible for specific immune responses to antigenic stimulation: this function has been described in Chapter 4 and its protective and harmful effects in the two subsequent chapters. Secondly, the **lymph nodes** and **spleen** also monitor the tissue fluid and blood respectively for abnormal constituents. To perform this second function they contain sponge-like areas of *reticular tissue* and *sinuses* rich in macrophages, through which the fluid filters. Such tissue, together with vascular sinusoids rich in lining macrophages in various non-lymphoid tissues, e.g. the liver and bone marrow, is traditionally grouped together as the *reticulo-endothelial system* (p. 55). The characteristic feature of such tissue is its richness in macrophages. It also contains fibroblasts and other, possibly heterogeneous, cells termed *reticulum cells*, the nature of which is uncertain. The lymph nodes and spleen are thus subject to abnormalities of the lymphoid cells proper and also of macrophages and cells associated with them in the reticular tissue and sinuses. **The thymus** differs from other mammalian lymphoid tissues in being the only known 'primary' lymphoid organ, concerned not with immune responses but with antigen-independent lymphopoiesis (p. 96), and it lacks also the filtering tissue of the lymph nodes and spleen. The **tonsils** and **Peyer's patches**, etc., are not sites of filtration of body fluids but are strategically placed in the wall of the alimentary tract to encounter microbial antigens either absorbed through the epithelium or transported by phagocytes, and to mount the appropriate immune responses.

The Spleen

Functions

As indicated above, the spleen is a composite organ consisting of: (*a*) units of **lymphoid tissue** termed *lymphoid follicles* or *Malpighian bodies* or collectively as the *white pulp*, and (*b*) the vascular network and sinuses termed the **red pulp**, which makes up most of the organ.

The spleen is not an essential organ, and indeed in adults it may be removed without any obvious impairment of health. In infants, however, there is evidence that splenectomy is followed immediately by increased susceptibility to infections by pyogenic bacteria. This is probably attributable largely to the capacity of the spleen to phagocytose micro-organisms in the blood before there has been time for the development of a specific immune response with production of protective antibody. Splenectomised animals, e.g. sheep, are abnormally susceptible to various parasitic infections, and it is known that, in both animals and man, the spleen is an important site of formation of antibodies in response to *intravascular* injection of antigens, and considerably less antibody is produced by splenectomised individuals. The spleen is of less importance than the lymph nodes in the response to antigens injected into the tissues.

The spleen plays an important physiological role in the removal from the blood of old or injured red cells, which are phagocytosed and digested by macrophages in the cords of the red pulp. The bilirubin formed from the breakdown of haemoglobin is secreted into the blood, to be extracted, conjugated and excreted by the liver cells, while the iron is re-utilised in haemoglobin synthesis in the marrow. The average life of the red cells and the number in the blood are not increased following splenectomy, and it is apparent that the phagocytic cells in the liver, marrow and other tissues also destroy old red cells. However, the macrophages in the red pulp of the spleen have a special function in extracting from the red cells various cytoplasmic inclusions, and also in removing the nuclei of any normoblasts which have gained entrance to the circulation, the cells then being returned to the blood. Loss of this function, which is known as 'pitting', is observed following splenectomy, when normoblasts and red cells containing Howell–Jolly bodies may be found in blood films (p. 456).

It is less certain that the spleen is an important site of physiological destruction of leukocytes and platelets, but splenectomy is commonly followed by a polymorphonuclear leukocytosis, sometimes of up to 30 000 per μl, a monocytosis, and a thrombocytosis which may reach 1×10^6 per μl. The polymorphs reach a peak level during the few days following splenectomy, the platelets 2–3 weeks later. The levels decline thereafter, but monocytes and platelets may remain above the normal ranges for months or even years.

Structure

The vascular arrangements of the spleen are of particular importance in relation to its two major functions. The larger arteries branch within the trabeculae, and give off arterioles of approx. 200 μm diameter which leave the trabecula and become ensheathed in a cuff of lymphoid tissue—the Malpighian bodies—to which they supply capillaries. At the periphery of the lymphoid tissue, each central arteriole divides into several penicillar arterioles, many of which show a fusiform swelling of the wall, termed an ellipsoid. The ellipsoid consists of an inner layer of prominent capillary endothelium surrounded by layers of large pale cells and a basement membrane. The red pulp consists of vascular channels termed *sinuses*, lined by elongated endothelial cells with their long axes parallel to that of the sinus. The sinuses traverse the continuous spongework, termed the *splenic cords*, of the red pulp. The sinus endothelial cells are supported by circular reticulin fibres: cells of

the blood and particulate material may pass between the sinuses and splenic cords through gaps between the endothelial cells. The vascular arrangements of the red pulp are not fully understood. Blood may pass from the central arterioles through the penicillar arterioles and thence directly along the sinuses to enter the trabecular veins—the so-called *closed circulation*. By a second pathway—the *open circulation*—the blood passes from the sinuses, which have incomplete walls, into the vascular network of the red pulp and then enters the venules. The distribution of the blood through these two pathways may be controlled by the ellipsoids, which are believed to be contractile, or by contraction of the distal ends of the sinuses. The splenic cords consist of stellate cells, many of which are macrophages, supported on a network of reticulin fibres: in fact, the cords form a continuous spongework through which blood can filter between the stellate cells, eventually draining into venules. The 'open' circulation through the splenic cords clearly provides opportunity for phagocytic removal of abnormal materials or cells from the blood, whereas the 'closed' circuit is a more direct route. In man, the spleen normally contains only 20–30 ml of blood although it can become enlarged and engorged with blood in various diseases.

Shrinkage of the spleen

Atrophy of the spleen occurs in old age, affecting both red and white pulp, and is sometimes a feature of wasting diseases. Hyaline thickening of the walls of the small arteries and arterioles of the spleen is very common and increases in incidence and severity with increasing age; it is by no means confined to subjects with chronic hypertension or generalised arteriosclerosis. The resulting ischaemia brings about splenic atrophy with some increase in reticulin. Splenic ischaemia is also a feature of *sickle-cell disease* (p. 469) and is due to blockage of sinuses by hypoxic sickle cells; infarcts and atrophy result, and eventually the spleen may be converted into a small fibrous remnant, often heavily pigmented by haemosiderin derived from phagocytosed red cells. Severe splenic atrophy is also a feature of some cases of *malabsorption syndrome* (p. 582), the mechanism being obscure.

Splenomegaly

As already stated, the two known major functions of the spleen are the production of specific immune responses and phagocytosis of abnormal materials in the blood. Accordingly, increased functional activity of the spleen, with hyperplasia of the lymphoid or macrophage cells, or of both, commonly results from antigenic stimulation or the presence of abnormal materials, for example micro-organisms, toxins or abnormal cells, in the blood. Splenomegaly is therefore a very common secondary phenomenon in a great many diseases. In general, enlargement of the spleen is attributable to its phagocytic role, and is due to hyperplasia and hypertrophy of the red pulp. Hyperplasia of the Malpighian bodies, with development of large germinal centres, occurs as an immune response in many diseases, and especially in infections. Another feature of the immune response in many diseases, particularly infections, is the development of large numbers of plasma cells, both in relation to the Malpighian bodies and throughout the red pulp, but these latter changes alone are seldom if ever sufficiently marked to give rise to significant splenic enlargement.

Because of its vascular nature and phagocytic role, the spleen is prone to blood-borne infection: it has, however, strong defences against pyogenic bacteria, and abscess formation is uncommon except for septic infarcts in pyaemia. However, bacteria are commonly arrested in the spleen and may be recovered from it in non-pyogenic generalised infections, as in typhoid and undulant fevers and in generalised tuberculosis. Colonisation of the spleen with great enlargement is brought about also by trypanosomes, and by micro-organisms which are capable of survival and multiplication within macrophages, as in leishmaniasis and histoplasmosis.

Moderate splenomegaly results also from chronic portal venous hypertension, as in cirrhosis of the liver or hepatic schistosomiasis.

In diseases of the blood, splenomegaly may result from accumulation and phagocytosis of abnormal cells or platelets; also the spleen may re-assume its fetal role of haemopoiesis, as in anaemia resulting from replacement of the haemopoietic marrow by fibrous tissue (myelofibrosis) or by neoplastic deposits. There is evidence also that splenic enlargement from various causes is sometimes accompanied by increased phagocytic activity (hypersplenism) leading to anaemia, leukopenia and thrombocytopenia (splenic anaemia). This is dealt with more fully on p. 509.

Like most other organs, the spleen may be the site of deposits of amyloid, and great enlargement may occur also in those metabolic diseases resulting in storage of abnormal amounts of various metabolites in the macrophages of the lymphoid and other tissues, e.g. Gaucher's disease. Splenic involvement is common in sarcoidosis, and in the various types of lymphoid and myeloid neoplasias—the leukaemias, Hodgkin's disease, etc.

Infections

Acute pyogenic infections

The earliest change in the spleen is congestion of the cords of the red pulp. As the number of circulating polymorphs increases, they accumulate progressively in the red pulp of the spleen, and in septicaemia, or severe localised pyogenic infections with a high leukocytosis, they may be present in the spleen in huge numbers. At post-mortem examination in such a case, the spleen is slightly enlarged (200–300 g), acutely congested and the splenic tissue is so softened that it looks and feels almost like a bag of fluid; the cut surface is pinkish or deep red, and the tissue is semi-fluid. These changes, sometimes termed 'septic spleen', are due to congestion, accumulation of polymorphs and marked terminal and post-mortem autolysis by the digestive enzymes released from degenerate polymorphs.

In fatal septicaemia, the bacteria may be recovered from the spleen, as from other organs, and the macrophages in the red pulp may contain bacteria, red cells, degenerate polymorphs and cell debris. However, microscopic examination of the septic spleen is seldom satisfactory owing to severe autolytic changes.

As already stated, abscess formation in the spleen is uncommon except when brought about by septic infarction in pyaemia. Involvement of the capsule produces perisplenitis, which may progress to perisplenic abscess.

Non-pyogenic bacterial infections

Moderate degrees of splenic enlargement commonly accompany generalised non-pyogenic bacterial infections, and are due to hyperplasia of both the lymphoid tissue and red pulp of the organ, together with granulomatous lesions brought about by arrest and proliferation of bacteria in the red pulp. As enlargement is due mainly to accumulation and local proliferation of macrophages, lymphocytes and plasma cells, together with increase in reticulin, the spleen is usually firm, and post-mortem autolysis is not nearly so marked as in pyogenic infections. Some examples are given below.

In **typhoid fever** splenic enlargement is an important feature, the weight sometimes reaching 500 g; it is usually deep red from congestion and not particularly soft: as elsewhere in typhoid, there is a virtual absence of polymorphs and accumulation of macrophages (many of which contain ingested red cells), lymphocytes and plasma cells. Typhoid bacilli usually occur in clumps in the red pulp, unaccompanied by any sign of damage in their neighbourhood, but sometimes there is necrosis around them.

Undulant fever is due to infection with small Gram −ve bacilli, the *brucellae*. There are three important species, *Br. abortus*, *Br. melitensis* and *Br. suis*, which commonly infect cows, goats and pigs respectively. Traditionally, infection results from drinking the milk of infected cattle or goats. A combination of pasteurisation and elimination of infection from dairy herds has considerably reduced the incidence in many countries. In this country, infection with *Brucella abortus* still occurs and is an occupational hazard of those who handle infected cattle, particularly in the veterinary profession: infection is also occasionally acquired in medical bacteriology laboratories.

The organisms, which are not easy to isolate in culture, colonise the macrophage system and cause lesions closely resembling tubercle follicles, sometimes with central necrosis: these occur in the lymph nodes, spleen and liver, all of which may be enlarged, but other organs may be affected, and in some cases there is a transient polyarthropathy. The clinical features vary greatly; there is usually fever, either acute or low grade with vague symptoms, malaise and weight loss. Bacteraemia commonly occurs, but is irregular and multiple blood cultures may be negative. Without treatment the condition usually subsides spontaneously but it may continue for months or even years. Diagnosis is dependent usually on either positive blood culture or demonstrating a high or rising titre of antibodies in the serum.

Tuberculosis. In acute miliary tuberculosis the tubercles are specially numerous in the spleen. They generally appear as minute grey points of about the size of Malpighian bodies, from which they may be distinguished by appearing to project slightly from the cut surface when viewed by oblique lighting. In less acute generalised tuberculosis in children, the spleen is occasionally studded with yellowish tubercles of 3–5 mm diameter. In chronic pulmonary and other forms of tuberculosis, a few tubercles of various sizes, and occasionally larger nodules, may be present in the spleen. Rarely the blood may present a very striking leukaemoid reaction difficult to distinguish from true leukaemia.

Protozoal infections

Massive splenic enlargement is seen in malaria and in kala-azar. In **malaria**, the spleen swells acutely during each attack of pyrexia, from acute congestion due to the accumulation of red cells containing the parasites. After repeated attacks, thickening of the stroma with induration may ultimately occur and in chronic cases the organ becomes firm, brownish-grey owing to accumulation of malarial pigment, and may weigh 1–1·5 kg. Some cases of so-called *tropical splenomegaly* (see below) are now thought to be due to chronic quartan malaria.

Kala-azar is the generalised type of leishmaniasis, in which there is widespread colonisation of macrophages by the leishmanial form of the protozoan *Leishmania donovani*. The vectors are various species of sandflies: in Indian kala-azar, man appears to be the only host and sandflies are infected by feeding on cutaneous lesions. In other affected areas of the world, canines and rodents act as reservoirs of infection. In the sandfly and in cultures, the parasite assumes a flagellate (leptomonad) form. *L. donovani* and other species of leishmania also cause localised cutaneous or muco-cutaneous infections in which the parasites are relatively few and the histology is similar to that of tuberculous lesions. The cell-mediated immune response appears to be of importance in determining whether the infection remains localised or becomes generalised.

In kala-azar there is anaemia, leukopenia and usually thrombocytopenia. The spleen is greatly enlarged, often exceeding 1·5 kg. It is firm and the red pulp is largely occupied by collections of macrophages which contain the leishmanial forms of *L. donovani*, known as *Leishman–Donovan bodies*. These occur also in the bone marrow and in the liver, and diagnosis can be made by sternal puncture, but if this fails, liver biopsy or splenic puncture may be required. The parasites are rounded or oval intracellular bodies of 2×3 μm. Each contains a nucleus and a rod-like kinetoplast.

Haematological disorders

The normal function of the spleen in destroying effete red cells, and probably also polymorphs and platelets, has been described on pp. 505–6. Numerous abnormalities of the red cells, as for example in various types of haemolytic and macrocytic anaemias, are accompanied by an increased rate of their destruction in the spleen, and as a consequence there is a great increase in the number of macrophages in the red pulp. The degree of splenomegaly depends on the severity and duration of the process, and is due partly to engorgement of the red pulp with red cells. Similarly in idiopathic thrombocytopenic purpura there is increased splenic destruction of the antibody-coated platelets, although splenomegaly is usually absent or slight. In contrast to these conditions, in all of which splenic hyperfunction is secondary to an abnormality of the blood cells concerned, splenomegaly from various causes may be accompanied by an increased rate of destruction of normal red cells, leukocytes and platelets. This is termed *hypersplenism*, or *splenic anaemia*, and is described below.

The haematological disorders accompanied by great splenomegaly, i.e. to about 2 kg, are chronic myeloid leukaemia, extramedullary haemopoiesis (p. 510) and sometimes chronic lymphocytic leukaemia. Moderate spleno-megaly, to about 1 kg, occurs in acute leukaemia, various haemolytic anaemias and polycythaemia vera. The changes in the spleen in these conditions have been described in the previous chapter.

Splenic anaemia and hypersplenism

The concept that certain disorders of the blood might be attributable to overactivity of the spleen was based on the observation that splenectomy is sometimes followed by improvement in the anaemia, leukopenia and thrombocytopenia (either singly or in any combination) commonly associated with splenomegaly. While it is possible that instances of primary hypersplenism occur in which there is no underlying disorder to account for the splenomegaly, most cases are secondary to splenomegaly due to various disease processes. The commonest of these is *portal hypertension* from hepatic cirrhosis or hepatic schistosomiasis, leading to congestive splenomegaly and sometimes splenic anaemia (the *Banti syndrome*). The anaemia is at first normocytic but after severe or repeated haemorrhage from oesophageal varices it may become markedly microcytic and hypochromic with a low MCHC. Reticulocytes are scanty and the anaemia responds only slowly to iron. The leukocyte count is generally low, often 2000–3000 per μl, and usually all types of white cell are proportionately affected. The platelets in some cases are about normal in number, in others distinctly decreased. Radio-isotope studies indicate excessive sequestration and destruction of red cells by the spleen, and imprints of the cut surface of the spleen sometimes show evidence of phagocytosis of both red and white cells.

In splenic anaemia the marrow shows a normoblastic hyperplasia and primitive cells tend to predominate.

The spleen in portal hypertension. The degree of splenic enlargement is usually much greater than in systemic venous congestion (p. 195); it is commonly about 500 g and seldom exceeds 1·5 kg. The capsule is thickened and often adherent to surrounding tissues. In some cases the organ is congested and blood readily flows out of the excised spleen, leaving the organ somewhat collapsed. In longer-standing cases the spleen is firm, and the Malpighian bodies are usually fibrotic and ill-defined, but may be quite distinct. In many cases siderotic nodules, the so-called Gandy–Gamna bodies, are present. These are organised haemorrhages of the size of pinheads or larger: they often have a yellowish centre surrounded by a brown zone due to deposition of haemosiderin.

Microscopy shows increase in reticulin fibres in the walls of the sinuses and in the reticulum of the red pulp, which may eventually progress to fibrosis. There is also an increase in the numbers of macrophages and fibroblasts in the red pulp and the venous sinuses are not as uniformly nor as greatly engorged and distended as might be expected. The trabeculae are thickened and prominent and recent haemorrhages or older haemosiderin-rich scars (see above) may be seen.

The walls of the dilated splenic and portal veins are often thickened and similar splenic changes, sometimes accompanied by hypersplenism, may result from portal vein thrombosis without cirrhosis. It remains unexplained why the Banti syndrome occurs in some cases of chronic portal hypertension and not in others.

Splenomegaly with extramedullary haemopoiesis. Great enlargement of the spleen may occur when the bone marrow is extensively destroyed by fibrosis, osteosclerosis or secondary carcinoma, especially of the prostate. The increase is due to the development of haemopoietic tissue in the red pulp. All the elements of marrow are represented, but in some cases megakaryocytes are present in marked excess. No doubt such extramedullary haemopoiesis is sometimes compensatory for marrow destruction but in cases of myelofibrosis the splenic abnormality is regarded by some authorities essentially as part of a myelo-proliferative disorder. The spleen may reach a huge size—e.g. 2·5 kg and may contain all the remaining haemopoietic tissue. The organ is of deep red or pinkish red colour but sometimes there are discrete somewhat firm red nodules (10 mm or more in diameter) in which the haemopoietic tissue is more abundant. The Malpighian bodies are indistinct, infarcts are usually absent and as a rule there are no adhesions.

In some cases the spleen is overactive in destroying red cells, and splenectomy may then be beneficial. It is, however, important to determine, for example by double isotope techniques, how much the spleen is contributing to red cell production and destruction.

As usual with extramedullary haemopoiesis, the blood picture is that of leuko-erythroblastosis (p. 453).

Other causes of splenomegaly

Amyloid disease. The spleen is commonly involved in generalised amyloidosis. Deposition may be mainly in the Malpighian bodies, which are changed to translucent rounded patches (Fig. 9.5, p. 234)—*Sago spleen*—or there may be diffuse involvement of the red pulp, in which case the spleen is most often enlarged, sometimes to over 1 kg. The occurrence of the two forms is unexplained, but diffuse involvement is said to be a feature of amyloidosis complicating syphilis.

Sarcoidosis. The spleen is commonly involved in sarcoidosis, although it is not usually enlarged, and frequently the lesions are not visible macroscopically: their histological features are the same as sarcoidosis elsewhere in the body (p. 182), i.e. follicles resembling those of tuberculosis, but showing little or no necrosis, and with multinucleate giant cells which often contain curious stellate and laminated inclusions. In some cases the spleen is extensively affected and moderately enlarged; the coalescent lesions are then visible macroscopically. Splenic anaemia may complicate the condition.

Disorders involving lipid storage

Storage of lipids in macrophages occurs in human disease in two groups of conditions.

(*a*) One group consists of hyperlipidaemias (pp. 20–21); it includes the familial forms of hyperchylomicronaemia, alpha-lipoprotein deficiency (in which unstable beta-lipoproteins are formed in excess), and hyperbetalipoproteinaemia. In these conditions and also in poorly controlled diabetes mellitus, in hypothyroidism, prolonged obstructive jaundice and in dietary hypercholesterolaemia, various grades of accumulation of cholesterol or its esters occur in macrophages (Fig. 17.1), not only in the spleen, lymph nodes, liver, bone marrow, etc., but also in the form of xanthomas in the skin and elsewhere. The increased incidence and severity of atheroma in these conditions is discussed on p. 317. Accumulation of sufficient lipid to cause splenic enlargement occurs only occasionally. Macrophages in the red pulp increase in number and in size and excess lipid is present either as cytoplasmic globules which react variously with fat stains, or in a masked state apparently combined with protein. For example, cholesterol may be present in the spleen in increased amount without doubly refracting esters being detectable in the cells. Although the deposit occurs secondarily to hypercholesterolaemia it is not known what actually determines the extent of deposition.

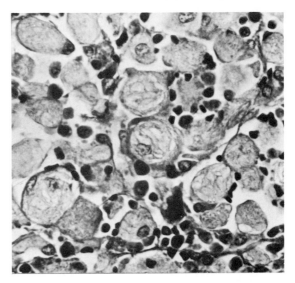

Fig. 17.2 Section of spleen in Gaucher's disease, showing the characteristic large cells with striated and vacuolated cytoplasm. × 440.

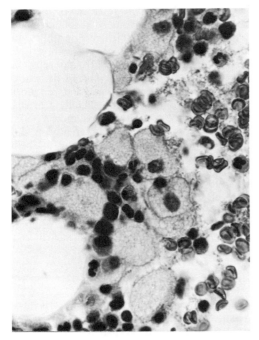

Fig. 17.1 Familial hyperbetalipoproteinaemia. Bone marrow biopsy showing foamy cells. × 540.

(*b*) In the second group we have rare diseases of familial and hereditary nature, such as those of the Gaucher and Niemann type, in which the lipid storage becomes excessive in various tissues and the enlargement of the spleen is very great. These conditions result from inborn abnormalities of lipid metabolism (p. 20). The composition of the lipids varies in different types.

Gaucher's disease. This uncommon condition was described by Gaucher in 1882. In its least rare form it becomes apparent in adult life, usually as slowly increasing and eventually extreme enlargement of the spleen and liver. This is due to accumulation of glucocerebrosides in macrophages which increase in number and size in the affected organs. Spleen weight may exceed 5 kg and microscopy shows huge numbers of macrophages termed **Gaucher cells**: they mostly have a single nucleus (but occasional cells

have two or three) and abundant cytoplasm which shows a characteristic streaky or irregularly vacuolated appearance (Fig. 17.2). Stains for fat are only weakly positive but the Gaucher cells are rich in acid phosphatase, the level of which may be raised in the plasma. The liver also is much enlarged by aggregation of Gaucher cells in the sinusoids. Involvement of the haemopoietic marrow may result in resorption of bone with widening of the marrow cavity, thinning of the cortex, and a tendency to pathological fractures. Displacement of haemopoietic elements by Gaucher cells may lead to a pancytopenia, but this may arise also from hypersplenism. Enlargement of lymph nodes, especially in the abdomen and mediastinum, is usual. In late cases Gaucher cells may form visible aggregates in the skin and also in the conjunctiva where they may be seen as wedge-shaped yellow-brown patches, termed *pingueculae*.

The adult form of Gaucher's disease described above is due to a deficiency of a lysosomal beta-glucosidase, resulting in accumulation of glucocerebroside derived from normal breakdown of red cells. The defect is consistent with long life, and death may eventually result from the effects of marrow replacement. It is transmitted as a Mendelian recessive factor and diagnosis of both the disease and the heterozygous carrier state, by the demonstration of beta-glucuronidase deficiency in leucocytes, has been described.

At least one other form of Gaucher's disease exists and becomes apparent in infancy. Glucocerebrosides accumulate not only in macrophages but also in neurones and death occurs in infancy or childhood from the effects on the central nervous system.

Niemann–Pick disease. This condition is an example of abnormal storage, chiefly of the phospholipid sphingomyelin, but also of cholesterol and other lipids. It is a very rare condition of early childhood which causes mental deficiency and is usually rapidly fatal. The storage of the lipid is very extensive, occurring in the specialised cells in the brain, intestinal mucosa, adrenals, lungs, pancreas, etc., as well as in macrophages in the spleen, liver, lymph nodes, bone marrow, etc. The accumulation of lipid enlarges the cells and gives their cytoplasm a foamy appearance. The lipid stains more readily with fat stains than in Gaucher's disease. The biochemical defect is probably an autosomal recessive trait and in some cases appears to be a deficiency of an enzyme involved in the breakdown of myelin. Occasionally similar lipid-storage diseases occur in which a different phosphatide accumulates, e.g. a cephalin, and it seems likely they are all founded on defects in the enzyme systems controlling lipid metabolism.

'Histiocytosis X'. This term is applied collectively to three uncommon conditions—Letterer–Siwe disease, Hand–Schüller–Christian disease and eosinophil granuloma of bone—of unknown aetiology, and characterised by apparently neoplastic proliferation of cells derived from the macrophage series.

These conditions are not related to any known abnormality in lipid metabolism, and plasma lipids are not raised. Lipids are, however, present in excess in the proliferated macrophages in longstanding cases, and particularly in Hand–Schüller–Christian disease and eosinophil granuloma.

Letterer–Siwe disease (non-lipid histiocytosis) develops most commonly in infants and usually runs a rapid and fatal course. It is characterised by hepatosplenomegaly, lymph-node enlargement and multiple nodules in the skin and bone marrow. There is usually fever, anaemia and sometimes leukopenia. The affected organs show massive replacement by proliferated macrophage-like cells; plasma cells, fibroblasts, eosinophil polymorphs and giant cells may be present, but usually in relatively small numbers. There is usually no storage of lipid in the macrophages, but this is sometimes observed in atypical cases running a more prolonged course.

Hand–Schüller–Christian disease occurs at all ages, but most frequently in children. The proliferated macrophages accumulate lipids, mainly cholesterol esters, and this is conspicuous in long-standing cases. The lesions are commonly infiltrated with eosinophils, lymphocytes, plasma cells and fibroblasts, and may eventually become extensively scarred: they occur particularly in the bones, but also in the skin, liver, lymph nodes, spleen and lungs. Exophthalmos or diabetes insipidus may result from lesions of the skull adjacent to the orbit or hypothalamus respectively.

In general, the course is much more prolonged than in Letterer–Siwe's disease, many patients surviving for 10 or more years, but in some instances, particularly when onset is in childhood, it is more acute.

Eosinophil granuloma of bone (p. 834), the third member of this group, is usually a solitary lesion arising most commonly in adolescents or adults, and is composed of a mixture of cells including lipid-laden macrophages, multinucleated giant cells, but predominantly of eosinophil polymorphs. It is not a cause of splenomegaly, and has a good prognosis, although progression to Hand–Schüller–Christian disease has been described in rare instances.

Although these conditions differ greatly in their behaviour, they are regarded by many as being closely related, and as forming a series in which eosinophil granuloma is the benign counterpart of the usually rapidly fatal Letterer–Siwe's disease, while Hand–Schüller–Christian disease lies intermediate. The aetiology is unknown, but accumulation of lipids appears to follow histiocytic proliferation, and is not the primary change.

Tumours

As in the lymph nodes, the commonest forms of primary neoplasia in the spleen are the various malignant lymphomas (p. 518). It is often not possible to determine the site of origin of a lymphoma, for many lymph nodes and sometimes the spleen, bone marrow, etc., are commonly involved when the patient is first seen. Occasional early cases do seem, however, to have originated in the spleen.

Benign tumours of the spleen, including fibroma, myoma, haemangioma and lymphangioma have been described, but all are rarities. *Cysts* of the spleen are occasionally seen. They are usually small and multiple, though one may reach a large size and form a fluctuant swelling on the surface. They contain a clear serous fluid, but there may be an admixture of altered blood. They are regarded as usually of lymphangiomatous origin.

Splenic metastases occur more frequently in sarcoma than in carcinoma, but even in the former they are not common. The spleen contrasts with the bone marrow and lymph nodes in its low frequency of secondary carcinoma.

Lymph Nodes

A brief description of the structure of the lymph nodes has been given in Chapter 4. They consist essentially of two parts, viz. the lymphoid tissue proper with its follicles and deep cortex (paracortex), and the lymph sinuses and medullary reticulum. The former is concerned in the production of immune responses, already described in some detail (pp. 84–113). The lymph sinuses and medullary cords not only house antibody-producing plasma cells, but are also involved in the destruction of organisms or damaged cells carried from the tissues, as the relatively slow lymph flow gives favourable opportunity for phagocytic action. In fact, the lymph node medulla and sinuses have much the same relation to the lymph as the splenic red pulp has to the blood. The macrophages in both react similarly. In addition to being active phagocytes for particulate material, they exhibit a great capacity for uptake and storage of substances present in solution.

Acute lymphadenitis

Experimental studies have shown that in normal circumstances lymph nodes are not very efficient in removing particulate elements from the lymph passing through them: for example, bacteria and similar-sized particles have been shown to pass rapidly from the peripheral lymphatics, through the regional nodes, and to reach the blood stream. However, within less than an hour of the establishment of an acute infection, the sinuses of the draining lymph nodes dilate, and neutrophil polymorphs migrate into them from the adjacent small blood vessels and aggregate particularly in the medulla where they provide a filter by actively phagocytosing bacteria in the draining lymph: the efficiency of the nodes in preventing spread of infection to the bloodstream is thus greatly increased. Unless the infection is rapidly overcome, the numbers of macrophages in the sinuses and medulla increase and they also participate in the phagocytosis of bacteria, degenerate polymorphs, cell fragments, etc., in the lymph.

In addition to the migration of polymorphs and monocytes, the lymph nodes draining a focus of acute infection show the other features of acute inflammation, including dilatation of the small blood vessels and inflammatory oedema: these changes are due to the local effects of bacteria or their toxins, or possibly endogenous mediators, carried in the increased flow of lymph from the focus of infection. Polymorphs are also carried in the lymph, and supplement those which have accumulated in the nodes by local migration. These inflammatory changes result in swollen, tender and sometimes painful lymph nodes, a common example being in the axillary nodes in acutely infected wounds of the hand.

Other changes in the lymph nodes in acute infections include those associated with immune responses, i.e. the formation of cortical germinal centres, 'blast' cell transformation and proliferation of lymphocytes in the deep cortex (p. 111).

Organisms that have invaded a lymph node are often destroyed by the leukocytes and the inflammation then resolves. They may, however, continue to multiply, with consequent suppuration which may spread to the surrounding tissues and, if superficial, discharge on the skin surface. Such changes may occur in the drainage area of infected wounds of various kinds, particularly when caused by streptococci, and sometimes by staphylococci.

In *lymphogranuloma inguinale*, a macrophage-granulomatous reaction with central necrosis and suppuration occurs in the inguinal lymph nodes (Fig. 17.3 and p. 917), and a closely similar lesion occurs in *cat-scratch disease*. Both are produced in the regional nodes, probably by chlamydiae (p. 188), which gain entrance through trivial superficial scratches in the skin.

Another infection which involves the lymph nodes in a suppurating and epithelioid cell granulomatous reaction is *tularaemia*, due to *Yersinia tularensis*, which infects many species of animals. It occurs in various parts of the Americas and Asia, but not in Western Europe.

In *plague* there is a severe inflammation with infiltration of polymorphonuclears, brought about by the bacilli which are present in enormous numbers; there is much haemorrhage and

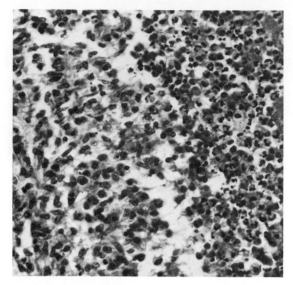

Fig. 17.3 An inguinal lymph node in lymphogranuloma inguinale, showing part of the macrophage granuloma (*left*) with central suppuration (*right*). × 320.

oedema in the nodes and in the tissue between them, and often considerable necrosis. The so-called bubo is simply an inflammatory mass consisting both of lymph nodes and the tissue

around them. In *anthrax* the lesion is mainly an inflammatory oedema with a varying amount of haemorrhage.

In *typhoid fever*, large numbers of macrophages accumulate in the sinuses and medullary cords of the lymph nodes draining the intestinal lesions (Fig. 17.4). The macrophages contain ingested cell debris and often erythrocytes. The nodes also contain plasma cells: haemorrhage, necrosis and autolytic softening may follow (Fig. 1.5, p. 5). As in other typhoid lesions, polymorphonuclear leukocytes are few or absent.

Infectious mononucleosis (glandular fever) is a virus infection which occurs sporadically and in small epidemics and affects chiefly children and young adults. It is characterised by swelling and tenderness of cervical lymph nodes, fever lasting a week or two and atypical lymphoid cells in the blood. The posterior cervical nodes are usually affected first, but other groups may be involved; splenic enlargement is not uncommon and rupture may follow a trivial injury. The disease is rarely fatal. In some cases sore throat is a prominent clinical feature and there may be actual ulceration of the mucosa. In others there is severe headache and a skin rash. At first there may be a neutrophil leukocytosis, but soon the characteristic blood picture appears, namely a leukocyte count usually of $10-20 \times 10^3$ per μl,

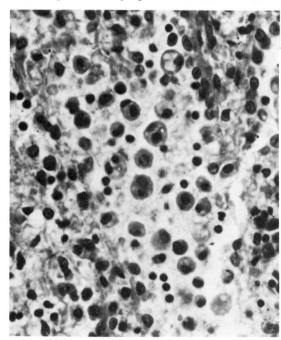

Fig. 17.4 A lymph node in typhoid fever, showing numerous macrophages in a sinus. Some of the macrophages contain ingested erythrocytes. × 520.

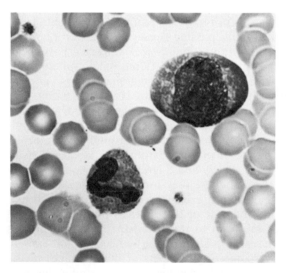

Fig. 17.5 Blood smear in infectious mononucleosis, showing an atypical lymphoid cell with enlarged irregular nucleus and abundant basophilic cytoplasm. It has the features of a lymphoblast, and is much larger than the adjacent polymorph. Leishman's stain. × 1400.

of which 50% or more are enlarged atypical lymphoid cells with an enlarged irregular, sometimes convoluted nucleus and an increased amount of basophilic cytoplasm (Fig. 17.5). The lymph nodes show enlargement of the germinal centres, but the most striking change is accumulation of large numbers of lymphoblasts in the deep cortex and sinuses. Mitoses are

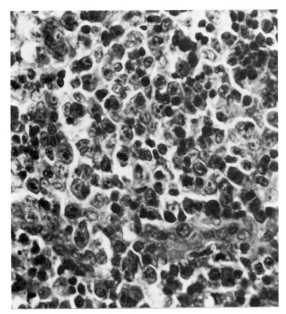

Fig. 17.6 Cervical lymph node in infectious mononucleosis, showing large numbers of lymphoblasts, among which mitoses were numerous. The Paul–Bunnell reaction was positive with a serum titre of 1 : 20 000. × 520. (Preparation provided by Dr. G. B. S. Roberts.)

frequent and the appearances are highly suggestive of a malignant lymphoma (Fig. 17.6). The architecture of the nodes is, however, preserved. In many cases liver function tests are abnormal, indicating a degree of hepatitis, and in some cases jaundice develops.

During infection, heterophil agglutinins for sheep red cells appear in the blood in some, but not all, cases. Their detection by the Paul–Bunnell test is in wide diagnostic use.

Following a chance observation of the development of antibody to Epstein–Barr virus (EBV, p. 265) in a technician during an attack of glandular fever, investigations of students at Yale University showed that the appearance of such antibody was a regular feature of infec-

tious mononucleosis. Moreover, leukocytes obtained during the illness can be cultured *in vitro* over a long period and can be shown, like those of the Burkitt lymphoma, to contain EBV antigen. Similar observations have since been made by other workers, and there appears a strong possibility that the EB virus is the causal agent of infectious mononucleosis. However, EBV antibody has been demonstrated in a high proportion of healthy individuals, and its incidence increases during childhood. This may possibly be related to sub-clinical attacks of infectious mononucleosis.

Curiously, although it is B lymphocytes which are stimulated to continuous growth *in vitro* by EBV, the large blast cells in the blood in infectious mononucleosis have been shown to have the surface markers of T lymphocytes: if they represent a T-cell response to the infection, then the large number appearing in the blood is surprising.

There is evidence of a second type of infectious mononucleosis, without sore throat or lymph node enlargement, but sometimes with hepatitis, associated with infection with cytomegalovirus; the Paul–Bunnell test is negative in such cases.

Measles. In measles, the lymphoid tissues show formation of multinucleated giant cells, termed Warthin–Finkeldey cells (Fig. 17.7).

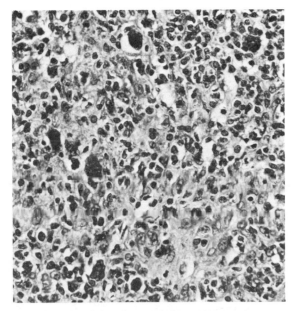

Fig. 17.7 Lymph node in the prodromal stage of measles, showing part of a germinal centre containing Warthin–Finkeldey giant cells. × 320.

They are sometimes observed in an appendix or tonsils which happen to have been removed during the incubation period of measles, and it is important not to mistake the changes for anything more sinister.

Chronic non-neoplastic lymph node enlargement

This occurs in a very large number of conditions and is, of course, a most important clinical sign. The causes may be classified as follows:

(*a*) Reactive hyperplasia, accumulation of lipid and pigments, etc.
(*b*) Chronic infections and sarcoidosis

Many enlargements of lymph nodes are of known cause and readily classified. Others are of unknown aetiology, and some have features which render difficult their classification as either neoplastic or reactive: the term *reticulosis* was usefully applied to this latter group, but has been used indiscriminately for any systematised cellular proliferation of the lympho-reticular tissue. *Malignant reticulosis* is still used for lympho-reticular neoplastic conditions, but the term *lymphoma* is now preferred.

(a) Reactive hyperplasia, lipid and pigment accumulations

Aggregation of macrophages in the peripheral and especially in the medullary lymph sinuses (formerly termed 'sinus catarrh') is brought about by the continued action of a mild irritant. It is often seen in the axillary nodes in chronic diseases of the breast, and must not be mistaken for secondary cancer. Lymph nodes draining a focus of chronic infection commonly show also the morphological changes of the immune response (p. 111). These combined changes constitute *reactive hyperplasia* of the lymph nodes. Chronic irritation of long duration leads to a thickening of the stroma; sinuses become obliterated, and ultimately there may be marked fibrosis with atrophy of the lymphoid tissue.

Accumulation of pigments, etc. Pigments of various kinds, carried to the nodes, are taken up by macrophages of the sinuses and medul-

lary cords, where they may persist indefinitely, as is seen in tattooing. The lymph nodes draining the areas affected by certain skin diseases show marked enlargement with accumulation and phagocytosis of melanin and of fat—so-called *lipomelanic reticulosis*. In cases of *anthracosis* carbon particles are dealt with in a similar way and they come to form black masses which replace the lymphoid tissue, with comparatively little stromal thickening. In *silicosis*, on the contrary, marked fibrosis results from the irritation caused by stone particles, and the nodes become enlarged and indurated. Where there has been local haemorrhage, haemosiderin may be seen in the related lymph nodes, and a remarkable accumulation of haemosiderin occurs in certain of the abdominal nodes in *haemochromatosis* and in transfusional siderosis (p. 243). Sometimes the amount is so great that the structure is quite obscured by the masses of pigment, and iron may constitute more than 10% of the dry weight of the nodes. Enlargement of the lymph nodes in lipid storage diseases and 'histiocytosis X' is mentioned on pp. 510–12.

(b) Chronic infections and sarcoidosis

Tuberculosis. Tuberculous disease of lymph nodes is a very much less common lesion than formerly. It appears first in the group of nodes draining the site of entry of the bacilli; thus the cervical, bronchial and mesenteric groups are the commonest to be involved, and the disease may spread to others. Infection of the bronchial nodes is nearly always due to lesions in the lungs; much less frequently due to spread downwards from the cervical nodes following tonsillar infection.

As elsewhere, tubercles in the lymph nodes may coalesce and then undergo extensive caseation. The process spreads until ultimately the whole node is destroyed and such nodes form large irregular masses matted together. This is a common feature of primary tuberculosis but is not usually seen with 're-infection' lesions (p. 178). Caseous lesions, known as *scrofula*, were formerly common in the cervical nodes, but have now become rare in countries where pasteurisation of milk has greatly reduced bovine tuberculosis. Such lesions, if untreated, may become adherent to the skin, ulcerate and discharge the softened caseous material, and secondary pyogenic infection may occur. Small sinuses thus formed may discharge intermittently for a long time, and disfiguring scarring results: this can be prevented by chemotherapy or surgical treatment. Even without treatment, the lesions usually subside: the caseous material undergoes calcification, while great thickening of the surrounding capsule occurs. In children, primary intestinal infection may cause great enlargement and caseation of the mesenteric lymph nodes—*tabes mesenterica*. Healing is usual and calcified mesenteric lymph nodes are still quite commonly encountered.

Sarcoidosis. This is a granulomatous condition of unknown aetiology (p. 182). There is enlargement of lymph nodes and a variable amount of surrounding fibrosis. The pulmonary hilar nodes are usually affected, although other deep and superficial nodes are commonly involved, and also the spleen, lungs and various other organs. The affected nodes may be greatly enlarged, greyish or pinkish, and the condition may readily be mistaken clinically for Hodgkin's disease. On microscopic examination the lesion is seen to consist of aggregates of

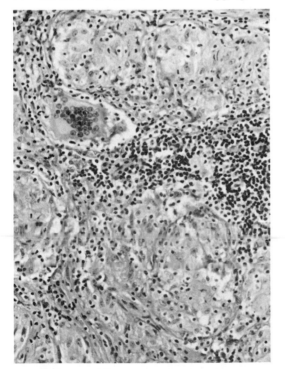

Fig. 17.8 Lymph node in sarcoidosis, showing tubercle-like epithelioid follicles and giant cells but no caseation. × 75.

epithelioid cells closely resembling those seen in tuberculous lesions. The epithelioid cells may form tubercle-like follicles without caseation (Fig. 17.8), although there may be a little central fibrinoid necrosis. Multinucleate giant cells may be present, and sometimes they contain curious stellate or conchoid bodies, which may be calcified. The tuberculin test is usually negative in cases of sarcoidosis, and there is evidence that this is due to depression of cell-mediated immunity: delayed hypersensitivity to other antigens, e.g. mumps virus, is also depressed, although the serum contains the usual blood-group and other antibodies, and there may be a raised level of serum IgG. In some cases, delayed hypersensitivity to tuberculin has been observed to diminish or disappear following the onset of sarcoidosis, and to re-appear following remission. The Kveim test, a granulomatous sarcoid reaction at the site of intradermal injection of a sterilised extract of sarcoidosis lesions, is useful in diagnosis.

Syphilis. Enlargement with induration of the regional nodes draining the primary sore has already been described (p. 183), and also the importance of spread of the spirochaetes by lymphatics and the blood. The skin rashes of the secondary stage are usually accompanied by moderate or slight general enlargement of lymph nodes. In the tertiary stage, gummas are comparatively rare in the lymph nodes.

Histoplasmosis most commonly causes a localised respiratory infection with eventual healing and calcification (p. 189). It may, however, cause a relatively acute generalised infection in which the macrophages in the spleen, lymph nodes, bone marrow, liver and elsewhere are colonised by huge numbers of *Histoplasma capsulatum* (p. 189). These organs are enlarged and the masses of colonised macrophages may show foci of necrosis similar to tuberculous caseation.

Toxoplasmosis. Infection with the protozoon, *Toxoplasma gondii*, may occur at any age and serological tests indicate that approximately 30% of adults in Europe have experienced infection, although very few have had an illness known or suspected to be toxoplasmosis. When, however, infection (usually clinically silent) occurs during pregnancy, the parasite may infect the fetus with serious results. Depending on the stage of pregnancy, these range from abortion, stillbirth, a live child with severe abnormalities, or an apparently normal child which may develop relatively mild disease within the first few weeks of age. The most serious effects of fetal infection are encephalomyelitis and choroido-retinitis (p. 702).

phages, scattered singly and in small groups throughout both the cortex and medulla (Fig. 17.9). The sinuses are stuffed with smaller cells of uncertain nature. Plasma cells may also be numerous. Tests for antibodies are exacting: the

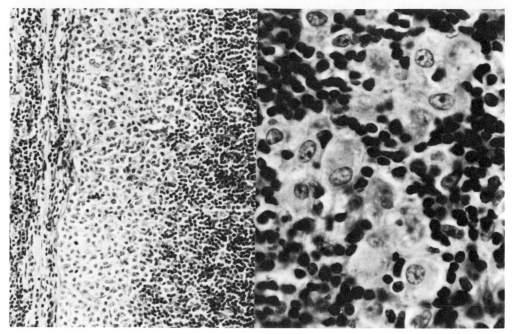

Fig. 17.9 Lymph node in toxoplasmosis. *Left*, a lymphoid sinus filled with pale cells of uncertain origin. × 165. *Right*, showing the large cells, probably macrophages, which are scattered singly and in small groups throughout the node. × 450.

Toxoplasmosis acquired after birth may present at any age, but most often in young adults. The commonest feature is lymph node enlargement, either localised or generalised, usually including upper cervical nodes. There may be no other symptoms or a febrile illness, and a wide variety of symptoms may also result from involvement of one or more organs including the lungs, heart and skeletal muscles. There are no typical blood changes. Histologically the main features of the affected lymph nodes are large cells, probably macro-

most satisfactory so far is a dye exclusion test; high or rising titres of antibody are suggestive of infection. Certain diagnosis depends on the inoculation of mice with fresh tissue mash, but this is seldom used.

The mode of human infection is uncertain. Hutchison has shown that, following infection of cats, oocysts develop in the intestinal epithelium and are shed into the lumen. They are resistant to drying, etc., and this may provide an important source of human infection by inhalation or ingestion.

The lymphomas

In view of their cellular variety and proliferative activity, it is not surprising that the lympho-reticular tissues give origin to a group of

tumours which vary greatly in their morphology and behaviour.

Although the exact histogenesis of these

tumours is often doubtful, there is good evidence that many of them originate from the lymphoid series of cells, while occasional tumours have features suggesting a derivation from the macrophage series. They are grouped together as the lymphomas. Most or all of these tumours will shorten the life-span of the victim, although they vary greatly in malignancy, some types causing death within a few weeks, others only after many years. With most lymphomas, the prognosis lies between these extremes, although surgical excision, x-irradiation and cytotoxic drugs in various combinations without doubt prolong life, and may effect cure in some cases.

Most lymphomas arise in the lymph nodes or other tissues rich in lymphoid cells or macrophages, such as the spleen, bone marrow, liver, skin and gastro-intestinal tract. Lymphocytes and macrophages are, however, almost ubiquitous in the body, and lymphomas can arise from virtually any tissue, including the central nervous system. Although some lymphomas resemble other malignant tumours in forming distinct tumour masses, they include also the lymphoid leukaemias, the cells of which tend to infiltrate the lymph nodes, bone marrow and various other organs diffusely, and also to circulate as single cells in the blood. It is not possible to draw a sharp distinction between the solid and leukaemic types of lymphoma, for the two patterns of growth are commonly associated. Indeed, enlargement of the lymph nodes, and sometimes of the spleen, commonly precedes the development of chronic lymphoid leukaemia (p. 493).

Classification

As with other tumours, the main purpose in classifying lymphomas is to provide an indication of how a particular example will behave and what form of therapy is likely to be most effective. Unfortunately we have not yet reached the logical stage where classification of all the lymphomas can be based on their cell of origin and morphological features, although rapid progress is now being made.

There is general agreement that *Hodgkin's disease* is a distinct entity, or at least group, different from other forms of lymphoma. The origin of the characteristic cells of Hodgkin's disease is still, however, undecided. The remaining lymphomas are sometimes called *the non-Hodgkin lymphomas*: most types occurring in adult life have been shown by tests for surface markers to have features indicative of *B-lymphoid cell origin*, and some of these, notably the *follicular lymphomas*, appear to arise from cells of the germinal centres. Both these and the remaining *non-follicular* or *diffuse lymphomas* can, with advantage, be broadly sub-divided into those of low-grade and high-grade malignancy, the individual sub-groups being based on the morphological features of the dominant cell type. Some examples of highly malignant diffuse lymphoma appear to be of T-lymphoid cell origin.

Hodgkin's disease

General features. Although this is the most common form of malignant lymphoma, its exact nature is still uncertain. The distinctive Reed–Sternberg cells and their mononuclear equivalents are widely regarded as the neoplastic elements, but opinion is divided on whether they are derived from lymphoid cells or from cells of the mononuclear phagocyte system.

The disease can develop at almost any age, although there is a peak incidence in early adult life and a second peak in the older age groups. The usual presenting feature is progressive and usually painless enlargement of lymph nodes, most often those of the cervical, inguinal or axillary groups. Early involvement of the abdominal or mediastinal nodes, the pharyngeal lymphoid tissue or the spleen is, however, not uncommon. It is unusual for extranodal sites to be primarily affected, although almost any tissue may be implicated by metastatic spread of the tumour. Constitutional symptoms are sometimes conspicuous, especially in advanced cases; they include an irregular low-grade pyrexia which occasionally assumes a periodic pattern (Pel–Ebstein fever), and an anaemia usually of normochromic normocytic type, sometimes accompanied by neutrophilia. Eosinophilia is less common. An important feature is an early depression of T-lymphocyte function with impairment of cell-mediated immunity. In consequence, patients are unusually prone to various infections, especially tuberculosis and zoster (p. 142), but also fungal and other 'opportunistic' infections by organisms of relatively low pathogenicity. The prognosis varies greatly from death in a few months to survival and good health for many years, even without treatment. The histological pattern and the extent of the disease process at the time of diagnosis have considerable prognostic significance.

Macroscopic changes. Initially the enlarged **lymph nodes** are discrete, soft and rubbery, with a greyish-pink cut surface. In some forms of the disease, however, fibrosis is present from the outset. As they become larger, the nodes tend to

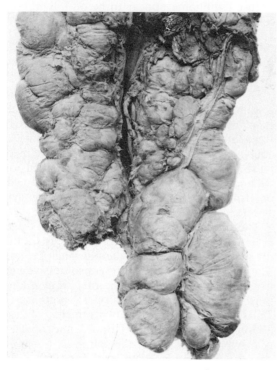

Fig. 17.10 A mass of fused retroperitoneal lymph nodes in Hodgkin's disease. The aorta (opened from behind) is surrounded by the enlarged nodes. × 0·7.

become firmer and bound together (Fig. 17.10), and they can produce serious pressure effects, for example on the trachea or mediastinal blood vessels. Foci of non-suppurative necrosis are also commonly observed in the lesions. **The spleen** is commonly involved and enlarged: the lesions develop in the Malpighian bodies, which become expanded and eventually confluent. This process ultimately produces the characteristic German sausage appearance of the cut surface, the pale patches of 'Hodgkin's tissue'

resembling flecks of suet (Fig. 17.11). Staging procedures in which splenectomy is carried out (see below) have shown, however, that the spleen may be involved without obvious enlargement, and that splenomegaly may occur in the absence of tumour involvement, presumably due to diffuse hyperplasia of the red pulp. Although the disease is often restricted at first to the lymphoid organs, almost

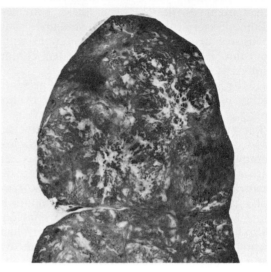

Fig. 17.11 Section of spleen in Hodgkin's disease, showing the characteristic pale irregular lesions involving the Malpighian bodies and extending into the red pulp. × 0·7.

any tissue may be affected at a later stage, the lesions appearing as infiltration and replacement of the normal tissue by patches of 'Hodgkin's tissue' with the appearances described above. Lesions occur especially in the **liver**, **kidneys** and **bone marrow**: involvement of the vertebrae may lead to pressure on the spinal cord with paraplegia: focal or diffuse lesions in the **lungs** are not uncommon (Fig. 17.12), especially if the mediastinal nodes are affected, and ulcerating tumour masses occur in the **gastro-intestinal tract**.

Microscopic appearances. The diagnosis is usually made readily by biopsy of an enlarged lymph node. The tissue of the node may be partly or completely replaced. The essential feature, without which the diagnosis cannot be made, is the presence of **Reed–Sternberg cells**. In its most characteristic form, this cell measures 40 μm or more in diameter, and has an

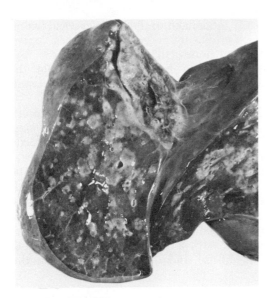

Fig. 17.12 Infiltration of the lung in Hodgkin's disease. The neoplastic tissue is white and solid: in this instance it is patchy, but sometimes it is more diffuse. × 0·3.

intricate double or bi-lobed nucleus, each component of which has a vesicular appearance due to condensation of chromatin peripherally, and a large central eosinophilic nucleolus (Fig. 17.13). The cytoplasm is abundant, usually faintly eosinophilic, and sometimes vacuolated. Reed–Sternberg cells may be much larger with

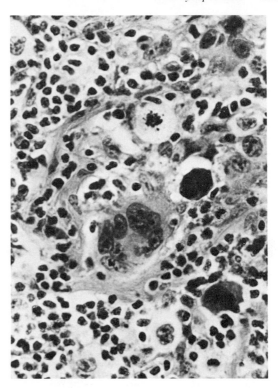

Fig. 17.14 Hodgkin's disease showing numerous neoplastic reticulum cells, including a multinucleated Reed–Sternberg cell. There was a mixed cell infiltrate in this case. × 450.

more complex or multiple nuclei (Fig. 17.14). Mononuclear cells with otherwise similar features are also present and appear to represent the main proliferating elements of the tumour: these neoplastic cells (termed here, without commitment on their origin, *neoplastic reticulum cells*) lie in a variable reactive cellular infiltrate which may be predominantly lymphocytic, or may be of *mixed cellular pattern*, including also plasma cells, macrophages, neutrophil and eosinophil leukocytes. Sometimes a sarcoid type of reaction with epithelioid cells and even Langhans' giant cells is seen and is liable to cause diagnostic difficulties. There is invariably some increase in reticulin fibres, particularly in the late stages, and abundant collagen is also formed in some variants of the disease.

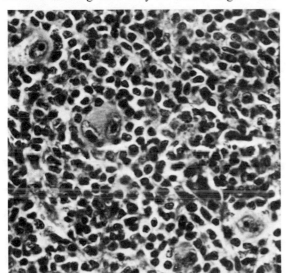

Fig. 17.13 Hodgkin's disease of lymphocyte-predominant type. Field chosen to show Reed–Sternberg cells, one of which shows the characteristic 'mirror-image' nuclei with large nucleoli. × 520.

Classification of Hodgkin's disease

For prognostic purposes, Hodgkin's disease has been sub-divided, on the internationally agreed

Rye classification, into four major types as follows.

(1) Lymphocyte-predominant (15% of cases). Formerly termed *Hodgkin's paragranuloma*, the important feature of this variant is the sparsity of Reed–Sternberg cells, lying among a cell infiltrate consisting mainly of mature lymphocytes (Fig. 17.13). There may, however, be small aggregates of macrophages and sometimes sarcoid-like follicles. Eosinophils and other reactive cells are scanty or absent and capsular thickening and reticulin deposition are minimal, although sometimes a nodular pattern develops (see below).

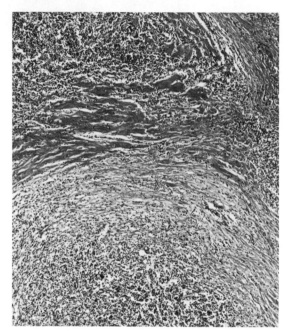

Fig. 17.15 Nodular sclerosing Hodgkin's disease in a lymph node. In this instance, the collagen dividing the 'Hodgkin's tissue' into nodules is abundant and the diagnosis is obvious. × 50.

(2) Nodular sclerosing type (40% of cases). In this type, the lymph node capsule is thickened and fine or coarse bands of collagen sub-divide the node into nodules of various sizes (Fig. 17.15). Within the nodules the neoplasm may show a mixed cellular reaction (see above) but lymphocytes are usually predominant. The Reed–Sternberg cells show extensive cytoplasmic vacuolation and are called *lacunar cells*: this feature is regarded by some as characteristic of this type of Hodgkin's disease, which

typically is confined to the lower cervical lymph nodes, mediastinum and sometimes upper abdominal nodes. In some instances the thymus appears to be first involved, and the condition has been misnamed *granulomatous thymoma*.

(3) Mixed-cellularity type (30% of cases) corresponds to some of the cases formerly classified as *Hodgkin's granuloma*. Typical Reed–Sternberg cells and their mononuclear equivalents, commonly showing mitotic activity, are numerous, and lie in a mixed cellular infiltrate of neutrophils, eosinophils, macrophages, plasma cells and lymphocytes (Fig. 17.14). Reticulin fibres are sometimes abundant, with early collagen formation but this is diffuse and does not result in nodularity.

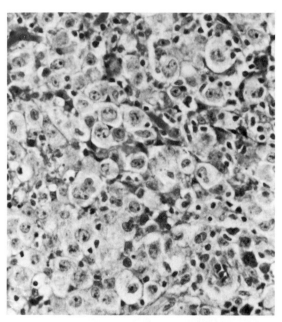

Fig. 17.16 Lymphocyte-depleted Hodgkin's disease. Most of the cells are neoplastic reticulum cells and lymphoctes are few. × 520.

(4) Lymphocyte-depleted type (15% of cases) includes cases previously classed as *Hodgkin's sarcoma*. The histological picture in such cases is dominated by Reed–Sternberg cells and their mononuclear equivalents (Fig. 17.16). Lymphocytes are sparse and other reactive cells, including eosinophils, are variable in number. Fibrous tissue varies greatly in amount, but in some cases is very abundant and diffuse.

Course of the disease

Hodgkin's disease often appears to start in a single lymph node or group of nodes, and may spread either by lymphatics or by the bloodstream to adjacent or distant tissues, both lymphoid and non-lymphoid. When limited to one area of the body, local ablation, e.g. by radiotherapy, is effective and sometimes apparently curative. Once the lesions are widely disseminated, systemic chemotherapy provides the only hope of controlling its otherwise relentless progress. The extent of the disease is thus

Table 17.1 Staging of Hodgkin's disease, based on the Ann Arbor system

STAGE I	Confined to a single lymph node or group of nodes.
STAGE II	Confined to upper or lower part of body, i.e. all lesions *either* above *or* below the diaphragm.
STAGE III	Involving lymph nodes above *and* below the diaphragm, with or without lesions in other tissues.
STAGE IV	Widespread involvement of one or more non-lymphoid tissues, with or without lymph node involvement.

critical in determining the prognosis and in planning therapy. To assess this accurately, clinical examination must be supplemented by at least bone marrow biopsy and abdominal lymphangiography, and many now advocate laparotomy with splenectomy and liver biopsy to detect and determine the extent of abdominal involvement. By these methods the disease can

be subdivided into four stages (Table 17.1). There can be little doubt that the more extensive the disease the worse, in general, is the prognosis, and most patients surviving for ten years or more were initially diagnosed in stage I. The prognosis can also be correlated with the histological type. In general, the outlook is most favourable when lymphocytes are abundant and Reed–Sternberg cells sparse. Thus the lymphocyte-predominant type is associated with a much longer survival than the lymphocyte-depleted type, while the mixed-cellularity type has an intermediate prognosis.

The histological type also correlates quite well with the clinical stage, most cases of lymphocyte-predominant Hodgkin's disease presenting in stage I. The great importance of staging, however, is best illustrated by the nodular sclerosing type. This shows no tendency to undergo transitions to other forms of the disease, and provided it is in stage I the outlook is good: indeed, most of the patients surviving for many years belong to this group. In stages II and III, however, this variant has a prognosis scarcely better than the mixed-cellularity type. Apart from the nodular sclerosing type, Hodgkin's disease is unfortunately prone to progress to a worse type, i.e. from lymphocyte-predominant to mixed-cellularity and to lymphocyte-depleted.

Lymphomas other than Hodgkin's disease

As indicated on p. 519, these varied tumours can be sub-divided according to their degree of malignancy, and also into follicular and diffuse

Table 17.2 Classification of the 'non-Hodgkin lymphomas'

Growth pattern	Low grade malignancy	High-grade malignancy
Follicular (all B cell)	Small cell ('centrocyte' or 'cleaved cell') Mixed cell ('centrocyte' and 'centroblast')	Large cell ('centroblast')
Diffuse	Small cell (B) (a) lymphocyte including CLL (b) 'cleaved cell' (c) 'lymphoplasmacyte' including WM	Large ('blast') cell (a) T cell, including ALL and ST (b) B cell, including BL and PBS (c) 'histiocytic lymphoma' including HMR
	Plasma cell (multiple myeloma)	

Abbreviations. ALL, acute lymphoblastic leukaemia; BL, Burkitt lymphoma; CLL, chronic lymphocytic leukaemia; HMR, histiocytic medullary reticulosis; PBS, plasmablastic sarcoma; ST, Sternberg's tumour; WM, Waldenström's macroglobulinaemia.

types according to their growth pattern. This forms the basis of the classification given in table 17.2, which includes also sub-divisions based on recent morphological observations and on the results of tests for B- and T-cell markers. In the present state of flux, any classification must be regarded as temporary.

Follicular lymphoma (Figs. 17.17–17.20) occurs mainly in old people. Although of low-grade malignancy, it often changes from an initial slowly progressive phase, which may last for as long as ten years, to a more aggressive form (see below). The prognosis is best when only a single group of nodes is enlarged, but often the disease is more extensive when the patient is first seen, involving the spleen, liver and bone marrow.

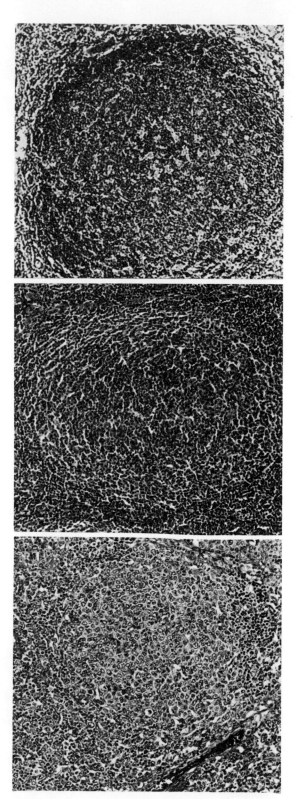

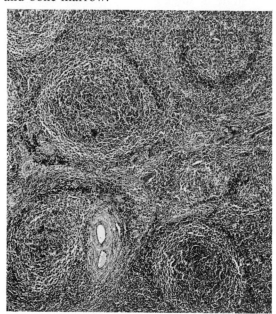

Fig. 17.17 Follicular lymphoma involving a lymph node. There are numerous follicles of roughly equal size. × 35.

Histologically the affected nodes contain numerous follicular structures (Fig. 17.17) which may closely resemble normal reactive germinal centres, but can usually be distinguished by their uniform size, spheroidal shape, their large number and widespread distribution through the node, and by their lack of macro-

Fig. 17.18 *Top*, a normal reactive germinal follicle. *Middle*, follicular lymphoma of small-cell type. *Bottom*, large-cell follicular lymphoma. × 100.

phages (Fig. 17.18). Two types of cell can be identified in the follicles, a small cell with a notched nucleus ('*cleaved cell*' or '*centrocyte*'), and a larger, more primitive blast cell ('*centro-blast*') with a larger, spherical, prominently nucleolated nucleus. Predominance of cleaved cells is usual and indicates a relatively good prognosis, while blast-cell predominance and a

high mitotic rate indicate a much more aggressive behaviour. The edges of the follicles are often ill-defined and there is a tendency for the lymphoma cells to spread out and eventually produce a diffuse pattern of growth.

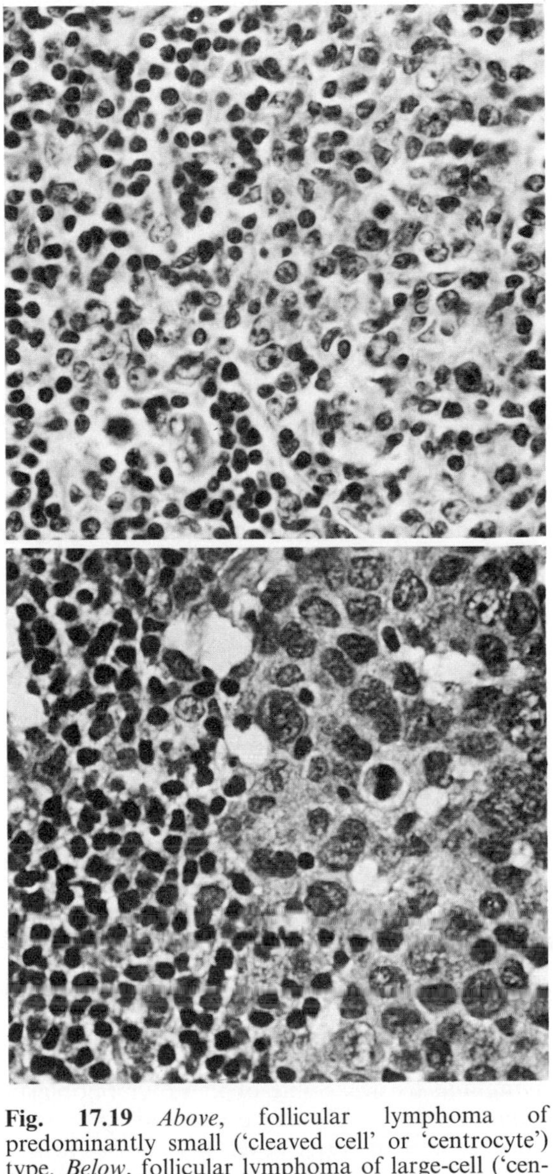

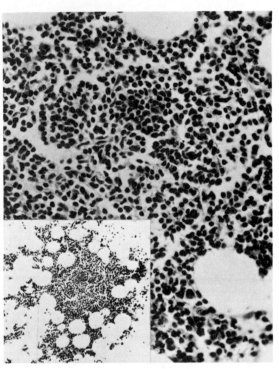

Fig. 17.20 Follicular lymphoma of small-cell type in a needle biopsy of the bone marrow. *Inset*, at low magnification, showing the follicular pattern.

Neoplastic follicles may be numerous in the bone marrow (Fig. 17.20) and occasionally cleaved cells appear in large numbers in the blood.

At least some of the diffuse lymphomas consisting of a mixture of cleaved and blast cell types result from diffuse spread of follicular lymphoma (see below).

Diffuse lymphoma of low-grade malignancy (Fig. 17.21). Most of the tumours in this group are disseminated widely, both in the lymphoid and non-lymphoid tissues (e.g. the bone marrow and liver), at an early stage. Generalised lymphadenopathy and hepatosplenomegaly are thus common presenting features. While the enlarged nodes cause pressure effects, local destructive changes are minimal and the tumour cells are usually sensitive to chemotherapeutic

Fig. 17.19 *Above*, follicular lymphoma of predominantly small ('cleaved cell' or 'centrocyte') type. *Below*, follicular lymphoma of large-cell ('centroblast') type. Each photograph shows the edge of a follicular lesion, the lymphoma cells being on the right, and adjacent lymphoid tissue, containing small lymphocytes, on the left. × 520.

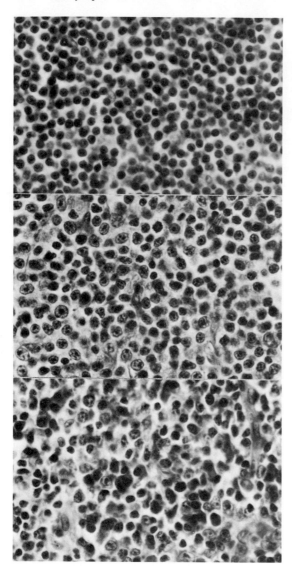

Fig. 17.21 Lymph nodes showing examples of diffuse lymphoma of low-grade malignancy. *Top*, lymphocytic type (from a case of chronic lymphoid leukaemia). *Middle*, 'centrocytic' type (also from a case of lymphoid leukaemia). *Bottom*, 'lymphoplasmacytic' type (Waldenström's macroglobulinaemia). × 520.

agents of low toxicity, such as chlorambucil: accordingly, the prognosis is relatively good. The *lymphocytic form* is the commonest member of this group. Histologically it is characterised by diffuse infiltration of the lymph nodes by small mature lymphocytes, with only very occasional large or nucleolated cells. Most

cases of this kind develop into chronic lymphocytic leukaemia (p. 494). Although this tumour is usually of B-cell derivation, plasma cell differentiation is never observed. In a closely-related variety of lymphoma, sometimes known as the *lymphoplasmacytic type*, plasma cell differentiation does take place and the affected lymph nodes are diffusely infiltrated by plasma cells, mature lymphocytes and intermediate cell forms. This pattern is almost always accompanied by the formation of monoclonal IgM and the clinical picture is that of *Waldenström's macroglobulinaemia*, discussed in greater detail on p. 499. Recently, *diffuse lymphoma* of *cleaved-cell type* has been described. The cleaved cells are of B-cell origin and, as indicated above, are believed to be germinal centre cells. Like follicular lymphoma, it is slowly progressive but apparently shows no tendency to transform to an aggressive phase (see above).

Diffuse lymphoma of high-grade malignancy (Fig. 17.22). These tumours, as Galton has pointed out, have a clearly identifiable primary focus, either in a lymph node or in an extranodal site. They are locally destructive and ultimately metastasise by lymphatics or the blood to distant sites involving both lymphoid and other tissues. In other words, they behave much like carcinomas and clinical staging procedures similar to those used in Hodgkin's disease are more relevant than in the diffuse lymphomas of low-grade malignancy.

It is often difficult to identify the cell type of these highly malignant tumours, for they are mostly blast cells which lack the morphological features and surface markers of lymphocytes or macrophages. In spite of their nuclear pleomorphism, however, a **lymphoblastic group** can be recognised morphologically, and while such tumours occur at all ages, they are the commonest lymphomas of childhood and adolescence except for Hodgkin's disease. They originate usually in a lymph node, but sometimes in the gastro-intestinal tract or other non-lymphoid tissues. Some of these lymphoblastic tumours do have surface markers suggesting their *T-cell nature*, especially those arising in the anterior mediastinum in childhood (Sternberg tumour); they may be of thymic origin and are liable to progress to *acute lymphoblastic leukaemia*.

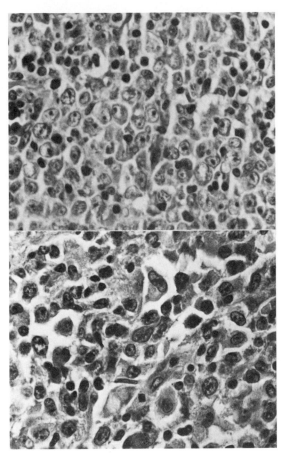

Other diffuse lymphoblastic lymphomas appear to be of *B-cell nature*, including some which apparently develop from follicular lymphoma and so show the features of germinal-centre cells ('centroblasts and centrocytes'). Burkitt's lymphoma (p. 265), which is of B-cell type, may arise from a particular type of germinal-centre cell, but the evidence is not strong.

Another group of diffuse lymphoblastic lymphomas consists of cells which have the cytoplasmic basophilia and abundant rough endoplasmic reticulum of plasma cell precursors, and in some instances synthesise immunoglobulin. These have been termed **plasmablastic sarcomas**: they arise both in lymph nodes and in extra-nodal sites, and are the commonest form of lymphoma originating in the gastro-intestinal tract.

Occasional lymphomas of aggressive blast-cell type have ultrastructural features and sometimes phagocytic activity suggesting that they are derived from the macrophage series of cells: they are somewhat illogically called '**histiocytic lymphomas**'. *Histiocytic medullary reticulosis* is an example. In this rapidly fatal condition the sinuses of the lymph nodes, spleen, liver and bone marrow are infiltrated by macrophage-like cells which tend to phagocytose erythrocytes, myeloid cells and platelets, thus producing a severe pancytopenia in the peripheral blood. This neoplasm has a curious geographical distribution, being rare in this country but quite common in East Africa and in the Far East.

Multiple myeloma appears usually in the bone marrow and is described on p. 496.

Fig. 17.22 Lymph nodes showing examples of highly malignant diffuse lymphomas. Both would formerly have been called 'reticulum-cell sarcoma'. Electron microscopy and immunohistology showed the lymphoma above to be of plasmablastic type, and the lower to be a 'histiocytic lymphoma'. × 520.

Lymph node tumour metastases

It must be emphasised that lymphocytic spread and formation of metastatic tumours in the lymph nodes is an extremely important feature of all forms of carcinoma (p. 282) with the exception of basal cell carcinoma of the skin. Usually the draining nodes are enlarged first, but eventually more distant nodal metastases commonly develop. Most types of sarcoma tend to spread especially by the bloodstream, but lymph node involvement is by no means rare, particularly in rhabdomyosarcoma and synovial sarcomas.

The Thymus

The development of the thymus and the advances in our understanding of its major role in the immune response are described briefly in Chapter 4, while the immunological deficiencies resulting from defective thymic development are considered in Chapter 5 (pp. 139–42). The changes in the thymus in myasthenia gravis, and their possible significance, are dealt with on p. 875, and the pathogenic role of thymus-derived lymphocytes in the auto-immune diseases on pp. 133–5. It remains to consider the condition known as *status thymico-lymphaticus*, and to provide a brief account of thymic tumours, all of which are rare.

Status thymico-lymphaticus

This term has been applied to cases of sudden death from some cause which is insufficient to account for the death of a normal individual, and in which necropsy has revealed neither adequate cause of death nor any constant abnormality apart from enlargement of the thymus and other lymphoid tissues. In such cases, death has resulted quite unexpectedly from a trivial injury, fright, general anaesthesia, immersion in cold water, etc. The distribution of lymphoid hyperplasia has varied from case to case, and has included the tonsils, follicles at the root of the tongue, groups of lymph nodes, and lymphoid tissue of the alimentary tract. Lymphoid follicles have also been described in abnormal situations, including the liver, kidneys and bone marrow. Hypoplasia has been reported in some cases in other tissues, notably the adrenal medulla and chromaffin system, the aorta and its major branches, and gonadal hypoplasia with alterations in the secondary sexual characters.

Normal weight of the thymus. In considering the size of the thymus, it must be appreciated that the organ reaches a maximal size in relation to body weight at about the time of birth; it continues to enlarge until around puberty, although its weight relative to whole body weight diminishes, and after puberty it undergoes involution, at first rapidly and then more slowly, its absolute weight declining. This involutionary process appears to be dependent on the steroid sex hormones produced by the gonads, and can be inhibited experimentally by castration of young male animals.

A second important consideration in assessing the significance of an enlarged thymus is the accumulation of adipose tissue which occurs in the organ during involution: this proceeds during adult life, until the adipose tissue far exceeds the thymic tissue proper, and crude thymic weights, without an assessment of the proportion of fatty tissue present, are liable to be misleading.

Finally, the thymus, like other lymphoid tissues, is sensitive to the action of glucocorticoid hormones, administration of ACTH, cortisol or cortisone, etc., causing shrinkage of the lymphoid tissues, including the thymus. The reduction in size of the lymphoid organs which occurs during severe illnesses is probable largely attributable to increase in secretion of endogenous corticosteroids as a result of stress. Accordingly, the thymus is larger at necropsy in cases of sudden death than in patients dying after a period of illness.

The total weight of the thymus, and the weight corrected to allow for the proportion of adipose tissue, were determined by Hammar (1926): the mean weights for individuals of various ages, dying suddenly without preceding illness, are given below in Table 17.3.

Thymic enlargement and sudden death. Considering the factors discussed above, it is not surprising that the thymus and other lymphoid tissues should appear unduly prominent in cases of sudden death, particularly in children, and the term status thymico-

Table 17.3   Age and thymic weights

	Thymic Weight (grams)	
Age (years)	*Total*	*Corrected for Fat*
Neonatal	13·26	12·33
1–5	22·98	19·26
6–10	26·10	22·08
11–15	37·52	25·18
16–20	25·58	12·71
21–25	24·73	4·95
26–35	19·87	3·87
36–45	16·27	2·98
46–55	12·85	1·48

lymphaticus was introduced on the basis that the enlarged lymphoid tissues predisposed in some way to sudden death from some minor injury or shock. Analysis of data collected by the Committee of the Pathological Society and Medical Research Council has been published by Young and Turnbull (1931) who concluded that an unduly large thymus is not, by itself, associated with a predisposition to sudden death, and that there is little, if any, association between the weight of the thymus and the amounts of lymphoid tissue elsewhere in the body. These views have been supported by other workers, and an analysis of Hammar's observations shows that, in those cases where the weight of the thymus exceeded the mean weight for the age group by more than two standard deviations, death was due not to some trivial incident, but to major trauma, drowning, carbon monoxide poisoning, etc.

In spite of the evidence against the significance of an enlarged thymus, lymph nodes, etc., in sudden death, most pathologists with a large necropsy experience have encountered occasional cases of sudden death from inadequate cause, and have noted thymic and other lymphoid enlargements. One possible explanation is an unsuspected state of adrenocortical hypofunction, which would account for the lymphoid hyperplasia and also for sudden death from minor causes. However, we know of no evidence to support this possibility, nor are we aware of a predisposition to sudden death in patients with known adrenocortical hypofunction, such as untreated Addison's disease or hypopituitarism, although in such conditions the lymphoid tissues may be enlarged.

Tumours of the thymus

Primary thymomas are of several types, all of which are rare.

Epithelial and lymphocytic tumours. Tumours containing both epithelial cells and lymphocytes are least uncommon. They usually consist of nodules, and may be predominantly epithelial, predominantly lymphocytic or may show widely differing ratios of the two cell types in different parts of the tumour and sometimes within single nodules. The epithelial cells may be plump and ovoid, spindle-shaped or rounded, or they may show acinar formation and resemble tumours of the endocrine glands, and two or more types of epithelium may be present in the same tumour. These tumours may be encapsulated, and intersected by dense fibrous stroma, or may extend locally to involve the adjacent tissues, including the major blood vessels, pleura, lung and pericardium. Most tumours are symptomless, and are detected incidentally by x-ray, or cause pressure symptoms, but not uncommonly a thymoma is accompanied by myasthenia gravis, or more rarely by systemic lupus erythematosus, hypogammaglobulinaemia or pure red-cell aplasia. The significance of these associations is not known, but it is noteworthy that the last two may respond to removal of the tumour, while the response of myasthenia gravis is more variable (p. 875).

Very rarely, tumours of mixed epithelial-lymphocytic type, or purely epithelial tumours, are anaplastic and more highly malignant, and squamous carcinoma has been observed.

Teratoma also occurs in the thymus, and may be wholly well-differentiated or have poorly-differentiated areas.

Seminoma of the thymus resembles closely the commoner testicular tumour, and is highly radiosensitive.

Lymphoid neoplasms may originate in the thymus. The condition sometimes termed *granulomatous thymoma* appears to be the nodular sclerosing form of Hodgkin's disease involving the thymus and often the mediastinal lymph nodes. *Sternberg's tumour* (p. 526) appears to originate, at least in some instances, in the thymus, which may be involved in various other forms of lymphoma.

18

Alimentary Tract

I The Oral Cavity and Pharynx

The lips and mouth

Inflammatory changes

The lips share with the tongue lesions resulting from severe iron-deficiency anaemia and from certain vitamin B deficiencies. In chronic microcytic anaemia with achlorhydria and koilonychia, there are characteristic changes in the labial mucosa resulting in cracks and fissures at the angles of the mouth—*angular stomatitis*—with desquamation, thinning of the epithelium and inflammatory cellular infiltrate in the lips—*cheilosis* and *perlèche*. The tongue is smooth and glazed with loss of the papillae—*atrophic glossitis*. Despite the anaemia, it often looks rather fiery red and may be very painful. In pernicious anaemia, atrophic glossitis is also a constant feature.

Similar changes occur in riboflavin deficiency and it is probable that the lesions in both cases are the result of defective intracellular respiration in epithelial cells that have normally a high turnover rate, in the first case from deficiency of the iron-containing cytochrome oxidase and in the second from lack of respiratory flavoprotein.

Herpes simplex. A common inflammatory lesion of the oral mucosa is that due to the virus of herpes simplex. Infection usually occurs in infancy or childhood and not infrequently the virus persists indefinitely in latent form in the neurons of the trigeminal ganglion. When virus reactivates within the trigeminal ganglion, it probably travels down the sensory fibres of the maxillary or mandibular nerves to produce inflammation with vesicles within the area of skin supplied by the nerve—usually labial herpes. Reactivation with labial sores is almost

invariable in lobar pneumonia, but occurs also in minor infections such as coryza, and it can also be provoked by exposure to cold or excessive ultraviolet light.

The primary lesions consist of groups of vesicles of 1–2 mm diameter on the mucosa; these rupture and form small shallow ulcers with a red margin and necrotic centre. In subsequent attacks lesions are located chiefly at the mucocutaneous junction; rupture of the vesicles leads to a painful crusted sore.

Measles. Koplik's spots are small inflammatory vesicles which appear on the buccal mucosa shortly before the morbilliform rash in the skin. The lesions consist of a central whitish area of thickened epithelium which undergoes necrosis and breaks down to form small shallow ulcers (Fig. 18.1). In lymphoid tissues the measles virus gives rise to multinucleated giant cells of characteristic appearance—Warthin–Finkeldey cells (p. 515).

Thrush is a superficial infection of the oral mucosa by the monilial fungus *Candida albicans*. It occurs chiefly in children and may be seen in epidemic form in nurseries. It consists of multiple whitish patches from which the fungus is easily recovered. These are irregularly distributed on the oral mucosa, and bleed on removal. In adults, candida infections of the oral mucosa occur in acute and chronic forms in such conditions as angular stomatitis, or injury from a chafing denture. They are, however, more liable to occur in patients who are debilitated or undergoing prolonged treatment with broad-spectrum antibiotics, steroids, or cytotoxic drugs. In these circumstances they may occur in severe form and extend to the oesophagus and other sites. Although it produces white patches on the oral mucosa, thrush is not usually included under the term 'leukoplakia' (see below).

Syphilis. A primary chancre may be contracted by kissing someone with the highly infective secondary syphilitic lesions in the mouth. The primary labial sore is often more exuberant than a typical genital chancre and the lesion commonly does not present an intensely indurated base, so that its true nature may be unrecognised. In the secondary stage the lips and oral mucosa may show the typical mucous patches and snail-track ulcers, and these are highly infective. In the tertiary stage, a gumma may develop in the tongue, usually posteriorly, where it presents as a deep punched-out ulcer with a yellowish grey wash-leather base. Gummatous ulceration of the hard palate leads to perforation into the nose.

Tuberculosis. Small shallow ulcers with undermined edges occur about the tip of the tongue in cases of chronic pulmonary tuberculosis.

Leukoplakia

This is a clinical term meaning the presence of white patches in a squamous epithelial mucous membrane. It may be due to epithelial thickening of various kinds. In the mouth it commonly results from chronic irritation, e.g. by pipe smoke or chafing dentures. The epithelium is thickened, the rete pegs are prolonged and the papillae contain a chronic inflammatory infiltrate. In some cases the epithelium becomes atypical with loss of polarity of the cells and invasive squamous carcinoma may develop. Leukoplakia of the mouth is thus, in some instances, a pre-cancerous lesion.

Pigmentation

Melanotic pigmentation of the lips and buccal mucosa occurs in Addison's disease (q.v.) as

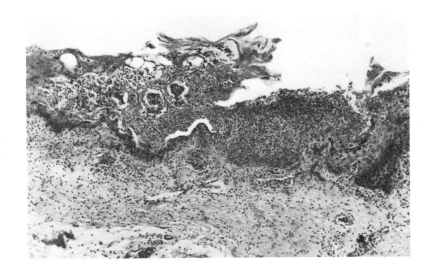

Fig. 18.1 Buccal mucosa in measles, showing a Koplik's spot, a small central area of ulceration with acute inflammatory reaction. At the margin epithelium is growing over the denuded surface. × 65.

brown patches of irregular distribution and of varying severity. In the absence of Addison's disease, marked patchy brown pigmentation of the lips involving both skin and mucosa, especially in an adolescent, raises the possibility of the Peutz–Jeghers syndrome (p. 590). In both conditions the pigment is seen in the basal cell layer.

Ingestion of various heavy metals gives rise to a pigmented line in the gums; blue in the case of lead, greyish-black with bismuth and purplish-grey with mercury. The metallic intoxication has to be of long duration to produce these lesions.

Benign tumours

Both *haemangioma* and *lymphangioma* may give rise to great enlargment of the lips and tongue and call for plastic surgery (Fig. 18.2). *Pleomorphic salivary adenomas* may arise in the lips, palate and fauces as well as in the more usual site in the major salivary glands (see below).

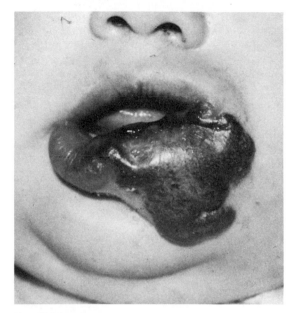

Fig. 18.2   Haemangioma of the lower lip.

Squamous papilloma is a common tumour of the oral tissues and may occur at all ages although it is most often seen in the elderly. In young persons it is sometimes viral in origin. There is in general less keratinisation than in the corresponding skin tumour. It rarely becomes malignant. A lesion which may simulate the papilloma macroscopically is the

fibroepithelial polyp occurring in the floor of the mouth. This consists of a small nodule of hyperplastic fibrous tissue covered by thinned or acanthotic epithelium. It is due to chronic irritation and is not neoplastic.

Granular-cell 'myoblastoma'. In spite of its name, this tumour is probably of neural origin and derived from Schwann cells: it occurs most commonly in the tongue but also in the skin, larynx, breast, etc. It is composed of elongated cells, with nuclei at intervals as in muscle fibres; the cytoplasm is acidophilic and is broken up into innumerable rounded granular masses, and striation is completely absent. The lesion is a true neoplasm and, though not well circumscribed, usually behaves as a benign tumour. It may, however, recur locally, and very rarely metastasise. A remarkable feature is the tendency of the overlying squamous epithelium to be markedly and irregularly hyperplastic (Fig. 18.3), so that an erroneous diagnosis of squamous carcinoma may be made, especially in such situations as the tongue or larynx.

Epulis is the term applied to tumours arising from the gingival margin. Some so designated clinically are inflammatory granulomatous masses, but true tumours also occur.

Congenital epulis is seen in two forms. The better-known arises usually from the maxillary gum margin and forms a soft polypoid mass consisting of cells closely resembling those of the so-called granular 'myoblastoma'. It is of interest that similar large granular cells occa-

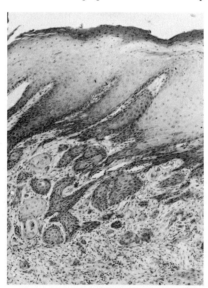

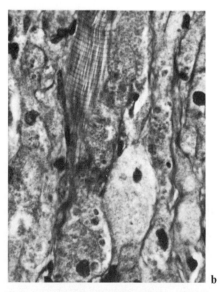

Fig. 18.3   Granular cell 'myoblastoma'. **a** The characteristic irregular hyperplasia of the overlying squamous epithelium. × 60. **b** The coarsely granular cytoplasm and small condensed nuclei of the elongated cells among the muscle fibres of the tongue. × 450.

sionally occur in tumours of the enamel organ (see Fig. 18.6). The other form is the rare, controversial melanotic tumour that occurs chiefly in the maxilla in the newborn or in early infancy and consists of masses of small darkly-staining cells resembling neuroblasts and larger paler cells resembling glia. Between these are tubules lined by cubical cells heavily pigmented with melanin granules which may have the rod-like morphology characteristic of retinal pigment. Despite the malignant-looking histology these tumours are clinically benign and do not recur after thorough removal.

The fibrous and bony epulis arises chiefly in connection with the maxilla. It consists of young fibrous tissue among which are irregular bony trabeculae and as there is always some inflammatory reaction it is difficult to distinguish from reactive lesions. The neoplastic nature of such an epulis may be displayed by destructive invasion of the maxilla and antrum and we have seen an example that looked histologically benign undergo repeated recurrence and finally metastasise to the lungs.

The giant-cell epulis or *giant-cell reparative granuloma* arises usually in the mandible in connection with the tooth sockets of the primary dentition. It consists of a loose spindle-celled tissue in which there are numerous multi-nucleated giant cells which closely resemble

those of giant-cell tumour of bone (Fig. 18.4). The surface is often ulcerated and inflammatory cellular reaction may be abundant in the superficial part. It rarely recurs after removal and although it is regarded by many as reactive rather than neoplastic, its true nature is still unknown.

Malignant tumours

Squamous carcinoma can arise anywhere in the mouth, but most often in the following situations. In the *lip* the disease occurs almost exclusively in the lower lip and in males. The lesion may begin as a patch of leukoplakia or as a warty excrescence which breaks down to form an indurated ulcer with rolled-over edges (Fig. 18.5). Spread to the submandibular lymph nodes is relatively late. Microscopically it is usually of well-differentiated keratinising type.

Squamous carcinoma of the *tongue* arises most often on the lateral margin of the anterior two thirds, beginning as a thickened patch of

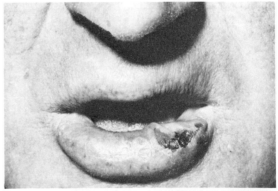

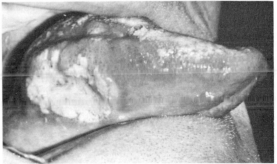

Fig. 18.5 *Above*, squamous carcinoma of the lip, presenting as an ulcer with raised edges. *Below*, squamous carcinoma of the side of the tongue, which has formed an irregular ulcer with a necrotic base. (Mr. I. A. McGregor.)

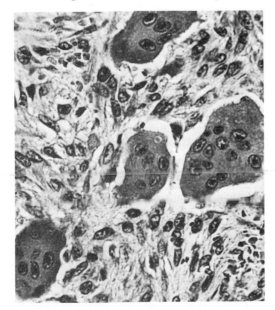

Fig. 18.4 Giant-cell epulis, showing multinucleated giant cells embedded in spindle-cell tissue. × 400.

leukoplakia and going on to a deeply excavated ulcer. Spread to the submandibular lymph nodes occurs commonly and usually early and extends quickly to involve the deep cervical nodes. Squamous carcinoma occurs in the *floor of the mouth* and in the *tonsil* and *pillars of the fauces*. Microscopically the growth is usually fairly well differentiated (Figs. 11.9 and 11.10, p. 278) but despite this it is radiosensitive. The rarer growths on the posterior third of the tongue resemble those on the tonsil and may be more anaplastic.

Lympho-epithelioma is an anaplastic squamous carcinoma, arising usually in the pharynx, and heavily infiltrated with lymphocytes. It tends to invade locally, commonly into the base of the skull, and to involve the cervical lymph nodes at an early stage: blood-borne metastases are also common. Evidence on whether the metastases are also infiltrated with lymphocytes is conflicting. Although these tumours are sensitive to radiotherapy, this is not usually curative.

Anaplastic carcinoma of the nasopharynx, including lympho-epithelioma, is particularly common in the Chinese. Such tumours have been shown to be associated with high titres of antibody to Epstein–Barr virus (pp. 265, 515).

Other malignant tumours are rare in the mouth. Various malignant lymphomas may, however, arise in the tonsils and other pharyngeal lymphoid tissues.

In the *soft palate* a distinctive type of *rhabdomyosarcoma* (p. 296) occurs in children. It is polypoid and consists of a number of blunt clubbed processes suspended from a narrow stalk. After simple operative removal, the tumour recurs locally, sometimes over a number of years, but ultimately spread takes place to the cervical lymph nodes and internal organs. Adequate local excision is therefore necessary.

Tumours of dental origin

Adamantinoma (ameloblastoma). This epithelial tumour is composed of masses and anastomosing strands of cells (Fig. 18.6). Those at the periphery are usually columnar and are believed to represent ameloblasts. The cells within are of more stellate or irregular form and occasionally are distended with granular material. The cell masses may be solid, but not infrequently the central portions undergo softening so that cysts are formed, which are often multiple. Such tumours were formerly called *epithelial odontomas*, but the terms *adamantinoma* and *amelo-*

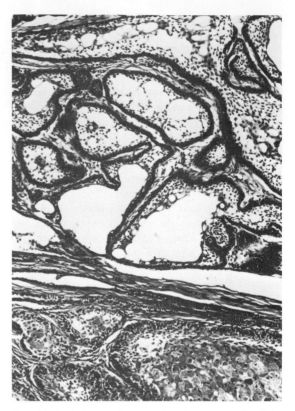

Fig. 18.6 Adamantinoma, showing spaces lined by epithelium, some of which contain a loose network of cells resembling the stellate reticulum of the enamel organ. The epithelial spaces in the lower part of the field contain granular cells. × 60.

blastoma are now used. They originate from the enamel organ, or from small masses of epithelial cells—'paradental remains'—which occur normally in the fetus in the vicinity of the developing teeth. While their behaviour may be benign, they are prone to repeated local recurrences and the more solid types sometimes invade and destroy the surrounding tissues.

Odontoma. The term is applied in a general way to any tumour-like mass developing in connection with the tissues which form the teeth. Such a lesion may arise at various stages of development, and may consist of one or several tissues; accordingly odontomas present considerable variety of structure. For example the tooth follicle may form a *dentigerous cyst*, containing one or more teeth or a large number of imperfectly developed teeth or denticles. In the cyst wall there may be calcium deposition and even formation of bone. Other examples of odontoma consist of various structures containing enamel and cement irregularly admixed and sometimes forming a hard irregular mass; the term *composite odontoma* is applied to such a structure.

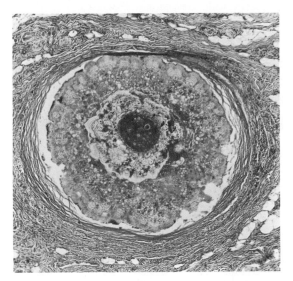

Fig. 18.7a Calculus obstructing duct of submaxillary gland. × 55.

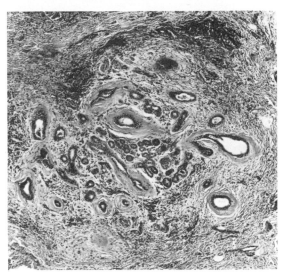

Fig. 18.7b Atrophy and fibrosis of submaxillary gland with chronic inflammatory infiltration, resulting from duct obstruction. × 55.

The salivary glands

Inflammation of the parotid and other salivary glands is most often due to the virus of **mumps**, which gives rise to an early viraemic phase. The chief lesion in mumps is an acute inflammatory swelling, mainly of the parotids, with oedema and interstitial mononuclear cell infiltration. Usually this subsides without permanent damage to the glands. It may be accompanied by orchitis and by pancreatitis, both of which are more prone to result in some degree of atrophy. Mumps virus is also a relatively common cause of aseptic meningitis (p. 694).

Suppurative parotitis occurs as a complication of prolonged febrile illnesses, infection usually reaching the gland by way of Stensen's duct. Infection is prone to occur if the duct is partially obstructed by a calculus.

Salivary calculi occur most often in the submaxillary gland. The calculus is round or elongated and may project from the orifice of the duct which it partially occludes. Salivary calculi are composed chiefly of calcium carbonate and phosphate. The obstruction thus caused is apt to lead to atrophy and fibrosis of the gland (Figs. 18.7*a* and *b*).

Sjøgren's syndrome occurs mostly in women of middle age. There is dryness of the mouth due to lack of saliva with consequent extensive dental caries. There may also be *kerato-*

conjunctivitis sicca. Many cases also suffer from chronic polyarthritis of rheumatoid type. The lacrimal, conjunctival and salivary glands are often swollen: they are extensively infiltrated by lymphocytes and plasma cells, the glandular acini are atrophic and may disappear, and the

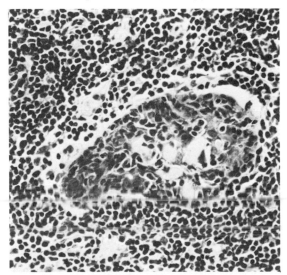

Fig. 18.8 The parotid gland in Sjøgren's syndrome, showing heavy infiltration with lymphocytes, loss of glandular tissue and proliferation of duct epithelium to form a cellular mass containing foci of pale-staining hyaline material. Note that the proliferated epithelium is also infiltrated with lymphocytes. × 320.

ducts show epithelial proliferation to form masses of cells, among which lie accumulations of homogeneous eosinophilic material (Fig. 18.8). Various auto-antibodies may appear in the serum, including antinuclear antibodies, precipitins to cellular constituents and rheumatoid factor. The syndrome is sometimes associated with chronic thyroiditis and its immunological accompaniments. The condition long known as Mikulicz's disease is now recognised as the same condition, with prominent lacrimal gland enlargement.

Uveo-parotid fever. This is one of the important lesions of sarcoidosis (p. 182) in which iridocyclitis and parotid swelling occur, sometimes involving the facial nerve and causing paralysis. The glands may be considerably enlarged due to the presence of chronic inflammatory infiltrates in which sarcoid follicles are found.

Salivary gland tumours

Pleomorphic salivary adenomas. This type of tumour, also called *mixed parotid tumour*, is commonest in the parotid gland, but occurs in the other major salivary glands and also in minor glands in the mouth, lips and palate. It may reach a large size and produce effects mainly by pressure. It appears well encap-

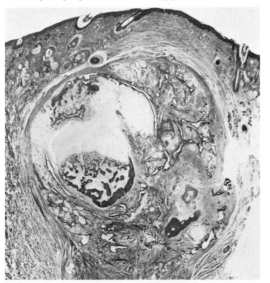

Fig. 18.9 A small pleomorphic salivary adenoma of the lower lip. The tumour is roughly rounded and sharply defined. The pale part of the mushroom-shaped area within it is cartilage, which shows formation of bone trabeculae, seen as dark areas. × 7.

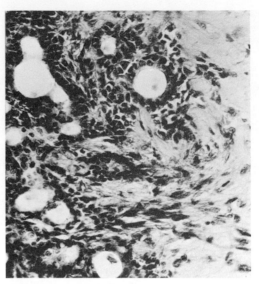

Fig. 18.10 Pleomorphic salivary adenoma, showing gland-like epithelial structures, from which cells appear to be streaming off into the connective tissue stroma. × 200.

sulated (Fig. 18.9), but microscopy commonly shows projections of tumour through the capsule, and complete removal requires excision of the tissue surrounding the tumour. Occasionally it becomes carcinomatous. Histologically, the tumour is found to consist both of epithelial elements and connective tissues, but the former are the essential elements. The epithelial cells are, in places, of a low columnar type and have an acinar arrangement, often with two layers of cells, but occasionally there is transition to squamous epithelium. Cells extend from the acini in solid strands which merge into the stroma, suggesting a transition between stroma and epithelial cells (Fig. 18.10). The epithelial cells appear to secrete mucinous material into the stroma around them. The stroma may remain mucoid, or cartilage may develop, which occasionally undergoes ossification (Fig. 18.9).

The nature of the cells which develop into chondrocytes is not known, and the stimulus for such differentiation is also obscure.

The range of structural variation among salivary tumours is extremely wide, and no histological classification is wholly satisfactory. It is worth distinguishing an **acinic tumour** with cells resembling those of the serous salivary glands and also a **muco-epidermoid type** in

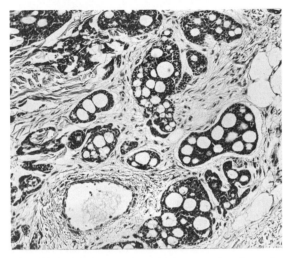

Fig. 18.11 Adenocystic carcinoma showing the characteristic architecture. × 90.

which large mucin-secreting cells mingle with cells of squamous appearance. The most important variant is the **adenocystic carcinoma** (*cribriform cylindroma*) (Fig. 18.11). This consists of solid masses of small darkly-staining cells among which lie tiny spaces containing clear fluid, either spherical, giving a sieve-like effect on section, or drawn out into little duct-like channels. The prognosis of this tumour type is substantially worse than that of other salivary

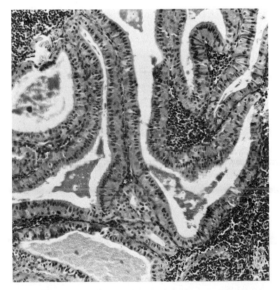

Fig. 18.12 Adenolymphoma of the parotid gland, showing the papillary architecture, with lymphoid stroma. × 130.

tumours. Despite initial slow growth, local recurrence after excision is the rule. Metastases to local lymph nodes are common in the later stages and blood spread is by no means rare. This type of tumour is relatively commoner outside the parotid than in it: it occurs also in the nose, external auditory meatus and skin (one form of hidradenoma). At all these sites except the last, where the necessary wide excision is usually possible, it has the same slow growth but poor ultimate prognosis.

Adenolymphoma. This is a type of adenoma which occurs in the parotid glands. It is seen especially in elderly men, is benign and occasionally bilateral. The epithelium is of tall columnar type, arranged as small glandular acini or as cysts with numerous small papillary ingrowths (Fig. 18.12). The stroma is lymphoid tissue with numerous germinal centres. These tumours are encapsulated and complete removal is usually not difficult.

Pharynx

Tonsillitis. Acute tonsillitis is a common cause of sore throat. Haemolytic streptococci are the commonest infecting agents and give rise to acute inflammatory swelling with purulent exudate in the tonsillar crypts—*follicular tonsillitis*. The infection occasionally extends more deeply and involves the whole tonsil and adjacent tissues with frank suppuration; this is known as *quinsy*. From such a lesion streptococcal cellulitis may spread widely into the neck—*Ludwig's angina*—or even into the mediastinum or may give rise to a retropharyngeal abscess.

Acute streptococcal tonsillitis occurring alone or in scarlet fever is the usual antecedent infection in rheumatic fever and post-streptococcal glomerulonephritis. Chronic enlargement of the tonsils and adjacent lymphoid tissue commonly results from colonisation by one or other of the many adenoviruses.

Vincent's angina is a painful necrotic ulcerating lesion on the fauces characterised by a patch of yellowish-white false membrane surrounded by an area of acute inflammation, and may be difficult to distinguish from diphtheria (p. 382). It is due to the symbiotic action of fusiform bacilli and the spirochaete *Borrelia vincenti*. Vincent's infection in its most severe form is probably responsible for the lesions on the cheek known as *noma* or *cancrum oris*, and it also gives rise to a severe ulcerative and necrotic gingivitis. A similar lesion is found in established scurvy, due to vitamin C deficiency. Great swelling, haemorrhage and ulceration of the gingivae are frequently seen in the acute leukaemias, particularly in the monocytic form, and necrotic ulceration occurs on the fauces, pharynx and larynx in various conditions characterised by extreme reduction in the number of circulating polymorphonuclear leukocytes, i.e. in *agranulocytosis* (p. 458).

Diphtheria is an acute inflammation which affects most frequently the fauces, soft palate and tonsils, but may also attack the nose, or the larynx and trachea; it occurs chiefly in young children, but may also affect adults. The causal organism, *Corynebacterium diphtheriae*, exists in three main forms, *mitis*, *intermedius* and *gravis*, and infections with the last type tend to be more severely toxic and also to show greater local inflammatory reaction. The organisms remain strictly localised at the site of infection and the systemic effects are due to the formation and absorption of a powerful exotoxin which may cause myocardial damage and toxic

fatty changes in the organs; the mechanism of cellular injury is outlined on p. 2. The local lesions are characterised by the formation on the affected surfaces of a false membrane composed of fibrin and leukocytes. In the fauces, palate and tonsils the stratified squamous epithelium becomes permeated by exudate which forms a fibrinous coagulum in which the epithelium is incorporated; it then undergoes extensive necrosis under the influence of the diphtheria toxin. The whole false membrane is dull greyish-yellow and it can be detached only with difficulty owing to the attachment of the dead epithelium to the underlying tissues. When it is removed a bleeding connective tissue surface is laid bare. In *gravis* infections, membrane formation may be less obvious but inflammatory congestion and swelling are more marked and the cervical lymph nodes may be much swollen.

Diphtheria of the nasopharynx and of the larynx is described on p. 382

Immunisation programmes are largely responsible for the present low incidence of diphtheria in many parts of the world.

Tumours of the pharynx are included with those of the oral cavity on pp. 531–4.

II Oesophagus

General considerations. The oesophagus is a muscular tube, lined by squamous epithelium and adapted to bear without injury the rapid passing of food over its surface. It has marked powers of resistance and is a rare site of primary bacterial invasion, but damage to the mucosa of the lower end from regurgitated gastric juice is fairly common. Oesophageal obstruction can arise from various lesions, the most important being carcinoma of the oesophagus and invasion by bronchial carcinoma.

Circulatory disturbances

Oesophageal varices. The submucosal veins in the lower oesophagus and cardia of the stomach communicate with both the portal and systemic venous systems. In cases of portal hypertension, most frequently due to *hepatic cirrhosis*, these veins become distinctly varicose

(Fig. 18.17): they may ulcerate, causing severe and often fatal haemorrhage.

Other causes of oesophageal haemorrhage. Rarely an *aortic aneurysm* ruptures into the oesophagus. A *foreign body*, for example a fish bone or safety pin, may become impacted transversely in the oesophagus, ulcerate through the wall, causing suppurative mediastinitis or empyema and subsequently lead to perforation of the aorta. A *carcinoma* of the oesophagus, especially of the soft and necrotic variety, may ulcerate into the aorta or other large vessel.

Inflammatory conditions

As already mentioned, primary infections of the oesophagus are rare in otherwise healthy individuals. Occasionally the lesion of diphtheria extends into, or arises primarily in, the oesophagus. In the rare but distinctive form of disseminated herpes simplex infection encountered in early infancy, the virus sometimes gains entry through the oesophagus. The characteristic lesion associated with South American trypanosomiasis (Chagas' disease) is described below.

'Opportunistic infections' (p. 140) may, however, occur in the oesophagus in states of debility or reduced immunity, and are often caused by organisms normally of low virulence. **Thrush** caused by the yeast-like fungus *Candida albicans*, is the most common infection of this type and is characterised by the formation of irregularly raised opaque whitish patches consisting of swollen and sodden epithelium infiltrated by the septate mycelial threads and

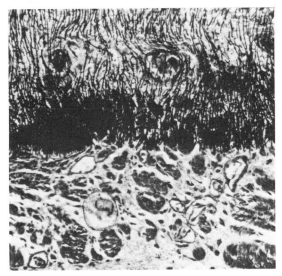

Fig. 18.13 Thrush of oesophagus, showing mycelial threads penetrating the wall. × 115.

spores of the fungus (Fig. 18.13). The infection may have spread from the mouth or throat and can extend more distally in the gastrointestinal tract or even invade the bloodstream to produce generalised lesions.

Oesophagitis can, of course, arise from non-infective causes. The most common example of this is **peptic oesophagitis** caused by regurgitation of gastric juice from the stomach (see below). Occasionally the self-administration accidental or otherwise, of irritating fluids is encountered and can give rise to serious and sometimes fatal lesions. Concentrated caustic soda, for example, produces extensive necrosis and sloughing of the oesophageal wall. More dilute solutions lead to superficial destruction followed by inflammatory changes. If the patient survives, scarring may result in fibrous stricture. Rarely the whole of the superficial layers of the oesophagus may become separated as a cast, without obvious cause; clinically this episode is accompanied by great pain and discomfort until the cast is completely separated (oesophagitis dissecans superficialis).

Peptic or reflux oesophagitis. Inflammatory changes and even frank ulceration may be produced at the lower end of the oesophagus by the reflux of acid gastric juice from the stomach. This may take place in severe toxic and infective conditions, particularly after operations, and cause haematemesis and even oesophageal perforation. Less severe forms of peptic oesophagitis are seen in about one-third of patients confined to bed for some time before death and give rise to a fiery-red oedematous mucosa with superficial ulcers, just above the cardiac orifice. Considerable digestion of the lower oesophagus may, however, take place after death, the wall then being discoloured, softened and shreddy, and often perforated. Recognition of true, antemortem oesophagitis depends upon the histological demonstration of inflammation or haemorrhage.

Hiatus hernia. The most important cause of peptic oesophagitis from the clinical viewpoint is, however, incompetence of the anti-reflux mechanism at the cardia associated with hiatus hernia, i.e. the herniation of part of the stomach through the oesophageal hiatus into the thoracic cavity. The mechanism preventing reflux of gastric juice depends upon three main components: (1) the intrinsic sphincter action of the lower end of the oesophagus, (2) the attachment of the cardio-oesophageal junction to the diaphragmatic hiatus and (3) the maintenance of the cardio-oesophageal angle, probably by a muscular 'sling' extending over the body of the stomach. Not all types of hiatus hernia lead to incompetence of this mechanism; for example, in the 'rolling' variety, in which part of the fundus of the stomach passes into the thorax alongside the cardia, reflux does not usually take place, although haematemesis and melaena are not uncommonly observed in this condition. It is in the 'sliding' type of hernia, which leads to obliteration of the cardio-oesophageal angle with upward displacement of the cardia, that reflux oesophagitis and its complications are most frequently observed.

The primary cause of hiatus hernia is not completely understood. It is certainly a common condition in the middle-aged and elderly although only symptomatic in a proportion of cases, and is usually attributed to increased intra-abdominal pressure coupled with laxity of the diaphragmatic hiatus. Obesity and pregnancy are thus common predisposing conditions and probably account for the higher incidence of hiatus hernia in women.

The principal symptoms, heartburn and regurgitation, are due to diffuse, superficial inflammation, congestion and ulceration caused by reflux of acid gastric juice into the lower oesophagus. Frank haematemesis and melaena are relatively uncommon complications, but chronic blood loss may lead to iron-deficiency anaemia. Perforation of the oesophagus is rare since the ulcers seldom penetrate the oesophageal muscularis. More often healing of the ulcerative lesions leads to the development of a fibrous stricture and dysphagia.

True **chronic peptic ulceration** of the oesophagus is uncommon. It occurs when the lower oesophagus is lined by columnar epithelium of gastric type (Barrett's syndrome). This may occur as a congenital abnormality but more often arises as a metaplastic change following recurrent reflux oesophagitis (Fig. 18.14).

Spontaneous rupture of the oesophagus

This unusual condition occurs in previously healthy men, usually when a heavy meal has been followed by violent vomiting. The lesion takes the form of a longitudinal slit, most often in the left posterior position, just above the diaphragm. The acid gastric contents are discharged into the pleural cavity directly or after first distending the posterior mediastinum. The appearance of the lesion indicates that it is essentially a longitudinal burst, brought about by sudden overdistension of the lower oesophagus in the act of vomiting, but the strongly acid gastric juice may also be a factor. In a number of the recorded cases peptic ulceration of stomach or duodenum has also been present.

Severe vomiting, usually associated with heavy alcohol intake, may also lead to brisk haematemesis as a result of laceration of the mucosa in the vicinity of the cardia. The damage, however, usually affects the gastric rather than the oesophageal mucosa. (Mallory-Weiss syndrome.)

Oesophageal obstruction

Obstruction of the oesophagus usually has an *organic* basis. In some instances, however, a primary organic lesion cannot be recognised and the obstruction is apparently due to muscular spasm.

Organic obstruction

This may arise in a number of different ways. (1) The lumen of the oesophagus may actually be occluded, usually by tumour, either benign or malignant, although occasionally by a foreign body. (2) Disease within the wall of the oesophagus may lead to stenosis of the lumen; again malignant tumours are most often implicated. Fibrous stricture may, however, arise as a complication of hiatus hernia, the swallowing of corrosive or scalding fluids, trauma, or as a congenital defect. (3) The oesophagus may be

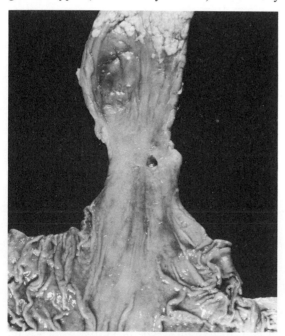

Fig. 18.14 Hiatus hernia with chronic peptic ulceration in the thoracic portion of the stomach.

compressed from outside, e.g. by a mediastinal tumour or cyst, aortic aneurysm, enlargement of the left atrium following mitral stenosis, congenital malformation of the great vessels, or pharyngeal diverticulum. (4) Diseases affecting the neuromuscular co-ordination of the oesophagus may interfere with normal deglutition. Progressive systemic sclerosis and Chagas' disease are suitably included in this group, and also disorders of the central nervous system which interfere with deglutition. Most of these diseases are discussed in the appropriate sections.

Progressive systemic sclerosis. This is regarded as a form of connective tissue disease (p. 878) which may produce widespread systemic lesions, the skin of the hands and face (acrosclerosis) and the kidneys being especially affected. Dysphagia is not uncommon, and is due to replacement of the oesophageal musculature by fibrous tissue which, if diffuse, leads to pronounced interference with peristaltic activity. Shortening of the oesophagus causing reflux oesophagitis may be an additional complication.

Chagas' disease (South American trypanosomiasis). The protozoon parasite (*Trypanosoma cruzi*) which causes this interesting disease appears to be capable of exerting a toxic effect on the autonomic ganglia of various viscera, especially the heart, oesophagus and colon. In the oesophagus, there may be widespread destruction of the ganglia of the myenteric plexus, leading to disturbance of peristalsis and the development of a clinical picture very similar to that of achalasia (see below).

'Functional' obstruction

The most important condition falling into this category is achalasia of the oesophagus, although other forms of functional disturbance have been described, e.g. diffuse spasm, sometimes associated with organic lesions of the gastro-intestinal tract, especially peptic ulcer, gall-bladder disease and hiatus hernia. Dysphagia may also occur at the upper end of the oesophagus in anaemic women (Kelly–Patterson or Plummer–Vinson syndrome, p. 485): the constriction can be visualised radiologically and by oesophagoscopy, and is sometimes described as an *oesophageal web*: since it is not seen at necropsy, and is usually

cured by treating the anaemia, it appears to be due to muscle spasm.

Achalasia of the oesophagus. In this condition, there is pronounced narrowing of the terminal part of the oesophagus with dilatation proximally. It usually develops in early adult life and leads to dysphagia and regurgitation of food; later there may be more serious obstruction. Oesophageal narrowing is usually at the diaphragmatic level and marked dilatation of

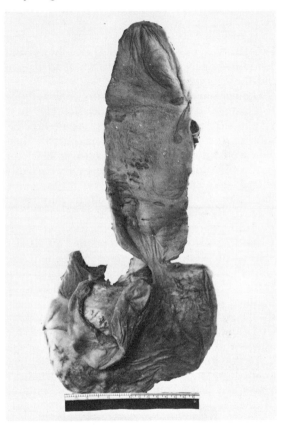

Fig. 18.15 Achalasia of oesophagus. Note the great dilatation with numerous superficial ulcers. × ¼.

the oesophagus results (Fig. 18.15), with compensatory muscular hypertrophy of the wall. The narrowing was formerly regarded as due to muscular spasm, hence the term 'cardiospasm' commonly applied to the disease; the present view, however, is that there is a primary disturbance of motility with defective transmission of peristaltic waves to the cardia and subsequent failure of relaxation of the cardiac sphincter. The cause of this disturbance remains uncertain. Degenerative changes have been described in the myenteric ganglia, and it is probable that the primary lesion in achalasia is an acquired abnormality of autonomic innervation; the close similarity to the oesophageal disturbance in Chagas' disease supports this hypothesis. Incision of the oesophageal wall through to the mucosa at the level of obstruction (Heller's operation) appears to be the most satisfactory form of surgical treatment in severe cases.

Diverticula

Two varieties of local dilatation are observed in the oesophagus, namely the *pulsion diverticulum* and the *traction diverticulum*.

The pulsion diverticulum is caused by forcible distension during the act of swallowing. It is usually not noticeable till early adult life but may be due to a congenital weakness or deficiency in the muscle of the inferior constrictor of the pharynx; it is therefore more correctly termed a *pharyngeal pouch* or *diverticulum*. Once a diverticulum has formed, as may result from repeated stretching of the deficiency in the wall during swallowing of food, it tends to become distended with food and gradually enlarges in a downward direction behind the wall of the oesophagus, tilting the tube forwards so that the mouth of the sac comes to lie in line with the upper pharynx. The sac ultimately becomes permanently distended by food and may compress and obstruct the adjacent oesophagus, with consequent severe dysphagia and weight loss.* Such a diverticulum is lined by mucous membrane supported by connective tissue, but its wall usually contains no muscle; occasionally ulceration may take place in it. A diverticulum may also occur anteriorly and bulge between the trachea and the oesophagus; but much more frequently the site is in the posterior wall at the junction of the pharynx and oesophagus.

The traction diverticulum of the oesophagus is produced by the contraction of connective tissue pulling the wall outwards, usually by the adhesion to the wall of the tube of a mass of calcified tuberculous lymph nodes or occasionally a mass of silicotic nodes. A pouch with a sharp apex is the result, and this is stretched and increased both by further scarring

and by the movements of the oesophagus. Ulceration of the diverticulum may occur and may lead to perforation, resulting in gangrenous mediastinitis which may extend to the pleura and other parts.

In rare cases a local diverticulum opposite the bifurcation of the trachea is due to a congenital abnormality, arising in the same way as a communication between the oesophagus and trachea (p. 543). The congenital diverticula are sometimes lined by columnar epithelium.

Tumours

Benign tumours. These are all rare. Lipoma, fibroma and leiomyoma may all occur, the last mentioned probably being the most common and occasionally reaching a large size. Benign tumours tend to project into the lumen as polyps.

Malignant tumours

Carcinoma of the oesophagus. Carcinoma is by far the commonest malignant tumour in the oesophagus and is comparatively frequent. It occurs usually after the age of forty-five, and is much commoner in men than in women. The commonest site is at the level of the bifurcation of the trachea, the lower and upper ends being next in order of frequency. There is, however, a distinct difference in the sites of incidence in the two sexes. About three-quarters of cases of cancer in the hypopharynx and upper end of the oesophagus occur in women, whereas over 80% of cancers elsewhere in the oesophagus occur in men.

Oesophageal carcinoma shows remarkable geographical variation in incidence. Although not uncommon in this country its incidence is much greater in certain parts of the U.S.S.R., and of Africa where it is suspected that the consumption of adulterated alcoholic beverages is a contributory factor. Fungal contamination of maize grown upon poor soil has also been incriminated. There is a remarkably high incidence in Curaçao, probably attributable to eating food that is too hot. Little is known about the causation of oesophageal cancer in Western Europe and North America apart

* 'Bloody' Judge Jeffries had a pharyngeal pouch, the discomfort of which may have contributed to the severity of his sentences.

from a possible association with heavy alcohol intake. There is also a relationship between iron-deficiency anaemia with dysphagia and post-cricoid carcinoma in women.

Naked-eye appearances. There are two chief types. The *scirrhous carcinoma* grows round the tube and induces a fibrous reaction, causing progressively severe stenosis. The *soft* or *encephaloid* type involves a greater length of the oesophagus, forms irregular projections into the lumen and thus tends to cause occlusion (Fig. 18.16). At the same time, the destruction of the muscular tissue by infiltration interferes with contraction. The tumour may spread

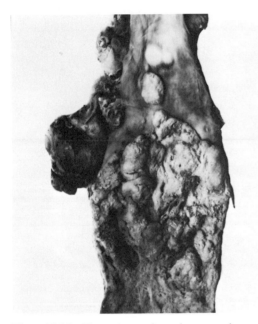

Fig. 18.16 Extensive ulcerating carcinoma in middle part of oesophagus.

upwards and downwards in the submucous tissue, and forms secondary nodules which raise the mucosa, giving an appearance of multifocal origin.

In addition to causing obstruction, the tumour may spread to the trachea or a bronchus, and ulcerate through the wall. Infected fluids then are likely to pass down the bronchi and cause aspiration pneumonia. Rarely ulceration into the aorta may result in fatal haemorrhage. Metastases also occur in the lymph nodes, and occasionally also in the internal organs, especially the liver; but death is usually caused by oesophageal obstruction.

Microscopic appearances. In nearly all cases the tumour is a poorly keratinised squamous carcinoma; rarely it resembles oat-cell bronchial carcinoma. Adenocarcinoma also has been described, but many examples are due to extension of a gastric carcinoma.

Sarcoma. This is rare. It resembles the softer varieties of carcinoma, but its growth may be more massive. In a few instances rhabdomyosarcoma of the oesophagus has been observed.

Congenital abnormalities

In addition to stenosis or dilatation, already mentioned, there may be various degrees of atresia of the oesophagus. The commonest of these is a condition in which the upper part forms a blind sac which is separated from the lower part, while the latter is patent and communicates with the trachea a short distance above its bifurcation. Sometimes the oesophagus is patent throughout, but there is a small communication with the trachea, through which food may pass into the trachea and cause a suppurative or necrotising pneumonia.

III Stomach

General considerations. The two most important pathological conditions in the stomach are peptic ulcer and carcinoma. Bacterial infection as a cause of serious disease in the stomach is comparatively rare. Gastric juice rapidly destroys most vegetative bacteria entering with food, and when digestion has been completed, and the stomach contents pass on to the intestine, the stomach soon returns to a state of virtual sterility. Nevertheless ingested tubercle, salmonellae, brucella and dysentery bacilli can all successfully evade the chemical barrier of the gastric secretion and no doubt more easily if there is defective acid secretion or stasis. Acute inflammation of the gastric mucosa is due to swallowing irritating fluids or food contaminated with bacterial, e.g. staphylococcal, toxins. It is also likely that the stomach can be affected by some of the enteroviruses and perhaps other viruses also.

Chronic gastritis of the acid-secreting mucosa has the features of an organ-specific auto-immune disease. Chronic inflammation also occurs in the antral mucosa and is of unknown cause.

Circulatory disturbances

Acute congestion occurs as part of the acute inflammatory changes produced by various kinds of ingested irritant, but its presence is often obscured by post-mortem autolysis.

Chronic congestion is seen in chronic systemic or portal venous congestion. The mucous membrane becomes swollen, purple or livid and towards the pylorus may be slate-grey, or minute brown points resulting from capillary haemorrhages may be present. Chronic inflammatory changes are often superadded. In long-continued portal hypertension there may be marked varicosity of the veins around the cardiac orifice as well as at the lower end of the oesophagus, and serious haemorrhage may

occur from them. Fig. 18.17 shows large varices produced in this way, which caused fatal haemorrhage.

Haemorrhages into the mucosa occur in various conditions, including chronic congestion, purpura, severe anaemia and infective fevers. Sometimes numerous haemorrhagic points 1–3 mm in diameter are scattered over the mucosa, especially in the fundus and they are often more marked along the summits of the folds. They are usually dark brown; occasionally the overlying mucous membrane becomes eroded with the formation of minute ulcers.

The term *haemorrhagic erosion* is applied to

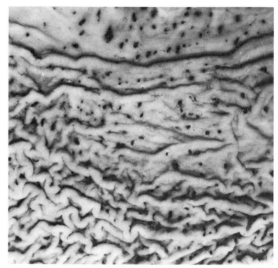

Fig. 18.18 Multiple minute haemorrhagic erosions of the gastric mucosa. × 0·75.

small ulcers of this type (Fig. 18.18). In some of the erosions the blood may have been removed by ulceration; occasionally, they become confluent and larger and merit the term 'acute ulcer'. A most important cause is ingestion of aspirin. Haemorrhagic erosions occur also in febrile conditions and are thus common in children. As elsewhere, small haemorrhages are seen in the wall of the stomach in septicaemias, due probably to toxic injury, or possibly to foci of bacterial multiplication.

Haemorrhage into the lumen of the stomach—haematemesis. Accumulation of blood in the stomach may result from lesions in its wall, or the blood may have come from the oesophagus or intestine.

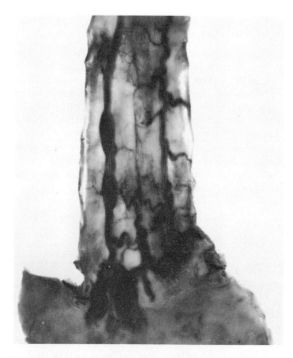

Fig. 18.17 Oesophagus and cardiac end of stomach, showing large dilated varicose veins from a case of cirrhosis of the liver. Death was due to haemorrhage from the large varicosity at the cardia.

The commonest causes of serious haemorrhage are peptic ulcer, either in the stomach or duodenum, and oesophageal varices (Fig. 18.17) due to portal hypertension, usually in hepatic cirrhosis. Carcinoma of the stomach frequently causes haemorrhage, but this is rarely severe. Haemorrhagic erosions (see above) are an important cause of gastric haemorrhage. Diffuse haemorrhage may occur from the mucous membrane without any discoverable lesion, or from apparently trivial local lesions. This is seen in haemorrhagic diatheses, in severe septic conditions, in yellow fever where it gives rise to 'black vomit', in acute liver failure, and occasionally without discoverable cause as an agonal event.

Blood effused into the stomach becomes mixed with its contents and acquires a brownish or almost black colour, or there may be fragments of brownish coagulum mixed with the fluid. In cases of rapidly fatal haemorrhage, however, the stomach may be filled by a large coagulum which forms a cast of the interior and the colour of the blood may be little altered. Such a condition may result when blood has passed down from the oesophagus, for example, in rupture of oesophageal varices. When there has been much haemorrhage into the stomach, altered blood is generally found in the small and large intestine.

Acute gastritis

Acute inflammation may be produced by the swallowing of irritants such as aspirin and other analgesics, hot fluids or strong alcohol. Acute fevers in children, viral infections and bacterial food poisoning may also be responsible, the latter usually taking the form of acute gastro-enteritis. The pathological changes have seldom been studied in biopsy material and post-mortem autolysis tends to efface the lesions, especially in the milder forms of gastritis. The most severe variety, known as *acute haemorrhagic gastritis* produces extensive oedema and focal erosion of the mucosa (Fig. 18.19), commonly associated with mucosal or submucosal haemorrhage. This has been observed especially following aspirin ingestion and in severely shocked patients; the mechanism is thought to be similar in both instances, viz. the back diffusion of hydrogen ions into the mucosa. In aspirin poisoning, acute ulceration may lead to haematemesis and even perforation (see above).

Bacterial gastritis is unusual, because gastric juice kills most vegetative forms of micro-organisms. Small mucosal ulcers may occur in typhoid and paratyphoid fevers; other salmonellae cause an acute illness with the clinical features of gastro-enteritis, but the histological changes in the stomach are not readily studied.

Tuberculous ulcers of the stomach, usually small and superficial, are a rare complication of pulmonary tuberculosis. In chronic gastritis, and particularly in chronic pyloric stenosis, with loss of acid secretion, various saprophytic bacteria, yeasts and fungi grow in the gastric contents, but rarely seem to invade the wall.

Phlegmonous gastritis, with extensive necrosis and suppuration in the wall of the stomach, occurs very rarely when bacteria, usually streptococci, penetrate into the submucosa through some local lesion, e.g. an injury caused by an ingested sharp foreign body.

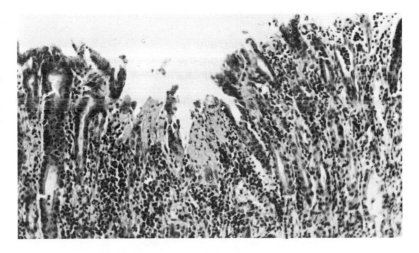

Fig. 18.19 Acute erosive gastritis. There is superficial loss of the surface epithelium with fibrinoid necrosis and polymorph infiltration. × 205.

Pseudomembranous gastritis can result from ingestion of irritant chemicals. It is rarely due to bacterial infection, but may occur in typhoid fever and septicaemias.

Corrosive poisons. Strong acids and alkalis cause extensive necrosis of the gastric wall, often with haemorrhage and changes in appearance of the necrotic tissue and blood which depend on the particular chemical swallowed. Chemicals which fix proteins, e.g. carbolic acid or mercuric chloride, may result in good preservation of the stomach at necropsy.

A large number of poisons of less intense action produce chiefly inflammatory changes accompanied by a varying amount of haemorrhage, superficial necrosis and pseudomembranous gastritis. These include weaker acids, such as oxalic acid or acetic acid, also various metallic salts. Arsenic (arsenious acid) causes an intense inflammation with white patches of tenacious mucus or exudate in which grains of the poison may still be present. Antimony causes a general acute inflammation, while in phosphorus poisoning there are usually haemorrhages and fatty degeneration in the mucosa. For details, however, special works on toxicology must be consulted.

Chronic gastritis

Chronic inflammatory changes in the mucosa of the stomach, with various degrees of loss of the specialised glandular tissue, are extremely common, although often clinically silent. The condition is, however, important when it affects the acid-secreting fundal mucosa diffusely and severely, for it then results in achlorhydria which predisposes to iron deficiency; moreover, secretion of intrinsic factor may be lost and this results in pernicious anaemia. There is also an association between chronic gastritis and gastric ulcer, and an increased incidence of gastric carcinoma.

As already explained, terminal and post-mortem digestion render the gastric mucosa unsuitable for detailed examination at necropsy. Safer techniques of performing gastric mucosal biopsy during gastroscopy, are, however, now providing valuable diagnostic material and contributing to elucidation of the natural history of chronic gastritis.

Diffuse chronic gastritis

In this form of gastritis, the changes may initially be focal, but in many cases they are progressive, and as the condition becomes more advanced, it extends to involve the whole of the **acid-secreting mucosa**. The mucosa of the antrum may show similar changes, but the occurrence of lesions in the two areas may be coincidental.

Pathological changes. Macroscopic examination of the gastric mucosa *in vivo* is of little value in diagnosing chronic gastritis. Microscopically, the condition may be divided into *superficial chronic gastritis*, *atrophic gastritis* of various degrees and *gastric atrophy*.

In *chronic superficial gastritis*, the necks of the gastric glands are increased in length, and the superficial lamina propria is infiltrated with lymphocytes and plasma cells, together with a few neutrophil and eosinophil polymorphs (Fig. 18.20b): the mucosa is of approximately normal thickness and the inflammatory changes are confined to its superficial part.

In *atrophic gastritis*, the inflammatory changes are similar to those of superficial chronic gastritis, but extend more deeply into the mucosa and are accompanied by various degrees of loss of the specialised (i.e. parietal and chief) cells of the mucosal glands. In its extreme degree, the changes affect the fundal mucosa diffusely and there is virtually complete loss of the specialised glandular cells (Fig. 18.20d). The glands appear fewer and their specialised cells are replaced by simple mucus-secreting epithelium similar to the surface mucosa (pseudo-pyloric metaplasia) or show intestinal metaplasia (see below). There is increase in the lamina propria, seen as widened areas of loose vascular connective tissue, heavily infiltrated with lymphocytes and plasma cells, between the glands. The mucosa is appreciably thinned and the rugae are not prominent. In less severe atrophic gastritis the changes are focal, affecting patches of mucosa in a part or the whole of its thickness, while the intervening areas of mucosa may show superficial gastritis, or may be normal.

In *gastric atrophy* the fundal mucosa is diffusely atrophic, with virtually complete replacement of parietal and chief cells by mucus-secreting glandular epithelium, and increase of loose vascular connective tissue in the lamina propria. The appearances resemble closely those of severe atrophic gastritis except for the much smaller numbers of lymphocytes and plasma cells in gastric atrophy.

A very common feature in both atrophic

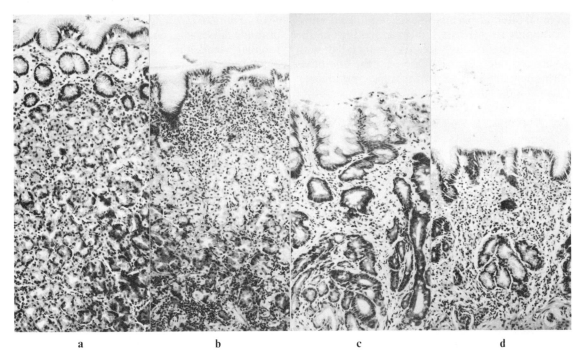

a   b   c   d

Fig. 18.20   Chronic gastritis of acid-secreting mucosa. All × 100. **a** Normal mucosa. **b** Superficial gastritis and atrophic gastritis affecting the deep part of the mucosa. **c** Complete loss of parietal and chief cells with intestinal metaplasia. **d** Complete atrophic gastritis. The remaining glands are of simple mucus-secreting type. In **b**, **c** and **d**, the full thickness of the mucosa is shown.

gastritis and gastric atrophy is *metaplasia* of the mucosal glands to resemble closely those of the intestine (Fig. 18.20c), with goblet cells, tall columnar cells bearing a brush border, and Paneth cells. The altered glands may show irregular cystic change, and there may also be abundant lymphoid nodules with germinal centres in the basal part of the mucosa and submucosa: the term 'follicular gastritis' has been applied when the lymphoid nodules are prominent, but they occur in variable numbers in the normal stomach.

Aetiology. The three types of chronic gastritis described above are merely different degrees of the same process. The destructive inflammatory changes begin superficially, and progress towards the base of the mucosa. At the stage of superficial chronic gastritis, the necks of the glands appear lengthened because there has been destruction of the specialised cells in the superficial part of the glands, and replacement by mucus-secreting cells of the type which normally line the surface and necks of the glands. As the change extends more deeply into the mucosa, the various grades of atrophic gastritis

are produced, and finally, when all or virtually all of the specialised cells have been destroyed, the inflammation subsides, leaving the appearances of gastric atrophy. This unitarian view is supported by the frequent finding of superficial chronic gastritis together with various degrees of atrophic gastritis in other areas of the same stomach, and of all grades of change between superficial chronic gastritis and gastric atrophy.

Diffuse chronic gastritis is widely regarded as one of the organ-specific auto-immune diseases: the evidence for this may be summarised as follows:

(1) *Auto-antibodies* are commonly present in the serum of patients with chronic gastritis, and their incidence increases with the extent of the gastric mucosal changes. Auto-antibody to a membrane lipoprotein of gastric parietal cells is detectable by immunofluorescence (Fig. 18.21) and by complement-fixation techniques: it is seldom present without chronic gastritis and reaches its highest incidence in patients with severe atrophic gastritis or gastric atrophy. The antibody is present in the serum of over 80% of patients in whom these severe grades of gastritis

have resulted in pernicious anaemia. Two auto-antibodies to intrinsic factor, a product of the gastric parietal cells, are also associated with severe chronic gastritis. One of these combines with the part of the intrinsic factor molecule which binds vitamin B_{12}, and the other with a

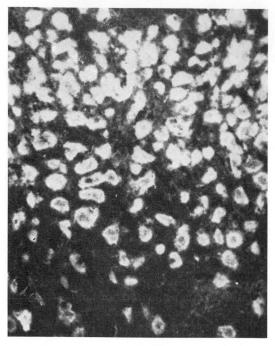

Fig. 18.21 Indirect immunofluorescence test for parietal-cell antibody. The parietal cells fluoresce brightly, indicating the presence of the antibody in the serum being tested.

site on the molecule distant from the B_{12}-binding site: they interfere respectively with binding of B_{12} by intrinsic factor, and with absorption of the complex from the ileum (p. 481). These latter antibodies are observed only occasionally apart from pernicious anaemia, in which their combined incidence is more than 50%.

(2) *Associated conditions.* The organ-specific auto-immune diseases tend to occur in association with one another (p. 133), and the common association of various grades of chronic thyroiditis and thyrotoxicosis with chronic gastritis supports the auto-immune nature of the latter. Moreover, the rarer members of the group— primary adrenocortical atrophy, and primary hypoparathyroidism—are frequently accompanied by chronic gastritis.

(3) *Familial tendency.* Like the other auto-immune diseases, chronic gastritis shows a familial tendency, and chronic thyroiditis commonly occurs in members of the same families.

(4) *Age and sex.* Like chronic thyroiditis, chronic gastritis occurs mostly in the middle-aged and elderly, and in women more often than men; the female sex preponderance is not, however, nearly so marked as in chronic thyroiditis or thyrotoxicosis.

(5) *Experimental chronic gastritis.* Attempts to induce chronic gastritis in animals by administering immunising injections of gastric mucosal preparations together with Freund's adjuvant have given equivocal results. Its induction has, however, been reported in monkeys, together with the development of cell-mediated immunity, and of antibodies, to gastric parietal cells.

The mechanism of the production of the changes in chronic gastritis has not been fully established. In general, auto-antibodies do not appear to play a major pathogenic role in the organ-specific auto-immune diseases, and it is more likely that a delayed hypersensitivity reaction against the specialised gastric glandular cells is largely responsible for the destructive changes, although the auto-antibodies might have a supplementary effect. Auto-antibodies to intrinsic factor also contribute towards the failure of absorption of B_{12} in pernicious anaemia. These antibodies have been demonstrated in the gastric juice of patients with this condition, and their presence there inhibits the function of any intrinsic factor produced by the atrophic mucosa.

Physiological disturbances. The degree to which the specialised gastric glands are lost or replaced in chronic gastritis correlates relatively well with the functional results observed clinically. Thus in superficial gastritis there is little functional upset; with progressing glandular atrophy varying degrees of hypochlorhydria develop, culminating eventually in complete achlorhydria as seen in severe atrophic gastritis. Even at this latter stage, some intrinsic factor is still secreted, and megaloblastic anaemia is not common. In the extreme gastric atrophy of pernicious anaemia, there is, however, absence of hydrochloric acid and pepsin, and near or complete absence of intrinsic factor, from the gastric juice.

Focal chronic gastritis

Chronic gastritis with the general features described above may occur focally in the fundal and antral mucosa, but often affecting especially the junctional zone between the two types of mucosa. While the aetiology is obscure, it seems likely that prolonged injury to the mucosa, e.g. by aspirin, alcohol, smoking and reflux of bile, results in increased desquamation of the surface epithelium and allows back diffusion of acid into the mucosa. Dyspeptic symptoms are common and acid secretion variable: the condition appears to predispose to gastric ulcer and possibly also to gastric carcinoma.

Peptic ulcer

Gastric ulcer

By far the most important type of ulceration found in the stomach is peptic ulceration, in which the action of gastric juice is primarily concerned. It is often referred to simply as gastric ulcer. Peptic ulceration is encountered, however, not only in the stomach but also in other parts of the alimentary tract exposed to gastric juice: it is especially common in the first part of the duodenum and is occasionally found in the lower part of the oesophagus. It is also seen in relation to heterotopic gastric mucosa, e.g. in a Meckel's diverticulum (p. 595) or at the umbilicus. Furthermore, in cases where gastrojejunostomy has been performed, peptic ulceration may take place in the part of the jejunal wall exposed to the action of gastric juice, especially when this is of high acidity. Apart from these circumstances, however, peptic ulceration distal to the duodenal bulb is rare.

Incidence. The incidence of the different types of peptic ulcer has changed considerably since the beginning of the century. Before that time the prevalent type was the acute perforating ulcer (Fig. 18.28) which was usually found in the anterior wall of the pylorus or duodenum and predominantly affected young women; it was frequently associated with a disease called 'chlorosis', a form of anaemia which has long since disappeared. After World War I gastric ulcer became much commoner in men and to a lesser extent in older women. At the present time, gastric ulcer is more common in men than in women at all ages up to 65, but thereafter the sex difference becomes less marked: on the other hand duodenal ulceration, which became more frequent at about the same time, is much commoner in men in all age groups and is between 4 and 10 times as common as gastric ulcer in the general population. Gastric ulcer was formerly considered to be a disease of the lower income groups, but it is doubtful if this is now the case, and duodenal ulcer had never shown any social differentiation. Both types of ulceration show a familial incidence.

Naked-eye appearances. Three main types of peptic ulcer are recognised, namely acute, subacute and chronic. Any such classification, however, is to some extent artificial since intermediate varieties occur.

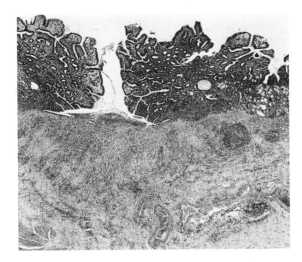

Fig. 18.22 A small acute peptic ulcer which has penetrated superficially into the submucosa. × 12.

(*a*) *Acute peptic ulcer.* This type involves only the mucosa and submucosa in the ulcerative process (Fig. 18.22); it is usually small, but may occasionally reach 1–2 cm diameter. The ulcers may be single, or may occur in large numbers and, unlike chronic ulcers, have a wide distribution. They rarely produce symptoms other than haemorrhage, which on occasion may be severe when a mucosal artery in the base of an acute ulcer is eroded (Fig. 18.29). This type of ulcer usually heals without a visible scar.

(*b*) *Subacute peptic ulcers* are usually fewer in number than the acute type, and not infrequently single. They extend down to the muscular coat, the superficial part of which may be involved; like chronic ulcers, they tend to be found on the lesser curvature of the stomach and they may represent a transition from the acute to the chronic type.

(*c*) *Chronic peptic ulcer*. Complete penetration of the muscular coat is regarded as the most important criterion of chronicity in a peptic ulcer (Figs. 18.25, 18.26). This type of ulcer is usually solitary; two apposed peptic ulcers are found in a small proportion of cases and there are practically never more than two in the stomach although there may be a duodenal ulcer as well. The commonest site in the stomach is the lesser curvature between 5 and 10 cm from the pylorus; the pyloric canal is the next most frequent site. Their occurrence in other sites is rare, and should make one look for some unusual cause.

Chronic ulcers are usually ovoid and larger than subacute or acute ones (Fig. 18.23), ranging from a few mm to several cm in diameter. The base of the ulcer may be formed by the outer part of the stomach wall, the floor being usually smooth and fibrous with induration of the surrounding tissues. More frequently, however, fibrous adhesions have developed over the ulcer and the base is firmly fixed to adjacent tissues; large ulcers often penetrate the gastric wall and erode into adjacent structures, usually the pancreas or liver. When this advanced stage has been reached, the ulcer margin is smooth with overhanging edges, the crater is deep and the floor is firm and nodular, being formed by a fibrosed layer of the eroded organ. Occasionally an ulcer may burrow into the large bowel, a gastro-colic fistula resulting. Perforation in the chronic type may be prevented by fibrous thickening and adhesions but, in about a third of cases, occurs obliquely through one margin of the ulcer beneath the overhanging edge and

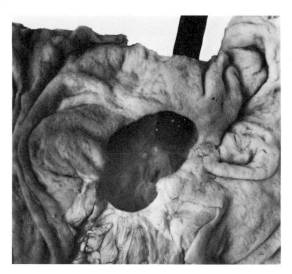

Fig. 18.24 Large chronic ulcer of duodenum just beyond the pylorus. The ulcer had perforated at the margin, as indicated by the pointer. × 0·8.

beyond the adhesions (Fig. 18.24). Erosion of a large artery in the floor of a chronic ulcer is not uncommon and may lead to fatal haemorrhage.

Duodenal ulcers

Peptic ulcers in the duodenum are similar to those in the stomach. The area affected by peptic ulceration is, however, remarkably restricted; over 99% of chronic ulcers arise within the first centimetre of the duodenum.

Acute ulcers may be single or multiple. They tend to be encountered in what might be

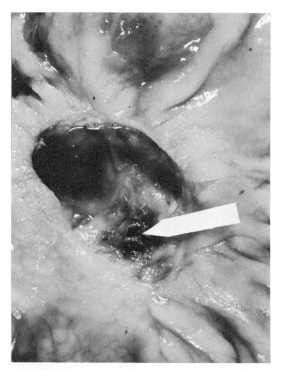

Fig. 18.23 A large chronic gastric ulcer, showing an eroded artery (*arrow*) from which fatal haemorrhage occurred. × 1·25.

regarded as 'stressful' situations. They are seen, for example, in patients with extensive burns, especially infants, and as a complication of lesions of the central nervous system or chronic debilitating disease both in adults and children.

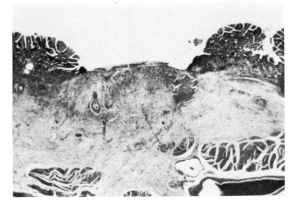

Fig. 18.25 Early chronic gastric ulcer, showing fibrous replacement of muscular coat. × 7.

Chronic ulcers may be as large as in the stomach (Fig. 18.24), especially those arising in the posterior wall of the duodenum. As a rule there is a single ulcer on the anterior or posterior wall, but in about 15% of cases two ulcers are present, and they may appose one another at a corresponding level ('kissing ulcers'). Severe haemorrhage usually occurs from ulcers on the posterior wall, which tend to erode the gastro-duodenal artery.

Microscopic appearances. The base of a peptic ulcer of the stomach or duodenum has a clean macroscopic appearance, presumably because of the digestive action of the gastric juice. Microscopically, the ulcer crater is lined by a thin layer of tissue showing the changes of fibrinoid necrosis, beneath which is a layer of granulation tissue showing some leukocytic infiltration. In chronic ulcers the muscle coat is interrupted and at either side of the ulcer merges into the fibrous tissue which forms the outer layer of ulcer lining and may extend for some distance beyond it. The muscle coat thus ends high up in the lateral walls of the crater (Fig. 18.26). In the floor, obliterative changes are frequently seen in the arteries. At the margin of the ulcer, the mucosal epithelium may show active regenerative changes; fragments of mucosa may also be 'buried' in fibrous tissue

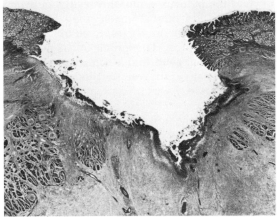

Fig. 18.26 Chronic gastric ulcer at later stage, showing breach of muscular coat. × 7.

during the ulcerative process, and give a false impression of malignant change (see p. 553).

Results and complications of peptic ulceration

(1) Healing and scarring. Acute peptic ulcers usually undergo healing and leave no visible scar. Healing is the rule also in the subacute type and it is common too in chronic ulcers, even when large, as is shown by the common necropsy finding of contracted stellate scars in the ulcer-prone sites. If the ulcer has been superficial, the scar may be merely a small depression with a smooth whitish surface; if, however, it has penetrated more deeply, there is often a radiating indrawing of the surrounding mucous membrane, so that a stellate appearance results (Fig. 18.27). Scarring of an ulcer at

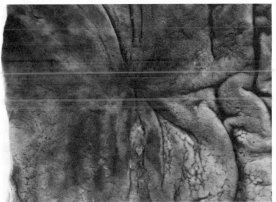

Fig. 18.27 Healed gastric ulcer with stellate scar. × 1.

or near the pylorus commonly results in **pyloric stenosis**, and the stomach may gradually become enlarged due to repeated retention of food and secretion. The muscle of the pylorus is apt to be thickened and oedematous, and the appearance may suggest scirrhous carcinoma; only microscopic examination can rule this out.

Stenosis of the adjacent duodenum or pyloric antrum by the scarring of chronic ulcers has similar effects, and ulcers higher up on the lesser curvature of the stomach may, by scarring and contraction, produce the deformity of '*hour glass*' stomach.

Since active peptic ulcers often cause spasm of the muscle coat, caution is necessary in the radiological diagnosis of fibrous stricture.

(2) Perforation. Perforation may occur, and, if rapid, it allows the stomach contents to escape into the general peritoneal cavity or, posteriorly, into the lesser sac. The pain, abdominal rigidity and symptoms of collapse which follow are caused by the acid gastric contents; these are virtually sterile at first, but without prompt surgical treatment, organisms soon flourish and **acute peritonitis** results. Air from the stomach comes to lie between the liver and diaphragm where it may cause loss of liver dullness to percussion and is visible radiologically. After successful surgical treatment of the perforation, there is a risk that infected material lodged between the liver and diaphragm may become sealed off by fibrinous exudate and cause a **sub-phrenic abscess** which may later infect the pleura. In other cases infection of the peritoneum may occur without actual perforation, and thus the peritoneal surface may be glued to adjacent parts by fibrinous exudate. This is more likely to happen posteriorly and in the region of the lesser curvature, where the movements of the stomach are less than in other parts. The inflammation may produce localised fibrous adhesions or rarely localised suppuration may result. Very rarely, bacterial invasion of a portal tributary may occur and secondary abscesses be produced in the liver (p. 632). The so-called **acute perforating ulcer**, formerly common but not often seen now, is usually single and situated in the anterior wall of the pylorus or duodenum. It is of 1·5 cm diameter or less, round or ovoid with a punched-out appearance and a terraced margin (Fig. 18.28), the mucosa being ulcerated

over a greater area than the muscle layer. Although any perforating peptic ulcer is, by definition, chronic (*v.s.*), the 'acute perforating' variety appears to penetrate the wall very rapidly.

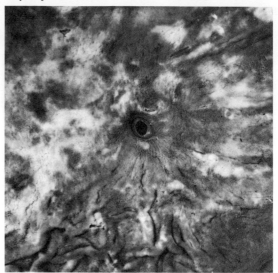

Fig. 18.28 Acute perforating ulcer. × 1.

(3) Haemorrhage. This is common and varies greatly in degree. Often there is oozing of blood from an acute or a chronic ulcer. The blood may be scanty and detectable in the stools only by chemical examination, or it may be abundant and give rise to 'coffee-grounds' vomit, or to 'tarry' stools. Sometimes a major artery may be eroded and a large, even fatal, haemorrhage take place. This may occur from a recent acute ulcer (Fig. 18.29) but is seen chiefly in large chronic ulcers which involve an artery lying outside the wall of the stomach, e.g. the left gastric artery. The artery becomes incorporated in the floor of the ulcer, and is in most cases obliterated by endarteritis (Fig. 13.2, p. 311), but sometimes this does not happen, and the wall of the vessel, weakened by the digestive process, ruptures. Occasionally a small aneurysm forms first. Usually, however, the artery is eroded rather than severed and its wall is so firmly incorporated in the scar tissue that contraction and retraction of the vessel cannot take place, so that bleeding is profuse and ceases only when the blood pressure has fallen and thrombus has formed at the site of erosion. For these reasons, resuscitation by transfusion should be attempted with due care

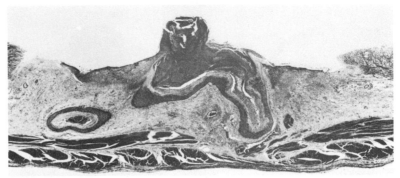

Fig. 18.29 Superficial acute ulcer of stomach which has eroded an artery and caused fatal haemorrhage. × 10.

not to raise the blood pressure too rapidly lest further bleeding be encouraged. Severe haemorrhage from duodenal ulcer is commonest when the ulcer is in the posterior wall. In a case of fatal haemorrhage one can usually find the eroded artery in the floor of the ulcer, its mouth partially occluded by thrombus.

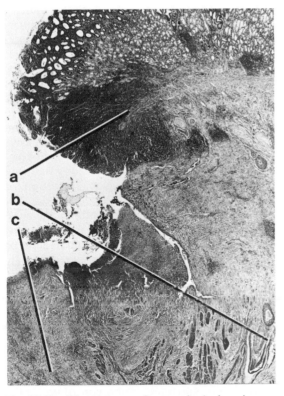

Fig. 18.30 Ulcer-cancer of stomach. A chronic peptic ulcer showing the characteristic complete breach of the muscle coat. A focus of early carcinoma was detected microscopically at **a** in the overhanging margin of the ulcer crater: **b** muscle coat: **c** fibrous base of ulcer.

(4) Development of carcinoma: ulcer-cancer. Although it cannot be doubted that carcinoma may arise in a chronic gastric ulcer, the frequency of this event has probably been overestimated in the past. One reason for this lies in the difficulty in distinguishing between a chronic peptic ulcer which has undergone malignant change and a carcinoma which has ulcerated. In the former case, it is necessary to demonstrate clear evidence of pre-existing chronic peptic ulceration, i.e. complete interruption of the muscular coat (Fig. 18.30).

The cancer begins at one margin of the ulcer crater (Figs. 18.30, 18.31) and tends to encircle it, spreading outwards into the submucosa and muscular coat, but not invading the fibrous ulcer floor to any extent. By contrast, a primary carcinoma often invades the muscular coat but practically never destroys it entirely and even in advanced cases remains of muscle are to be found between cancer cells. Another important point is that irregular growth and displacement of epithelium at the margin of a peptic ulcer may give a false impression of malignant change.

Taking these factors into consideration, it is unlikely that cancer develops in more than 1% of chronic gastric ulcers, although it is probable that there is an increased tendency for carcinoma to develop in a stomach bearing a chronic peptic ulcer. Carcinomatous change does not arise in chronic duodenal ulcers.

Aetiology of peptic ulcers

Although it is convenient to discuss the causes of peptic ulceration in general, chronic gastric and duodenal ulcers differ in many respects, including age and sex distribution, occupational incidence and familial tendency; their causes may therefore differ. It may also be necessary

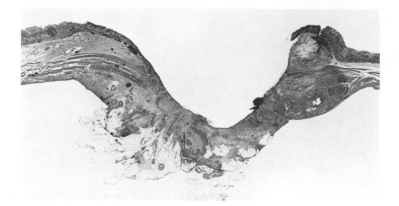

Fig. 18.31 Ulcer-cancer of stomach. Carcinoma has arisen in the margin of the ulcer on the right, which now has become raised up above the level of the mucosa. × 2.

to distinguish between acute and chronic ulcers in this respect. In any case, no single factor is clearly responsible and causation is complex.

The possible importance of genetic factors in the pathogenesis is reflected in the familial incidence (p. 549), and in the relationship between duodenal ulcer and individuals who do not secrete blood-group substances into the gastric juice and belong to blood group O. Environmental factors, however, must be responsible for the varying incidence of peptic ulcer during this century and for 'epidemics' of the disease which may be localised or affect certain age groups in the community. Geographical variations in incidence also emphasise the importance of environment. Peptic ulcer is essentially a disease of developed, industrialised communities. Factors such as dietary habits, the ingestion of drugs (especially aspirin) and occupational or social 'stresses' may be important. Cigarette smoking is also a contributory factor, especially in gastric ulcer, and may account for the association between peptic ulcer and chronic bronchitis.

It seems necessary to explain firstly the development of a mucosal lesion, and secondly why it does not heal like a wound made in a normal stomach. Local ischaemia due to thrombosis, embolus or vascular spasm has been postulated as a cause of the initial injury, but lacks supporting evidence.

The only entirely consistent finding associated with peptic ulceration is the presence of gastric acid, which is undoubtedly responsible for the special features of this disease. Peptic ulcer does not develop in patients with histamine-fast achlorhydria and is caused by interference with the capacity of the gastro-intestinal mucosa to resist digestion by gastric acid, due either to impaired mucosal resistance or to hypersecretion of gastric juice, or possibly both. The nature of the mucosal defence mechanism is complex and depends among other things upon the secretion of mucus, the maintenance of normal epithelial cell turnover rates and the presence of inhibitors of gastric secretion. Interference with these factors appears to be of particular importance in the pathogenesis of **gastric ulcer**. In this disease, gastric secretion may be normal but is often reduced due to the presence of chronic gastritis. Indeed there is some evidence to suggest that gastric ulcers tend to develop during certain phases in the evolution of chronic gastritis, which impairs the defensive capacity of the mucosa. Aspirin, smoking, 'stress', etc., may exert their effects by reducing mucosal resistance, increasing acid secretion, or both.

By contrast, gastric hypersecretion appears to be of major significance in the pathogenesis of **duodenal ulcer**, and there is a tendency for affected individuals to have an increased parietal-cell mass. The cause of this hypersecretion, which is often nocturnal, is not entirely clear. It is probably mediated by vagal stimulation, and without doubt emotional stress can aggravate peptic ulcer symptoms. Furthermore, acute peptic ulcer sometimes complicates lesions of the central nervous system.

Although the extent to which humoral stimulants of gastric secretion contribute to the pathogenesis of peptic ulcer in general is uncertain, there is no doubt that the circulation of such substances in excessive quantities is capable of invoking a fulminating ulcer diathesis. Such a situation is observed in the Zollinger–

Ellison syndrome (p. 968) the central feature of which is the development of single or multiple pancreatic islet-cell tumours which secrete gastrin, a polypeptide and potent stimulant of gastric secretion. These pancreatic tumours may be associated with tumours of other endocrine glands such as the parathyroids, pituitary, adrenals, etc. (the multiple endocrine adenoma syndrome) and it has been suggested that this represents a widespread disturbance of polypeptide hormone synthesis. In these syndromes, peptic ulceration takes place not only in the common sites but also in unusual areas, e.g. the greater curvature of the stomach and distal duodenum. There is evidence that a raised level of blood calcium promotes an increase in gastric secretion, and this may account for the high incidence of peptic ulceration in patients with hyperparathyroidism.

Dilatation of the stomach

This occurs in two forms, one due to obstruction and the other without obstruction. The first results from either scarring due to gastric or duodenal ulcer, carcinoma at the pylorus or occasionally from fibrous adhesions outside the stomach at the pyloric region. A degree of congenital stenosis of the pylorus (p. 559) may produce a similar result. In these conditions, dilatation is associated with hypertrophy of the gastric musculature which, owing to the dilatation, often appears less than it actually is.

In the second form inflammatory change, atony of the muscle and fermentative changes may be concerned, and any one of these may lead to the others; thus deficiency of gastric juice due to gastritis may lead to abnormal retention of food in the stomach allowing fermentation to take place, and atony of the muscle will have a similar result. Atonic dilatation, which may be a chronic condition, occurs after acute fevers and may also be associated with neurasthenia or hysteria: the stomach may reach an enormous size and become displaced downwards in the abdominal cavity—*gastroptosis*. The duodenum may become kinked and share in this atonic, dilated state.

A well-recognised form—*acute dilatation of the stomach*—occasionally occurs after abdominal operations; in the absence of sepsis, excessive handling or trauma is probably the cause (c.f. paralytic ileus, p. 585). It may also be a feature of diabetic coma and may be relieved by intubation. In chronic dilatation, the contents of the stomach may show an abundant growth of yeasts, sarcinae, hyphomycetes, etc., leading to fermentation, with the formation of lactic and butyric acids and considerable evolution of gas. There is little growth of bacteria unless there is marked reduction or absence of hydrochloric acid such as is common in cases of carcinoma.

Tumours

Benign tumours

Epithelial benign tumours are rare. Mucosal polyps occur, but are usually chronic inflammatory lesions, not true neoplasms. The commonest benign tumour is the *leiomyoma*, which is sometimes multiple: it arises from the muscular layer and projects into the lumen. Although usually small, it may show a characteristic type of clean punched-out ulceration and can produce very brisk bleeding. Some well-differentiated 'leiomyomas' invade locally and even metastasise: it is therefore important to ensure that excision is complete. Lipoma, fibroma and neurofibroma associated with generalised neurofibromatosis, and a glomus tumour (p. 298) may also occur.

Gastric carcinoma

Carcinoma is by far the most important tumour in the stomach, both numerically and clinically, and is also one of the commoner internal malignant tumours in man. There is considerable geographical variation in its incidence, which has shown a slight fall in this country in recent years. It still, however, remains the commonest internal carcinoma in many countries, with a particularly high incidence in Iceland, Finland and Japan. Men are affected more often than women in the ratio of 2 : 1, and the disease is commoner in the poorer economic groups. The maximum incidence is between 50 and 70 years of age. The five-year survival rate is of the order of 10%.

Aetiology. No specific cause for the development of carcinoma has been identified but certain predisposing factors are recognised. Some families have an unusually high incidence of gastric cancer and **genetic influences** may be involved in a proportion of cases, perhaps indirectly, as in the association with pernicious anaemia. It has been established that, in caucasians, blood group A is associated with a significantly higher incidence of gastric cancer than other blood groups, in contrast to the reputed high incidence of peptic ulcer in those of group O. It is also likely, from the variations in the incidence of gastric cancer between communities, that **environmental factors**, such as the diet and methods of cooking, are important. Specific dietary factors have not been incriminated, but the repeated heating of fats to temperatures used in cooking can lead to the formation of potent carcinogenic or co-carcinogenic agents. The constituents of the soil and the extent of background radiation have been investigated to explain geographical variations in incidence but nothing substantial has emerged; the presence of chromium in soil has been suggested as of possible importance.

Precancerous lesions. Of *local gastric factors*, the importance of *gastric ulcer* has already been discussed (p. 553). There remains the possible relationship of *chronic gastritis* to carcinoma. Certainly the two lesions co-exist in a high percentage of cases and there is a notable degradation of cell type and replacement of the superficial mucosa by cells of intestinal type, especially in the pyloric antrum. The aetiological relationship remains unsettled, but the incidence of gastric carcinoma in patients with pernicious anaemia, adequately maintained on vitamin B_{12}, is about three times that in the general population in a comparable age group.

Macroscopic appearances. The pylorus and the pyloric antrum are the most common sites of carcinoma (85%) which thus differs in distribution from gastric ulcer. Also, carcinoma occurs in any part of the stomach while 94% of gastric ulcers are restricted to the vicinity of the lesser curvature.

Five main types of gastric carcinoma are recognised.

Fungating carcinoma not infrequently arises in the fundus of the stomach and growth is directed mainly towards the lumen to form large friable masses which readily undergo necrosis and ulceration. The gastric wall, is, however, eventually penetrated and spread to adjacent structures takes place.

Scirrhous carcinoma is commonest in the

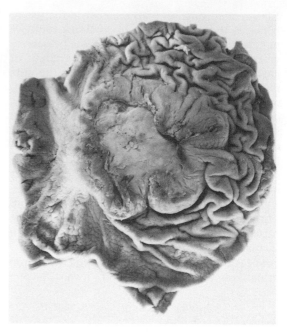

Fig. 18.32 Scirrhous carcinoma of stomach, with thickened, raised margin and ulcerated base.

pyloric region, and is characterised by deep infiltration of the gastric wall with marked induration but without obvious protrusion into the lumen. Ulceration is frequent (Fig. 18.32), but does not completely penetrate the muscular layer as occurs in a chronic peptic ulcer. Confusion between the two may, however, occasionally arise. The surrounding muscle is often thickened and hypertrophied and the

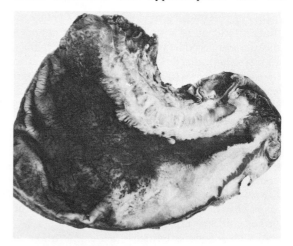

Fig. 18.33 Mucoid carcinoma at pylorus, showing great infiltration and thickening of the wall (anterior part of stomach viewed from behind). × 0·5.

growth frequently encircles the pylorus, causing stenosis. Extension into the duodenal mucosa is very rare.

Mucoid cancer, like the scirrhous type, usually arises in the pyloric region and is characterised by a diffuse mode of spread in the wall of the stomach, which is markedly thickened (Fig. 18.33) and, because of accumulation of mucin, has a translucent appearance. This type of cancer also tends to invade, and grow extensively in, the peritoneal cavity, embedding the abdominal viscera in masses of translucent, gelatinous material.

A less common fourth type is recognised,

duodenal muscle coat is not unusual. The duodenal mucosa is rarely invaded, whereas the oesophageal mucosa is often involved by tumours of the fundus or cardia. The gastric serosa is penetrated early, with direct extension to surrounding structures such as the greater omentum, lesser omentum, liver, pancreas, spleen, diaphragm and abdominal wall. Invasion of the peritoneum may lead to *transcoelomic spread*. Numerous minute nodules may be scattered throughout the peritoneal cavity and the greater omentum may come to form a hard, palpable contracted mass. Peritoneal spread may also be detectable by rectal

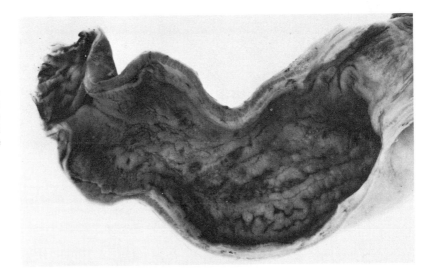

Fig. 18.34 Diffuse carcinoma of stomach. Note the general thickening of the wall without a localised tumour mass and with little ulceration. × 0·7.

namely *diffuse scirrhous carcinoma* (Fig. 18.34). It appears to arise deep in the mucosa and diffuse infiltration of the gastric wall takes place, often without apparent involvement of the mucosal surface. The wall of the stomach is commonly grossly thickened and stiffened (*leather-bottle stomach* or *linitis plastica*), and extension into the oesophagus proximally is not unusual; more rarely some spread into the duodenum distally may occur.

Superficial spreading carcinoma, which involves only the mucosa and submucosa, is recognised by American authors, particularly in relation to peptic ulcer, but is not well documented in this country.

Spread of gastric carcinoma. Local spread is usually prominent. The muscularis is infiltrated most extensively in the scirrhous and diffuse types and involvement of the oesophageal and

examination. The ovaries are not infrequently involved via the peritoneum. If the tumour is of the 'signet-ring' cell type with prominent connective tissue reaction, bilateral ovarian metastases are referred to as 'Krukenberg tumours' (p. 916).

Lymphatic spread is early and frequent. From the primary focus in the mucosa, the growth spreads to the wide network of submucosal lymphatics (Fig. 18.35) and through the muscularis to the serosal lymphatics and thence to the para-gastric lymph nodes which are usually the first to be involved. Extension may take place into the mucosa from the submucosal lymphatics to form numerous nodules, giving a false impression of multifocal origin. Lymphatic spread is often extensive, especially in *diffuse scirrhous cancer*, involving lymphatics in the omentum, mesentery and wall of the intestine; it may take the form of diffuse

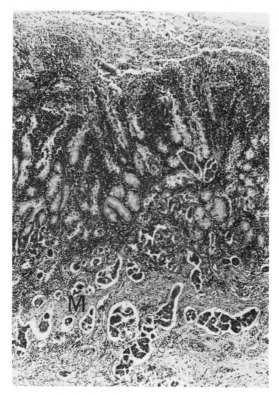

Fig. 18.35 Stomach wall, showing infiltration of lymphatics by carcinoma cells, which, in places, are growing upwards through the muscularis mucosae (*M*) into the mucosa. Note the severe chronic gastritis. × 30.

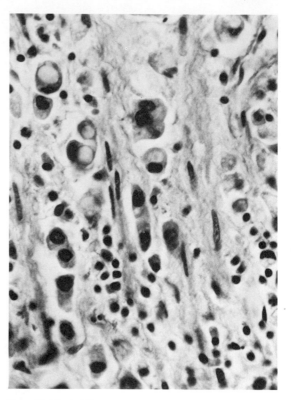

Fig. 18.36 Diffuse type of carcinoma in muscular coat of stomach. The cells are irregularly scattered, some containing mucous globules and others showing atrophic change. × 600.

permeation without formation of tumour nodules. Lymph node metastases are usual in the upper abdomen, and more distant nodes may also be involved.

Spread occurs by the portal venous blood usually resulting in early metastasis to the liver, and eventually to the lungs, and various other organs, including the brain and bones, may be involved. Blood spread is less common in mucoid cancer, and is unusual in the diffuse scirrhous type, although in the latter the liver is sometimes involved by lymphatic permeation.

Microscopic appearances. In most cases the growth is an **adenocarcinoma** with more or less differentiation towards an acinar structure. Some, however, are composed of solid masses of anaplastic cells. Mixed patterns are observed in both scirrhous and fungating tumours. In the mucoid type, the cells are bathed in extracellular mucin. In the diffuse scirrhous type the cells often occur singly or in small groups throughout the thickness of the gastric wall: they may be small and difficult to recognise, but some of them have the characteristic '*signet-ring*' appearance (Fig. 18.36) in which the droplets of mucin confirm their identification as cancer cells.

Associated conditions. Achlorhydria or hypochlorhydria is usual in gastric carcinoma, and in many cases is due to the chronic gastritis which precedes or accompanies the tumour. When carcinoma has developed secondarily to chronic gastric ulcer, hydrochloric acid is likely to be present but may be reduced in amount.

The absence of hydrochloric acid, aided by stasis due to pyloric obstruction and infection of necrotic tumour tissue, leads to the growth of micro-organisms of various kinds—torulae, sarcinae, lactobacilli, etc. Bacteria are rarely profuse unless there is complete achlorhydria. The presence of lactic acid produced by micro-organisms in the stomach is suggestive, although not diagnostic, of gastric cancer.

Secondary bacterial infection of the ulcerating tumour may account, in part, for the *cachexia* and *anaemia* observed clinically in gastric cancer. Anaemia may be either microcytic or normocytic; in the former, blood loss is partly responsible. Macrocytic anaemia is rare, and due to atrophic gastritis, i.e. pernicious anaemia.

Cancer of the stomach is sometimes accompanied, or even preceded, by the appearance in the skin of multiple warty hyperkeratotic patches, especially about the folds or flexures. This has been named *acanthosis nigricans*. It is seen more commonly in relation to carcinoma of the gastro-intestinal tract than elsewhere.

Although examination of exfoliated gastric mucosal cells has proved disappointing in the diagnosis of early gastric cancer, cytological examination of mucosal brushings obtained during endoscopy is more promising.

Other malignant tumours of the stomach

Various types of sarcoma may arise in the stomach, but these constitute less than 5% of malignant neoplasms of the stomach.

Leiomyosarcoma (p. 296) is perhaps the commonest of these. It tends to be more localised than carcinoma and usually takes the form of a fungating large mass projecting into the lumen. Ulceration and necrosis are common.

Malignant lymphoma may develop as a localised mass or a more diffuse infiltrative growth, causing enormous thickening of the whole gastric wall. When it is localised to the stomach, the prognosis after surgery is better than for carcinoma.

Congenital abnormalities

The most important of these is **stenosis of the pylorus**. It is not uncommon, symptoms appearing usually about two to three weeks after birth, and by obstruction and persistent vomiting may lead to death. The condition is often satisfactorily treated by operation. The obstruction is due to thickening of the wall at the pylorus, and this may extend back over a considerable distance, gradually fading off; or it

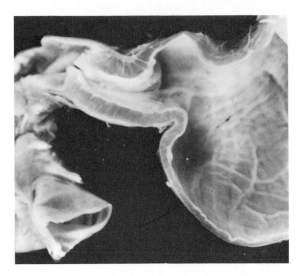

Fig. 18.37 Congenital stenosis of pylorus. The anterior wall at the pylorus has been cut away to show the greatly hypertrophied muscle at the pyloric antrum. × 1·2.

may be more localised and in the form of a definite band (Fig. 18.37). The thickening is essentially due to hypertrophy of the muscle, the circular fibres especially being increased, whilst the lumen is narrowed to a varying, sometimes marked, degree. It is usually regarded as a hypertrophy produced by spasmodic contraction at the pylorus, but the nature of the exciting agent or neuromuscular abnormality is not known. Investigations on the incidence among families and in the twins of affected infants has led to the suggestion that there is a genetic predisposition, and it has been claimed to be due to a Mendelian recessive gene. Against this, however, the incidence in affected families is less than the expected 1 in 4, the condition is about six times commoner in male than in female infants, and is reported to be disproportionately common in firstborn infants. Relief of the obstruction by incision of the hypertrophied muscle is usually necessary. Occasionally some degree of congenital pyloric stenosis may persist into adult life, and if symptoms are produced the condition is liable to be confused with carcinoma.

Diverticula occur in connection with the stomach, either in the pyloric portion or in the region of the fundus, but they are rare. Occasionally the stomach is somewhat narrowed about the middle, a certain degree of so-called 'hour-glass' contraction being produced. Such a condition, however, occurs more frequently as the result of cicatrisation from an old gastric ulcer (p. 552). Persistent vomiting and failure of a neonate to thrive may also be due to congenital deficiency in the enzymes necessary for the metabolism of the sugars—galactose, lactose or sucrose—and these rare conditions may be mistaken for congenital pyloric stenosis.

IV The Intestines

Introduction

The pathology of the intestine is influenced considerably by the normal presence of bacteria in its lumen: lesions of the intestinal wall, whether due to ischaemia, neoplasia or of unknown cause, e.g. Crohn's disease and ulcerative colitis, are prone to undergo secondary bacterial infection, with the usual forms of inflammatory response. In addition, various pathogenic bacteria and parasites find a suitable environment in the intestine, and infection is much more important than in the stomach. Extensive mucosal lesions, particularly in the small intestine, can result in malabsorption syndromes, and a large number of conditions can cause intestinal obstruction. Finally, carcinoma is very common in the colon and rectum, but rare in the small intestine.

Although the small and large intestines each have their own specific diseases, these are relatively few, and most pathological processes affect them both similarly. For that reason the intestine is considered as a whole in most of the account which follows.

Inflammatory conditions

The pH of the intestinal contents and their high nutritional value provide conditions favourable to the growth of many kinds of bacteria. Not surprisingly, therefore, bacterial infection is the commonest cause of inflammation in the intestinal tract; although viral infection is probably more common than is generally realised, and bacterial toxins, e.g. staphylococcal enterotoxin, chemical agents, e.g. arsenic, and physical agents, e.g. ionising radiation, may also be responsible for inflammatory changes. As indicated above, damage to the intestine of whatever cause is likely to be exploited by the resident bacterial flora, and this must be taken into account in the histological interpretation of inflammatory lesions; thus conditions which are not primarily of an inflammatory origin, e.g. ischaemic lesions, may be confused both grossly and histologically with inflammatory disorders.

As in other organs, inflammatory states in the intestinal tract may be acute or chronic, and vary greatly in severity from a simple 'catarrh' at one end of the spectrum to severe necrotising and ulcerative lesions at the other. Some intestinal infections are known to be caused specifically by particular species of micro-organisms: others can be due to various bacteria or are, as yet, of unknown cause.

Ischaemia and inflammation

In most instances, ischaemic damage is due to partial or complete occlusion of the major mesenteric arteries. Complete occlusion usually leads to haemorrhagic infarction and gangrene of variable extent limited to the areas supplied by the artery involved (Fig. 18.64, p. 585). Narrowing of the mesenteric arteries, usually resulting from degenerative vascular disease in elderly individuals, does not, as a rule, produce pathological change unless there are also hypotensive episodes, e.g. in cardiac failure, which aggravate the intestinal ischaemia. The effects depend upon the duration of the ischaemic episode and vary from full thickness necrosis with subsequent gangrene to slight mucosal damage which heals completely. Occasionally more extensive mucosal and submucosal necrosis takes place and subsequent healing leads to fibrous thickening of the bowel wall, sometimes with stricture formation. In addition, bacterial infection of the damaged mucosa produces inflammatory change so that the ischaemic lesion resembles inflammatory bowel disease, although its true origin may be revealed by the presence in the bowel wall of haemosiderin-laden macrophages indicating sites of previous haemorrhage. The term 'ischaemic colitis' has been applied to such lesions which occur especially in the watershed zone between the areas supplied by the superior and inferior mesenteric arteries, i.e. in the vicinity of the splenic flexure of the colon.

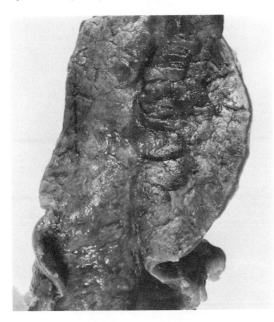

Fig. 18.38 Ischaemic colitis in an elderly woman. The lesion was multifocal in the transverse and descending colon. The area illustrated shows pseudomembranous inflammation, but there were older lesions with submucosal fibrosis and narrowing. Although ischaemic, the exact causation of such lesions is not clear (*see text*).

There is also a group of ischaemic intestinal lesions in which major vascular obstruction does not appear to be implicated since the pathological changes tend to be patchy and can involve both the small and large intestine in apparently, random fashion. Such lesions, which are sometimes extensive, develop in various clinical circumstances, including states of shock following surgical operations or myocardial infarction, uraemia and cardiac failure. The clinical picture is that of severe circulatory collapse associated with abdominal pain, diarrhoea and blood loss per rectum: the condition is usually fatal. The generic term **ischaemic enterocolitis** has been given to this group. In its most severe form, usually known as **acute necrotising enterocolitis** the intestinal mucosa shows extensive haemorrhage and necrosis (Fig. 18.38), which may involve the entire thickness of the bowel wall. In less severe cases, necrosis is limited to the superficial mucosa, which is incorporated into a fibrinopurulent surface exudate, hence the term **pseudomembranous enterocolitis**. Fibrin thrombi have been demonstrated in the mucosal blood vessels in the various forms of the disease, and disseminated intravascular coagulation (p. 227) may be involved in its pathogenesis. In some cases pathogenic bacteria such as *Staphylococcus aureus* and *Clostridium welchii* can be detected in the intestinal lesions, but this is probably due to secondary infection of ischaemic tissue. This does not necessarily mean that these organisms are incapable of producing intestinal inflammation *de novo*: prophylactic antibiotic therapy prior to surgical operations can predispose to both primary and secondary 'superinfections' of the intestinal tract. Moreover *Cl. welchii* is thought to have been responsible for some fortunately uncommon forms of necrotising enterocolitis, such as the epidemic disease 'darmbrand' described by German workers, a condition observed in primitive tribes in New Guinea ('pig-bel') due to the ingestion of infected porcine offal, and the fatal condition 'necrotising jejunitis' reported in East African children.

Pseudomembranous forms of enterocolitis can arise from other causes, e.g. in bacillary dysentery (p. 576), the stercoral ulceration complicating intestinal obstruction (p. 585) and mercuric chloride poisoning. Recently it has been shown that administration of certain antibiotics, e.g. lincomycin and clindamycin, can produce a pseudomembranous colitis which is sometimes fatal. The cause of this is unknown; it is not apparently a bacterial superinfection, and a viral aetiology has been suggested.

Conditions of uncertain aetiology

Gastro-enteritis of infancy

This infection, which can become epidemic in nurseries, carries a high mortality, usually attributable to fluid and electrolyte depletion resulting from diarrhoea and vomiting, in infants under two years of age. Despite this, the pathological changes are seldom impressive, although intestinal mucosal biopsies have shown epithelial damage associated with some increased leukocytic infiltration in the lamina propria and moderate degrees of villous atrophy (p. 581). Indeed, villous atrophy may persist for some weeks after the acute episode and produce transient malabsorption. In fatal cases the liver often shows marked fatty change. The pathogenesis is sometimes uncertain but some serological types of *Escherichia coli* (for example 0111, 055 and 0119) are commonly blamed. Recently, virus particles have been demonstrated by electron microscopy, both in duodenal biopsies and in the faeces, in a substantial proportion of cases in which pathogenic bacteria have not been isolated. The identity of these viruses is uncertain but they resemble reoviruses, and have been christened **rotaviruses** in view of the 'cart wheel' morphology of the particles.

Crohn's disease (regional enteritis)

Although this is a relatively uncommon condition it is becoming increasingly recognised as a cause of both small bowel and colonic lesions. Most commonly, however, the terminal part of the ileum is primarily involved.

Clinical features. Young adults of both sexes are most commonly affected, and there is some evidence of familial incidence, although this is not striking. The symptoms are ill-defined at first, mild diarrhoea and vague abdominal pain being the usual complaints. Later, signs of subacute or chronic intestinal obstruction develop and necessitate operative intervention. The disease runs a prolonged course, with long remissions, and recurrence after operation occurs in about 50% of cases. Serious consequences can

result from repeated and extensive involvement of the small intestine.

Naked-eye appearances. The changes are most often observed in the distal ileum, which is usually involved for a distance of 12 to 20 cm from the ileo-caecal valve. 'Skip lesions' separated from the main lesion by apparently healthy bowel are sometimes found, and distal extension into the caecum and ascending colon is common. The colon may also be involved

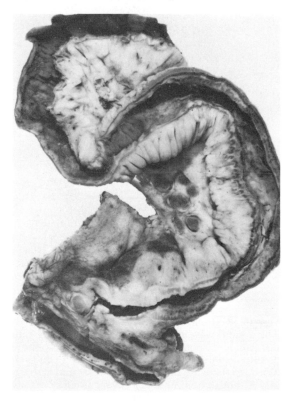

Fig. 18.39 Crohn's disease, showing diffuse thickening of the wall of the lower part of the ileum, with narrowing of its lumen.

primarily, especially in the older age groups, and it is probable that many cases of segmental or right-sided forms of colitis, previously classified as cases of ulcerative colitis (p. 564), are examples of Crohn's disease. The lesion is characterised by intense oedematous thickening of the bowel wall, the submucosa being especially involved, and there is marked narrowing of the lumen (Fig. 18.39). Ulceration of the oedematous mucosa is invariable and often assumes a linear form to produce the typical 'cobblestone' appearance (Fig. 18.40). Fistulae

which resemble closely those of sarcoidosis: they may occur in all the layers of the bowel wall and even in the mesentery and mesenteric lymph nodes. Sometimes they arise in relation to lymphoid aggregates, but more often they are found in and around lymphatic channels (Fig. 18.41). It is notable, however, that lymphatic obstruction and dilatation are almost invariably found in early cases, and lymphatic

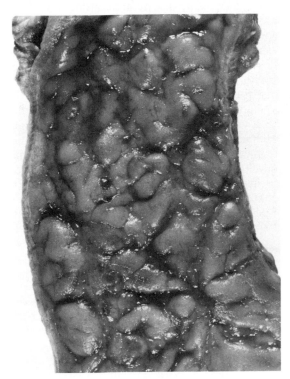

Fig. 18.40 The ileum in Crohn's disease, showing the 'cobblestone' appearance of the fissured, oedematous mucosa.

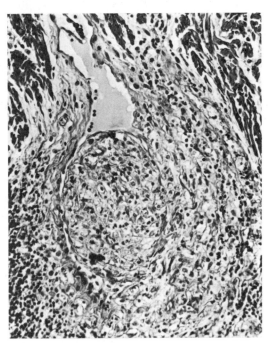

Fig. 18.41 Crohn's disease, showing a granulomatous lesion occluding a lymphatic in the muscle coat of the ileum. × 200.

penetrating the entire thickness of the bowel wall, and sometimes involving adjacent organs, are characteristic. The mesentery is usually thickened and oedematous and the regional lymph nodes conspicuously enlarged.

Microscopic appearances. It is characteristic of Crohn's disease that the inflammatory changes, although non-specific, extend throughout the entire thickness of the bowel wall and are thus described as being transmural (c.f. ulcerative colitis, p. 565). The most constant change is focal lymphocytic infiltration, usually most prominent in the submucosa. Of greater diagnostic value, however, is the presence, in about 60% of cases, of epithelioid-cell granulomas

obstruction is thought to be of primary importance in the pathogenesis of the disease. Certainly this accounts for the marked oedema which is always most conspicuous in the submucosa (Fig. 18.42) and is mainly responsible for the thickening of the bowel wall and mesentery in the early stages of the disease. Fibrotic changes, however, become increasingly prominent in more chronic cases. The mucosal changes, such as ulceration and subsequent metaplasia to pyloric type glands, are mainly due to secondary infection of the lesions, although the epithelioid-cell follicles are occasionally found in the lamina propria, particularly in the colon. A further change of diagnostic value is the presence of fissures which arise from ulcer bases and may penetrate the whole thickness of the bowel wall. Microscopically, they are lined by granulation tissue with foci of suppuration due to secondary bacterial infection.

Aetiology. There is no convincing evidence that Crohn's disease is related to sarcoidosis (p. 182), which rarely affects the intestinal tract. It is of interest, however, that as in sarcoidosis, abnormalities of cell-mediated immunity have been reported and in some instances the disease has been found to respond to the therapeutic use

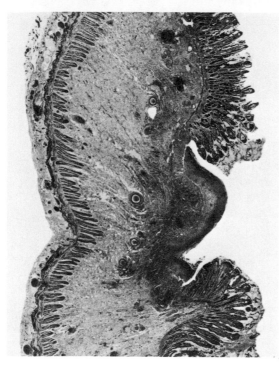

Fig. 18.42 Crohn's disease showing oedematous thickening, especially of the submucosa, with focal inflammatory infiltration and ulceration. × 12:

of immunosuppressive drugs such as azathioprine. Recently it has been demonstrated that intestinal lesions in Crohn's disease contain an infective agent which can be transmitted to experimental animals, although there is a long incubation period before lesions appear and the results are as yet unconfirmed (Mitchell and Rees, 1970; Cave, Mitchell and Brook, 1973). Nevertheless there is a possibility that Crohn's disease is caused by exposure of susceptible individuals to a particular type of microorganism, possibly a virus, and that suscepti-

bility is determined by some immunological peculiarity.

Complications. Intestinal obstruction, initially due to oedema and later to fibrosis of the bowel wall, may ultimately necessitate operative treatment, but the risks of fistula formation in relation to the surgical wound and of recurrence of the disease are considerable. Perianal fistulae are not uncommon, and are sometimes an early feature of the disease, especially the colonic form, and it is of diagnostic importance that the granulomas may be found in these lesions. Hypochromic anaemia due to blood loss is common, and occasionally a macrocytic anaemia caused by interference with vitamin B_{12} absorption, which takes place exclusively in the ileum, is encountered. Other features of malabsorption syndrome may develop, especially in diffuse jejuno-ileal forms of the disease (p. 580). As in ulcerative colitis, systemic complications may occur. These include arthritis, uveitis and skin lesions.

Ulcerative colitis

Although no specific cause is known for this common condition it behaves as a distinct clinical and pathological entity, the incidence of which appears to be rising.

Clinical features. The disease mainly affects young adults of both sexes and is characterised by episodes of diarrhoea with the passage of blood per rectum. Malaise, anorexia and weight loss vary greatly in degree. Most cases follow a chronic relapsing course with exacerbations and remissions. Some are mild and possibly self-limiting, but a few run a more severe, continuous course and fulminating rapidly fatal forms are by no means rare.

Naked-eye appearances. Ulcerative colitis typically involves the sigmoid colon and rectum (proctitis) either alone or in continuity with the remainder of the colon. The entire colon is affected in about half of the cases, and in such instances the terminal ileum may also be involved. Although classically a disease of the distal half of the colon, the proximal colon, with or without the terminal ileum, may be principally affected. It is now recognised, however, that many such 'segmental' or 'right-sided' forms of colitis are examples of Crohn's disease

(p. 562) and others may have an ischaemic origin.

In its early phases, as seen for example through the sigmoidoscope, the colonic mucosa is deeply congested, velvety in appearance and bleeds easily (Fig. 18.43). Punctate erosions herald the onset of ulceration, which usually

sacculation produces a characteristic radiological appearance.

In fulminating cases, loss of mucosa is accompanied by dilatation of the colon and sometimes perforation.

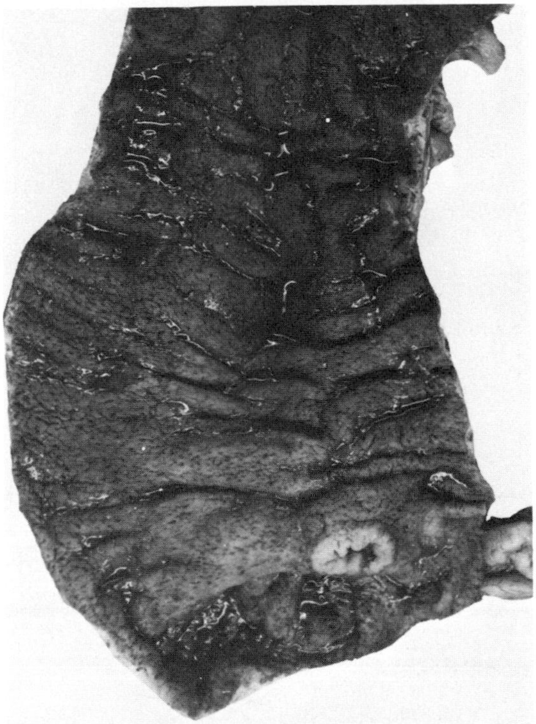

Microscopic appearances. Unlike Crohn's disease, it is the mucosa which is primarily

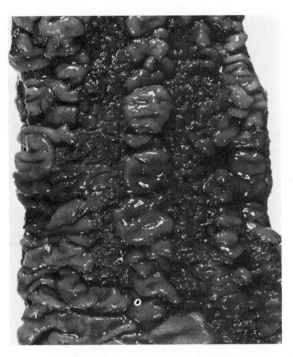

Fig. 18.43 The caecum in early ulcerative colitis. Intense congestion, haemorrhage and multiple pinpoint ulcers of mucosa. The appendicular orifice is shown, and in this case is not affected. × $\frac{2}{3}$.

Fig. 18.44 The colon in chronic ulcerative colitis. The mucosa is extensively ulcerated and the surviving portions are swollen and hyperplastic with many undermined bridges of mucosa. × $\frac{4}{5}$.

begins in the rectum or sigmoid and is found initially at the tips of the mucosal folds overlying the longitudinal muscle bands. Later the ulcers coalesce, giving rise to large irregular areas of mucosal denudation associated with extensive muco-purulent discharge and haemorrhage. Between the ulcers, especially in chronic cases, the surviving mucosa becomes swollen and hyperplastic (Fig. 18.44) and in some instances numerous polypoid excrescences are seen, a condition known as *pseudo-polyposis*. Attempts at healing take place during remissions, but fibrous thickening and stenosis of the lumen are relatively uncommon. During relapses, the colon is spastic and the early loss of the normal

involved in ulcerative colitis. During active phases it is congested and densely infiltrated with leukocytes, especially plasma cells. The formation of *crypt abscesses* (Fig. 18.45a), characterised by the accumulation of neutrophils, eosinophils, red cells and mucus within crypt lumina, is a conspicuous feature, although by no means specific for ulcerative colitis. The epithelial lining of the crypts degenerates and ultimately breaks down, releasing infected material into the lamina propria mucosae. This lesion is a prelude to the appearance of frank ulceration (Fig. 18.45b), which is produced by the coalescence of ruptured crypt abscesses in the deeper parts of the mucosa. Ulceration seldom extends more deeply than the submucosa

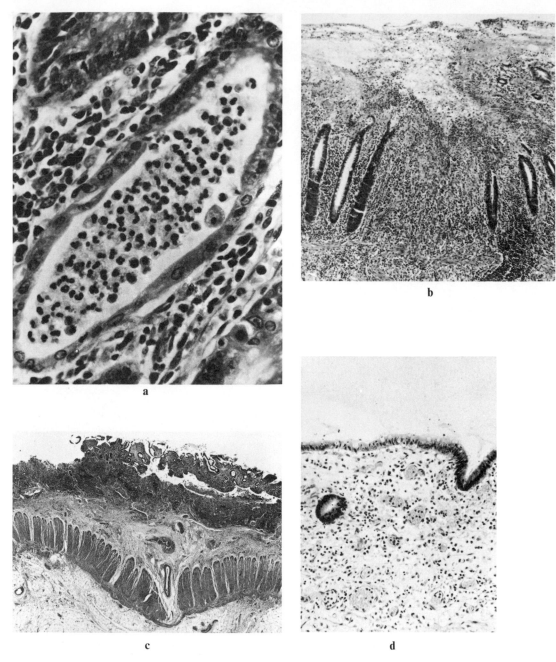

Fig. 18.45   Ulcerative colitis. **a** Crypt abscess. × 425. **b** Early mucosal ulceration with purulent exudate. × 70. **c** Chronic stage: complete loss of mucosa on the left, with undermining of surviving mucosa on the right. × 13. **d** Healing stage showing granulation tissue covered by a simple mucosa. × 115.

and the base is formed by vascular granulation tissue (Fig. 18.45c) containing large numbers of plasma cells and lymphocytes, the latter becoming increasingly conspicuous in chronic cases.

The pseudo-polyps observed in chronic cases consist of islands of surviving hyperplastic mucosa and tags of granulation tissue; true polypoid adenomas (p. 591) are rare. Re-epithelialisation of ulcerated areas may take place (Fig. 18.45*d*) but regeneration is seldom complete. An increase in the number of Paneth cells in the crypts of Lieberkühn is noted especially in the proximal parts of the colon; the significance of this is uncertain.

It has been suggested by Morson that it might be possible to identify those cases in which carcinoma is likely to develop by demonstrating pre-malignant changes in rectal biopsies. These changes usually develop in a flat (as opposed to a polypoid) mucosa and include nuclear pleomorphism, hyperchromatism, loss of polarity and abnormal mitotic activity in the epithelial cells.

Complications. The most urgent of **local complications** is perforation of the colon, which may occur in fulminating cases. An association between steroid therapy and perforation has been claimed, but remains unproved. Peri-anal fistulae may be troublesome in some cases. Although simple fibrous strictures are uncommon, it is now recognised that the development of carcinoma of the colon is a considerable risk. It occurs most commonly in cases in which the entire colon is involved, the onset is early in life and the disease has been present for 10 years or more; the risk is such as to provide an indication for total colectomy in some instances.

The various **systemic complications** include fever and leukocytosis, and debilitating diarrhoea with haemorrhage and exudation leads to protein depletion and anaemia. Arthritis, iridocyclitis and skin lesions, such as erythema nodosum and pyoderma gangrenosum, are seen in a proportion of cases. There appears to be an association between joint disease, especially ankylosing spondylitis, and chronic inflammatory disease of the intestine. Liver disease, of which chronic pericholangitis is the most characteristic and frank cirrhosis the most severe, is not infrequent in ulcerative colitis.

Aetiology. The cause of ulcerative colitis remains an unsolved problem. No specific micro-organism has been isolated, although it is notable that certain types of colonic infection, especially amoebiasis (p. 577) may closely resemble ulcerative colitis pathologically. A search for *Entamoeba histolytica* and other known pathogens should always be undertaken in suspected cases. The possibility that ulcerative colitis has an immunological basis is gaining increasing acceptance. The finding of antibodies to human colonic epithelium in the serum of patients has not, however, been universally confirmed; and the auto-immune hypothesis of causation must be regarded as speculative at the present time.

Various 'non-specific' inflammatory lesions

Phlegmonous enteritis. This rare condition is similar to that described in the stomach (p. 545). It is usually due to the entrance of pathogenic streptococci into the submucosa, especially of the caecum and ascending colon. The organisms probably gain access to the submucosa through a superficial lesion and spread widely, causing extensive suppuration and necrosis. The resultant thickening of the bowel may lead to obstructive features. The precipitating causes of this disease are obscure.

Non-specific ulcers of the intestine. Solitary ulcers of a non-specific nature are occasionally encountered both in the small bowel and colon. In most instances the causation is unknown. Recently, however, it has been suggested that administration of enteric-coated tablets of potassium chloride in association with the diuretic chlorothiazide is responsible in some instances.

Solitary ulcer of the rectum. This term is used to describe a recurrent ulcerative condition, which usually affects young adults and presents a distinctive appearance in rectal biopsies. The mucosa shows variable inflammatory change with irregular superficial ulceration, and fibro-muscular thickening of the lamina propria. There is also displacement of crypt epithelium into the submucosa with subsequent cyst formation. These changes are thought to be the result of chronic mucosal trauma, possibly self-induced, and have also been described in association with rectal prolapse and in the vicinity of haemorrhoids. The main importance of the ulcer is that it may be mistaken for invasive rectal carcinoma.

Functional disorders of the colon. In clinical practice it is by no means uncommon to encounter patients who have symptoms associated with constipation and excessive mucus secretion, although organic lesions cannot be demonstrated.

'Mucous colitis', in which membranous structures composed of inspissated mucus are passed by the bowel, is probably a variant of this syndrome.

Although a variety of names has been attached to such states, the term 'irritable colon syndrome' is most commonly employed, and finds justification in the fact that the colon may be found to exhibit unusual irritability or hypermotility. The causation is obscure—indeed this syndrome may possibly include more than one disease entity—although previous organic disease, for example dysentery, psychological disturbance and dietary indiscretion might be of aetiologic significance.

Appendicitis

Acute appendicitis

This lesion is of the highest importance on account of its frequency and the serious results which often follow. Individuals of either sex and of virtually any age may be affected but the disease is commonest in children and young adults.

Naked-eye appearances. The condition occurs in three forms: simple acute appendicitis, suppurative or phlegmonous and gangrenous appendicitis. The first two of these types may be regarded as different degrees of severity of the same condition; the third has special features of its own. Perforation may occur in both suppurative and gangrenous types.

In all cases, the whole thickness of the wall is involved. In the earlier stages of *acute appendicitis*, the appendix is swollen, tense and markedly congested, and there may be a little fibrin on the surface (Fig. 18.46). When the appendix is cut into, the mucosa bulges owing to the swelling, and purulent-looking material may exude from the lumen.

In other cases the changes are of greater severity. The primary inflammatory lesion may increase in intensity and lead to a small abscess in the wall, and this may perforate. There may occur also more general suppuration and necrosis with multiple abscesses and perforations. The presence of a concretion in the lumen (see below) may predispose to perforation because, in acute appendicitis, the swollen wall becomes stretched over the concretion with consequent ischaemia and gangrene.

Gangrenous appendicitis. In the course of acute appendicitis, gangrene may affect the distal portion, sometimes in relation to a concretion in the lumen, or it may occur in patches. In some cases it appears to be due to thrombosis of the veins in the meso-appendix, which, aided by the inflammatory condition, leads to haemorrhage and arrests the circulation. But in other cases gangrene develops early and rapidly and affects the whole appendix apart from any vascular lesion. The two factors determining

gangrene are obstruction at the outlet of the appendix and distension with faecal material. Experimentally a closed portion of small intestine filled with faecal material becomes gangrenous within a short time, and many cases of so-called fulminating, i.e. gangrenous, appendicitis are of this nature. The great danger of

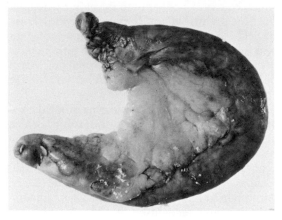

Fig. 18.46   Acute appendicitis, showing swelling of the appendix with congestion and deposition of fibrin on the serous surface.

gangrenous appendicitis is the early development of general peritonitis due to mixed bacterial infection, including anaerobes.

Microscopic appearances. In most cases of acute appendicitis, there is an acute inflammatory reaction involving the entire thickness of the appendicular wall, with a fibrinopurulent exudate on the peritoneal surface. It seems likely that this inflammatory reaction originates from a focus of mucosal ulceration, possibly in the deeper parts of the epithelial crypts with subsequent extension into the lamina propria (Fig. 18.47). Several foci of inflammation are sometimes observed, but the changes are usually most marked in the distal part (i.e. the blind end) of the appendix. Sometimes the inflammation is localised and can easily be missed on cursory examination. In some patients with an appendicitis-like syndrome the only changes seen are pus cells in the appendicular lumen, associated with some foci of polymorph infiltration in the superficial parts of the mucosa, or the occasional crypt abscess. The clinical significance of such limited forms of appendicitis is debatable since similar changes are sometimes seen in appendices removed prophylactically during the course of some other operation, e.g. hysterectomy.

Clinical features. Acute appendicitis presents typically as colicky abdominal pain in the um-

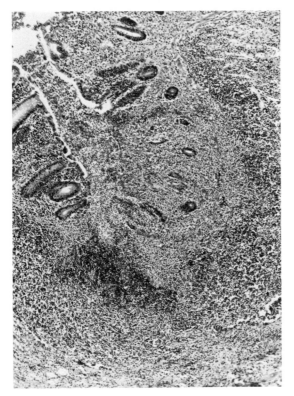

Fig. 18.47 Acute appendicitis, showing a local ulcerative lesion in mucosa with commencing abscess formation beneath. × 60.

bilical region, due to spasmodic contractions of the inflamed appendix. This is followed by a continuous 'burning' pain, tenderness and rigidity of the abdominal muscles, in the vicinity of the appendix. These latter features are due to irritation of the parietal peritoneum by the inflamed appendiceal serosa, and they may be inconspicuous or absent when the appendix is retrocaecal. Vomiting, pyrexia, increased pulse rate and leukocytosis are inconstant features.

The diagnosis of acute appendicitis is often difficult and gangrenous appendicitis may be accompanied by remarkably slight clinical upset. The results of delay in removing an acutely inflamed appendix (see below) are so serious that exploratory laparotomy is often necessary in cases where the diagnosis is anything but certain.

Results. Acute appendicitis gives rise to important complications. In some cases there is merely a slight amount of fibrinous exudate on the surface, which does not spread and may afterwards give rise to local adhesions. In others, a localised collection of pus may form around the appendix—*appendix abscess*—which in many cases shows perforation of the wall. Sometimes an escaped concretion is present in the pus. The suppuration may spread upwards alongside the caecum and ascending colon and between the surface of the liver and the diaphragm. Alternatively, an abscess may develop in, or extend into, the pelvic cavity. Cases of this kind may run a prolonged course. In other cases, a fatal generalised peritonitis may result. This is specially apt to occur at an early stage in gangrenous appendicitis. Other complications of appendicitis are due to infection of the veins. There may be a local septic phlebitis, and from this emboli may be carried to the liver, where they set up secondary abscesses. Rarely, a spreading thrombosis with secondary suppuration may extend up the portal vein—*portal pylephlebitis* (p. 632).

Aetiology. Although the lesions of acute appendicitis are due to bacterial infection, the factors which trigger it off are still largely unknown. There is even uncertainty about which organisms primarily invade the tissues, although there is no doubt that the important effects are caused by coliform bacilli, streptococci and occasionally anaerobic species, all of which are present in the lumen. It seems certain, however, that *obstruction* of the appendicular lumen is involved in many cases and, as already mentioned, gangrenous appendicitis is often produced in this way. Less easy to explain is the cause of the obstruction: foreign bodies and intestinal parasites, e.g. *Oxyuris vermicularis*, have been blamed from time to time, but they can only be found in some cases. A more promising suggestion is that obstruction is caused, particularly in childhood, by swelling of the appendicular lymphoid tissue, due possibly to viral infection, or, as has recently been demonstrated, by infection with *Yersinia enterocolitica*, an organism also known to produce acute mesenteric lymphadenitis (which incidentally can mimic acute appendicitis clinically). The part played by faecal concretions, or faecoliths, which are hard masses of faeces mixed with mucus and occasionally calcium salts, is difficult to assess, since these are commonly found even in normal appendices. As explained above, a concretion is likely to cause ischaemia and gangrene in an acutely inflamed appendix. It is notable that appendicitis, like diverticular disease (see below), is essentially a disease of developed societies, and it might well be that, as Burkitt has claimed, refined diets lacking in roughage are also of importance in its pathogenesis.

Chronic appendicitis and mucocele of the appendix

Fibrous thickening of the wall of the appendix, especially in young people, may be a consequence of acute inflammation. Occasionally, fibrosis may be the result of persistent chronic infection—the so-called *chronic appendicitis*—and there may be no history of an acute attack. It is conceivable that mild attacks of abdominal pain in the region of the appendix are due to this ('appendicular dyspepsia'). It should be emphasised, however, that in older individuals asymptomatic appendicular fibrosis is extremely common and can almost be regarded as a normal ageing process.

A common result of a localised lesion of the appendix is obliteration of the lumen at that

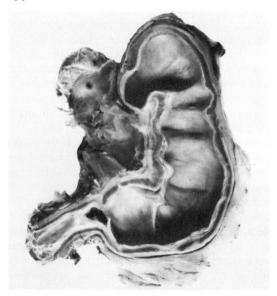

Fig. 18.48 Chronic appendicitis with obliteration at proximal end and mucocele of the distal portion.

point, whilst elsewhere the mucosa may be comparatively well preserved. Such a condition may be readily explained by the commonly focal nature of acute appendicitis. When localised obliteration is present dilatation of the distal portion of the tube may follow (Fig. 18.48). This may be slight, or there may be a cyst-like enlargement or **mucocele**. Another not uncommon result, owing to the distension acting on a localised lesion in the muscle, is the production of a diverticulum, which may project on the surface of the appendix. Occasionally rupture of a mucocele occurs and results in its mucoid contents leaking into the peritoneum. Reactive phenomena follow and the thick mucus is invaded by young connective tissue cells and by new blood vessels; this is known as *pseudo-myxoma peritonei*. It is a serious complication when the escape of mucus continues, and adhesions form with collections of mucus between. The microscopic appearances may simulate those of a mucoid carcinoma.

Diverticular disease

A diverticulum consists of protrusion of the mucous and submucous coats through the muscle of the wall, and since the sac has no muscle coat, it is properly called a 'false diverticulum', in contrast to a true diverticulum, e.g. Meckel's (p. 595), which has a complete layer of muscle like the bowel.

(a) Small intestine. Diverticula are uncommon in the small bowel. The duodenum is most often involved, followed by the jejunum and ileum in that order. The diverticula may be single or multiple and are invariably found along the mesenteric border of the bowel in close relationship to the entry-sites of the blood vessels. They may measure 3 cm or more in diameter.

Pathological effects. Small-bowel diverticula are seldom encountered before adult life; they probably cause abdominal symptoms more often than is generally realised. Frank inflammatory change, haemorrhage and obstruction are, however, rare complications; more often a malabsorptive disturbance related to the 'blind-loop syndrome' (p. 583) is the principal feature. The latter is caused mainly by abnormal and excessive bacterial proliferation in the diverticula. Bacterial uptake of vitamin B_{12} before it

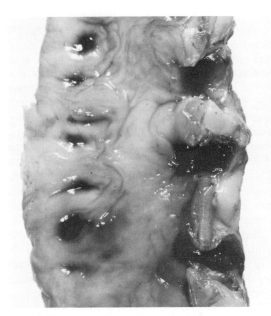

Fig. 18.49 Part of the sigmoid colon cut open to show the mucosal surface in diverticulosis. There are two longitudinal rows of diverticula: those on the right have been opened and can be seen to herniate through the muscle coat of the bowel.

the appendices epiploicae. Small depressions at first, they enlarge and become spherical or flask-shaped (Fig. 18.49), usually less than 1 cm in diameter. Diverticula frequently contain inspissated faeces and it is notable that muscle hypertrophy and thickening of the peri-colic fat are commonly observed in the adjacent bowel.

Pathological effects. Inflammatory change in the diverticula (*diverticulitis*) is the common cause of clinical symptoms, which are usually encountered in the older age groups. Acute inflammation leads to a syndrome resembling appendicitis with localisation of pain to the left side of the abdomen. This condition may progress to peri-colic abscess formation and even to free perforation into the peritoneal cavity and acute peritonitis. The development of fistulae between the colon and adjacent organs, especially the bladder, is not uncommon. More chronic diverticulitis leads to fibrous thickening of the colonic wall with some degree of intestinal obstruction, and the lesion may be mistaken macroscopically for carcinoma. There is no evidence that diverticular disease is a precancerous condition. Rarely severe rectal haemorrhage occurs, probably due to erosion of blood vessels in the diverticular wall.

Aetiology. It is generally accepted that diverticula are caused by high pressure within the bowel lumen leading to protrusion of the mucosa through points of weakness in the bowel wall. The latter are usually related to the entry of blood vessels from the mesocolon. Recent studies suggest that, at least in the colon, diverticula are associated with the generation of localised areas of unusually high intraluminal pressure by abnormal segmental contraction of the bowel musculature, and that the muscle hypertrophy related to diverticula is a morphological expression of this effect. It is notable that diverticular disease is mainly restricted to developed societies and the consumption of refined foods lacking in roughage may be the most important aetiological factor.

can reach its main absorptive site in the distal ileum leads to vitamin B_{12} deficiency and megaloblastic anaemia, and it is probable that bacteria are also responsible for the steatorrhoea which is sometimes observed. Oral broad-spectrum antibiotics lead to improvement in both vitamin B_{12} and fat absorption.

(b) Colon. Multiple diverticula of the colon are very common in later adult life: in this country about one person in ten is affected, although in only 20% of cases does the condition produce symptoms. The sigmoid colon is most often involved, although diverticula may occur at a higher level, including the caecum. Characteristically they lie in two rows between the mesenteric and the anti-mesenteric taeniae and are related to the entry of blood vessels into the colonic wall. They commonly extend into

Specific bacterial infections

Many inflammatory conditions of the intestines, both acute and chronic, are produced by bacilli of the typhoid-coli group. These organisms affect chiefly the small intestine with special localisation in the lymphoid tissue. The food-poisoning bacilli (*Salmonella typhimurium* and others) cause acute diffuse catarrhal inflammation of the small or large intestine, and the paratyphoid organisms sometimes have a similar effect; the dysentery bacilli affect chiefly the large intestine and cause both acute and chronic lesions. In all these cases, and also in cholera, infection is acquired by ingesting the specific micro-organisms in food or water contaminated by the excreta of cases of the disease or of carriers of the infection. Contamination by handling of food, or by the activities of flies, gives rise to sporadic cases or small outbreaks, but major epidemics are virtually always due to seepage of sewage into water supplies. An additional source of infection in food poisoning by *Salmonellae* is the soiling of food by the faeces of infected mice or rats. Other organisms which produce important effects are the anthrax bacillus, actinomyces, and the tubercle bacillus, and it is known that many viruses that produce no apparent lesion of the gut are nevertheless excreted in the faeces and are invasive when ingested, e.g. poliomyelitis virus, Coxsackie virus.

The enteric fevers

This term is used to describe the illnesses caused by acute infections with *S. typhi* (typhoid fever) or *S. paratyphi* (paratyphoid fever).

Typhoid fever

This disease is caused by the Gram-negative bacillus *Salmonella typhi*. Corresponding with the clinical illness there are inflammatory changes in the lymphoid tissue of the bowel, leading to destructive effects which are followed by healing.

Course. After an incubation period of about two weeks, the ingested organisms, which have invaded the lymphoid tissues of the small intestine, enter the bloodstream. There is then progressive fever of insidious onset, sometimes with a 'staircase' rise; after a further week the characteristic rose spots appear in the skin. In the first week of the fever the organisms from the blood can usually be cultured, thus confirming the diagnosis. Thereafter they persist in the liver and biliary passages and re-enter the small intestine in large numbers from the bile so that they are then readily detected in the faeces.

About the end of ten days, immunity begins to develop and the organisms disappear from the blood stream, but during the bacteraemic phase they may settle in various sites and later produce localised lesions. It is significant that the gallbladder bile is invariably infected during the early phase, and the wall of the viscus may become inflamed, producing a typhoid cholecystitis with serious secondary effects. These phases in the distribution of the organisms are of decisive importance in the bacteriological diagnosis of the disease. The course may be modified considerably by previous immunisation, and diagnosis may then be difficult both clinically and bacteriologically.

Naked-eye appearances. Re-infection of the lymphoid tissue of the gut by organisms in the bile leads to the development of lesions which are usually most marked in the Peyer's patches of the distal ileum, although solitary lymphoid follicles more proximally or distally are also affected. The lymphoid patches initially show an inflammatory swelling which is followed, usually about the tenth day of the illness, by necrosis and subsequent ulceration (Figs. 18.50, 18.51). Healing usually begins about the end of the third week and is complete by the fifth week in uncomplicated cases. The ulcers have a

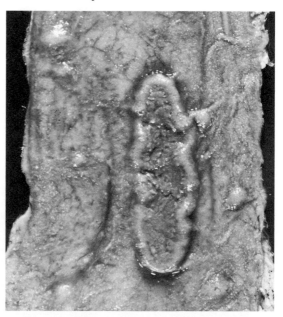

Fig. 18.50 The lower ileum in typhoid fever, showing necrosis and ulceration of the Peyer's patches and solitary lymphoid follicles.

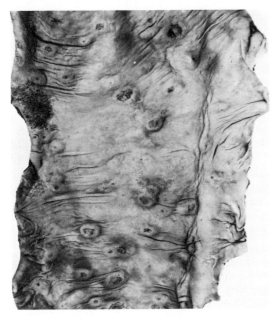

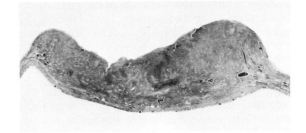

Fig. 18.52 Peyer's patch in the early stage of typhoid fever, showing the marked inflammatory swelling and commencing necrosis. × 5.

Fig. 18.51 Colon in typhoid fever showing swelling and ulceration of the lymphoid follicles.

yellowish-brown or black colour, correspond in shape and extent to the lymphoid patches, and tend to have soft, shreddy, undermined margins. Healing of these ulcerated lesions leaves a smooth silky scar which never shows any tendency towards stricture formation. Severe haemorrhage sometimes occurs from these necrotic ulcerated lesions, although a more serious complication resulting from extensive necrosis is perforation of the small bowel with usually fatal generalised peritonitis. Clinically this latter event is seldom accompanied by the dramatic symptoms associated with gastro-duodenal perforation, possibly because the alkaline intestinal contents have less irritant effect on the peritoneal cavity.

Microscopic appearances are characteristic. The enlargement of the Peyer's patches (Fig. 18.52) is due to congestion, oedema and the infiltration of inflammatory cells, predominantly lymphocytes, plasma cells and macrophages. Haemorrhage and fibrinous exudation often contribute to the inflammatory swelling. This inflammatory reaction may extend deeply to involve the muscularis propria (Fig. 6.3, p. 153) and even the serosal coat. Neutrophil polymorphs are notably absent from the lesions except in secondarily infected ulcerated surfaces. Progressive lesions usually show

patchy necrosis with extensive nuclear karyorrhexis and the surrounding macrophages, sometimes called typhoid histiocytes, typically ingest the nuclear debris as well as extravasated red cells. The development of necrosis may well represent a delayed hypersensitivity reaction to bacterial antigens. The **mesenteric lymph nodes** are commonly enlarged and show changes closely similar to those in the Peyer's patches (Figs. 17.4, p. 514 and 1.5, p. 5). The development of focal necrosis can lead to softening and rupture of the lymph node with subsequent peritonitis.

Associated lesions. As in the tissue lesions, there is a comparative absence of neutrophil polymorph reaction in the peripheral blood and bone marrow. Similarly the spleen, although commonly enlarged, contains few neutrophils, contrary to what might be expected in a severe bacterial infection. Typhoid fever is associated with a great variety of lesions which are widely distributed and may arise during the course of the disease or later: they are due to endotoxaemia (p. 148) and bacteraemia. **Endotoxaemia** may be responsible for the fever and produces degenerative changes in several organs, e.g. myocardial damage, which may precipitate heart failure, and focal necrosis of the abdominal muscles (Zenker's degeneration), which is characteristic. The liver and kidneys also show toxic injury. Typhoid endotoxaemia probably also impairs resistance to invasion by other bacteria and the well recognised development of laryngitis, bronchitis (sometimes an early symptom) and pneumonia may well be due to this. **Bacteraemia** brings about acute enlargement of the spleen and probably accounts for the characteristic rose-coloured spots in the skin. Of epidemiological importance is the establishment of persistent infection with or without inflammatory change in the gallbladder and less often in the urinary tract. This is the pathological basis of the *carrier state*, since patients thus affected excrete bacilli in the faeces or in the urine for varying periods and are commonly the source of outbreaks of typhoid fever. Other lesions produced by circulating bacilli include endocarditis, meningitis and arthritis. Recurrent periostitis and perichondritis involving the costal and laryngeal cartilages are also well recognised complications.

Paratyphoid infections

Infections caused by the paratyphoid organism are not uncommon, paratyphoid B being the most frequent of the enteric fevers in West Europe. In some cases the disease has the general features of typhoid, though usually less severe. There is a similar involvement of the lymphoid tissue, especially the Peyer's patches and solitary follicles of the small intestine, with swelling of mesenteric nodes and spleen; but the necrotic and ulcerative processes are less marked and usually limited to a small part of the intestine. In other cases a generalised mucosal inflammatory reaction is found, and there is little implication of the lymphoid tissue; sometimes enteritis is associated with marked gastritis. The 'carrier' condition may result also from paratyphoid infections, as has been described above in typhoid fever.

Food poisoning

This term is widely applied in a restricted sense to include acute gastro-enteritis due either to **infection** with *Salmonellae* other than those which cause enteric fever, or to ingestion of bacterial toxins. The *Salmonellae* most commonly responsible are *S. enteritidis* and *S. typhimurium*, harboured by rats and mice respectively, but a very large number of other *Salmonellae* cause local outbreaks in all parts of the world. Characteristically, acute gastro-enteritis, with fever, vomiting and diarrhoea, develops 12–24 hours after eating contaminated food. The inflammation is catarrhal and affects the ileum or colon most severely; in most cases, recovery is complete within 3–4 days, but death can result from water and electrolyte depletion. Blood culture is usually negative although in

fatal cases the organisms may be recovered from the spleen.

The commonest cause of **toxic food poisoning** is *staphylococcal enterotoxin* in foods contaminated by *Staph. aureus*: this toxin is highly resistant to heat and produces acute gastro-enteritis within 1–6 hours. It is rarely fatal.

Botulism. Small outbreaks of botulism occur in North America and other countries where home bottling or canning is popular. The organism, *Clostridium botulinum*, grows in inadequately cooked fruit or vegetables, or in sausages, and produces the most powerful toxin known. Within 12–36 hours of its ingestion, muscular weakness and paralysis develop, particularly in the muscles of the eye, pharynx and neck. Death commonly results from respiratory paralysis and aspiration pneumonia. Alimentary symptoms are slight, and constipation is more usual than diarrhoea.

Cholera

This disease is caused by *Vibrio cholerae* or its subtypes and is a classical example of a waterborne infection capable of causing explosive epidemics. Profuse watery diarrhoea is the outstanding clinical feature and the stools are often described as having a colourless 'rice-water' appearance. Diarrhoea leads to the loss of about 30 litres of fluid during an illness lasting 3–6 days, and the depletion of water and electrolytes, especially sodium and potassium, is extremely severe and often fatal.

Until recently it was considered that the pathological basis for the severe diarrhoea was an acute inflammation of the small intestine, especially its distal part, and occasionally of the large bowel in addition. Intestinal biopsies have failed, however, to demonstrate loss of the integrity of the surface epithelium, and *Vibrio cholerae*, which is present in large numbers in the intestinal lumen, is now known to cause diarrhoea by producing an exotoxin which increases the net flow of fluid and electrolytes from the plasma into the lumen of the gut, particularly in the jejunum. The mechanism differs from that of inflammatory exudation, and the fluid has a low protein content. It is probable that cholera toxin exerts its effect by stimulating adenyl cyclase activity, thus increasing adenosine monophosphate which affects the equilibrium of fluid and electrolytes between the mucosal cell and gut lumen. Oral administration of glucose and electrolyte solutions has been shown to be of great therapeutic value. Although the organisms are largely confined to the intestinal tract, they can become established in the gallbladder and lead to a carrier state which, although usually of short duration, may last as long as four years. It has also become apparent that the number of cases of cholera is far exceeded by the number of individuals who become infected and excrete the vibrio without developing the disease.

The **El Tor vibrio**, first isolated in Sinai, is closely related to *V. cholerae* and has been responsible for recent outbreaks of a cholera-like illness in various parts of the world.

Tuberculosis

Intestinal tuberculosis was formerly common, but in many countries the incidence is now low, partly because infection of milk by bovine tubercle bacilli has been eliminated, and partly as a consequence of the falling incidence of pulmonary tuberculosis. Three main forms of intestinal tuberculosis are recognised.

(a) Primary infection. The small bowel was formerly a common site for the primary tuberculous complex in children who had ingested cow's milk containing bovine tubercle bacilli. As elsewhere, the site of entrance of the organisms is inconspicuous, although this probably means that the lesion has been minute and has not spread, rather than that the bacilli have invaded without producing any lesion. The prominent change is produced in the mesenteric lymph nodes, which become greatly enlarged and caseous (tabes mesenterica). In favourable circumstances, the condition remains localised, and the calcified mesenteric nodes still quite often observed in adults represent the result of intestinal infection in early life. Occasionally, however, the disease spreads from the nodes to the peritoneal cavity leading to tuberculous peritonitis (p. 598).

(b) Secondary infection. Intestinal lesions used to be a common complication of open pulmonary tuberculosis, especially in children. This secondary form of intestinal tuberculosis, caused by swallowing sputum containing tubercle bacilli, causes ulcers of the intestine, but

with only slight involvement of the mesenteric lymph nodes.

The small intestine is the common site of the lesions, which usually occur in the Peyer's patches or solitary lymphoid follicles. Initially, caseating tubercles develop in the mucosa and the submucosa, and subsequent mucosal breakdown leads to the formation of small ulcers, which become progressively enlarged by direct spread of the organisms to adjacent parts of the mucosa. Ultimately large ulcers are produced and these tend to extend by spread of infection along the lymphatics, transversely to the longitudinal axis of the bowel; sometimes indeed they encircle the gut (Fig. 18.53). The larger

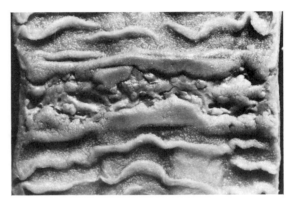

Fig. 18.53 Tuberculosis of the ileum causing transverse ulcers.

ulcers have an irregular outline, undermined edges and raised nodular margins (Fig. 18.54). The floor is uneven or granular and may be coated by caseous material, but tubercles are rarely visible. The serous coat overlying the ulcer is often thickened and opaque and the presence of visible tubercles along the lines of serosal lymphatics may be of diagnostic value. Histologically, the tuberculous lesions are similar to those observed elsewhere; the ulceration is seen to extend through the mucosa into the submucous layer and there may be varying degrees of fibrous replacement of the muscular coat. Tubercles are usually found throughout the entire thickness of the bowel and in the related mesenteric lymph nodes. These, however, are seldom as grossly affected as in the primary form.

Tuberculous ulceration rarely causes gross haemorrhage, and perforation into the peritoneal cavity is uncommon. The formation of fistulae

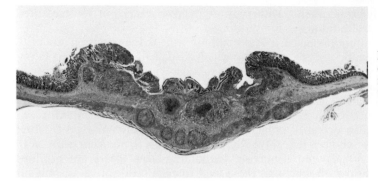

Fig. 18.54 Small tuberculous ulcer of small intestine with thickened and irregular margins and floor. Note the tubercles in the serous coat. × 6.

between adjacent loops of bowel, initiated by the development of adhesions, may, however, lead to short-circuiting of bowel contents and malabsorption: the effects thus contrast with those of typhoid ulceration. The peritoneum may show frank tuberculous lesions (p. 598) or simply multiple fibrous adhesions which may cause mechanical obstruction of the bowel.

(c) **'Hyperplastic caecal tuberculosis'.** This is an uncommon tuberculous lesion, now rare in Europe and North America. It consists of gross fibrous thickening of the wall of a length of the caecum or ascending colon with ulceration of the surface and caseating tubercle follicles. Because it causes obstruction and is sometimes palpable, the lesion may be clinically suggestive of carcinoma. Pathologically, it may be confused with Crohn's disease affecting the caecum, and demonstration of tubercle bacilli by microscopy, culture or animal inoculation is important. Hyperplastic caecal tuberculosis is usually secondary to pulmonary disease.

The **appendix** is occasionally affected in cases of intestinal tuberculosis. The changes are of the usual kind, and in a proportion of cases a faecal fistula develops post-operatively. More often this sequence is attributable to Crohn's disease.

The dysenteries

The term dysentery was originally used clinically to denote conditions of severe inflammation and ulceration of the colon, attended by diarrhoea, tenesmus and the passage of blood and mucus in the stools. Two main types of dysentery are distinguished, namely, *bacillary* and *amoebic*.

Bacillary dysentery

Bacillary dysentery is produced by bacilli of the *Shigella* group, of which there are several varieties, distinguishable by their serological and fermentative reactions. The mildest type is usually caused by *Shigella sonnei*, and in children is often called ileocolitis; more severe infections are caused by *Sh. flexneri*, and the most severe tropical form by *Sh. dysenteriae* (*Sh. shigae*), which produces a powerful exotoxin. The lesion is essentially inflammation of variable intensity in the colon, though the lower end of the ileum is sometimes also affected.

In mild cases the main features are intense mucosal inflammation with oedema, haemorrhage and excess mucus secretion. There may be some fibrinous exudation on the mucosal surface, but this is much more marked in severe cases in which there is extensive pseudomembrane formation with mucosal necrosis, and subsequent ulceration. The ulcers extend in an irregular manner and tend to have shredded margins. It is usual for healing to take place after the acute phase and the re-epithelialised ulcers assume a smooth and even appearance in contrast to the surrounding mucosa. The disease may, however, be prolonged and relapses are quite frequent. Such subacute or chronic cases are characterised by repeated ulceration and healing and can lead to polypoid mucosal irregularity with fibrous scarring and subsequent stenosis of the bowel. Bacillary dysentery may also be complicated by pyogenic bacterial infection of the portal venous system and focal suppuration in the liver.

Microscopically, the colonic mucosa shows intense inflammatory reaction in the lamina propria and polymorphs can be seen surrounding the mucosal crypts and invading the epithelial surfaces. The appearances resemble early ulcerative colitis (p. 564). The presence of polymorphs admixed with red cells and mucus in the faeces is of presumptive diagnostic value.

Amoebic dysentery

This is caused by *Entamoeba histolytica*. The disease is only rarely acquired in temperate climates, but is common in tropical and subtropical countries, a fact not easily explained since entamoeba cysts are found in the faeces of a small proportion of people in this country who have not been abroad.

Naked-eye appearance. The organisms, swallowed in the cystic stage in food or water, are freed in the gut by digestion of the cyst wall, and enter the wall of the large intestine through the mucosa to settle in the submucous tissue where they liberate a proteolytic enzyme causing tissue necrosis. Accordingly, the first lesion visible to the naked eye is the formation of swollen congested patches in the mucosa, the central parts of which become soft and somewhat yellowish as necrosis occurs (Fig. 18.55). The mucosa then gives way and an ulcer is

formed with shreddy and undermined margins. Such ulcers, as they spread, become confluent first in their deeper parts, so that a probe may be passed under the mucosa from one to the other; the bridges then give way and the ulcerated areas are greatly increased. Accordingly a considerable part of the bowel may have lost its mucosa, while in the intervening parts fragments of mucosa in process of disintegration and separation are present (Fig. 18.56). Gangrene of the mucosal patches may be superadded.

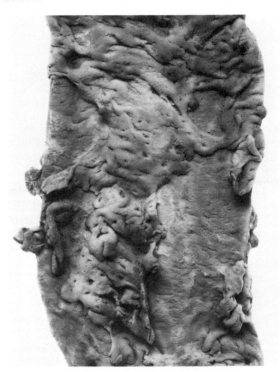

Fig. 18.56 The colon in chronic amoebic dysentery, showing irregular smooth areas where the mucosa has been destroyed.

Microscopically the most prominent feature is an intense inflammatory oedema, which is accompanied by remarkably little leukocytic infiltration. Subsequent necrosis takes place in the tissues around the entamoebae which multiply and spread in the submucous tissue and thus necrosis extends. Amoebae are found in the base and at the margins of ulcers (Fig. 18.57), chiefly in the submucosa but also extending more deeply. Occasionally they can be seen within small intestinal veins (Fig. 18.58). The mucosa overlying submucous lesions

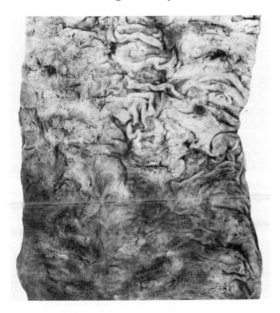

Fig. 18.55 The colon in early amoebic dysentery, showing irregular swelling of the mucosa, but, as yet, no obvious ulceration.

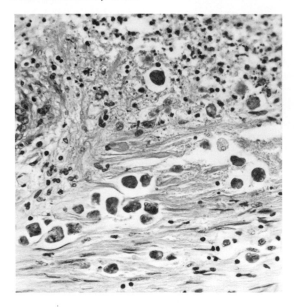

Fig. 18.57 Section through the base of an amoebic ulcer of the colon. The amoebae are seen lying in spaces with no surrounding inflammatory cellular reaction. × 200.

commonly becomes secondarily infected and shows changes similar to those of ulcerative colitis (p. 565). In suspected cases of the latter disease, it is thus most important to examine the stools for the presence of amoebae (see below).

Results and complications. When the acute stage of amoebic dysentery has passed off, at-

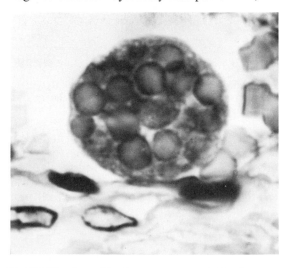

Fig. 18.58 Amoebic dysentery: an entamoeba containing red cells is seen in a venule in the base of an ulcer of the colon. × 1100.

tempts at healing may occur. The necrotic tissue is thrown off and the epithelium grows over the denuded areas. But the process is often interrupted, and just as in bacillary dysentery, the disease may become protracted and pass into a chronic condition. Overgrowth of fibrous tissue is apt to occur in the deeper coats with resulting narrowing of the bowel at places. Enterostomy or faecal fistula in the presence of active amoebic infection may be followed by spread of amoebae into the skin, where they produce a severe necrotising ulceration. The passage of entamoebae to the liver in the portal blood gives rise to amoebic hepatitis and in some cases a tropical abscess is produced (p. 634).

Diagnosis. In the acute phase the stools contain blood and mucus but, in contrast with bacillary dysentery, pus is absent. The mucus is thus clear and in it vegetative amoebae showing active movements are readily found on microscopic examination of a fresh preparation, examined without delay on a warm stage; the ingestion of red cells by the amoebae is diagnostic. In the chronic phase, vegetative forms are absent, and the diagnosis depends on the detection of cysts in the faeces or from the base of ulcers seen on sigmoidoscopy.

Actinomycosis

As a path of entry for the streptothrix *Actinomyces israelii*, the intestine comes next to the mouth in order of frequency. The lesions are found in the wall of the large intestine, and sometimes ulcers with suppuration of the submucous coat have been present usually with extension beyond the wall of the gut, especially in the region of the caecum and in the tissues around the rectum. More commonly, the organism seems to gain entrance to the appendix, from which it spreads to give rise to an inflammatory mass containing multiple abscesses. In the peritoneum, loculated abscesses between the coils of intestine may discharge into the bowel. Diagnosis can usually be made by finding colonies of *Actinomyces* on microscopic examination. Secondary actinomycotic abscesses may occur in the liver, and suppurative pylephlebitis due to secondary invasion by other pyogenic organisms has been recorded.

Intestinal schistosomiasis (bilharziasis)

This disease, which is common in various tropical and subtropical parts of Africa and other countries, is produced by the dioecious trematode, *Schistosoma mansoni*. The adult parasites lodge in the tributaries of the portal vein (Fig. 18.59), especially those in the colonic wall, and the females there lay ova which escape into the surrounding tissues. The ova give rise

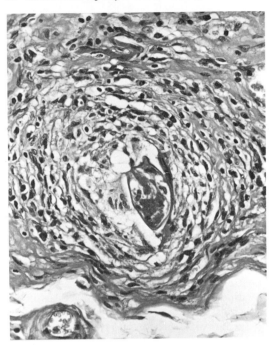

Fig. 18.60 Ovum of *S. mansoni* with surrounding granulomatous reaction in the wall of the colon. × 300.

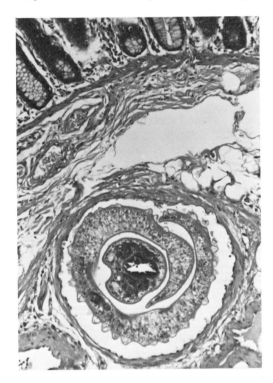

Fig. 18.59 Schistosomiasis. Wall of colon, showing *S. mansoni* adults in cross section. The female lies in the gynaecophoric canal of the male. × 200.

to much irritation and lead to lesions in the large intestine, especially in the rectum (Fig. 18.60), similar to those caused in the bladder by the *Schistosoma haematobium* (p. 804). The eggs are oval, measuring about 140 μm in length, and have a small lateral spine near one end. The reaction is chronic inflammation, with macrophage granulomas around the ova and granulation tissue formation progressing to fibrosis in the mucous and submucous coats, resulting in nodular and polypoid projections of the mucosal surface (Fig. 18.61). Ulceration with haemorrhage occurs, and sometimes there is gross fibrous thickening of the wall.

Similar chronic inflammatory lesions may be observed in other tissues, particularly the liver and

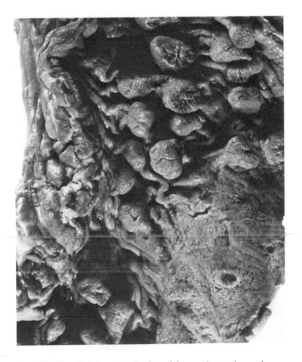

Fig. 18.61 Schistosomiasis of large intestine, showing multiple polypoid nodules projecting from mucosal surface.

lungs. In the liver, they develop in relation to the portal tracts and lead to a condition sometimes referred to as 'pipe-stem cirrhosis' (Fig. 19.41, p. 635); portal hypertension with splenomegaly arises from obstruction of the portal radicles. Unlike the urinary type, intestinal schistosomiasis does not appear to predispose to the development of carcinoma; even so, it is an all too frequent cause of chronic ill-health in the tropics.

The life-cycle of the parasite is similar to that of *S. haematobium* (p. 804).

Inflammatory stricture of the rectum

The least rare cause of this is probably *lymphogranuloma inguinale* (p. 917) which, in women, tends to spread by the lymphatics from the genitalia to the rectum and peri-rectal tissues.

As elsewhere, the rectal lesion is a chronic inflammation with necrosis and suppuration. Ulceration may extend round the whole circumference and scarring then results in stricture. The lesion may also result in recto-vaginal fistula, or discharge on to the perineum.

The malabsorption syndrome

The products of digestion of food are absorbed almost exclusively from the small intestine, and accordingly most pathological processes in the small intestine, if at all extensive, interfere with this important function to some degree. The absorption of some nutrients may be restricted to certain relatively well-defined parts of the small bowel; iron, for example, is absorbed mainly from the duodenum and vitamin B_{12} from the distal ileum. Depending thus upon the extent, site or nature of the disease process, the absorption of some constituents of the diet may be affected more than others. In severe cases, all nutrients including protein, fat, carbohydrates, vitamins, minerals and even water may fail to be adequately absorbed. Failure to absorb fat is the most prominent feature in most cases and on it depend some of the other deficiencies.

Clinical features. The clinical manifestations of malabsorption vary accordingly. The most common symptom is chronic diarrhoea; the stools are pale, bulky and foul-smelling and contain an excess of fat (**steatorrhoea**) and of nitrogenous material. In severe cases, loss of weight, muscle wasting, dehydration and hypotension are prominent features. Hypoglycaemia, with a low glucose tolerance curve (p. 964) indicates failure of carbohydrate uptake. Hypoproteinaemia, associated with oedema, may be the result not only of impaired amino-acid absorption, but also of protein leakage into the bowel lumen (**protein-losing enteropathy**)—a feature of many gastro-intestinal diseases. Vitamin deficiencies are common, and symptoms of beri-beri, pellagra, scurvy and rickets in children, may be presenting features of the syn-

drome. Anaemia frequently dominates the clinical picture; usually it is microcytic and attributed to iron deficiency but macrocytic anaemia following failure to absorb vitamin B_{12} or folic acid is by no means unusual. It is rare for all of those features to be noted together, and any one deficiency may predominate; biochemical tests, however, usually reveal more extensive malabsorption than is clinically evident.

Peroral intestinal biopsy. This technique, now widely used, has proved of considerable value in the diagnosis and investigation of malabsorptive disturbances. Biopsy makes it possible to assess not only the morphological state of the mucosa but also the enzyme content of the absorptive epithelium and the bacterial content of the intestinal lumen.

Under the dissecting microscope, the normal jejunal mucosa has tall, slender finger-shaped villi interspersed with occasional broader leaf-shaped villi, which are more conspicuous in the duodenum. The villi measure about 400 μm in height and usually account for about 70% of the total mucosal height. In tropical residents, however, the villi are more often leaf-shaped and may even fuse to form short ridges. Histologically, moreover, they appear shorter and broader than their temperate counterparts. The cause of this geographical variation in jejunal morphology is not known.

The absorptive epithelial cells clothing the villi are formed in the crypts of Lieberkühn and gradually ascend the villi before becoming extruded into the lumen after a life-span of about 3 days. It is now known that these cells are the principal source of the digestive enzymes of the succus entericus, and that the final stage in the digestion of many nutrients takes place in the vicinity of the innumerable microvilli which form the epithelial surface. Malabsorptive disturbance may be caused by deficiency of intestinal enzymes, especially the disaccharidases.

Villous atrophy (Fig. 18.62) is the commonest pathological change in mucosal pattern. In the *partial* form (PVA) the villi show extensive fusion with the formation of long ridges or convolutions; histologically they appear shorter and broader than normal, although the crypts are enlarged and hyperplastic. The villous epithelium often shows degenerative change, and there is little doubt that the fundamental disturbance is a shortening of the life-span of these cells with compensatory hyperplasia of the generative crypt cells. There is often increased cellular infiltration in the lamina propria mucosae, plasma cells being most conspicuous. In the more severe *subtotal* form (SVA) villous fusion is more advanced and the mucosa appears completely flat both histologically and under the dissecting microscope. Epithelial degenerative changes are also more prominent.

Villous atrophy is not a specific change. It is however, characteristic of the two major primary malabsorption disorders, namely tropical sprue and coeliac disease, the latter being by far the commonest cause of severe villous atrophy in this country. Less often it is found following gastro-enteritis in childhood and in association with malignant lymphoma and skin diseases, especially dermatitis herpetiformis. Some

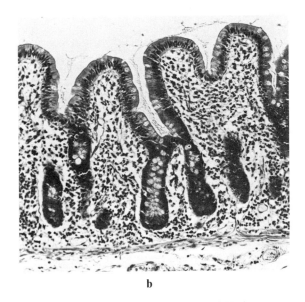

b

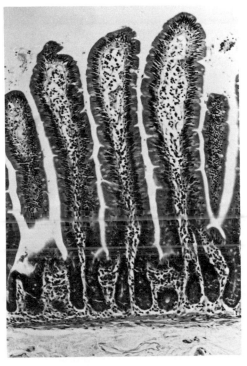

a

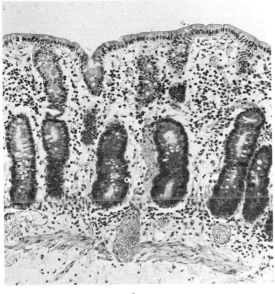

c

Fig. 18.62 Villous atrophy of jejunum: **a** normal jejunal mucosa; **b** partial villous atrophy; **c** subtotal villous atrophy. × 150. (Material obtained by peroral biopsy.)

degree of villous atrophy is also commonly associated with some forms of hypogammaglobulin-aemia, although this has been attributed to complicating giardiasis. In the tropics, kwashiorkor is a recognised cause of villous atrophy. Minor villous changes have also been described in many other diseases, although the association is inconstant and of dubious significance.

In malabsorptive states, intestinal biopsy may reveal other important pathological changes. The lesions of Whipple's disease (see below) and amyloidosis (p. 234) are unmistakable and congenital agammaglobulinaemia can be recognised by absence of plasma cells in the lamina propria. In the rare intestinal lymphangiectasia, there is diffuse dilatation of mucosal lymphatics which is associated with fat malabsorption, lymphopenia and protein-losing enteropathy (p. 580). Congenital absence of β-lipoprotein produces a complex syndrome in which there is a curious spiny abnormality of red cells (acanthocytosis), cerebellar dysfunction, retinal abnormality and fat malabsorption. Distension of villous epithelial cells by neutral fat, in an otherwise normal intestinal biopsy, is the diagnostic feature. It is unusual for Crohn's disease or tumour to be detected by biopsy techniques, although the rare, so-called Mediterranean type of intestinal lymphoma produces a typical appearance (p. 591). Intestinal parasites capable of causing malabsorption, e.g. *Giardia lamblia*, can be readily detected by intestinal biopsy as well as in the stools.

Classification of the causes of malabsorption is to some extent unsatisfactory, since in any one case several different mechanisms may be operating. Two main groups are, however, recognised mainly on the basis of the intestinal biopsy changes: (*a*) the *primary malabsorption disorders* in which there is diffuse villous atrophy of uncertain causation, and (*b*) *secondary malabsorption* which may complicate various diseases.

Primary malabsorptive disorders

This group includes *coeliac disease* (idiopathic steatorrhoea or gluten enteropathy), *tropical sprue* and the rare *Whipple's disease*.

Coeliac disease. This term is used to describe one of the most important causes of intestinal malabsorption in this country and includes both the childhood form of the disease and the adult condition formerly called idiopathic steatorrhoea. In this disease, malabsorption is characteristically associated with severe diffuse abnormalities of the intestinal mucosa, and withdrawal of the wheat protein gluten from the diet brings about both clinical and morphological remission. The mucosal abnormality takes the form of villous atrophy which is most marked, usually with almost complete disappearance of the villi, i.e. subtotal, in the proximal jejunum, and becomes progressively less severe, with only partial villous atrophy distally. Associated with this is pronounced plasma cell infiltration in the lamina propria and a marked increase in the number of lymphocytes between the surface epithelial cells. In some cases, especially those with a poor response to therapy, there is collagen deposition beneath the epithelial surface, but American workers regard this as a disease entity ('collagenous sprue') distinct from coeliac disease. Withdrawal of gluten leads to a reversal of the mucosal changes, initially in the distal small bowel and later in the upper jejunum which, particularly in adults, may never revert entirely to normal. It seems clear that gluten is in some way responsible for the mucosal damage, but the mechanism involved is not known. Coeliac disease has a familial tendency and patients have a strikingly high incidence of histocompatibility antigen HLA–A8. While an inherited enzyme defect cannot be discounted as a causative factor, it seems more likely that coeliac disease is caused by a genetically-determined abnormal immune response to gluten. Certainly the nature of the mucosal inflammatory reaction is consistent with this and a variety of immunological abnormalities, including auto-immune phenomena and impaired immune responses to exogenous antigens, have been described. Splenic atrophy is also a common complication (p. 506). There is an increased incidence of neoplasia of the alimentary tract, especially malignant lymphoma of the small bowel, possibly associated with a defect in the immunological surveillance mechanism (p. 268).

Tropical sprue is a disease encountered in certain areas in the tropics and sub-tropics, Africa being an exception. There is malabsorption resulting in severe emaciation and chronic diarrhoea, and anaemia which is often macrocytic may arise from deficiency of B_{12}, folate or both. Villous atrophy, usually partial and less often subtotal, is the characteristic change found at jejunal biopsy. This lesion, and the malabsorptive disturbance, are relieved by removal of the patient from the tropical environment and by oral broad-spectrum antibiotics, but a gluten-free diet has little or no beneficial effect. Folic acid may also cause some improvement. The cause of the disease remains uncertain, but it is likely that abnormal bacterial colonisation of the upper small bowel is implicated.

Whipple's disease. This rare and interesting disease affects mostly adult males in middle age. Malabsorption is usually the presenting feature, although other signs and symptoms such as generalised lymphadenopathy, arthropathy, skin pigmentation and chronic cough may be encountered. Jejunal biopsy is diagnostic: the mucosal lamina propria is stuffed with large granular macrophages containing material staining strongly with the periodic acid-Schiff technique for mucopolysaccharides (Fig. 18.63). The

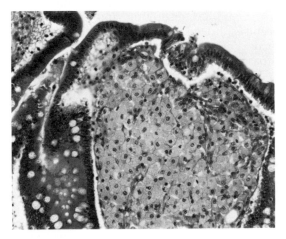

Fig. 18.63 Whipple's disease of small intestine, showing infiltration of the mucosa with granular macrophages. × 230.

regional lymph nodes, and occasionally other tissues, e.g. brain and heart valves, contain similar cells. Neutral fat accumulates in lymphatic channels. Electron microscopy has demonstrated that the abnormal macrophages contain unidentified bacteria and bacterial debris. Moreover, the disease responds to oral antibiotics. It would, however, be premature to assert that Whipple's disease is a form of specific infection, especially in view of the unusual age and sex incidence of the condition.

Secondary malabsorption

Numerous disease processes are capable of interfering with absorption. Most of these are discussed elsewhere, and only a brief account will be given here. Classification is most rationally based upon the mechanism thought to be mainly involved in causing malabsorption, although it should be appreciated that more than one mechanism may be operating in any individual disease.

(a) Chronic intestinal disease may cause malabsorption if extensive areas of the mucosa are affected. Examples of this include regional enteritis, tuberculosis, tumours, (especially malignant lymphoma), connective tissue disorders such as systemic sclerosis, radiation damage and amyloidosis.

(b) Abnormal bacterial proliferation in the small bowel interferes not only with the absorption of vitamin B_{12} but also to some extent with fat absorption. It results from stasis in the intestinal lumen, especially that produced by short-circuit operations which leave stagnant loops of bowel (**the blind-loop syndrome**). Stasis occurs also in jejunal diverticulosis (p. 570), in chronic intestinal obstruction, and in the blind loop resulting from some techniques of partial gastrectomy; malabsorption may complicate these conditions.

(c) Other mechanisms which may cause malabsorption include *biochemical defects* such as disaccharidase deficiency, agammaglobulinaemia and abetalipoproteinaemia; *endocrine disturbances*, including the carcinoid syndrome (p. 590) and the Zollinger–Ellison syndrome (p. 968); *lymphatic obstruction*, congenital or acquired, e.g. as a result of tuberculosis or tumour; *circulatory disturbance*, especially mesenteric vascular insufficiency; and *drug therapy*, e.g. phenindione, neomycin.

(d) Inadequate digestion must always be considered as a cause of malabsorption and may be due to disease of the liver and biliary tract or to pancreatic deficiency. Malabsorption following gastro-jejunostomy, alone or with partial gastrectomy, is largely a consequence of disordered digestion. There is inadequate mixing of food with pancreatic enzymes or bile as a result of interference with the normal anatomical relationships.

Intestinal Obstruction (Ileus)

Interference with the passage of the intestinal contents may be complete or incomplete, slowly or suddenly produced; it may occur in the small or in the large intestine and it may be brought about in a variety of ways, **mechanical**, **nervous** or **vascular**.

The following are the chief mechanical causes of intestinal obstruction:

(a) Constriction from outside—for example, by a hernial sac, by special conditions such as volvulus or intussusception, or by fibrous peritoneal adhesions. This is the commonest cause of acute mechanical obstruction.

(b) Stenosis caused by thickening and contraction of the wall is produced by diverticular disease, ischaemic stricture, Crohn's disease, tuberculosis and, of course, primary or secondary malignant tumours, most commonly carcinoma of the colon. The obstruction from these causes is ordinarily incomplete and chronic, but an acute state may be added by the impaction of inspissated faecal masses in the narrowed portion of bowel.

(c) Actual obstruction of the lumen. This may result from impaction of a large gallstone or other foreign body or by the growth of a tumour into the lumen, usually malignant but sometimes a benign polyp.

(d) Pressure from outside, for example by a large tumour in the pelvis; obstruction is not often complete from such a cause.

The *nervous type* of intestinal obstruction is called **paralytic** or **adynamic ileus** and may occur after handling of the intestines at operation, or it may result from peritonitis. The principal *vascular* lesions producing intestinal obstruction are occlusion of the mesenteric vessels by embolism or thrombosis. In the type of mechanical obstruction seen in group (*a*) above, vascular obstruction is commonly superadded and the subsequent course is then modified. When the blood supply is intact the obstruction is said to be **simple**, when it is impaired the term **strangulation** is applied.

The results of intestinal obstruction

The site of the obstruction plays an important part in determining both the effects and the prognosis. High intestinal obstruction is in general more acute in onset, more rapid in its progress and more likely to be complete than low intestinal obstruction which is usually of slow onset, is often incomplete and is less rapidly fatal.

Acute obstruction. When a portion of the small intestine is suddenly obstructed, e.g. by passing under a fibrous band, the part above contracts actively for a time and then passes into a condition of paralytic distension. There are probably both increased secretion from the wall and diminished absorption, and thus the bowel becomes distended with fluid contents in which there is abundant growth of bacteria. The fluid is passed back to the stomach by antiperistalsis and is vomited. Its exact composition depends on the site of the obstruction, but since nearly 8 litres of fluid are secreted into the gut daily, of which all but 100 ml are normally reabsorbed, the volume of fluid available for loss by vomiting or by pooling in the gut is obviously considerable.

If the obstruction is at the *pylorus* or *duodenum* the fluid lost is predominantly acid in reaction with a high Cl^- content. This results in a depletion of plasma chloride, and the urinary excretion of chlorides is then diminished or absent. Since sodium, the ion which normally balances the Cl^- ion, is not lost, carbonic acid is retained to take the place of the lost chloride and the plasma bicarbonate content therefore rises. This state of *alkalosis* is shown clinically by drowsiness and slow shallow respiration and can be demonstrated on analysis by a rise in the CO_2 combining power. A further complication is the development of *tetany* due to a fall in the ionised serum calcium, as a result of the alkalosis. Extracellular potassium deficiency may be superadded—*hypokalaemic alkalosis*. If the fluid loss is great enough, oliguria and extrarenal uraemia may follow, the blood urea being markedly raised terminally.

Obstruction in the *jejunum* results in the loss by vomiting of a fluid which contains saliva, gastric juice, bile, pancreatic juice and succus entericus. This leads to depletion of Na^+, K^+, and Cl^-. The CO_2 combining power remains normal, without marked disturbance of the acid-base balance. Although in high obstruction there is a tendency towards acidosis, it is the loss of fluid and electrolytes that leads rapidly to a fall in blood volume, dehydration, haemoconcentration and finally death. Fluid and electrolyte replacement is therefore essential to prolong life until surgical intervention can be undertaken.

Chronic obstruction. In low intestinal obstruction the absorptive area of the gut proximally is extensive, and depletion of water and electrolytes is often delayed. Ultimately, however, dehydration due to vomiting does take place and the vomitus becomes brown and foul-smelling—the so-called faecal or stercoral vomit. The dominant and dangerous factor in this form of obstruction is distension of the gut with fluid and with gas mainly derived from swallowed air. Prolonged increase of intraluminal pressure impairs the viability of the bowel wall, with subsequent diffusion of toxic bacterial products into the peritoneal cavity where they are absorbed and produce toxaemia and death. Relief of distension by intubation is thus critically important and sustains life until surgical intervention can be undertaken. The fluid lost by intubation is predominantly alkaline and this leads to acidosis and a low CO_2 combining power. Parenteral infusion of normal saline should thus be supplemented by lactate or carbonate. A further complicating factor is potassium depletion which leads to weakness and muscular paresis and may superimpose a state of adynamic ileus on the existing obstructive lesion (see below). In this context it must be appreciated that potassium is an intracellular ion and the plasma level does not reflect accurately the state of the cells. Caution must therefore be exercised in interpreting the biochemical analysis of the plasma as a basis for potassium replacement. In partial chronic obstruction, prolonged intermittent gut distension leads to hypertrophy of the bowel muscle proximal to the obstructive lesion. Also the pressure of faecal accumulation impairs mucosal viability and predisposes to bacterial invasion which leads to the formation of a mucosal exudate and ultimately to mucosal breakdown and ulceration. This so-called *stercoral ulceration* can take place some distance proximal to the obstruction and sometimes leads to perforation and faecal peritonitis. The effects of chronic stricture, especially in the colon, are aggravated if the regurgitation of faecal material proximally is prevented, for

example by an all too competent ileo-caecal valve (closed loop obstruction). In this situation stercoral ulceration is likely to occur in the caecum even when the stricture is in the distal colon, and the caecum may rupture.

Vascular causes. Apart from strangulation these are chiefly embolism or thrombosis of the superior mesenteric artery, but thrombosis of the mesenteric veins will produce the same result. This is sometimes seen when a thrombus occluding the portal vein extends backwards to obstruct the mouths of the splenic and superior mesenteric veins. Haemorrhagic infarction with gangrene of a segment of bowel quickly supervenes (Fig. 18.64), and death follows from toxic absorption and peritonitis.

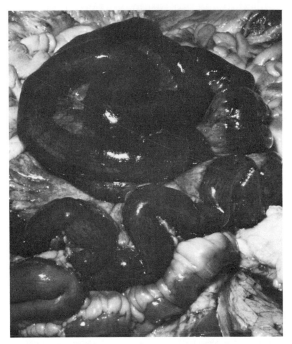

Fig. 18.64 Haemorrhagic infarction of the small intestine due to thrombosis of the superior mesenteric artery. The infarcted bowel is black and would soon have become gangrenous.

Paralytic ileus. In this condition the motor activity of the bowel is impaired without the presence of a physical obstruction. Sometimes it is due to over-activity of the sympathetic nervous system, and may then be relieved by antagonistic drugs, but in other cases toxic damage to the bowel muscle causes the paralysis. Lowering of the potassium level of the plasma greatly aggravates the condition. It is seen most often in association with peritonitis or it may follow operations on the abdomen, frequently of a minor nature. It may result also from intestinal infections or severe toxaemia. The whole intestine may be implicated and there may be a great distension of the bowel. The condition is serious and if untreated will result in death in much the same way as in acute mechanical obstruction. Following intubation and drainage of the distended bowel, its contractility may return, particularly if electrolyte and fluid balance can be restored.

Hernia

The term really means a rupture, but it is applied to any protrusion of a portion of viscus outside its natural cavity. Protrusion of the bowel usually occurs in a pouch of the peritoneum, which projects on the surface of the body, forming an *external hernia*. The term *internal hernia* is applied when the swelling does not present to an external surface. In the occurrence of hernia two prime factors are concerned, *local weakness* and *increased pressure*, the latter being usually brought about by muscular exertion, coughing or straining at stool. The local weakness is usually congenital, notably at the umbilicus or the inguinal canal; occasionally it results from the stretching of the scar of an operation wound—*incisional hernia*.

External hernias. The commonest are the *inguinal*, *femoral* and *umbilical*. Others, less common, are the *ventral*—through any portion of the abdominal wall other than the sites mentioned—*obturator*, etc. The inguinal herniae are of two varieties, the indirect, where the hernia follows the inguinal canal lateral to the inferior epigastric artery, and the direct, which passes medial to the latter vessel and comes through the external abdominal ring. The femoral hernia passes under Poupart's ligament medial to the femoral vessels. Examples of **internal hernia** are seen when the protrusion occurs through an aperture in the diaphragm, through the foramen of Winslow, or into a pouch in the jejunoduodenal fossa, the pouch then passing behind the peritoneum. In the ordinary external hernias, the contents are usually part of the small intestine, though in the larger ones omentum or other structures may be present. So long as it is possible to return the contents into the abdominal cavity, the hernia is termed **reducible**. When this is impossible owing either to the bulk of the contents or to adhesions which have formed, the hernia is said to be **impacted.**

The most serious result of hernia is strangulation, seen when the circulation in the protruded bowel is interrupted. This may occur by the addition of a fresh loop of bowel to the sac or by accumulation of faeces and gas. Strangulation may develop when the hernia is first formed, a portion of bowel being forced into a tight aperture; this is not uncommon in a femoral hernia. The changes following strangulation have already been described (p. 584).

Intussusception

In this condition one portion of the bowel is invaginated into the portion below. This usually has serious consequences and presents clinically as an acute surgical emergency. An exception to this is the multiple form observed quite often at necropsy, particularly in children dying from various causes, and presumably due to irregular bowel contraction around the time of death (agonal intussusception). The clinically important forms are also most often observed in infancy and early childhood. This is probably because the intestinal lymphoid tissue, especially in the distal ileum, is prone to undergo swelling in childhood, and because it protrudes into the intestinal lumen, is propelled distally by peristaltic activity. Viruses of the echo or adenovirus groups may be responsible for the lymphoid swelling and have been isolated from the intestinal contents and mesenteric lymph nodes in children with intussusception. An inverted Meckel's diverticulum projecting into the intestinal lumen also predisposes to intussusception, and in adults polypoid intestinal tumours are the usual cause.

Naked-eye appearances. In intussusception of the ordinary type three layers of bowel are seen on section, two layers formed by the doubling of the invaginated length of bowel, and one layer consisting of the wall of the bowel into which the invagination has occurred. Thus it consists of an entering tube, a returning tube and an ensheathing tube (Fig. 18.65). The commonest site is at the ileo-caecal valve, and usually the valve forms the apex of the intussusception and is passed along the large intestine. The

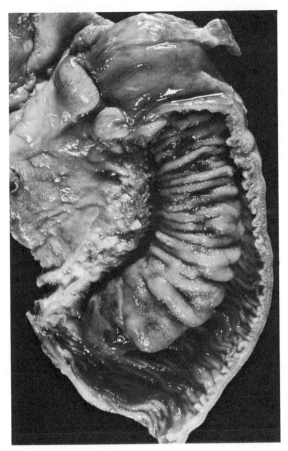

Fig. 18.65 Intussusception of the small intestine. The ensheathing section of gut has been cut open to show the invaginated loop, which is passing downward. The invaginated loop shows early haemorrhagic necrosis at the apex (near lower margin of excision) and near the entrance (at the top of the photograph).

apex may ultimately reach the rectum, and the whole lesion forms a fairly firm sausage-shaped mass, which is palpable during life. This type of intussusception is called **ileo-caecal**. More rarely the small intestine is passed through the orifice into the colon—**ileo-colic** type—and there may also be combinations of these two types with more complicated invaginations. For example, the ileo-caecal valve may be passed along for only a short distance, so that the tip of the appendix may be still visible, and then coils of the small intestine may be passed down through the valve and firmly impacted. Intussusception occurs in other situations, for example, in the small intestine or the transverse colon, but it is comparatively rare. Intussusception of

the appendix has been recorded, but it is very rare; it occurs chiefly in children.

Results. The important effects of intussusception are interference with the blood supply and mechanical obstruction of the bowel. The vessels of the invaginated part are stretched and also compressed; venous obstruction, oedema and extensive haemorrhage result. Accordingly the passage per anum of a mixture of blood and mucus is a common sign of intussusception, but pure blood may be passed. The haemorrhagic, ischaemic bowel becomes infarcted and gangrenous. At the point of entrance of the invaginated bowel into the ensheathing bowel, the serosal surfaces of the two, which are in contact, may become glued together by fibrinous exudate and prevent peritonitis. The gangrenous invaginated loop may then slough off and the fibrinous serosal adhesions organise. In this way, natural amputation and union may restore the continuity of the gut and effect cure. In most unoperated cases, however, death occurs from obstruction or from diffuse peritonitis. When a favourable result follows without operation, portions of sloughs from the dead bowel may be passed for a considerable time after the intussusception has occurred.

Volvulus

This is a condition in which a loop of bowel is twisted or rotated through 180° or more, so that obstruction and a varying degree of strangulation result (Fig. 18.66). It is most apt to occur when a loop has a long attachment and the ends are comparatively close together; rotation is then facilitated. Most cases involve the sigmoid colon, and the occurrence of the volvulus is aided by a long mesocolon and by a loaded sigmoid due to constipation. Usually the upper part of the sigmoid passes forwards and downwards to lie in front of the upper part of the rectum. Once the twist has occurred, passage of faeces is prevented. The bowel becomes more and more distended, the venous return is interfered with and the wall becomes congested, haemorrhagic and ultimately gangrenous. In some cases a portion of bowel is found to be enormously distended, filling a large part of the abdominal cavity. Volvulus of the small intestine may occur also, but it is less common; the favouring conditions are the same, and sometimes the approximation of the

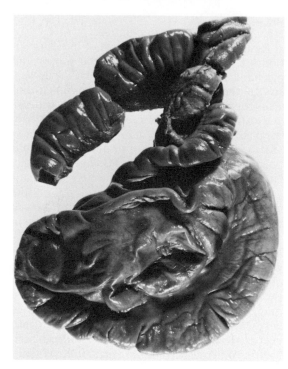

Fig. 18.66   Volvulus of sigmoid colon.

ends of the loop is due to local adhesions around calcified mesenteric lymph nodes. In children, however, volvulus of the small bowel is much commoner than in adults. More rarely two loops of intestine become intertwined and then the symptoms are very severe.

Intestinal obstruction by foreign bodies

The most common cause of this type of obstruction is a large composite gallstone, which has entered the duodenum through a fistulous track developing between gallbladder and bowel; commonly there is little or no history of symptoms to indicate cholelithiasis. The calculus passes along the intestine but may become impacted at some point. Even the largest stone is smaller than the diameter of the fully relaxed bowel, so muscle spasm must contribute to the impaction, which usually occurs about a metre proximal to the ileocaecal valve. Unmasticated food may act similarly, for example obstruction of the ileum by a mass of dried fruit. Gastro-enterostomy predisposes to the passage of large masses of undigested food into the intestine, and thus to obstruction.

Hirschsprung's disease

This is a rare congenital condition characterised by an enormous accumulation of faeces in the greatly enlarged colon which comes to occupy much of the swollen abdomen. There may be periods of weeks or months without defaecation, and repeated attacks of obstruction. The distension may extend as far as the caecum, but at first affects mainly the lower colon. The grossly hypertrophied and dilated colon tapers rather abruptly into a narrow rectal segment joining sigmoid to anus. There is congenital absence of the para-sympathetic ganglion cells of both Auerbach's and Meissner's plexuses for a distance of 5–20 cm below the dilated sigmoid, i.e. corresponding to the narrow segment of rectum. In consequence there is overaction of the sympathetic, which normally inhibits the propulsive contraction of the intestinal wall and stimulates contraction of the internal anal sphincter. The disease is thus one of neuromuscular incoordination. While lumbar sympathectomy has proved helpful in some cases, the results have not always been permanent and excision of the defective narrow segment and anastomosis of the sigmoid to the anus has proved more effective.

Tumours of the Intestines

Small intestine

For reasons which are obscure, the small bowel has a surprisingly low incidence of clinically important tumours. Epithelial neoplasms of the small bowel, for example, account for less than 2% of all intestinal (including colonic) tumours.

Nevertheless the tumours that do arise form an interesting group.

Carcinoid tumour (argentaffinoma)

This arises from certain specialised cells, which, although located within the epithelial surface of the gastro-intestinal tract, are thought by many to be of neural crest origin. These cells belong to a widely distributed family of cells subserving an endocrine function and sometimes referred to as **apud cells**, an acronym derived from the property common to all cells of the system, namely, **a**mine-**p**recursor **u**ptake and **d**ecarboxylation. Most members of the group, however, also produce polypeptide hormones. While tumours arising from these endocrine cells have been given the generic name **apudoma**, those occurring in the gut are more commonly called **carcinoid tumours**, since in the appendix (their commonest site of origin) they are clinically benign despite an appearance of infiltration resembling carcinoma. Both in the appendix and in the ileum, which is also a common primary site, carcinoid tumours arise from the most distinctive intestinal representative of the apud system, namely the *argentaffin cell*, so named because of its capacity to form cytoplasmic deposits of metallic silver from silver salts. This histologically demonstrable property is related to its secretion of 5-hydroxytryptamine (5HT). Carcinoids only rarely occur in the stomach and large intestine, and in these sites they may arise from a different member of the apud sys-

tem, since the cells often fail to show the argentaffin reaction and only deposit the silver when an external reducing agent is applied (argyrophilia). Carcinoid tumours are usually found by chance in or near the tip of appendixes removed surgically, often for acute appendicitis. Although sometimes only a few millimetres in diameter, they can occlude the distal lumen of the appendix and have a distinctive yellowish-brown colour.

In the small intestine, especially in the lower ileum, carcinoids are commonly multiple. They form small button-like swellings in the mucosa, one or more of which shows deep penetration of the muscular wall which may be locally hypertrophied (Fig. 18.67). Lymphatic invasion is often widespread in the affected segment. Ileal carcinoids are not benign like those in the appendix, and as a consequence both intestinal obstruction (Fig. 18.68) and metastases to the mesenteric lymph nodes and liver occur; characteristically these secondary deposits grow exceedingly slowly.

Microscopically, carcinoid tumours consist of small clear cells, closely packed in alveolar

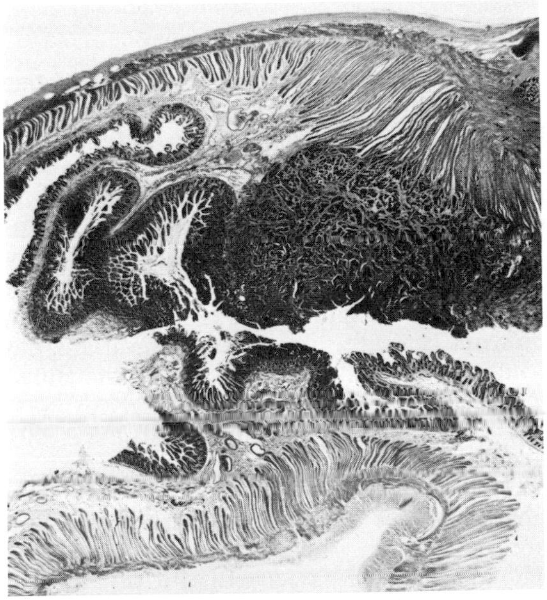

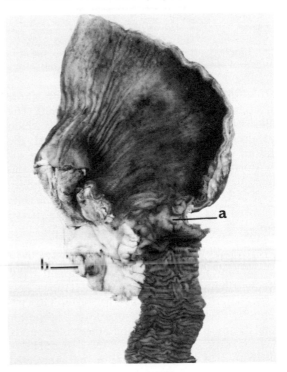

Fig. 18.67 Carcinoid tumour of ileum, seen as the darkly-stained tissue invading the circular muscle coat, which is greatly hypertrophied, and causing stenosis. There were hepatic metastases and the carcinoid syndrome developed. × 2·5.

Fig. 18.68 Carcinoid tumour of ileum causing obstruction. Note the dilatation and hypertrophy of the bowel above the tumour **a** and secondary deposit in the mesenteric lymph node **b**.

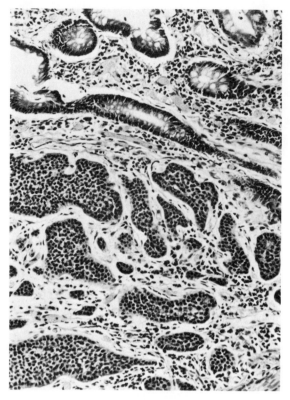

Fig. 18.69 Carcinoid tumour of ileum, showing clumps of small polygonal epithelial cells infiltrating the mucosa. × 125.

formation (Fig. 18.69), throughout the whole thickness of the appendicular or ileal wall. The yellowish colour is due to lipids, some of which are doubly refracting. As stated above, the tumour cells contain granules which reduce silver salts—hence called argentaffin cells. In the appendix, carcinoid tumours are commonly related to old inflammatory lesions and the cells are often associated with proliferated nerve fibres.

The carcinoid syndrome. Large hepatic secondary growths of carcinoid tumours are sometimes, but not invariably, accompanied by attacks of flushing of the face, diarrhoea and bronchospasm. There may also be pulmonary stenosis. These effects are due to the secretion of large amounts of 5HT and other compounds by metastatic tumour cells in the liver. 5HT is inactivated by amine oxidase in the liver cells, and so long as the tumour is confined to the drainage area of the portal circulation systemic effects are not produced. Hepatic metastases, however, set free 5HT into the systemic cir-

culation. 5HT is a potent vasodilator, and smooth-muscle stimulant; it may also stimulate fibroblastic proliferation and so cause the subendocardial fibrosis in the right atrium and ventricle and the pulmonary stenosis which is a late feature of the syndrome. The left side of the heart is less often involved, since 5HT is inactivated also in the lungs. Excessive diversion of tryptophane to the metabolism of massive secondary deposits may induce symptoms of pellagra. 5HT is converted by the enzyme amine-oxidase to 5-hydroxyindoleacetic acid (5HIAA), which is excreted in the urine where its quantitative estimation affords a valuable clinical test for the presence of large argentaffin tumours. The flushing attacks are often precipitated by alcohol or sympathetic stimulation: they are not due to 5HT, but probably to kallikrein, which is also secreted by the tumour cells, and activates the kinin system (p. 43).

Carcinoid tumours of the bronchi (p. 447) secrete 5-hydroxytryptophane, possibly because they lack the enzyme decarboxylase required to convert this substance to 5HT. Carcinoids of the stomach may also secrete histamine in addition to 5HT and kallikrein. Colonic carcinoid tumours rarely give rise to the syndrome.

Other tumours of the small intestine

Connective tissue tumours. Members of this group, such as leiomyoma, lymphangioma and lipoma, are quite common but seldom cause symptoms unless they protrude into the intestinal lumen and produce intussusception. Occasionally a leiomyoma ulcerates and leads to intestinal blood loss and iron-deficiency anaemia. *Leiomyosarcoma*, the only malignant tumour of this group that is at all common, presents clinically like its benign variant but tends to recur after operation and sometimes metastasises to the liver.

The Peutz–Jeghers syndrome. This interesting hereditary disorder is transmitted as a Mendelian dominant of high penetrance. Multiple polypi of highly differentiated structure are found in the small intestine, especially the jejunum, and are associated with pronounced melanotic pigmentation of the lips and oral mucosa which is the key to diagnosis. The polyps cause recurring attacks of intussusception and sometimes iron deficiency anaemia due to blood loss, but rarely if ever undergo malignant transformation; indeed they are perhaps better regarded as hamartomatous (p. 297) rather than truly neoplastic in nature.

Carcinoma. This is surprisingly uncommon in the small bowel, being rather less frequently encountered than lymphoid tumours. Length for length, the proximal parts of the small bowel are more often affected than the distal. In appearance and behaviour carcinomas of the small intestine are very similar to those of the colon (p. 593). Intestinal obstruction and the effects of haemorrhage are the most common modes of presentation, but diagnosis is not often made early enough to allow curative excision. The causal factors are unknown, although occasionally carcinoma arises as a complication of a primary malabsorptive disorder.

Lymphoid neoplasms. Although generalised forms of lymphoma may metastasise to the intestinal tract, it is important to realise that lymphomas may arise primarily in the small intestine, where they are at least as common as carcinomas. These primary intestinal lymphomas, which may be multiple, ulcerate deeply (Fig. 18.76) and frequently cause perforation, less often intestinal obstruction; most are lymphoblastic lymphomas of B lymphocyte derivation; indeed many show extensive plasma-cell differentiation. Malabsorption is sometimes a feature, and it has been suggested that coeliac disease predisposes to the development of lymphoid neoplasia, and occasionally carcinoma. Malabsorption can, however, result from neoplasia, as in the peculiar form of intestinal lymphoma described in young adults mainly of East Mediterranean origin. The entire mucosa of the small bowel is swollen by a diffuse pleomorphic infiltrate of plasma cells, lymphocytes, eosinophils and undifferentiated lymphoid cells. The neoplastic condition called *α-chain disease* is probably a variant of this 'Mediterranean lymphoma', the distinctive feature being that the tumour cells, which tend to be more differentiated, produce the heavy chain of IgA immunoglobulin (p. 499).

Large intestine

Although connective tissue tumours and lymphomas are rare in the large intestine, both benign and malignant epithelial tumours are all too common and constitute a major problem in terms of management and prevention.

Benign neoplastic polyp

This term is used to include all benign epithelial colonic tumours. They present a spectrum of pathological features. At one end is the **polypoid adenoma** which is globular in shape, has a smooth surface and is usually pedunculated (Fig. 11.6, p. 275): it has a wide distribution in the colon and consists histologically of neoplastic glands which show a variable degree of epithelial de-differentiation as revealed by nuclear hyperchromatism and loss of polarity. In contrast, the **villous papilloma** is usually an extensive sessile growth with a frond-like structure (Fig. 11.5, p. 275) and shows a predilection for the rectum: the fronds are lined by mucin-secreting epithelium; indeed excessive mucin secretion may be associated with potassium loss per rectum with resulting muscular weakness due to hypokalaemia. Many neoplastic polyps, however, show a mixed villous and adenomatous structure. In spite of their name, benign neoplastic polyps as a group show a tendency to malignant transformation. This is supported by the degree of epithelial de-differentiation observed in many of them and by the high frequency of finding one or more polyps in colons excised for carcinoma; the association of polyps with carcinoma is particularly strong in *polyposis coli* (see below). More direct evidence is provided by early carcinomatous change with invasion found in some neoplastic polyps (Fig. 18.70). Nevertheless, simple excision of a benign polyp by transection of the base is usually curative providing that it can be shown histologically that the pedicle or base is free of neoplastic epithelium. It is sometimes claimed that the villous papilloma carries a greater risk of malignant change than the other types of neoplastic polypi. Possibly, however, this is related to tumour size, for neoplastic polypi of less than 1 cm in diameter are rarely found to have undergone malignant change, and villous papillomas are often much larger than this before they are detected clinically.

Polyposis coli. This hereditary disorder is usually transmitted by either sex as a Mendelian dominant but in some families either

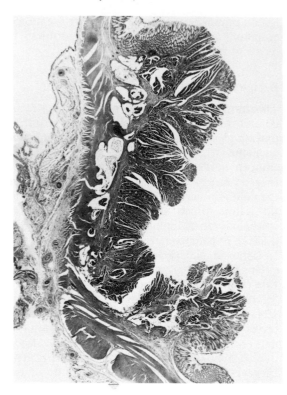

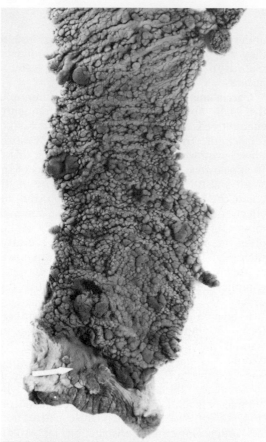

Fig. 18.70 Villous papilloma of rectum. There is early malignant infiltration of the wall by mucoid carcinoma. × 3.

with very poor penetrance or as a recessive character. It is characterised by the development of hundreds of adenomatous polyps in the large intestine (Fig. 18.71). The condition does not usually appear until late childhood or early adult life. Since each of the many polyps appears to share the predisposition to become malignant, the onset of carcinoma of the colon is almost inevitable, usually about 15 years after the development of symptoms of polyposis.

Other polypoid lesions are encountered in the large bowel, and are not to be confused with the true tumours already described. The **metaplastic polyp** is a small, raised, pale, sessile lesion not infrequently encountered in middle or later adult life. Histologically there is localised papilliform hyperplasia of the epithelium lining the surface and upper parts of the crypts. This lesion lacks the hyperchromatism of the polypoid adenoma and does not appear to be premalignant. In childhood, globular polypoid lesions, sometimes quite large, are encountered in the rectum: histologically they consist of

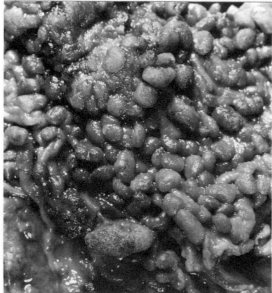

Fig. 18.71 Polyposis coli. *Above,* innumerable small polyps and several larger ones are present. Two small cancers have developed just above the anal margin. × 0·5. *Below,* showing the appearance of the individual polyps. × 2·5.

intensely inflamed mucosa in which the crypts are markedly dilated and cystic, and are frequently ulcerated. Usually referred to as **juvenile polyps**, they do not show epithelial de-differentiation and are probably inflammatory in nature. Apart from polyposis coli, true adenomatous polyps are seldom observed in children. Finally, mention must be made of the condition known as **benign lymphoid polyposis of the rectum**, in which multiple polypi, consisting of masses of lymphoid tissue, showing numerous germinal centres and covered by normal rectal epithelium, develop in the rectum especially in young women. The condition is of unknown causation but, as the name implies, does not have malignant potential.

Carcinoma of the large intestine

This is one of the commoner malignant tumours. It occurs mainly among older people. The rectum is the commonest site, especially in males; next follows the sigmoid colon, the caecum and ileo-caecal valve and the flexures. The overall incidence is about the same for males and females.

Aetiology is largely unknown, although carcinoma of the large bowel is principally a disease of urban communities. As already explained, benign neoplastic polyps (especially polyposis coli) and ulcerative colitis are predis-

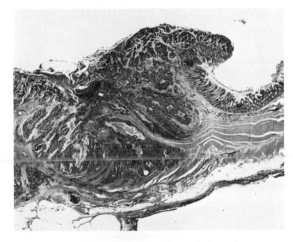

Fig. 18.72 A longitudinal section of the colon passing through the edge of an ulcerated carcinoma. The muscular coat (right) proximal to the tumour is hypertrophied; the tumour has a raised margin and an ulcerated centre (left) and has penetrated through the wall to the serosa. × 5.

posing conditions. In ulcerative colitis, and in polyposis coli, carcinoma tends to develop 10–15 years after the onset and thus may affect relatively young individuals.

Naked-eye appearances. When carcinoma begins in an adenomatous polyp, infiltration of the stalk and base occurs so that the tumour appears like a button fixed to the bowel wall; subsequently the centre breaks down leaving a necrotic ulcer with raised everted ('rolled') edges (Fig. 18.72). The base is then fixed to the muscular coat, which is ultimately breached by progressive ulceration. Spread in the submucous and subserous lymphatics also occurs so that the tumour gradually encircles the bowel wall. The majority of cancers of the colon are scirrhous, and cause contraction and stricture; some, however, are soft and fungating, and others are mucoid and gelatinous. The more slowly growing types especially tend to encircle the bowel, forming a ring-shaped growth and thus producing narrowing or complete obstruction. The bowel above the obstruction undergoes great, sometimes enormous dilatation, while its wall becomes hypertrophied (Fig. 18.73). The pressure of the contained faeces interferes with the nourishment of the mucosa and a pseudomembranous inflammation may be superadded. In other cases, the wall becomes thinned and so-called stercoral ulceration may follow, and may undergo perforation with resulting peritonitis. The softer type of cancer forms an irregular mass which in its turn may bring about obstruction by projecting into the lumen (Fig. 18.74). The mucoid type may, as in the stomach, lead to widespread infiltration and thickening of the wall, and may give rise to secondary tumours in the peritoneum.

Microscopic appearances. Practically all intestinal cancers are adenocarcinomas, some being highly differentiated, while others are anaplastic and the arrangement of the cells is irregular (Fig. 11.12, p. 279). This is the usual variety that complicates ulcerative colitis.

Spread and prognosis. These tumours tend to spread circumferentially in the wall of the large intestine and also directly through the wall to the serosa. Occasionally extensive spread occurs in the peritoneal cavity. Lymphatic spread, with metastases in the mesocolic lymph nodes, often occurs quite early, while blood spread to the liver or elsewhere is usually relatively late. Using *Duke's staging*, patients in which the

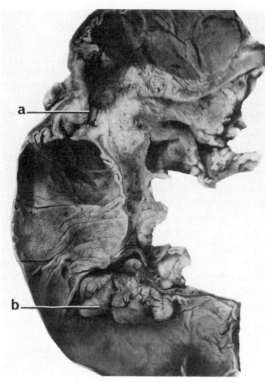

Fig. 18.73   Carcinomatous stricture **(a)** of the colon: note proximal hypertrophy of the colon wall. There is also a polypoid adenoma **(b)** distil to the carcinoma.

tumour is confined to the intestine (stage A) have a cure rate approaching 100%, unless the tumour has penetrated the whole thickness of the wall (stage B), when the cure rate falls to 70%. Lymph-node metastases (stage C) reduce the cure rate to approximately 30%.

Colonic carcinomas are among the tumours which secrete a glycoprotein (**carcino-embryonic antigen** or **CEA**) which is produced also by normal fetal endodermal tissues (p. 268). Detection of CEA in the serum has not provided a reliable diagnostic test, for it is present in trace amounts in the serum of normal subjects and in increased amounts in various types of cancer, in inflammatory bowel disease and in some other non-neoplastic conditions. Nevertheless, assay of CEA may be helpful in the management of patients with carcinoma, for the level falls after removal of the tumour and a subsequent increase suggests recurrence or metastases.

Other malignant tumours

Smooth muscle tumours, some of which are malignant, are rare. Malignant lymphomas occur, particularly in the caecum and rectum, but

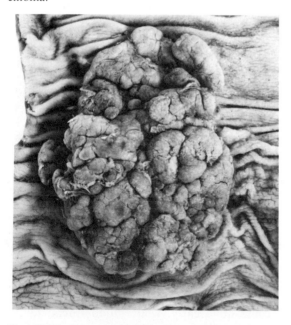

Fig. 18.74   Large polypoid adenocarcinoma of the descending colon. × 1.

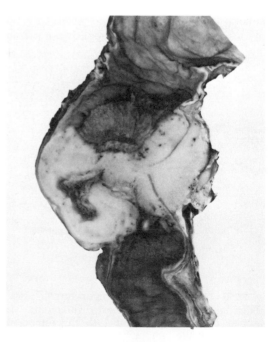

Fig.   18.75   Lymphosarcoma   of   the   ileo-caecal region.

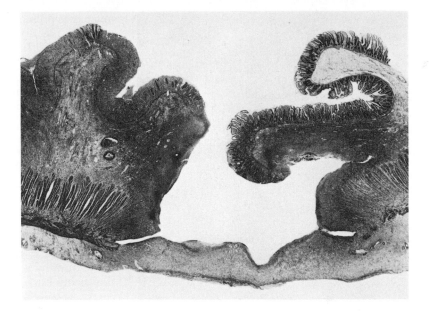

Fig. 18.76 Lymphosarcoma of small intestine, showing deep but sharply localised ulcerative penetration of the wall. × 6·5.

are less common than in the small intestine. They may form a large mass and cause obstruction (Fig. 18.75) or ulcerate and sometimes perforate.

Tumours of the anal canal

Malignant tumours are uncommon. Most are *squamous carcinomas*, often with a 'basaloid' pattern, i.e. resembling rodent ulcer: some show a mixture of squamous and mucin-secreting elements (*muco-epidermoid carcinoma*). These tumours all tend to metastasise to both pelvic and inguinal nodes, and the prognosis is then poor. *Malignant melanoma* also occurs

in the anal canal, where it is almost always fatal.

Secondary tumours of the intestines

Apart from invasion by peritoneal and lymphatic spread, intestinal metastases are extremely uncommon, though metastatic melanoma is seen occasionally, and also the lymphoid neoplasm *struma reticulosa* of the thyroid (p. 963) has a notable tendency to metastasise to the gut. The peritoneum is a common site for secondary carcinoma (p. 599) and the bowel may become invaded from the serous surface and its lumen considerably contracted.

Congenital Abnormalities

The commonest of these is the **Meckel's diverticulum**, which represents the proximal end of the omphalomesenteric duct. The diverticulum usually measures about 2–3 cm in length, and is narrower than the small intestine (Fig. 18.77). Occasionally it is adherent at the umbilicus and in some cases a fistula is present; or again, there may be obstruction at the proximal end, sometimes merely by a fold, and accumulation

of mucus occurs so that an *enterocyst* results. A Meckel's diverticulum rarely leads to any serious results, but when it is adherent it may cause volvulus of the small intestine or, even more serious, strangulation. Acute inflammation of a Meckel's diverticulum presents features similar to those of acute appendicitis, and requires similar surgical treatment. Sometimes heterotopic acid-secreting gastric

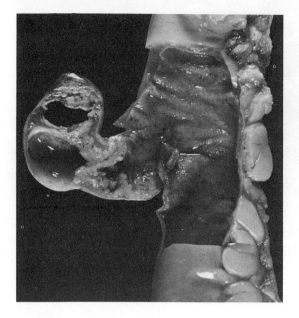

Fig. 18.77 Meckel's diverticulum. In this instance there was pancreatic tissue in the wall and a cystic space.

mucosa is present and may lead to peptic ulceration of the diverticulum with perforation or haemorrhage. In the adult the diverticulum occurs usually about a metre above the ileo-caecal valve, and at about half that distance in young children. Carcinoma has very rarely been observed to develop in the apex of a Meckel's diverticulum.

Stenosis or actual **atresia** may occasionally occur in the intestines. In the small intestine, the commonest site is at the orifice of the common bile duct or at the ileo-caecal valve. Part of the intestine may be absent, usually along with other malformations. The commonest site of atresia, however, is at the lower end of the rectum. Sometimes a dimple in the skin, representing the anus, is separated from the lower end of the rectum by a thin layer of tissue—the condition being known as **imperforate anus**. In other cases, however, there may be atresia of the lower end of the rectum, the lower end of the bowel sometimes communicating with the bladder or urethra in the male and with the vagina in the female.

V The Peritoneum

Acute peritonitis

Because it contains the gastro-intestinal tract, with its heavy bacterial flora, the peritoneal cavity is liable to bacterial infection, and because of its potential volume and large surface area, acute bacterial infection of the whole peritoneal cavity is a severe, often fatal condition. It is therefore not surprising that the cavity is guarded by potent defence mechanisms. Like other serosal membranes, there are a large number of readily available macrophages in or on the endothelial lining. These cells are particularly numerous in the omentum, in which they are aggregated in visible 'milk spots'. Even the mild irritation of perfusion by 'physiological' solutions, as in peritoneal dialysis, releases huge numbers of macrophages into the cavity. This phenomenon does not, of course, exclude the usual emigration of polymorphs and subsequently monocytes from the venules in the inflamed peritoneal surfaces. A

second important defence mechanism is localisation of an infected focus by the omentum and adjacent viscera. These tissues become glued together by fibrin deposition on their surfaces and so tend to wall off the site of infection from the rest of the cavity.

Causes. Acute bacterial peritonitis is nearly always due to infection from one of the abdominal viscera, in most instances the gastro-intestinal tract. Any breach in the integrity or viability of the wall of the tract is likely to cause local or general peritonitis. The list of causes is thus long. The commonest of all in this country is acute appendicitis, but perforation of a peptic ulcer and acute diverticulitis are also frequent causes. Others include perforation of typhoid ulcers, usually in the ileum; rupture of the large intestine proximal to an obstruction or in acute ulcerative colitis; penetrating abdominal wounds; perforation of an ulcerated tumour of the intestine, particularly a lymphoma; devitalisation of the gut due to mesenteric vascular thrombosis; or strangulation of part of the gut by herniation, volvulus, etc.

Acute peritonitis can also arise from an acutely infected gallbladder, either by rupture of the wall or spread of the bacteria through it. Acute haemorrhagic pancreatitis, acute salpingitis and acute cystitis may also result in peritonitis. Haematogenous peritonitis is relatively uncommon.

Appearances. The features of acute peritonitis depend on the types of bacteria responsible and the nature of the causal lesion. When the infection is due to escape of bacteria from the gut, the infection is likely to be a mixed one, although one or other species of bacteria may predominate. *Escherichia coli* infection is extremely common, either alone or associated with the other species. Various streptococci, including anaerobes, and *Clostridium welchii*, *Bacteroides*, and various Gram −ve bacilli are all encountered. Pneumococcal peritonitis used to be encountered in young girls, but is not often seen now in this country.

When virulent bacteria enter the peritoneum, or when heavy infection occurs, as in perforation of an ulcer or gangrenous appendicitis, general peritonitis is likely to result. With less virulent bacteria or more gradual infection, the spread may be limited, either by rapid elimination of the bacteria or by formation of fibrinous adhesions around the infected site.

In **generalised peritonitis**, the surfaces are inflamed and the exudate varies in amount and appearance. In haemolytic streptococcal peritonitis, formerly a common puerperal infection, there may be only a little serous or haemorrhagic exudate. With coliform bacilli and the other bacteria mentioned above, exudate is usually more abundant and turbid or frankly purulent, and there is usually a deposit of fibrin on the serosal surfaces. When peritonitis has resulted from perforation of a peptic ulcer, there may be accumulation of air beneath the diaphragm, detectable by radiography: the leakage of acid gastric juice results in a haemorrhagic exudate, and this is seen also when there has been leakage of bile. In acute haemorrhagic pancreatitis the affected surfaces show fat necrosis and the exudate is haemorrhagic: the changes may be generalised or limited to the lesser sac.

The appearances of **localised peritonitis** depend on the causal organisms and the site affected. If infection is mild, it may resolve without suppuration, although there may be residual adhesions; this is seen when gonococcal salpingitis progresses to pelvic peritonitis. Frequently, however, local acute peritonitis results in suppuration as, for example, when an acutely inflamed appendix becomes surrounded by omentum, loops of gut, etc., and a peri-appendicular abscess results: this may occur also in relation to an acutely inflamed diverticulum, or when perforation of a peptic ulcer occurs in the lesser sac.

General peritonitis may be overcome, and yet leave residual foci of infection, e.g. a collection of pus in the pelvis or between the liver and diaphragm (subphrenic abscess) walled off by adhesions between adjacent structures.

Effects. Acute generalised peritonitis is an extremely serious, often fatal condition, firstly

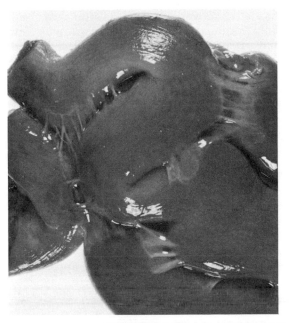

Fig. 18.78 Fibrous adhesions between loops of small intestine, resulting from organisation of fibrin deposited during acute peritonitis.

because the cavity is so large and has such a great surface area from which toxins are absorbed, and secondly because the intestines bathed in bacterial toxins are very likely to develop paralytic ileus (p. 586). These factors result in severe toxaemia and also gross dehydration and disturbance of electrolyte and acid–base balances from loss of fluid into the peritoneal exudate, the paralysed gut, and by vomiting. The result is a combination of endotoxic and hypovolaemic shock which is very likely to be fatal unless effectively treated. In many instances, bacteraemia or septicaemia develops.

The organs show evidence of toxic change, and in particular there is usually focal or zonal necrosis of liver cells.

Recovery may be complicated by residual abscesses, as mentioned above, or by organisation of deposited fibrin to form fibrous adhesions between loops of gut (Fig. 18.78) and the parietal peritoneum, etc.: such adhesions carry a risk of subsequent intestinal obstruction by kinking of the gut or internal hernia.

Chronic peritonitis

As stated above, abscess formation may result from localised or generalised peritonitis, and may persist for weeks or months unless drained. As elsewhere, the persistent abscess becomes enclosed in dense fibrous tissue, which may interfere with the function of the loops of intestine usually forming the wall.

Tuberculous peritonitis is much less common than formerly: it may be general or localised. The origin of the generalised type may be a caseous lymph node in tabes mesenterica, or the bacilli may reach the peritoneum from a tuberculous Fallopian tube, either directly through its covering or by way of its abdominal opening. In other cases where no gross lesion can be found, the infection is probably by the bloodstream, a small focus forming from which dissemination afterwards occurs. The appearances vary widely in different cases. There may be an eruption of minute grey tubercles all over the peritoneum, with or without a sero-fibrinous effusion. The omentum is often extensively involved and forms a large mass across the upper part of the abdomen. In other cases, there may be caseation, either in scattered foci or diffusely. Lastly, cases are encountered in which the tubercles are comparatively scanty and where the chief result is formation of adhesions, sometimes with serous effusion between them. When chronic tuberculous peritonitis is associated with ulcers of the intestine,

ulceration between adjacent loops of the bowel may lead to the formation of multiple fistulae, and may result in the malabsorption syndrome.

Non-bacterial peritonitis

As already mentioned, acute peritonitis results from the irritant effect of gastric juice or bile when these escape into the peritoneal cavity, and also from leaking pancreatic enzymes in acute pancreatitis. All these conditions are likely to be complicated by the supervention of bacterial peritonitis.

There are a number of miscellaneous conditions in which chronic peritonitis or fibrous thickening of the peritoneum occurs in the absence of bacterial infection.

The former use of *talc* to lubricate surgical gloves led, in some instances, to the development of a granulomatous peritoneal reaction with consequent fibrous adhesions. Peritoneal involvement by *carcinoma*, e.g. from the stomach, colon or ovary, often results in an inflammatory exudate and adhesions (see below). The term *chronic hyperplastic peritonitis* is sometimes used to describe hyaline fibrous thickening of the visceral peritoneum, often over the liver and spleen, but sometimes also the omentum and mesentery. It is usually accompanied by ascites. The term 'sugar-iced liver' (Zuckergussleber) has been applied: in appearance, it resembles the hyaline pleural plaques attributable to inhalation of asbestos, and indeed this may be the cause in some cases. Hyaline thickening involving all the serous sacs is sometimes called *Concato's disease*, while involvement of the pericardium and hepatic peritoneum is termed *Pick's disease*. Very striking thickening of the posterior peritoneum may also occur in the carcinoid syndrome, possibly due to a desmoplastic effect of 5HT (p. 590).

Retroperitoneal fibrosis

In this condition, there is extensive formation of fibrous tissue retroperitoneally. It tends to cause trouble by constricting the ureters. While the aetiology is not known, the condition has been associated with Riedel's thyroiditis, and also with taking the drug methysergide.

Ascites

Serous effusion into the peritoneum occurs in cases of general oedema of both the cardiac and renal types, and is sometimes abundant; some fluid may accumulate also in severe anaemias and wasting diseases. The most severe ascites, however, results from portal obstruction, and the accumulation of fluid often leads to enormous distension of the abdomen: the commonest cause is cirrhosis of the liver, and in cases which develop primary liver cancer, thrombosis of the portal vein often occurs, the ascitic fluid then accumulating very rapidly and becoming bloodstained. Ascites *may* sometimes result from conditions outside the liver which lead to pressure on the portal vein, such as tumour growth, chronic inflammation with contraction, etc., but it does not necessarily follow them, and in portal vein thrombosis with cavernous transformation there may be little or no ascites. Ascites is always most severe and intractable

peritoneum—for example, disseminated carcinoma or tuberculosis; in such cases there is usually an inflammatory reaction and the fluid is at least partly an inflammatory exudate, though the protein content is relatively small. Polymorphonuclear leukocytes are then found, and not infrequently there is blood in the fluid.

Tumours

Primary tumours of the peritoneum are rare, and in most cases they take origin not from the serous layer but from some adjacent structure. For example, *lipoma* may arise from the *appendices epiploicae*; *fibroma* takes origin from the connective tissue and sometimes from the sheaths of the nerves in *neurofibromatosis*; and *lymphangioma* occasionally arises from the lymphatics of the mesentery. *Mesothelioma* of the peritoneum presents features like those of

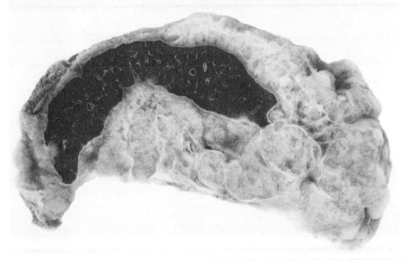

Fig. 18.79 Section of the spleen embedded in a large mass of mucoid carcinoma.

when the site of obstruction is intrahepatic, as in portal cirrhosis. Thus endophlebitis of the hepatic veins (Chiari's syndrome) is accompanied by pronounced ascites. In the above conditions the fluid is a transudate and there is no formation of fibrin in the peritoneum, but in cases of portal cirrhosis it is not uncommon for a mild infection to become superadded, and occasionally this is tuberculous. Ascites may also result from some lesion of the

mesothelioma of the pleura but is less frequent, and the same caution in the interpretation of the appearances is required. In both situations there is an association with inhalation of asbestos (p. 447).

Secondary tumours of the peritoneum are comparatively frequent, especially from gastric and ovarian carcinoma. They may be extremely numerous and very minute, often producing a haemorrhagic and inflammatory reaction; or there may be larger nodules and diffuse infiltration. The omentum is very frequently involved and becomes contracted into a hard irregular mass. In some cases of cancer the chief lesion is a very diffuse infiltration with thickening of the serous layers, but with little nodular formation; by such a process the mesentery may become greatly thickened and shrunken. This often results from *linitis plastica* of the stomach, and is accompanied by marked ascites. In mucoid carcinoma the peritoneum is sometimes overgrown by enormous soft translucent tumour masses (Fig. 18.79). Metastases of melanoma are not infrequent and the peritoneum may be studded with enormous numbers of small black nodules; these tend to be specially numerous in the omentum and mesentery.

As in the other serous cavities, the lining cells may desquamate and multiply in ascitic fluid, sometimes developing bizarre morphological features which make them very difficult to distinguish from cancer cells.

Extensive lymphatic permeation by carcinoma is often readily seen in the peritoneum (Fig. 18.80).

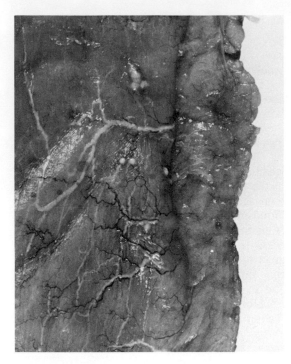

Fig. 18.80   Permeation of lymphatics in the serosa of the small intestine by gastric carcinoma cells. × 2·5.

19

Liver, Biliary Tract and Exocrine Pancreas

The Liver

General considerations

The liver subserves a very large number of important physiological functions, being involved in the intermediary metabolism of proteins, carbohydrates and fats, in the synthesis of a number of plasma proteins such as albumin and fibrinogen, the production of various enzymes, the formation and secretion of bile, the detoxication of endogenously produced waste products or exogenously derived toxins and drugs, and in the storage of proteins, glycogen, various vitamins and metals. Accordingly, the liver is liable to injury from a variety of causes, and injury to it may have profound metabolic effects on the host.

Injury from metabolic disturbances. In experimental animals specific dietary deficiencies can produce fatty liver and liver cell necrosis. Similarly in man, protein malnutrition, e.g. in kwashiorkor, can produce marked fatty change and there is evidence that malnutrition may considerably exacerbate other forms of injury. Specific enzyme deficiencies may cause various hepatic storage diseases (p. 607) or failure of biliary secretion (p. 651).

Injury from toxins and poisons. The liver cell is especially liable to injury because of its function of taking up and dealing with many metabolites, toxic substances, drugs and poisons. The vast number of chemicals used industrially and pharmacologically provide an ever-increasing hazard to the liver, particularly as it has been shown that certain chemicals are harmless to most individuals, but can cause extensive liver damage in individuals with a special susceptibility, as yet unpredictable. The liver also receives blood draining the gastro-intestinal tract, and is exposed to poisons and toxins absorbed from the gut.

A wide spectrum of hepatotoxic effects may be produced by the numerous drugs now in clinical use (p. 642). Meanwhile it is important to appreciate that a careful history of any administration of drugs or exposure to chemicals is an essential part of the investigation of patients with liver disease.

Lesions of the biliary tract affect the liver in two ways. Biliary tract obstruction if sufficiently prolonged results in secondary biliary cirrhosis, and the bile ducts are also the most common route of bacterial infection of the liver.

Certain virus infections damage the liver severely, causing acute hepatitis with extensive necrosis of liver cells. The most important of these, because of their ubiquity, are infectious hepatitis (virus A) and serum hepatitis (virus B).

Hypoxia. Owing to their active and complex metabolism, liver cells are readily injured by hypoxia, as in shock, venous congestion or anaemia.

Tumours. Primary tumours of the liver are relatively uncommon in this country though of great frequency in parts of Africa and the Far East; they are commonly associated with cirrhosis. The liver is a common site of *metastatic carcinoma*, particularly from primary tumours of the gastro-intestinal tract.

Pathological effects of disturbed hepatic function

Disturbances of function resulting from lesions of the liver and biliary tract are varied and complex in their effects. They may be considered under three major headings: Hepatocellular failure (p. 630), portal hypertension (p. 629) and biliary obstruction (p. 626). These are described more fully later in this chapter, as indicated, but brief summaries of their main features are helpful at this point.

Hepatocellular failure arises when total liver cell function falls below the minimum required to maintain a physiological state. It results from loss of a large number of liver cells from various causes, and/or from impaired function of liver cells, usually attributable to chronic interference with hepatic blood flow; both factors may be involved, especially in hepatic cirrhosis. The more important effects include: (*a*) *changes in nitrogen metabolism* with a rise in the blood level of toxic nitrogenous compounds produced by bacteria in the gut and normally metabolised by the liver cells; these compounds affect especially the central nervous system, causing hepatic encephalopathy which consists of neuro-psychiatric and locomotor disturbances, delirium, convulsions and sometimes 'hepatic coma'; (*b*) *failure to remove bilirubin* from the blood, to conjugate it and excrete it in the bile; (*c*) *failure to produce plasma proteins* in normal amounts, particularly albumin, but also fibrinogen, prothrombin and various other clotting factors; (*d*) *hormonal disturbances* attributable to interference with hepatic metabolism of various steroid and other hormones; (*e*) *circulatory disturbances* of obscure nature, with

cyanosis and a hypervolaemic hyperkinetic circulation.

Portal hypertension. This is caused by obstruction to the portal blood flow through the liver. As a result, veins which provide an anastomosis between the portal and systemic systems enlarge and some of the portal blood is shunted directly into the systemic circulation instead of through the liver. Some of these dilated anastomotic channels, notably in the submucosa of the oesophagus, may rupture and bleed; furthermore the bypassing of the liver increases the blood level of toxic compounds absorbed from the gut, thus aggravating the effect of hepatocellular failure on the central nervous system.

Biliary obstruction. This results from obstruction of the common hepatic or common bile duct or from stagnation of bile in the biliary canaliculi without major duct obstruction. The effects include: (*a*) re-absorption of conjugated bilirubin into the blood, producing *obstructive jaundice*; (*b*) re-absorption of other constituents of bile, such as bile acids and cholesterol; (*c*) malabsorption of fats and fat-soluble vitamins because of the lack of bile salts in the intestine, producing steatorrhoea and effects arising from the deficiency of vitamins A, D, E and K; (*d*) prolonged cholestasis resulting in liver cell necrosis and eventually in cirrhosis. Secondary bacterial infection of the biliary tract—*ascending cholangitis*—is an important complication of major duct obstruction.

Circulatory Disturbances

The total hepatic blood flow is approximately 1·5 litres per minute, three-quarters of the blood being supplied by the portal vein and one-quarter by the hepatic artery. Thus, although hepatic arterial blood has a higher oxygen saturation (95%) than portal vein blood (85%), the latter provides approximately 70% of the hepatic oxygen requirement in normal circumstances. Mixing of the two blood supplies takes place in the liver sinusoids. The internal vascular arrangements of the liver are such that the centrilobular liver cells are supplied by relatively poorly oxygenated blood, and they

are therefore more susceptible to any degree of local or systemic hypoxia.

Hepatic arterial obstruction

The hepatic artery is rarely severely obstructed by disease. Fatal infarction has followed accidental ligation of the main trunk or its branch to the right lobe, but in other instances adequate collateral circulation has prevented such an outcome. Obstruction of smaller intrahepatic branches is usually without effect because of adequate collateral circulation.

However, local infarction may occur in polyarteritis nodosa and has also been described in acute bacterial endocarditis.

Portal venous obstruction

The normal portal venous pressure is 7 mm of mercury, and the most important effect of portal venous obstruction, whatever the site or cause, is *portal hypertension* (p. 629). Impairment of the portal venous blood flow can arise from obstruction of the hepatic veins, hepatic sinusoids, intrahepatic portal vein radicles, or of the portal vein itself. The commonest and most important cause of obstruction is hepatic cirrhosis. Other intrahepatic causes include congenital hepatic fibrosis (p. 641), schistosomiasis (p. 635) and metastatic or primary carcinoma in the liver. Obstruction of the portal vein itself is uncommon. It can result from: (*a*) umbilical sepsis in the neonatal period; (*b*) portal pylephlebitis associated with intra-abdominal sepsis; (*c*) pressure of enlarged lymph nodes in the porta hepatis or direct invasion by tumour; (*d*) myeloproliferative disorders predisposing to thrombosis; (*e*) after splenectomy, especially in a patient with a normal pre-operative platelet count; and (*f*) spontaneously and especially in subjects with portal hypertension.

The effects of *complete portal vein obstruction* depend on the site. If it is in the portal vein alone, nothing dramatic happens, but when it extends to occlude the ostium of the splenic vein, then the blood cannot drain via the splenic and gastro-oesophageal anastomoses and venous infarction of the bowel follows. In cases of longstanding portal thrombosis, new vascular channels are formed in the portal fissure, so that a cavernous type of tissue is formed. Closure of a branch of the portal vein may sometimes be followed by 'red infarction' (Fig. 19.1), especially when venous congestion is also present. Such lesions, however, are not complete infarcts but are due to sinusoidal engorgement and atrophy of liver cells (p. 211).

Hepatic venous obstruction

Obstruction of the major hepatic veins, clinically producing the Budd–Chiari syndrome, is rare. In many instances it is due to endophlebitis with superadded thrombosis, the aetiology being unknown. Compression by tumour

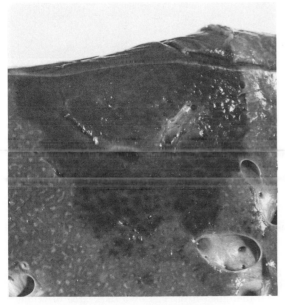

Fig. 19.1 Subcapsular 'red infarct' of the liver.

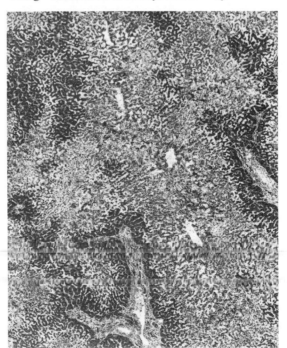

Fig. 19.2 Liver in Budd–Chiari syndrome due, in this instance, to carcinomatous obstruction of the inferior vena cava; there is extensive centrilobular hepatocyte necrosis and haemorrhage, and prominent sinusoidal dilation. × 28.

masses or direct spread of tumour in the hepatic vein or the terminal inferior vena cava may predispose to thrombotic venous occlusion, and spontaneous thrombosis of these vessels may occur in myeloproliferative blood dyscrasias or in thrombophlebitis migrans. Intense engorgement of the liver results, with sinusoidal dilatation, centrilobular congestion and haemorrhage, and atrophy and necrosis of liver cells (Fig. 19.2). Ascites is usually severe, and death results from hepatocellular failure.

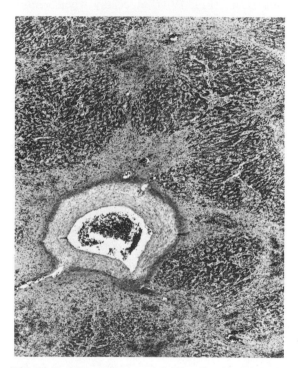

Fig. 19.3 Liver in veno-occlusive disease. There is extensive centrilobular hepatocyte loss with replacement fibrosis and marked intimal fibrosis of the central vein branch. × 28.

Veno-occlusive disease of the liver occurs in Jamaica and certain other tropical countries, probably as a result of drinking various plant or herbal medicines—'bush teas'. The active agents are alkaloids of the pyrrolizidine group present in plants of the genera *Senecio* (ragwort), *Crotalaria* and *Heliotropium*. Liver damage also occurs in animals that eat these plants, and has been produced experimentally by this means. The hepatic vein radicles show sub-intimal oedema and progressive fibrosis, which may proceed to complete occlusion. This produces sinusoidal congestion and haemorrhage with accompanying liver cell necrosis (Fig. 19.3). Death may result from liver failure in acute cases, but a chronic stage may develop with centrilobular fibrosis and nodular hyperplasia progressing to cirrhosis. A similar condition may result from irradiation of the liver, and has also been associated with certain drugs, e.g. urethane.

Venous congestion. In acute cardiac failure, the liver is enlarged, often tender, and histologically there is sinusoidal dilatation and congestion in the centrilobular areas. In chronic cardiac failure the changes are more marked (p. 193), with liver cell necrosis resulting from the continued effects of hypoxia and compression by the dilated sinusoids. Clinically there may be mild jaundice, moderate or sometimes marked elevation of the serum transaminase levels and also a reduced rate of hepatic inactivation of various drugs. In very longstanding cases of congestive cardiac failure, centrilobular hepatocyte loss may be fairly extensive and replacement fibrosis takes place, accompanied by a degree of portal fibrosis (Fig. 8.3, p. 194):

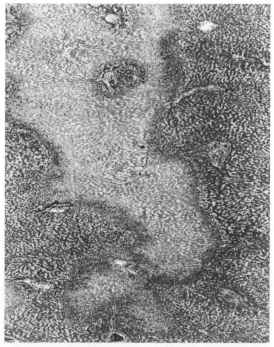

Fig. 19.4 Liver in shock. The pale areas are due to ischaemic necrosis of hepatocytes, and are separated from the intact liver cells by a dark area of cellular reaction. × 32.

although still called 'cardiac cirrhosis' (p. 194), this seldom, if ever, progresses to a true cirrhosis. The prognosis in hepatic venous congestion is that of the cardiac disease causing it.

Hepatic changes in shock

In cardiac, hypovolaemic and bacteraemic shock the circulation through the liver is impaired. This results from a fall in both hepatic arterial and portal venous blood flow as part of the general circulatory failure. This may result in extensive ischaemic hepatocyte necrosis (Fig. 19.4) with a related acute inflammatory cell infiltration. Biochemically these changes are reflected by elevation of serum bilirubin and often by increase in serum transaminase levels which are sometimes as high as in acute viral hepatitis.

Degenerations and Metabolic Disorders

Atrophy

The chief cause of general atrophy of the liver is starvation, in which it becomes shrunken and brown. This is seen in lesser degree in senility. The cells, especially in the central part of lobules, are shrunken, and often contain granules of lipofuscin (p. 244).

Pressure atrophy occurs around tumours and cysts in the liver, in amyloidosis, and focal atrophy is widespread in cirrhosis. The so-called cough furrows occurring in chronic bronchitis consist of antero-posterior grooves on the upper surface of the liver. They are due to the pressure of diaphragmatic contraction during coughing and are of little importance.

Hyperplasia and hypertrophy

These occur commonly as a compensatory process, the cells both multiplying and enlarging, and often becoming multinucleate. These processes are prominent where there has been extensive liver cell necrosis, e.g. in viral or drug-induced hepatitis (Fig. 19.5), and in cirrhosis. The changes are often focal and the surrounding liver tissue may be stretched and the cells atrophied. Hyperplasia and hypertrophy occur in the residual liver following experimental partial hepatectomy. Even when as much as two-thirds of the liver are removed, the weight of the organ may be restored within a few weeks. In fact, restoration occurs so rapidly that attempts to study diminished hepatic function by this method have usually failed.

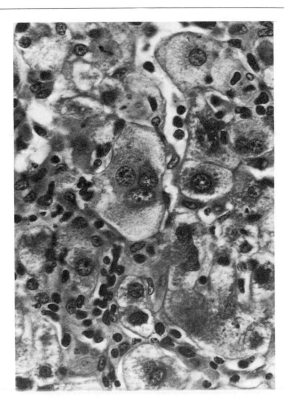

Fig. 19.5 Multinucleated liver cells, in the stage of recovery after acute hepatitis. × 450.

Fatty change

A general account of disturbances of fat metabolism has been given on pp. 15–19. Because of their central role in fat metabolism, the liver cells are particularly prone to undergo fatty change, i.e. to accumulate in their cytoplasm droplets consisting mainly of neutral fat. In addition to the causes of general fatty change—hypoxia, starvation and wasting diseases, and numerous chemicals, and bacterial toxins—fatty change in the liver may also result from chronic malnutrition, alcohol abuse, in obesity, and in a rare condition known as acute fatty liver of pregnancy.

The mechanisms of fatty change in alcohol abuse (p. 619), in obesity (p. 18) and in pregnancy (p. 641) are dealt with separately. In the other causes listed above, present evidence suggests that the fatty change is attributable largely to reduced synthesis of lipoproteins in the hepatocyte endoplasmic reticulum. Fatty change in chronic malnutrition has been the subject of continuing controversy, and is a topic of some importance because of the prevalence of malnutrition in many parts of the world.

Severe malnutrition gives rise to a syndrome termed *kwashiorkor*, which affects infants and young children in many parts of southern and central Africa, in tropical America, and extensively in the Far East. The syndrome is a complex one, attributable to a diet severely deficient in high-grade protein, less deficient in total calories, and with additional features due to vitamin deficiencies. Growth is impaired, the liver is grossly fatty (Fig. 19.6), the pancreas is atrophic, the plasma albumin is low and there is nutritional oedema. On the basis of experimental work in rats it was suggested that the fatty liver of kwashiorkor was due to dietary deficiency of lipotropic factors, particularly choline. There is no evidence for this in man, however, and it seems likely that the fatty liver is the result of failure of the hepatocytes to synthesise adequate lipoprotein due to protein deficiency in the diet, perhaps aggravated by inadequate carbohydrate intake. There is no evidence to suggest that the fatty liver in malnutrition subsequently progresses to cirrhosis.

The liver in obesity. In pathological obesity (p. 18), fat is deposited mainly in adipose tissue, and does not accumulate in other types of cell. The liver, however, is exceptional in this respect. The accumulation of fat usually begins and is greatest in the liver cells round the portal tracts (Fig. 1.17, p. 17); thence it extends inwards, and in severe cases involves all the liver cells. The fat appears first as a few small globules which run together, and ultimately the cell becomes distended with a single large globule of fat, while the nucleus is flattened and pushed to one side. In extreme cases almost every liver cell is distended with a fat globule, the microscopic appearance coming almost to resemble adipose tissue. When there is great accumulation of fat the liver becomes much enlarged, greasy and yellow.

The gross fatty change in the liver in pathological obesity results from the special role of the liver cells in normal fat metabolism. Not only do they take up a high proportion of dietary fat absorbed from the intestine and fatty acids released from the depots, but they are active in the synthesis of fat from glucose and amino-acids. The relative importance of these processes will depend on the amounts of carbohydrate, fat and protein in the diet, but the essential cause is a caloric intake which exceeds the body's requirements.

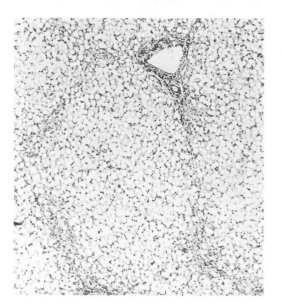

Fig. 19.6 Fatty liver in kwashiorkor. In addition to vacuolation of each liver cell by a large globule of fat, there is an increase in connective tissue in the form of fine strands running through the parenchyma. × 40. (Preparation kindly lent by Professor R. S. Patrick.)

Haemosiderosis

Haemosiderin pigment gives a blue staining reaction with prussian blue stain (Perls' reaction). The normal adult liver contains 0·08% dry weight of iron, but more than half of this is in the form of ferritin, and the amount of haemosiderin is not sufficient to give a prussian blue reaction (p. 241). In infancy the liver normally gives an iron reaction and this becomes more marked in wasting conditions of children.

Excess iron deposition occurs (*a*) in idiopathic haemochromatosis (p. 628); (*b*) in conditions of excessive blood destruction, e.g. haemolytic anaemias of all types; (*c*) following haemorrhage with replacement transfusion (transfusional siderosis); (*d*) in alcoholic liver disease; and (*e*) from ingestion of excessive amounts of iron, either in medicines or in the diet. This is common in the South African Bantu whose staple porridge is prepared in iron pots. Excessive iron deposits in the liver usually appear first in the Kupffer cells and then as brownish-yellow granules within the liver cells, especially at the periphery of lobules. Subsequently there may be diffuse hepatocellular deposition.

Amyloid disease

In this condition the liver becomes larger, firmer and elastic and is often palpable during life. The structural changes and causation have already been dealt with (pp. 233–7). Amyloid disease does not produce jaundice, nor, as a rule, ascites; but the latter may occur as part of the general oedema in the nephrotic syndrome due to accompanying amyloid disease of the kidneys and the hypoproteinaemia is possibly aggravated by the liver damage. The amyloid is irregularly deposited in perisinusoidal spaces and compresses neighbouring hepatocytes (Fig. 9.4).

Glycogen storage diseases

Glycogen storage diseases result from a number of enzyme defects, which were elucidated largely by Cori. Six of these are known and are associated with excessive glycogen accumulation in various tissues (pp. 21–3). Hepatic involvement occurs in five of these, the intracellular site of glycogen storage depending on the particular enzyme deficiency. Marked hepatosplenomegaly results, and cirrhosis may supervene in Type IV.

Excessive accumulation of glycogen occurs also in other forms of metabolic disturbance, e.g. in diabetes mellitus. The histochemical recognition of glycogen is described on p. 22.

Lipid storage diseases

In these conditions abnormal amounts of *lipids* (other than triglyceride fats) accumulate, mainly in cells of the mononuclear-phagocyte system, the Kupffer cells being consistently involved in Gaucher's disease (cerebroside accumulation) and Niemann–Pick disease (sphingomyelin). Hypercholesterolaemic lipid storage diseases rarely affect the liver.

Accumulation of *acid mucopolysaccharides* occurs in the liver cells and Kupffer cells in Hurler's syndrome (gargoylism).

Liver Cell Necrosis

Necrosis of liver cells, of greater or lesser extent, occurs in many diseases of the liver, and also in many other conditions, such as severe infections, wasting diseases and cardiac failure, in which liver cell injury is neither the most important nor the most characteristic feature. Infarction (p. 211) needs no further description here.

Necrosis may affect: (*a*) single scattered liver cells which die one by one (*necrobiosis*) and are recognised as shrunken, deeply eosinophilic, granular cells with a pyknotic nucleus; (*b*) small groups of hepatocytes not related to any particular part of the liver lobule—*focal necrosis*; (*c*) large numbers of hepatocytes, but occurring in a particular part of the lobule—*zonal necrosis*: this is further subdivided according to whether the lesions are *centrilobular, mid-zonal or peripheral* in affected lobules; (*d*) extensive parts of the liver—*massive hepatic necrosis*; this may sometimes involve almost the whole organ and should be considered as a separate entity. Why various aetiological agents affect one zone rather than another zone is not understood.

Focal liver cell necrosis

The lesions consist of irregularly distributed microscopic foci of necrotic liver cells, sometimes with a related inflammatory cell reaction, and in which there may be evidence of reticulin fibre collapse, resulting from autolysis of dead liver cells. Such foci are common in severe toxaemias particularly those resulting from infections within the portal drainage area, e.g. typhoid fever, peritonitis and severe bacillary dysentery. Focal and single cell necrosis are seen also in acute viral hepatitis (p. 611).

Zonal liver cell necrosis

Centrilobular necrosis is caused by certain chemicals and drugs, e.g. chlorinated hydrocarbons and paracetamol; it is sometimes seen in streptococcal and pneumococcal infections (Fig. 19.7), is a marked feature in circulatory shock (p. 226), and may also occur in patients with hyperpyrexia.

Peripheral lobular necrosis is uncommon. It is seen in phosphorus poisoning in which the initial lesion is an intense peripheral fatty infiltration (p. 18). Necrosis of cells develops 3 to 4 days later, and in patients who survive the acute poisoning the liver is often atrophic with persis-

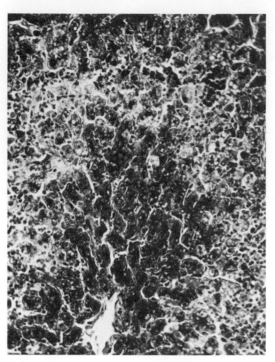

Fig. 19.8 Necrosis of mid-zonal type. The necrotic part, which appears pale, occupies the intermediate zone, though closer to the portal tracts. × 140.

tent periportal fibrosis—the *atrophic phosphorus liver*. Peripheral necrosis also occurs in eclampsia (p. 641). Peripheral 'piecemeal' necrosis is a well-marked feature in chronic active hepatitis (p. 617).

Mid-zonal necrosis is also uncommon, but is consistently present in fatal cases of yellow fever, and may occasionally be seen in fatal acute peritonitis (Fig. 19.8).

Massive liver cell necrosis

This consists of confluent necrosis of all or nearly all the parenchymal cells in large areas of the liver, often more severe in the left lobe. When almost the whole of the parenchyma is destroyed, death results from fulminant hepatic failure.

Massive liver cell necrosis may occur as an unusual complication in acute viral hepatitis. It is thought to be commoner in Type B. Certain chemicals used therapeutically and in industry produce massive liver cell necrosis in a small proportion of individuals at risk. With some of these agents there is a relationship between the

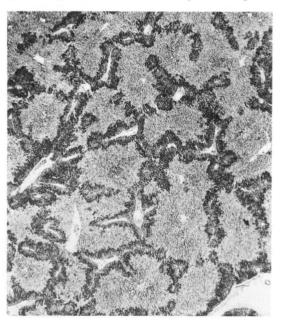

Fig. 19.7 Centrilobular necrosis and peripheral fatty change. A case of streptococcal peritonitis. × 15.

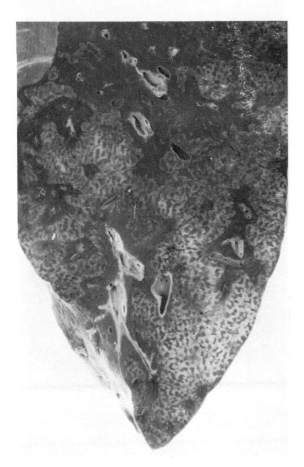

usually approaches 70%. When death occurs within a few days, before autolysis of the dead liver cells, the liver is approximately normal in size and is strikingly yellow owing to bile-staining. Subsequently the dead cells disappear, the affected areas of the liver become shrunken, soft, and red due to sinusoidal congestion and local haemorrhage (Fig. 19.9). If the patient survives for weeks or months, proliferation of the surviving parenchyma produces pale nodules varying in size to over a centimetre, and scarring occurs in the areas of liver cell loss. These changes result in a shrunken nodular liver (*multiple nodular hyperplasia* or *post-necrotic scarring*). The variation in size of nodules and the breadth of intervening fibrous tissue bands are much greater than in cirrhosis (Fig. 19.10). The prognosis is still poor, and death may result from a recurrence of massive

Fig. 19.9 Massive necrosis of liver, three weeks after the onset of jaundice. Note the irregular dark areas from which the dead liver cells have been absorbed, and the portions showing persisting liver structure which were deeply jaundiced. These latter areas had undergone necrosis shortly before death.

dosage and the extent of hepatic necrosis, but with others there appears to be some form of individual idiosyncrasy of unknown nature. The therapeutic substances include a number of monoamine oxidase inhibitors which are hydrazine derivatives, halothane and increasingly common in this country, paracetamol which is frequently used in suicide attempts. Industrial agents include chlorinated hydrocarbons such as carbon tetrachloride and tetrachloroethylene, chlorinated naphthalenes and certain nitrobenzene compounds. The poisonous mushroom *Amanita phalloides* is fatal chiefly owing to massive hepatic necrosis. Massive liver cell necrosis results in clinical acute (fulminant) hepatic failure in which the mortality rate

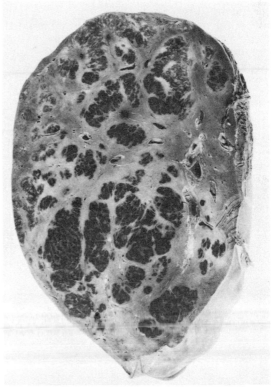

Fig. 19.10 Massive necrosis of liver with fatal recurrence. The pale areas consist of fibrous tissue, the liver cells having undergone necrosis in the initial attack and subsequent autolysis. The dark areas consist of tissue in which the liver cells survived the initial attack, but were destroyed in a rapidly-fatal recurrence. × 0·9.

necrosis, from chronic hepatocellular failure, or from portal hypertension. Some of the chemicals causing massive necrosis may also cause acute renal failure due to tubular necrosis.

Histologically the patterns of massive necrosis due to viral hepatitis, drugs or chemicals are indistinguishable. Initially there is extensive liver cell death, with only a few surviving hepatocytes near portal areas, and with little inflammatory cell reaction (Fig. 19.11). Subsequently there is extensive autolysis of dead cells with consequent collapse of the reticulin framework (Fig. 19.12). There is a moderately intense mononuclear cell infiltrate, and after a few days early fibrosis and hepatocyte regeneration may be noted.

It is not clear why massive hepatic necrosis may occur in some cases of viral hepatitis, usually a fairly benign condition, or following therapeutic doses of various drugs in certain susceptible individuals. In the 1940s Himsworth

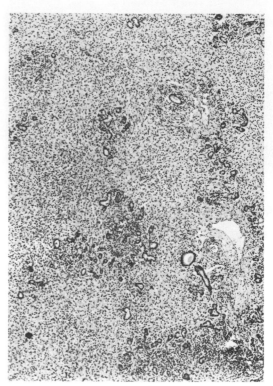

Fig. 19.12 Massive necrosis of liver; portion of red area from which the liver cells have completely disappeared and the lobules consist of dilated capillaries. Early formation of new bile ducts is seen around the portal tracts. × 60.

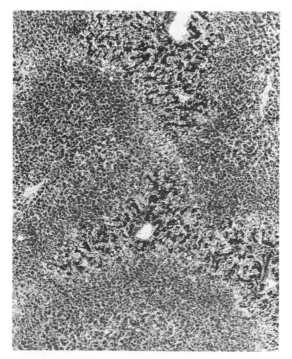

Fig. 19.11 Massive liver cell necrosis in paracetamol overdosage: surviving hepatocytes are darkly stained and surround portal areas. × 60.

and others showed that diets lacking in sulphydryl-containing amino acids (cystine and methionine), and vitamin E could produce massive hepatocellular necrosis in rats. Subsequently it was demonstrated that the protective effect of these amino acids was dependent on their contamination with trace amounts of selenium, and combined deficiency of selenium and vitamin E regularly produced hepatocellular necrosis in rats. However, such deficiencies do not produce liver injury in other species and there is no evidence to suggest that they are of importance in massive necrosis in man. While there are reports that acute viral hepatitis may run a more severe course in malnourished people, there is little evidence that malnutrition is a factor in massive hepatic necrosis in this country.

Hepatitis

Hepatitis literally means any inflammatory lesion of the liver. In practice the term is not used for focal lesions, such as an abscess, but only when there is diffuse involvement of the liver. This may be either acute or chronic, and in some instances acute and chronic hepatitis may be present simultaneously.

Hepatitis may be further classified on an aetiological basis, and some types are best dealt with under separate headings, e.g. alcoholic hepatitis, drug-induced hepatitis, and chronic hepatitis in Wilson's disease, haemochromatosis and biliary disease. Cirrhosis represents a late, irreversible and progressive stage of chronic hepatitis, and it also will be discussed separately (p. 621). In this section we propose to deal with *acute hepatitis* due to the A and B hepatitis viruses, and to other virus and virus-like infections; and *chronic hepatitis*, often of unknown cause, and sub-classified into chronic persistent and chronic active types.

Acute viral hepatitis

This is an acute infection characterised by diffuse hepatitis with widespread liver cell necrosis. There are two common types, but other 'non-A, non-B' types are being recognised.

Type A or infectious hepatitis which is a naturally acquired infection, has an incubation period of 15–40 days, and occurs endemically and as epidemics. Evidence that the causal agent is a virus is based on epidemiology, the infectivity of bacteria-free materials from affected patients, and the development of protective antibodies.

Type B or serum hepatitis has an incubation period of 50–180 days, and is most frequently transmitted by blood and blood products, but may be acquired naturally from an infected person. Virus-like particles of specific antigenicity—hepatitis B associated antigen (HB Ag)—have been demonstrated in affected persons, and their significance will be discussed later.

Clinical and biochemical features

The clinical and biochemical features of Types A and B are very similar, but Type B is regarded as being more severe and is more often fatal. Other differences are summarised in Table 19.1.

Table 19.1

	Type A	Type B
Mode of spread	Oro-faecal and parenteral	Parenteral: ? oro-faecal; ? sexually
Incubation period	15–40 days	50–180 days
Age affected	Younger age groups	Any age
Clinical episode	Mild: mortality rate 5%	Severe: mortality rate 10–20%
Serological markers	Not identified	HB Ag and HB Ab
Prophylaxis	Immune serum of value	? anti-HB immunoglobulin
Transmissible experimentally	Marmoset	Chimpanzee

The early clinical features comprise severe nausea, anorexia, intolerance of fat, often retching, vomiting and fever. A 'serum-sickness like' syndrome may be seen with arthralgia and occasionally skin rashes. There is often epigastric pain, and the liver is enlarged, tender and the site of a dull ache. Jaundice develops 3 to 9 days after this prodromal illness, reaches a peak in 10 days and during this time, the stools are pale and the urine dark. The spleen is palpably enlarged in a third of patients. These features subside in 2–6 weeks but full clinical recovery may take several weeks. An initial leukopenia is seen in the pre-icteric stage, succeeded by a lymphocytosis with, in a small proportion of cases, atypical lymphocytes resembling those found in infectious mononucleosis. The serum bilirubin level is between 80 and 250 μmol/litre (4–12 mg/100 ml) and this is mainly in the conjugated form. Serum alkaline phosphatase levels do not usually exceed 30 King–Armstrong (KA) units/100 ml. Serum aspartate aminotransferase (SGOT) and alanine aminotransferase (SGPT) levels may reach levels greatly in excess of 1000 iu/litre early in the disease and then fall rapidly with the onset of jaundice. The one-stage prothrombin time is usually prolonged, and this measurement provides the best single indication of the severity of the hepatitis.

Most patients recover completely from an

attack. Mortality rates are lower in Type A than in Type B, but may vary in different communities and outbreaks from 1 to 20%. In very severe cases, death results acutely from fulminant liver failure due to massive hepatic necrosis. The hepatitis may progress, sometimes with fluctuations in severity, and cause death from liver failure in 3–8 weeks: this occurs more frequently in females. In some cases jaundice is deeper and persists for weeks or even months— **prolonged cholestatic hepatitis**—but eventually with complete recovery. The relationship of viral hepatitis to chronic active hepatitis (p. 617) and cirrhosis (p. 624) are discussed later. The so-called *post-hepatitis syndrome* with vague features—undue fatigue, dyspepsia and hepatic pain—occurs in a small number of patients.

Pathological changes

There is diffuse hepatic involvement, with acute degenerative changes in scattered hepatocytes leading to irregularity and disruption of trabeculae. This is accompanied by a predominantly mononuclear cell infiltrate of the portal tracts and parenchyma, Kupffer cell reactive hyperplasia, and varying degrees of hepatocyte regenerative activity (Fig. 19.13).

There is great variation in the degree of injury of individual liver cells: many cells appear normal, but there may be single or focal hepatocellular necrosis. The cells may be enlarged, with granular cytoplasm tending to be

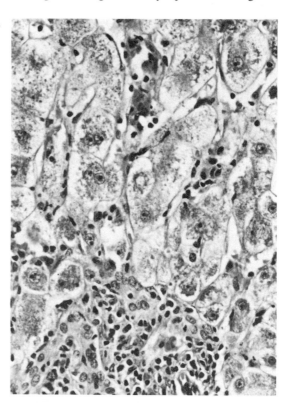

Fig. 19.14   Liver in viral hepatitis, showing ballooning of liver cells, and the remains of a group of shrunken, hyaline cells (*upper centre*). × 465. (Professor R. S. Patrick.)

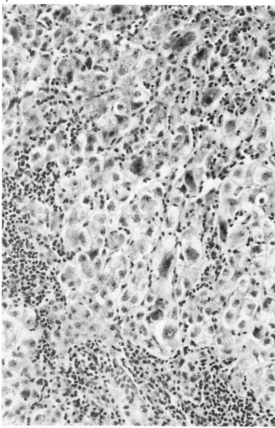

Fig. 19.13   Liver in viral hepatitis. Scattered liver cells are shrunken, hyaline and pyknotic; others are ballooned. Cellular infiltrate, predominantly lymphocytic, is heavy in the portal areas (*lower and left margins*) and lighter within the parenchyma. × 185. (Professor R. S. Patrick.)

condensed round the nucleus—*ballooning degeneration* (Fig. 19.14); others show acidophilic degeneration, with shrinkage of the cells, increased cytoplasmic eosinophilia, pyknosis and eventually extrusion of the nucleus, producing the so-called acidophilic or

'*Councilman-like*' *body* (Fig. 19.15). With necrosis and eventual lysis of single cells or groups of cells, there is disruption of liver cell plates, but the reticulin framework remains intact. An inflammatory infiltrate, mainly of lymphocytes, occasional plasma cells and a few polymorphs, is intimately related to the foci of liver cell necrosis, and is also a regular finding

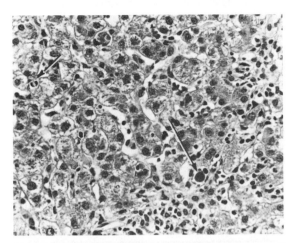

Fig. 19.15 Liver in viral hepatitis: mononuclear cell infiltrate of portal tracts and parenchyma and with a 'Councilman-like' body (*arrow*)—note extruded pyknotic nucleus beside the hyalinised hepatocyte; note also mitotic figure (*arrow—upper left*). × 220.

in the portal tracts. Kupffer cells show reactive hyperplasia, many contain phagocytosed cellular debris, bile pigment and lipofuscin granules, and they contribute to the striking increase in cellularity so characteristic of the histological appearance. Biliary stasis is usually not severe but intracytoplasmic bile pigment granules and occasional bile thrombi are seen. Electron microscopy shows irregular swelling of the endoplasmic reticulum to form vesicles, and detachment of the membrane-associated ribosomes. Enlarged autophagic vacuoles containing altered mitochondria and organelle debris (phagosomes) are seen, but none of these electron microscopic changes is specific.

The acute liver cell injury is brief, and before the attack has subsided clinically, hypertrophy and hyperplasia are seen among surviving hepatocytes with the formation of binucleate and multinucleate cells (Fig. 19.5).

In unusually severe cases there may be more extensive loss of liver cells, sometimes affecting especially the centre of the lobules—

centrilobular confluent necrosis (Fig. 19.16). When this is extensive the picture is that of *massive hepatic necrosis* (p. 608). Bridging necrosis may occur between centrilobular areas and portal tracts. This change is associated with the risk of death from liver failure in weeks or months: it occurs especially in middle-aged women, and has been termed *subacute hepatic*

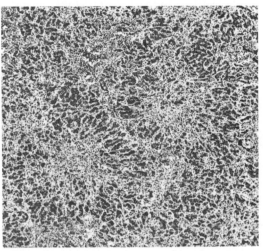

Fig. 19.16 Liver in viral hepatitis, showing centrilobular loss of liver cells. × 45. Accidental death on 7th day of illness.

necrosis. In those cases which progress to chronic active hepatitis (p. 617), the portal tracts are more markedly involved, there is evidence of 'piecemeal necrosis' of adjacent hepatocytes and fibrous tissue extends intralobularly, eventually progressing in some cases to cirrhosis. In those patients who develop **cholestatic hepatitis** there is a marked degree of cholestasis, and there is evidence of damage to bile ducts with necrosis of their epithelial lining cells.

Aetiology and epidemiology

Type A. The aetiological agent in Type A hepatitis has not yet been fully characterised. Recently, however, 27 nm particles, which seem to be specifically aggregated by convalescent sera, have been observed in the faeces of infected persons. There is evidence that it is a DNA virus. This material has also proved infectious in the marmoset (a South American primate), the only experimental animal in which it has previously been possible to transmit Type A hepatitis. In human volunteers the disease has been transmitted by the oral and parenteral routes. The highest natural incidence occurs in children under 15, boys and girls being equally affected, with a higher frequency in the lower socio-economic classes. It is estimated that 50–75% of the community may be infected during epidemics, but most of them develop only anicteric or subclinical disease. Faeces and blood become infected 3–4 weeks after exposure to the virus, and remain infective for about 3 weeks. Specific immunity is established after recovery from Type A hepatitis. Active immunisation is still not possible, but passive immunisation with pooled human IgG has been shown to prevent clinical disease.

Type B. Blumberg and his co-workers in 1964 first described a lipoprotein complex in the blood of an Australian aborigine, using as antibody the serum of a much transfused haemophiliac. This complex they called *Australia (Au) antigen*, and subsequently it was shown by them and by others to be particularly associated with cases of serum hepatitis. It has also been variously referred to as *serum hepatitis (SH) antigen*, and *hepatitis associated antigen (HAA)*, but the generally accepted term is **Hepatitis B antigen (HB Ag)**.

HB Ag is demonstrable by various serological techniques of differing sensitivities—agar diffusion precipitation, complement fixation, immuno-electrophoresis, passive haemagglutination and inhibition, immuno-electron microscopy, and radio-immunoassay. The electron microscopic appearances of the antigen are

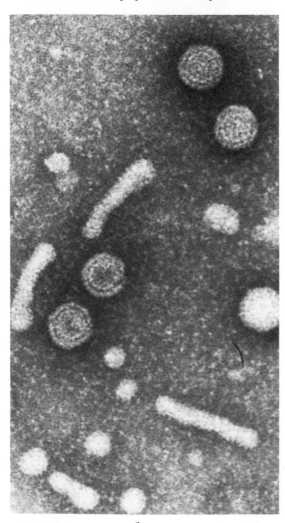

a

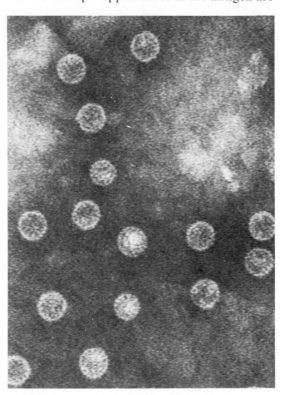

b

Fig. 19.17 Electronmicrographs showing the morphological forms of the HB Ag. **a** This shows the small spheres and tubular structures (20 nm diameter) together with the larger double-shelled Dane particles (42 nm diameter). The small spheres, tubules and outer coat of the Dane particle consist of HB_s Ag. The inner part of the Dane particle is HB_c Ag. × 300 000. **b** A preparation of purified core particles—HB_c Ag. × 300 000. (Dr. June Almeida.)

shown in Fig. 19.17. Antigenicity is associated with the surface (HB_s Ag or surface antigen) and with the core (HB_c Ag or core antigen). The core of the Dane particle is now regarded as the nucleocapsid of the virus; it has been shown to contain DNA polymerase and twin-stranded DNA and is almost certainly the causal agent of Type B hepatitis. Antibody to HB_c develops in Type B hepatitis and persists in the serum. Complement fixation and radio-immunoassay techniques are likely to prove the screening tests of choice for epidemiological studies in this disease. HB_c Ag, however, is still available in only small amounts and in a few centres, and blood is tested routinely for evidence of infectivity by detection of HB_s Ag.

The main significance of the discovery of HB Ag has been as follows: (*a*) it allows of the screening of potential blood donors and may thus reduce the incidence of direct transmission of serum hepatitis; (*b*) it has resulted in specific diagnostic and retrospective tests for the disease and this has already greatly increased our knowledge of the epidemiology of the disease and of its clinical behaviour; (*c*) it has provided useful information on the possible relationship of Type B hepatitis to chronic liver disease; and (*d*) it has raised the possibility of active and passive immunisation, and perhaps eradication of the disease.

There is evidence that HB Ag is not sero-logically homogeneous and various antigenic determinants have been described—'a' common to all; 'e' closely associated with, but probably not part of, the core; 'd' and 'y', which are mutually exclusive; 'W' and 'R' and others. The significance of these awaits further studies, although evidence is accumulating that the presence of 'e' is associated with chronic liver damage.

The agent is transmissible in man by the parenteral and oral routes, possibly venereally, and by mosquito bites. Males are infected more frequently than females. The results of infection vary greatly. Firstly, there may be no clinical evidence of disease, and the subject may or may not become a symptomless carrier; secondly, clinical hepatitis may develop from which the patient makes a full recovery with elimination of HB Ag; thirdly, persistence of infection may be associated with chronic active hepatitis, and lastly, there may be persistence of HB Ag with no evidence of chronic liver disease. The mechanisms which determine these outcomes of infection are not yet fully understood. The incidence of carriers shows

marked geographical variation, being as high as 20% or more in some tropical areas while in this country the figure is less than 0·1%.

Infection may be transmitted by as little as 2×10^{-6} ml of (HB Ag +ve) blood, serum or plasma of carriers, and also by small amounts of blood products, including fibrinogen and thrombin. Infection is common in drug addicts, and in recent years outbreaks of Type B hepatitis, often usually severe, have been described among patients and staff in renal dialysis units.

Using immunofluorescent techniques, direct electron microscopy and immuno-electron microscopy, HB_c Ag has been demonstrated in hepatocyte nuclei, in spherical particles of 20 nm. Cytoplasmic deposits, mainly of HB_s Ag, have also been described in HB +ve patients with chronic liver disease and in asymptomatic carriers, but not in acute hepatitis. These deposits may be stained by orcein, by aldehyde thionine, or by immunofluorescent techniques and on occasion may produce a characteristic 'ground glass' hepatocyte appearance on routine haemalum and eosin or Masson's stain (Fig. 19.18).

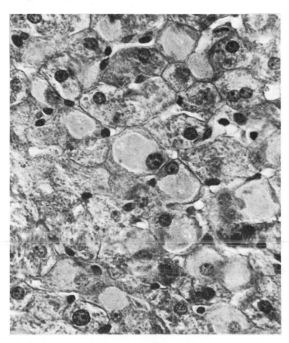

Fig. 19.18 'Ground glass' hepatocytes in a liver biopsy from an asymptomatic carrier of HB_s Ag. The Ag inclusion forms a smooth homogeneous spherical particle in the cell cytoplasm. (Masson's trichrome.) × 450.

Hepatitis due to other viruses

Acute hepatitis may occur as an unusual complication of *rubella* or of *herpes simplex* in infancy and childhood, but rarely in adults. In *infectious mononucleosis* due to the Epstein–Barr virus, abnormal lymphoid cells may accumulate in the portal tracts and sinusoids, and a mild form of clinical hepatitis may occur with focal liver cell necrosis and slight cholestasis. *Cytomegalovirus* hepatitis is a feature of the generalised form of infection with this virus, which occurs in neonates infected *in utero*. In older children and adults, this virus can cause hepatitis closely resembling acute viral hepatitis (Type A or B) which may sometimes occur as part of an illness resembling infectious mononucleosis.

Yellow fever, caused by a Group B arbovirus, occurs sporadically and in epidemics in certain parts of Africa and tropical America. The disease occurs in monkeys and is transmitted to man by the bite of *Aedes aegyptii* and certain other mosquitoes. It varies in severity from a mild unsuspected febrile illness to a fatal combination of fulminant massive hepatic necrosis, acute renal failure and marrow depression with leukopenia and thrombocytopenia. The hepatic lesion consists of mid-zonal necrosis and fatty infiltration in mild cases. Acidophilic or hyaline liver cell necrosis is prominent, producing the classical Councilman body. The kidneys show proximal tubular necrosis.

Chronic hepatitis

Chronic hepatitis may be conveniently, if arbitrarily, defined as inflammation of the liver continuing without improvement for at least six months. It has been subdivided into a relatively benign form, **chronic persistent hepatitis**, in which the inflammation is confined to the portal areas, and a more aggressive form, **chronic active hepatitis**, in which there is portal and parenchymal involvement with progressive fibrosis culminating in cirrhosis. These definitions are based on morphological criteria, and have replaced former terms such as subacute hepatitis, lupoid hepatitis, juvenile cirrhosis, etc. Chronic hepatitis occurs also in alcoholic liver disease, Wilson's disease and haemochromatosis; it may also be drug-induced. The clinical and pathological features of chronic hepatitis will first be outlined, and possible aetiological mechanisms will then be discussed.

Chronic persistent hepatitis

This is regarded as a mild disease, with a benign course, and characterised clinically by symptoms of fatigue, malaise, vague upper abdominal pain and sometimes intolerance of dietary fat. The liver may be tender and slightly enlarged. Biochemical tests show a moderate elevation of aminotransferase levels, and levels of IgG within the normal range.

The pathological changes in the liver comprise a moderately intense mononuclear cell infiltrate of the portal tracts, with a normal lobular architecture, intact limiting plates (i.e. margin between hepatocytes and portal tracts), little or no significant increase in portal fibrous tissue and only minimal parenchymal cell necrosis (Fig. 19.19).

This entity is thought to be a sequel to a subclinical or clinical attack of acute viral hepatitis. Although progression to cirrhosis has

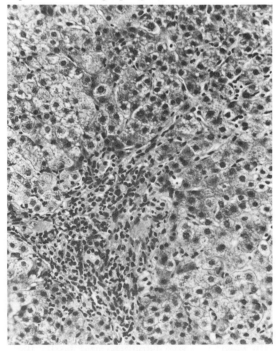

Fig. 19.19   Chronic persistent hepatitis. There is a mononuclear cell infiltrate confined to the portal tract in the lower left quadrant with little or no involvement of the hepatic parenchyma. × 205.

not been reported, development of the picture of chronic active hepatitis has been described in a few cases, and cases of chronic active hepatitis have changed to a pattern of chronic persistent hepatitis following treatment.

Chronic active hepatitis

Without treatment, this condition usually progresses to cirrhosis, although some cases may subside spontaneously. There is a female to male preponderance of more than 3 to 1, and while more than half the patients are aged between 10 and 30 years, the disease can occur in older women. The onset may be acute and indistinguishable from an acute viral hepatitis, or it may be insidious with non-specific symptoms of anorexia, fatiguability, vague upper abdominal pain, and often amenorrhoea. There may be evidence of hepatocellular failure, but the disease tends to fluctuate in severity. There is hepatomegaly, and often splenomegaly which precedes the development of any portal hypertension.

Additional features include arthralgia, skin rashes, pleural effusions, thrombocytopenia, leukopenia and proteinuria attributable to glomerular lesions; they occur in various degrees and combinations. Some patients also may have chronic inflammatory bowel disease, chronic thyroiditis, Sjøgren's syndrome, and other diseases of possible auto-immune aetiology.

Biochemical tests show elevations of aminotransferase levels, usually over 100 iu/litre. The occurrence and degree of jaundice varies; when present it is usually associated with moderate rise of the serum alkaline phosphatase level. Hyperglobulinaemia, predominantly of IgG, is a frequent finding. In the later stages, more advanced changes of hepatocellular dysfunction and cirrhosis are manifest, e.g. hypoalbuminaemia and prolongation of the prothrombin time.

The liver may be of normal size or enlarged. For a long time the surface is smooth but eventually it becomes nodular. There is a dense infiltrate of lymphocytes and plasma cells in the portal tracts, but unlike that in chronic persistent hepatitis, these extend into the lobules, infiltrating between individual and groups of hepatocytes and producing irregularity of the limiting plate between the portal tracts and par-

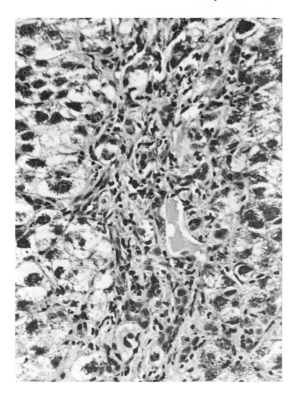

Fig. 19.20 Chronic active hepatitis. The centre of the field is occupied by an enlarged portal area with irregular margins, and the adjacent liver cells show feathery degeneration. There is an infiltrate of lymphocytes in the portal area and among the liver cells. × 350.

enchyma (Fig. 19.20), where the liver cells show feathery degeneration: they are swollen, with irregularly vacuolated cytoplasm, and nuclear enlargement or pyknosis. This progresses to 'piecemeal necrosis', i.e. individual loss of liver cells, with the formation of fibrous septa which extend out to distort the lobular architecture (Fig. 19.21). Eventually the parenchyma becomes broken up into irregular-sized nodules, bounded by fibrous tissue, and the picture is that of *macronodular cirrhosis* (Fig. 19.26).

Spontaneous remission may occur, and a similar change may be produced by treatment with corticosteroids and azathioprine. The prognosis, however, is variable. Approximately 50% of patients survive longer than 5 years, but recent reports suggest that this figure is improved by better therapeutic management.

The aetiology of chronic active hepatitis remains in some dispute. In some cases the onset of chronic active hepatitis is indistinguish-

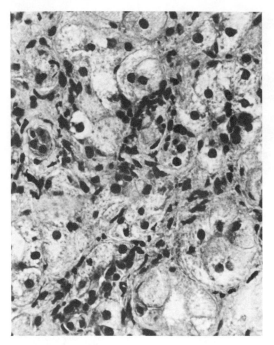

Fig. 19.21 Chronic active hepatitis. Connective tissue has extended irregularly through the parenchyma. Note the lymphocytic infiltration and feathery degeneration of the liver cells. × 560.

able from that of acute viral hepatitis. The recognition of HB Ag has shown that a small group (probably less than 5%) of patients with Type B hepatitis progress to chronic active hepatitis with persistence of HB$_s$ Ag in the serum. While chronic liver disease may possibly ensue from Type A hepatitis, this must be rare.

Various auto-antibodies are commonly present in the serum of patients: these include antinuclear factor and smooth muscle antibodies in over 60% of cases, while a positive LE-cell test, rheumatoid factor or mitochondrial antibody are less frequent. None of these antibodies is specific for chronic active hepatitis. HB Ag and serum auto-immune markers tend to be inversely related. While these features indicate auto-immunity to various cell constituents, their aetiological significance is unknown.

The elevations of serum immunoglobulin levels, the lymphocyte and plasma cell infiltrate in the liver, and the clinical response to immuno-suppressive therapy also suggest an immunological basis. The peculiar female preponderance, the development of the disease in only a small percentage of HB Ag associated hepatitis patients, its rare occurrence in association with certain drugs (oxyphenisatin and methyldopa) and most recently its association with histocompatibility antigens HLA–A1 and 8, also indicate that host factors are important. The interplay between host immune mechanisms and possible viral, drug or other aetiological agents remains to be defined.

In our experience chronic active hepatitis is not common, and this agrees with the small number of deaths from cirrhosis which we have encountered in young women. In its typical form it does not appear to be the explanation for many cases of cryptogenic cirrhosis (p. 625), in most of whom there is either little evidence of pre-cirrhotic illness or a rather vague history of ill-health without the various additional features of chronic active hepatitis. In some, however, immunological abnormalities and histological features similar to that found in chronic active hepatitis may be demonstrable.

Alcoholic Liver Disease

The changes in the liver brought about by high alcohol consumption include *fatty liver*, *alcoholic hepatitis*, *hepatic fibrosis* and *cirrhosis*. Fatty change alone is considered to be a reversible disorder although when it is very severe, cholestasis and hepatocellular failure may develop; alcoholic hepatitis is considered to be the precursor of cirrhosis. Excess alcohol consumption alone has now been shown to produce these hepatic lesions in man without any other nutritional abnormality, and their degree and severity are related to the amount and duration of alcohol abuse. This is supported by the recent description of the production of the entire spectrum of alcoholic liver injury in baboons on a nutritionally adequate diet. There is also evidence that malnutrition and lipotropic deficiencies in experimental animals enhance the effects of alcohol on the liver, but it is not clear how much this contributes to the production of the liver lesions in man.

Alcoholic fatty liver

Under controlled conditions, alcohol administration has been shown to produce hepatic fatty change in all human subjects. After a single dose of alcohol, the fatty acids which accumulate in the liver are derived from fat depots, whereas with chronic alcohol intake they are predominantly of dietary origin, mobilisation of fat from adipose tissues being inhibited in this state, probably by acetate circulating as an end product of alcohol metabolism.

The relationships between alcohol metabolism and accumulation of fat in the hepatocyte are outlined in Fig. 19.22. The main pathway of alcohol breakdown is by its oxidation by alcohol dehydrogenase (ADH) in the cell sap. This results in the generation of hydrogen ions, and is reflected by an increase in the reduced nicotinamide adenine dinucleotide: nicotinamide adenine dinucleotide ratio (NADH : NAD), with a resultant change in reduction–oxidation (redox) potential. Recently it has been shown that some alcohol is also metabolised by microsomal enzymes in the smooth endoplasmic reticulum (SER), this pathway being known as the microsomal ethanol oxidising system (MEOS): it is dependent on the reduced form of NAD phosphate (NADPH), or an NADPH generating system. Normally it is thought that the ADH : MEOS ratio for alcohol metabolism is approximately 3 : 1, but in chronic alcohol abuse with an increase in SER a greater amount may be metabolised *via* the MEOS.

This increase in the SER is a well recognised feature of alcoholic liver damage, and it seems likely that induction of a number of

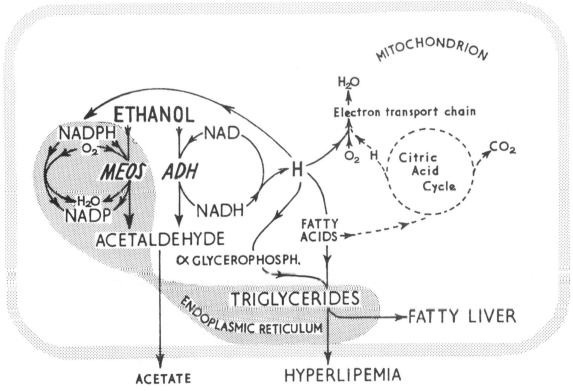

Fig. 19.22 Alcohol metabolism and fatty change in the liver cell, schematic representation. ADH = alcohol dehydrogenase; MEOS = microsomal ethanol oxidising system. Pathways that are decreased by alcohol are represented by interrupted lines. See text pp. 619–20. (Modified after and printed with permission from Professor C. S. Lieber.)

microsomal enzyme systems may accompany this increase in SER and contribute to some of the other effects of alcohol on hepatocyte fat metabolism. In addition, the mitochondria are damaged by alcohol: they become swollen, sometimes markedly so, producing giant forms with disorganisation of the cristae, associated with increased fragility and permeability of the mitochondrial membrane.

The cumulative effects of these changes on hepatocyte fatty metabolism are as follows: (*a*) increased lipogenesis *per se*; (*b*) accumulation of fatty acids, mainly because the NADH : NAD redox changes inhibit their oxidation *via* the citric acid cycle; this is aggravated by the direct damage to mitochondria. In addition there is an increase in the concentration of α-glycerophosphate and this results in trapping of fatty acids in the hepatocytes. These fatty acids are then esterified in the endoplasmic reticulum to triglycerides, some of which accumulate in the hepatocytes. In addition, however, increased lipoprotein synthesis occurs in the SER and some of these triglycerides are thus transported into the circulation, producing hyperlipidaemia; (*c*) cholesterol esters also accumulate, and there is evidence that this is partly due to increased cholesterol production in the SER and partly to a reduced cholesterol catabolic rate.

These mechanisms thus combine to produce hepatic fatty change, which can be detected after only two days of excess alcohol. Similarly, stopping alcohol results in a rapid mobilisation of the stored fat.

Alcoholic hepatitis and cirrhosis

It is now generally accepted that gross fatty change without necrosis does not lead to cirrhosis. Thus in severe prolonged protein malnutrition, as in kwashiorkor, the liver is grossly fatty (Fig. 19.6) and yet there is no evidence that this progresses to cirrhosis, although there may be some residual fibrosis. The biochemical events that lead to the development of alcoholic hepatitis and cirrhosis are therefore still not understood. It is, however, agreed that alcoholic hepatitis sometimes progresses to cirrhosis.

In alcoholic hepatitis there is fatty change together with focal hepatocellular necrosis, ballooning of hepatocytes, polymorphonuclear

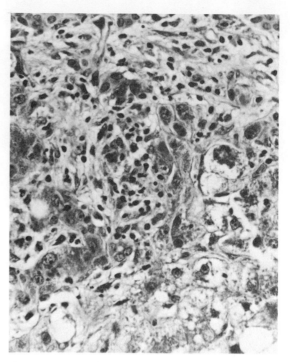

Fig. 19.23 Alcoholic liver disease—fatty infiltration, ballooning of hepatocytes and liver cell necrosis with a related polymorphonuclear cell reaction are present. × 336.

leucocytic infiltration of the parenchyma (Fig. 19.23), and the appearance of an amorphous eosinophilic material (*Mallory's hyaline*) which forms in the liver cytoplasm (Fig. 19.24), characteristically in centrilobular zones; it has a fibrillar

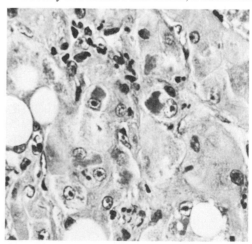

Fig. 19.24 Alcoholic liver disease. Mallory's hyaline is seen as irregular dark cytoplasmic inclusions. × 345. (Professor R. S. Patrick.)

pattern and may represent an accumulation of microfilaments in damaged hepatocytes. Accompanying these changes there is progressive fibrosis, initially round central vein radicles—so-called *sclerosing hyaline necrosis*. In some instances the changes progress rapidly with more marked necrosis and fibrosis, intense polymorph infiltration, peripheral leucocytosis and progressive ascites and hepatocellular failure.

With continuing alcoholic hepatitis there is progressive fibrosis and scarring, fibrous septa extend out from portal areas, and eventually a regular *micronodular cirrhosis* is established (Fig. 19.25). If there is still further parenchymal cell loss and fibrosis, the end-stage liver may show a macronodular or irregular cirrhosis and in these later stages fatty change is usually less marked.

The pathogenic mechanisms involved in the hepatitis and cirrhosis remain unclear. Delayed hypersensitivity reactions to alcohol, to altered hepatic proteins or to Mallory's hyaline have been suggested, but with only scant evidence, while other workers have postulated that there may be superimposed viral or bacteriological infection. Genetic factors may be important, possibly determining differences in the rate of alcohol metabolism. The importance of additional causal factors is indicated by the well-established observation that only 10–15% of chronic alcoholics develop cirrhosis.

Cirrhosis

Definition. Cirrhosis is a condition in which the hepatic parenchyma is changed into a large number of nodules separated from one another by irregular branching and anastomosing sheets of fibrous tissue. It results from long-continued loss of liver cells, with a persistent inflammatory reaction accompanied by fibrosis and compensatory hyperplasia. The progressive loss and regeneration of liver cells occurs focally and leads to disruption of the normal lobular architecture, so that the portal tracts and hepatic veins are spaced irregularly in the nodules of surviving parenchyma, as well as being embedded in the fibrous septa. The condition is irreversible and the fibrosis and distortion of lobular architecture interfere with the flow of blood through the liver, with the result that, in most cases, loss of liver cells continues, even in the absence of the original cytotoxic agent (e.g. alcohol) and death usually results from hepatocellular failure, portal hypertension or a combination of both.

It is important to emphasise that the changes of cirrhosis affect the whole liver. Localised scarring caused, for example, by syphilitic gummas, is not included within the term cirrhosis; nor are mild degrees of more generalised hepatic fibrosis unaccompanied by loss of lobular architecture.

Pathological features

The liver may be of normal size or enlarged, where there is fatty change of the liver cells or excessive development of hyperplastic regenerating nodules. Usually, however, it shrinks as the disease progresses, due to loss of liver cells exceeding regeneration, and terminally may weigh less than 1 kg. The surface is diffusely nodular and on section the parenchyma is seen to be divided up everywhere into rounded nodules, separated by bands of fibrous tissue (Figs. 19.25 and 19.26). The colour varies considerably, depending on whether or not there is severe fatty change, on the presence or absence of jaundice, and on the degree of congestion. Recently-divided liver cells are deficient in lipochrome, and the nodules are thus often paler than normal liver parenchyma.

Microscopy of the nodules shows loss of lobular architecture, the portal tracts and central veins having lost their regular spacing. This is associated with foci of liver cell atrophy and loss, and foci of hypertrophy and hyperplasia, so that in some parts of a nodule the cells are small, and in others they are enlarged and include binucleate forms (Fig. 19.27).

The fibrous tissue runs in septa between parenchymal nodules: it may contain fine or dense collagen fibres, and varies in its vascularity

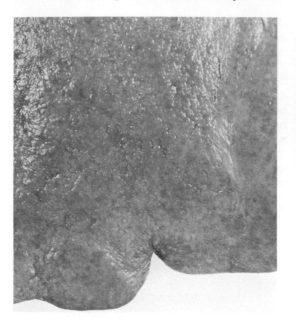
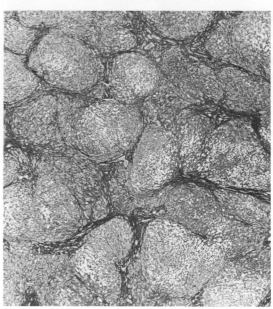

Fig. 19.25 Micronodular cirrhosis. *Left*, showing the fine uniform nodularity of the liver surface. × 0·75. *Right*, microscopy shows regular nodular regeneration: the hepatocytes in many of the nodules show marked fatty change. (Gordon and Sweet's reticulin.) × 20.

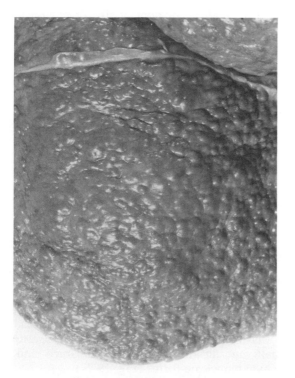
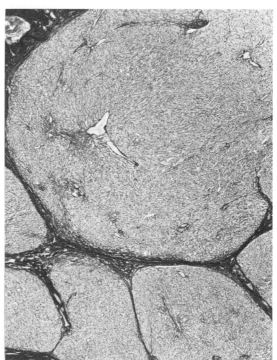

Fig. 19.26 Macronodular cirrhosis. *Left*, surface view, showing the coarse irregularity, with considerable variations of nodular size. × 0·75. *Right*, microscopy shows the variation in nodular size. (Gordon and Sweet's reticulin.) × 20.

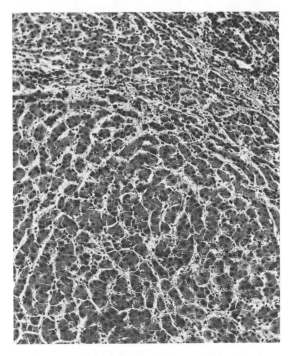

Fig. 19.27 Early cirrhosis of liver, showing hypertrophy of the liver cells in part of a nodule, and stretching and atrophy of the adjacent cells in upper part of field. × 90.

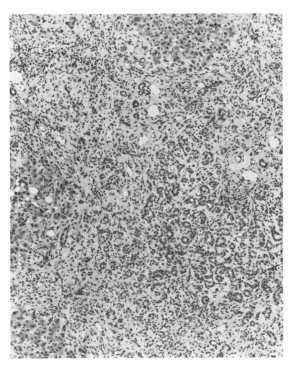

Fig. 19.28 Hepatic cirrhosis. Ductular proliferation in fibrous septa. × 83.

depending on the duration of the cirrhotic process. It tends to involve the portal tracts, but also envelops central veins. Some nodules are seen to be partially divided by incomplete septa extending into them. Collagen develops in relation to damaged liver cells, which presumably stimulate its production by fibroblasts or the perisinusoidal cells of Ito. Fibroblasts are not, however, conspicuous in early experimentally-induced cirrhosis. Commonly, single and small groups of liver cells are entrapped within the fibrous septa. Increased numbers of small bile duct elements are also present in the fibrous tissue so-called 'ductular proliferation' (Fig. 19.28). Cholestasis is not usually marked (except in biliary cirrhosis, p. 625), but is seen focally in some cases and may develop terminally in hepatocellular failure.

Lymphocytes, and less commonly plasma cells, infiltrate the connective tissue and less frequently the parenchymal nodules. The infiltrates vary considerably in degree from case to case, and may be focal.

Although cirrhosis is the result of necrosis of liver cells, it is a slow process, the cells dying one by one, and necrotic cells are not usually seen in biopsy material unless there has been recent circulatory collapse, e.g. as a result of haemorrhage. In necropsy material, there is often extensive recent liver cell necrosis, attributable to terminal failure of the circulation.

Feathery degeneration of liver cells (p. 617) may be observed especially at the margins of the nodules, and this, particularly if associated with heavy lymphocytic infiltration, is an indication that the cirrhotic process is actively progressing.

Classification of cirrhosis

The differentiation of cirrhosis into various types is not entirely without clinical significance, and elucidation of the causes of cirrhosis, and thus eventually its prevention, are dependent on distinguishing between various types. Cirrhosis may be classified on an aetiological basis or on the morphological appearances of the liver.

The morphological divisions are into a **micronodular** or regular cirrhosis in which the nodules are of approximately the same size, i.e. up to 1 mm in diameter; a **macronodular** or irregular cirrhosis in which the nodules are of variable size and may range up to 1 cm in diameter; and a **mixed** type in which both small and large nodules are present (Figs. 19.25, 19.26). The value of this classification is debatable. In our experience the correlation between aetiological factors and post-mortem hepatic morphology is poor. In the end-stage liver the distinctive morphological features of most aetiological types have largely disappeared. Furthermore the same aetiological factor may produce different morphological patterns. However, it is becoming increasingly apparent that examination of liver biopsy material reveals features which correlate with aetiological factors, and it now seems appropriate to give an aetiological classification and describe the pathological features most commonly found in each type. Such a classification is given in Table 19.2.

Table 19.2   Classification of Cirrhosis

Acquired

Alcoholic

Post-hepatitic or post-viral

Of unknown aetiology

Cryptogenic
Indian childhood cirrhosis

Biliary cirrhosis

Primary (also classifiable as of unknown aetiology)
Secondary.

Congenital

Inborn errors of metabolism

Haemochromatosis
Thalassaemia
Wilson's disease
Alpha 1—antitrypsin deficiency
Galactosaemia
Type IV glycogen storage disease
Tyrosinosis
Fructose intolerance.

In our experience in this country, alcoholic comprises 20–25% of all cases of cirrhosis, post-viral 15–20%, 50–55% are cryptogenic and the remainder form a miscellaneous group.

The features of some of these will now be briefly outlined.

Alcoholic cirrhosis

The pathological features have already been described (p. 620). Alcoholic cirrhosis is commoner in men than in women, and develops mainly between 40 and 70 years of age, although recent changes in these patterns reflect alterations in social drinking habits.

The degree of fatty change in the liver tends to diminish as the disease progresses. Reduction in size of the liver, if present, is usually slight, the weight being 1200 g or more. The early pattern of the cirrhosis is micronodular (Fig. 19.25), but with progressive collapse and liver-cell loss the end-stage liver may show a mixed or a predominantly macronodular appearance.

The margins between nodules and fibrous septa are in most places fairly regular, the septa are narrow and composed of mature connective tissue, bile duct proliferation is slight, and lymphocytic infiltration is usually not heavy. The presence of Mallory's hyaline (Fig. 19.24) is a useful diagnostic marker; it is seen also in Wilson's disease, Indian childhood cirrhosis, and in primary biliary cirrhosis, but in alcoholic liver disease it occurs especially in centrilobular hepatocytes.

Hepatic encephalopathy is less common than in post-viral cirrhosis. Additional features which may be present include muscle wasting, anaemia, vitamin B and C deficiency, polyneuritis, alcoholic gastritis and peptic ulceration, chronic pancreatitis, Dupuytren's contracture, and the mental changes of chronic alcoholism.

It is important to recognise this type of cirrhosis because it progresses more slowly than most other types, and improvement may result from abstinence from alcohol.

Post-viral (post-hepatitic cirrhosis)

The liver is usually smaller than in alcoholic cirrhosis, and fatty infiltration is slight or absent. It may be reduced to about 1 kg and the pattern of cirrhosis is usually macronodular (Fig. 19.26). The lobular architecture is not completely lost, and can be detected in parts of some of the nodules. The liver cells vary considerably in size, multiple and large nuclei being common, and in places the margin between nodules and fibrous septa is irregular. The septa are thicker than in alcoholic cirrhosis, are often composed of younger, more cellular connective tissue, and are often, but not always, heavily infiltrated with lymphocytes. Bile duct proliferation is usually marked.

Post-hepatitic cirrhosis is commoner in women than in men, and occurs usually at a younger age than alcoholic cirrhosis, although the range is wide. In those cases which result from chronic active hepatitis (p. 617), many of the additional features of this condition may persist. For example, the spleen is often palpable at an early stage, there may be skin rashes, arthropathy, leukopenia, etc., the serum IgG may be high and there may be various auto-antibodies. The disease has a poor prognosis, progressive portal hypertension and hepatocellular failure usually being more rapid than in alcoholic cirrhosis. There is also a higher incidence of liver cell carcinoma, especially where there is associated persistent HB antigenaemia.

Cryptogenic cirrhosis

Morphologically this group is a heterogeneous one. Most cases show a macronodular pattern, but micronodular and mixed macro- and micronodular patterns are also observed.

Biliary cirrhosis

Long-continued cholestasis, whether of extra- or intrahepatic origin, can lead to cirrhosis. Two varieties are recognised.

(a) *Primary biliary cirrhosis* in which a non-suppurative destructive process of unknown aetiology affects intrahepatic bile ducts.

(b) *Secondary biliary cirrhosis* resulting from prolonged mechanical obstruction of the larger biliary passages.

Primary biliary cirrhosis. This is an uncommon condition, occurring predominantly in middle-aged women, the female preponderance being 8 or 9 to 1. Clinically, the onset is insidious, frequently with pruritus and sometimes with a period of vague ill-health before jaundice appears. There is frequently a marked degree of hepatomegaly. The level of jaundice may fluctuate, and is initially usually mild. The serum level of conjugated bilirubin is usually disproportionately low when compared with the increase in alkaline phosphatase. Serum transaminase levels are mildly raised and cholesterol levels may be markedly elevated. After a duration varying from months to many years, death results from liver failure or complications of portal hypertension. In longstanding cases malabsorption develops, and there may be osteomalacia and osteoporosis. There may also be features of secondary hypersplenism with varying degrees of leukopenia, thrombocytopenia and anaemia.

Although the clinical and biochemical features are those of obstructive jaundice, the large intrahepatic and extrahepatic bile ducts are patent. The most conspicuous change is an infiltration of lymphocytes and plasma cells in and around the epithelium of the smaller (50 μm or less) intrahepatic bile ducts. The epithelium shows degenerative changes in some areas and becomes heaped up in others (Fig. 19.29), and there is gradual destruction and loss of

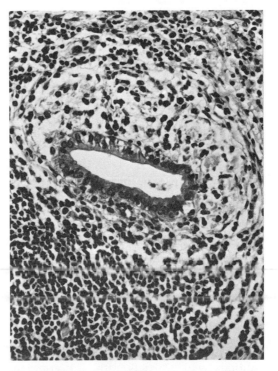

Fig. 19.29 Primary biliary cirrhosis. Showing an intrahepatic bile duct with surrounding inflammatory reaction. The duct epithelium is unduly basophilic with vacuolation of the cells along the upper margin. × 350.

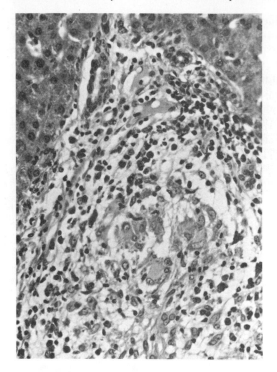

Fig. 19.30 Primary biliary cirrhosis, showing a miliary granuloma with formation of giant cells, lying in a portal area which is heavily infiltrated with lymphoid cells. × 350.

these smaller bile ducts. Macrophage granulomas resembling sarcoid follicles are found in about one-third of the cases and may be intimately related to bile ducts (Fig. 19.30). Later there is extension of the chronic inflammatory cell infiltrate to lie among the periportal parenchymal cells, and this is accompanied by portal fibrosis and cholestasis, usually most marked in the periphery of the lobules. Eventually irregular loss and nodular regeneration of liver cells complete the picture of cirrhosis, which is usually of a micronodular pattern. Mallory's hyaline may be seen in 25% of cases.

Aetiology. In this disease the initial lesion is an inflammatory destructive process involving septal and interlobular bile ducts. Later, parenchymal cell necrosis is superadded, probably due to cholestasis, and progresses to cirrhosis. In nearly all cases the serum contains, in high titre, an antibody which reacts with a non-organ specific mitochondrial antigen. Demonstration of this antibody by indirect immunofluorescence provides a valuable confirmatory diagnostic test. The lymphocytic and plasma-cell infiltration of the portal tracts and bile duct epithelium, the occurrence of the mitochondrial antibody and the commonly elevated serum IgM levels, raise the probability that immune reactions are involved in this disease. Sensitisation to an antigen present in bile has been demonstrated in some patients, but its significance is not yet known.

Secondary (obstructive) biliary cirrhosis. Unrelieved obstruction to the outflow of bile from the liver from any cause results, in time, in secondary biliary cirrhosis. The rate of development of cirrhosis is extremely variable, and depends partly on the degree of obstruction. In some cases, and particularly when obstruction is due to gallstones, an ascending bacterial cholangitis is superadded and, if severe, leads to

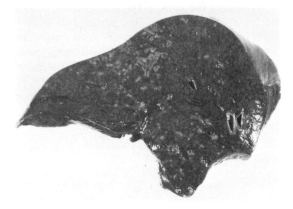

Fig. 19.31 Cut surface of liver in extrahepatic obstruction showing numerous abscesses of various size resulting from an ascending cholangitis.

necrosis and abscess formation (Fig. 19.31). In obstruction due to neoplasms, e.g. cancer of the head of the pancreas, the period of survival is limited and death often results before cirrhosis has developed.

The early changes following biliary obstruction consist of cholestasis, bile accumulation developing in the hepatocytes, bile canaliculi and Kupffer cells, particularly in the centrilobular zones (Fig. 19.32), and in the small bile ducts. Subsequently the larger bile ducts become dilated and filled with concentrated bile. After weeks or months a progressive inflammatory reaction develops in the portal tracts, which become oedematous and infiltrated with lymphocytes, plasma cells and significant numbers of polymorphs (Fig. 19.33). Bile duct proliferation develops, and there is fibroblast pro-

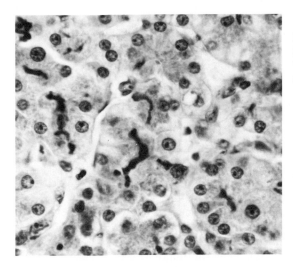

Fig. 19.32 Centrilobular cholestasis in early extrahepatic obstruction. × 390.

liferation and development of fibrous septa extending irregularly between and into lobules and linking up with adjacent portal tracts. Periductal fibrosis is often also a feature.

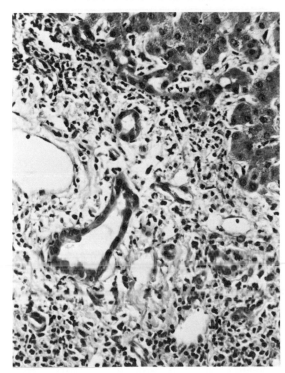

Fig. 19.33 Extra-hepatic obstruction with oedema of the portal area, a prominent neutrophil infiltrate some of which are closely related to the bile ducts, and early ductular proliferation. × 250.

Single or small groups of liver cells become pigmented and swollen, with the cytoplasm appearing as wispy strands—feathery degeneration. Aggregates of such necrotic cells may form distinct '*bile infarcts*'. Rupture of canals of

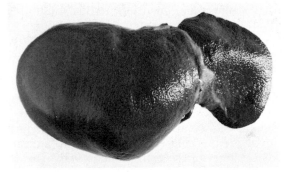

a

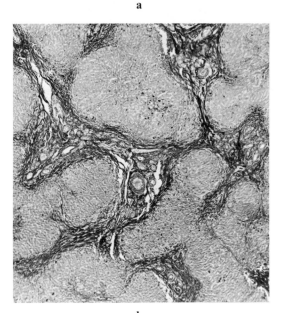

b

Fig 19.34 Secondary biliary cirrhosis. The liver of a child with congenital atresia of the biliary tract. (**a**) Uniform fine nodularity of the surface. × ⅔. (**b**) Fine cirrhosis with cholestasis. × 25. (Dr. A. M. Mac-Donald.)

Hering may occur at the periphery of lobules, with escape of bile to form *bile lakes*. Biliary granulomas may also be a feature. Loss of liver cells and fibrosis result eventually in disturbance of lobular architecture, and together with the development of regenerating nodules, progress to a micronodular cirrhosis. Possibly because the cholestasis interferes with their function, the hepatocytes show marked hyperplasia, and consequently the liver is enlarged: it is also firm from the increase in fibrous tissue, deeply jaundiced and the surface is usually finely nodular. Portal hypertension may eventually supervene, but death results more often from liver failure or intercurrent infection.

The cirrhosis appears to be due to the harmful effect of retained bile upon liver parenchymal cells; in some cases this is aggravated by the occurrence of ascending bacterial cholangitis. In man, the best example of pure obstructive biliary cirrhosis without infection is seen in congenital biliary atresia (Fig. 19.34) which may involve either the extrahepatic or intrahepatic biliary tree. In the extrahepatic variety there is marked jaundice and death occurs within a few months of birth. Patchy atresia of smaller intrahepatic bile ducts sometimes has a more prolonged course with survival into early adult life: secondary biliary cirrhosis develops, as described above, but is of a finer, more truly monolobular pattern.

Congenital cirrhosis

Many of the metabolic abnormalities listed in Table 19.2 can cause cirrhosis in childhood. In addition, there are other causes of cirrhosis in childhood, e.g. *Indian childhood cirrhosis* which is common in 1–3-year-olds in that country and is of unknown aetiology; biliary cirrhosis may result from congenital intra- or extrahepatic biliary atresia, and from mucoviscidosis.

Wilson's disease (Hepato-lenticular degeneration). This is a familial disease affecting young people, in which cirrhosis of the liver is associated with bilateral degeneration of the lenticular nuclei. It is an inherited disorder of copper metabolism determined by a pair of autosomal recessive genes and characterised in some cases by an abnormally low level of the copper-binding serum α-globulin (caeruloplasmin). Consequently copper is absorbed from the gut in excess and is carried in the plasma in loose combination with serum albumin from which it is too easily deposited in the tissues, especially the liver and brain, and in the kidneys where it leads to amino-aciduria by defective tubular absorption. It is unlikely, however, that loss of aminoacids plays any part in the development of the hepatic lesions. The liver proteins have a high affinity for copper and this leads to deposition of copper in the liver in greatly increased amounts. Treatment with penicillamine is of value in chronic cases. The cirrhosis is of macronodular type, with a dense chronic inflammatory cell infiltrate of fibrous septa and evidence of piecemeal hepatocellular necrosis, fatty infiltration and prominent glycogen vacuolation of nuclei. In the later stages Mallory's hyaline is seen in some cases. The changes in the nervous system are described on p. 662.

Idiopathic haemochromatosis. A general account of this disease, and of other conditions causing gross iron overload, is given on pp. 242–3. The liver is the major organ affected, but iron deposition and fibrosis of the pancreas and other viscera is also present. The cirrhosis is usually micronodular, less commonly macronodular. Excess iron deposits are present in hepatocytes, Kupffer cells, fibrous septal macrophages and in bile duct epithelium. Increased amounts of lipofuscin are also present in hepatocytes.

The degree of cirrhosis and the intensity of iron deposition are not closely correlated. However, the iron deposition is considered to be fibrogenic, and removal of iron by repeated venesection has been reported to produce resolution of the cirrhotic pattern. Primary carcinoma of the liver may develop in both treated and untreated patients.

Pathogenesis of cirrhosis

Cirrhosis results from long-continued loss of liver cells, accompanied by compensatory liver cell hyperplasia and nodule formation, and by a continuing inflammation and progressive replacement fibrosis, i.e. chronic hepatitis. It is, in fact, the outcome of prolonged hepatocellular necrosis, the cause of which is, more often than not, unknown. It is likely that the disturbance of lobular architecture, with interference with the blood flow by regenerating nodules and fibrous septa, results in ischaemia irregularly affecting the intrahepatic microcirculation; consequently there is a gradual and progressive loss of hepatocytes (which are very susceptible to ischaemia) and so a vicious spiral is established. In experimental animals the liver, when repeatedly damaged, e.g. by carbon tetrachloride, has remarkable powers of recovery by regeneration of the central necrotic zones within 10–14 days; if the doses of poison are closely spaced, complete regeneration does not occur and the lesion progresses to cirrhosis (Fig. 19.35).

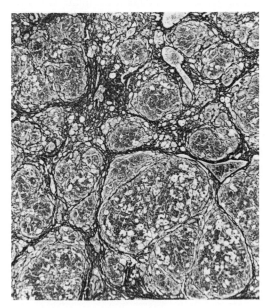

Fig. 19.35 Cirrhosis produced in a rat by repeated inhalation of carbon tetrachloride (see p. 11). (Gordon and Sweet's reticulin.) × 40.

The possible aetiological factors in human cirrhosis have already been enumerated, but in over 50% of cases in this country none of these factors can be incriminated and the aetiology remains unknown. Whereas in secondary biliary cirrhosis the progression to cirrhosis is predictable, in alcoholic abuse only 10% of patients develop cirrhosis. Similarly, in acute viral hepatitis only a small percentage, probably less than 5, progress to cirrhosis. In some patients there is an intervening period of continuing clinical hepatitis, morphologically manifest as chronic active hepatitis. In others no such intermediate phase is clinically apparent, but after some years of well-being the patients present with manifestations of the complications of cirrhosis: presumably these patients have had sub-clinical chronic active hepatitis.

In cryptogenic cirrhosis there is, by definition, no history of any previous acute liver disease nor is there any clinically apparent stage of their morphologically progressive chronic hepatitis. While some such cases are probably the result of an episode of viral hepatitis, more sensitive tests for evidence of previous hepatitis A and B virus infection must be developed before this relationship can be elucidated.

In previous editions of this book there was much discussion of the role of malnutrition in the pathogenesis of cirrhosis. It is now generally accepted that, in spite of apparently contrary experimental evidence in rats, malnutrition *per se* is not a cause of cirrhosis in man, although it may be a contributory factor and may aggravate the effects of alcohol abuse and of viral hepatitis.

The sequence of events in the development of cirrhosis seems likely to be as follows: liver cell necrosis and loss from whatever cause; variable degrees of architectural collapse; compensatory liver cell hyperplasia and nodule formation; a continuing acute or chronic inflammatory response; interference with intrahepatic microcirculation; progressive replacement fibrosis. Predisposing host factors, such as known metabolic defects, may explain some cases, but in others the nature of such factors is not clear. The progression from an acute to a chronic hepatitis may be due to persistence of the aetiological agent, as has been shown in some cases of Type B virus hepatitis, or may be the result of auto-immunisation or some other cytotoxic immunological reaction, as has been postulated in some cases of chronic active hepatitis and in primary biliary cirrhosis. Similarly the factors responsible for initiating hepatic fibrosis also remain obscure, but the importance of the fibrosis in the progression of the cirrhosis and in the development of the secondary effects of cirrhosis is not in doubt. Fibrosis is a feature of chronic inflammation of any sort and so is to be expected in chronic hepatitis.

Effects of cirrhosis

Cirrhosis has two important effects, portal hypertension and hepatocellular failure. It is the major cause of these two conditions, particularly when they occur together.

Portal hypertension is due to interference with the normal blood flow through the liver. Hepatic and portal venous pressure and wedge-pressure measurements indicate that the hepatic venules are seriously obstructed: this is due to compression by hyperplastic nodules and constriction by fibrous tissue. The same effects may also interfere with the small portal branches. As a result of these intrahepatic changes, much of the portal blood bypasses the liver and enters the systemic veins, and some of the blood which does enter the liver passes through it and merely perfuses fibrous tissue and not liver cells.

Hepatocellular failure is due in part to loss of liver cells, which gradually outstrips regeneration as cirrhosis progresses, and in part to the reduction in effective hepatic blood flow resulting from the haemodynamic changes just described. The overall effects are thus a reduction of functional hepatic cell mass.

The association of portal hypertension and hepatocellular failure in cirrhosis gives rise to the additional feature of ascites, and oesophageal and gastric varices can also rupture and bleed, thus aggravating the features of hepatocellular failure.

Apart from biliary cirrhosis, which is associated with cholestasis, jaundice is usually no more than latent or mild in cirrhosis. It increases, however, as hepatocellular function fails and is then a bad sign. A sudden increase in bilirubin may be a result of acute hepatic necrosis, either of unknown cause or resulting from circulatory collapse following haemorrhage, e.g. from oesophageal varices.

Liver cell carcinoma arises in approximately 10–15% of cirrhotic patients in this country, the incidence varying in different types of cirrhosis (p. 639). It is an example of the tendency of long-continued hyperplasia to progress to neoplasia.

Hepatocellular Failure (Liver Failure)

Although the liver has a large functional reserve and a high regenerative capacity when injured, liver insufficiency, manifested by failure of the liver cells to perform adequately their various functions, occurs both in patients with severe acute liver injury and in advanced cases of chronic liver disease. Acute hepatic failure occurs in severe viral hepatitis, as an adverse reaction to certain drugs, as a result of drug overdose or poisoning by certain hepatotoxic chemicals, in massive liver cell necrosis of unknown cause, and occasionally in severe fatty infiltration of the liver. In the acute form the hepatic failure results directly from the parenchymal cell injury and is a manifestation of the degree of hepatocellular damage. Chronic liver failure is most often due to cirrhosis. It may occur even in patients with a relatively large amount of surviving liver tissue, and is attributable in part to the interference with hepatic blood flow which results from the disturbed architecture and fibrosis of the liver. Acute or chronic hepatic failure may be precipitated by factors such as gastro-intestinal bleeding, the use of diuretic or narcotic drugs, bacterial infection, paracentesis, portacaval shunt and other surgical operations.

Because of the multiple functions of the liver, acute or chronic hepatic insufficiency gives rise to a complex syndrome, which includes neurological disturbances, jaundice, defects of blood coagulation and renal failure. Additional features include ascites and oedema, endocrine and circulatory disturbances, but these occur mainly in chronic failure. The mechanisms involved in these manifestations of liver failure are discussed below.

Neurological disturbances comprise mental disturbances with apathy, disorientation or excitement, a coarse flapping tremor and muscular rigidity, and finally coma. These are accompanied by characteristic changes on the electro-encephalogram and by a number of biochemical abnormalities. All these features are reversible, and morphological changes have been observed only in the astrocytes, the nuclei of which are enlarged, sometimes to 25 μm in diameter; the chromatin is condensed around the nuclear membrane, and the nucleolus is unduly conspicuous. In occasional cases, however, progressive brain damage may occur.

The neurological disorder is attributed to a failure of the liver to detoxify nitrogenous bacterial metabolites absorbed from the gut, due to liver cell loss and/or porta-systemic bypass of the liver. An increased nitrogen load will also follow a bleed from varices into the gastro-intestinal tract. It has been suggested that the liver cells produce factors essential for normal neuronal function, but these have not yet been identified. In most cases there is an increased level of ammonia in the blood, and there is good evidence that this contributes significantly to hepatic coma. However, this is not the sole factor involved, for blood ammonia levels do not correlate closely with the clinical state. Other metabolic products of intestinal bacteria have also been implicated, and increases in serum aromatic amino acids and/or a decrease in branched-chain amino acids may be of importance. In addition, there may be an increased cerebral sensitivity to nitrogenous compounds, possibly due to interference with oxidative metabolism via the citric acid cycle and consequent ATP depletion. These factors may be further aggravated by the hypotension, anoxia and electrolyte disturbances which accompany hepatic failure.

Jaundice is usual in acute hepatocellular failure, its severity reflecting the degree of hepatocellular damage. In very severe cases, however, death may result before jaundice has become conspicuous. In chronic failure the degree and type of jaundice depends upon the nature of the liver disease. In secondary biliary cirrhosis, obstructive jaundice precedes and accompanies the development of hepatic dysfunction. In other cirrhoses, jaundice is a late but bad prognostic sign, and is usually only of mild or moderate degree. The precise mechanisms of the hyperbilirubinaemia are uncertain, but are considered to be most likely due to failure of hepatocytes to excrete bilirubin.

Coagulation defects result primarily from defective synthesis of a number of coagulation factors by the liver, notably prothrombin, fibrinogen and factors V, VII, IX and X. There may also be thrombocytopenia (accompanied sometimes by anaemia and leukopenia) due to hypersplenism, and, particularly in acute failure, disseminated intravascular coagulation with consumption of clotting factors.

Renal failure may develop in both acute and chronic hepatic failure. Acute renal failure may result from hypotension due to bleeding from oesophageal varices. Impairment of renal function without morphological damage may also occur terminally in hepatic failure: this is characterised by reduced glomerular filtration rate and progressive oliguria, but without a fall in urine osmolarity. The mechanisms remain uncertain; disturbances of renal cortical perfusion, chemical or bacterial toxic effects, or deficiency of natriuretic factors having been postulated.

Ascites and oedema. Ascites does not result from hepatocellular failure unless there is also portal hypertension, as in cirrhosis. In chronic liver failure there is diminished production of plasma albumin, with a consequent fall in plasma osmotic pressure. The portal hypertension increases the intravascular hydrostatic pressure in the microvasculature of the gut, and in addition there is leakage of hepatic lymph because of obstruction to its outflow from the liver. Secondary hyperaldosteronism (p. 222) occurs in some cases, and may, by inducing sodium retention, aggravate the oedema and ascites. The causation of secondary hyperaldosteronism, and why it occurs in some cases and not others, is not clear. Peripheral oedema is due mainly to the fall in plasma osmotic pressure.

Endocrine disturbances. In chronic liver failure there is, in both sexes, a tendency to depression of libido, sterility and loss of body hair. In men, the testes are frequently atrophic, and occasionally one or both breasts are enlarged (*gynaecomastia*). These effects result from failure of hepatic inactivation of oestrogens, which have a stimulating effect upon the breast and may also suppress the production of pituitary gonadotrophin, thus explaining the testicular atrophy. The exact mechanisms of the menstrual irregularities, secondary amenorrhoea and breast atrophy which occur in women are not clear. Two well-known vascular changes in liver failure are exaggerated mottling, due to patchy congestion, of the skin of the palms—the so-called '*liver palms*'—and the development in the superior vena caval drainage area of small leashes of dilated vessels in the superficial dermis, radiating out from a central arteriole—the '*spider naevus*'. Both these features may occur in normal pregnancy and probably have a hormonal basis.

Circulatory disturbances. A hyperkinetic circulation characterised by peripheral vasodilatation and an increase in circulation rate, cardiac output and blood volume may be associated with hepatic failure. This may possibly result from circulating vaso-active substances or may be due to impaired sympathetic responsiveness.

Cyanosis with arterial hypoxia is not uncommon and finger clubbing develops in a small percentage of patients.

Other features. In hepatocellular failure, particularly when acute, the breath has a peculiar sweetish smell termed '*foetor hepaticus*', possibly due to failure of the liver to detoxicate substances absorbed from the gut. *Fever* is also common in acute failure, but profound *hypothermia* has been described in chronic failure. *Bacteraemia*, particularly with coliform organisms, is also a complication. General ill-health with anorexia, wasting and vomiting is common.

Non-Viral Infections of the Liver

The common virus infections of the liver are dealt with on p. 611 *et seq*. Accordingly this account deals with infections by bacteria and protozoa, and infestation by metazoan parasites.

Pyogenic infections. Because of improvements in diagnostic facilities and the earlier use of antibiotics, pyogenic infection of the liver is less common than it used to be, and when it does occur it is usually due to extension of bacteria within the biliary duct system—**ascending cholangitis.** *Escherichia coli*, either alone or with other bacteria, is the commonest causal organism. Bile duct obstruction is the most important predisposing cause, and because bacterial infection commonly accompanies stones, obstruction by a stone is especially liable to be complicated by suppurating cholangitis. The process extends into the liver tissue, giving rise to multiple abscesses in which the pus is characteristically bile-stained.

Multiple abscess formation in the liver results from suppurative phlebitis affecting the veins around a septic focus in the abdomen or pelvis, e.g. acute appendicitis, diverticulitis of the colon, or infected haemorrhoids: the infection may reach the liver by septic emboli or by **portal pylephlebitis**. Umbilical sepsis in the neonate sometimes spreads to the intrahepatic portal vein radicles *via* the umbilical vein.

Abscesses may also develop in the liver in septicaemia or pyaemia, but these are less frequent and less important than in various other organs.

Actinomycosis. Actinomycosis occurs in and around the appendix, from where it may extend to the liver by the portal venous system or by direct spread. Multiple abscesses form in the liver separated by granulation and fibrous tissue, and produce a honeycomb appearance. The abscesses contain thick greenish-yellow pus, and the characteristic yellowish or greyish sulphur granules, which comprise aggregates of the branching filament of the causal organism—*Actinomyces israelii* (p. 187).

Leptospirosis. The spirochaete *Leptospira icterohaemorrhagiae* causes endemic chronic renal infection in rats, and can survive in water or damp conditions for some time after excretion in rat urine. It can penetrate the intact human skin or may gain entry via the respiratory or oral routes, and after an incubation period of 10–15 days causes an intense febrile illness **(Weil's disease)** with conjunctivitis, renal tubular damage, a haemorrhagic tendency, jaundice, focal myocardial and skeletal muscle necrosis and often a mild lymphocytic meningitis. The disease occurs chiefly in sewer workers, agricultural workers and fish handlers. Various other leptospira, including *L. canicola* from dogs, can cause a similar but usually milder disease in man.

Liver biopsy may show liver cell degeneration, prominent mitotic activity of the hepatocytes and sometimes focal necrosis, cholestasis and haemorrhages. In some cases, however, the changes are slight. After death, the liver cells are often rounded and separated from one another (Fig. 19.36); this may be a post mortem change but it is seen when necropsy has been performed within a few hours of death, and is sometimes helpful in suggesting the diagnosis.

The mortality rate is about 15%. Death may occur in the first week, when haemorrhagic consolidation of the lungs may be the most conspicuous lesion. Later, death is usually due to renal failure, which in these patients is almost always accompanied by evident hepatic involvement.

Syphilis. The liver is frequently affected in both congenital and acquired syphilis. In **congenital syphilis**, the commonest lesion is a diffuse interstitial pericellular fibrosis, proliferating fibroblasts extending between the sinusoidal

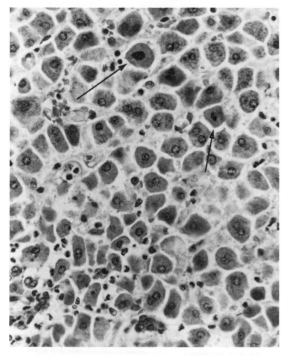

Fig. 19.36 Liver in Weil's disease: post-mortem liver showing separation and rounding up of hepatocytes, proliferative activity (*arrows*) and focal liver cell necrosis with a related inflammatory cell exudate (*lower left*). × 400.

endothelium and the liver cells producing compression or ischaemic atrophy of the hepatocytes. A dense interstitial mononuclear cell infiltrate is also present. Miliary gummas are not uncommon. These are minute foci of necrosis in which the hyaline remnants of necrotic liver cells are surrounded by inflammatory cells. Rarely, large gummas occur in congenital syphilis. In fatal cases, spirochaetes are usually abundant throughout the liver. In **acquired syphilis**, a diffuse hepatitis, sometimes with miliary granulomata, may occur in the secondary stage. Hepatic gummas were a common feature of tertiary syphilis before effective treatment became available. They were typically rounded, might be multiple and became very large ($>$10 cm). They presented the usual features of central necrosis and peripheral fibrosis which might extend as dense radiating bands into the surrounding parenchyma. Healing usually occurred even without treatment, and scarring was extensive, producing gross distortion of the liver—*hepar lobatum* (Fig. 19.37). The adjacent tissues usually became

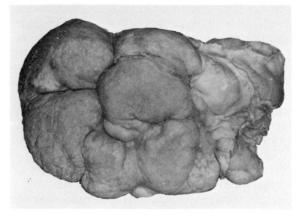

Fig. 19.37 Hepar lobatum. The liver is greatly deformed as a result of deep scarring from tertiary syphilis. × $\frac{1}{3}$.

adherent to the liver. Amyloid disease, sometimes irregular in distribution, was also a common complication.

Relapsing Fever. This is a spirochaetal disease, caused by various species of *Borrelia*. Large epidemics have occurred in the past and sporadic outbreaks are encountered in various parts of the world. The species of parasite and its vectors differ in different places. In Europe, *Borrelia recurrentis* or *B. obermeieri* are transmitted by lice or ticks, the spirochaete gaining entrance through scratches. In parts of Africa *B. duttoni* is transmitted by tick bites and the reservoir is in rodents and other animals. After an incubation period of 1–2 weeks a febrile illness develops and lasts for about a week, during which *Borreliae* are present in the blood, cerebrospinal fluid and urine. The attack of fever may recur once or more. The liver is congested with centrilobular necrosis, the kidneys show tubular degeneration with fatty change, the spleen is enlarged with foci of necrosis and there may be petechial haemorrhages in the skin and internal organs. Severe cases are deeply jaundiced and may die of liver failure.

Tuberculosis. Tuberculous lesions are less common in the liver than in most other organs. In generalised tuberculosis miliary tubercles occur, and are distributed irregularly in the parenchyma: sometimes they are large enough to be visible to the naked eye and may have a caseous bile-stained centre. Rarely, a few large caseous lesions result from blood spread, and may be distinguishable from gummas only by the finding of tubercle bacilli. Tuberculous cholangitis is extremely rare, and probably results from ulceration of a tuberculous nodule of the liver into a bile duct.

Other causes of tubercle-like granuloma in the liver. Lesions resembling tubercle follicles occur in the liver in several non-tuberculous conditions. They consist of aggregates of epithelioid cells, often with one or more multinucleated giant cells which may contain various cytoplasmic inclusions, and show little or no central necrosis. Such lesions occur in most cases of sarcoidosis and brucellosis, and are seen frequently in tuberculoid leprosy and histoplasmosis; they occur sometimes in secondary syphilis and in chronic berylliosis due to inhalation of beryllium compounds. Tubercle-like follicles are seen also in rather less than 50% of liver biopsies from patients with early primary biliary cirrhosis and around impacted ova in schistosomiasis. Occasionally granulomas are found incidentally in the liver in individuals not obviously suffering from tuberculosis or any of the above conditions: their significance is unknown.

Protozoal parasites

Hepatic amoebiasis. This is a complication of amoebic dysentery (p. 577), brought about by amoebae entering colonic venules and passing by the portal vein to the liver, which they then colonise. Liver lesions may be the presenting clinical feature, or may occur only many years after the colonic lesions have apparently subsided.

In the liver they multiply in the sinusoids, releasing a proteolytic enzyme which digests the liver tissue producing a cavity—the so-called '**tropical abscess**'. For reasons unknown, there is usually a single 'abscess', most often in the upper part of the right lobe and measuring up to 15 cm in diameter. It may ulcerate through the diaphragm into the lung and discharge *via* the

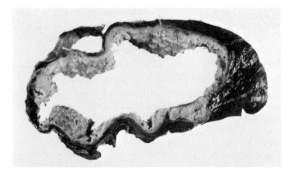

Fig. 19.38 Sagittal section of right lobe of liver, extensively replaced by a large amoebic 'abscess': some surviving liver parenchyma on the right.

bronchus, or less commonly, may rupture into the pericardial or peritoneal cavities.

Macroscopically, the lesion has a compressed fibrous capsule, with an irregular shaggy necrotic inner wall and the cavity contains thick glairy fluid, often chocolate-coloured or showing admixture of blood (Fig. 19.38). On microscopic examination the contents include

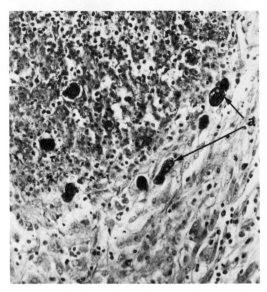

Fig. 19.39 Amoebic abscess of liver showing numerous amoebae **a** in the necrotic margin of a small recent lesion. × 200.

necrotic liver cells, granular debris and a varying number of red cells. Only a few neutrophils are present and the lesion is thus not really an abscess. *Entamoeba histolytica* may be demonstrable in the inner aspects of this necrotic wall (Fig. 19.39), but are rarely present in the fluid.

Malaria. In the incubation period, malarial parasites develop within hepatocytes but they do not bring about permanent hepatic damage. In the stage of blood infection, colonised erythrocytes are phagocytosed by Kupffer cells, which show marked hypertrophy and hyperplasia and contain abundant dark brown granules or 'malarial pigment'.

Kala-azar (visceral leishmaniasis). The liver is usually enlarged, and there is hyperplasia of the Kupffer cells which are distended by large numbers of Leishmann–Donovan bodies. There may be some intralobular fibrosis, but cirrhosis does not result.

Metazoal parasites

Schistosomiasis. Infestation with *Schistosoma mansoni*, in which the adult worms colonise the veins of the colon, is prevalent in Egypt and various other parts of Africa, in the West Indies and parts of South America. *S. japonicum* infestation occurs in Japan, China and the Philippines, and the worms are present in the veins of the small intestine. Both species produce large numbers of ova, some of which enter the portal venous circulation and impact in the liver. Adult worms may also colonise the larger portal vein branches, and deposit their eggs in the adjacent liver tissue. The life cycles of the parasites are similar to that of *S. haematobium* (p. 804), which only rarely involves the liver.

The worms evoke both an antibody response and cell-mediated immunity in the host. In experimental animal infections there is evidence that the adult worms are protected by a coating of mucopolysaccharide which may be of host origin, and which acts as an immunological barrier and prevents hypersensitivity reactions. When ova are laid in the tissues, however, they lack this coating and stimulate a delayed hypersensitivity reaction characterised by accumulation of epithelioid macrophages and eventually dense fibrosis.

The morphological features of the human disease are, in general, consistent with similar immunological phenomena, but these have not been proved (Fig. 19.40). Where there is extensive fibrosis of portal areas, the picture is that of 'pipe-stem' fibrosis, with irregular attenuated fibrous septa extending into the parenchyma (Fig. 19.41), but cirrhosis does not result. Portal

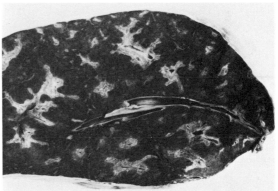

Fig. 19.41 Liver in schistosomiasis, showing the pale areas of fibrous tissue around the portal veins.

hypertension may develop with marked enlargement of the spleen and there may be haemorrhage from oesophageal varices. Hepatocellular function is well maintained, and relief of portal hypertension by porta-caval anastomosis is much more permanently successful than in cirrhosis.

Hydatid disease. Hydatid is the cystic stage of *Echinococcus granulosus*, a small (3–6 mm long) tapeworm, and occurs most commonly in sheep, but also in cattle, pigs and men. Infection results from swallowing the ova shed in the faeces of dogs, which harbour the adult worm in the small intestine. Dogs become infected by eating the offal of infected sheep, cattle or pigs, thus enabling the life cycle to be completed. The disease in man results from close contact with

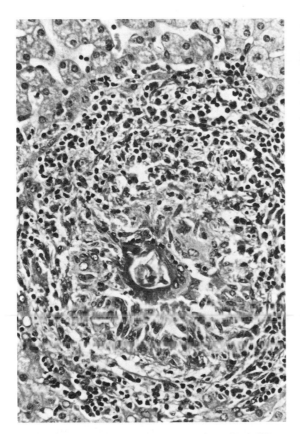

Fig. 19.40 *Schistosoma mansoni* infestation of liver, with a granulomatous reaction surrounding an ovum impacted in a portal vein branch. × 250. (Preparation kindly lent by Mr. C. Campbell.)

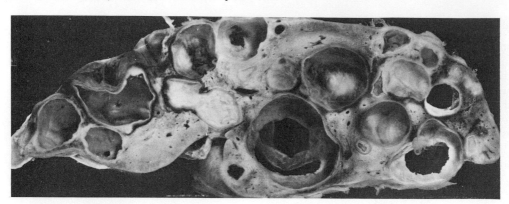

Fig. 19.42   Liver in hydatid disease, with multiple sharply circumscribed cysts replacing much of the organ. (Professors R. A. Joske and M. N.-I. Walters.)

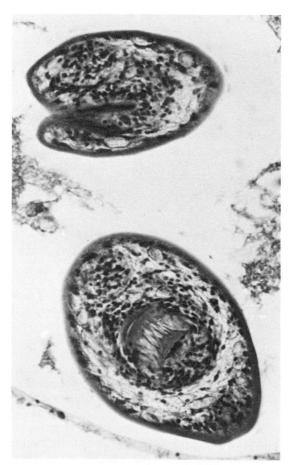

Fig. 19.43   Scolices of *Echinococcus granulosus* showing their rows of hooklets by which they become attached to the brood capsule. (Professor R. A. Joske and Dr. L. R. Matz.)

infected dogs and possibly from eating contaminated vegetables. It is commonest in sheep-farming communities, notably in Australia, New Zealand and South America: in the United Kingdom it is uncommon except in parts of Wales.

The ingested ova have a chitinous coat which is digested by gastric juice, liberating the embryos. They invade the veins of the gastro-intestinal tract and reach the liver *via* the portal vein, where most of them lodge. A few may pass into the pulmonary or systemic circulation, producing cysts in the lungs and other organs, e.g. muscles, kidneys, spleen and brain.

The commonest type of hydatid is a cyst of up to 20 cm diameter, usually multilocular due to the presence of daughter cysts, and with a thick wall comprising the inner germinal layer and an outer non-nucleated hyaline laminated layer, which in turn is surrounded by a layer of host granulation tissue; sometimes the liver is the site of a mass of small cysts, each approximately 6 mm in diameter (Fig. 19.42). Brood capsules bud from the germinal layer, and scolices are formed within the brood capsule from buds which develop on its inner surface (Fig. 19.43). The cysts contain straw-coloured fluid and rupture of brood capsules into this releases their scolices which form 'hydatid sand'.

The cysts occur most commonly in the right lobe of the liver. The symptoms are those of a slowly expanding lesion. The parasites may die in the cystic stage, which then undergoes calcification. The diagnosis is made radiologically or on scintiscanning of the liver, and by the demonstration of hypersensitivity to an intradermal injection of hydatid antigen (the *Casoni test*).

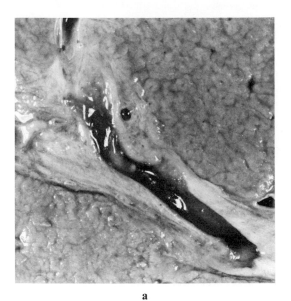

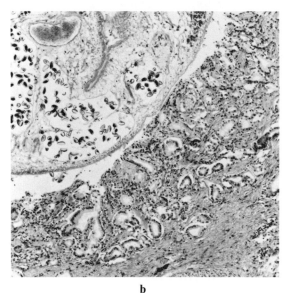

a   b

Fig. 19.44 Liver infestation by *Clonorchis sinensis*. **a**, fluke lodged in bile duct, which shows thickening of its wall and surrounding fibrosis. **b**, microscopic appearances with fluke in lumen, and the proliferation of duct-like elements in the wall of the bile duct. × 177.

Clonorchiasis and fascioliasis result from invasion of the biliary tree by the larvae of the Chinese liver fluke (*Clonorchis sinensis*) and the sheep fluke (*Fasciola hepatica*) respectively. Clonorchiasis results from eating inadequately cooked or raw fish. It can produce biliary obstruction and ascending cholangitis, and is characterised by marked proliferation of bile-duct-like elements (Fig. 19.44). Portal hypertension may develop, and there is a high incidence of cholangiocarcinoma. Fascioliasis is characterised by a cholangitis.

Ascariasis, i.e. infestation of the intestine by the round worm *Ascaris lumbricoides* is widely distributed throughout the world, but is particularly prevalent in Africa and the Far East. It commonly affects children, and in over a third of cases is associated with direct invasion of the common bile duct, producing obstruction and cholangitis.

Tumours

Benign tumours

Benign tumours of the liver are rare, comprising approximately 5% of all hepatic neoplasms. They include: (*a*) **liver cell adenomas**, which bear a close microscopic resemblance to normal liver tissue, the cells forming regular trabeculae two or three cells thick. Bile canaliculi are present and appear normal but bile ducts are absent. These tumours are usually very vascular and are not always encapsulated. An increased incidence due to the use of oral contraceptive pills and sex hormone therapy has recently been reported; (*b*) **bile duct adenomas** are very rare and are usually an incidental finding. These are less than 1 cm in diameter, and are composed of small bile duct elements in a fibrous stroma. Intrahepatic bile duct **cystadenomas** are also rare, but sometimes large tumours; (*c*) **haemangiomas**, usually cavernous, dark purple owing to the contained blood, and sharply demarcated from the surrounding hepatic tissue, are not uncommon. Most are less than 2 cm in diameter, but some are larger. They are usually superficial and may be mistaken for infarcts by the casual observer.

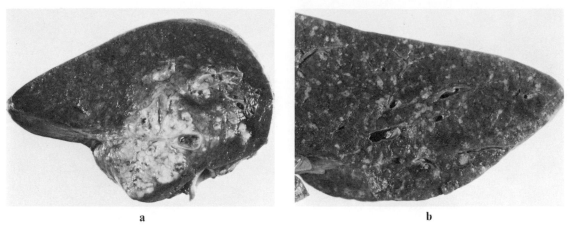

Fig. 19.45 Hepatocellular carcinoma. **a**, arising as a single large mass and with evident permeation of surrounding portal vein branches. **b**, arising as multicentric foci throughout the liver.

Malignant tumours

Liver cell carcinomas (malignant hepatomas) account for approximately 85% of primary malignant tumours of the liver, cholangiocarcinomas for approximately 5–10%, and the remainder consist of relatively rare tumours including haemangiosarcomas, hepatoblastomas, and mesenchymal tumours.

Liver cell carcinoma

This tumour shows marked geographic variation in incidence. In this country it is present in less than 1% of all necropsies, whereas in parts of Africa and Far East Asia it may be 5–6 times more common.

There has been considerable discussion about the relation of cirrhosis to carcinoma. We

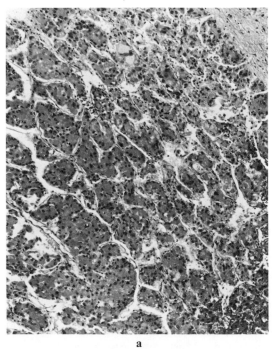

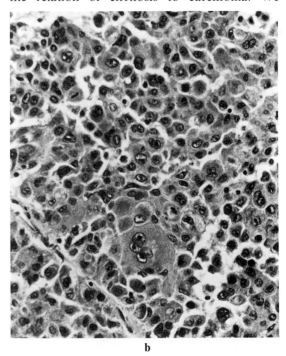

Fig. 19.46 Hepatocellular carcinoma. **a**, trabecular arrangement with endothelial lined sinusoids separating the aggregates of tumour cells. × 77. **b**, individual tumour cells resembling hepatocytes and with some binucleate and giant cell forms. × 250.

believe that cancer develops secondarily to the liver cell hyperplasia of cirrhosis, the compensatory proliferation, for some reason, becoming neoplastic. Where the tumour arises in a cirrhotic liver, foci of aberrant, dysplastic cells are not infrequently seen in regenerating nodules indicating an intermediate stage, and malignant transformation may also be multifocal. Liver cell carcinoma is a complication of macronodular cirrhosis, the average frequency in our own series being 12%, but it is much more frequent in males (17·5%) than in females (4·5%) with cirrhosis. Conversely, in our series of primary liver carcinoma, cirrhosis was present in more than 75%. In the South African Bantu and in the Far East where liver cell carcinoma is extremely common, there is also a high incidence of cirrhosis; but in addition, tumour appears to supervene more frequently in the cirrhotic liver, the frequency approaching 40–50%.

Macroscopically the tumour may form a single large mass (Fig. 19.45*a*) which may appear to be encapsulated, with central necrosis, haemorrhage and irregular bile-staining. In other cases multiple tumour nodules are present (Fig. 19.45*b*), and there is also a type in which extensive nodular infiltration involves a considerable part of the liver. Extensive permeation of intrahepatic portal vein branches is a common feature; extrahepatic metastases occur in less than half the cases, mostly in the lungs and lymph nodes.

Microscopically the tumour cells closely resemble hepatocytes, their arrangement being more or less trabecular, and with intervening sinusoids (Fig. 19.46). True acini are not found. Canaliculi, sometimes containing bile, may be seen.

The aetiological factors in hepatocellular carcinoma are not clear. The relationship to cirrhosis has already been discussed. A high incidence of liver tumours has been produced experimentally in rats by feeding with mouldy peanuts and this has been attributed to *aflatoxins* which are products of the mould *Aspergillus flavus*. These and other mycotoxins and plant toxins may contaminate stored foods and cereals, and this has been proposed to explain in part the geographical variation in incidence. Chemical carcinogens, notably *o*-aminoazotoluene and *p*-dimethylaminoazobenzene (butter yellow) produce liver tumours in experimental animals, the incidence being increased by a diet low in protein or deficient in cystine and methionine. Accordingly protein deficiency may be synergistic in promoting the development of liver cell cancer in man, and may in part also explain geographical variation in incidence. Recent attention has been focussed on the possible role of nitrosamines, compounds which can be synthesised from nitrites and secondary amines in the gastrointestinal tract, and which produce experimental liver tumours. Nitrites (and nitrates) are common food additives, and the possibility that some nitrosamines are carcinogenic for man is raised. The nature of the relationship of alcohol abuse to liver cell carcinoma remains uncertain; but there is growing epidemiological evidence of an association between HB Ag and liver cell carcinoma.

Cholangiocarcinoma

Primary tumours composed of cells resembling biliary epithelium (Fig. 19.47) are much less common than liver cell tumours. They are not

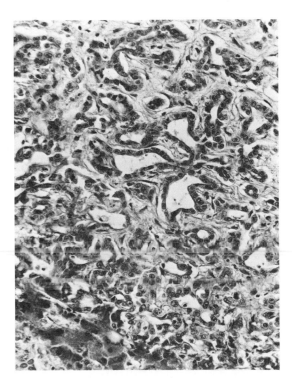

Fig. 19.47 Cholangiocarcinoma—an adenocarcinomatous pattern resembling bile ducts, with a related fibrous reaction. × 200.

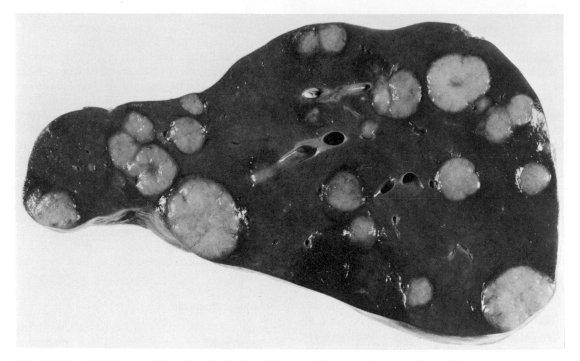

Fig. 19.48   Multiple secondary deposits in liver from a primary carcinoma of oesophagus.

usually associated with cirrhosis, and there is no difference in sex incidence. In the Far East, where these are relatively frequent, about 65% of cases are associated with infestation by the liver flukes *Clonorchis sinensis* or *Opisthorchis viverrini*.

Hepatoblastoma and haemangiosarcoma

These are both very rare. Hepatoblastomas are congenital tumours of childhood and are composed of mixtures of epithelial and mesenchymal elements. Haemangiosarcomas are angioformative tumours, possibly arising from Kupffer cells: there is current interest and concern over their postulated association with exposure to vinyl chloride monomer (p. 256).

Secondary tumours

The liver is a very common site of secondary carcinomas of all kinds, notably from the gastro-intestinal tract, lung and breast. Secondary carcinoma may develop as one or two main masses, but often the whole organ is permeated by tumour nodules (Fig. 19.48). The liver becomes enlarged and its surface is beset with nodular elevations, some of which may show umbilication owing to central necrosis. The organ may come to weigh 5 kg or more. Intrahepatic cholestasis and jaundice may develop from pressure on bile duct radicles.

Sarcomas also frequently metastasise to the liver, and may produce marked hepatomegaly: Leukaemic infiltration and metastatic spread by malignant lymphoid neoplasms are common.

Other Disorders of the Liver

Liver diseases in childhood: congenital malformations

Many of the forms of liver disease which can occur in childhood are dealt with elsewhere.

They include the congenital forms of cirrhosis, Indian childhood cirrhosis, biliary cirrhosis due to bile duct atresia or as a complication of mucoviscidosis, congenital syphilitic infection and the various metabolic storage diseases in which there may be hepatic involvement. There remain a few miscellaneous conditions which merit a brief description.

Neonatal giant-cell hepatitis. Multinucleated giant cells may be a feature of liver damage in children, and they are conspicuous in an acute hepatitis which may develop in the fetus or within the first 2 weeks of life. The aetiology is uncertain; a genetic predisposition has been postulated and a number of viruses have been suggested. There is extensive fibrosis and disturbance of the lobular pattern: the prognosis is poor, the survivors usually developing cirrhosis.

Other viral infections. Disseminated herpes infection may produce widespread and large foci of liver-cell necrosis, and the liver may also be involved in congenital rubella infection and in cytomegalovirus disease. Transmission of the B hepatitis virus from mother to fetus can occur and sometimes produces an acute hepatitis.

Cystic disease of the liver. Congenital cysts in the liver are rare and are usually associated with cystic disease of the kidneys; the latter condition, however, occurs much more commonly alone. The cysts vary greatly in size and number; the liver may be studded with them, there may be only a few, or they may comprise microscopic hamartomatous lesions—*von Meyenberg complexes*. They usually contain a clear fluid, have a cuboidal epithelial lining, and probably originate from the bile ducts.

Congenital hepatic fibrosis. This is regarded by some workers as a form of cystic disease of the liver. It may be familial and is sometimes accompanied by cystic disease of the kidneys. Bands of dense fibrous tissue extend irregularly throughout the liver, but the normal lobular architecture between these is preserved. Within the fibrous bands there are numerous mature bile duct elements lined by cuboidal epithelium (Fig. 19.49). Affected individuals present in childhood or early adult life with portal hypertension, and when this is relieved surgically the prognosis is usually good because hepatocellular function is normal (c.f. cirrhosis). However, there appears to be an increased susceptibility to cholangitis.

Focal nodular hyperplasia. This is a benign hamartomatous lesion in which there is a focal aggregation of large irregular non-capsulated liver cell nodules, and which may be mistaken for tumour. The lesion is usually functionally and histologically benign, although a few instances of portal hypertension have been reported where the lesion has arisen in the region of the porta hepatis.

Liver disease in pregnancy

Pregnancy may modify the clinical course of certain hepatic diseases. *Massive hepatic necrosis* may be more severe, and unexplained (but possibly viral) acute fatal massive necrosis may occur in the last trimester.

A benign form of **intrahepatic cholestasis** may recur with each pregnancy and is probably due to increased levels of steroid hormones.

Acute fatty liver of pregnancy occurs usually in the last trimester, and is commonly fatal. There is widespread fatty accumulation in hepatocytes, but of an unusual appearance (Fig. 19.50). A similar morphologic appearance may occur with tetracycline toxicity, and the lesions appear to result from depressed hepatocyte protein synthesis with resultant accumulation of fat.

Liver in eclampsia. The liver is not usually

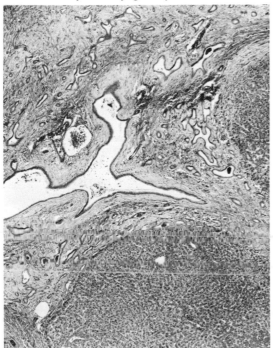

Fig. 19.49 Congenital hepatic fibrosis: wide fibrous septum within which are numerous mature bile duct elements, some of which contain inspissated bile. × 31.

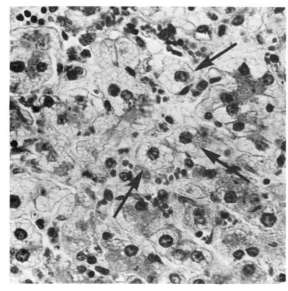

Fig. 19.50 Acute fatty liver of pregnancy: the hepatocytes are enlarged and contain multilocular droplets of fat arranged circumferentially round the nucleus (arrows). × 400.

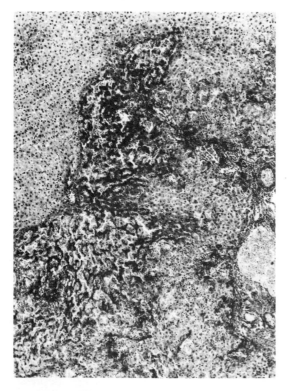

Fig. 19.51 Liver in eclampsia, showing necrotic liver cells (darkly stained), fibrin and haemorrhage. × 75.

injured in eclampsia, but in fatal cases there are often foci of periportal necrosis and haemorrhage with fibrin thrombi within related portal capillaries and sinusoids (Fig. 19.51). Centrilobular necrosis and haemorrhage, if present, are manifestations of shock. These lesions are ischaemic and due to hepatic involvement in the disseminated intravascular coagulation now regarded as probably of aetiological significance in pre-eclampsia and eclampsia.

Drugs and the liver

The liver plays a central role in the metabolism of many drugs, and drug-induced hepatic injury is now one of the commonest forms of iatrogenic disease. Indeed, in any patient presenting with obscure liver disease or with unexplained jaundice, the possibility of a drug-induced lesion should always be considered. Many of the pathological features which have already been described in this chapter can be reproduced by drugs—hepatocellular injury and necrosis; hepatitis, both acute and chronic; and jaundice by various mechanisms. It is not proposed to list the drugs which have hepatotoxic side-effects but merely to outline those hepatic disease patterns which they may mimic and to give examples of those drugs which may produce them.

Drug reactions can be divided into: (*a*) those which are predictable, i.e. they occur in most individuals taking the drugs in sufficient amount, and the severity is related to the dose of the drug; and (*b*) those which are unpredictable, i.e. they occur in only a proportion of individuals taking the drug, may not be dose-related and appear to be idiosyncratic.

In the first category are: (i) hepatocellular necrosis due to various drugs with a direct hepatotoxic effect, e.g. paracetamol; and (ii) intrahepatic cholestasis due to synthetic androgens and oestrogens. Idiosyncratic reactions include: (i) acute hepatitis, sometimes with death from hepatic failure, caused, for example, by halothane and methyldopa. With methyldopa, and also with a laxative, oxyphenisatin, progression to a condition resembling chronic active hepatitis has been described; (ii) intrahepatic cholestasis caused, for example, by chlorpromazine and other drugs of the phenothiazine group.

Jaundice is a feature in most of these patients. In addition, it must be remembered that an unconjugated bilirubinaemia may occur as a result of intravascular haemolysis, which also may be drug induced, and from interference with hepatocyte conjugation of bilirubin, for instance by novobiocin.

In addition to these effects of drugs, recent evidence of an association between hepatic adenomas and the use of the contraceptive pills has been mentioned above. There are a few cases in the literature claiming an association between androgens and hepatocellular carcinoma, and mycotoxins may play a significant causal role (p. 639) in these tumours. Many chemicals and toxins used in industrial plants may have hepatotoxic and possibly carcinogenic effects. The need for continued surveillance of such effects cannot be too strongly emphasised and a careful occupational and drug history should always be taken in cases of hepatic disease.

The Gallbladder and Bile Ducts

Function of the gallbladder

The relatively watery bile from the liver is stored in the gallbladder and concentrated by the absorption of water and electrolytes. Accordingly, with the addition of mucin from the mucosa, gallbladder bile becomes thick and mucoid. The normal structure of the mucosa is well suited to this absorptive function (Fig. 19.52). This concentrating ability of the gallbladder facilitates its radiological examination, in that certain iodine-containing compounds taken orally or administered intravenously are excreted and concentrated in the bile and, being radio-opaque, allow the gallbladder and the extrahepatic biliary system to be visualised.

The gallbladder bile is discharged into the duodenum in response to the entry into the duodenum of food, particularly fatty foods. When the food enters the duodenum the gallbladder discharges a proportion of its contents, and thereafter only small quantities are passed at intervals: there is always a relatively large amount of bile retained in the gallbladder. Between these periods of discharge there is probably a steady flow of hepatic bile into the gallbladder where it is concentrated.

The release of the bile into the duodenum is due to contraction of the gallbladder accompanied by relaxation of the sphincter of Oddi. This is mediated humorally by cholecystokinin which is secreted by the duodenum in response to the presence there of fatty food.

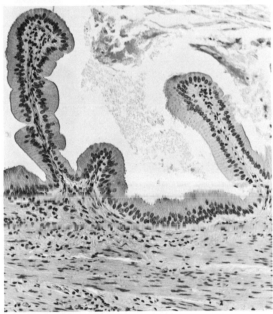

Fig. 19.52 Normal human gallbladder, showing delicate villous folds of mucosa covered by tall columnar epithelium. × 180.

Gallstones (Cholelithiasis)

Gallstones are formed from constituents of the bile—cholesterol, bile pigments and calcium salts—in various proportions, along with other organic material. They form usually in the gallbladder, but may also develop in the extrahepatic biliary tree and occasionally within intrahepatic ducts.

There is marked geographic variation in

incidence, cholesterol stones being uncommon in developing countries. There is a very high incidence in North American Indians. Gallstones are commonest in late adult life, in women, especially multiparous, and in association with diabetes and obesity. There is also an increased tendency to stone formation in patients who have undergone ileal resection.

Pathogenesis

The exact mechanisms of stone formation remain debatable, and it seems likely that changes in the composition of the bile, local factors in the gallbladder and biliary tract infection are predisposing causes.

Composition of the bile. Cholesterol is the main constituent of gallstones. It is synthesised in the liver and excreted in the bile, where it is kept in solution by the formation of micelles comprising cholesterol, phospholipids and bile salts. The phospholipids, also insoluble in water, are mainly (96%) lecithins and small amounts of lysolecithin and phosphatidyl ethanolamine. The bile acids are synthesised in the liver from cholesterol, the most important ones being cholic acid and chenodeoxycholic acid: they are secreted in the bile as conjugates of the amino acids glycine and taurine, the glycine/taurine conjugate ratio being 3 to 1. In the colon the primary bile acids are dehydroxylated to form the secondary bile acids, deoxycholic and lithocholic acid. These major bile acids, together with other minor ones, constitute the bile acid pool, approximately 2–4 g in man, and more than 85% of this is reabsorbed daily from the gut and re-cycled.

The primary bile acids act as detergents in the bile and thus help to keep the cholesterol and phospholipids in true solution as mixed micelles. The ratio of cholesterol to bile acids and phospholipids determines cholesterol solubility.

Gallstones tend to form when there is a relative excess of cholesterol to bile acids and phospholipids—so-called '*lithogenic bile*'. This may result either from increase in cholesterol or decrease in the bile-acid pool: these changes may occur in gallbladder disease, but their mechanism is not clear.

Local factors in the gallbladder. These must have some part to play in the actual precipitation of stones. Not all patients with cholesterol stones secrete lithogenic bile. The parts played in stone formation by the gallbladder mucosa, the mucus and glycoprotein which it secretes, and the effects of local stasis are not known. There may also be a feedback effect on bile composition from the gallbladder and lithogenic bile shows a return to more normal composition following cholecystectomy.

Infections. It is doubtful whether infection plays a significant role in the pathogenesis of the majority of gallstones. The bile is sterile in most patients with stones, and no consistent pattern of bacterial infection has been demonstrated. Infection, however, may enhance the effects of local factors already mentioned and thus contribute to increase in size of stones and the formation of additional and mixed ones.

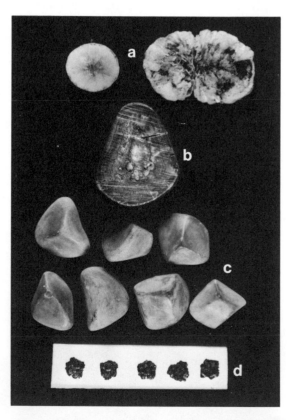

Fig. 19.53 Types of gallstones. **a** Two cholesterol stones; **b** Combination stone: a cholesterol core coated by laminated surface deposits of mixed composition; **c** multiple faceted mixed stones; **d** bile-pigment stones.

Types of stone

Stones can be classified as *mixed or laminated, pure, and combination or compound cholesterol* stones (Fig. 19.53).

Mixed or laminated gallstones. These, the commonest type, are always multiple and often very numerous (Fig. 19.53c). They are sometimes associated with and secondary to a solitary cholesterol stone. They vary greatly in size—from 1 cm or more in diameter to the size of sand grains, are irregular in form and often faceted. On section they have a distinctly laminated structure, dark brown and paler layers alternating. These layers consist chiefly of cholesterol and bile pigment respectively, both containing also an admixture of calcium salts and organic material. The layers are thicker at the angles. The faceting is due to growth of the stones in contact with one another. Their colour varies greatly from white, grey, brownish-yellow, pinkish, brown or almost black according to the nature of the covering layer and the stage of oxidation of the bile pigment. Mixed gallstones occur in very variable numbers; occasionally there may be hundreds of

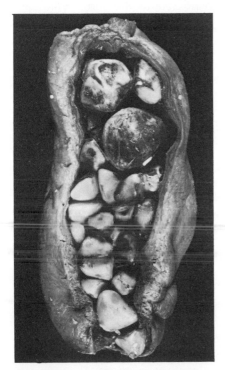

Fig. 19.54 Gallbladder filled with numerous gallstones of mixed type.

small stones. They may lie free in the bile, which may be mixed with inflammatory exudate or pus, or they may be tightly packed together within a contracted gallbladder with thickened wall (Fig. 19.54).

The cholesterol stone. This is usually solitary, oval, and may reach over 3 cm in length. It is pale yellow or almost white, soapy to the touch and of low specific gravity, often floating in water. Some are almost transparent with a frankly crystalline surface (Fig. 19.53a). When broken across, the stone shows a crystalline structure composed of sheaves of cholesterol crystals which radiate outwards from the centre. The latter is sometimes dark owing to the incorporation of bile pigment between the crystals, but there is no break in the continuity of their formation, and no trace of lamination. Some specimens of solitary cholesterol stones, however, have a laminated cortex (i.e. concentric deposits) composed of bile pigment and calcium salts, the pigment causing the darker markings (Fig. 19.53b). This is due to a secondary deposit, which occurs when the gallbladder wall becomes inflamed by superadded bacterial infection. Stones of this class may be called *combination* or *compound cholesterol stones*. They constitute the largest gallstones. Occasionally a contracted gallbladder contains two or three barrel-shaped combination cholesterol stones placed end to end.

Bile pigment stones. Such stones are comparatively rare; they are usually multiple, black, irregular in form or occasionally somewhat stellate (Fig. 19.53d). They are composed chiefly of bile pigment, and may be friable or hard. They are often present in chronic haemolytic anaemias and are due to excess of bile pigment in the bile, but are encountered also occasionally in the absence of increased red cell destruction. The gallbladder usually appears normal.

Calcium carbonate stones. These also are rare. They are multiple, small, pale yellowish and fairly hard.

Cholesterosis of the gallbladder

This unimportant condition results from the patchy deposition of doubly refractile cholesterol esters within mucosal macrophages. This produces distinct yellowish flecking of the mucosa giving the appearance of so-called

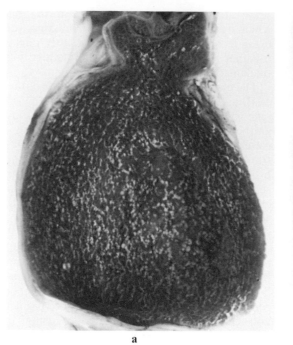 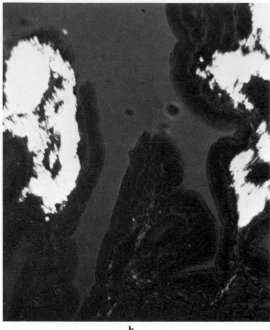

a   b

Fig. 19.55   Cholesterosis of gallbladder. **a**, the characteristic macroscopic pattern of 'strawberry gallbladder'. **b**, deposits of cholesterol esters in papillae, viewed by polarised light. × 90. (Professor W. A. Mackey.)

'strawberry gallbladder' (Fig. 19.55). The lipid deposits may increase in size to form polypoidal nodules. It is associated with cholesterol stones, solitary or mulberry, in one-third of cases.

Cholecystitis

Inflammation of the gallbladder is one of the commonest causes of abdominal pain, and frequently necessitates cholecystectomy.

Acute cholecystitis

Acute cholecystitis is nearly always associated with the presence of stones. It has been shown repeatedly that in the early stages of acute cholecystitis, bacteria cannot usually be cultured from the gallbladder. It is therefore thought that the initial inflammation is chemically induced. Obstruction to the outflow of bile due to a stone results in the bile becoming hyperconcentrated and this produces an irritant effect with consequent inflammation. Secondary bacterial infection may then occur, aggravating the inflammatory reaction. The organisms are thought to reach the gallbladder

via the lymphatics, and are most commonly *Esch. coli.* or *Strep. faecalis.* Acute cholecystitis may occur in the absence of stones but is then usually associated with a source of infection elsewhere.

Pathologically, acute cholecystitis may be merely a mild catarrhal inflammation, or more severe—fibrinous, pseudo-membranous, haemorrhagic or suppurative. These more severe types occur especially when there is continued obstruction of the cystic duct either by stone or by superadded inflammatory oedema and exudate. The lumen may then become filled with pus—*empyema of the gallbladder*. Abscesses may also form in the wall, or there may even be necrosis or gangrene of the wall with rupture into the peritoneal cavity. In recurrent attacks, the related local inflammation may result in the development of adhesions around the gallbladder: also the disease may pass into a chronic stage.

Chronic cholecystitis

This may result from repeated attacks of acute cholecystitis. In many patients, however, the disease is one of insidious onset, accompanied by

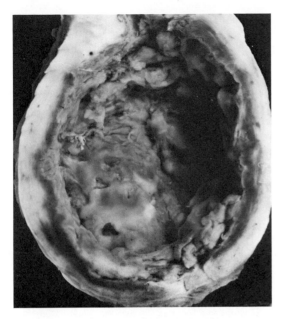

Fig. 19.56 Chronic cholecystitis, showing great thickening of wall. The gallbladder was packed with small rounded stones.

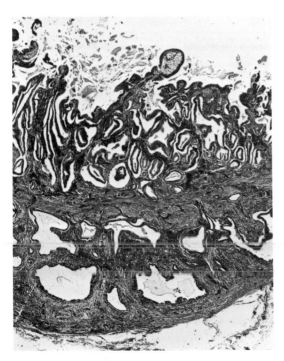

Fig. 19.57 Chronic cholecystitis showing extensive penetration of fundus of gallbladder by epithelial-lined spaces lying between muscle and serosa. (Rokitansky–Aschoff sinuses.) × 20.

dyspeptic symptoms or biliary colic. Gallstones are almost always present. The gallbladder wall is shrunken and shows marked fibrous thickening (Fig. 19.56). The lining is irregular, and there may be distinct pouches, especially when numerous stones are present. The contents may be clear, turbid or frankly purulent. The lining epithelium sometimes extends normally as downgrowths between the muscle bundles to form gland-like structures known as *Rokitansky–Aschoff sinuses*. This becomes much more marked in some cases of chronic cholecystitis, and there may be multiple complex epithelial overgrowths within the wall, which have occasionally been mistaken for adenocarcinoma (Fig. 19.57). Previously referred to as 'cholecystitis glandularis proliferans', the condition is now known as *adenomyomatosis of the gallbladder* and is benign. It may rarely occur in the absence of stones, and produce inflammation and symptoms resembling biliary colic.

Complications of cholelithiasis and cholecystitis

Gallstones and infections of the gallbladder are so intimately related that the complications associated with them are best considered together. Some of these have been referred to already.

Gallstones, single or multiple, may lead to no noticeable symptoms—so-called silent stones. When a stone becomes impacted in Hartmann's pouch or in the cystic duct, great distension of the gallbladder results: the bile pigments are absorbed and the contents become clear and mucoid—mucocele of the gallbladder (Fig. 19.58). In the presence of infection, however, the contents become turbid or purulent—empyema of the gallbladder. Inflammation of the wall may progress to necrosis, with escape of the contents into the peritoneal cavity producing localised or generalised peritonitis.

Stones may also obstruct the common bile duct, producing biliary colic, extrahepatic obstruction and jaundice (p. 626). If the stone remains loose in the duct, the jaundice may be intermittent. Secondary bacterial infection is common, resulting in ascending cholangitis. In only a small proportion of cases does obstruction of the bile duct by stones lead to secondary biliary cirrhosis.

In chronic cholecystitis the wall becomes thickened and may be contracted over a mass

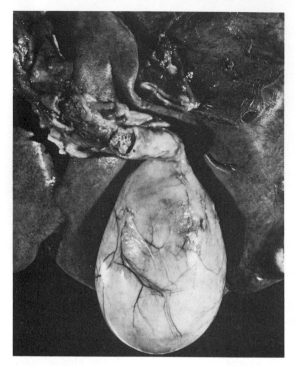

Fig. 19.58 Mucocele of the gallbladder. A stone is impacted in the cystic duct producing distension of the gallbladder, the contents of which have become clear and mucoid. Note how this accentuates the vascular markings on the serosa.

of closely packed stones: there are often adhesions around the gallbladder and a stone or stones may ulcerate in one of several directions. A large stone of the compound cholesterol type may, for example, ulcerate through into the duodenum or less frequently into the colon. It may pass along the bowel, or may become arrested at some part of the small intestine, chiefly by contraction of the muscular coat, and may produce acute intestinal obstruction, which is then termed *gallstone ileus*. Ulceration into the portal vein with the setting up of portal pyaemia has been recorded.

Lastly, the irritation produced by gallstones may lead to carcinoma of the gallbladder, or, more rarely, of the large ducts.

Tumours of the biliary tract

Benign tumours, such as fibroma, lipoma and papilloma, are all very rare. Rarely, a large papilloma may obstruct the outflow with much distension of the gallbladder.

Carcinoma is uncommon, and gallstones are an important factor in its causation, being present in fully 80% of cases of cancer. The commonest site is the fundus and next is the neck of the gallbladder. It is usually of the slowly-growing, infiltrating type, but sometimes it is a soft growth with a tendency to necrosis. Occasionally the gallbladder may be practically destroyed and its cavity represented by a small irregular space in which gallstones may be present. It may invade the liver (Fig. 19.59) and may also give rise to numerous metastases. In most cases the growth is an

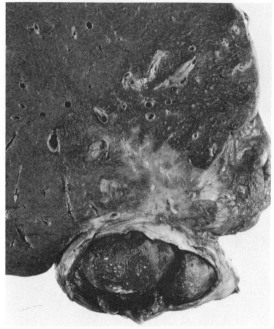

Fig. 19.59 Carcinoma of the gallbladder spreading directly into the overlying liver.

adenocarcinoma, sometimes a cancer of spheroidal cell or the mucoid type. Squamous carcinoma, arising secondarily to metaplasia of the lining epithelium, also occurs.

Carcinoma occurs also in the *large bile ducts* and is usually a small and slowly growing tumour. The two commonest sites are the lower end of the common bile duct (Fig. 19.60) and the junction of the cystic and hepatic ducts, the latter being more frequent; this site is also commonly involved by secondary lymphatic spread from carcinoma of the gallbladder.

Of the very many individuals who develop gallstones, less than 2% develop carcinoma of the gallbladder; the incidence of bile-duct carcinoma

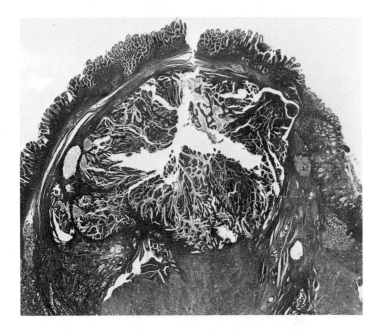

Fig. 19.60 Primary carcinoma of the ampulla of Vater causing obstructive jaundice. × 6.

is also low, although it is often not possible to determine whether a tumour around the ampulla has originated from bile duct or pancreas.

Congenital anomalies of the gallbladder and bile ducts

A large number of abnormalities of the gall-bladder have been described and may affect its size, shape, position, relation to the liver, etc. Gallstones may occur more frequently at a younger age in association with these anomalies.

Varying degrees of extrahepatic *biliary atresia* may occur and may result in secondary biliary cirrhosis (p. 628). The rare *choledochal cyst* comprises a sac-like dilatation of a part or all of the biliary tract, and is associated with jaundice and cholangitis.

Jaundice

Staining of the tissues with bilirubin or bilirubin complexes is known as *jaundice* or *icterus*. When the serum level of these pigments rises above 34·2 μmol/litre (2 mg/100 ml), generalised jaundice develops. According to the severity and duration of the condition the skin presents various degrees of yellow staining up to deep orange colour and in very chronic cases it becomes olive-green owing to formation of biliverdin. The internal organs also are pigmented except the brain and spinal cord, which are not usually affected. In *icterus gravis neonatorum*, however (p. 651), there may be bile staining of areas in the central nervous system, usually localised to the grey matter of the basal nuclei—the so-called *kernicterus*—but sometimes affecting the cortex (p. 662). The presence of the pigment in the blood in a case of marked jaundice is readily shown by the colour of the serum. Bile pigment may also be excreted in the urine and in the sweat; the tears, however, are not coloured, nor are the saliva, gastric juice or secretion of the bile-duct epithelium.

When the cause of the jaundice has been removed the skin may remain stained for some time after the serum bilirubin level has returned to normal, owing to the strong affinity of the elastic tissue for bilirubin. A rise of serum bilirubin from the normal level of 3·4–13·7 μmol/litre (0·2–0·8 mg/100 ml) up to 34·2

μmol/litre (2 mg/100 ml) is not usually accompanied by visible jaundice, but is sometimes called 'latent jaundice'. The term 'localised jaundice' is seldom used but it is seen around a bruise, the escaped haemoglobin being broken down to bilirubin.

Before considering further the features and types of jaundice, it is necessary to give an outline of the normal bile pigment metabolism.

Bile pigment metabolism

More than 80% of the bile pigment is derived from the breakdown of effete mature red cells. Approximately 6 g of haemoglobin are broken down daily, mainly in macrophages, in man chiefly in the spleen, bone-marrow and liver, and the steps have already been described (p. 239). The remaining 20% is derived in part from non-haemoglobin haem-containing pigments, e.g. myoglobin, catalase and cytochromes, and in part from ineffective erythropoiesis during red cell maturation. Excessive production of this latter erythropoietic component may occur in thalassaemia, congenital porphyria and in dyserythropoietic or shunt hyperbilirubinaemia (p. 479). Approximately 300 mg of bilirubin are produced daily.

Following release from macrophages, bilirubin (sometimes called **unconjugated bilirubin** to distinguish it from bilirubin glucuronides—see below) circulates in the plasma and is preferentially taken up by the hepatocytes. Within these cells it is transported by bilirubin-binding 'z' and 'y' proteins to the endoplasmic reticulum where it is conjugated with glucuronic acid, a reaction catalysed by the enzyme uridine diphosphate glucuronyl transferase. Both mono- and diglucuronide conjugates are formed, and possibly also sulphate and carbohydrate conjugates whose importance is uncertain. These conjugates are water soluble, and are referred to as **conjugated bilirubin**; they are rapidly excreted directly into the bile canaliculi and hence pass into the bile. Conjugated bilirubin is converted in the intestine into **stercobilinogen**, the normal brown faecal pigment. A small fraction of the stercobilinogen is re-absorbed from the gut, and most of this passes back to the liver where it is re-excreted into the bile—the entero-hepatic circulation of bile pigment. A minute amount (1–3 mg daily) of the re-absorbed stercobilinogen is excreted in the urine as **urobilinogen**.

To understand the clinical, biochemical and morbid anatomical features of the different types of jaundice, it is necessary to appreciate that unconjugated bilirubin is water-insoluble and remains in solution in the plasma only as a rather firm complex with albumin. Consequently, it does not readily pass through capillary walls, and its increase in the plasma is not accompanied by bilirubinuria. Nevertheless, unconjugated bilirubin is capable of staining the tissues, although the form in which it escapes from the plasma remains unknown. Another feature of unconjugated bilirubin is its solubility in lipids, which may explain the bilirubin-staining of the brain in neonates with high plasma levels of unconjugated bilirubin. The brain damage which may result is due to the toxic effects of bilirubin on nerve cells. By contrast, conjugated bilirubin is water-soluble, and increased levels in the plasma are always accompanied by its appearance in the urine: it is relatively insoluble in lipids and causes neither staining of, nor damage to, the central nervous system.

The biochemical estimation of serum bilirubin employs the **van den Bergh reaction**. When Ehrlich's diazo reagent, a mixture of sulphanilic acid and sodium nitrite, is added to a solution of bilirubin, the pigment becomes diazotised to give a blue-violet compound which can be assayed colorimetrically. Conjugated bilirubin gives an *immediate* or *direct* reaction, and the *total* bilirubin is then measured after treatment with alcohol which splits the unconjugated or indirect-reacting bilirubin from its bilirubin–albumin complex.

Classification of Jaundice

Jaundice may result from:

(1) Increased bilirubin production.
(2) Interference with hepatic uptake of bilirubin.
(3) Interference with hepatic conjugation of bilirubin.
(4) Interference with hepatic excretion of bilirubin.
(5) Combinations of 2–4 resulting from reduction in functional hepatic cell mass.

While it is of diagnostic and therapeutic importance to determine which of the above five factors is responsible for the development of jaundice, in practice it is found that more than one factor is often concerned. For example, the anaemia resulting from increased red cell destruction may cause liver cell injury, as also does prolonged obstruction of the biliary tract, whether or not accompanied by infection. Thus jaundice is frequently attributable to more than one factor, and diagnosis of the underlying condition is sometimes very difficult.

(1) Increased bilirubin production

(a) Haemolytic (acholuric) jaundice. Increased red cell destruction, either acute or chronic (see p. 465), results in the production in the macrophage system of increased amounts of bilirubin, up to 1·5 g daily. Normally, the liver is capable of extracting, conjugating and excreting such large amounts of bilirubin, and jaundice is often latent or mild. The agent causing the haemolysis may, however, also damage the liver, or the anaemia resulting from haemolysis may depress liver function, and in these circumstances jaundice is more pronounced. In infants, the rate of red cell destruction is relatively high, and the liver is deficient in the enzymes necessary for conjugation of bilirubin, particularly when birth is premature. Accordingly, *icterus neonatorum* is a common condition, and is likely to be especially severe in infants with haemolytic anaemia due to maternal iso-antibodies (p. 473). Exchange blood transfusions may be necessary to keep the plasma bilirubin below 340 μmol/litre (20 mg/100 ml), the level at which there is a real danger of brain damage from kernicterus.

In haemolytic jaundice, most of the bilirubin in the plasma is unconjugated, and thus bile pigment is absent from the urine (*acholuric jaundice*). The amount of urobilinogen in the urine is, however, usually much increased and its estimation is used in the investigation of haemolytic states. The faeces are dark from the excessive amounts of bile pigment excreted.

(b) Dyserythropoietic (shunt) hyperbilirubinaemia. This is associated with ineffective or abnormal red cell maturation resulting in the premature destruction of these erythrocytes in the marrow: there is an unconjugated bilirubinaemia but with a normal peripheral blood red cell survival time. The disease is rare, familial and the mode of inheritance is not defined.

(2) Interference with hepatic uptake of bilirubin

Gilbert's disease. Although rare, this is the commonest form of familial non-haemolytic acholuric jaundice. It is apparently due to a 'dominant' defect of a single autosomal gene which impairs either transport of bilirubin to the liver, or uptake of bilirubin by the liver. Mild intermittent acholuric jaundice results. The condition is, however, rather poorly defined.

(3) Interference with hepatic conjugation of bilirubin

(a) Physiologial or neonatal jaundice. This is associated with a relative deficiency of glucuronyl transferase in the neonatal liver, a situation which may be aggravated by prematurity. The jaundice usually improves 2–3 weeks postpartum as the enzyme attains normal levels.

(b) Inherited defective bilirubin conjugation. In the very rare *Crigler-Najjar* syndrome the deficiency of glucuronyl transferase results in very high levels of unconjugated bilirubin. Kernicterus within the first two years of life is the usual cause of death.

(4) Interference with hepatic excretion of bilirubin

(a) Intrahepatic inherited. In the rare *Dubin–Johnson* syndrome, there is a partial failure of the liver cells to secrete conjugated bilirubin into the bile canaliculi, and as a consequence conjugated bilirubin is regurgitated into the blood and intermittent jaundice results. The other constituents of the bile are secreted normally, and the serum alkaline phosphatase level is not raised. A curious feature is accumulation of granules of brown pigment in hepatocyte lysosomes, as yet of uncertain nature but possibly melanin-like. Little or no disability results from this syndrome, which is believed to be due to a single gene defect with 'dominant' transmission. A second, and genetically related condition, is the *Rotor syndrome* in which there is failure to secrete conjugated bilirubin but no accumulation of brown pigment in the liver cells.

In a further rare condition—*benign idiopathic recurrent intrahepatic cholestasis*—multiple recurrent attacks of cholestasis occur in the absence of large duct obstruction, the jaundice persisting for some months, but without producing any evidence of progressive or permanent liver damage.

(b) Intrahepatic acquired. This occurs in primary biliary cirrhosis (p. 625), and also as a complication of therapy with certain drugs (p. 642).

Drug-induced cholestasis occurs as an idiosyncrasy in a small proportion of patients taking phenothiazine derivatives, notably chlorpromazine, and appears unrelated to dosage. It is reversible, at least in most cases, on discontinuing the drug. Cholestasis results also from administration of methyl testosterone and certain other C17-alkyl-substituted testosterones, and does not depend upon idiosyncrasy, being produced regularly by a sufficient dosage of such compounds.

(c) Extrahepatic biliary obstruction. (Obstructive, regurgitation or retention jaundice). Major duct obstruction is caused chiefly by gallstones lodging in the common bile duct, and by carcinoma of the head of the pancreas or of the lower end of the common bile duct. Less commonly, it arises from scarring of bile ducts due to previous inflammation and ulceration by gallstones, and from accidental injury or ligation of the common bile duct during operations in this area. Other causes include congenital malformations of the major duct system, and involvement of the ducts in tumours or tuberculosis affecting the lymph nodes and surrounding tissues in the portal fissure.

When due to gallstones, the obstruction may be sudden and complete, or intermittent if the stone or stones move along the common bile duct; it is often accompanied by biliary colic. In carcinomatous involvement or scarring of the ducts, obstruction, and hence jaundice, are usually of more gradual onset, progressive and often painless. As in all forms of obstructive jaundice the serum **alkaline phosphatase** is greatly raised.

Apart from jaundice and its effects, major duct obstruction, particularly if caused by gallstones, is likely to be complicated by superadded suppurative cholangitis, and in unrelieved obstruction the patient does not usually survive long enough to develop secondary biliary cirrhosis (p. 626).

(5) Reduction in functional hepatic cell mass (hepatocellular or toxic jaundice)

This type of jaundice results from damage to liver cells, e.g. by viruses, bacterial toxins or hepatocellular chemicals. It is a feature of the various forms of viral hepatitis (p. 611) and leptospirosis (Weil's disease), where the organisms are actually present in the liver, and it occurs occasionally in typhus, pneumonia, septicaemia, relapsing fever, smallpox, etc. It is seen also in some forms of snake bite, in poisoning with various chemicals and toxins—trinitrotoluene, phosphorus, amanitine and amanita toxin from various fungi, etc. Except in biliary cirrhosis, jaundice is usually a late complication of hepatic cirrhosis, and is then likely to be attributable to liver cell necrosis and hepatocellular failure.

Two factors are concerned in the production of hepatocellular jaundice: (*a*) damage to the liver cells may interfere with the passage of bile along the bile canaliculi: in other words, a degree of intrahepatic cholestasis arises. Focal necrosis or swelling of the liver cells, and disorganisation of the columns of liver cells and fibrosis (as in cirrhosis), may thus cause focal cholestasis; (*b*) removal of unconjugated bilirubin from the blood, its conjugation and discharge into the bile canaliculi, may all be impaired as a result of liver-cell injury. The relative importance of these two factors varies in different cases, and may also change, as liver-cell injury progresses, in the individual case.

The Exocrine Pancreas

The pancreas is composed of two kinds of tissue with distinct functions. Firstly, the **acinous or exocrine glandular tissue**, which produces the digestive secretion of the gland, of pH 7·5–8·0 and containing bicarbonate, amylase and lipase which are secreted in their active form, and trypsinogen and chymotrypsinogen which are converted to the active enzymes trypsin and chymotrypsin in the duodenum. Secondly, the **islets of Langerhans or en-**

docrine glandular tissue, which secrete several hormones—insulin and glucagon, which are of importance in carbohydrate metabolism, and gastrin, which is important in the control of gastro-intestinal secretion and motility. The pathology of the islets is dealt with in Chapter 24.

Exocrine pancreatic function can be assessed by measuring the volume and enzyme content of pancreatic juice obtained by duodenal aspiration following a standard small meal of gruel—the Lundh test. Evidence of structural pancreatic abnormalities may be seen on plain x-ray films of the abdomen or by a barium meal; special radiological procedures include hypotonic duodenography, angiography, radio-isotope scanning, and more recently ultrasonography and endoscopic cannulation of the pancreatic duct. In acute pancreatitis some enzymes are released into the circulation and may be measured in serum and urine.

Degenerative changes

Focal necrosis occurs in infections, fatty change in various poisonings, and sometimes amyloid change from the usual causes. Lipomatosis occurs in obesity, and is often a marked feature when the glandular tissue becomes atrophied, e.g. after obstruction of the duct. Atrophy of the gland accompanies fibrotic lesions and obstructions of the duct, described below; it occurs also in wasting diseases, and to a lesser degree as a senile change. Abnormal smallness of the pancreas without any other change occurs in some cases of diabetes in young subjects, but its nature and significance are doubtful. Pigmentation from deposition of granular haemosiderin, sometimes considerable, is common in haemochromatosis (p. 628) and may be accompanied by diabetes. When the pancreatic tissue is injured in various ways, it is attacked by its own enzymes, and necrosis results. Thus small circumscribed areas of dull yellowish necrotic tissue are a common necropsy finding. They are seen especially after operations on the pancreas, in acute and chronic pancreatitis, and in obstruction of the ducts; they are often accompanied by patches of necrosis in the fat around the pancreas (Fig. 19.61b). Fine fibrosis and dilatation of the pancreatic ducts and acini may occur in uraemia ('*uraemic pancreatitis*').

Experimentally the administration of ethionine to rats has resulted in pancreatic degeneration and necrosis, apparently by antogonising methionine and interfering with protein synthesis.

Pancreatitis is classified into acute and chronic forms, which are now believed to be two distinct entities. Acute pancreatitis rarely proceeds to the chronic form, even when it is of the recurrent variety. Chronic relapsing pancreatitis is a further variant.

Acute pancreatitis (acute haemorrhagic necrosis of the pancreas)

In most cases this condition is essentially an acute necrosis with haemorrhage in greater or lesser degree; in the later stages secondary infection leading to *suppuration* and even to *gangrene* may occur. These changes characterise stages in the condition rather than distinct varieties. In cases dying very rapidly after the onset of symptoms there may be patchy necrosis of the pancreas with only a light haemorrhagic speckling, indicating that necrosis precedes thrombosis and haemorrhage, but in others of longer duration the whole organ may be deep purple-black owing to diffuse interstitial haemorrhage.

Clinical features. This is a not uncommon clinical emergency. It occurs most frequently after the age of 40, is commoner in women, and its most frequent clinical associations are biliary tract disease, alcoholism, obesity and trauma. In more than 50% of cases, gallstones or chronic cholecystitis are present. The frequency of alcohol abuse varies, being as high as 30–40% in some series, but in Scotland the associated frequency is approximately 20%. There is no correlation, however, with the pattern or dosage of alcohol intake. Surgical trauma, closed abdominal trauma or trauma as a result of endoscopic cannulation of the pancreatic duct, may all precipitate an attack. Less common clinical associations include pregnancy, hyperparathyroidism, hypothermia, pancreatic tumours, hyperlipoproteinaemia (particularly Friedrichsen's types I and V) and polyarteritis nodosa. A number of drugs have also been suspected as causal agents including corticosteroids, azathioprine and thiazides, and in the West Indies acute pancreatitis may follow scorpion bites, due to an unidentified toxin.

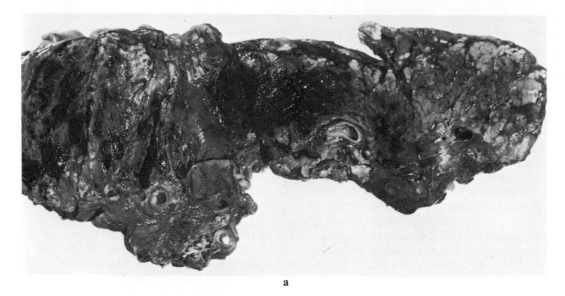

a

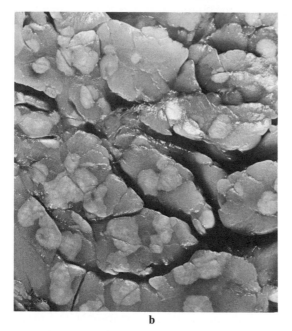

b

Fig. 19.61 **(a)** Acute haemorrhagic pancreatitis. × 0·6. **(b)** Part of the greater omentum from the same case, showing pale patches of fat necrosis. × 1·7.

The disease comes on suddenly with abdominal pain, vomiting and collapse, and may simulate gastro-duodenal perforation. Shock may be marked, with hypotension, and sometimes may lead to acute renal failure. Hypocalcaemic tetany and hyperglycaemic coma may complicate the picture. There is a marked degree of hypoxia with arterial Po_2 levels of less than 60 mm of mercury, and thus the patients are bad operative risks. Amylase and lipase are released into the circulation and their measurement in the serum, and of amylase in the urine, are of diagnostic value. Recurrent acute pancreatitis should lead to careful investigation for possible causal factors, such as gallstones or alcohol abuse, for correction of these will usually prevent further episodes.

The peritoneal cavity generally contains bloodstained serous fluid, and numerous patches of *fat necrosis* result from the liberation of pancreatic lipase from the damaged parenchyma; the fat is split, the glycerol being absorbed, while the firm yellowish-white patches represent fatty acids. These patches are specially numerous in the region of the pancreas and in the greater omentum (Fig. 19.61*b*), but occur elsewhere. The haemorrhage into the pancreas and tissues around may be so extensive that a dark mass is seen through the peritoneum of the lesser peritoneal sac. The cut surface of the pancreas varies; in some cases it is almost uniformly haemorrhagic, in others there is a mixture of dull yellowish areas of necrosis with haemorrhage between and around (Fig. 19.61*a*), and sometimes necrosis predominates.

On **microscopic examination**, necrosis, haemorrhage and inflammation are associated in varying proportions. Haemorrhage may be the outstanding feature, the whole tissue of the gland being infiltrated with blood, while diffuse necrosis of the acini is seen at places. Many of the small veins and capillaries contain packed red cells owing to extreme loss of plasma; later their walls become necrotic and this may play a part in causing haemorrhage. In other cases there are areas of well-defined necrosis, affecting all the tissues, both glandular and interstitial, and accompanied by heavy neutrophil polymorph infiltration (Fig. 19.62). The

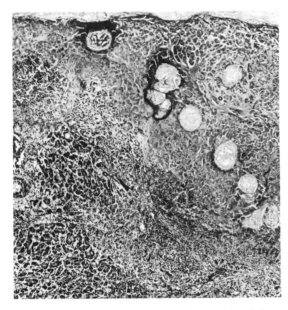

Fig. 19.62 Acute pancreatitis. The pale-staining necrotic area with fat necrosis is seen top right, with surviving pancreas below. × 38.

inflammatory reaction seems to occur later, and is most marked in the less acute cases. All the appearances may be interpreted as the result of some toxic agent, which kills the parenchyma and also acts on the vessels, leading to thrombosis and haemorrhage. Superadded bacterial infection is common and may be severe, progressing to suppuration with abscess formation or gangrenous pancreatitis, often with generalised peritonitis.

The aetiology of acute pancreatitis is not clear. It is thought to be due essentially to liberation of activated endogenous proteolytic enzymes either as a result of damage to the parenchyma or perhaps from rupture of distended ducts. The free enzymes are presumed to

result first in acute inflammatory oedema, and later necrosis of the vessel walls, sludging of red cells, haemorrhage, thrombosis and necrosis of the parenchyma.

Pancreatic enzymes can be activated by bile, acid gastric or duodenal juice, and by bacteria. Cases have been reported in which obstruction of the ampulla of Vater, usually by a gallstone, has resulted in bile passing along the pancreatic duct, and it has been shown that spasm of the sphincter of Oddi, which can be induced by hydrochloric acid, can have a similar effect. However, in most instances of acute pancreatitis the bile and pancreatic ducts have been found to open separately into the duodenum and this mechanism cannot operate. The reflux of duodenal contents along the pancreatic duct resulting from raised intra-abdominal pressure has also been postulated. Increased secretion of pancreatic juice in the presence of partial or complete block of the pancreatic duct (e.g. by squamous metaplasia or due to a local duodenitis) could also result in local release of proteolytic enzymes. Squamous metaplasia is not frequent, but may produce partial blockage of the ducts in some cases of acute pancreatitis. The vascular thrombi seen microscopically have been claimed by some workers to be primary, producing local ischaemic damage and thus causing the acute attack. However, it seems just as likely that the vascular occlusion is a secondary manifestation. The aetiology of acute haemorrhagic pancreatitis is obviously enigmatic.

Suppurative pancreatitis may occur apart from secondary infection in acute pancreatitis, and is then usually caused by passage of bacteria along the ducts, or by direct spread from a local focus of infection, e.g. from an infected pancreatic tumour, or inflammatory diseases of the duodenum. Pancreatitis may occur as a rare complication of mumps and is thought to be due to viral infection of the organ.

Chronic pancreatitis

It is important to distinguish between *acute recurrent pancreatitis*, which does not necessarily lead to pancreatic deficiency, and *chronic pancreatitis*, which is usually progressive. Two clinical varieties of chronic pancreatitis are recognised: (*a*) a chronic pancreatitis in which the manifestations are usually those of malabsorption and/or

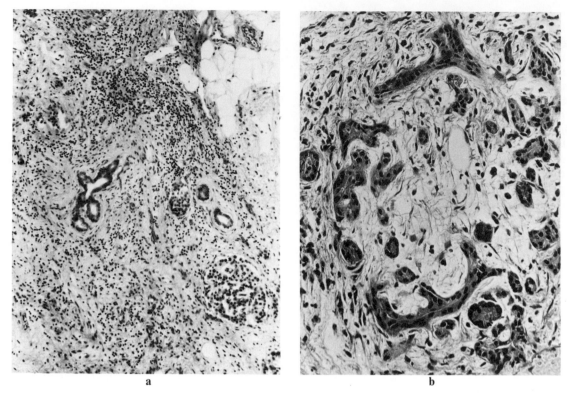

a   b

Fig. 19.63   a Chronic pancreatitis with diffuse fibrous replacement of exocrine pancreas: a surviving islet is present (*lower right*) and there is a chronic inflammatory cell infiltrate of the interstitium. × 100. **b** Chronic pancreatitis: surviving acinar elements in fibrous tissue showing compression and distortion. × 250.

diabetes; and (*b*) a chronic relapsing pancreatitis in which there are intermittent recurrent attacks of abdominal pain associated with exacerbations of the disease, but which pursues a progressive course.

Chronic pancreatitis is fairly common, but its aetiology is often obscure. It may be associated with pancreatic duct obstruction by carcinoma of the head of the pancreas or in the periampullary region, or by pancreatic calculi. Chronic alcohol abuse appears to be a factor in many cases, and there is a resultant association with hepatic cirrhosis. In haemochromatosis, diffuse fibrous replacement of the pancreas is accompanied by iron deposition in both the exocrine and endocrine elements. Areas of fibrosis in the pancreas may be produced, as in other organs, by arteriosclerosis. A form of diffuse interstitial pancreatitis has also been described in congenital syphilis.

In chronic pancreatitis the gland becomes firmer. Sometimes it is enlarged, but more frequently shrunken and atrophic. The histological changes comprise fibrosis and atrophy of the glandular elements (Fig. 19.63). The fibrosis may be chiefly between the lobules—*interlobular*—or there may be a more diffuse fibrosis between the acini—*intralobular*. In the connective tissue, the small ducts may be unduly prominent, and some of these may be newly formed in the same way as the small bile ducts in cirrhosis of the liver. The islets of Langerhans suffer less than the glandular acini, but they also may be implicated in the fibrosis when it is intralobular in distribution, and thus diabetes may result. The histological distinction between chronic pancreatitis and carcinoma of the pancreas may be very difficult.

Obstruction of pancreatic ducts

Obstruction of the main duct may be caused by a pancreatic calculus, occasionally by a gallstone filling the ampulla of Vater, by scarring, or by pressure of a tumour, most frequently cancer of the head of the pancreas. Obstruction leads to irregular dilatation of the large ducts. The smaller ducts may be similarly affected and may occasionally show cyst-like distension. The result, as in other organs, no doubt depends on whether the obstruction is constant or intermittent, but two changes are prominent: atrophy of the exocrine cells and overgrowth of the connective tissue. In long-standing cases only shrunken remains of the parenchyma are found in the connective tissue. Sometimes the atrophy is accompanied by extensive replacement of the gland by adipose tissue without loss of shape (lipomatosis). The islets of Langerhans are not affected by the atrophic process, but, on the contrary, they are more prominent and appear more numerous than usual, owing to the shrinking of the other tissues. Even when the exocrine tissue has almost gone, groups of virtually unchanged islets remain. Similar results follow experimental ligation of the pancreatic duct in animals; here also the persistence of the islets is outstanding. This explains why diabetes does not, as a rule, follow ligation of the main duct.

In view of the effects of pancreatic duct obstruction, it is curious that pancreatic tissue of normal microscopic appearance is sometimes seen in teratomas: it seems most unlikely that such tissue could have a patent duct system.

Pancreatic calculi

These are small concretions composed of calcium carbonate and a little phosphate, which form in the pancreatic ducts, though their occurrence is rare. They seldom exceed 5 mm, and they may be numerous and minute. They are irregularly rounded or elongated, whitish and usually hard. In addition to causing obstruction in varying degree, they may lead to secondary bacterial infection, with acute or chronic inflammatory change as the result.

Cysts

The most important variety is the single 'pancreatic cyst' which forms a large rounded swelling, sometimes of over 10 cm diameter. The cyst usually contains a colourless fluid, clear or slightly turbid, though sometimes there may be an admixture of altered blood. The pancreatic enzymes are present in the fluid for a time, and may be detected by the usual tests; later, however, they disappear. The formation of such a cyst has been observed after injury, and this is regarded as the usual cause. The layer of peritoneum over the pancreas is torn and there then occurs an escape of blood and pancreatic secretion into the lesser peritoneal sac, the fluid becoming localised by adhesions. The condition is thus really a *pseudo-cyst* which is situated outside the pancreas. A similar condition may follow an attack of pancreatitis, but the cause is often obscure. A cystic form of adenoma sometimes occurs in the pancreas. In *Lindau's disease* (p. 731), cysts may occur in the pancreas along with haemangiomas in the cerebellum. Hydatid cysts also occur in and around the pancreas.

Cystic fibrosis (Fibrocystic disease of the pancreas)

Formerly known as fibrocystic disease of the pancreas, this disease is due to a generalised abnormality of exocrine gland secretion involving pancreas, bowel, lungs, biliary tree and sweat glands. In the newborn it may give rise to intestinal obstruction and sometimes perforation—meconium ileus and meconium peritonitis—caused by luminal impaction of inspissated meconium. In older children respiratory infections, and eventually bronchiectasis, are common. Biliary obstruction, due to inspissated secretions in the bile ducts, may lead to segmental hepatic fibrosis and secondary biliary cirrhosis. Failure of pancreatic exocrine secretion produces a malabsorption syndrome (p. 583). There is an increased sodium chloride content of the sweat both in affected individuals and in presumed heterozygotes, and this provides a useful diagnostic test and a test for studies of the genetic inheritance of the disease.

The inheritance is autosomal recessive, but apparently with some genetic heterogeneity. It is not uncommon, occurring in approximately one per 2000 live births in caucasians. The precise aetiology is unknown, postulated mechanisms including defective function of cholinergic autonomic nervous control, absence of an enzyme, or some other type of inherited metabolic disorder. The pancreas is small, firm and gritty, the cysts rarely being visible to the naked eye. On section the acini and ducts are dilated and filled with tough yellowish eosinophilic secretion which contains abundant mucin (Fig. 19.64). Subsequent fibrosis, both in the head practically always leads to obstruction of the main ducts, with exclusion of the pancreatic secretion from the intestine, and usually the common bile duct also is obstructed, causing jaundice.

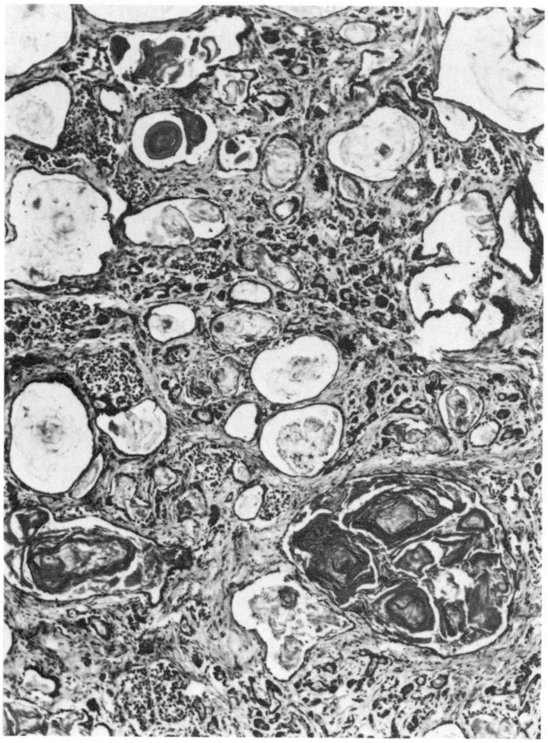

Fig. 19.64 Fibrocystic disease of the pancreas. The ducts are filled with eosinophilic laminated secretion; the acini are either markedly atrophied or much dilated. × 50. (Professor G. L. Montgomery.)

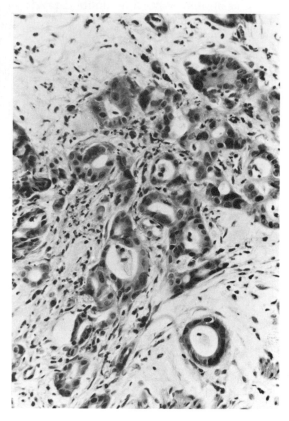

Fig. 19.65 Adenocarcinoma of pancreas, showing a regular acinar pattern and with a related scirrhous reaction.

inter- and intra-lobular, may lead to loss of the normal lobulation. Rarely hepatic cholestasis and biliary cirrhosis may develop.

Tumours

Apart from carcinoma, tumours are rare in the pancreas. Fibroma, lipoma, lymphangioma, adenoma and cystadenoma have been described; the last mentioned may reach a considerable size.

Carcinoma of the pancreas nearly always occurs in the head, less frequently in the body, rarely in the tail; it is usually a scirrhous adeno-carcinoma, which may mimic the pancreatic acinar structure (Fig. 19.65), but sometimes the cells are quite irregularly arranged. The growth,

Carcinoma of the pancreas is one of the most commonly obscure forms of malignant disease clinically, and is one in which bizarre symptoms such as unexplained venous thrombosis, peripheral neuropathy and myopathy may be the presenting ones.

It usually appears in the sixth decade and is twice as common in men as in women. The incidence has increased greatly and in some American surveys of alimentary tract cancers, it ranks second in frequency only to cancer of the large intestine. It is sometimes accompanied by anomalies of carbohydrate metabolism, and is twice as common in diabetics as in the general population. The possibility of pancreatic cancer should therefore be considered in late-onset unstable diabetes, or development of instability in a previously stable diabetic.

Tumours of the islet-cells are described on p. 967, in the account of disorders of the endocrine part of the pancreas.

Congenital abnormalities

Variations in the configuration of the pancreas and in the arrangement of its ducts are not uncommon. Occasionally the tissue of the head surrounds the adjacent part of the duodenum as a circular band, and stenosis may be produced. This is known as 'annular pancreas'. Foci of ectopic pancreatic tissue also occur, and may be single or multiple. The commonest site is the submucous tissue of the jejunum, though occasionally they occur in the duodenum and even in the stomach. Ectopic pancreas is sometimes found in the apex of a Meckel's diverticulum and also in an ordinary 'false diverticulum' of the small intestine. In the latter situation it has been supposed that its presence may cause the diverticulum.

20

The Nervous System

I The Brain

Introduction

The nervous system is composed of two types of tissue both of which are involved in varying degree in disease processes. The first consists of the highly specialised nerve cells and their processes together with the neuroglial cells, all of which are of neuro-ectodermal origin: the second comprises the meninges, the blood vessels and their supporting connective tissue, and phagocytic cells, all derived from mesoderm and similar in many respects to corresponding tissue found in other systems of the body. Some diseases of the nervous system are similar to those observed in other organs—for example, inflammation, diseases of the blood vessels and tumours. Others are primary diseases of the neuron involving its cell body, its axon or its myelin sheath and in this group the aetiology is often obscure although certain virus infections, metabolic disturbances and nutritional deficiencies, particularly of the vitamin B group, may cause direct damage to nerve cells. Even in those diseases where the primary damage is to the neuron, the most conspicuous pathological abnormalities are often reactive changes in the neuroglia, the microglia or the blood vessels. Indeed quite severe derangement of neuronal function may occur in the absence of obvious structural abnormalities in neurons.

Applied anatomy

The arrangement of the meninges and the distribution of the cerebrospinal fluid (CSF) are intimately concerned with the spread of pathological processes. The dura mater acts as the periosteum to the cranial bones but it can be stripped from the skull by haemorrhage or exudation into the potential *extradural space*, the former secondary to tearing of a meningeal

blood vessel by a fracture and the latter from spread of an infective process in the adjacent bone. The dura and the outer surface of the arachnoid are normally in contact but the *subdural space* can readily be distended by blood or exudate in some pathological processes. The arachnoid forms a continuous sheet in contact with the dura, while the pia follows the windings of the convolutions of the brain. The space between them, known as the *subarachnoid space*, is broken up by delicate trabeculae of connective tissue into a series of intercommunicating spaces filled with CSF. Apart from the cisterna magna and the cisterns at the base of

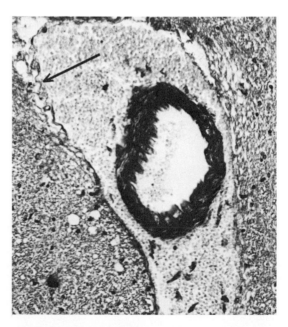

Fig. 20.1 Haemorrhage into Virchow–Robin space. The blood shows the relation of the small artery to the brain tissue. Note the pia (*arrow*). (A. C. L.) × 100.

the brain, the subarachnoid space is broadest in the sulci. The major cerebral arteries and veins run in the subarachnoid space, and from the arteries small *nutrient* vessels pass into the cortex. The nutrient arteries to the basal ganglia and other deep structures enter the base of the brain at the *perforated spots.*

As an artery penetrates the brain it carries the pia with it, the resulting potential perivascular space (often known as the Virchow–Robin space) between the vessel wall and the invaginated pia being continuous with the subarachnoid space (Fig. 20.1). As the vessels become smaller the two layers fuse to form a reticular perivascular sheath which can be followed as far as precapillary vessels but not to the capillaries themselves. The foot processes of astrocytes form a cuff in apposition to and completely surrounding the Virchow–Robin space and the capillaries of the brain.

Micro-organisms and their toxins readily diffuse throughout the subarachnoid space, which may become filled with inflammatory exudate. The inflammatory process may then spread into the brain around the nutrient blood vessels which are often seen to be surrounded by collections of leukocytes. The ventricular system communicates with the subarachnoid space by means of the exit foramina in the roof (Magendie) and lateral recesses (Luschka) of the fourth ventricle. Cerebrospinal fluid passes freely through these foramina and, in certain disease processes, so also do blood, pus, micro-organisms or, more rarely, tumour cells. The circulation of the CSF is dealt with in greater detail in relation to hydrocephalus (p. 669).

Examination of the CSF often provides valuable information about diseases of the nervous system. Specimens are ordinarily obtained by lumbar puncture but ventricular or occasionally cisternal puncture may sometimes be indicated. The pressure of the CSF should always be measured, as either an increase or a decrease may be of diagnostic value. Microbiological, serological, cytological and biochemical investigations on the CSF are routine procedures. As the changes may be many and varied, only the most important are given in the accounts which follow.

Normal CSF is clear and colourless, does not coagulate and has a specific gravity of 1·006. It contains about 150–400 mg/litre protein, about 2·75–5·5 mmol/litre (50–100 mg/ml) glucose, and approximately 128 mmol/litre sodium, and 128 mmol/litre chloride. A few mononuclear cells may be found in normal fluid but rarely more than 4 per μl. (See Table 20.1, pp. 708–9.)

The Reactions of the Nervous System to Disease

Neurons

Neurons are extremely complex cells and, since they exhibit great metabolic activity and require a continuous supply of oxygen and glucose, they are highly sensitive to alterations in their environment. As mitotic division of neurons ceases within a few weeks after birth, dead cells cannot be replaced, and the alterations observed within nerve cells are generally of a degenerative nature.

Primary degenerations

These include the structural changes produced directly by toxic action or impairment of oxygen supply.

Necrosis of neurons is produced by a variety of noxious processes, e.g. ischaemia, anoxia, hypoglycaemia and acute viral infections. The neuron shrinks and its triangular shape becomes accentuated, Nissl granules disappear and the cytoplasm becomes more eosinophilic, and the nucleus becomes pyknotic and fragments. Sometimes the necrotic nerve cells are attacked and removed by phagocytes (*neuronophagia* see below) but more commonly, particularly in infarcts, they undergo autolysis and disappear. A moderate diffuse loss of neurons may be very difficult to recognise histologically unless there are some reactive glial changes.

Another common degenerative change in neurons is simple **atrophy**. This occurs in many of the slowly progressive degenerative diseases of the nervous system such as motor neuron disease (p. 714). The nerve cells appear smaller than normal and lipofuscin accumulates in the cytoplasm. The cells ultimately disappear. Atrophy of neurons also occurs as an age-related phenomenon.

There are many other but less common intrinsic degenerative changes in neurons, e.g. the appearance of inclusion bodies in certain viral infections and in Parkinsonism, neurofibrillary degeneration in some types of dementia, and distension of the cytoplasm with lipid-laden lysosomes in certain inborn errors of metabolism, but these will be dealt with later in the chapter.

Abnormalities may also be brought about in neurons if the functioning of their intracellular oxidation–reduction enzyme systems is impaired as a result of some deficiency state, particularly in association with vitamin B deficiency. Deranged metabolism of this type underlies the pathogenesis of disorders apparently so diverse as peripheral neuropathy, Korsakoff's psychosis, Wernicke's encephalopathy, pellagra and beri-beri, and subacute combined degeneration of the cord.

Wernicke's encephalopathy. This is attributed to thiamine deficiency, but patients with it are likely to be deficient also in other components of the vitamin B complex. The deficiency may be of long duration as in chronic alcoholism or prolonged malnutrition, or it may be acute and occur as a complication of persistent vomiting. Wernicke's encephalopathy caused by acute vitamin deficiency is probably considerably commoner than is generally recognised, but chronic alcoholism remains the commonest underlying cause in well-nourished communities. The disorder was rather common among prisoners of war in the Far East during the Second World War and was attributed to dietary deficiencies.

Clinically the disease presents as an acute or subacute disorder characterised by disturbances of consciousness, ophthalmoplegia and ataxia with, if untreated, terminal coma. The blood pyruvate level is raised and, if the deficiency state is of considerable duration, a peripheral neuropathy is likely to be present. Pathologically there are, in acutely fatal cases, numerous petechial haemorrhages in the mamillary bodies, in the floor and walls of the third ventricle, around the aqueduct, and in the floor of the fourth ventricle. The various nuclei of the thalamus may also be involved. In subacute cases, macroscopic abnormalities may be restricted to slight granularity and loss of definition in the affected areas. Histologically there is dilatation and proliferation of capillaries, small haemorrhages, distinct pallor of staining of the parenchyma, and varying degrees of reactive change in astrocytes and microglia. Neurons are relatively spared.

Quite dramatic improvement may follow the administration of the vitamin B group, but good clinical recovery is unlikely if the mamillary bodies are already structurally damaged before treatment is initiated. The mamillary bodies become small and shrunken and often have a brownish discoloration on section. Such patients usually have a persistent psychosis of Korsakoff type.

Hepatolenticular degeneration. This is a rare condition in which the changes are very striking: it occurs mainly in adolescents and young adults, shows a familial tendency, and is probably due to an autosomal recessive character which determines an inborn error of copper metabolism (see p. 628). The main changes in the brain are in the putamen and caudate nucleus, which become soft, shrunken, and ultimately cystic. The neuronal loss is accompanied by a fibrillary gliosis and the occurrence of large astrocytes with strikingly vesicular swollen nuclei. These are Alzheimer astrocytes and in hepatolenticular degeneration they may be widely distributed throughout the grey matter. The lesions in the nervous system are due to metabolic disturbances dependent partly on the deposition of copper. The greenish-brown discoloration of the cornea near the limbus, known as Kayser–Fleischer rings, is due to deposition of copper. The resulting symptoms are mainly muscular tremors and spasticity. The condition is associated with cirrhosis of the liver, which is also due to the defect in copper metabolism mentioned above.

Acquired hepatocerebral degeneration is also recognised. The acute forms are associated with massive liver-cell necrosis when the principal abnormality in the brain is the occurrence of Alzheimer astrocytes. A chronic form is seen in individuals with a large porto-systemic venous shunt as occurs in cirrhosis (p. 630). Alzheimer astrocytes again appear in the brain but there may also be microcystic degeneration in the caudate nucleus, the putamen, and the deeper layers of the cortex.

Kernicterus. When severe jaundice occurs in infancy it carries the risk of brain injury: necrosis of neurons and bile staining are seen particularly in the hippocampus and basal nuclei (hence *kernicterus* or *nuclear jaundice*) and sometimes in the cerebral cortex, and are followed by gliosis. If not fatal, the brain injury is likely to cause choreo-athetosis, spasticity and often mental deficiency.

Pathogenesis. The condition is particularly likely to occur when the plasma level of *unconjugated* bilirubin exceeds 250 μmol/litre (15 mg/100 ml), and by far the commonest cause of this in full-term infants is haemolytic anaemia due to fetal-maternal Rh incompatibility (p. 473). Other causal factors include functional immaturity of the liver in premature infants, liver injury of various kinds and genetically determined defects of bilirubin conjugation (p. 651). Hypoxia during labour or at birth, or due to severe anaemia, may be contributory factors and the administration of excess vitamin K (for haemorrhagic disease of the newborn) tends to aggravate haemolysis and so may increase the jaundice.

In the fetus, bilirubin is excreted by the placenta, and so jaundice is likely to become severe after birth. This can be prevented by exchange blood transfusion which, by removing antibody and replacing the sensitised fetal red cells by compatible cells, is especially effective in preventing kernicterus in Rh incompatibility. With increasing age, the blood–brain barrier becomes more efficient, and kernicterus very rarely develops in adults.

Secondary degenerations

Secondary degeneration can be defined as changes occurring in one part of a neuron as a result of damage to another part. The commonest of these is **Wallerian degeneration** which occurs in its most typical form when axons in a peripheral nerve are transected. The axon distal to the point of transection shrinks, becomes varicose and granular, and then breaks up into fragments which are later absorbed. The myelin sheath reacts at the same time and the complex lipids are broken down into simpler lipids and, ultimately, neutral fat. Products of myelin degeneration may be seen three or four days after damage to the axon and thereafter the fatty globules are gradually absorbed by phagocytes. The Schwann cells proliferate to form cords of cells within endoneural tubes. Degeneration of the central part of the axon usually extends for only a short distance proximal to the level of transection. The sequence of changes in the nerve cell is described below. An essentially similar degeneration occurs in axons within the central nervous system when they are transected. The lipids produced by the degeneration of myelin are absorbed by microglia and when large tracts are affected, these cells persist for a considerable time.

In peripheral nerves, axonal sprouts from the proximal stump proliferate rapidly and, unless the cut ends of the nerve lie in close apposition, form a **traumatic neuroma** (p. 77). If they are in apposition, however, the axons grow along the degenerated part of the nerve where they may ultimately make contact with motor endplates and terminal sensory organelles. Regeneration of axons with restoration of function does not occur in the central nervous system.

Wallerian degeneration of the long tracts in the spinal cord will be dealt with in more detail later (p. 710) but it should be observed here that two principal staining techniques are used to demonstrate loss of myelin. The first of these—the Marchi technique—is used as a positive technique to demonstrate recent or active breakdown of myelin as the unsaturated fatty acids formed during this process are stained black, while normal myelin remains unstained. In the later stages, however, when most of the breakdown products have been removed, the demyelinated areas remain pale with conventional stains for myelin, e.g. the Weigert–Pal method and its modifications. Negative techniques of this type are used also to demonstrate loss of myelin in conditions other than Wallerian degeneration, e.g. multiple sclerosis (see p. 706).

The other form of secondary degeneration occurs in the body of the nerve cell when its axon has been destroyed or injured—**retrograde degeneration**. When a motor nerve, for example the hypoglossal, is cut across, changes begin to appear in the related nerve cell bodies two or three days afterwards, and reach their maximum about two weeks later. The Nissl granules gradually lose their configuration and break down into small dust-like particles, some of which disappear. The process, which is called **central chromatolysis**, is associated with considerably increased nucleic acid and protein synthesis. It appears first round the nucleus and then extends to the periphery. The whole cell becomes pale-staining and at the same time somewhat swollen; its nucleus becomes eccentric in position, and may even form a slight bulging on the surface of the cell. If the axon regenerates, the nerve cell body may return to normal. If it does not, or if the axon is damaged close to the cell body, the cell dies. Essentially similar destruction of fibres within the central nervous system, however, is followed by gradual disappearance of the corresponding nerve cell bodies. This has been found to be the case, for example, in the motor neurons in the cortex when the pyramidal fibres have been interrupted, and also in the thoracic nucleus when the posterior spino-cerebellar tract has been interrupted.

Another form of secondary degeneration is trans-neuronal or trans-synaptic atrophy. This occurs in neurons whose principal afferent connections have been destroyed: examples are atrophy of the neurons in the external geniculate body after lesions in the retina or optic nerves, or in the nucleus gracilis and nucleus cuneatus when the posterior columns of the spinal cord have degenerated. Trans-synaptic degeneration is sometimes 'retrograde', i.e. it can occur in cells which make synaptic connections with cells which have been destroyed.

Atrophy

Diffuse atrophy of the brain is usually due to a progressive loss of neurons, particularly within the cerebral cortex. When the process is advanced, the convolutions become more rounded and firmer than normal and the sulci widened, so that there is an excess of CSF in the subarachnoid space. The pia-arachnoid, especially over the vertex, is thickened and opalescent and the sulci appear to be filled with semi-gelatinous material.

The full extent of the atrophy is often not apparent until the meninges have been stripped from the surface of the brain. As the neuronal loss is accompanied by the disappearance of their axons and myelin sheaths, the white matter also becomes reduced in amount and this is accompanied by enlargement of the ventricles. The histological changes underlying atrophy vary with the many different causes, e.g. senile and pre-senile dementia, ischaemia, subacute encephalitis and, to a more limited degree, as part of the changes in old age, but the two constant abnormalities are loss of neurons and neuroglial overgrowth.

Neuroglia

The neuroglia includes astrocytes, oligodendrocytes and ependymal cells, all of which are of neuro-ectodermal origin.

Astrocytes. The astrocytes, which form the astroglia, and constitute the principal supporting tissue of the central nervous system, are stellate cells with numerous fine branching processes, which lie in a mucopolysaccharide ground substance. Protoplasmic astrocytes and fibrillary astrocytes may be distinguished; the latter have fibres in their cytoplasm, which join cell to cell, and their processes are longer and straighter. In normal conditions the protoplasmic astrocytes are found mainly in the grey matter, the fibrillary astrocytes in the white matter and subpial glial layer. Both forms are attached to the walls of capillaries and other small vessels by one or more processes with swellings at their ends, the so-called 'sucker feet'. Similar expansions unite with the fibres of the pia.

In general, the reactions of astrocytes resemble those of fibroblasts. They are less susceptible to noxious processes than neurons but where the process is severe, as in an infarct or an acute inflammatory lesion, they undergo necrosis and disintegration. In less severe injury or when adjacent to an area of tissue necrosis, astrocytes enlarge, proliferate and produce glial fibrils in increased amount. This process is known as *gliosis* and it occurs in almost all conditions where damage is inflicted on any part of the central nervous system. Where gliosis is recent and active, many enlarged cell bodies are seen, but in the late stages the cell bodies disappear and all that can be seen is a dense network of glial fibrils. The brain tissue is then firmer than normal and may have a grey translucent appearance.

Oligodendrocytes. The oligodendrocytes are small cells so named because of their few short protoplasmic processes. They are extremely numerous and occur as perineuronal satellites in the grey matter, and as rows of closely apposed nuclei in relation to myelinated nerve fibres where they constitute the interfascicular oligodendroglia.

Developing axons invaginate into oligodendrocytes which then form the characteristic laminated myelin sheath. Oligodendrocytes play an important role in the maintenance of myelin, and in some of the leukodystrophies (p. 707), loss of interfascicular oligodendrocytes appears to precede obvious degeneration of myelin. Very little is known about the causes or significance of reactive changes in the oligodendrocytes apart from the *acute swelling* which occurs in many acute toxic processes and the proliferation of perineuronal satellites around degenerating neurons. The latter process is known as *satellitosis* and has to be distinguished from neuronophagia (see below).

Ependyma. The ependyma is a single layer of columnar cells lining the ventricular system and the central canal of the spinal cord. Cilia are attached to their free, i.e. ventricular, surface immediately deep to which there is a line of small oval bodies known as blepharoplasts. Processes from the deep surface of the cells merge with the underlying neural tissue.

Ependymal cells show few reactive changes. Thus when the ventricles distend as in hydrocephalus, the ependyma is stretched and then broken, but the ependymal cells do not proliferate to fill the defects. A common but nonspecific reaction of the ependyma to chronic irritation is the appearance of numerous small excrescences on its surface, the condition being known as a **granular ependymitis**. However, this is consequent on focal proliferation of groups of subependymal astrocytes and not to reactive changes in the ependymal cells themselves (Fig. 20.2).

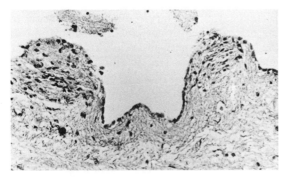

fig. 20.2 Granular ependymitis in the floor of the fourth ventricle. × 112.

Microglia

The microglial cell is small, with an elongated hyperchromatic nucleus, scanty cytoplasm and delicate cytoplasmic processes. They may be regarded as the homologues of the histiocytes of ordinary connective tissue (p. 56), and belong to the mononuclear-phagocyte system.

Microglia do not appear in the central nervous system until the vessels are formed, and they are few in number until shortly before birth, when they invade the neural tissue from the pia. They are often closely related to blood vessels.

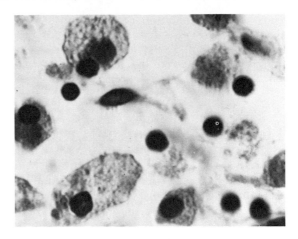

Fig. 20.3 Lipid-laden phagocytes in a cerebral infarct. × 750. A.C.L.

Although normally inconspicuous, microglia play an important part in disease. In the presence of tissue destruction they become enlarged and spherical and phagocytose debris, particularly lipid, to become lipid phagocytes (Fig. 20.3). Some then migrate into the perivascular spaces but others remain in the damaged area for a long time. In other conditions, e.g. subacute encephalitis, the microglial cells increase in length but do not become spherical: they are then referred to as *rod cells*. Another important function of the microglia is the phagocytosis of neurons which have undergone necrosis as in hypoxic brain damage or virus infections. The effete nerve cell becomes obscured by a group of enlarged elongated microglial cells, and often also by polymorphonuclear leukocytes, this process being known as *neuronophagia* or neuronophagy. This has to be distinguished from satellitosis by oligodendroglia (*vide supra*).

In many disease processes, macrophages are derived from emigration of blood monocytes as well as from local microglia.

The meninges and blood vessels

While gliosis readily occurs when there is any damage to the brain, production of fibrous tissue is seen only in more severe lesions where the blood vessels and their sheaths are involved. For instance, when suppuration occurs within the brain, fibroblastic proliferation and activity along with the formation of new blood vessels, leads to the production of a distinct capsule around the abscess cavity. Gliosis occurs also and this combined glial and fibroblastic reaction is often referred to as a *gliomesodermal reaction*. Proliferation of capillary blood vessels is the rule in infarcts and other anoxic lesions and in relation to rapidly growing cerebral tumours. The reactions of the meninges to disease will be considered in the section on meningitis (p. 683).

The Pathology of an Intracranial Expanding Lesion

Diverse pathological processes, such as tumour, haematoma, or a massive recent cerebral infarct, have in common the feature of increasing the bulk of the brain. As the brain is enclosed within the rigid cranium, there is very little free space to accommodate these various *expanding lesions* with the result that they ultimately produce an **increase in intracranial pressure**. An essentially similar state is produced by an extracerebral intracranial expanding lesion such as an extradural or subdural haematoma or a meningioma. There is, however, a stage of spatial compensation during which the intracranial pressure remains within normal limits. This compensation is brought about principally by a reduction in the volume of CSF both within the ventricles and within the subarachnoid space, possibly by a reduction in the volume of blood within the cranium, and less commonly by actual loss of brain tissue. When all the available space has been utilised there is a critical point at which a further slight increase in the volume of the intracranial contents causes an abrupt increase of intracranial pressure with subsequent and often rapid deterioration in the patient's condition. Near this critical point, arteriolar vasodilatation consequent on a short period of increased arterial P_{CO_2} may be sufficient to produce this effect. Clearly the compensatory mechanisms will fail more rapidly when the lesion is expanding rapidly, e.g. an intracerebral haematoma, than one of similar size that has developed slowly, e.g. a meningioma. Indeed in the latter instance there is often also local pressure atrophy and loss of brain tissue. Expanding lesions also cause distortion of the brain and it can hardly be emphasised too strongly that distortion and displacement of the brain and any associated increase in intracranial pressure are often of greater significance with regard to the immediate survival of the patient than the nature of the lesion or the amount of cerebral tissue destroyed by it.

The sequence of changes in the brain caused by a supratentorial intracerebral expanding lesion follows a fairly standard pattern. As the lesion expands so also does the hemisphere. The CSF fluid in the subarachnoid space is displaced and the convolutions become flattened against the dura, the sulci are progressively narrowed and the surface of the brain, when exposed *post mortem*, is dryer than normal. Cerebrospinal fluid is also displaced from the ventricular system with the result that the lateral ventricle on the same side as the lesion becomes smaller while the contralateral ventricle may become larger. Further expansion of the affected hemisphere leads to distortion of the brain and a shift to the opposite side of the midline structures, viz. the interventricular septum, the anterior cerebral arteries and the third ventricle (Fig. 20.4). Such displacement is readily seen radiologically by air encephalography or carotid arteriography. Then, depend-

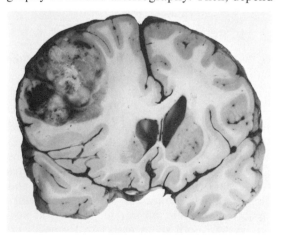

Fig. 20.4 Increased intracranial pressure due to frontal lobe tumour. Note displacement of the lateral ventricles, mid-line shift and supracallosal hernia.

ing to some extent on the site of the expanding lesion, internal herniae develop. Thus the cingulate gyrus frequently herniates under the free margin of the falx cerebri above the corpus callosum—the so-called **supracallosal** or **subfalcine hernia** (Fig. 20.4). However, the most important hernia associated with a supratentorial expanding lesion is a **tentorial hernia**, viz. protrusion of the medial part of the ipsilateral temporal lobe

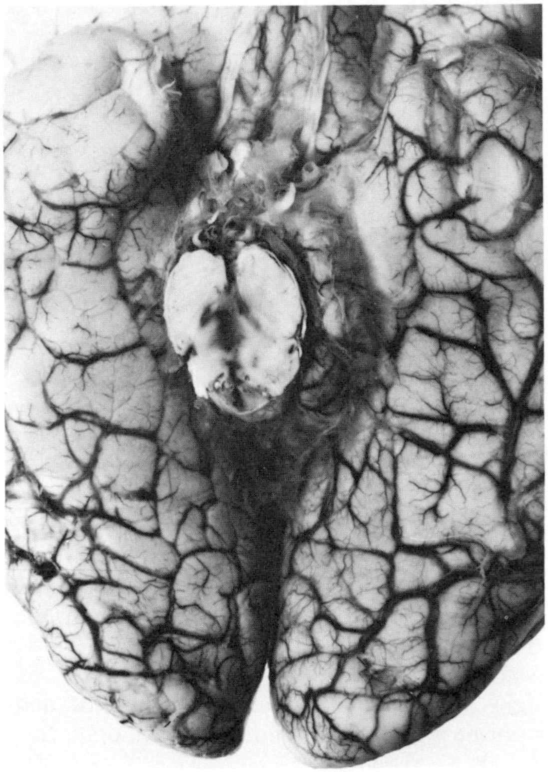

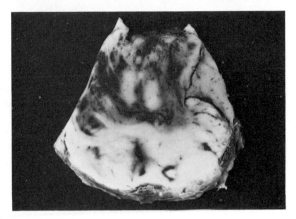

Fig. 20.6 Increased intracranial pressure, and secondary haemorrhage into the pons.

Other features associated with a tentorial hernia are caudal displacement of the brain stem, compression of the third and sixth cranial nerves with resultant disturbances of eye movement and pupillary reflexes and, less commonly, infarction of the ipsilateral medial occipital cortex due to selective compression of the posterior cerebral artery over the tentorium. A common terminal event in raised intracranial pressure is haemorrhage into the midbrain and pons (Fig. 20.6), usually involving the tegmentum adjacent to the midline. The precise pathogenesis of this haemorrhage is obscure but it is presumably a combination of caudal displacement of the brain stem, obstruction to venous drainage and to stretching and spasm of arteries.

Similar abnormalities are brought about by extracerebral intracranial expanding lesions, although flattening of the ipsilateral convolutions is often not so pronounced. If the increase in volume of the brain is more diffuse, as in generalised cerebral oedema, both lateral ventricles and the third ventricle are reduced in size. There may also be bilateral tentorial herniae. A frequent clinical sign of raised intracranial pressure is *papilloedema* due to compression of the retinal vein where it traverses the subarachnoid space in the optic nerve sheath.

A supratentorial expanding lesion may also cause a **tonsillar hernia (cerebellar cone)**, viz. impaction of the cerebellar tonsils in the foramen magnum (Fig. 20.7) but this type of hernia is more constant when the lesion lies below

Fig. 20.5 Increased intracranial pressure due to a supratentorial tumour. Note displacement of brain stem and medial and downward displacement of the parahippocampal gyrus—a tentorial hernia. The deep groove indicates the position of the edge of the tentorium.

through the tentorial opening (Fig. 20.5). The herniated parahippocampal gyrus compresses and displaces the midbrain which is pushed against the contralateral rigid edge of the tentorium. The pressure may be sufficient to produce a distinct groove (Kernohan's notch) on the surface of the midbrain at this point. Compression of the aqueduct may then block the free flow of CSF from the lateral ventricles and this further increases the intracranial pressure.

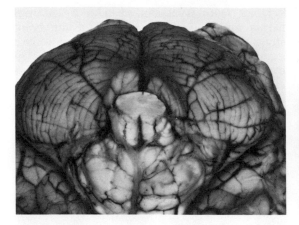

Fig. 20.7 Increased intracranial pressure. Tonsillar hernia resulting from a diffuse glioma of the pons.

the tentorium cerebelli. The tonsils compress the medulla oblongata and interfere with the function of the vital centres adjacent to the floor of the fourth ventricle. The hernia, by obstructing the flow of CSF through the fourth ventricle and the exit foramina, may in turn further increase the intracranial pressure so that a vicious circle is set up.

In a patient with an intracranial expanding lesion, lumbar puncture can precipitate cerebellar coning or tentorial herniation, with serious consequences. Even if only a small amount of CSF is withdrawn, more is likely to leak into the extradural space via the puncture wound in the meninges. Lumbar puncture is therefore contra-indicated in all cases where an intracranial expanding lesion is suspected.

Prolonged increase in intracranial pressure

may result in erosion of certain parts of the skull and these changes can often be seen on radiological examination. The most common examples are erosion of the posterior clinoid processes and, in children, thinning of the inner table of the skull over the convolutions, the so-

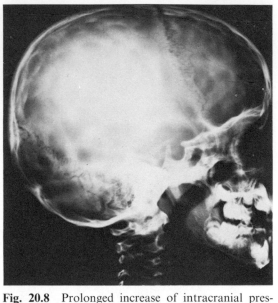

Fig. 20.8 Prolonged increase of intracranial pressure. Note thinning of the inner table of the skull.

called convolutional markings or beaten-brass appearance (Fig. 20.8).

The clinical features of a raised intracranial pressure include headache, vomiting, a raised systolic blood pressure with a slow pulse and high pulse pressure, and diminished consciousness passing into coma. Ophthalmoscopy reveals papilloedema.

Hydrocephalus

Definition. Hydrocephalus denotes an increase in the amount of CSF, and by far the commonest cause of **primary hydrocephalus** is obstruction to the flow of CSF. **Secondary hydrocephalus** is an increase in CSF which is compensatory to loss of neural tissue, e.g. from cerebral atrophy, when the hydrocephalus is unimportant since there is no increase in the total volume of the intracranial contents and so no rise in intracranial pressure. The increase of

CSF may be in the ventricles, the subarachnoid space or in both. Primary hydrocephalus can be either **communicating** or **non-communicating** in type. In the former, CSF is still able to pass from the lateral ventricles to the subarachnoid space while, in the latter, it is unable to do so owing to the site of the obstruction. The two types may be distinguished during life by cerebral pneumography by injecting air either into the lumbar subarachnoid space or directly into the ventricles. The air extends wherever there is free communication, and can be seen as dark areas on the x-ray plate. By varying the position of the patient's head the air can be made to pass from the ventricles to the subarachnoid space in cases of communicating hydrocephalus, or in the reverse direction if air has been introduced by the lumbar route. This technique can also be used to locate the site of obstruction in the ventricular system, or in the subarachnoid space. A more accurate technique is to introduce a radio-opaque fluid into the lateral ventricles after withdrawing an equivalent volume of CSF.

The source and circulation of cerebrospinal fluid

The main source of CSF is the choroid plexuses of the ventricles but some may be formed on the surface of the brain and spinal cord, for it is known that ionic exchange between blood and CSF can occur widely and is not restricted to the choroid plexuses. Dandy was the first to show convincingly that the CSF is derived from the choroid plexuses by demonstrating experimentally (*a*) that obstruction of one foramen of Monro in the dog caused enlargement of the corresponding lateral ventricle and, (*b*) that if, in addition to obstruction, the choroid plexus was removed, the ventricle became smaller than that on the normal side. The total volume of the CSF is about 120–150 ml and it is renewed several times per day. When, however, it is able to escape freely, as in a fracture of the base of the skull, the amount formed may be greatly increased. The mechanism of production is by secretion, and the fluid formed in the lateral ventricles passes by the foramina of Monro to the third ventricle and then by the aqueduct of Sylvius to the fourth ventricle. It then passes through the foramina of Magendie and Luschka in the roof and lateral recesses respectively of the fourth ventricle to reach the subarachnoid space of the cisterna magna and basal cisterns. Thereafter it spreads through the subarachnoid space over the surface of the brain and spinal cord and is absorbed into the blood through the arachnoid granulations (arachnoid villi) which project into the dural venous sinuses (Fig. 20.82).

Primary hydrocephalus

This is most often caused by obstruction to the free flow of CSF. Obstruction is most likely to occur where the channel is narrow, e.g. in the aqueduct or at the exit foramina of the fourth ventricle, but obstruction may also occur in the subarachnoid space itself. Dandy demonstrated this by placing a strip of gauze soaked in iodine around the brain stem; the resulting inflammation produced thickening of the meninges and obliteration of the subarachnoid space with the subsequent development of hydrocephalus.

Obstruction to the flow of CSF results in expansion of that part of the ventricular system which lies proximal to the obstruction. Thus, if the obstruction is in the third ventricle, both lateral ventricles enlarge symmetrically; if at the exit foramina in the roof of the fourth ventricle, the entire ventricular system enlarges; if in the subarachnoid space around the brain stem, the entire ventricular system again enlarges but the hydrocephalus in this instance, in contrast to the two preceding examples, is of communicating type (see above).

It is convenient to divide obstructive hydrocephalus into *congenital* and *acquired* types but the separation of the two varieties is not always clear-cut. Other possible causes of primary hydrocephalus are increased production or impaired absorption of CSF. Increased production is rare but may contribute to the hydrocephalus associated with a secreting papillary tumour of the choroid plexus (Fig. 20.75). Decreased absorption of CSF is theoretically possible, but its occurrence in man has been questioned.

(1) Congenital

This condition may be present at birth in such degree as to interfere with parturition. More often it is only slight at birth and afterwards increases. The head may become enormously enlarged and tends to become quadrangular, the vertex becomes flattened and the frontal bone projects over the orbits. The sutures are greatly widened and the fontanelles much enlarged, their closure being long delayed. There is a corresponding enlargement of the brain, the convolutions being broadened and flattened and the sulci shallow. The accumulation of fluid in the lateral ventricles may be so great that the brain around them may be less than a centimetre wide (Fig. 20.9). If the third ventricle is involved its floor can become greatly ballooned and extremely thin. It is remarkable how the brain can adapt itself to its altered shape and although considerable interference with mental function is usual, in a very few cases the child may be surprisingly intelligent.

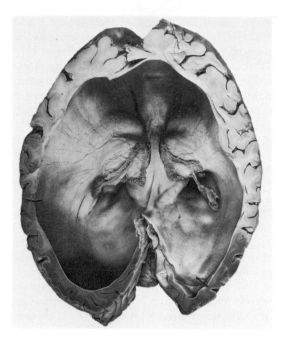

Fig. 20.9 Section of brain in congenital hydrocephalus, showing enormous dilatation of the lateral ventricles.

One of the commoner causes of congenital hydrocephalus is the **Arnold–Chiari malformation** (Fig. 20.10): this consists of a tongue-like prolongation of the inferior cerebellar vermis through the foramen magnum and lying dorsal to the greatly elongated medulla. The lower part of the fourth ventricle thus lies in the upper part of the vertebral canal and the foramen magnum is blocked by the misplaced tissue from the posterior fossa. Cerebrospinal fluid can flow out of the main exit foramina in the fourth ventricle—the hydrocephalus is, therefore, of communicating type (p. 668), but as the CSF is unable to re-enter the cranial cavity, it cannot reach the main sites of reabsorption. The entire ventricular system thus becomes grossly enlarged. A meningomyelocele (see

p. 721) is an almost invariable accompaniment of the Arnold–Chiari malformation, and other features include a small posterior fossa, a poorly developed tentorium cerebelli and fusion and 'beaking' of the colliculi.

Other relatively common congenital abnormalities which give rise to hydrocephalus are faulty development of the aqueduct of Sylvius

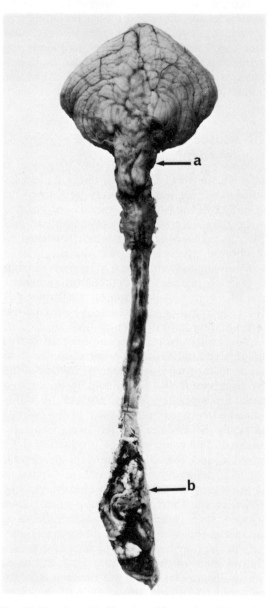

Fig. 20.10 Arnold–Chiari malformation. The inferior part of the cerebellum protrudes as a tongue-like mass (**a**) through the foramen magnum. There is also a meningomyelocele (**b**).

and atresia of the foramina of Luschka and Magendie: in the former, hydrocephalus is confined to the third and lateral ventricles; in the latter there is in addition enlargement of the aqueduct and of the fourth ventricle. The ballooning of the roof of the fourth ventricle in these cases is usually so severe as to cause distortion of the inferior surface of the cerebellum.

Congenital hydrocephalus occurs also in the absence of any apparent developmental malformation. One cause of this is intra-uterine meningitis or ventriculitis, e.g. due to toxoplasmosis in which the inflammatory process produces obliterative changes in the subarachnoid space or in the ventricular system, particularly in the aqueduct. It seems likely, too, that some cases of hydrocephalus which are apparently congenital in type are in fact a consequence of neonatal meningitis or subarachnoid haemorrhage resulting from cerebral birth injury, either of which may evoke a fibroblastic reaction leading to obliteration of the subarachnoid space and obstruction to the flow of CSF.

(2) Acquired

Any expanding lesion within the skull can obstruct the flow of CSF but the nature of the lesion, e.g. a tumour, an abscess, a haematoma or a granuloma is much less important than its location. Even a small lesion, if it lies in a vital site, e.g. adjacent to a foramen of Monro or close to the aqueduct, will cause hydrocephalus, whereas larger lesions elsewhere in the cerebral hemispheres may not interfere with the circulation of CSF. In general, expanding lesions in the posterior fossa are particularly prone to cause hydrocephalus because they readily compress the aqueduct and the fourth ventricle. Common examples are a tumour of the acoustic nerve, a meningioma or a tumour within the fourth ventricle. Acquired obstruction of the exit foramina or the subarachnoid space is almost always due to meningitis; this may be acute, as in an acute purulent meningitis, or subacute, as in tuberculous meningitis, since, in both, the subarachnoid space is at least partly occluded by exudate. If the inflammation does not resolve, fibroblastic proliferation proceeds to obliteration of the subarachnoid space particularly in the basal cisterns (Fig.

20.11) and around the midbrain which is closely embraced by the rigid tentorium cerebelli. Such an occurrence is common in the later stages of tuberculous meningitis and sometimes is a late result of acute purulent meningitis particularly

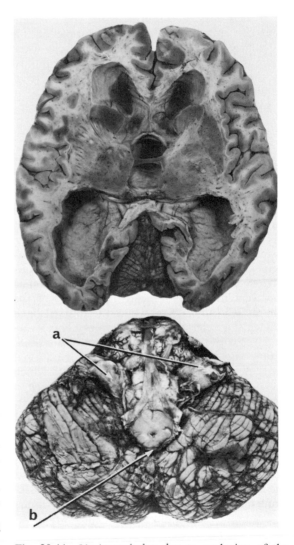

Fig. 20.11 Hydrocephalus due to occlusion of the foramina of Luschka (**a**) and Magendie (**b**) by fibrous adhesions.

if there has been some delay in instituting effective treatment.

A relatively uncommon cause of hydrocephalus occurring after early childhood is progressive gliosis around the aqueduct. The aetiology of this is obscure but it is probably a hamartomatous proliferation of astrocytes.

Secondary hydrocephalus

Symmetrical enlargement of the ventricles may be secondary to a generalised reduction in the amount of brain tissue, as in senile dementia or general paralysis of the insane. If there is only local loss of cerebral tissue, the adjacent ventricle enlarges; a frequent example of this is enlargement of one lateral ventricle when there is an old infarct in the territory supplied by the ipsilateral middle cerebral artery (Fig. 20.24).

In recent years, there has been increasing recognition of an uncommon syndrome characterised by dementia, a disturbance of gait, and hydrocephalus in the absence of conventional clinical evidence of increased intracranial pressure. The syndrome is usually referred to as '**normal pressure hydrocephalus**' but a more appropriate term would be intermittent hydrocephalus, since monitoring of the ventricular fluid pressure has shown that although the pressure is basically normal, there may be significant rises during sleep. A proportion of patients with this syndrome improve if a ventricular shunt operation is undertaken.

Head Injuries

In the United Kingdom trauma is responsible for more deaths in all age groups under 45 than any other single cause, and brain damage resulting from a head injury is the most important factor contributing to death or serious incapacity due to trauma. In civilian practice the great majority of head injuries are of the *non-missile* (*blunt*) type where the unfixed head suddenly accelerates or decelerates. This is associated with transient deformation of the skull, which may fracture, and linear or rotational movements of the brain within the skull which produce focal contusions and diffuse damage to nerve fibres in varying degree. These may be referred to as **immediate impact damage**, and the clinical manifestations may range from mild concussion to coma persisting until death. Other damage directly attributable to impact may be **delayed**, i.e. the process is initiated at the moment of impact but its clinical manifestations may not become apparent for some hours or even days: the commonest of these are intracranial haemorrhage and brain swelling. Other sequelae of a head injury include brain damage attributable to raised intracranial pressure and distortion of the brain, ischaemic or hypoxic brain damage, or infection.

(1) Immediate impact injury

Fracture of the skull

There is a tendency to exaggerate the importance of a fracture of the skull, since many patients with simple fractures of the skull may have suffered no significant brain damage, whereas about 20% of fatal head injuries do not have a fracture. A fracture, however, does indicate that the blow has probably been of considerable force and that there is a greater likelihood of brain damage. There are some specific features associated with fractures which are important. Thus a fracture may be depressed, causing local pressure on the brain and providing a potential source of subsequent intracranial sepsis. Any fracture at the base of the skull may also provide a potential route of entry for micro-organisms from the nasal passages, the paranasal sinuses or the middle ear. The presence of such a fracture may be shown by a CSF rhinorrhoea or otorrhoea. Other complications of a fracture are laceration of a meningeal artery leading to the formation of an extradural haematoma (see below), or injury to the carotid artery within the cavernous sinus giving rise to a carotico-cavernous fistula.

Contusions and lacerations

These are the classical features of focal brain damage directly attributable to impact. They may occur at the site of impact, particularly if there is a depressed fracture, but in any blunt head injury they tend to occur at the frontal poles, on the orbital gyri, at the temporal poles and on the inferior and lateral surfaces of the anterior halves of the temporal lobes (Fig.

20.12). This distribution is due to the fact that it is in these regions that movement of the brain within the skull brings the surface of the brain into contact with bony protuberances in the base of the skull. Contusions are usually asymmetrical and they may be more extensive on the side opposite the one that has suffered the impact: thus severe frontal contusions may occur

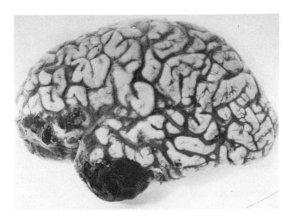

Fig. 20.12 Acute head injury: contusions at frontal and temporal poles.

in association with an occipital impact. These contusions are often called *contre-coup*. Contusions may be superficial, when they tend to be restricted to the crests of gyri, but they may extend through the full thickness of the cortex into the adjacent white matter and be associated with some intracerebral haemorrhage and oedema. Old healed contusions are represented by golden-brown shrunken scars which have such a characteristic distribution and appearance that it is often possible to state with certainty at necropsy that a patient has experienced a head injury some time in the past.

Diffuse brain damage

There is now considerable evidence to suggest that nerve fibres can be torn at the moment of impact as a result of shear strains produced by movement, particularly rotational, of the brain within the skull. This type of brain damage may occur in the absence of conventional contusions, and if the patient dies soon after the injury the only macroscopic abnormalities in the brain may be haemorrhagic lesions in the corpus callosum and in the dorso-lateral

quadrant of the rostral brain stem (Fig. 20.13) adjacent to one or both superior cerebellar peduncles. Some patients with this type of brain damage who experience no further complications of their injury may survive in a persistent vegetative state for many months or even a year or more. At necropsy the brain may appear remarkably normal on external examination apart from small healed contusions. In sections

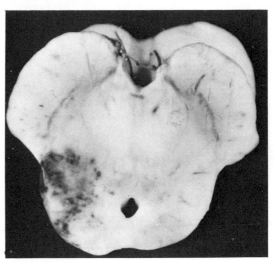

Fig. 20.13 Immediate impact injury. There is a haemorrhagic lesion in the dorso-lateral quadrant of the midbrain.

the ventricles are enlarged because of a reduction in the white matter and there are usually small shrunken cystic lesions in the corpus callosum and in the dorso-lateral quadrant of the rostral brain stem, i.e. in the situations where haemorrhagic lesions occur in patients who die shortly after their injury. The principal histological abnormality in these patients is Wallerian-type degeneration in the cerebral and cerebellar hemispheres, the brain stem and the spinal cord. The clinical features of diffuse brain damage are often referred to as primary brain stem injury, but in such cases the damage is not restricted to the brain stem.

(2) Delayed impact injury

Intracranial haemorrhage

Extradural haematoma most often results from haemorrhage from the middle meningeal

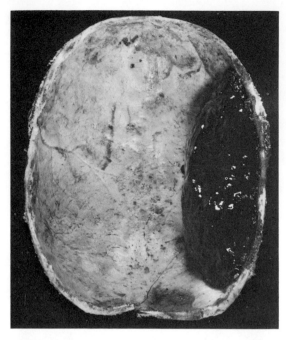

Fig. 20.14 Extradural haemorrhage complicating fracture of the skull. The specimen shows the under-surface of the vault of the cranium from which the dura has been removed.

artery and, as the haematoma develops, it gradually strips the dura from the skull to form a large ovoid mass (Fig. 20.14) that progressively compresses the temporal lobe. Although the tear in the meningeal artery is directly attributable to a fracture of the skull in about 80% of patients with extradural haematoma, the initial injury is often apparently mild. Thus many cases experience a lucid interval of some hours before developing headache and becoming drowsy. As the haematoma enlarges the patient lapses into coma and dies from the effects of raised intracranial pressure unless the haematoma is evacuated. Occasionally extradural haematomas occur in the frontal or the parietal regions, or within the posterior fossa. Extradural haematoma may occur in the absence of a fracture of the skull, particularly in children.

Subdural haematoma. In contrast to the localised nature of an extradural haematoma, haemorrhage into the subdural space produced by laceration of small 'bridging' veins or of larger veins running into the main venous sinuses tends to spread diffusely over one or both hemispheres.

Acute subdural haematoma is a common necropsy finding if death has occurred soon after a head injury. The haematoma is often thin and may not have contributed significantly to the patient's death since such patients often have fairly severe and extensive contusions and lacerations of the brain. In some cases, however, an acute subdural haematoma may attain a considerable thickness and unless surgically evacuated can produce coma and death as a result of raised intracranial pressure. Some patients with acute subdural haematoma experience a lucid interval similar to that classically associated with extradural haematoma.

Chronic subdural haematoma presents weeks or months after what may have seemed at the time to have been a trivial head injury. Indeed many patients deny any history of head injury. The precise aetiology of chronic subdural haematoma is not clear but the clot becomes encapsulated in a membrane and slowly increases in size, probably as a result of repeated small haemorrhages into it. Since chronic subdural haematoma is particularly common in older age groups in whom there is already some cerebral atrophy and since the haematoma expands very slowly, it may attain a considerable size—often 2–3 cm thick—before symptoms appear. In untreated cases, however, death is usually due to brain damage secondary to increased intracranial pressure (Fig. 20.15). Chronic subdural haematoma is not uncommonly bilateral.

Intracerebral haematoma usually occurs in association with contusions of the brain with the

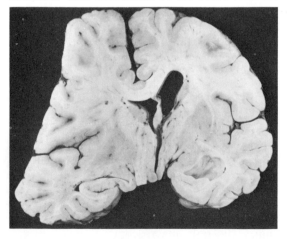

Fig. 20.15 Severe distortion of the brain caused by a chronic subdural haematoma.

result that haematomas are most common in the frontal and in the temporal lobes. They are often multiple and vary greatly in size. They may also occur deep within the hemispheres where they are presumably due to shearing strains affecting small vessels at the moment of impact.

(3) Other types of brain damage

Not all of the brain damage found in patients who have died as the result of a head injury is directly attributable to impact. If the patient has developed an intracranial haematoma, much of the brain damage, particularly in cases of extradural haematoma, is due to *raised intracranial pressure* and distortion of the brain (p. 674). A further factor which may contribute to a high intracranial pressure is oedema of the brain around contusions or occasionally diffuse cerebral oedema. The latter is particularly common in young children and may be precipitated by convulsions.

Hypoxic brain damage is frequently observed in the brains of patients dying as a result of a blunt head injury. Some of the causes of this are well recognised, e.g. cardiorespiratory arrest or status epilepticus, the latter being particularly frequent in children. Other hypoxic brain damage may be a direct consequence of raised intracranial pressure, but there remains a fairly large group of cases who develop focal infarction in the cerebral cortex or in the basal nuclei, the pathogenesis of which is not clearly understood. A further fairly common complication of a head injury is **infection** due to the spread of micro-organisms through a compound fracture or a fracture of the base of the skull. The infection usually presents as meningitis and it is not necessarily restricted to the early post-traumatic period because a small traumatic fistula from the subarachnoid space to one of the major air sinuses in the base of the skull may persist. Intracranial abscess is a rarer complication and is usually secondary to a penetrating injury.

Clinical implications of head injury

Since the pathogenesis of brain damage due to a head injury is complex, the clinical spectrum is wide. Immediate impact damage is the beginning of an evolving process which may range from progressive improvement without complications, as is the case in the vast majority of patients with so-called concussion, to death. The period of disturbed consciousness and the interval between the injury and the return of continuous memory—post-traumatic amnesia—are probably closely related to the degree of diffuse brain damage: if this is mild, the patient may only be transiently dazed; if it is severe the patient will remain in a persistent vegetative state until death. On the other hand quite severe immediate impact damage of focal type, i.e. contusions, may have relatively mild clinical effects since it is well recognised that patients with quite severe cerebral contusions may survive with little or no cerebral dysfunction. But even if the initial injury appears only trivial, there is the possibility of delayed, or secondary, brain damage as a result of intracranial haematoma, raised intracranial pressure, ischaemic brain damage or infection. Thus in a personally studied series of 151 patients with fatal non-missile head injuries, who had been referred to a neurosurgical unit because their neurological state had been causing concern, 58 were found to have talked some time after their injury, i.e. they had apparently recovered in some measure after their injury, only to deteriorate and die later. The management of head-injured patients has therefore to be based on the knowledge that delayed brain damage occurs quite frequently, and that at least some of this is potentially preventable.

Head injury is an important cause of symptomatic **epilepsy**. About 10% of patients admitted to hospital with a non-missile head injury develop fits. These tend to occur in the first week after injury (*early epilepsy*) or are delayed until 2–3 months or more after the injury (*late epilepsy*). Early epilepsy occurs more commonly after severe or complicated head injuries, although children under 5 may develop epilepsy after apparently trivial injuries. Factors predisposing to late epilepsy include a depressed fracture and an acute intracranial haematoma. Fits are less liable to recur in patients with early epilepsy than in those who develop late epilepsy. With missile head injuries, the incidence of epilepsy is about 45%.

Trauma to the spinal cord

Injuries of the *spinal cord*, like those of the brain, are of all degrees of severity. In cases of fracture-dislocation, bullet wounds, etc., the cord may be directly lacerated, or even torn across. Apart from such extreme cases, the cord may be damaged by acute flexion or extension of the neck, when haemorrhage may occur outside or inside the dura or within the spinal cord

itself. There may also be infarction of the cord. Haemorrhage occurs especially immediately dorsal to the grey commissure, and tends to extend upwards and downwards through several segments. In cases of haemorrhage into the cord, or haematomyelia, the blood is broken down and ultimately an elongated pigmented encapsulated cavity may result, which may simulate syringomyelia (p. 716).

Circulatory Disturbances

Cerebrovascular disease falls into two principal categories—spontaneous intracranial haemorrhage and ischaemic brain damage. Both are often referred to as 'strokes'.

Spontaneous intracranial haemorrhage

The two common causes of spontaneous intracranial haemorrhage are primary intracerebral haemorrhage and subarachnoid haemorrhage from a ruptured aneurysm.

Intracerebral haemorrhage

The great majority of primary intracerebral haematomas develop in patients with hypertension. About a century ago Charcot came to the conclusion that the haemorrhage occurred from miliary aneurysms on small perforating cerebral arteries but this has only become generally accepted in recent years as a result of postmortem micro-angiographic studies which have clearly demonstrated the existence of microaneurysms on these arteries. They are usually multiple, tend to occur on arteries less than 25 μm in diameter and may attain a diameter of 2 mm. They occur mainly in hypertensive subjects over the age of 50. In contrast, microaneurysms are rare in normotensive individuals although a few can be demonstrated in some people over the age of 65.

The commonest site for a hypertensive

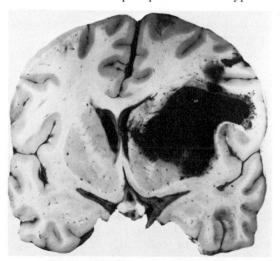

Fig. 20.16 Large haematoma in basal ganglia, resulting from chronic hypertension.

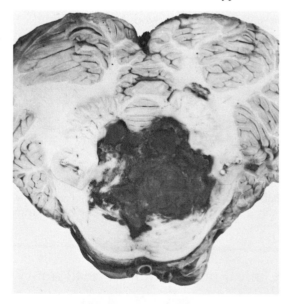

Fig. 20.17 Hypertensive haemorrhage into pons.

intracerebral haematoma is in the region of the basal ganglia and the internal capsule (Fig. 20.16). Other fairly common sites are the pons (Fig. 20.17) or the cerebellum. Subcortical haematomas also occur but they are rare. The haematoma usually increases in size rapidly, causes severe local destruction of tissue, and produces a sudden rise in intracranial pressure and subsequent distortion and herniation of the brain (p. 667). The haematoma may rupture into the ventricles or through the surface of the brain directly into the subarachnoid space. The clinical onset is usually sudden and patients with large intracerebral haematomas rarely survive for more than a few days, death often being precipitated by secondary haemorrhage into the brain stem as a result of raised intracranial pressure.

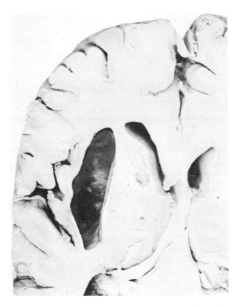

Fig. 20.18 Old apoplectic cyst on left side of brain. The cyst is centred on the external capsule and the outer part of the lentiform nucleus.

The appearance of the haematoma at necropsy varies with its duration. A recent haematoma is composed of ordinary dark coloured clot. If the haematoma is not large enough to be rapidly fatal, its periphery has a brownish colour after about a week and there are early reactive changes in capillaries and astrocytes in the adjacent brain. This brownish colour then spreads throughout the entire haematoma while gliosis leads to the formation of a poorly-defined capsule. If the patient survives, the clot is ultimately completely absorbed and replaced by xanthochromic fluid to form a so-called *apoplectic cyst* (Fig. 20.18).

Ruptured intracranial aneurysm

Aneurysms occur on the major arteries at the base of the brain in about 1–2% of the adult population, and they are not uncommon incidental findings at necropsy. They are often referred to as **congenital** or **berry aneurysms**, but the developmental abnormality is not the aneurysm but a defect in the medial coat of the artery at the bifurcations of the larger cerebral arteries within the subarachnoid space. Subsequent degeneration of the internal elastic lamina, probably due to early atheroma, may be a prerequisite for the development of the aneurysm. The arterial wall at the bifurcation then commences to bulge and an aneurysm forms which may vary in size from a small blister 2–3 mm in diameter to a large sac measuring as much as 2–3 cm across.

The commonest sites for these aneurysms are on the middle cerebral artery within the Sylvian fissure, at the junction of the anterior communicating artery with an anterior cerebral artery, and at the junction between the internal carotid artery and the posterior communicating artery. Aneurysms may also occur on the basilar artery and its branches. About 10–15% of patients who present with symptoms due to an aneurysm are found to have multiple aneurysms, usually two or three but sometimes five or more.

Most aneurysms rupture at their fundus to produce **subarachnoid haemorrhage**. This may be limited to the immediate vicinity of the aneurysm but frequently there is severe and extensive haemorrhage into the subarachnoid space. When an aneurysm ruptures, blood may also track into the brain to produce an **intracerebral haematoma** (Fig. 20.19), and if its fundus is embedded in brain tissue—a not uncommon occurrence—intracerebral haemorrhage may occur without any subarachnoid haemorrhage. Anterior communicating aneurysms tend to burst into the frontal lobe while posterior communicating aneurysms and middle cerebral aneurysms commonly rupture into the temporal lobe. Thus patients with ruptured intracranial aneurysms may have the clinical and

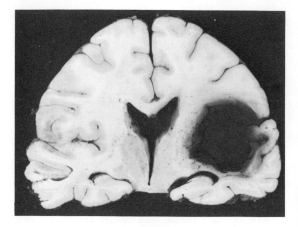

Fig. 20.19 Ruptured aneurysm. Haemorrhage from an aneurysm on the middle cerebral artery has produced a haematoma in the Sylvian fissure and in the adjacent brain.

pathological features of an acute expanding lesion in addition to subarachnoid haemorrhage. Such intracerebral haematomas often in turn rupture into the ventricles.

Another complication of a ruptured aneurysm is **infarction**, most commonly in the region of the brain supplied by the artery on which the aneurysm is situated. This is probably partly attributable to arterial spasm, and the swelling which occurs in a recent infarct (p. 680) may cause further displacement and distortion of the brain.

In many fatal cases of ruptured intracranial aneurysm there is a history of a previous small subarachnoid haemorrhage and in such cases examination of the brain may reveal the presence of altered blood pigment in the meninges adjacent to the aneurysm.

Rarer causes of intracranial aneurysm are those produced by infected emboli (mycotic aneurysms) and atheroma.

It should be emphasised that subarachnoid haemorrhage and ruptured intracranial aneurysm are not synonymous terms; the former may be the result of an acute head injury or haemorrhage from a vascular malformation (see below) or it may be subsequent to a primary intracerebral haemorrhage tracking into the ventricles or through the surface of the brain; moreover, a ruptured aneurysm may cause an intracerebral haematoma or a cerebral infarct without any significant subarachnoid haemorrhage.

Other causes of spontaneous intracranial haemorrhage

Probably the commonest of these is haemorrhage from a **vascular malformation.** These may range in size from small capillary angiomas to massive lesions composed of a plexus of large often thick-walled vascular channels (Fig. 20.20). More commonly they occur on the surface of the brain or the spinal cord but they are sometimes restricted to the

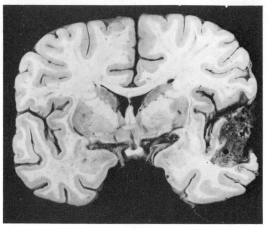

Fig. 20.20 Vascular malformation. There is a plexiform mass of vessels in the superficial part of the temporal lobe.

deeper structures of the brain. When a vascular malformation ruptures it may produce a massive intracerebral haematoma which is rapidly fatal but a more frequent result is mild subarachnoid haemorrhage. Many of these lesions are compatible with long survival, perhaps punctuated with episodes of subarachnoid haemorrhage.

Other causes of spontaneous intracranial haemorrhage include haemorrhage into tumours or haemorrhagic diseases. Thus cerebral haemorrhage is a not infrequent terminal event in patients with acute leukaemia.

There remains a group of patients who suffer spontaneous intracerebral haemorrhage who are not hypertensive. The pathogenesis of this type of lesion is not clear but it may be related to the occasional micro-aneurysm which may be found in normotensive subjects, to degenerative vascular disease or to a rupture of a small vascular malformation within the brain.

Ischaemic Brain Damage

The brain receives its blood supply from the internal carotid and vertebral arteries, frequently referred to as the *extracranial* cerebral arteries, from which the major *intracranial* cerebral arteries arise. A **cerebral infarct** occurs when the blood flow to any part of the brain falls below the critical level necessary to maintain the viability of brain tissue: it is essentially *focal* in nature, in contrast to the *diffuse* selective neuronal loss that may occur in various hypoxic states not necessarily due to reduction of cerebral blood flow (p. 682), and may be restricted to a small discrete lesion in the grey or white matter or may affect a large part of the brain. The reduction in blood flow may be of such a degree as to result only in the death of the most susceptible cells, *viz.* the neurons, but usually it is more severe, producing necrosis also of the neuroglial cells and, slightly less commonly, of microglia and blood vessels also. Occlusion of a cerebral artery is not a prerequisite for a cerebral infarct: indeed an episode of severe hypotension or transient cardiac arrest may cause cerebral infarction in the absence of any occlusive arterial disease, but more usually there is stenosis and/or occlusion of a major extracranial or intracranial cerebral artery. The critical reduction in the blood flow to a particular region of the brain needs to extend over a period of only several minutes to produce an infarct. If this reduction is transient, blood flow through the infarct may return to normal. When the cerebral circulation is already compromised by pre-existing arterial stenosis, infarction is particularly liable to occur in any state of generalised circulatory insufficiency, such as hypotension due to a myocardial infarct.

The principal local causes of an *inadequate cerebral blood flow* are intrinsic structural abnormalities in the arteries, embolism or spasm. By far the commonest abnormality is *atheroma.* this may result only in stenosis, but the artery may become occluded by the formation of thrombus on an atheromatous plaque. Other vascular diseases leading to a reduced arterial lumen with or without thrombosis are *arteritis* (polyarteritis nodosa, giant cell arteritis, tuberculous meningitis and syphilitic endarteritis). A cerebral artery may also be blocked by an *embolus* which usually comes from vegetations on the mitral or aortic valve cusps in cases of subacute bacterial endocarditis or from mural thrombus in patients with auricular fibrillation or a myocardial infarct. Transient neurological symptoms, the so-called 'transient ischaemic attacks' are often attributable to small cholesterol emboli from atheromatous plaques in the carotid or vertebral arteries. Spasm of intracranial cerebral arteries is probably only of significance in association with a ruptured intracranial aneurysm or in acute head injuries.

An infarct may occur in almost any part of the brain although the middle cerebral arterial territory is most frequently involved. The size of the infarct depends to a considerable extent on the degree of occlusive arterial disease and the available collateral circulation. Collateral channels exist between the major cerebral arteries on the surface of the brain and by way of the circle of Willis, but similar channels do not exist within the brain. An infarct may therefore affect an entire arterial territory or only part of it, while if the blood flow through two adjacent arterial territories is affected, infarction may be restricted to the boundary zone between them.

Arterial obstruction

Occlusive arterial disease leading to a cerebral infarct may lie within the skull or in the neck. The commonest intracranial site of occlusion is the middle cerebral artery. The commonest site of occlusion of the extracranial cerebral arteries is at the origin of an internal carotid artery and, if the collateral circulation is or becomes inadequate, the usual site of infarction is in the distribution of the middle cerebral artery on the same side. In some cases thrombosis extends along the internal carotid artery into the middle and anterior cerebral arteries to produce infarction of a large part of the cerebral hemisphere. When the vertebral arteries are the more severely involved, ischaemic changes occur characteristically in the brain stem, the cerebellum and the part of the cerebral hemispheres supplied by the posterior cerebral arteries, i.e. the occipital lobes. Cerebral infarction is often the result of a combination of systemic circulatory insufficiency and stenosis of the extracranial or intracranial cerebral arteries, or of both, and it has been suggested that stenosis of the extracranial cerebral arteries is more often a major factor than stenosis of the intracranial arteries. Although occlusion of the internal carotid artery in the neck is usually secondary to atheroma, it may also occur after closed injuries to the neck.

Structural changes in a cerebral infarct

A cerebral infarct may be pale or haemorrhagic (Fig. 20.21): this depends (*a*) on whether or not some blood flow has been restored through the

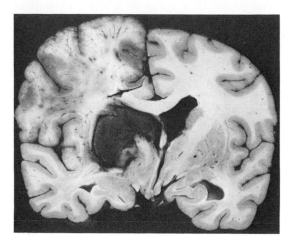

Fig. 20.21 Recent infarct in left cerebral hemisphere. The basal ganglia show the features of haemorrhagic infarction; the posterior part of the frontal lobe above the Sylvian fissure shows those of pale infarction. Note that the affected hemisphere is swollen and that there is displacement of the mid-line structures to the right.

infarct and (*b*) on whether or not necrosis of vessel walls has occurred, thus allowing the extravasation of blood into the necrotic tissue. An intensely haemorrhagic infarct may superficially resemble a haematoma but the distinctive feature of an infarct is the preservation of intrinsic architecture. A pale infarct less than 24 hours old may be difficult to identify macroscopically, but thereafter the dead tissue becomes slightly soft and swollen and there is a loss of the normal sharp definition between grey and white matter. At this stage histological examination will show ischaemic necrosis of neurons, pallor of myelin staining and sometimes polymorphonuclear leukocytes in relation to necrotic vessel walls. If the infarct is large, it may swell to the extent of producing

the typical features of an acutely expanding lesion and raised intracranial pressure (see p. 666). Within a few days the infarct becomes distinctly soft and the dead tissue disintegrates: hence a cerebral infarct is often referred

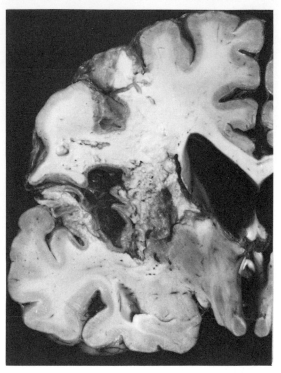

Fig. 20.22 Infarct of a week's duration in the left cerebral hemisphere. The dead tissue is distintegrating and there is already some shrinkage of the affected cortex.

to as a '*softening*' (Fig. 20.22). Microscopic examination at this stage will show phagocytes filled with globules of lipid produced by the breakdown of myelin (Fig. 20.3), enlarged astrocytes, and early capillary proliferation. Eventually the dead tissue is removed, lipid phagocytes become scanty, a fibrillary gliosis occurs and the lesion ultimately becomes shrunken and cystic. The cysts are often traversed by small vessels and glial fibrils (Fig. 20.23). If the infarct has been of the haemorrhagic type, a proportion of the phagocytes will contain haemosiderin. Shrinkage of the affected region is usually accompanied by enlargement of the adjacent lateral ventricle (Fig. 20.24). In the case of an old cortical infarct, the overlying meninges are somewhat thickened and opaque

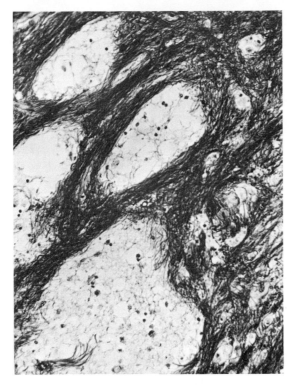

Fig. 20.23 Thickened neuroglia and spaces containing fluid in an old infarct. × 140. (A. C. L.)

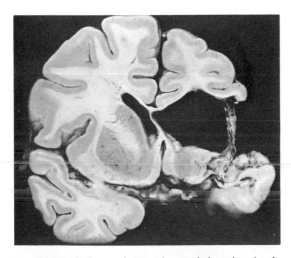

Fig. 20.24 Infarct of several years' duration in the right cerebral hemisphere. The dead tissue has been completely removed. The lateral ventricle is separated from the surface of the brain by a narrow web of tissue composed of leptomeninges, ependyma and a few glial fibrils.

and underneath there is usually an adherent layer of brownish-yellow cortical tissue composed of enlarged astrocytes and occasional lipid phagocytes. Beneath this the cortex is usually cystic and traversed by strands of thick astrocytic fibres. A consequence of infarction is Wallerian degeneration in the nerve fibres that have been destroyed. Thus if the infarct involves the internal capsule, there is progressive degeneration and shrinkage of the corresponding pyramidal tract in the brain stem and in the spinal cord.

Other aspects of ischaemic brain damage

A diminished blood supply to the brain may lead to loss of nerve cells without frank infarction. The neuroglia in such circumstances retains its vitality with the result that focal neuronal loss is accompanied by a fibrillary gliosis. This process is analagous to the ischaemic atrophy with fibrosis which occurs as the result of arterial narrowing in the kidneys and other organs. Areas of sclerosis produced in this way are a prominent feature in dementia of arteriopathic type, and they are common also in general arterial disease, especially in old people.

Venous obstruction

The most important form of this occurs as a result of thrombosis in one of the sinuses. Two types of thrombosis are usually distinguished, *marantic* and *infective*: in the latter there is often suppuration within the sinus. *Marantic thrombosis* is most frequent in poorly nourished children during the course of acute infections, e.g. gastro-enteritis; but it may occur in adults in conditions of cachexia, e.g. malignant tumours, or as a complication of infective fevers. Impaired circulation and possibly bacterial infection of mild virulence may be causal factors. The commonest site is the superior longitudinal sinus, and, when obstruction is complete, intense engorgement of the superficial veins occurs. There may also be irregular zones of intensely haemorrhagic infarction in the parasaggital parts of the cerebral hemispheres. In cases of thrombosis of the straight sinus, similar haemorrhagic areas are present in the walls of the third ventricle. *Infective thrombosis* is the result of direct spread of organisms from an adjacent infective lesion (p. 683).

Cerebral hypoxia

Neurons are particularly susceptible to hypoxia, and consciousness is lost within a few seconds of complete oxygen deprivation. Their supply of oxygen depends on the cerebral blood flow which in turn depends on the cerebral perfusion pressure, i.e. the difference between the systemic arterial pressure and the cerebral venous pressure. Since the most important factor maintaining an adequate oxygen supply to the brain is the cerebral blood flow, there are inbuilt protective mechanisms to preserve it. This mechanism is known as autoregulation which can be defined as the maintenance of a relatively constant blood flow in the face of changes in perfusion pressure. Autoregulation is brought about mainly by changes in the cerebrovascular resistance—when arterial pressure falls, cerebral arterioles dilate; when arterial pressure increases, cerebral arterioles constrict. Autoregulation may be impaired in chronic hypertension, in hypoxic or hypercapnic states, and in a wide range of acute conditions producing brain damage, e.g. head injuries and strokes, but when it is normal, the cerebral blood flow may be maintained within normal limits even when the systemic arterial pressure falls to as low as 50 mmHg provided the subject is in the prone position. At arterial pressures lower than this, cerebral blood flow falls rapidly.

Because of the susceptibility of neurons to hypoxia, the vital factor with regard to the ultimate clinical outcome in many medical emergencies, e.g. cardiorespiratory arrest, a severe episode of hypotension, carbon monoxide or barbiturate intoxication or status epilepticus, is whether or not satisfactory resuscitation can be achieved before the occurrence of irreversible hypoxic brain damage. Hypoglycaemia has an essentially similar effect because neurons require glucose as well as oxygen for their metabolism. The neuronal damage varies in its distribution; thus it tends to be *focal* and accentuated in the boundary zones between major arterial territories when there is a severe but transient episode of hypotension, whereas it is *diffuse* in more generalised disturbances of the supply of oxygen and glucose to the brain as in cardiac arrest, status epilepticus, carbon monoxide poisoning and hypoglycaemia.

Many patients who suffer severe hypoxic brain damage of the diffuse type die very soon after the episode, and the brain may appear entirely normal macroscopically. Indeed it may still appear normal macroscopically even if the patient has survived deeply comatose for a few days. Provided the patient has survived for more than about 12 hours, however, microscopic examination will disclose widespread and severe neuronal necrosis. There are minor variations in the distribution of the neuronal necrosis but the neurons in the brain that are selectively susceptible to oxygen deprivation are those in the Ammon's horns (hippocampus), in the third, fifth and sixth layers of the cerebral cortex, particularly within the sulci, and in certain of the basal nuclei, and the Purkinje cells in the cerebellum.

With the passage of a few days, the dead neurons disappear and reactive changes in astrocytes, microglia and capillaries become intense. If the patient survives for more than a few weeks, the affected regions become shrunken and cystic as in a conventional infarct.

Bacterial Infections of the Nervous System

Since the brain and spinal cord are relatively well protected from microbes, infections of the nervous system are not particularly common. But once micro-organisms have gained access to the nervous system, the infection may spread rapidly by way of the CSF pathways. The severity of the clinical illness depends on the virulence of the infecting agent and the susceptibility of the host, but many micro-organisms which are relatively non-pathogenic elsewhere in the body may cause serious and often fatal infection of the nervous system.

Inflammation of the meninges—**meningitis**—and inflammation of the brain—**encephalitis**—will be considered separately since, although both are usually present in any severe inflammatory process, one is almost always much more severe than the other.

Meningitis

Meningitis may involve the dura—**pachymeningitis**; or the pia and the arachnoid—**leptomeningitis**. The latter is by far the commoner, and is usually referred to simply as meningitis.

Pachymeningitis

Acute inflammation of the dura is practically always due to extension of inflammation from the bones of the skull. The underlying infection may be chronic suppurative otitis media or mastoiditis, or the infection may be a sequel to a depressed fracture of the skull. When pyogenic organisms spread from the bone, suppuration occurs between bone and dura and an *extradural abscess* may form. The dura becomes swollen, softened and infiltrated with pus, and if the infection spreads to its inner aspect, pus will accumulate in the subdural space: the infection can then spread widely over the hemisphere to form a *subdural abscess*. The organisms may also spread to the arachnoid, setting up either localised or general leptomeningitis. Further effects of spread, such as the production of cerebral abscess, are described below. The dura is occasionally the site of gummatous lesions in syphilis (p. 690), but it is rarely affected by tuberculosis except in the case of direct spread, for example, from the petrous bone or from the vertebral column.

Leptomeningitis

This is produced by the spread of microorganisms throughout the subarachnoid space where they provoke an inflammatory reaction as a result of which exudate is added to the CSF. This is a medium in which many microorganisms can multiply freely.

Causes. These are many and varied. The commonest causes of acute purulent meningitis are *Neisseria meningitidis* (meningococcus), *Streptococcus pneumoniae* (pneumococcus) and the haemophilus group. *Escherichia coli* is fairly common in infants. Some viral diseases of the nervous system and also the presence of blood in the subarachnoid space are accompanied by many of the clinical features of acute meningitis. Less frequent causes of meningitis are *Mycobacterium tuberculosis*, the ordinary pyogenic cocci, the bacilli of the coli-typhoid group, the anthrax bacillus, *Treponema pallidum*, leptospirae and various fungi.

Routes of infection

(*a*) *Infection by the bloodstream.* Most cases of meningitis are of haematogenous origin. In meningococcal meningitis (*cerebrospinal fever*), for example, infection is spread by droplet infection from carriers who harbour the micro-organism in the nasopharynx. Spread is favoured by poor hygienic conditions, especially overcrowding, and thus the disease tends to occur in epidemic form among recruits in overcrowded barracks, refugees in camps, etc. In susceptible persons the meningococci pass from the nasopharynx to the meninges by the bloodstream and during epidemics cases of fatal meningococcal septicaemia can occur without meningitis, death sometimes occurring within a few hours of infection. A characteristic feature of meningococcal septicaemia is the occurrence of a haemorrhagic rash from which the old name 'spotted fever' is derived (Fig. 20.25).

(*b*) *Infection by spread from an adjacent*

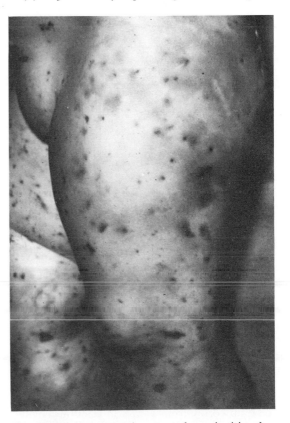

Fig. 20.25 Acute meningococcal meningitis, showing the haemorrhagic rash.

lesion. Infection may spread to the subarachnoid space from suppurative inflammation in the middle ear or in any of the air sinuses in the base of the skull, or through an open depressed fracture. Some cases of pneumococcal meningitis in young children may also be due to the direct spread of *Streptococcus pneumoniae* from the middle ear. It should be emphasised that acute leptomeningitis is a not infrequent complication of a fracture of the base of the skull as a result of direct spread of organisms from air sinuses or the nasopharynx.

(*c*) *Iatrogenic infection* happens occasionally, by the introduction of micro-organisms at operation or by lumbar puncture with non-sterile instruments. This is a rare occurrence but as the infecting agents are introduced directly into the subarachnoid space, a generalised meningitis rapidly ensues.

Structural changes. Exudate accumulates in the subarachnoid space and is most easily seen where the space is wide, i.e. within sulci (Fig. 20.26) and at the base of the brain, where it ac-

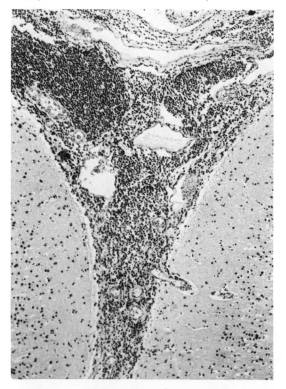

Fig. 20.26 Acute pneumococcal meningitis: section of cerebral cortex from a case of acute meningitis, showing distension of the subarachnoid space with polymorphonuclear leukocytes. × 55.

cumulates around the optic chiasma and in adjacent cisterns. It varies markedly in appearance, even in the same type of infection. There may merely be excess of turbid fluid in the sulci, or the exudate may be abundant, yellowish and fibrinous or purulent.

The inflammation frequently extends in to the ventricles: they contain turbid fluid and a varying amount of fibrinous exudate is seen on their walls and on the choroid plexuses. Some degree of internal hydrocephalus is a common result. Exudate also tends to be abundant in the spinal subarachnoid space, particularly on the dorsal surface of the cord.

In anthrax infection of the meninges, the exudate is serous and contains a considerable admixture of blood—in fact the effused blood may be so abundant as to simulate subarachnoid haemorrhage. In meningitis due to the yeast *Torula histolytica* (*Cryptococcus hominis*), the exudate is notably gelatinous (p. 703).

Diagnosis. The CSF must be examined as soon as possible whenever meningitis is suspected since this is the only means by which the diagnosis can be established and the causal agent identified. Lumbar puncture is often essential even when there is some clinical evidence of raised intracranial pressure (p. 668). The CSF presents varying degrees of turbidity and may even be distinctly purulent. Microscopic examination shows it to contain numerous polymorphonuclear leukocytes. The protein content is raised and the sugar reduced or absent (Table 20.1, pp. 708–9). The causal organisms are often apparent, although in some cases they can be obtained only by culture. In early acute meningitis, particularly in children, the first specimen of CSF may be normal in every respect. This is difficult to explain, but a subsequent lumbar puncture only 24 hours later may show all the features of an acute florid meningitis.

Treatment. Vigorous early treatment with the appropriate antibiotic often results in resolution of the infection with little or no residual damage. If treatment has been inadequate or has been commenced too late for resolution of the inflammatory exudate to occur, the disease may pass into a subacute or chronic phase. Formerly this was not uncommon in young children, particularly with meningococcal meningitis, and the disease was then referred to as *posterior basal meningitis*. The meninges become thickened and oedematous and the exudate organises leading to obliteration of the foramina in the roof of the fourth ventricle and/or some degree of obstruction in the subarachnoid space, and consequent hydrocephalus (p. 671). Various cranial nerves may be involved with resulting paralyses. Similar chronic changes can occur in the spinal meninges with widespread involvement of nerve roots. Organisms are usually scanty in such chronic cases. Closely similar structural changes may be brought about by the tubercle bacillus (see p. 686) and by *Haemophilus influenzae*.

Encephalitis

Most cases of encephalitis are caused by virus infections of the nervous system (p. 693). Bacterial encephalitis is usually suppurative (i.e. a *brain abscess*) but non-suppurative encephalitis may result from extension of inflammation from an active meningitis. The degree to which this occurs varies greatly. In some cases it is striking how little leukocytic infiltration may be present along the blood vessels; in others the perivascular spaces are crowded with leukocytes which may extend a considerable distance into the brain substance, while exudate, haemorrhage and foci of cortical infarction may be present. In tuberculous meningitis there is usually marked involvement of the cortex due to obliterative arteritis and thrombosis in many of the arteries in the subarachnoid space. Similarly the spinal cord is almost invariably implicated to some extent in meningitis.

Brain abscess

The causative organisms vary greatly, anaerobic strains of streptococci, diphtheroids and coliforms, etc., being encountered in addition to the common pyogenic cocci. The organisms reach the brain, as in meningitis, by direct spread or by means of the blood stream.

Direct spread of organisms. This is usually a consequence of pyogenic infection in the bones or sinuses of the skull or of a compound fracture. In our experience the commonest and most important cause is extension of infection from a chronic suppurative otitis media or mastoiditis. The bone is eroded by a chronic osteitis

and infection reaches the dura and may produce a local pachymeningitis, an *extradural abscess*, or a *subdural abscess* (p. 683). The inflammation extends to the leptomeninges and a generalised meningitis may ensue but more frequently the inflammation is limited by local adhesions. The organisms may then cause superficial destruction of the cortex before extending more deeply into the brain, but more often the subsequent abscess is separated from the surface of the brain by an intact layer of cortex; in fact, in some cases of middle ear disease, the caries may not even have reached the surface of the bone. The precise route of infection in these cases is open to doubt but it may be via small blood vessels or their perivascular spaces. It is to be noted that the emergent veins from the bone drain into a venous sinus, into which the veins of the brain also discharge, providing a possible route of infection

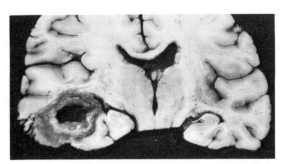

Fig. 20.27 Cerebral abscess. There is an encapsulated abscess in the left temporal lobe, secondary to chronic suppurative otitis media.

If middle ear infection spreads upwards through the tegmen tympani, it comes to the under surface of the temporal lobe, and thus the abscess occurs in this lobe (Fig. 20.27). If the disease has spread from the mastoid antrum, or from the middle ear to the posterior aspect of the petrous bone, the abscess occurs in the cerebellum; in such cases the sigmoid sinus may become implicated and may be thrombosed. In some cases with chronic middle ear disease, abscesses may be found both in the temporal lobe and in the cerebellum.

As elsewhere, an abscess in the brain becomes limited by a pyogenic membrane which, unless the infection extends very rapidly to involve the meninges or ventricles, soon becomes a well-defined capsule composed of young connective tissue, new capillaries, proliferated astrocytes and lipid phagocytes: i.e. there is a gliomesodermal reaction. In the adjacent cerebral tissue there are varying degrees of oedema, reactive gliosis and infiltration by inflammatory cells, the latter being particularly prominent in the perivascular spaces. Plasma cells often predominate. These changes are commonly silent clinically and, by the time the patient presents with symptoms, the abscess is likely to contain thick greenish-yellow pus commonly with a foul odour because of the mixed bacterial flora. The abscess can exist for a considerable time in a virtually latent state but localised extension to form a multilocular abscess is not uncommon. Without effective treatment, spread to the ventricles or the subarachnoid space often occurs as a terminal event.

Otitis media and mastoiditis. Disease of the middle ear, mastoid antrum and air cells is the result of infection spreading along the Eustachian tube from the pharynx, especially in children, but also in adults. Not infrequently it starts as a complication of streptococcal tonsillitis, but in infants pneumococci are often concerned. Other organisms are soon superadded. Acute suppurative inflammation of the lining of the tympanic cavity develops and, if this progresses, the mucous membrane is destroyed and replaced by a layer of granulation tissue; commonly the tympanic membrane is perforated allowing access of a very mixed bacterial flora. The bone becomes eroded by osteitis and infection may reach the dura, giving rise to local pachymeningitis, acute leptomeningitis, cerebral abscess, sinus thrombosis, etc. A similar sequence of events may follow acute suppuration in the frontal sinus, the resulting abscess being in the frontal lobe, but this is more rare.

Sinus thrombosis. This is the result of an extension of pyogenic infection to the wall of a sinus, and occurs most frequently in the sigmoid sinus in cases of mastoid or middle ear disease. The first effect is the production of acute phlebitis with secondary formation of thrombus on the damaged intima. The thrombus itself may then become infected. Once thrombosis has started it tends to spread, and it may pass into the internal jugular vein. The oldest part of the thrombus may thus become purulent, but if the process of ordinary thrombosis continues to spread this may prevent the detachment of infected portions. Accordingly, while septic emboli may become detached, and cause secondary abscesses in the lungs, this occurs only in a relatively small proportion of cases of septic sinus thrombosis.

Haematogenous abscesses. These occur most frequently in the parietal lobes but they may be found in any part of the brain and they are not infrequently multiple. When solitary they may attain a large size and develop a thick gliomesodermal capsule before being diagnosed. The source of the septic embolus may be anywhere in the body but the primary site is often in the lung as a result of septic involvement of small pulmonary veins. There is a particularly close association between suppurative bronchiectasis and brain abscess, but fortunately most cases of bronchiectasis can now be adequately controlled by antibiotics. Individuals with congenital cyanotic heart disease are particularly prone to develop a brain abscess. Multiple small acute abscesses occur in pyaemia, while in a patient dying with subacute bacterial endocarditis numerous small perivascular inflammatory foci are almost invariably found in the brain. Such lesions may sometimes be seen as minute haemorrhagic foci but frequently they are identifiable only on microscopic examination.

Yeasts and fungi are rarer causes of haematogenous brain abscess (p. 703).

Tuberculosis

Involvement of the nervous system is a not uncommon feature of tuberculosis. It usually presents as subacute meningitis but less commonly it takes the form of one or more large caseating lesions—tuberculomas—embedded in the brain. These latter may present clinically as expanding lesions.

Tuberculous meningitis

This is always preceded by an active tuberculous infection in some other organ in the body, usually the lung. In the meninges it causes both the formation of tubercles and an exudative inflammation. The bacilli may reach the meninges from the bloodstream as in generalised miliary tuberculosis, or, less commonly, by direct spread from tuberculous disease in any of the bones related to the central nervous system (e.g. vertebrae).

Another mode of infection is from small haematogenous caseous lesions in the cortex which are secondary to active tuberculous disease elsewhere in the body. Such cortical foci often contain abundant tubercle bacilli, and it has been suggested that such small foci are a commoner cause of tuberculous meningitis than direct haematogenous infection of the meninges. Another possible source of infection is miliary tubercles in the choroid plexus.

Tuberculous meningitis is most likely to occur in association with the primary complex and was, therefore, most frequently encountered formerly in young children in whom miliary spread had occurred. This preponderance is now rather less as the primary complex is no longer so restricted to this age group. The disease can also arise as a complication of adult fibrocaseous tuberculosis but miliary tuberculosis in the adult does not invariably lead to tuberculous meningitis.

Structural changes. When the bacilli reach the meninges they spread in the perivascular connective tissue of the arteries which become ensheathed in a cellular reaction in which tub-

ercles develop as small grey nodules along the lines of the vessels. These tubercles are rounded aggregations of cells with central caseation (Fig. 20.28) rather than typical follicles; epithelioid cells are poorly developed and giant cells are usually scanty or absent, except in subacute cases. There is a generalised inflammatory reaction in the pia-arachnoid, often with a fibrinous exudate (Fig. 20.29), containing at first many polymorphonuclear leukocytes, which are soon

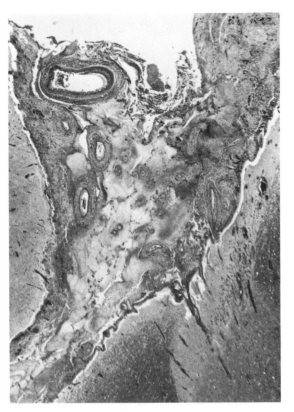

Fig. 20.29 Tuberculous meningitis. Chiasmal cistern, showing soft fibrinous exudate filling the subarachnoid space, with cellular exudate in the walls of vessels. × 8.

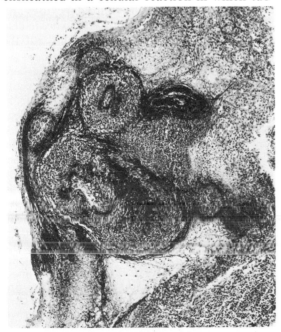

Fig. 20.28 Tuberculous meningitis showing serofibrinous exudate in the subarachnoid space and cellular exudate, most abundant around vessels. Caseation is beginning. × 48.

replaced by lymphocytes, monocytes and desquamated arachnoidal cells. Leukocyte emigration is abundant not only in the meninges but also around nutrient vessels as they extend into the brain tissue (Fig. 20.29). Necrosis and caseation affect also the unaggregated cells in the exudate, so that in certain areas both fibrin and cells are blended into a homogeneously eosinophilic mass. The presence of necrotic and caseous exudate on the wall of an artery causes a reactive endarteritis, which leads to great thickening of the intima and not infrequently actual occlusion; caseous necrosis of the wall may follow. Focal infarction of the superficial grey matter is therefore quite often present. Obliterative endarteritis is more marked in chronic cases and is very pronounced in cases in which antibiotics have prolonged life but failed to effect a cure (Fig. 20.30).

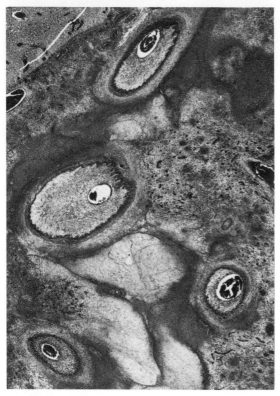

Fig. 20.30   Cerebral arteries in chronic tuberculous meningitis, showing severe obliterative endarteritis. × 15.

The inflammatory process often also extends into the proximal parts of cranial and spinal nerves to produce focal neurological signs.

Post-mortem appearances. The dura is usually tense, and the convolutions are markedly flattened and somewhat dry in appearance, as the result of hydrocephalus and raised intracranial pressure. The abundant exudate at the base of the brain obscures the optic chiasma, anterior surface of the pons, etc. Occasionally the meningitis may be more localised (Fig. 20.31) perhaps representing spread from a blood-borne cortical focus. The exudate may be soft

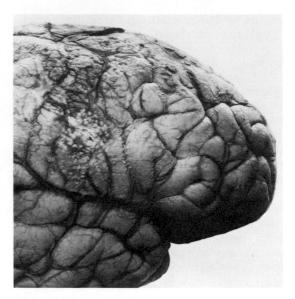

Fig. 20.31   Tuberculous meningitis: localised eruption of tubercles on surface of hemisphere in region of Sylvian fissure.

and yellowish, with much fibrin, or the chief change may be more an inflammatory oedema with greyish opacity and thickening of the meninges. The ventricles are enlarged and tubercles may often be found in the choroid plexuses and also in the lining of the ventricles. Exudate also tends to be particularly abundant around the spinal cord.

Tubercles are most readily seen in the congested areas just beyond the exudate, especially between the frontal lobes and extending from the Sylvian fissure (Fig. 20.32). A hand lens greatly assists the search for them. In adults, the disease may run a relatively chronic course, the meninges being greyish, opaque and rather firm from fibroblastic proliferation, often with implication of the roof of the fourth ventricle. Tubercles may be found only with difficulty; in fact, occasionally the true nature of the case can be determined only by microscopic examination.

The CSF in tuberculous meningitis is under increased pressure. It is often clear but more frequently has an opalescent appearance. A fine fibrin web may appear on standing. The number of cells is raised, often being 200 per μl or even higher; the majority are lymphocytes as a rule, with a small proportion of macrophages, but polymorphonuclears may be quite numerous and may occasionally exceed the lymphocytes, especially in the earliest stages. The polymorphonuclears often show signs of

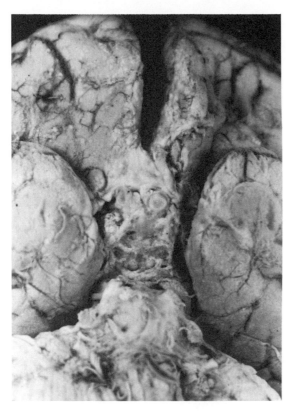

Fig. 20.32 Tuberculous meningitis, showing exudate which obscures structures at base of brain. A few tubercles can be seen on the frontal lobes.

degeneration. The protein is increased but in variable amount, and the glucose and chlorides are diminished, the latter due to the persistent vomiting which reduces the general body chlorides. Tubercle bacilli can usually be found on microscopic examination of the centrifuged deposit or of the fibrin web which forms in the fluid. They may be scanty and difficult to find and, as they grow only slowly in culture, it is essential to treat immediately with the appropriate antibiotics all suspected cases in which the general picture is strongly suggestive of the diagnosis. Delay in starting treatment may allow the pathological changes to progress to a point from which complete resolution and restoration to normal are impossible.

Tuberculosis of the cranial dura mater is very rare. Infection of the spinal dura mater from tuberculosis of the vertebrae is, however, not uncommon, the resulting caseous exudate causing compression of the cord.

Tuberculomas

The occurrence of tuberculomas in the brain is nowadays uncommon in Europe. They are, however, frequently seen in East Africa, India and South America where they can account for as many as 20% of all intracranial expanding lesions. They are often multiple, are encountered especially in young subjects, and their commonest sites are the cerebellum (Fig. 20.33),

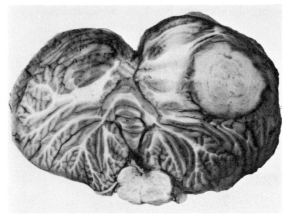

Fig. 20.33 Tuberculoma in cerebellum.

medulla, pons and mid-brain. Their consistence is usually firm and they present a dull yellowish centre which is surrounded by a pinkish-grey capsule, though sometimes there may be a considerable degree of vascularity at the periphery.

Syphilis

Syphilitic lesions of the central nervous system were formerly both frequent and serious. They fall conveniently into two groups. The first includes lesions found in the late secondary and in the tertiary stages, which involve the ordinary connective tissues and the blood vessels; these comprise meningitis, gummas and endarteritis, and various combinations of these. In the second group are tabes dorsalis and general paralysis; these occur much later than the tertiary stage, and in them the nervous tissue is involved from the outset.

Syphilitic meningitis

At a relatively early period syphilitic meningitis may involve either the dura or the leptomeninges, or both. Syphilitic *leptomeningitis* is commonest at the base of the brain, where it causes a diffuse thickening of the meninges with, as a rule, superficial involvement of the brain. The affected meninges are swollen and gelatinous, with patches of necrosis, the condition being then known as *gummatous meningitis*. Various cranial nerves, especially the optic and oculomotor nerves, become implicated. The process may obstruct the foramina of the fourth ventricle and give rise to hydrocephalus.

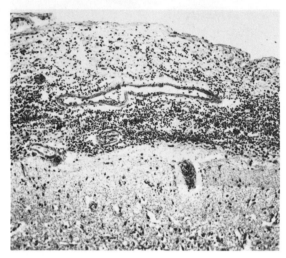

Fig. 20.34 Syphilitic leptomeningitis, showing thickening and lymphocytic infiltration of the meninges. × 50.

Microscopic examination reveals proliferation of connective tissue cells accompanied by abundant infiltration of lymphocytes and plasma cells (Fig. 20.34); reactive endarteritis is a common accompaniment (Fig. 20.35) and may cause focal infarction in the adjacent cortex. Cellular infiltration occurs round the small penetrating vessels and there is gliosis in the outer layers of the cortex.

Corresponding lesions occur in the spinal cord. Arterial changes are prominent and infarction may follow from lack of blood supply. The rare condition of *hypertrophic cervical pachymeningitis* is produced mainly by syphilis. In this condition the dura becomes markedly thickened, and generally adherent to the arachnoid. The leptomeninges also become thickened, a varying amount of gliosis occurs in the spinal cord, and the nerve roots may be compressed or invaded by the dense connective tissue and undergo atrophy.

Gummas occur in the meninges and are to be regarded as an extension and intensification of

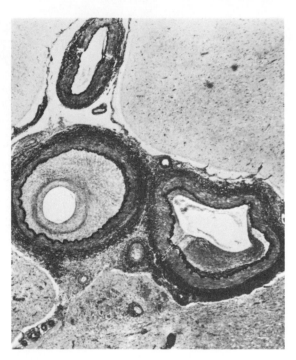

Fig. 20.35 Syphilitic endarteritis of the anterior cerebral arteries. There is also a well-marked syphilitic meningitis. Multiple small infarcts were present in both hemispheres. × 28.

meningitis. Not infrequently they are multiple. When originating in the leptomeninges, they extend inwards and have a somewhat rounded or irregular shape; the central parts may be diffusely necrotic or multiple foci of necrosis may be present. Gummas originating in the dura are usually flattened and may cover a large part of a hemisphere (Fig. 20.36). The meninges become adherent, and there may be superficial infarction of the brain, probably from endarteritis. A gumma growing from the outer aspect of

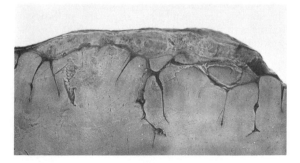

Fig. 20.36 Section of hemisphere showing a large gummatous mass arising in the dura. × ½.

the dura affects chiefly the bone, leading to erosion; or it may grow inwards and press on the brain.

General paralysis of the insane (GPI)

This disease is a subacute encephalitis with widespread lesions in the nervous system; the resulting symptoms are motor and sensory as well as psychiatric. Like tabes dorsalis it is a late or quaternary syphilitic condition, occurring some years after the period at which tertiary manifestations are encountered. Occasionally, as a sequel to congenital syphilis, it may appear about the age of ten or somewhat later. *Treponema pallidum* has been found in the brain and is irregularly distributed, being present in some areas in large numbers, whereas in others it cannot be demonstrated. The Wassermann reaction is usually positive in both blood and CSF.

Structural changes. In an advanced stage of the disease the dura mater is usually abnormally adherent and somewhat thickened. There are often unilateral or bilateral chronic subdural haematomas. The arachnoid over the hemisphere shows thickening and opacity, while, particularly in the frontal lobes, the gyri are atrophied and the sulci are widened and contain an excess of rather gelatinous CSF. Sometimes the pia-arachnoid cannot be stripped from the surface of the convolutions in the normal way, and small portions of the grey matter are removed along with it, leaving a worm-eaten appearance on the surface of the convolutions particularly over the frontal lobes. The ventricles are enlarged as a result of cerebral atrophy and there is a granular ependymitis (Fig. 20.2, p. 665).

On *microscopic examination*, the cortical grey matter is much more cellular than normal, due mainly to an increase of neuroglial cells. The small nutrient vessels stand out more prominently, surrounded by lymphocytes and plasma cells. There is a general increase of glial fibres, while the astrocytes are enlarged and branched, constituting the well-known 'spider-cells'. These cells are specially abundant in the superficial parts of the cortex (Fig. 20.37) and around the small vessels. The microglial cells also are enlarged and increased in number, and many contain granules of iron pigment. There is also loss of neurons. Gliosis may also be present in

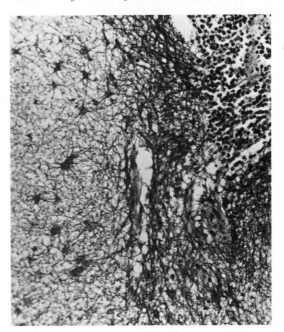

Fig. 20.37 Cerebral cortex in general paralysis of the insane, showing giant astrocytes and subpial felting. Syphilitic meningitis is also present. × 230.

the subjacent white matter and in other parts of the brain. There may be degeneration in the spinal cord, a degree of lateral sclerosis being not uncommon, and occasionally the typical lesions of tabes dorsalis are superadded (see below), the combined disorder being known as *taboparesis*.

In cases in which the disease has been arrested by treatment, e.g. by malarial pyrexia or by chemotherapy, the signs of active inflammation disappear and gliosis, both general and subpial, together with loss of nerve cells, indicate the previous damage.

Cerebrospinal fluid. There is usually an increase in the cell content of the CSF, the number of cells being 50 per μl or more. They are chiefly lymphocytes, but small proportions of macrophages and plasma cells also are present. There is a considerable increase of the protein, the level of IgG is usually raised, and the fluid almost invariably gives a positive Wassermann reaction. The Lange colloidal gold test usually gives a paretic reaction.

Tabes dorsalis or locomotor ataxia

This disease of the lower sensory neurons is characterised by degeneration of the posterior roots of spinal nerves and their upward prolongations in the spinal cord. *Tabes dorsalis*, like GPI, is a late result of syphilis. The Wassermann test is positive in both blood and CSF in most cases, and when the symptoms of tabes appear, a previously negative Wassermann reaction may become positive, indicative of renewed activity of the syphilitic process. *Treponema pallidum* has been found in the cord in only a few instances. Occasionally tabes and GPI occur together, though one is usually more marked than the other.

Tabes is much commoner in men than in women (in a proportion of about 9:1), and usually a period of about ten years intervenes between the primary syphilitic infection and the appearance of symptoms, though both shorter and longer intervals are observed. Rarely, it has developed as a result of congenital syphilis, the symptoms then commencing in childhood— juvenile tabes. The disease usually starts in and affects the lumbar segments of the cord and gradually fades off in an upward direction, so that the upper thoracic roots may be practically normal. In a small proportion of cases, however, tabes affects chiefly the region of the cervical enlargement (*cervical tabes*).

Structural changes. In the common type of tabes, the posterior columns in the lumbosacral region of the cord are somewhat shrunken and greyish; the pia-arachnoid over them is thickened. The posterior roots proximal to the dorsal root ganglia appear wasted and many have a distinctly grey tint contrasting with the white colour of the anterior roots, these changes gradually diminishing in the upper segments of the cord. The posterior columns are shrunken and rather grey and the overlying meninges are thickened.

Microscopically, in sections of the lumbar enlargement of a severe case, the posterior roots proximal to the ganglia exhibit considerable degeneration and loss of fibres, as indicated by the pale staining, and this degeneration becomes still more marked in the root fibres inside the cord. The posterior horns also lose myelinated fibres and thus appear pale (Fig. 20.38). The posterior columns show marked degeneration and gliosis, though there are usually a considerable number of non-degenerated fibres just behind the commissure; these represent endogenous or commissural fibres which are not affected. At higher levels

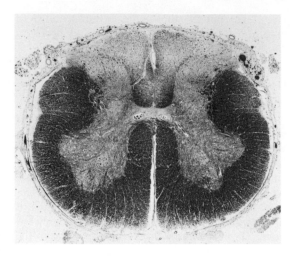

Fig. 20.38 Tabes dorsalis: section through lumbar enlargement of cord, showing the degeneration in the posterior roots and dorsal columns. × 8. (Weigert–Pal method.)

the posterior root fibres gradually become less affected, until ultimately they appear healthy. At this level the degenerated fibres of the posterior columns have become separated from the posterior horns by a layer of healthy fibres, which represent the root fibres which have entered the cord above the level of the actual disease. In the *cervical form* of tabes the posterior roots show similar degeneration and the outer parts of the posterior columns are then chiefly involved. The degeneration in tabes does not extend higher than the nucleus gracilis and the nucleus cuneatus, that is, the upper terminations of the long fibres of the posterior columns.

Changes occur also in sensory neurons in the higher parts of the central nervous system. Atrophy of the optic discs and optic nerves is common, as is also the *Argyll–Robertson phenomenon*, in which there is a loss of the light reflex while contraction of the pupils in accommodation is retained. Degenerative changes may be present also in the sensory cranial nerves and in their nucei—the trigeminal, auditory, glossopharyngeal and vagus. Similar changes in the sympathetic system may explain the severe attacks of pain and sickness—the '*gastric crises*'—which are sometimes a marked feature of the disease, though the lesions in the vagi also may be concerned in their production.

Clinical features. These widespread lesions are necessarily attended by marked disturbances of sensory function. The afferent fibres first affected are chiefly those from the deeper structures, muscle sense being impaired early, loss of co-ordination and ataxia resulting. The sensation of pain, especially in the deeper structures, is affected before tactile sensation, though the latter also becomes impaired and paraesthesia is common. Severe shooting pains in the limbs—*'lightning pains'*—also occur, and there is often a 'girdle sensation', or feeling of constriction, round the trunk at a level corresponding to the upper limit of the disease. The lesions in the posterior root fibres necessarily interrupt the reflex arc and accordingly the tendon reflexes disappear; absence of the knee-jerk is thus a well-recognised clinical sign.

The *cerebrospinal fluid* shows fairly constant changes. The cells are increased, often to 50 per μl or more; they are chiefly lymphocytes but large macrophages may be found. The protein is normal or slightly raised and there is usually an increase of globulin. The Lange colloidal gold test as a rule gives a luetic reaction, and the Wassermann reaction is usually positive (see Table 20.1, pp. 708–9).

Other effects. In addition to interference with the sensory functions and irritation of the sensory nerves, various trophic disturbances are common. Thus in the skin, zoster and pemphigoid eruptions are encountered, and a fairly common lesion is a perforating ulcer which starts in the sole of the foot, passing deeply into the tissue, and is of a very intractable nature. Important lesions occur in the joints and bones constituting what is known as 'Charcot's disease'. The hip-joint and the knee-joint are those most commonly affected, though the ankle joint and more rarely the joints of the upper extremities may be affected. Charcot's disease occasionally occurs in association with other diseases of the spinal cord and the pathological changes are described on p. 861.

The precise pathogenesis of the lesions of tabes is uncertain. Tabes occurs in only a small proportion of cases of long-standing syphilis, and we do not know what factors, in addition to the presence of syphilis, are important in determining the site of the lesions.

Virus Infections of the Nervous System

Virus infections of the nervous system produce meningo-encephalitis but the majority of patients with acute virus infections of the nervous system present as cases of **aseptic meningitis** or of **encephalitis**. In some types of encephalitis due, for example, to the polioviruses or other enteroviruses, the most severe lesions occur in the spinal cord, where there is selective involvement of motor neurons: in such cases the term *paralytic disease* is often appropriate clinically. Aseptic meningitis is the commonest clinical illness but relatively little is known about its pathology since it is rarely fatal. Encephalitis, on the other hand, usually causes severe and frequently fatal brain damage.

Acute virus diseases of the nervous system have long been recognised but only relatively recently have **persistent virus infections** of the nervous system, e.g. subacute sclerosing panencephalitis (p. 700), and **slow virus infections**, e.g. kuru (p. 701), been widely recognised as being important in man.

Pathogenesis

Most viruses reach the nervous system by way of the bloodstream, i.e. there is a viraemia, often after primary viral multiplication in lymphoid tissue. They may gain access to the body by various routes, e.g. infection of the skin or mucous membranes (herpes simplex virus), by way of the alimentary tract (enteroviruses), infection through injured skin (B virus), or introduction through the skin by the bite of an arthropod (arboviruses). A few viruses may reach the nervous system by travelling along peripheral nerves (rabies virus). Polioviruses readily travel along nerves in the experimental situation, but the natural route of infection in man is by way of the bloodstream.

The clinical features of virus infections of the nervous system frequently occur late in the course of the infection when viraemia is subsiding and circulating antibody has appeared. This has led to the concept that at least a proportion of the brain damage is brought about by the reaction of antigen and antibody in the walls of cerebral arterioles and venules.

Viruses which show a particular predilection for the nervous system are often referred to as *neurotropic viruses*, but only a small proportion of individuals infected by a potentially neurotropic virus develop clinical evidence of disease of the nervous system.

General features of virus encephalitis

The reactions of the brain and spinal cord to virus infections tend to be similar in all types of virus encephalitis but, as will be seen in the brief accounts of specific virus diseases below, they vary both in their intensity and distribution throughout the nervous system.

There may be no macroscopic abnormalities in the nervous system in a fatal case of acute virus encephalitis but in some varieties there may be congestion, swelling, softening, or focal haemorrhage in the more severely affected regions. If the patient lives for some time after the acute illness, the areas that have borne the brunt of the damage may be shrunken and cystic. In the acute stage the most prominent and widespread abnormality on microscopic examination is the presence of lymphocytes, large mononuclear cells and plasma cells in the meninges and around small vessels (often referred to as *perivascular cuffing*), in all parts of the brain and spinal cord. The next most characteristic feature is necrosis of nerve cells and neuronophagia, when the dead neurons become engulfed by hypertrophied microglia and other macrophages, and less commonly by polymorphonuclear leukocytes. In the more florid types of encephalitis, necrosis may not remain restricted to nerve cells but may spread to involve grey and white matter, e.g. in herpes simplex encephalitis. In certain forms of encephalitis, e.g. herpes simplex encephalitis and subacute sclerosing panencephalitis, intranuclear inclusion bodies may be found in neurons or astrocytes. Another feature of encephalitis is focal or diffuse hypertrophy and hyperplasia of microglial cells.

In aseptic meningitis, abnormalities are virtually restricted to infiltration of the subarachnoid space by mononuclear cells and perivascular cuffing in the superficial layers of the cortex.

Essentially similar abnormalities are found in the CSF in all acute virus infections of the nervous system. It is often under increased pressure and there is characteristically an increase of leukocytes (50–200, usually lymphocytes, plasma cells and large mononuclear cells) and of protein (0·7–2 g/litre, 70–200 mg/100 ml) whereas the sugar content is normal.

Aseptic meningitis

Although usually not a severe illness, this is the commonest acute viral infection of the nervous system. It is therefore an important cause of morbidity, especially in children. It is caused by many viruses but those most frequently implicated in Britain are the *enteroviruses* and *mumps virus*. Enterovirus meningitis is a summer disease and is often seen as an epidemic in which one or perhaps two enteroviruses predominate. The virus is spread by the faecal–oral route. In mumps meningitis, which does not show the striking seasonal incidence of enterovirus meningitis, there is no accompanying parotitis in about 50% of cases.

One type of virus aseptic meningitis, termed *lymphocytic choriomeningitis*, is rare but of great interest. The natural hosts of the causal virus are mice and the infection is transmitted to man by the inhalation of dust or by fomites contaminated by mouse faeces. In mice the disease is a generalised infection with marked and widespread lymphocytic infiltration, the liver and kidneys being more severely affected than other organs: there is also a mild meningo-encephalitis. Immunological reactions show that infection with lymphocytic choriomeningitis virus in mice is distinct from other virus infections. In infected colonies the young mice harbour the virus but show only a low level of antibodies to it and do not develop disease. If non-infected mice are placed in such a colony, or are inoculated with the virus, they develop disease with full production of antibodies and cell-mediated immunity to the virus. These observations suggest that mice infected with virus during fetal life develop immunological tolerance to it and in this situation the virus is harmless, and that in mice infected later in life, the lesions result from immunological reactions with the viral antigen. Further studies have lent strong support to these suggestions, and there is now good evidence that the choriomeningitis is mediated by a delayed hypersensitivity reaction to the virus. There is evidence also that mice infected *in utero* may, in later life, gradually lose their tolerance: they then develop glomerular lesions due to the deposition of virus–antibody complexes, i.e. immune complex disease (pp. 126, 756).

Viruses of the herpes group

The nervous system may be affected by at least four viruses in the herpes group—herpes simplex, varicella-zoster, B virus of monkeys and cytomegalovirus. All are DNA viruses of similar morphology.

Herpes simplex virus

Herpes simplex virus affects the nervous system in one of three ways. The most severe manifestation is *acute necrotising encephalitis* which appears to be the commonest type of acute encephalitis in Western Europe at the present time. The others are encephalitis associated with disseminated herpes simplex virus infection in infants, and aseptic meningitis.

Acute necrotising encephalitis. This is a fulminating and often rapidly fatal type of encephalitis. Its most characteristic feature is selective, bilateral but asymmetrical involvement of the temporal lobes. In a fatal acute case there is usually flattening of the convolutions and raised intracranial pressure, while the more severely affected temporal lobe is soft, swollen and often focally haemorrhagic (Fig. 20.39). There is often also an ipsilateral tentorial hernia (see p. 667). Necrosis usually occurs also in the insulae and in the cingulate gyri. Microscopic examination shows diffuse infiltration of the meninges and perivascular spaces by lymphocytes and plasma cells: where necrosis has occurred, plasma cells stream out from the

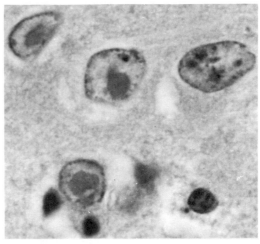

Fig. 20.40 Acute necrotising encephalitis. Note the presence of intranuclear inclusion bodies. H and E. × 1200.

perivascular spaces into the brain tissue. In the temporal lobes there is total necrosis of the cortex and the adjacent white matter and there are varying degrees of microglial hyperplasia. In the cortex adjacent to the zones of necrosis, intranuclear inclusion bodies may be found within neurons in a proportion of cases (Fig. 20.40). Neuronophagia is distributed widely throughout the brain and spinal cord. The diagnosis of herpes simplex encephalitis during life rests on the isolation of virus from a brain biopsy taken through a burr-hole in the skull.

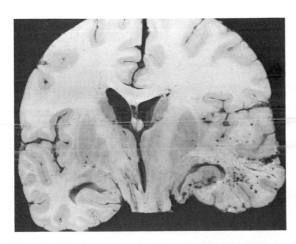

Fig. 20.39 Acute necrotising encephalitis due to Herpes simplex virus. Within the swollen right temporal lobe there are many small haemorrhagic foci.

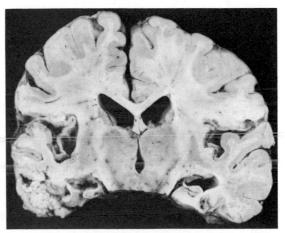

Fig. 20.41 Acute necrotising encephalitis. This patient survived for several weeks. The affected regions are now shrunken and focally cystic. The left temporal lobe is more severely affected than the right one.

Virus cannot usually be isolated from the CSF. If the patient survives the acute phase, the necrotic tissue becomes shrunken and cystic (Fig. 20.41).

Zoster

This is a disease of adults, caused by the same virus that causes varicella. During the illness there is often a rise in the antibody titre against the virus to levels above those commonly seen in varicella. Adults with zoster sometimes infect susceptible children, typical varicella resulting. The reverse, however, does not occur, and it is now believed that zoster is the result of recrudescence of a latent infection with varicella virus in a partially immune subject. In its ordinary form zoster results from an acute inflammatory lesion of a posterior root ganglion, most commonly the lower cervical and dorsal ganglia. In one type of zoster the Gasserian ganglion is affected. Along the course of the nerve related to the affected ganglion, pain and hyperalgesia occur and are followed by erythema and the formation of vesicles which contain a serous fluid, sometimes with admixture of blood. The lesion of the posterior root ganglion is an acute

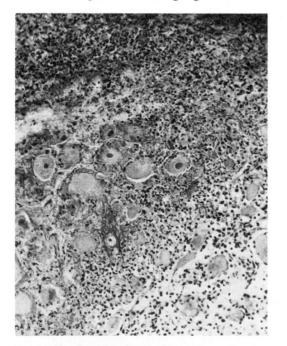

Fig. 20.42 Section of posterior root ganglion in zoster, showing inflammatory infiltration and destruction of nerve cells. × 160.

inflammation, accompanied by infiltration of lymphocytes which may form dense aggregations, and by haemorrhage, while the nerve cells are injured in varying degree; inflammatory change is present also in the capsule of an affected ganglion (Fig. 20.42). Many of the nerve cells involved in the lesions undergo necrosis while in other parts they are practically unaffected. The inflammatory process may extend into the spinal cord at the level of the affected ganglion, where it is often restricted to the dorso–lateral quadrant. Central chromatolysis in anterior horn neurons is not uncommon.

As a result of the damage to the nerve cells, secondary degeneration shown by Marchi's method can be traced along the nerve fibres to their peripheral distribution, and also proximally through the posterior nerve roots and for a distance upwards in the posterior columns of the cord. At a later period secondary fibrosis occurs in the various structures which have been damaged.

What produces reactivation of the latent virus is not clear, but physical trauma to the affected part seems to be a fairly frequent precipitating factor. A high incidence of zoster has also been reported in association with malignant lymphomas. Immunological imbalance may therefore be a factor, and in some patients with malignant lymphoma, particularly those treated with cytotoxic drugs and corticosteroids, the lesions may become disseminated and lead to a generalised varicelliform rash. In such cases there may also be a multifocal necrotising encephalomyelitis.

B-virus encephalomyelitis

B virus is a natural parasite of monkeys and in them behaves very similarly to herpes simplex virus in man, causing stomatitis and viraemia. Transmission to man is by a monkey bite or by contamination of a skin wound by saliva or tissues from an infected monkey. In man the disease takes the form of an acute encephalomyelitis with paralysis of cranial nerves and the respiratory muscles, usually progressing to coma and death within one to two weeks. Histological examination shows a multifocal necrotising encephalitis affecting grey and white matter, sometimes with a particular predilection for the spinal cord.

Cytomegalovirus

Involvement of the nervous system by cytomegalovirus is mainly due to infection acquired *in utero*. Neonatal cytomegalovirus encephalitis may be severe and run an acute course when there is a severe disseminated necrotising encephalomyelitis with selective involvement of periventricular tissue. Cytomegalic inclusions may be found in various types of cell. Survivors are often mentally retarded, and in such cases the principal abnormalities in the brain are hydrocephalus and periventricular calcification. Infection early in pregnancy may lead to developmental malformations such as microgyria (p. 721).

Enteroviruses

The most important enteroviruses are the polioviruses, the Coxsackie viruses and the ECHO viruses. All are small RNA viruses. They are a frequent cause of aseptic meningitis but they may also cause paralytic disease, acute anterior poliomyelitis being classically associated with the polioviruses. Occasionally, however, it may be produced by other enteroviruses, particularly Coxsackie A7 virus. Indeed in countries where a vigorous poliovirus vaccination programme has been undertaken, Coxsackie virus may now be a commoner cause of paralytic disease than the polioviruses. Overt paralysis probably occurs in no more than about 1% of individuals infected with poliovirus.

Acute anterior poliomyelitis

This is an acute inflammatory condition affecting chiefly, though not exclusively, the anterior horns of the spinal cord, and leading to destruction of the motor neurons, with corresponding paralysis and atrophy of the related muscles.

Epidemiology and virology. Before the introduction of poliovaccine, this was probably the commonest acute encephalomyelitis caused by a neurotropic virus. It may occur sporadically but also in both major and minor epidemics. Three strains of poliovirus have been distinguished. Most cases of paralytic poliomyelitis are caused by type I virus: immunity to one type does not protect against the others. A similar paralytic illness may be caused by other enteroviruses.

Until comparatively recently poliomyelitis was a disease affecting, in urban communities, young children almost exclusively, whereas in sparsely populated rural areas there were proportionately more cases in older subjects. Although the infectivity rate of poliovirus is high, most of those infected develop either no symptoms or a mild febrile illness. Only a few develop severe neurological lesions, which may appear after a brief temporary remission of fever. There is good evidence that this recrudescence of infection may be determined by factors such as muscular fatigue during the initial stage of the illness or by local tissue damage, e.g. by intramuscular injections, such as those used in the immunisation of children by combined prophylactics, especially those containing alum. In developing countries with poor hygiene and living standards there is a high proportion of young children among the cases, since the majority of adults are immune as a result of previous non-paralytic and subclinical infections acquired during childhood. The rise in the proportion of adult cases in recent years is a reflection of improved hygiene, which has resulted in a greater number of people escaping infection in childhood and thus constituting an increased element at risk among the higher age groups. Adults are also more likely than children to develop paralysis when infected with poliovirus. This change in incidence has not been shared by more primitive communities.

In man the natural route of infection is by the mouth and the virus multiplies in the alimentary tract. It is often present in the nasopharyngeal secretions of a person suffering from the disease but is most readily isolated from the faeces, where it may persist for long after the disease has been overcome. There is an early viraemia and the infection reaches the central nervous system by crossing the blood–brain barrier.

Structural changes. The virus displays a remarkable predilection for the neurons in the ventral horns of the spinal cord, especially in the lumbar and cervical enlargements, and it attacks these in an asymmetrical manner. Macroscopic examination in an acute case reveals little beyond congestion of the meninges over the affected part of the cord, and of the ventral horns with, in severe cases, some softening and haemorrhage.

Microscopic examination reveals an extensive inflammatory infiltration of the leptomeninges, with lymphocytes, plasma cells, and some polymorphonuclear leukocytes, but no fibrin. The infiltrate extends along the nutrient vessels, especially the anterior spinal arteries and their branches (Fig. 20.43).

In the anterior horns, where inflammation is usually most marked in the medially placed cell groups, there is much congestion and oedema along with the cellular infiltration; some of the

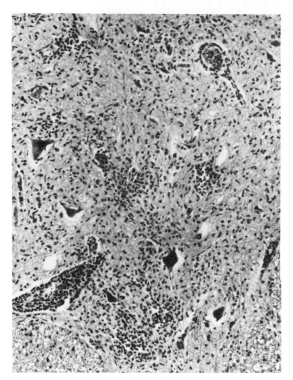

Fig. 20.43 Ventral horn of lumbar cord in poliomyelitis fatal on the 5th day. Note the perivascular cuffing, the general inflammatory infiltration and neuronophagia of dead nerve cells.

minute vessels may be thrombosed and small capillary haemorrhages are not uncommon. The nerve cells are affected in varying degree. Some undergo acute necrosis, and are removed by phagocytes—neuronophagia (Fig. 20.44). If the nerve cell dies, disintegration of its axon and myelin sheath follows. Other nerve cells show varying degrees of chromatolysis, though it is remarkable how little altered some of them are, even when surrounded by inflammatory change. There may be little change in the adjacent white matter beyond perivascular leukocytic infiltration.

The lesions are usually much more widespread in the nervous system than might be thought on the basis of clinical signs.

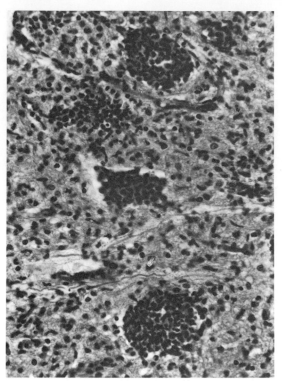

Fig. 20.44 Ventral horn of lumbar cord in acute poliomyelitis (5th day). Each of the dense cellular aggregates is a dead neuron which is obscured by polymorphs and microglia (neuronophagia).

Sometimes the virus affects severely the motor nuclei in the medulla, causing acute bulbar paralysis. There are also lesions in the cerebral cortex, characteristically localised to the motor and pre-motor areas, but there is no generalised involvement of the cortex as in other types of virus encephalitis.

Effects. The more acute changes usually pass off in a few days, but the infiltrate of lymphocytes and plasma cells may persist for some months. Many of the motor neurons which are only partially damaged recover; accordingly, considerable diminution in the amount of the paralysis may occur at a later stage. The destructive lesions in the cord are followed by absorption of the degenerated material and by proliferation of the neuroglial cells, with subsequent gliosis. Gradually the affected parts shrink, and if the lesion has been a severe one, the ventral horns become very small. The anterior nerve roots also become wasted. The permanently affected muscle fibres soon give the reactions of degeneration and undergo rapid wasting, the classical histological feature being bundles of atrophied muscle fibres among fibres of normal size (Fig. 22.70, p. 873). Owing to the unopposed action of the unaffected muscles, deformities of the limbs, including various forms of club-foot, etc., are brought about. The bones in the affected limbs may show atrophy, being reduced both in thickness and in density (Fig. 1.33, p. 30).

Rabies

It is generally accepted that rabies virus reaches the central nervous system by travelling along peripheral nerves. Rabies is still a major problem in Central and Eastern Europe, in India and in some parts of North and South America. Its incidence in Western Europe is increasing and, after having been free of the disease for many years, occasional cases have recently occurred in Britain although there is no reason to believe that there is yet a reservoir of infection there. The major reservoirs of the virus are the fox, the skunk and the jackal, although the majority of human cases can be traced to the bites of rabid dogs. Vampire bats seem to be important in maintaining the circulation of the virus in some regions. The incubation period of the disease in man is usually between one and two months. Rabies in man may be of the restless type, corresponding to the 'furious' rabies of dogs, or, much less commonly, of the paralytic type. The old name *hydrophobia* is based on the frequency with which spasm of the muscles of deglutition on attempting to drink water is a prominent and early symptom.

Microscopically, rabies encephalitis is predominantly a polio-encephalitis since perivascular cuffing by lymphocytes and plasma cells and microglial hyperplasia occur principally in grey matter. Neuronophagia is common, as are larger aggregates of proliferated microglial cells. The pathognomonic histological feature of rabies, however, is the **Negri body**, which is a large sharply defined, rounded or oval acidophilic cytoplasmic inclusion body. They may lie anywhere within the cytoplasm of a neuron, including its dendrites, and two or more may be seen in the one cell. The largest bodies are usually seen in the pyramidal cells of the hippocampus and in Purkinje cells in the cerebel-

lum. Virus particles have not been identified in Negri bodies, and it has been suggested that they store nucleoproteins until a proper template for virus assembly is formed. Negri bodies are found only after infection with 'street' virus and do not occur after the virus has become 'fixed' by laboratory passage.

The principal regions of the nervous system affected by inflammatory changes in the classical type of rabies are dorsal root ganglia, the lower brain stem, and the hypothalamus. In the paralytic form, abnormalities are more severe in the lower parts of the spinal cord and the medulla oblongata.

Arboviruses

The only shared attributes of arboviruses are that they are transmitted from host to host by blood-sucking insects (**ar**thropod–**b**orne **vir**uses), and that they are all probably RNA viruses. They multiply in both vertebrate and invertebrate hosts. An arthropod vector is infected by ingesting blood from the vertebrate reservoir and, after an incubation period, the virus reaches the salivary gland of the arthropod. The virus is then inoculated into a new host and, after an interval during which viral proliferation occurs, there is a period of viraemia during which a further arthropod may become infected. Man is not the natural host for any arbovirus but, during periods of epizootic spread among the natural hosts, he may become infected.

Several arboviruses can cause severe encephalitis in man, e.g. *St. Louis encephalitis*, *Eastern and Western equine encephalomyelitis* and *Japanese B encephalitis*, all of which are mosquito-borne. The structural changes are in general those of a disseminated encephalitis (p. 694), sometimes with focal necrosis in vessel walls. Tick-borne arboviruses are responsible for *Russian spring summer encephalitis* and *louping ill*.

Encephalitis lethargica

This was the first pandemic encephalitis in modern times, and its sudden appearance, rapid pandemic spread and subsequent disappearance are not the least of its mysterious features since its cause was never established. It is however generally accepted that the disease was a virus encephalitis. A small epidemic with a mortality rate of about 50% occurred in Vienna in the winter of 1916–17. The disease then spread through Western Europe, and the epidemic reached its peak in Britain in 1924. It had virtually disappeared from there by 1926.

Clinical features. The symptoms were those of a general affection of the brain—headache, pyrexia, drowsiness and delirium; there was usually a general weakness of muscular power, with marked disturbance of sleep rhythm and extreme lethargy by day. In addition, there were local symptoms due to implication of the oculomotor, facial and other nerves, and sometimes there was nystagmus. The mortality varied in different epidemics, but averaged about 25%. Among a high proportion of the non-fatal cases, however, a more or less permanent residual neurological syndrome occurred, including tremor, rigidity and loss of associated movements. This was known as post-encephalitic Parkinsonism. Immobile facial expression, excessive salivation and emotional disturbances of various kinds also occurred and, in children, a loss of inhibitions with a tendency to violent actions.

At necropsy following death in the acute stage, there was usually marked congestion of the meninges, especially over the pons and medulla and the base of the brain, and occasionally minute haemorrhages were present. Intense congestion was found throughout the brain stem, basal ganglia and cortex, and minute haemorrhages and even points of softening were often present in the floor of the fourth ventricle.

Microscopic examination shows the features typical of encephalitis. In severe acute cases, damage to vessels and nerve cells is the outstanding feature as shown by intense congestion, haemorrhages both into the perivascular sheaths and adjacent tissues, and sometimes by actual thrombosis: occasionally part of a vessel wall may appear swollen and hyaline. Many nerve cells show chromatolysis and other signs of acute degeneration, but neuronophagia is slight; nevertheless many nerve cells are destroyed. Perivascular cuffing by leukocytes, chiefly lymphocytes along with a few plasma cells, develops rapidly and becomes the most prominent feature in less acute cases (Fig. 20.45). Infiltration of similar cells occurs in the meninges. These abnormalities are usually most pronounced in the brain stem.

The histological changes of *post-encephalitic Parkinsonism* are chiefly centred in the substantia nigra in the cerebral peduncles where there is considerable loss of neurons. Associated with this there is free pigment in the parenchyma, occasional pigment-containing phagocytes, and some gliosis. Frequently some of the residual pigmented neurons contain large intracytoplasmic inclusion bodies

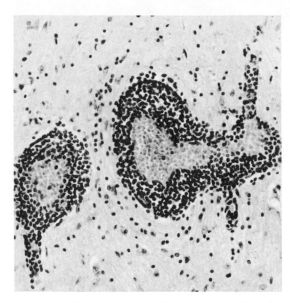

Fig. 20.45 Section of posterior part of medulla in encephalitis lethargica, showing the extensive perivascular infiltration by lymphocytes and plasma cells. × 170.

known as Lewy bodies. Similar inclusion bodies occur in the pigmented nuclei of the pons. Essentially similar histological abnormalities occur in *idiopathic Parkinsonism*, the principal macroscopic abnormality being depigmentation of the substantia nigra.

Subacute sclerosing panencephalitis

First described in children as subacute inclusion body encephalitis, and later as subacute sclerosing leukoencephalitis, subacute sclerosing panencephalitis (SSPE) is a **persistent virus infection** of the nervous system caused by the measles virus. It is a rare condition occurring principally between the ages of 4 and 20 years. The disease is a subacute encephalitis, usually fatal in from 6 weeks to 6 months: the early period of the disease is characterised by personality changes and intellectual deterioration, the middle period by periodic involuntary movements, and the terminal period by profound dementia and decerebrate rigidity.

The mechanism and sequence of events whereby a patient develops SSPE some years after apparently uncomplicated measles have not yet been clarified but it appears to be due to reactivation of measles virus which has remained latent in the brain since the time of primary infection. There are high levels of both IgM and IgG classes of antibodies to measles virus in the blood and CSF, and this suggests that there is a continuous or repeated antigenic stimulus over a period of time and that there is synthesis of antibody in the central nervous system. Complete measles virus has been isolated from brain tissue obtained by biopsy in cases of SSPE.

At necropsy, the brain may appear almost normal, but the white matter is often abnormally firm. Microscopic examination shows the features of a subacute encephalitis with widespread cuffing of vessels throughout the brain with lymphocytes and plasma cells. Neuronophagia is common, and varying numbers of residual neurons contain intranuclear inclusion bodies. There is also considerable gliosis in the white matter.

Subacute spongiform encephalopathy

The discovery and investigation of **kuru** has been one of the most dramatic occurrences in the entire field of diseases of the nervous system in the past two decades. It is subacute degenerative disease of the brain characterised by microcystic degeneration in grey matter referred to as status spongiosus, associated with which there is loss of neurons and a great excess of hypertrophied astrocytes, and selectively severe degeneration of the cerebellar system. Kuru is restricted to the Fore tribe and their tribal neighbours in the Eastern Highlands of New Guinea. Its peculiar importance is that it was the first progressive degenerative disease of the nervous system of man to be transmitted to another animal, first the chimpanzee but later to other primates, by injecting extracts of brain tissue from patients with the disease. It is therefore now classified as a **slow virus infection** although the agent, which is filterable and capable of replicating, has not been identified. It is now generally accepted that cannibalism was the primary mode of transmission, and the incidence of the disease has subsided since this practice ceased.

In more recent years, a second progressive degenerative disease of the nervous system, **Creutzfeldt–Jakob disease** which is a progressive dementia of world-wide distribution, again characterised by status spongiosus and astrocytosis, has been transmitted to primates. Kuru and Creutzfeldt–Jakob disease along with two transmissible diseases of the nervous system in animals—*scrapie* of sheep and *mink encephalopathy*—are now classified as *subacute spongiform encephalopathies*. All appear to be due to slow viruses, have an exceptionally long incubation period, and have an unremitting and always fatal progressive course. The transmissible agents have so far not been shown to be antigenic in that antibody has not yet been demonstrated.

Progressive multifocal leukoencephalopathy

The precise nosological position of this condition has still to be determined but there is a remarkably consistent association of polyoma-type viruses with the disease. As its name implies, progressive multifocal leukoencephalopathy (PML) is characterised by multiple foci of degeneration in the brain, particularly in the white matter. The most characteristic macroscopic feature is the presence of multiple small grey foci distributed widely but usually asymmetrically in the white matter. These foci can coalesce to form large grey areas which may become frankly cystic. Histological examination shows multiple foci of demyelination associated with which there are lipid phagocytes, abnormal oligodendrocytes containing large hyperchromatic nuclei within which ill-defined inclusion bodies occur, and usually large and bizarre astrocytes. The precise relationship of polyoma-type viruses to PML has not yet been established but since the vast majority of patients who develop the disease already have disseminated disease of the lymphoreticular system, usually a malignant lymphoid neoplasm or leukaemia, it has been suggested that the virus may normally produce a latent infection in man and that it may attack the brain when some other factor such as immunological deficiency, cytotoxic drug therapy or immunosuppressive treatment is superimposed.

Other Infections of the Nervous System

Protozoal infections

The commoner protozoa which cause infections of the nervous system are *Toxoplasma gondii* and some amoebae. Various trypanosomes produce a meningo-encephalitis with no specifically identifying histological abnormalities: sleeping sickness, well known in central Africa, is an example.

Toxoplasmosis. For congenital toxoplasmosis to occur, the woman must experience a primary infection during pregnancy. Infection in early pregnancy may lead to abortion, a little later to a stillborn infant, and still later to a live-born child with clinical manifestations of the disease. The latter, however, may not appear until the early weeks of life. In babies who survive the congenital or neonatal infection, there is often residual mental retardation, epilepsy and chorioretinitis. In fatal cases there is extensive granulomatous destruction of the brain (Fig. 20.46) and often hydrocephalus. Parasites may be found in the granulomas (Fig. 20.47), both extracellularly and in large endothelial cells (pseudocysts).

Amoebiasis. *Primary amoebic meningo-encephalitis* is a relatively recently recognised disease of man, caused by free-living amoebae traditionally regarded

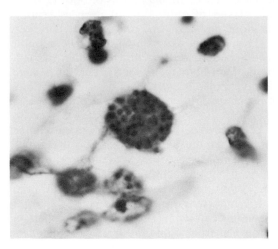

Fig. 20.47 Congenital toxoplasmosis. A large central pseudocyst containing many parasites: a few are also seen in the cell below (from same case as 20.46). × 900.

as being non-pathogenic in man. Numerous cases have now been reported from all parts of the world, the amoebae usually belonging to the Naegleri group. It appears that the amoebae reach the nasal sinuses when exposed to contaminated water, and that they then spread through the olfactory plate into the skull. The disease takes the form of an acute meningo-encephalitis, most patients dying within about a week. At necropsy there is a fibrinopurulent exudate in the subarachnoid space, necrotising vasculitis and necrosis in the superficial parts of the cortex. Amoebae are found in the exudate, and the diagnosis is made during life by identifying amoebae in the CSF. The amoebae do not appear to cause a systemic infection.

Amoebic abscess. Although uncommon, amoebic abscess in the brain is one of the most frequently encountered fatal complications of amoebic dysentery (p. 577). The abscess may not appear until many years after the first attack of amoebic dysentery. They are usually single abscesses that contain reddish-brown or pinkish creamy fluid, and act as rapidly expanding intracranial lesions (p. 666).

Cerebral malaria is almost always due to *Plasmodium falciparum*. In fatal cases there are numerous petechial haemorrhages throughout the brain.

Metazoal parasites

Cysticercosis may involve the brain. The larvae of *Taenia solium* may reach the brain where they usually produce multiple small cysts measuring up to

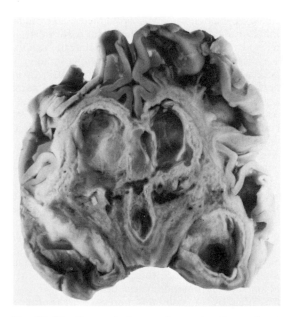

Fig. 20.46 Congenital toxoplasmosis. Coronal section of brain of a 2 months' old infant. Note the enlarged ventricles with necrotic lining, and extensive cystic and gelatinous degeneration of the hemispheres.

about 1 cm in diameter. They are a cause of epilepsy where cysticercosis is prevalent. The larva exists as a mural nodule in the cyst, which usually becomes surrounded by a collagenous capsule. When the larva dies, the cyst may become calcified. **Hydatid cysts** may also occur in the brain (p. 635). **Schistosomiasis** may be a cause of granulomas in all parts of the central nervous system including the spinal cord.

Fungal infections

Fungal infections of the nervous system are invariably secondary to infection elsewhere in the body but lesions at the portal of entry may be small and readily overlooked. The brain, therefore, may appear to be the only organ involved. In other cases, infection of the nervous system may simply be one of the manifestations of a systematised infectious process. Some fungi, e.g. *Cryptococcus neoformans* and *Coccidioides immitis*, may produce disease in man in the absence of predisposing factors other than increased exposure to a particular fungus. Apart from cryptococcosis (torulosis), these infections are extremely rare in Britain. On the other hand there is an ever increasing incidence of *opportunistic infections*, with fungi which normally have little or no pathogenicity for man, but become more pathogenic if the natural defences of the body are lowered, e.g. by debilitating or immunodeficiency diseases, or the prolonged use of antibiotics, or cytotoxic or immunosuppressive agents.

Cryptococcosis. The commonest clinical presentation of infection with *Cryptococcus neoformans* (p. 190) is as a subacute meningitis. The exudate in the subarachnoid space is usually rather gelatinous and within it there are usually masses of encapsulated cryptococci. Flask-shaped cysts filled with cryptococci in the superficial layers of the cortex are frequently found. Inflammatory changes in the brain and subarachnoid space are often remarkably mild

but occasionally there is a granulomatous reaction very similar to that seen in tuberculous meningitis.

Opportunistic fungal infections. These are caused mainly by *Candida albicans*, *Aspergillus fumigatus* and *Nocardia asteroides*. They generally produce multiple abscesses of variable size (Fig. 20.48). In the

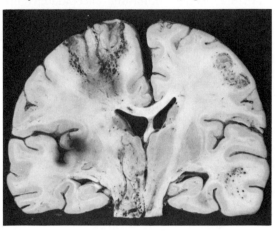

Fig. 20.48 Opportunistic fungal infection. There are several acute haemorrhagic lesions. The causal fungus was *Candida albicans*.

acute stages the abscesses may resemble haemorrhagic infarcts but later they usually become encapsulated. Candida may also cause a florid meningitis. Histological examination usually discloses abundant fungus, particularly at the edges of the abscesses. Accurate identification, however, depends on culture. *Mucormycosis* is a rarer opportunistic infection. It has a particular predilection for uncontrolled diabetic patients. Infection usually commences in the paranasal sinuses and spreads directly into the anterior fossa of the skull to produce selective involvement of the frontal lobes.

Demyelinating Diseases

This is a convenient term to bring together a number of disorders characterised by loss of myelin unrelated to specific fibre systems or particular arterial territories. The group includes **acute** conditions associated with considerable cellular exudation, and **chronic** disorders, in which there is conspicuous fibrillary gliosis in the demyelinated areas, but forms intermediate in both clinical and pathological

features are not very rare. Examples of the chronic type are **multiple** or **disseminated sclerosis**, where the lesions are focal and not specially perivascular, and **diffuse cerebral sclerosis** where the process is more generalised but may affect certain areas of the brain more severely than others. In the acute disorders the demyelination is usually strikingly perivascular and may develop with astonishing rapidity as in **acute disseminated encephalomyelitis**, which usually occurs as a complication of an acute virus infection, or in **acute haemorrhagic leukoencephalitis**, a condition in which the aetiology is still unknown.

An acute demyelinating encephalomyelitis (**experimental allergic encephalomyelitis**, or **EAE**) is readily produced in animals by injection of homogenised neural tissue emulsified in Freund's adjuvant. The disease develops after a latent period of 10 days or more, and is believed to be due to the development of an immune response to neural tissue antigen in the inoculum and a subsequent immunological reaction with the animal's own neural tissue. EAE has been very extensively investigated in guinea pigs, rats, mice, rabbits and several other species. The antigen is a basic protein and is common to neural tissue of many species. The presence of antibody in the serum does not correlate well with the occurrence of the disease, and there is strong evidence to suggest that the lesions result from a delayed hypersensitivity reaction in which sensitised lymphocytes and possibly macrophages react directly with neural tissue. However, there is also evidence suggesting that early changes in the CNS precede the infiltration of lymphocytes and macrophages, and the pathogenic mechanism is not completely understood.

The changes of EAE vary somewhat depending on the experimental detail and the animal species. Typically, acute demyelination, inflammatory oedema and cell infiltration occur around venules in the brain and cord. In the guinea-pig, cellular infiltration is pronounced and demyelination slight. The changes in some experimental species are similar to acute disseminated encephalomyelitis in man, and the normal incubation period of 10 days or so between the predisposing virus infection and the onset of neural changes suggests that an immunological process may be involved. Although EAE can be induced by one injection of antigen in Freund's adjuvant, its production in monkeys without the use of Freund's adjuvant requires many injections, and it is very likely that the acute demyelinating encephalitis which occurs in man as a complication of *vaccination against rabies* is the equivalent of EAE and results from the repeated injection of the rabbit spinal cord preparation used for the prophylactic injections.

Acute disseminated encephalomyelitis

This disease, known also as **post-infectious encephalitis** or **acute perivascular myelinoclasis** because of the rapid occurrence of perivascular demyelination, occurs as a sequel to various acute virus diseases such as measles, rubella, or varicella, to certain presumably viral respiratory infections, or to primary vaccination (**post-vaccinial encephalitis**) or anti-rabic inoculation. Post-vaccinial encephalitis occurs mainly in older children and adults, about ten days after primary vaccination.

The focal lesions in the nervous system are mainly around small venules throughout the brain and spinal cord, but often affecting the ventral half of the pons, the deeper layers of the cerebral cortex, the thalamus and the white matter of the cerebral hemispheres with particular severity. The characteristic histological features are a conspicuous excess of cells around venules comprised mainly of lymphocytes and macrophages in addition to occasional plasma cells, and perivenular loss of myelin (Fig. 20.49). This demyelination takes place with great rapidity, being sometimes almost complete within four days. Axons show only slight damage, nerve cells adjacent to the

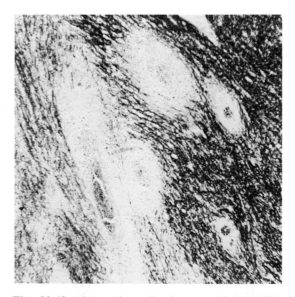

Fig. 20.49 Acute demyelinating encephalomyelitis following measles. A section showing perivascular demyelination in the white matter of the brain. (Loyez stain: myelin stained block). × 60.

perivascular demyelination may show mild degenerative changes and there may be a slight increase of mononuclear cells in the leptomeninges. The lesions are therefore quite different, both in character and distribution, from those of acute viral encephalitis due to the presence of any known virus in the central nervous system.

It is now generally accepted that acute disseminated encephalomyelitis represents an immunological reaction in the CNS: from its similarity to experimental allergic encephalomyelitis, it seems likely that the predisposing virus infection leads to the development of an immune response against neural tissue antigen, and that the resulting sensitised lymphocytes, and possibly free antibody, react with the neural tissue to bring about the lesions.

Acute haemorrhagic leukoencephalitis

This relatively uncommon disease may also occur as a sequel to any one of several possible viral infections but it may have its onset during apparently perfect health. It frequently has a rapid, fulminating course, death occurring within a few days. At necropsy the brain is swollen and congested and there are numerous petechial hemorrhages restricted almost entirely to the white matter, the naked-eye appearances being very similar to those observed in cerebral fat embolism.

Histological examination shows varying degrees of necrosis of the walls of venules and arterioles, perivascular haemorrhage and loss of myelin, often with emigration first of polymorphonuclears and later of mononuclear cells, cerebral oedema and an inflammatory exudate in the leptomeninges. The grey matter is relatively spared. The disease, therefore, has several features in common with acute disseminated encephalomyelitis but although some consider that acute haemorrhagic leukoencephalitis is simply a particularly acute form of this disease, the different distribution of the focal lesions suggests that the pathogenesis may not be the same.

Multiple or disseminated sclerosis

This disease is characterised by the presence of patches (usually referred to as *plaques*) of de-

myelination and gliosis in the central nervous system. It occurs most frequently in early adult life, though cases are encountered at an earlier and later period. The disease characteristically follows an episodic course, periods of partial remission alternating with acute exacerbations, but in the later stages it tends to become relentlessly progressive. Less frequently it is of steadily progressive character from its onset. A common early symptom is an acute unilateral optic neuritis which progresses to some degree of optic atrophy.

Structural changes. The abnormal plaques are scattered in an irregular manner throughout the

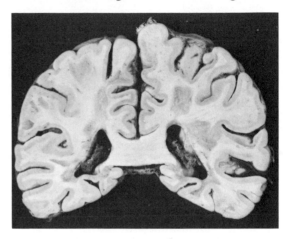

Fig. 20.50 Multiple sclerosis. There are several well-defined large grey plaques of demyelination in each cerebral hemisphere.

spinal cord and brain. The plaques are typically grey and rather translucent in appearance, in marked contrast to the normal white matter from which they are usually sharply demarcated (Fig. 20.50). They vary in consistency, being sometimes firmer and sometimes less firm than the normal tissue. As there is little or no contraction, the affected parts are not distorted. Smaller lesions are usually spherical or oval but larger plaques often have an irregular shape which may result either from the confluence of several small plaques or from extension of a previously smaller lesion. Recent lesions are often yellowish and rather soft, and in the more acute cases, may constitute a large proportion of the lesions. Plaques vary greatly in size and number in individual cases. They are usually most easily seen in the white matter of the cerebral hemispheres, particularly at the angles of the lateral ventricles and at the junction of the cortex with the white matter; but they may be seen also within the cortex and central grey matter. They are also common in the brain stem, particularly around the aqueduct and adjacent to the fourth ventricle (Fig. 20.51), and in the spinal cord. If there is a history of retrobulbar neuritis, a plaque can usually be found in the optic nerve and they have been observed also in other cranial and spinal nerve roots.

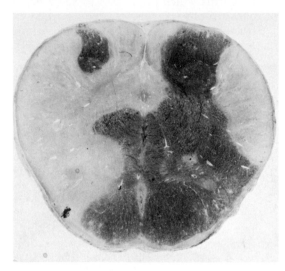

Fig. 20.51 Multiple sclerosis. Section through the lower part of the medulla. The demyelinated plaques appear pale. (Weigert–Pal method.)

In sections stained by the Weigert–Pal method, a most striking feature is the complete disappearance of myelin from the affected areas and the sharp line of demarcation from the adjacent healthy tissue (Fig. 20.51). In older plaques there is a great increase in glial fibres and the vessel walls are thickened, but they often appear less cellular than the surrounding tissue owing to loss of oligodendrocytes. In contrast, recent plaques contain a great excess of cells; some are lipid-containing macrophages, others are perivascular lymphocytes and plasma cells. At this stage demyelination may be less sharply demarcated than in older lesions. Although the myelin sheaths are so extensively destroyed, many of the axis cylinders persist and continue to transmit impulses for a long period. Eventually, however, there may be much destruction of axis cylinders, especially in the spinal cord, with consequent Wallerian

degeneration in the distal part of the axon. Nerve cells, in general, show little abnormality even when included in a plaque.

The CSF in multiple sclerosis may at times contain a slight excess of lymphocytes, and there may also be an increase of protein; but these changes are often absent. Lange's colloidal gold test gives a *'paretic' reaction* in about one-third of cases, rather more give atypical curves. The level of IgG in the CSF is usually raised, particularly when the disease is active.

Aetiology. The aetiology of multiple sclerosis is not known but there is evidence suggestive of a transmissible agent or an auto-immune process, or both. Epidemiological surveys point to some environmental factor acquired in the early years of life. Thus there are high incidence areas in the higher latitudes of the Northern and Southern Hemispheres, and low incidence areas in lower latitudes. Yet people who migrate from one area to another after about the age of 14 years retain the incidence of their country of origin. Evidence supporting an auto-immune process includes the similarity between the acute stages of multiple sclerosis and experimental allergic encephalomyelitis but plaques of demyelination are not normally produced in the latter nor is it spontaneously an episodic disease. Nevertheless antibodies that cause demyelination *in vitro* have been found in both experimental allergic encephalomyelitis and in multiple sclerosis. The finding of gamma globulin in multiple sclerosis plaques has also been considered as evidence supporting an immune aetiology. Most patients with multiple sclerosis have unusually high levels of measles antibodies in their serum and CSF and this is also in keeping with their having some immunological peculiarity.

There has always been much speculation about the aetiology of multiple sclerosis but now that it is well recognised that viruses can persist within cells for many years, the possibility exists that the disease is brought about by a cell-mediated immune response. If this is so, the 'incubation period' must be long, since the onset of the disease is commonest between the ages of 20 and 40.

Neuromyelitis optica is the name given to a disease of adults characterised by rapid loss of vision and the occurrence of extensive demyelinating lesions in the optic nerves, cerebral white matter and especially in the spinal cord. The disease is commonly preceded by fever, it runs a more acute course than that of multiple sclerosis and the lesions are more severely destructive, but a proportion of cases recover.

Diffuse cerebral sclerosis

This is rather a complex group of diseases which have in common *diffuse demyelination* and *gliosis* in the white matter of the cerebral hemispheres and sometimes also in the cerebellum, the brain stem and the spinal cord. Most are hereditarily determined and occur in early life when they are referred to as the **leukodystrophies**: indeed if it were not for apparently non-familial cases with an onset in adult life and showing some changes of inflammatory type in addition to demyelination, all types of diffuse cerebral sclerosis would probably be classed as leukodystrophies. The latter have also been referred to as *dysmyelinating diseases* on the basis that the myelin is biochemically abnormal before it degenerates.

Sudanophilic cerebral sclerosis

In this type of diffuse sclerosis, myelin breakdown is similar to that which occurs in any disease process associated with the destruction of myelin, i.e. the myelin breaks down into simple lipids, mainly cholesterol esters and neutral fat, which stain with ordinary fat stains, e.g. the Sudan dyes.

Sudanophilic cerebral sclerosis is commoner than the other types of diffuse sclerosis and it occurs both in childhood, when it may be familial (i.e. a leukodystrophy), and in adult life as a sporadic disease. It is a progressive disease, characterised by mental deterioration, blindness and spastic paralysis. In subacute cases, death occurs within a few months, but more frequently the patient survives for one or two years. The brain exhibits widespread degeneration of the white matter notably in the occipital lobes (hence the common occurrence of visual impairment early in the disease), but any part of the cerebral hemispheres, cerebellum or brain stem may be affected. Typically, the subcortical arcuate fibres are spared and stand out as a conspicuous white band in the affected areas. In Weigert–Pal preparations, the demyelination is seen to be less sharply demarcated than in disseminated sclerosis and shades off marginally into normally stained white matter. In the affected areas microglial cells stuffed with sudanophilic lipid are abundant while the degree of fibrous gliosis varies with the duration of the disease. Loss of axis cylinders is usually severe but, apart from occasional neurons showing central chromatolysis, the grey matter is normal.

There is an increasing awareness of the association of adrenal atrophy with this type of diffuse sclerosis in males. Obvious signs of adrenal failure may precede the onset of the neurological illness, may coincide with it, or may remain subclinical. The disease is known as **adrenoleukodystrophy** and the single most reliable test to establish the diagnosis is adrenal biopsy since the characteristic feature is the presence of ballooned vacuolated cortical cells which contain linear lamellar bodies with distinctive ultrastructural features. Similar ultrastructural cytoplasmic inclusions occur in the brain. It has been suggested that the overwhelming majority of males with sudanophilic cerebral sclerosis are in fact instances of adrenoleukodystrophy, and that cases occurring in males without adrenal atrophy and in females may represent a variant of multiple sclerosis. The term *Schilder's disease* has been used in the past for diffuse sclerosis of sudanophilic type. If the term has to be retained, it should probably now be restricted to cases of adrenoleukodystrophy.

Metachromatic leukodystrophy

In contrast to the commoner sudanophilic type, myelin is not broken down into neutral fat and cholesterol esters but into metachromatic material containing sulphatides which stains brown when stained by cresyl violet or thionine in an acid solution.

Metachromatic leukodystrophy is a rare familial disease occurring mainly in children between 2 and 5 years old, but not confined to this age group. It is progressive and tends to run a course of one or two years. The brain feels unusually firm and the white matter may be somewhat greyer and more translucent than normal: the subcortical arcuate fibres are usually not spared.

Histological examination demonstrates widespread loss of myelin in the white matter, the fibre systems which mature last often being the most severely affected. The demyelinated areas contain large quantities of intracellular and extracellular metachromatic material which is also PAS positive. The metachromatic material can only be demonstrated satisfactorily in frozen sections since much of it dissolves in the course of normal histological processing. Sudanophilic lipid is present only in small amounts in perivascular phagocytes. Metachromatic material is not restricted to white matter since it may also be demonstrable in neurons and peripheral nerves. It may also be present in the urine and many somatic tissues, e.g. liver, pancreas, adrenal and kidney.

The enzyme defect in metachromatic leukodystrophy is an insufficiency of arylsulphatase A. A useful diagnostic test is the demonstration of this deficiency in circulating leukocytes.

A rarer type of leukodystrophy is *Krabbe's disease*.

Table 20.1 The Cerebrospinal Fluid in health and

	Normal	Acute pyogenic meningitis	Tuberculous meningitis	Acute virus infection with meningo-encephalitis
Pressure (horizontal posture)	60–150 mmH$_2$O	Increased—probably to 200 mm or more	Increased to as much as 300 mm or more	Increased sometimes to 250 mm
Appearance	Clear and colourless	Turbid or frankly purulent	Clear or slightly opalescent. A fine fibrin coagulum may form	Clear or slightly opalescent
Cell content per μl	0–4 leukocytes (all mononuclears)	Markedly raised 500–5000 polymorphs at first, mononuclears later	Increased up to 500 lymphocytes; some polymorphs at first	Increased 50–500 lymphocytes, some polymorphs at first
Protein g/litre	0·2–0·45	0·5–2·0 average; up to 10 g	0·5–3·0 usually; if spinal block present, may rise to over 10 g	0·5–2·0; 0·5–1·0 in paralytic polio
Sugar (mg/100 ml mmol/litre)	50–80 (2·8–4·4)	Absent or greatly reduced	Decreased to 20–30 (1–1·5)	Normal
Bacteriology	Sterile	Causative organisms present; type confirmed by culture	Tubercle bacilli in fibrin coagulum or in deposit. Positive cultures usually obtained	Sterile
Lange's colloidal gold test	Normal, i.e. 0000000000	May be normal or meningitic, i.e. 0012344320	Normal or meningitic	Normal or meningitic. Weak paretic or luetic in poliomyelitis
Wassermann Reaction	Negative	Negative	Negative	Negative

There is a deficiency of the enzyme galactocerebroside B-galactosidase. The striking histological feature is the presence of large multinucleated histiocytes known as globoid cells.

Neuronal storage diseases

In this group of diseases there is abnormal accumulation of certain metabolites within neurons. As in storage disorders mainly affecting other systems in the body (pp. 19–23), the neuronal storage diseases are genetically determined, they usually manifest themselves within the first 10 years of life and often in infancy, they are due to a deficiency in one or more lysosomal enzymes which usually results in the block of one or more catabolic pathways, and the metabolite which cannot be further degradated accumulates in the neuronal cytoplasm. Thus the abnormal neuron has a ballooned appearance, the storage material can be demonstrated histochemically, and electron microscopy demonstrates abnormal cytosomes, viz. lysosomes containing non-metabolisable residues. Some of these cytosomes have highly distinctive morphological features diagnostic of a specific storage disorder.

There is a certain similarity in the clinical and pathological features of all neuronal storage disorders although there may be features specific to individual diseases. In the early stages, the storage leads to neuronal dysfunction. Ultimately the cell dies and disappears and there is atrophy of the brain and gliosis in grey and white matter. Thus there is retardation or progressive deterioration of mental and motor functions, apathy, lassitude, spastic or flaccid paralysis, fits, often visual disturbances and ultimately coma and death.

The terminology of these diseases has had to be greatly modified in the last decade. In the past, various sub-divisions were based on certain clinical and pathological similarities, e.g. the amaurotic family idiocies but, as a result of the information now available about the intrinsic metabolic defects, some of these groupings cannot now be sustained. There are about 20 known storage diseases which involve neurons: in many the neuronal disorder is the most prominent feature of the disease but in others there is also involvement of other tissues.

One of the commonest neuronal storage disorders is the disease long known as **Tay–Sachs disease**, the classical infantile type of amaurotic family idiocy. A particularly characteristic sign of this disease, but not restricted to it, is the cherry red spot at the macula consequent on involvement of the retina in the disease process. Since the abnormal metabolite is ganglioside GM$_2$, this condition is now best referred in certain diseases as obtained by lumbar puncture

General paralysis of the insane	Tabes dorsalis	Multiple sclerosis	Subarachnoid haemorrhage	Complete spinal block (Froin's syndrome)
Normal	Normal	Normal	Raised often to 300 mm or more	Low: CSF may have to be actively withdrawn
Normal	Normal	Normal	Frankly bloodstained: on centrifugation, supernatant is yellow	Yellow, opalescent and tends to clot
Up to 100 (lymphocytes)	Up to 50–100 (lymphocytes)	Slight increase to 20–100 (lymphocytes)	Many red cells	Slight increase of mononuclear cells
0·5–1·0	0·3–0·6	0·3–0·6	Normal in the early stages. Slight rise later	More than 5
Normal	Normal	Normal	Normal	Normal
Sterile	Sterile	Sterile	Sterile	Sterile
Paretic, i.e. 5544321000	Luetic, i.e. 123321000	Paretic, rarely luetic or may be normal	Normal	Meningitic
Positive	Positive in 80% of cases	Negative	Negative	Negative

to as GM_2 gangliosidosis. The missing enzyme is hexosaminidase A and the abnormal cytosomes with highly distinctive ultrastructural features are known as membranous cytoplasmic bodies. There are also other types of gangliosidosis with similarities to and differences from GM_2 gangliosidosis.

Other lysosomal storage disorders involving the nervous system include infantile Gaucher's disease (deficiency of B glucosidase), Niemann–Pick's disease (deficiency of sphingomyelinase), type II glycogenosis (Pompe's disease, deficiency of acid maltase), the mucopolysaccharidoses and certain syndromes previously classified as types of amaurotic family idiocy (e.g. Batten's disease) which do not appear to be biochemically related to GM_2 gangliosidosis.

Other inborn errors of metabolism involving the nervous system

Phenylketonuria and galactosaemia are the most important of these because the ill effects can be prevented or mitigated by exclusion of the harmful substances from the diet.

In **phenylketonuria**, inherited as an autosomal recessive, absence of the active enzyme phenylalanine hydroxylase leads to accumulation of phenylalanine in the blood and excretion of phenylpyruvic acid in the urine. Epileptiform seizures, severe mental deficiency and some failure of myelination are the principal findings.

In **galactosaemia** there is hepato-splenomegaly, cataract and mental retardation associated with inability to metabolise galactose owing to absence of the enzyme galactose-1-phosphate uridyl transferase; consequently galactose-1-phosphate accumulates in toxic amounts and is excreted in the urine.

Despite the severe mental derangement no specific pathological abnormality has been recognised in the brain in these serious disorders.

The dementias

Schizophrenia and the involutional psychoses show no constant pathological changes and in consequence are described as functional disorders. Other cases of dementia are secondary to certain organic brain diseases such as general paralysis of the insane, deeply-seated slowly-growing tumours, diffuse cerebral sclerosis and occlusive vascular disease. Of these the last, *arteriopathic dementia*, is the commonest and in it the brain is small and the ventricles large, atheroma of the large and small arteries is widespread and severe, and numerous small infarcts can often be found.

There remains a group of primary organic dementias, usually relentlessly if slowly progressive, in which there are fairly specific pathological changes in the brain. Common to all is cortical atrophy, the gyri becoming rounder and firmer than normal and the sulci widened, and secondary hydrocephalus.

Alzheimer's disease and senile dementia. These two types of dementia show the same pathological features but Alzheimer's disease is the term used when the onset is pre-senile, i.e. before the age of 60. The pathological findings in both types resemble a gross exaggeration of those of the normal ageing processes in the brain. Death usually occurs a few years after the onset of the disease. Cortical atrophy is widespread but more conspicuous at the frontal and temporal poles. Histological examination reveals a generalised loss of neurons, reactive gliosis and vast numbers of senile (Alzheimer) plaques in the cortical grey matter. The plaques are composed of masses of small argyrophilic granules and filaments often with a core of amyloid material. In addition, there are tangles of coarse neurofibrils (Alzheimer's neurofibrillary change) in many of the larger nerve cells of the cerebral cortex.

Pick's disease is classed as a pre-senile dementia. Cortical atrophy from loss of neurons is particularly intense in the frontal and temporal lobes, giving the brain a distinctive naked-eye appearance. The consequent degeneration of axis cylinders probably accounts for the loss of myelin, reactive gliosis and considerable shrinkage of the underlying white matter. Some of the surviving neurons are greatly swollen by a globular mass of intracellular argyrophilic material.

Huntington's chorea. This disease of middle adult life is characterised by coarse choreiform movements, progressive mental deterioration and, in some cases, striatal rigidity. It is believed to be inherited by an autosomal dominant gene. In addition to widespread cortical atrophy, there is selective atrophy and loss of nerve cells in the caudate nucleus and the putamen.

II The Spinal Cord

The tissue of the spinal cord is similar to that of the brain but the relative frequencies of various lesions are very different. Specific diseases of the spinal cord are described later but so-called *transverse lesions* and the consequent ascending and descending Wallerian degeneration within the cord will be dealt with first.

Transverse Lesions

These occur when the full thickness of the cord is involved by intrinsic or extrinsic lesions. The effects may be produced slowly by pressure on the cord by extrinsic tumours in the extradural space, e.g. metastatic carcinoma (Fig. 20.52) or lymphoid neoplasm, or in the subdural space, e.g. meningioma (Fig. 20.85, p. 729) or Schwannoma. Intrinsic tumours, e.g. astrocytoma and ependymoma, are rarer causes. Tuberculosis of the vertebral bodies although uncommon in Britain is still frequently encountered in various parts of the world. It leads to angular curvature of the spine and tuberculous granuloma, both of which can cause pressure on the cord; this may be so severe that infarction of the cord may occur at this level. Acute transverse lesions may be due to *trauma*, usually a fracture-dislocation of the vertebrae, *infarction* when the circulation through the anterior spinal artery is impeded, *haemorrhage*, usually from a vascular malformation, *acute myelitis* (see below) or acute *demyelination* as in neuromyelitis optica (p. 706).

An inevitable consequence of a total or partial transverse lesion of the cord, besides the local damage, is the development of **ascending and descending Wallerian degeneration** in the respective tracts of the spinal cord. Degenera-

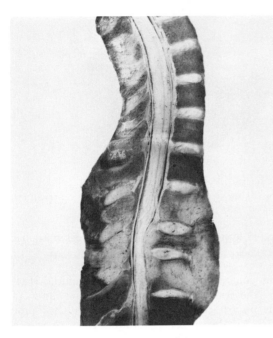

Fig. 20.52 Sagittal section of the vertebral column in lower cervical–upper dorsal region, showing metastatic tumour pressing on the cord.

tion occurs in those fibres that are separated from their cell bodies by the lesion and, when recent, is best demonstrated by the Marchi technique. The degenerating fibres appear black from about a week after onset (Fig. 20.53). The method is applicable until the degenerated myelin has disappeared—that is, for several months. In the case of long-standing lesions of the spinal cord, Weigert's method or one of its

modifications, which stain the normal myelin black, should be used; accordingly, when the degenerated myelin has become absorbed, the affected tract appears as a pale area (Fig. 20.55).

Ascending degenerations

If we take as an example a comparatively recent lesion at the level of the lower dorsal region, the following ascending degenerations are found in a section taken a few segments above the lesion (Fig. 20.53). There is degeneration in the posterior columns (with the exception of a small area dorsal to the grey commissure where there are chiefly commissural fibres) and in the spino-thalamic and spino-cerebellar tracts. At a higher level, however, in the cervical region, the degeneration in the posterior columns is practically confined to the gracile tracts (Fig. 20.54) as the cuneate tract is composed mainly of ascending fibres that have joined the cord above the level of the lesion. Degeneration of the affected axons extends up to the nucleus cuneatus and nucleus gracilis in the medulla. Ascending degeneration in the posterior spino-cerebellar tract extends up to the inferior cerebellar peduncle and into the cerebellum, and in the anterior spino-cerebellar tract to the middle lobe of the cerebellum. In old lesions, loss of myelin (Figs. 20.55 and 20.56) and reactive gliosis are conspicuous only in the posterior columns since the inflow of normal myelinated fibres at higher levels masks the relatively slight

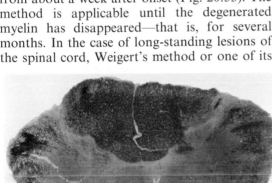

Fig. 20.53 Immediately above the lesion. The whole of the posterior columns and antero-lateral ascending tracts are degenerating.

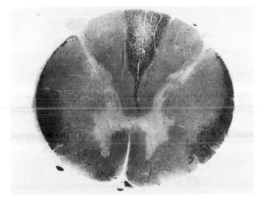

Fig. 20.54 Cervical region. There are fewer degenerating fibres because of the inflow of fibres above the level of the lesion.

Figures 20.53 and 20.54 Ascending degeneration above a recent transverse lesion in the lower dorsal region, stained by Marchi's method: the degenerating fibres appear black.

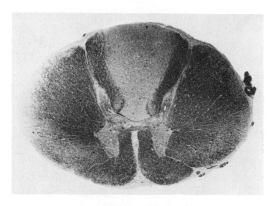

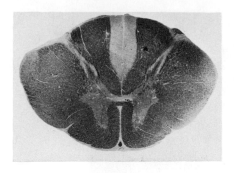

Fig. 20.56   Cervical region. Degeneration appears to be confined to the gracile tract.

Fig. 20.55   A short distance above the lesion.

Figures 20.55 and 20.56   Ascending degeneration above an old transverse lesion in the dorsal region, stained by the Weigert–Pal method. The degenerated fibres appear pale.

loss of myelin in the spino-cerebellar and spino-thalamic tracts.

Descending degenerations

These are encountered in two chief conditions, (*a*) when there is a transverse lesion in the cord, and (*b*) when the lesion is at a higher level. In a section taken from below a recent *transverse lesion* of the cord the most marked degeneration is in the crossed (lateral) and uncrossed (anterior) pyramidal tracts unless the lesion is low in the cord where the uncrossed tract is no longer present.

The commonest example due to a *lesion at a higher level* is destruction of the motor fibres in the internal capsule. In such a case there is degeneration of the crossed pyramidal tract on the opposite side (Fig. 20.57) and of the uncrossed pyramidal tract on the same side. As the direct pyramidal tract does not usually extend lower than the first thoracic segment, degeneration in that site will not appear in sections below this level (Fig. 20.58).

When there is compression of the spinal cord by a gross lesion so as to block the subarachnoid space the CSF below the block becomes altered. A great increase of protein occurs and the fluid coagulates rapidly after withdrawal; it is often yellow (xanthochromia). The cells may or may not be increased; any increase is on the part of the mononuclears. These changes are grouped under the term 'Froins' syndrome' (see Table 20.1, pp. 708–9).

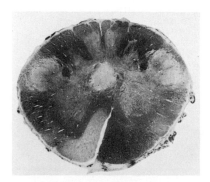

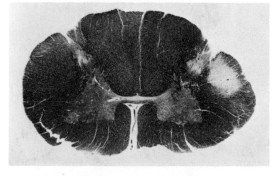

Fig. 20.57   Medulla. The pyramid on one side is degenerated.

Fig. 20.58   Thoracic region. The crossed pyramidal tract on one side is degenerated.

Figures 20.57 and 20.58   Descending degeneration. Transverse sections through medulla and spinal cord showing descending degeneration from an old lesion of one internal capsule. Stained by Weigert–Pal method: degenerated fibres appear pale.

Prolapsed intervertebral disc

A very common cause of compression of the cord or of nerve roots is a prolapsed intervertebral disc. The intervertebral disc consists of a central nodule of semifluid matrix, the nucleus pulposus, surrounded by a circle of fibrous tissue and fibrocartilage, the annulus fibrosus. The posterior segment of the annulus is thinner and less firmly attached to bone and, following unusual stress, part of the matrix of the nucleus pulposus may herniate through it (Fig. 20.59). The lesion may occur, however, after slight

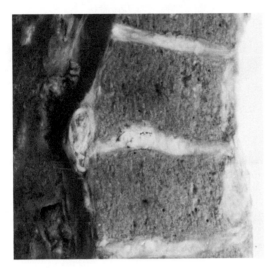

Fig. 20.59 Sagittal section of vertebral column, showing ruptured disc protruding beneath the posterior longitudinal ligament.

injury and the symptoms produced depend on the direction taken by the material extruded from the nucleus pulposus. The herniated material usually tracks postero-laterally around the expansion of the posterior longitudinal ligament, appearing at one side and compressing spinal nerve roots in the intervertebral foramen. Clinically, disc protrusion in the lumbar spine is most common and L5 S1, L4 L5 and L3–L4 disc spaces are affected in that order of frequency, the cervical spine at the C5–6 and C6–7 level being less often involved. If the protrusion is slight, localised pain is produced by irritation of the posterior longitudinal ligament; if larger, there may be root pain due to pressure on nerves leaving the spinal canal giving rise to the clinical signs and symptoms of sciatica. A single posterior disc protrusion may cause compression of the cord or obstruction of the anterior spinal artery, but this is only rarely severe enough to give rise to a transverse lesion. When there are several protrusions, as in cervical spondylosis, the resulting compression may impair the circulation and variable degrees of ischaemia of the spinal cord may result. There may be cavitation of the cord and loss of nerve cells in the severely affected areas, the condition being known as *spondylotic myelopathy*. Even in cervical spondylosis, however, nerve root compression is commoner than myelopathy.

Acute myelitis

This uncommon condition, by definition an acute inflammation of the cord, is more a clinical syndrome than a precise pathological entity. It is usually of acute or subacute onset and is characterised by flaccid paralysis and sensory loss, either of which may be total or partial, below the level of the lesion. A considerable part of the cord may be affected—*diffuse myelitis*; or the lesion may be confined to one or two segments—*transverse myelitis*. The terms, however, tend to be used for any pathological process other than external pressure or tumour which causes intrinsic damage to the grey and white matter of the cord. There are various causes.

Aetiology. Acute demyelination (p. 703), and infarction of the cord due to failure of circulation through the anterior spinal artery, are probably the commonest causes. In some cases of infarction of the lumbo-sacral cord in adults, there are numerous hyalinised vessels within the cord: this condition is known as *subacute necrotic myelitis*. Other causes of transverse myelitis are acute disseminated encephalomyelitis (p. 704), spontaneous haematomyelia (probably from a vascular malformation) and, more rarely, infections.

Structural changes. The appearances of the cord vary with the underlying pathological process. In general, however, the affected part of the cord is swollen and soft, the normal architectural markings are blurred and there may be foci of haemorrhage.

If the patient survives the acute stage, there may be considerable restoration of function. More often the affected part of the cord becomes shrunken, cystic and gliosed, there is ascending and descending degeneration, and the patient is permanently paraplegic.

Lesions of the motor neuron

The main acute lower motor neuron disease, *acute anterior poliomyelitis*, has already been considered (p. 697). Chronic progressive degenerative disease of the motor neurons is usually referred to as motor neuron disease.

Motor neuron disease

Lower and upper neurons are usually involved together, as in most cases there is a combination of atrophic and spastic conditions and the term *amyotrophic lateral sclerosis* is applied. In a comparatively small group the changes are chiefly, but not entirely, in the motor cells of the anterior horns or the cranial nerve nuclei; the conditions known as *progressive muscular atrophy* or *progressive bulbar palsy* then result. These three variants of *motor neuron disease* occur in middle and late adult life, much more frequently in men than in women, and their aetiology remains unknown.

Progressive muscular atrophy. In cases where atrophic changes are the outstanding feature, the lesion is mainly a progressive degeneration of the neurons in the anterior horns. It usually starts in the cervical enlargement in the neurons related to the small muscles of the hand. The affected muscles show fibrillary twitchings and, gradually, atrophy with corresponding weakness follows. The thenar and hypothenar eminences become markedly wasted, the interossei also become affected, and the hand assumes a characteristic claw-like form. Involvement then extends to the muscles of the arm and shoulder girdle; terminally the symptoms of bulbar paralysis may appear. In one type of the disease the wasting appears first in the muscles of the shoulder girdle. In the anterior horns corresponding to the wasting, the process is a progressive atrophy of the neurons. Some of them have disappeared, while many of those remaining show stages of atrophy. Gliosis occurs but is usually not marked. The anterior spinal roots become wasted and appear grey and thin to the naked eye, while in the related muscles the atrophy corresponds to the loss of the neurons and is patchy in distribution (Fig. 22.70, p. 873).

Amyotrophic lateral sclerosis. In the cases classified as progressive muscular atrophy, there is usually some loss of myelinated fibres entering the anterior horns, and in the crossed pyramidal tracts; this indicates some involvement of the axons of the upper motor neurons. In cases, however, where spasticity is prominent and occurs early there is much more extensive involvement of the upper motor neurons and this is designated amyotrophic lateral sclerosis. In addition to the atrophic changes in the anterior horns, there is widespread sclerosis and loss of myelin in the lateral and anterior white columns, most marked in, but not confined to, the pyramidal tracts (Fig. 20.60).

The changes in the pyramidal fibres, as a rule, start first and are most marked at their lower extremities, the process then extending upwards. Atrophic changes, corresponding to those in the anterior horns, occur in the motor cells of the cerebral cortex and here also many disappear. The sclerosis of the pyramidal tracts may extend to a lower level in the cord than that at which the anterior horns are implicated.

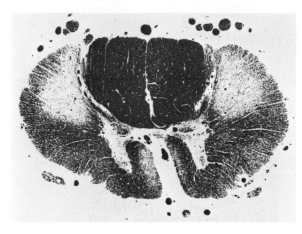

Fig. 20.60 Amyotrophic lateral sclerosis. Section of the spinal cord, showing degeneration in the lateral and anterior columns and preservation of the posterior columns. There is selectively severe involvement of the crossed pyramidal tracts. (Weigert–Pal method.)

Progressive bulbar paralysis. This variant of motor neuron disease may appear first, or may follow spinal involvement. It is characterised by progressive paralysis and wasting of the muscles of the tongue, lips, jaws, larynx and pharynx; death often occurs by involvement of the respiratory centre, or by foreign matter entering the lungs through the paralysed larynx. The lesions are in the medulla and are essentially of the same nature as those in the cord. They are usually most marked in the hypoglossal and spinal accessory nuclei, but occur also in the nuclei of the vagus and seventh nerves, and in the nucleus of the motor part of the fifth. Along with the changes in the brain stem there is a varying involvement of the nerve cells in the anterior horns and in the pyramidal fibres.

No sharply dividing line can be drawn between these variants of motor neuron disease. They merely emphasise that in any one case, the early stages of the disease may have a different distribution. In the terminal stages there is often widespread involvement of motor neurons in the brain stem and in the spinal cord, and involvement of the lateral and ventral white columns in the spinal cord.

Friedreich's ataxia. This disease, in which there is atrophy in both motor and sensory tracts, often af-

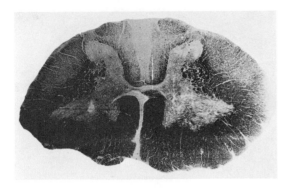

Fig. 20.61 Section of cord in Friedreich's ataxia, showing degeneration in posterior and lateral columns. (Weigert–Pal method.)

fects more than one member of a family, hence it is sometimes called **familial ataxia**; rarely it occurs in successive generations. Isolated cases of the disease are also encountered. It usually begins in the years before adolescence and the chief symptoms are ataxia with muscular weakness. Lateral curvature of the spine and talipes equinus are often present, and nystagmus and disturbances of speech also are common. In such cases, the spinal cord is found to be relatively thin and there is degeneration in the posterior and lateral columns (Fig. 20.61). The posterior roots also show degeneration, especially the fibres within the cord, and involvement of the roots and posterior columns may be present in the cervical region as well as lower down; the cells in the posterior root ganglia, however, are little altered. In the lateral columns the pyramidal fibres are degenerate, the degeneration being most marked below and diminishing in an upward direction. The posterior spino-cerebellar tracts are similarly affected, and the cells of the thoracic nucleus show degenerative changes. There may be some degeneration also in the anterior spino-cerebellar and spino-thalamic tracts. The nature of the disease is obscure. Family studies have shown that Friedreich's ataxia and *Marie's hereditary cerebellar ataxia* are probably varieties of an essentially similar disorder; the two conditions sometimes overlap and intermediate forms occur, but each affected family presents its own variant. Friedreich's ataxia is frequently associated with a chronic progressive myocarditis, in which focal coagulative necrosis of the muscle fibres is followed by replacement fibrosis.

Other lesions of the spinal cord

Subacute combined degeneration

This type of degeneration formerly occurred in a high proportion of cases of inadequately treated pernicious anaemia, but since highly effective purified preparations of cyanocobalamin have been available this complication is now much less common. Similar lesions have been found much more rarely in other chronic diseases, such as malabsorption syndromes, leukaemia, diabetes and carcinoma. Subacute combined degeneration may develop in the 'pre-anaemic stage' of pernicious anaemia, associated with chronic gastritis and megaloblastic erythropoiesis. The administration of vitamin B_{12} in adequate doses is completely effective in preventing the development of neural lesions in cases of pernicious anaemia.

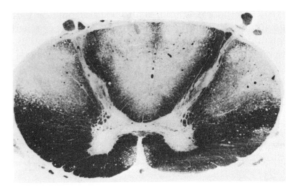

Fig. 20.62 Subacute combined degeneration, showing conspicuous degeneration in both lateral and posterior columns. (Weigert–Pal method.)

The anatomical changes consist of degeneration in the dorsal and lateral columns of the spinal cord (Fig. 20.62). The change appears to start, and to be most severe and extensive, in the lower thoracic region and then extends upwards and downwards. In the involved segments the degenerate myelin is removed by phagocytes which migrate to the perivascular sheaths. In untreated cases there is practically no glial proliferation and the degenerated areas present an open spongy appearance. With long survival on B_{12} treatment, however, some gliosis eventually occurs. The degeneration in the motor tracts may ascend through the internal capsule and degenerative changes may be seen in the Betz cells of the cortex. There is no evidence that anaemia in itself produces the lesions mentioned; in fact, it may be preceded by them. The symptoms depend on the tracts involved. If they are mainly the posterior columns, ataxic symptoms are prominent, while involvement of the lateral columns leads to spastic symptoms. In view of its progressive, disabling nature, and the arresting effects of B_{12} therapy, early diagnosis is of the utmost importance.

Syringomyelia

This term is applied to a space or spaces within the cord, containing fluid and enclosed by neuroglia. There is considerable controversy at the present time over the nature and pathogenesis of syringomyelia. Teaching in the past was that syringomyelia had to be distinguished from hydromyelia (dilatation of the central canal of the spinal cord), and that syringomyelic cavities first appear dorsal to the central canal. It may be that this type of syringomyelia does exist, but there is an increasing body of opinion that syringomyelia is caused by CSF being propelled through a valve-like opening between the caudal extremity of the fourth ventricle and the central canal, i.e. the cavity is in fact a greatly distended central canal. Individuals with this type of syringomyelia also tend to have a mild developmental abnormality at the cranio-cervical junction, the cerebellar tonsils protruding further through the foramen magnum than usual. Whatever its pathogenesis, however, the structural abnormalities in the cord are fairly stereotyped. The cavity usually extends through several

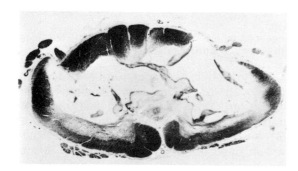

Fig. 20.63 Syringomyelia: upper part of cervical enlargement. (Weigert–Pal method.)

segments of the cervical cord (Figs. 20.63 and 20.64) and, as it enlarges, the cord becomes swollen and feels somewhat soft. On microscopic examination the tissue lining the cavity is composed of enlarged astrocytes and coarse astrocytic fibrils which are rarefied in the tissue around the central cavity. Occasionally syringomyelia occurs in association with tumours affecting the spinal cord.

Effects. These are due principally to destruction of the structures in the cord by the enlarging cavity but pressure may also play a part. The first fibres to be affected are the decussating sensory fibres conveying the sensations of heat and pain: the resulting defect,

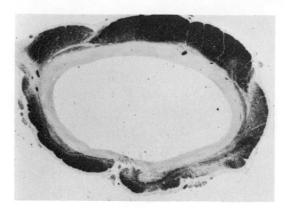

Fig. 20.64 Syringomyelia: junction between cervical and thoracic portion. (Weigert–Pal method.)

known as dissociated anaesthesia, is a selective insensibility to heat and pain in the region corresponding to the involved segments of the spinal cord. Trophic disturbances affect the joints, bone and skin. A neuropathic arthritis occurs, closely similar to that in tabes (p. 861), but, as syringomyelia is usually in the cervical region, it is the joints of the upper limbs which are chiefly involved. The trophic lesions of the skin are various and include vesicles, ulceration and painless whitlows. As the cavity enlarges it ultimately affects the lateral white columns leading to spastic paraplegia, the ventral grey horns leading to neurogenic atrophy of muscles, and the posterior white columns leading to even greater disturbances of sensation.

Dietary-induced disorders

In human nutritional disease, a pure deficiency of only one factor is very rarely encountered: variation in the clinical picture can then be explained by the presence of various deficiencies, one or more of which may be responsible for the most conspicuous abnormalities. **Pellagra**, for example, appears to be caused by deficiency of the B_2 complex but chiefly of nicotinic acid. Cutaneous lesions, glossitis, diarrhoea and mental changes make up the classical clinical picture, some cases show also a peripheral neuropathy very similar to that observed in beri-beri, and others exhibit a form of postero-lateral degeneration of the spinal cord which is not identical with that produced by lack of B_{12}. In cases of chronic **ergotism** somewhat similar changes are observed in the spinal cord, and these are apparently the result of toxins produced by the fungus in rye. The term **lathyrism** is applied to a disease occurring especially in India among people whose diet consists mainly of pulse. It occurs sometimes in epidemics, chiefly in males in times of famine. The chief symptoms are spasticity affecting the extensor and adductor muscles of the lower limbs, but sensory symptoms also are present.

Both lateral and posterior columns of the cord are affected, but the exact changes are not definitely known.

A similar condition produced by a diet of dwarf peas (*cicerism*) is attributed to a toxic action of the pea protein; this can be prevented by choline or methionine (Diaz). The production of 'hysteria' in dogs and ferrets by flour treated with nitrogen trichloride (agene) has been traced to the development of a toxic amino-acid derivative, methionine sulphoximine, from the gluten and gliadin of wheat and from the zein of maize. The significance of these observations in human pathology is not yet clear.

Acute decompression sickness (caisson disease)

This occurs when an individual is subjected to a rapid reduction in environmental pressure. It is thus a hazard for deep water divers who are brought back to atmospheric pressure without sufficiently gradual decompression, to workers in compressed air, and occasionally to aviators and others subjected to sub-atmospheric pressures.

Symptoms may come on during return to atmospheric pressure or up to more than a day afterwards. In its mildest form the disorder consists of pain in one or more large joints ('bends' or 'divers cramps'), but bone necrosis may subsequently become apparent (p. 813). In more severe cases, there are complex disturbances, including haemoconcentration and hypovolaemia, sludging of red cells, thrombocytopenia and activation of clotting and fibrinolytic mechanisms. Profound circulatory disturbance occurs and may cause death. Some of the features of decompression sickness are explicable on the basis that nitrogen, which dissolves slowly in the tissues and blood, comes out of solution and forms bubbles on reduction of the environmental pressure, and therefore of the pressure within the body. Other features are not well explained, but may be due to the surface effects of blood or cell/gas interfaces on proteins, platelets, plasma membranes, etc., i.e. an indirect effect of bubbles in the blood and tissues.

This condition is included here because in more serious cases the central nervous system, and particularly the **spinal cord**, is commonly affected. It has been suggested that, because of its high solubility in lipid (including myelin), large amounts of nitrogen under pressure dissolve in the nervous tissue, particularly the white matter, during compression and come out of solution to form bubbles there on too rapid decompression. However, the formation of bubbles in the white matter of the cord has not been demonstrated, and another theory is that, because of its venous drainage, the cord is highly susceptible to pressure fluctuations in the thorax and systemic veins. Such fluctuations occur in acute decompression sickness due to plugging of the alveolar capillaries with bubbles (and sometimes fat emboli).

Spinal cord involvement results in paraplegia, which usually passes off, although permanent disability may result. The cord lesions resemble multiple microscopic foci of infarction.

The likelihood of developing decompression sickness depends on many factors, including individual variations, and although the condition can be prevented by ensuring that decompression is gradual, calculated rates of decompression must include wide safety margins.

III The Peripheral Nerves

Although the terms *neuritis* and *polyneuritis* have often been used in the past to describe virtually all disorders of the peripheral nerves, there is only rarely a true inflammatory process within the nerve. Thus the terms *neuropathy* or *polyneuropathy* are often more appropriate. The neuropathies fall into three major categories, viz. those with (*a*) primary degeneration of the nerve cell (parenchymatous neuropathy), (*b*) dysfunction of the Schwann cell, or (*c*) alterations in the blood supply to the nerve. A true, i.e. inflammatory, neuritis also occurs and is considered after the neuropathies.

Parenchymatous neuropathies

Parenchymatous neuropathies usually affect several nerves more or less symmetrically, i.e.

they are polyneuropathies. The first manifestation of the primary abnormality in the nerve cell is degenerative change in the most distal part of the fibre as shown by dissolution of the axon and destruction of the myelin sheath. The myelin is broken up into globules, which undergo phagocytosis: these globules stain with Sudan dyes and are positive with the Marchi reaction (Fig. 20.65). This Wallerian-type

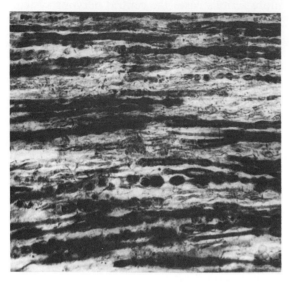

Fig. 20.65 Longitudinal section of peripheral nerve in alcoholic neuropathy showing degeneration of myelin sheaths. (Marchi method.) × about 400.

degeneration then extends proximally—the so-called 'dying-back' process. Ultimately, the most severely affected part of the nerve may become soft and develop a slightly yellow tint. In general the longest and largest fibres are affected first with the result that the earliest neurological disturbance appears in the distal parts of the limbs: the most characteristic are paraesthesiae, muscle weakness, loss of vibration sense and diminished two-point discrimination. Histological examination of the proximal part of an affected nerve may show very few abnormal fibres although they may be very numerous in its distal part. In some cases where muscle weakness is considerable, abnormalities in the nerves may be restricted to the small distal radicles actually within the muscle. As the motor fibres degenerate the muscle end-plates lose their innervation and the muscle fibres undergo neurogenic atrophy (see p. 873). If some healthy nerve fibres remain, attempted

regenerative phenomena to re-innervate motor end plates are shown by the presence of collateral and ultraterminal axonal sprouting. As the degeneration extends proximally, central chromatolysis becomes apparent in the motor neurons in the ventral horns of the spinal cord and in the neurons in the dorsal root ganglia.

The causes of parenchymatous peripheral neuropathy are many and varied. Probably the commonest is **nutritional deficiency**, beri-beri being the most important disease in this group.

Beri-beri. In this disease the essential lesion is a polyneuropathy, which results from the absence or deficiency of vitamin B_1 (thiamine), and is usually caused by a diet consisting exclusively of over-milled cereals, especially rice. The disease, which is encountered principally among rice-eating populations, occurs in two forms. In one—the 'dry' form—the peripheral nerves are chiefly affected. Degenerative changes are often prominent in the ventral horns of the spinal cord and in the dorsal root ganglia. The levels of pyruvate in the blood and CSF are raised. In the other, or 'wet' form, the disturbances are mainly cardiac; the heart becomes dilated, especially the right ventricle, there is general venous congestion, and oedema usually becomes a marked feature. Degenerative changes have been found in the vagi, in the phrenic nerves, and in the sympathetic system. It may be that the cardiac dilatation is secondary to the lesions in the nerves, but the possibility of a primary change in the cardiac muscle cannot be excluded.

Polyneuropathy can readily be produced in fowls and pigeons by feeding them with milled or polished rice. In the experimentally produced disease rapid recovery takes place when the birds are fed on diets containing the necessary vitamin. The essential pathogenesis is the failure of neural tissue to complete the oxidation of carbohydrate in the absence of co-carboxylase which normally is produced by phosphorylation of thiamine. Consequently carbohydrate metabolism ceases at the pyruvate level and this substance accumulates in blood and tissue.

Since the body's requirements of thiamine are proportional to the amount of carbohydrate metabolised, the deficiency of thiamine is exaggerated by a predominantly carbohydrate diet, and the severity of the results on neural tissue are attributable to its dependence on carbohydrate oxidation. *In vitro* the metabolic defect of homogenised affected tissue is rectified very speedily by the addition of co-carboxylase, and *in vivo* by the administration of the precursor, vitamin B_1. Substitution of undermilled for milled rice has caused beri-beri to disappear in many places but it has not been established that beri-beri in man is due *solely* to the lack of thiamine, and deficiencies in other members of the vitamin B group may well contribute. Protein deficiency is thought to be partly responsible for the 'wet' form of the disease (p. 221).

Other metabolic disturbances. Deficiency of nicotinic acid or vitamin B_{12} are other causes of peripheral neuropathy, while a deficiency of various members of the vitamin B group is probably the principal cause of the peripheral neuropathy associated with chronic alcoholism. This is brought about partly by the restricted diet and partly by deficient absorption from the alimentary canal because of associated gastro-intestinal disturbances.

Various chemicals may produce a parenchymatous polyneuropathy. Examples are *tri-orthocresyl phosphate*, dinitrobenzene and carbon disulphide or certain drugs such as isoniazid. Some metabolic or toxic derangement is probably the cause of carcinomatous neuropathy (see p. 720) while an endogenous metabolic defect is the cause of the neuropathy in acute porphyria.

In **acute porphyria**, there is usually a history of attacks of colicky abdominal pain followed by the onset of weakness in legs and arms and sometimes mental disturbances, an association of symptoms suggestive of lead poisoning. The essential lesion is a polyneuropathy, but in spite of paraesthesiae, there is little true sensory loss. In severe cases, paresis may progress rapidly to complete quadriplegia and death. Some run a relapsing course, and others recover completely, though the metabolic abnormality may persist. The condition may be precipitated by drugs, especially allyl-barbiturates, but there is often a hereditary predisposition and the metabolic pigment abnormality may be present in healthy siblings; in some families, the disorder is transmitted as a Mendelian dominant. The diagnosis depends on the recognition of the abnormal chromogen, porphobilinogen, and other pigments in the urine, which darkens on exposure to light, uroporphyrin III being the usual pigment in idiopathic cases. Since these pigments are pharmacologically inert, the actual cause of the symptoms is still obscure. In chronic congenital porphyria, on the other hand, the pigment excreted is uroporphyrin I and photosensitisation is a prominent symptom. Recently a number of cases of the idiopathic disease with neurological symptoms have been recorded in which uroporphyrin I was excreted.

Schwann cell dysfunction

In neuropathies due to dysfunction of the Schwann cell, the characteristic abnormality is *segmental demyelination*, i.e. demyelination of an axon between two nodes of Ranvier. Many segments in a single fibre may be affected and there appears to be no predilection for their distal parts. Segmental demyelination affects nerve conduction but a particularly interesting feature is that remyelination may occur. The regenerated myelin, however, usually forms a thinner sheath than normal, while the formation of extra nodes means that the internodal distance becomes reduced. This type of nerve damage contributes to the neuropathy in individuals with diabetes mellitus, and occurs particularly in post-diphtheritic paralysis and in lead poisoning.

Vascular and ischaemic changes

These account for the third major group of neuropathies. In contrast to the types already

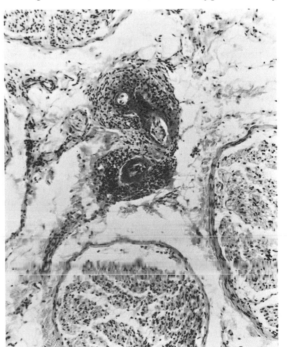

Fig. 20.66 Transverse section of the sciatic nerve in polyarteritis nodosa, showing an acute arterial lesion. × 170.

described, the cause is usually local with the result that the distribution is not symmetrical although sometimes several nerves are affected. Probably the commonest cause is pressure such as in 'crutch palsy' or 'Saturday night paralysis'. The duration of the disability depends on the degree of ischaemia produced by the pressure. Abnormalities in the vasa nervorum account for the peripheral neuropathy commonly seen in polyarteritis nodosa (Fig. 20.66): the term **mononeuritis multiplex** is often used because of the presence of multiple individual lesions in various nerves. The ischaemia may be sufficient only to produce transient dysfunction but there may be frank infarction with subsequent Wallerian degeneration of the affected fibres. In peripheral vascular disease of the lower limbs, caused usually by atheroma, there may be a pronounced reduction in the number of nerve fibres and a progressive increase of fibrous tissue in peripheral nerves.

True peripheral neuritis

The peripheral nerves may also be affected by an inflammatory process—*true peripheral neuritis*—and as the interstitial tissue in the nerve is more severely affected than the nerve fibres themselves, the term *interstitial neuritis* is often appropriate. This type of neuritis may result from the extension of any type of local tissue inflammation, e.g. wounds, abscesses, bedsores, arthritis, etc., into the nerve. The latter becomes swollen and congested and there is an interstitial inflammatory exudate. A similar though ill-understood process may be responsible for the neuritis that follows exposure to cold and wet as in **Bell's palsy** of the facial nerve.

Interstitial neuritis may also be *chronic* from the outset. A striking example of this is seen in *leprosy*, where the bacilli enter the supporting sheaths of the nerves, and give rise to interstitial proliferation of connective tissue followed by atrophy of nerve fibres, leading to paralytic and trophic disturbances. Interstitial neuritis may be produced also by syphilis, notably in the cranial nerves at the base of the brain. In any form of meningitis, the inflammatory change may spread to and affect the emerging nerves or roots. There is described also a senile form of chronic neuritis, in which there is sclerosis of the interstitial tissue with involvement of the

nerve fibres. This is the result of advanced arterial disease, which interferes with the blood supply and causes fibrous atrophy.

Acute infective polyneuritis, often known as the Landry–Guillain–Barré syndrome, is the most important type of true neuritis. Its incidence is greatest in young adults and it usually follows a mild 'non-specific' febrile illness. There is symmetrical progressive ascending paralysis usually commencing in the lower limbs and then spreading to the arms, the trunk, and the cranial nerves. Sensory disturbance is absent or only mild. Provided the patient can be tided over the acute phase, if necessary with the aid of artificial ventilation, a progressive slow recovery over a period of weeks or months is to be expected. Sudden death occurs in a proportion of cases and this is often attributable to a true myocarditis. In a fatal case the main *structural alterations* are seen in the proximal parts of spinal nerve roots where there is oedema of the nerve, infiltration by lymphocytes and plasma cells, and various degrees of damage to myelin and axons. The cerebrospinal fluid shows a highly characteristic dissociation of protein and cell count, the protein rising to as much as 8g/litre while the cell count remains normal. This disease has been likened to the experimental allergic neuritis produced in animals by injecting homogenates or extracts of nerve tissue incorporated in Freund's adjuvant. This experimental disease has much in common with experimental allergic encephalomyelitis (p. 704), and the human disease may be caused by an auto-immune reaction of the delayed hypersensitivity type. The presence of antibody reactive with neural tissue has been detected in patient's serum early in the disease, but it did not react specifically with peripheral nerve.

Pathological changes in the nervous system in association with malignant tumours

The nervous system may be implicated by malignant tumours arising elsewhere by direct or metastatic invasion of the brain, cord and peripheral nerves, or by compression of the cord by extradural deposits. Abnormalities may also occur in the nervous system without its being directly implicated by metastatic tumour. The commonest of these derangements is *peripheral neuropathy* which may be predominantly motor or sensory, or of mixed type. The most conspicuous histological abnormalities in the cases with sensory symptoms are loss of neurons in the dorsal root ganglia and degeneration of the dorsal roots, posterior columns and peripheral nerves. In predominantly motor neuropathies, histological changes are usually slight although there may be a varying degree of atrophy of muscle fibres. Other conditions in this group are a *myasthenic syndrome*, a *diffuse encephalomyelitis* characterised by intense perivascular cuffing by lymphocytes, and *subacute cerebellar atrophy* characterised by an extensive loss of Purkinje cells and degeneration of the dentate nuclei and of the long tracts—motor and sensory—in the spinal cord. These changes are found most often in, but are not confined to, cases of *bronchial carcinoma*. The neurological symptoms not infrequently ante-date local ones caused by the tumour itself. In long-standing malignant lymphomas, and in widespread involvement of the lympho-reticular tissues by other conditions, e.g. carcinomatosis and sarcoidosis, the brain may show many irregularly disposed areas of demyelination and an unusually severe degree of astrocytic hyperplasia. The term *progressive multifocal leukoencephalopathy* is applied to this condition (p. 701).

Congenital abnormalities of the nervous system

Defects of the brain are of considerable variety and the anatomical changes are often of a complicated nature; we can only summarise the main facts. *Anencephaly* is a condition in which there is deficiency of the cranial vault with absence of the brain, although there is often a small sac with remains of cerebral tissue on the exposed base of the cranial cavity, the base also being deficient in size. The condition, which is incompatible with life, is not infrequently associated with non-closure of the spinal canal or *rachischisis*.

Occasionally there is a deficiency in the cranial bones and a sac-like protrusion is present. This occurs in the line of a suture, is often median in position and as a rule occipital; or it may be lateral, e.g. at the side of an orbit or the nose. The sac is lined in some instances by the meninges and contains only CSF—**meningocele**. In other cases the sac is lined by neural tissue and sometimes, when the defect is posterior, may contain a considerable part of the cerebrum—**encephalocele**. The term **micrencephaly** means a congenital smallness of the brain. There is deficiency in the convolutions, and the sulci, especially the secondary, are imperfectly formed; the state is associated with a greater or lesser degree of idiocy. The whole brain may be abnormal, but as a rule the cerebellum and brain stem are less affected than the hemispheres. Sometimes again, there is a local defect in growth, often associated with a small size of the convolutions or *microgyria*. There is no doubt that micrencephaly is a primary defect in the growth of the brain, though its cause is not known, and it is not due to early closure of the sutures, as was once supposed. The term **porencephaly** is applied when part of the brain is replaced by a collection of fluid, covered by meninges and sometimes in communication with the ventricles. In the *primary type*, which results from failure of growth of the brain, the edges of the defect are usually smooth. The condition is occasionally bilateral and sometimes accompanied by other defects. In the *secondary form*, the lesion is supposed to be the result of encephalitis, e.g. toxoplasmosis, or of interference with the blood supply during intra-uterine life, and a somewhat similar condition may result from injury at the time of birth.

Spinal cord defects. A fairly common abnormality is non-closure of the spinal canal, or **rachischisis**, in which there is a local deficiency in the arches of the vertebrae, while the opening is covered posteriorly by soft tissues. The term **spina bifida** is applied to such a condition; a distinct rounded projection is usually present over the site of the defect, which is then known as *spina bifida cystica*. When there is no such projection the term *spina bifida occulta* is applied.

The commonest position of spina bifida is in the lumbo-sacral region, and in all cases the spinal cord extends to a lower level than the normal; in other words, it remains in the position it normally occupies only in the earlier stages of development. The cord and meninges are variously disposed in different cases. In the commonest form, the spinal cord is adherent to the posterior wall of the sac and the term **meningomyelocele** is applied. The dura mater is absent in the sac, and at the apex of the latter there is often an area where the skin is deficient. At this point there is a smooth membrane in which the spinal cord is incorporated, the cord being open posteriorly, and sometimes one or two small depressions are present, the latter indicating the upper and lower terminations of the central canal. The spinal nerves are spread out on the inner lining of the sac. In another rare form, the space containing the fluid is a distension of the central canal of the spinal cord and is lined by the epithelium of the ependyma. In this variety, which is called **myelocystocele** or **syringomyelocele**, the spinal cord has been closed in posteriorly, and thus the abnormality has arisen at a later period of development than the previous form. In a third variety, which is the least common, the sac is lined by a hernial protrusion of the arachnoid, while the spinal cord is in its normal position in relation to the vertebrae. This is called **meningocele**. In all three varieties the dura mater is absent locally. In spina bifida the sac contains CSF. In the first variety, the fluid is in the subarachnoid space in front of the spinal cord; in the second, it is in the dilated canal of the cord, and in the third, it is in the subarachnoid space behind the cord.

The more severe forms of meningomyelocele are almost invariably associated with hydrocephalus and the Arnold–Chiari malformation (p. 670).

In **spina bifida occulta**, where there is no swelling to indicate the defect, the skin over the part usually shows abnormalities in appearance, and not infrequently there is excessive growth of hair on it. Here, also, the cord extends to a lower level in the spinal canal than normally.

Tuberous sclerosis. In this disorder multiple foci of hyperplasia of neuroglia and nerve cells occur in the cortex of the brain and in the subependymal tissue, in association with rhabdomyoma of the heart muscle (p. 377), adenoma sebaceum and other congenital abnormalities. In a few cases one or more of the glial foci give rise to a distinctive giant-celled type of astrocytoma.

Tumours of the Nervous System

Many tumours of the central nervous system arise intrinsically in neural tissue, i.e. they are neuro-ectodermal tumours. Others arise from the meninges (meningioma) or from cranial and spinal nerve roots (Schwannoma). The brain is also a common site of metastatic carcinoma, and finally there are many relatively rare tumours which implicate the nervous system.

The incidence of these various tumour types will vary according to whether this is based on necropsy reports from a general hospital, or on biopsies and autopsies in a neurological institute. Of a total of about 1500 consecutive primary tumours of the nervous system encountered over a 10-year-period in the Institute of Neurological Sciences, Glasgow, approximately 1000 were neuro-ectodermal, 250 were meningiomas, and 65 were Schwannomas. During the same period some 400 cases of metastatic carcinoma in the brain were encountered but this figure does not reflect its true incidence since not all patients with suspected cerebral metastases are referred to neurosurgical or neurological wards.

Tumours of neuro-ectodermal origin

These consist of all the tumours which arise from the primitive medullary epithelium. In the central nervous system these cells are represented firstly by the neuroglia, i.e. astrocytes, oligodendrocytes and ependymal cells, and secondly by nerve cells. Tumours related to the neuroglial cells are known collectively as the **gliomas** and constitute the great majority of neuro-ectodermal tumours.

The gliomas

Some gliomas are mature tumours composed of cells that have a fairly close resemblance to astrocytes, oligodendrocytes or ependymal cells, the respective tumours being called *astrocytoma*, *oligodendroglioma* and *ependymoma*. Secondly, there are tumours in which only a proportion of the cells are of this type, the others being pleomorphic and less well differentiated: these are referred to as the *anaplastic* variants of these tumours.

As in other tissues, the general rule usually applies that the more primitive or undifferentiated the cells are, the more rapid is their growth, but in contrast to tumours in other systems the terms 'benign' and 'malignant' have a new connotation. All the tumours in this group, whether cytologically benign or malignant, infiltrate the adjacent brain tissue and are never truly sharply demarcated or encapsulated. Paradoxically the rapidly growing anaplastic forms appear to be the better demarcated, because they also compress and push aside surrounding tissues. Further, neuro-ectodermal tumours *do not metastasise to other organs*, except in very rare cases, usually after craniotomy. They may however be disseminated by the CSF to other parts of the nervous system. The terms 'benign' and 'malignant' therefore refer in this context purely to the degree of cellular differentiation and rate of growth.

Astrocytoma. This is by far the commonest type of glioma. A 'benign', i.e. well-differentiated, astrocytoma is a slowly growing whitish tumour, usually poorly defined at its margin where it merges with the surrounding tissue. The consistence of the tumour varies with the number of glial fibres in it; if abundant, it is tough, almost rubbery; if scanty, it is soft. Cystic change is not uncommon (Fig. 20.67). The cerebellar astrocytoma of childhood has a notable tendency to become grossly cystic.

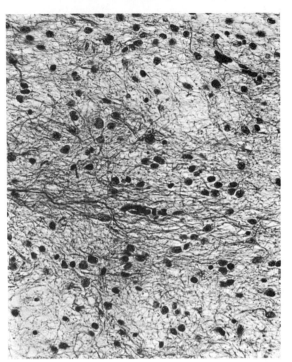

Fig. 20.68 Astrocytoma of relatively low cellularity showing well formed glial fibrils. (PTAH). × 260.

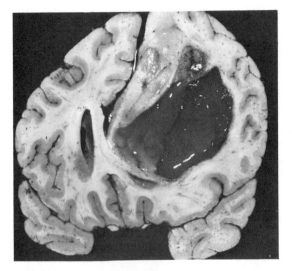

Fig. 20.67 Cystic astrocytoma in right frontal lobe. Tumour tissue is identifiable adjacent to the upper pole of the cyst.

In a *fibrillary astrocytoma*, microscopic examination shows unevenly distributed and often loosely arranged elongated cells separated by glial fibrils (Fig. 20.68). Even in the absence of gross cystic change there are often numerous microcysts. Sometimes the brain tissue is diffusely permeated by tumour astrocytes, often with remarkable preservation of nerve cells and fibres. The edge of this type of tumour often defies recognition with the naked eye. It is referred to as *diffuse astrocytoma* (sometimes known as gliomatosis) and is a particularly common type of astrocytoma in the brain stem and spinal cord. Other rarer forms of astrocytoma are composed of protoplasmic astrocytes or swollen, so-called gemistocytic astrocytes.

All astrocytomas display a marked propensity to become anaplastic: this may be restricted to one part of the tumour or it may be multifocal. To the naked eye the anaplastic areas are haemorrhagic and necrotic and often appear to have a relatively well-defined edge. The microscopic features of these areas are similar to those of glioblastoma multiforme.

The term **glioblastoma multiforme** may be

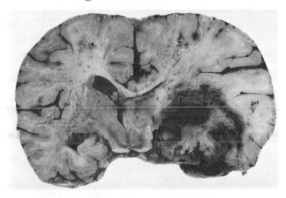

Fig. 20.69 Glioblastoma multiforme of temporal lobe. Note the well-defined margin and haemorrhagic areas within the tumour. There is a pronounced midline shift, virtual obliteration of the lateral ventricle and a supracallosal hernia.

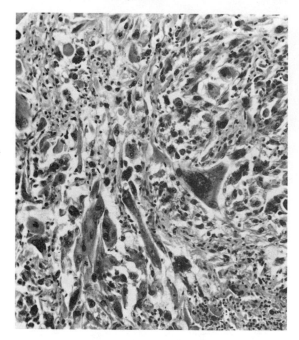

Fig. 20.70   Glioblastoma multiforme showing many aberrant giant cells. × 110.

used for astrocytomas that are highly anaplastic throughout. Such tumours occur in adults, most frequently in the cerebral hemispheres, forming a rapidly growing, apparently relatively well-defined mass with extensive necrosis and haemorrhage. It produces considerable distortion of the brain and often a rapid increase in intracranial pressure (Figs. 20.4, 20.69).

Microscopically a glioblastoma multiforme is richly cellular in the areas that are not necrotic and there are great variations in cell type ranging from closely packed masses of small anaplastic cells to bizarre giant cells (Fig. 20.70). Mitoses are often frequent and glial fibrils extremely scanty. Small vessels in and around the tumour may show curious bud-like or 'glomeruloid' endothelial proliferations (Fig. 20.71). Necrosis is pronounced within the tumour and frequently slightly elongated cells form a palisade around necrotic foci (Fig. 20.72).

Ependymoma. This not uncommon tumour is most frequently encountered in children, most often in the fourth ventricle but it may also occur in the other ventricles. The tumour cells

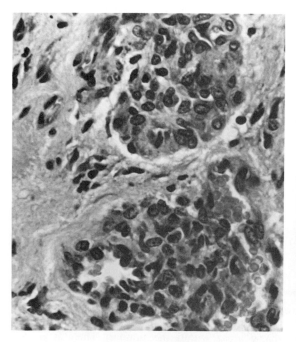

Fig. 20.71   Glomeruloid endothelial proliferation in glioblastoma. × 390.

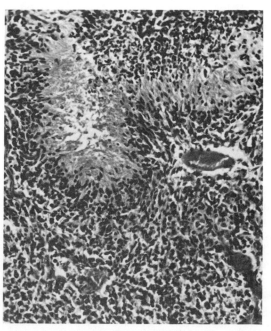

Fig. 20.72   Glioblastoma multiforme, showing a common pattern of central necrosis with peripheral palisading of spindle-shaped cells. × 130.

often have a distinctly epithelial appearance and they are characteristically orientated around small blood vessels but are separated from them by an eosinophilic fibrillary band (Fig. 20.73). Less frequently columnar cells form small canaliculi (Fig. 20.74), and near the free edge of these cells there may be small rod-shaped blepharoplasts. Ependymomas may also

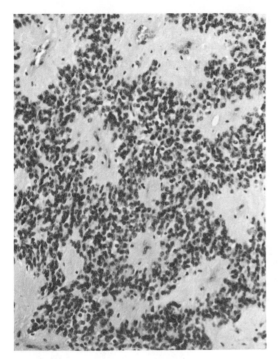

Fig. 20.73 Ependymoma. Note the perivascular fibrillary halo that is particularly characteristic of ependymoma. × 125.

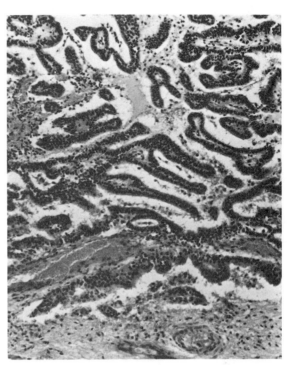

Fig. 20.75 Papillary tumour of the choroid plexus, showing delicate papillary processes covered by cubical epithelium. × 100.

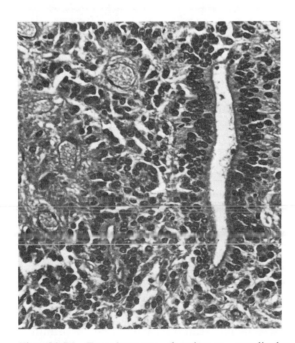

Fig. 20.74 Ependymoma showing a canaliculus lined by columnar ciliated cells. × 230.

become anaplastic as shown by the occurrence of cellular pleomorphism and poor differentiation, haemorrhage and necrosis. Closely related to the ependymoma is the *papillary tumour of the choroid plexus*. This is again most frequently seen in children when it forms a rounded bulky tumour usually in one lateral ventricle. The papillae have a vascular connective tissue core covered by columnar epithelium very similar in appearance to normal choroid plexus epithelium (Fig. 20.75). It frequently causes hydrocephalus.

There is also a curious type of tumour arising from the filum terminale, known as *myxopapillary ependymoma*. It is a slowly growing, markedly gelatinous tumour that occurs in adults, and gradually ensheathes the nerve roots of the cauda equina and the caudal part of the spinal cord. The stroma consists of a central vascular core surrounded by very mucoid connective tissue and covered in places by a cubical epithelium (Fig. 20.76); elsewhere the covering cells may form a network between the papillae. This tumour may cause pressure

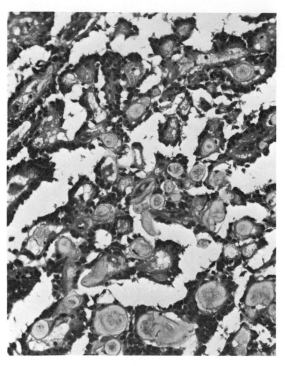

Fig. 20.76 Myxopapillary ependymoma, a papillary structure with very gelatinous stroma, covered by a mainly cubical epithelium. × 125.

atrophy of the adjacent bones and may even invade them; it is then liable to be mistaken for a chordoma (p. 850).

Oligodendroglioma. In our experience this glioma is rarer than ependymoma. It occurs in the cerebral hemispheres, is a slowly growing, rather gelatinous tumour, and commonly exhibits numerous small foci of calcification which may be seen radiologically. The cells are uniform, small and rounded, like those of the oligodendroglia, with somewhat clear cytoplasm and distinct cell-membranes (Fig. 20.77). Cell processes are small and difficult to demonstrate. As with other gliomas, anaplastic change may occur in these tumours.

The principal characters of the commoner

gliomas have now been described but many clearly defined variants have not been mentioned. It would be wrong to suggest that every glioma can be easily assigned to a specific category. Indeed a comprehensive microscopic examination of any glioma may result in the identification of various types of tumour and the name applied comes to depend on the most

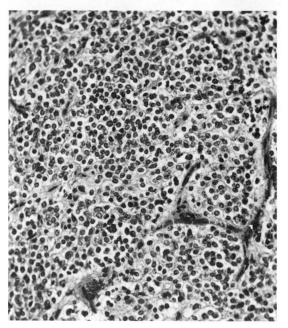

Fig. 20.77 Oligodendroglioma. The tumour is very cellular, the cells being round or oval with distinct cell boundaries. × 125.

prominent element. Furthermore each main division tends to exist as a spectrum; at one end there is a mature well-differentiated tumour composed of cells similar to normal glial cells in many respects, while at the other there is a highly anaplastic and poorly differentiated tumour. As all gliomas infiltrate into the adjacent brain, particularly the better differentiated types, total surgical excision is rarely feasible: radiotherapy is also at best palliative and the ultimate prognosis for a patient with a glioma is usually poor.

Tumours of the neuron series

These include tumours composed of primitive cells, namely *medulloblastoma*, *neuroblastoma* and *retinoblastoma* (p. 743), and tumours containing large ganglion cells, namely *ganglioneuroma* and *ganglioglioma*. The latter types, however, occur very rarely within the central nervous system.

Medulloblastoma. This not uncommon tumour of childhood is composed of undifferentiated primitive cells. It is a rapidly growing cellular tumour, restricted to the cerebellum where it forms a soft greyish-white mass protruding into the fourth ventricle. Commonly it spreads over the surface of the cerebellum as a thin sheet that obscures the normal surface architecture. Seeding of tumour cells by the CSF may result in diffuse implantation but sometimes only small secondary nodules develop on the nerve roots of the cauda equina.

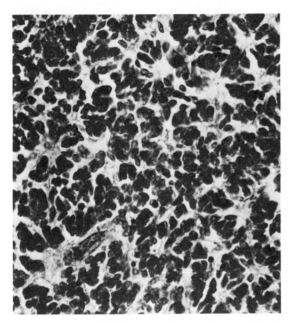

Fig. 20.78 Medulloblastoma. The cells are small and closely packed, but form poorly defined rosettes. × 285.

Microscopically, its cells are either spherical with little cytoplasm and no fibrils, or somewhat triangular, like short carrots, and arranged around blood vessels and also as circles and rosettes without a central cavity (Fig. 20.78).

Neuroblastoma and ganglioneuroma. These, in general, are tumours derived from ganglion cells or their precursors in sites outwith the central nervous system. The majority arise in the adrenal medulla or in sympathetic ganglia but they may also arise in the more distal groups of the parasympathetic system. *Neuroblastoma* (sometimes known as sympathicoblastoma) is a primitive, highly malignant tumour whereas *ganglioneuroma* is a mature benign tumour: tumours of an intermediate or mixed character are also encountered.

Neuroblastoma. This is essentially a tumour of childhood, the majority being encountered in children under 4 years of age. The commonest sites are the adrenal medulla and the retroperitoneal tissues. A neuroblastoma of the adrenal gland forms a bulky soft cellular and haemorrhagic tumour with extensive necrosis, which destroys the adrenal, spreads rapidly to the upper abdominal lymph nodes, to the liver and notably to the skeleton, secondary tumours in the skull being especially frequent.

On *microscopic examination*, the cells are small, round or oval, with little cytoplasm. In many parts they are irregularly arranged, while in places they may form small ball-like masses of cells which sometimes show further differentiation into rings or rosettes, the central part of the ring being occupied by a large number of fine fibrils which give, somewhat imperfectly,

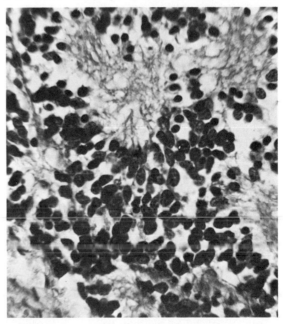

Fig. 20.79. Neuroblastoma. Many of the cells are carrot-shaped and are arranged in well-defined rosettes, the centres of which contain the fine fibrils prolonged from the tapering cells. × 425.

the staining reactions of nerve fibrils with silver impregnation. The cells surrounding such rosettes are radially arranged, tail-like prolongations of the cytoplasm projecting into the centre to form the fibrillary network (Fig. 20.79). These structures are closely similar to the clumps of neuroblasts which grow out to

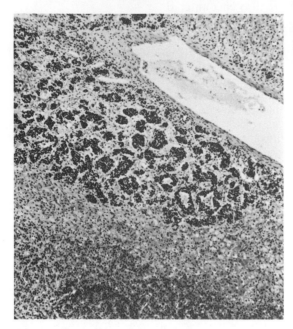

Fig. 20.80 Adrenal medulla of an infant of 9 months, showing masses of undifferentiated neuroblasts. × 60.

form the sympathetic system, as can be well seen in the fetal adrenal when it is becoming invaded by neuroblasts to form the medulla of the gland. Rests of undifferentiated neuroblasts are occasionally found in the adrenal medulla in infancy (Fig. 20.80). In some neuroblastomas, often referred to as ganglioneuroblastomas, some neuroblastic differentiation, as shown by the formation of cells resembling immature neurons, may occur.

Ganglioneuroma. This tumour affects older age groups than neuroblastoma and occurs more often in the posterior mediastinum than in the abdomen. A ganglioneuroma is usually firm, encapsulated like a simple tumour and of rounded or irregular outline. On microscopic examination, it is found to contain well-formed ganglionic nerve cells, irregularly arranged in a finely fibrillar stroma, and also smaller cells of various forms (Fig. 20.81). There are usually also a large number of nerve fibres both myelinated

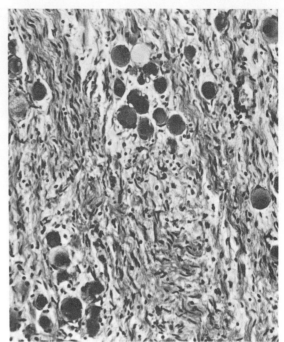

Fig. 20.81 Ganglioneuroma of adrenal, showing abundant mature ganglion cells and non-myelinated nerve fibres.

and non-myelinated, and some naked axis cylinders. The tumour is as a rule benign, but occasionally it is associated with a cellular malignant neuroblastoma.

Neuroblastoma is rare in the central nervous system. So also are tumours containing well-formed ganglion cells, but here the term *ganglioglioma* is more accurate than ganglioneuroma as neoplastic proliferation of neuroglia is an intrinsic component of the tumour.

The common embryological background of these various tumours derived from the sympathetic rudiment is emphasised by the fact that certain neuroblastic and ganglionic tumours in infancy unconnected with the adrenals, e.g. in the thorax, may secrete pressor substances, notably dopamine and noradrenaline, causing severe hypertension. These are excreted in the urine respectively as homovanillic acid and vanillyl mandelic acid (VMA).

Tumours of the meninges

The common tumour of this class is the *meningioma*, which takes origin from the arachnoid granulations (Fig. 20.82).

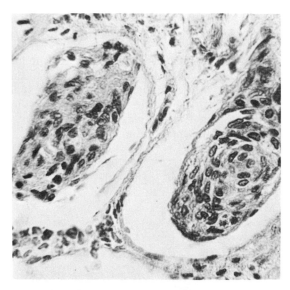

Fig. 20.82 Two arachnoidal granulations lying in small dural veins.

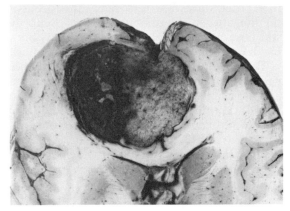

Fig. 20.84 Large meningioma between frontal lobes.

Meningiomas vary greatly in character, some being relatively hard or gritty, others less fibrous and softer. In certain situations they may grow to a remarkable size before causing symptoms. They are solid lobulated tumours, well demarcated from the brain tissue in which they excavate a bed, and are, as a rule, firmly attached by a broad base to the dura. They are benign, and thus can generally be successfully removed surgically. They tend to be related to major venous sinuses and commonly arise parasagitally (Fig. 20.83) or on the base of the skull, where they may originate in the region of the olfactory groove and grow into the fissure between the frontal lobes (Fig. 20.84). Another common site is the sphenoidal ridge. Rarely a meningioma may arise from the tela choroidea and appear as an intraventricular tumour. Frequently a meningioma infiltrates the overlying bone like a malignant tumour and gives rise to considerable thickening of the bone in relation

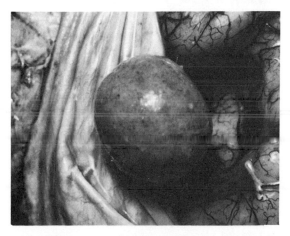

Fig. 20.83 Meningioma attached to dura mater, showing the typical depression of the cerebral cortex from which the tumour is readily withdrawn. × 1·4.

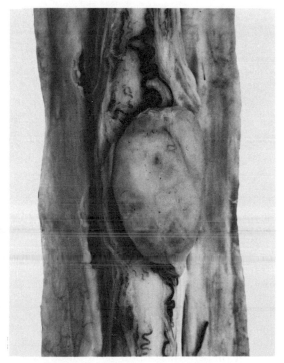

Fig. 20.85 Spinal meningioma compressing the cord. × 1·5.

to it. Metastases are very rare; most occur in the lungs when the tumour has spread into the soft tissues of the scalp after craniotomy, but a few have followed invasion of a venous sinus.

The *spinal meningiomas* correspond in their general characters, but, owing to their situation, are of smaller size (Fig. 20.85). They are intradural tumours which arise most frequently on the postero-lateral aspect of the cord, and the disturbances at first are chiefly sensory—pain, paraesthesia, etc. At a later period various effects up to complete paraplegia may result from pressure on the cord.

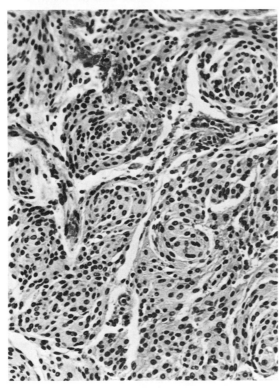

Fig. 20.86   Section of meningioma of common cellular type showing the arrangement of cells and fibres in whorls. × 220.

Microscopically the meningiomas show considerable variation in histological structure, the most common variety being composed of a fibro-cellular tissue with a somewhat whorled appearance owing to the concentric arrangement of the cells (Fig. 20.86). The centres of some of the whorls contain small blood vessels, but others undergo hyaline change and become calcified, resulting in a hard gritty mass con-

taining numerous spherical calcified particles—*psammoma bodies* (Fig. 20.87). In the more cellular varieties the whorls are composed of rather plump spindle-shaped cells resembling endothelium, but all degrees of transition to the fibrous type are encountered. The cellular type of tumour which invades the overlying bone, giving rise to hyperostosis, may subsequently spread into the surrounding tissues.

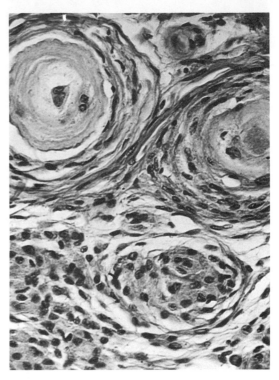

Fig.   20.87   Meningioma,   showing   fibrocellular masses with concentric arrangement and formation of psammoma bodies. × 350.

Sarcoma very occasionally arises from the meninges and extends widely over its surface. Occasionally a primary *melanoma* occurs as a diffusely spreading tumour in the meninges.

Tumours of vascular origin

Tumours of vascular origin are uncommon, forming about 2% of cerebral tumours. They are divided into (1) *angiomatous malformations*, and (2) the *haemangioblastomas* or true neoplasms of blood-vessel elements. The former are not true tumours but are similar to vascular hamartomas elsewhere. They may be chiefly capillary, venous, or arterio-venous, and their principal importance is as a cause of intracranial haemorrhage (p. 678).

The true vascular tumours, which occur most frequently in the cerebellum, are composed of

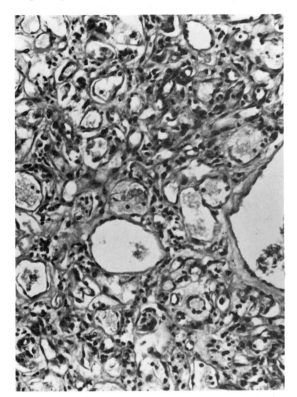

Fig. 20.88 Haemangioblastoma of the cerebellum in a case of Lindau's disease. × 130.

vascular channels or spaces (Fig. 20.88), among which there is a large accumulation of lipid-laden cells with an abundant network of reticulin fibres between them. There is a marked tendency to cyst formation; transudation of fluid occurs into the tissue and forms a space or spaces containing fluid and lined with compressed neuroglia, the tumour being represented by a mural nodule. A peculiar syndrome in which one of the latter tumours is present is known as Lindau's disease. In association with the haemangioblastoma there may be capillary angiomatosis in other parts of the nervous system and in the retina; there are also lesions which are not of vascular nature—cysts in the pancreas (p. 657) or kidneys, and adenomas in the kidneys or adrenals.

Tumours arising in developmental defects

Dermoid and epidermoid cysts, which present clinically as tumours, are occasionally found in connection with the meninges, especially at the base of the brain, in the vertebral canal, and in the bones of the skull. An epidermoid cyst is well encapsulated, and has a whitish and rather shining appearance (pearly tumour) and a somewhat crumbling character. The wall is thin and is composed of cells of squamous epithelial type from which keratinised squames are shed into the interior where they accumulate, together with crystals of cholesterol, and thus distend the cyst. In dermoid cysts, hairs and sebaceous glands are present. Midline dermoid and epidermoid cysts in the posterior fossa and in the vertebral canal are sometimes connected to the skin surface by a sinus. The opening on the skin may be very small but the sinus provides a route by which the cyst may become

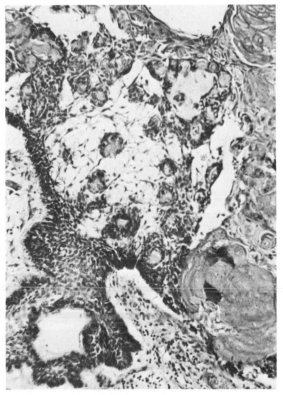

Fig. 20.89 Craniopharyngioma, showing partly squamous, partly 'adamantinomatous' structure. Note the stellate reticulum within the epithelial bands. × 130.

infected. Inclusion epidermoid cysts in the region of the cauda equina can result from repeated lumbar puncture during childhood.

A somewhat similar tumour, partly cystic, partly solid, is found in children and adults in the region of the pituitary stalk, compressing the gland in the sella turcica and pressing upwards into the third ventricle. Probably these suprasellar growths arise from nests of epidermoid cells derived from the pars tuberalis and they are known as **suprasellar cysts** or **craniopharyngiomas**. Their lining epithelium is in part squamous, but there is also a partial differentiation towards stellate reticulum resembling enamel organ (Fig. 20.89), and the name **adamantinoma** is sometimes applied. The wall is usually partially calcified. The chief clinical features are disturbances of vision and of hypophyseal function (p. 946). True Rathke pouch cysts are intrasellar.

Teratomas are rare intracranial tumours, their chief site being the pineal, where, in boys, their occurrence may be associated with precocious sexual development. They may be well differentiated but more often are of the germinoma type, the histological features being very similar to those of seminoma (p. 887).

Metastatic tumours

Metastatic tumours are very common in the brain and the possibility must be considered that a cerebral tumour which clinically appears to be primary may in fact be a metastasis. This occurs most commonly with bronchial carcinoma. Metastatic deposits are typically multiple

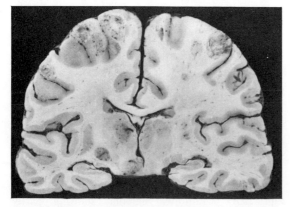

Fig. 20.90 Metastatic carcinoma. Numerous deposits of tumour are present in each cerebral hemisphere.

and are sharply circumscribed (Fig. 20.90). The tumour cells have a tendency to spread along the perivascular spaces, so that vessels may be ensheathed by them. Not infrequently metastatic carcinoma spreads diffusely throughout the subarachnoid space, often producing the clinical features of a subacute meningitis. This is known as meningeal carcinomatosis, and in such cases it is usually possible to identify tumour cells in the CSF. The brain may also be infiltrated directly or compressed by tumours arising in the nasopharynx, or by a chordoma growing from the basisphenoid. Secondary tumours within the dura of the spinal cord are rare, but extradural spinal metastases are common.

Effects of tumours

Intracranial tumours produce local and general effects on the brain. The latter are due mainly to raised intracranial pressure and the characteristic features are headache, vomiting, papilloedema, and blunting of the intellect. The increase in pressure is brought about by the size of the tumour, by the frequent occurrence of cerebral oedema around it, and, when the tumour is in a situation to block the free flow of CSF fluid, by hydrocephalus. The morphological changes brought about in the brain by any intracranial expanding lesion have been fully considered on p. 666. Local effects depend on the site of the tumour and include, for example, focal (Jacksonian) epilepsy, paralysis and defects in the visual fields.

Tumours of nerve roots and peripheral nerves

These may be solitary or multiple, the latter being especially associated with neurofibromatosis, a disorder inherited as an autosomal dominant. Some of these tumours have many of the features of a fibroma: they are generally believed to originate principally from the cells of the endoneurium or perineurium and they may be referred to as *neurofibromas*. In others the cells are arranged in a distinctive pattern with their nuclei forming a palisade across the bundles of long spindle cells; these tumours are thought to arise mainly from Schwann cells and are therefore termed *Schwannomas*. This group of tumours, however, ranges from a discrete paraneural Schwannoma at one end of the spectrum to a poorly delineated plexiform neurofibroma at the other.

Schwannoma. This is typically a rounded or lobulated, often partly cystic, well circumscribed and encapsulated tumour arising in relation to a nerve; they may be intracranial, intraspinal or peripheral. Within the cranium the commonest site of origin is the vestibular portion of the auditory nerve, but they also occur in association with the trigeminal nerve. An acoustic Schwannoma ('**acoustic neuroma**') takes origin just within the internal auditory meatus, which it invariably expands; and the enlargement may be visible radiologically. The tumour fills the cerebello-pontine angle (Fig. 20.91) and produces severe distortion and

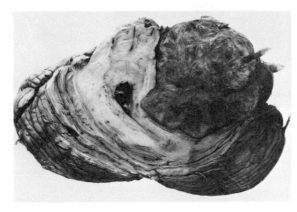

Fig. 20.91 Large Schwannoma of the auditory nerve in the cerebello-pontine angle, which has caused great displacement of the adjacent structures.

displacement of the adjacent brain and some degree of hydrocephalus from compression of the fourth ventricle. When bilateral, they are usually associated with von Recklinghausen's disease. In the spinal canal, Schwannomas occur as intradural tumours on the dorsal nerve roots, mostly in the thoracic region. Their main effect is to compress the spinal cord, but they may extend through the intervertebral foramen to produce a much larger intrathoracic portion. On peripheral nerves they may occur as isolated single nodules or they may be multiple. The nerve fibres tend to be spread over the surface, especially at one side, and are not incorporated in the tumour.

Microscopic examination shows the tumour to be composed of fibro-cellular bundles in a whorled pattern; within the fasciculi, the cells are closely arranged in parallel fashion with their rod-shaped nuclei forming a characteristic 'palisade' (Fig. 20.92). In other areas the tumour may be of looser texture or even cystic and contain large numbers of fat-laden foamy cells between the fasciculi. The softer and more

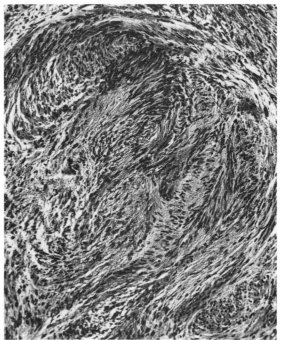

Fig. 20.92 Schwannoma of acoustic nerve, showing whorling and palisading of cells. × 100.

cellular tumours are prone to repeated local recurrence with progressive anaplasia, and may become frankly sarcomatous.

Neurofibroma. In some cases, a group of nerves, a plexus or the sciatic nerve and its branches, may be affected diffusely, and show numerous irregular thickenings with oval or beadlike swellings in their course (Fig. 20.93). There is also the form known as the *plextform* or *racemose* type, where the nerves of a region, usually the scalp or the neck, show irregular tortuous thickenings which often give rise to firm elevations with a somewhat convoluted appearance.

Histological examination shows the nerve to be expanded by large elongated and spindle-shaped cells often separated by mucoid matrix (Fig. 20.94). Residual nerve fibres can be identified in neurofibromas.

In **neurofibromatosis** ('**von Recklinghausen's**

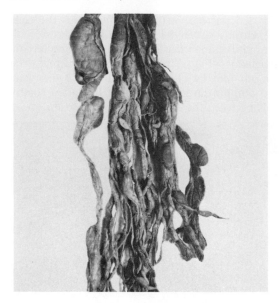

Fig. 20.93 Diffuse neurofibromatosis of sciatic nerve and its branches. Note the numerous nodules of various sizes and forms.

disease'), nodules of various sizes, sometimes numbering hundreds, occur along small nerve branches, especially of the skin, but also in some cases along the visceral branches of the sympathetic. In this disease, tumours sometimes arise also on the spinal nerves and their roots, within the spinal canal, leading to compression of the spinal cord. The connective tissue of the nodules varies in character but is often of dense hyaline nature; nerve fibres can be traced running through it. Neurofibromatosis is often associated with multiple pigmented patches in the skin.

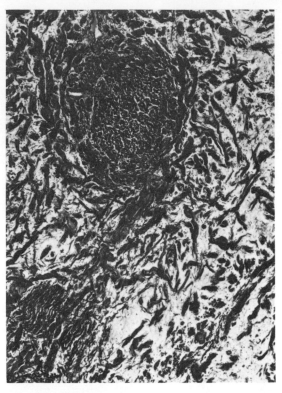

Fig. 20.94 Plexiform neurofibroma showing nerve fibres and loosely arranged interlacing connective tissue bundles. × 120.

Lastly, there is occasionally a localised general thickening of the tissues, with nodulation and folding of the skin—a sort of local elephantiasis, to which the name *elephantiasis neuromatosa* has been applied.

IV The Eye

Introduction

The pathological changes which occur in the eye and the orbital structures are in many respects similar to those described in other systems of the body. However, owing to the particular anatomical and functional properties of the eye, there are some common ocular disease processes which merit separate consideration. Emphasis is therefore placed on the inflammatory, neoplastic and degenerative disorders, corneal scarring, glaucoma and degenerative retinopathies, in order to provide suitable examples of pathogenic mechanisms which lead to blindness. The progress of many ocular diseases is followed *in vivo* by a variety of clinical techniques, e.g. slit-lamp microscopy, ophthalmoscopy, angiography and electrophysiological analysis, so that a unique facility exists for clinico-pathological correlation and this permits an insight into the pathogenesis of many disorders.

Applied anatomy

The structure of the eye is shown dia-gramatically in Figs. 20.95 and 20.96. Visual acuity depends upon a transparent focusing system (the cornea and lens), transparent media (the aqueous and vitreous) and a normal

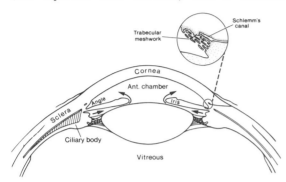

Fig. 20.95 Schematic diagram of the structures of the anterior segment of the eye to show the principal route of aqueous outflow.

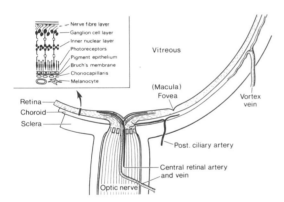

Fig. 20.96 Schematic diagram of the structures of the posterior segment of the eye to show the vascular supply to the choroid, retina and optic disc.

photoreceptor and neural conducting mechanism. The metabolism of the cornea and lens is maintained by the circulation of the aqueous fluid, which is produced in the ciliary processes and leaves the anterior chamber via the outflow apparatus situated in the inner peripheral cornea adjacent to the root of the iris—the iridocorneal angle. The outflow apparatus is a filtering system consisting of a series of fenestrated collagenous plates (trabeculae) which are covered by endothelial cells with phagocytic potential—this tissue is limited externally by an endothelial monolayer which lines the circum-

ferential outflow canal of Schlemm (drained by episcleral collector channels). The pressure within the eye is normally 15–20 mmHg and depends upon the relative rates of aqueous production and outflow. Any marked variation in pressure—*ocular hypotension* or *hypertension*—whether acute or chronic causes an imbalance in vascular perfusion leading to ischaemic damage to the sensitive neural tissues within the eye.

The retina and the pigment epithelium are maintained by blood flow via two separate arterial systems. The inner two-thirds of the thickness of the retinal tissue are supplied by the branches of the central retinal artery while

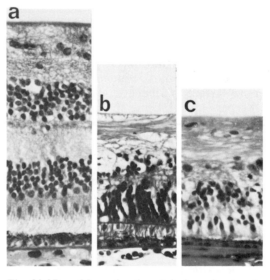

Fig. 20.97 **a** Normal retina; **b** ischaemic atrophy of the inner retina due to occlusion of the central retinal artery; **c** ischaemic atrophy of the outer retina due to posterior ciliary artery occlusion. × 240.

the outer third (the photoreceptor layer) is maintained by the choriocapillaris, which is supplied by the posterior ciliary arteries. Although the optic nerve is supplied by the central retinal artery and the meningeal arteries, the optic disc or papilla is nourished by blood vessels which are derived from the adjacent (peripapillary) choroid. Because of this vascular arrangement, distinctive patterns of ischaemic damage can occur in the visual sensory system according to the anatomical site of the vascular occlusion or impairment (Fig. 20.97).

Infections

The eye can be invaded primarily from the exterior, or by spread of infection from the adjacent orbital tissues or through the bloodstream. The tissue response to various pathogens is, in general, similar to that observed in other body tissues. In the eye, infections are of particular importance, firstly because a small infective lesion (e.g. of the cornea) can impair vision irreversibly and secondly, because the lens and vitreous are avascular protein-rich structures ideal for the proliferation of many pathogenic bacteria. An ulcer of the cornea due to pyogenic bacterial infection may measure only a few millimetres in diameter, but if it progresses to perforation, to ocular hypotonia and to endophthalmitis, removal of the eye will be necessary. While numerous types of micro-organisms can cause eye disease, the following are of particular significance.

Viral infections most commonly involve the external surface of the eye, the adenoviruses and herpes simplex being the most important. The **adenoviruses** (types 3 and 8) cause a conjunctivitis in which there is a hyperplasia of lymphoid tissue in the oedematous and hyperaemic conjunctival stroma (*follicular conjunctivitis*); this disease often occurs in epidemic form, and can involve the cornea. In **Herpes simplex** virus infection, *damage to the cornea* is more important than the associated conjunctivitis: the virus infects the epithelium of the cornea, which it destroys in a particular finger-like or *dendritic* pattern. Herpes keratitis tends to recur and spread to the corneal stroma, inducing neovascularisation and infiltration by lymphocytes, plasma cells and monocytes from the corneal periphery; disorganisation of the corneal lamellae leads to fibrotic scarring and opacity. Destruction of the stroma of the cornea is aggravated by the release of collagenases from the damaged corneal epithelial cells and the stromal keratocytes. When scarring impairs vision or when ulceration and secondary bacterial infection threaten an endophthalmitis, it is often necessary to replace the involved cornea by a homotransplant (see p. 139).

Trachoma-inclusion conjunctivitis or TRIC infection is caused by chlamydiae (p. 188). Infection with *Chlamydia trachomatosis* is common in the tropical zones and '**trachoma**', which is responsible for blindness on a massive scale.

The organism initially infects the conjunctival epithelium and it can be identified in smears of these cells by the presence of characteristic intracytoplasmic inclusion bodies formed by proliferation of elementary bodies. The superior tarsal conjunctiva is involved by a dense chronic inflammatory infiltrate containing lymphoid follicles which commonly extends on to and destroys the superficial cornea. The healing stage is associated with extensive corneal and conjunctival scarring.

Chlamydia oculogenitalis causes a milder inclusion conjunctivitis in the temperate zones. The lesion is confined to the lower tarsal conjunctiva where there is a low-grade chronic inflammatory infiltration in the stroma. The inclusion bodies observed in the epithelium in this type of TRIC infection can only be distinguished from those of *Chl. trachomatosis* by an immunofluorescent technique.

Bacteria. Primary infections of the conjunctiva and cornea by pyogenic organisms (e.g. gonococcus, Gram +ve cocci, haemophilus, moraxella and pseudomonas) were previously common and serious causes of corneal ulceration, but are now of minor significance in communities in which topical broad-spectrum antibiotics are readily available. Suppurative corneal ulceration, however, is still of importance as a secondary complication of pre-existing corneal disease, e.g. traumatic abrasion, viral and chlamydial infection, advanced glaucoma and is facilitated by the inappropriate use of steroids.

Histological examination of pyogenic ulceration of the cornea (Fig. 20.98) reveals a massive leukocytic infiltration in the disintegrating corneal stroma. Initially the dense membrane which lines the posterior corneal surface (*Descemet's membrane*), provides resistance to bacterial spread, but toxin diffusion induces migration of polymorphs into the iris and lower part of the anterior chamber (*hypopyon*) and irido-corneal adhesion results. Ultimately Descemet's membrane prolapses into the corneal deficit (to form a *Descemetocoele*) and, when this ruptures, bacterial penetration is unhindered and abscess formation occurs in the anterior chamber, lens and vitreous.

The eye may be affected in systemic microbial infection, e.g. tuberculosis, syphilis and brucellosis, and usually the uveal tract (the iris, ciliary body and choroid) is involved primarily

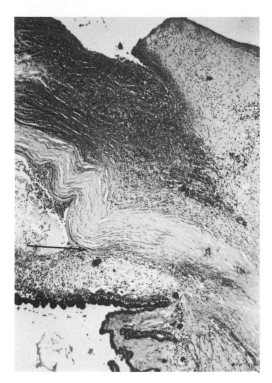

Fig. 20.98 A pyogenic ulcer of the cornea with inflammatory exudation into the anterior chamber and adhesion between the iris and the cornea (*arrow*). × 40.

(*uveitis*). A chronic inflammatory process in the choroid (*choroiditis*) can lead to focal destruction and reactionary proliferation of the pigment epithelium and degeneration in the adjacent retina, which either fuses with the choroid or may be detached by exudation of protein from damaged blood vessels in the choroid and retina. In the iris (*iritis*) and ciliary body (*cyclitis*) the inflammatory process leads to exudation of protein and inflammatory cells into the anterior and posterior chambers and clumps of inflammatory cells adhering to the posterior corneal surface (keratic precipitates) are a classical clinical sign of *iridocyclitis*.

In syphilis and tuberculosis there is widespread destruction of the choroid, ciliary body and iris and the adjacent structures. A similar pattern of tissue destruction is observed in sarcoidosis, fungal infection, protozoal (toxoplasmosis, p. 702) and metazoal (toxocara) infestation, although in the last two examples, the retina is the tissue more severely affected.

It should be noted that many cases of chronic uveitis are of unknown aetiology, although evidence is accumulating to incriminate a hypersensitivity reaction. The inflammatory infiltration in the uveal tract is predominantly lymphocytic, but the end-result is similar to that described above in the chronic bacterial infections, and ophthalmoscopy reveals punched out areas of depigmentation of the fundus. Involvement of the ciliary body leads to ocular hypotension, reactionary fibrosis in the vitreous body, choroidal and retinal oedema and lens degeneration. Contraction of the fibrotic vitreous and exudation into the

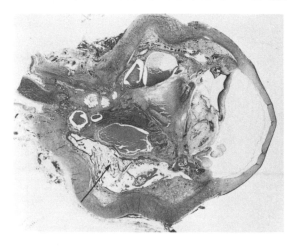

Fig. 20.99 Shrinkage and disorganisation of the eye following inflammation (phthisis bulbi). The retina is detached and the choroid is thickened by oedema and ossification (*arrow*). × 4.

subretinal space detaches the retina and the end-stage is a striking shrinkage of the eye with massive subretinal fibrosis and secondary ossification (*phthisis bulbi*) (Fig. 20.99). Conversely, ocular hypertension or secondary glaucoma (p. 740) can result from occlusion of the iridocorneal angle by post-inflammatory adhesions between the iris and the cornea (*anterior synechiae*) or by infiltration of the outflow apparatus by inflammatory cells.

Auto-immune disease

Auto-immune reactions occur in the eye in two established disease entities, *lens-induced uveitis* and *sympathetic ophthalmitis*.

(1) Lens-induced uveitis. Traumatic breakdown of lens tissue releases lens protein into the anterior chamber or the vitreous and in some circumstances this gives rise to a granulomatous reaction with giant cells due to a complex hypersensitivity reaction involving both auto-antibodies and also delayed hypersensitivity. The inflammatory reaction destroys the lens and the adjacent uveal tissue.

(2) Sympathetic ophthalmitis. Trauma to one eye which involves damage to or incarceration of either the iris or the ciliary body in the overlying scleral wound may be followed by a

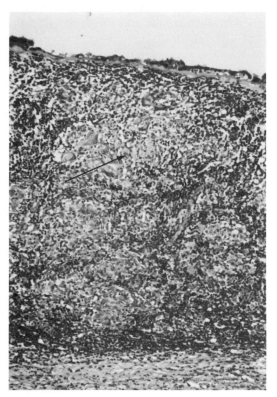

Fig. 20.100 The choroid in sympathetic opthalmitis; the tissue is infiltrated by a giant-cell granulomatous reaction (*arrow*). × 370.

giant-cell granulomatous uveitis in the opposite eye (Fig. 20.100). This secondary inflammatory process may arise months or years after the original injury and results in extensive damage to the second or 'sympathising' eye.

It is widely believed that release of uveal antigens from the injured eye stimulates a cell-mediated auto-immune response and that the second eye is the target organ of a delayed hypersensitivity reaction. If the first eye is preserved, it too is damaged by a giant-cell

granulomatous reaction in the remaining uveal tissue. Although rare, the risk of occurrence of this condition after eye injury often raises difficulties over the decision between surgical repair and enucleation of the injured eye, which in the latter case will abolish the risk of sympathetic ophthalmitis.

Vascular disease

Retinal ischaemia and haemorrhage. The pattern of ischaemic disease in the ocular tissues can often be related to the anatomy of the blood supply (p. 735). Complete occlusion of the central retinal artery by atheroma, thrombus or embolism, results in ischaemic atrophy of the inner two-thirds of the retina, while occlusion of the posterior ciliary arteries causes atrophy of the photoreceptor layer (Fig. 20.97). The outer plexiform layer is a zone in which there is inadequate resorption of exudates from damaged capillaries. Exudates which consist predominantly of plasma protein are seen by ophthalmoscopy as discrete pale yellow areas in the retina and are described as

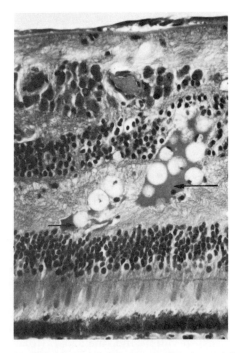

Fig. 20.101 A proteinaceous exudate (*arrow*) in the inner nuclear and the outer plexiform layers; lipid-laden macrophages are prominent. × 300.

hard exudates; resorption by lipid-laden glial macrophages may take several months (Fig. 20.101). The hard exudate is therefore a clinical manifestation of retinal ischaemia and another

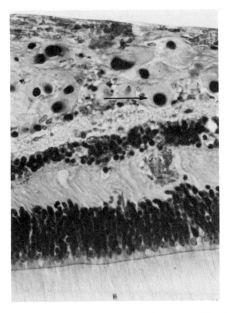

Fig. 20.102 A micro-infarct in the nerve fibre layer of the retina in which the swollen ends of axons (*arrow*) are seen as large darkly-staining round masses surrounded by paler areas. × 300.

feature is the so-called *soft exudate* which is an ill-defined small white area resembling cotton wool in the inner retina. On histological examination, the cotton wool spot is seen as a micro-infarction of the nerve fibre and ganglion-cell layers of the retina. The damaged segment becomes oedematous and contains the swollen ends of disrupted axons (*cytoid bodies*) (Fig. 20.102). Acute focal ischaemia in the retina is most commonly caused by angiospastic arteriolar disease and is a feature of malignant hypertension. When arteriolar disease is so severe that it leads to haemorrhage, the blood tracks within the nerve fibre layer to produce the flame haemorrhages seen on ophthalmoscopy. Accumulation of blood in the outer plexiform layer is derived from the rupture of capillaries and so-called blot haemorrhages are observed.

Haemorrhages are most prominent when venous outflow is impaired by thrombotic occlusion of the central retinal vein. The clinical consequences of venous occlusion are sometimes less serious than those of arterial occlusion, because dilatation of collateral venous channels relieves the pressure in the retinal venous system. Retinal oedema often persists and cystic degeneration, particularly in the region of the macula, leads to loss of central vision (Fig. 20.103).

One of the important responses to retinal ischaemia is vasoproliferation from the blood vessels around the ischaemic area. Although this process is potentially beneficial within the retina, penetration by the delicate newly-formed vessels into the vitreous is a common source of haemorrhage and contraction of fibrovascular scar tissue leads to retinal detachment. A related feature of retinal ischaemia is the release of a chemically unidentified and as yet hypothetical '*vasoproliferative factor*' which is thought to induce angioblastic proliferation on the anterior surface of the iris with consequent occlusion of the iridocorneal angle and

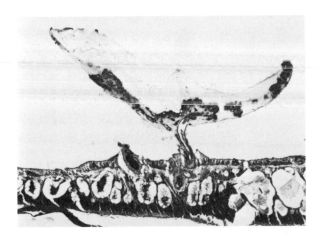

Fig. 20.103 The retina in ischaemic vascular disease due to central retinal vein occlusion. A tree-like growth of blood vessels extends into the vitreous and there is advanced cystic degeneration in the macula. × 40.

obstruction of aqueous outflow (secondary closed angle glaucoma). This factor is also considered to be the immediate cause of neovascularisation on the retinal surface.

The pathological processes described above are exemplified in **diabetic retinopathy** which can be regarded as an insidious focal ischaemic arteriolar disease complicated by additional degenerative changes in the capillary walls, including basement membrane thickening and pericyte degeneration. The formation of aneurysmal dilatations in the weakened capillaries (micro-aneurysms) is an important feature of diabetes although the same process also occurs in other forms of vascular insufficiency.

Senile macular degeneration. In elderly patients, hyalinisation of the choriocapillaris, with dystrophic calcification and rupture of Bruch's membrane in the macular area, can result in focal sub-retinal haemorrhage and fibrovascular proliferation. The pigment epithelium proliferates and contributes to the submacular fibrous mass (Fig. 20.104). The overlying photoreceptors degenerate and loss of central vision is a serious consequence of this disease.

Retinal detachment. Vascular insufficiency is considered to be an important factor in atrophic degenerative disease in the peripheral retina where microcyst formation and ischaemic chorioretinal scars are often observed. Tears through weakened areas in the retina lead to separation of the photoreceptors from the pigment epithelium by the spread of fluid from the vitreous and the consequent progress of the retinal detachment leads *pari passu* to a loss of visual field.

Glaucoma

Glaucoma is a generic name for a group of diseases in which the intra-ocular pressure increases to a level which impairs the vascular perfusion of the neural tissue and causes blindness. The rise in pressure is usually due to obstruction to the outflow of aqueous which can occur at either of two sites, thus giving rise to *closed-angle* and *open-angle glaucoma*.

Closed-angle glaucoma. This may be *primary* or *secondary*. The *primary form* occurs in middle-aged and old people who have a narrow iridocorneal angle and a shallow anterior chamber. In such individuals the iris and lens may come into contact and this interferes with the outflow of aqueous: pressure builds up behind the iris, which becomes bowed anteriorly, resulting in further obstruction and rising intra-ocular pressure. This vicious circle causes glaucoma of acute onset, presenting as ocular congestion, corneal oedema and pain.

Narrowness of the iridocorneal angle is attributable partly to normal individual variation, and partly to the ageing process of shrinkage of the eye and enlargement of the lens. When these factors are marked, they predispose the individual to glaucoma (Fig. 20.105).

Secondary closed-angle glaucoma has many causes, but in enucleated eyes the most common is the fibrovascular proliferation and adhesion between the iris and cornea (Fig. 20.98) which may follow inflammation, trauma and ischaemic retinal disease (Fig. 20.106).

Open-angle glaucoma (clinically, *chronic simple glaucoma*) is an insidious disease in the

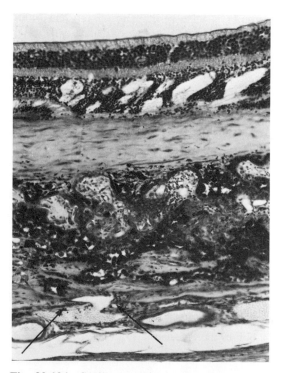

Fig. 20.104 Senile macular degeneration, in which there is a sub-macular mass formed by fibrovascular tissue and proliferating pigment epithelium. Bruch's membrane (*arrows*) is penetrated by a vessel from the choroid. × 100.

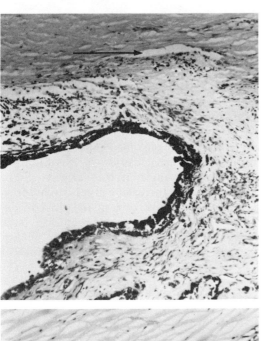

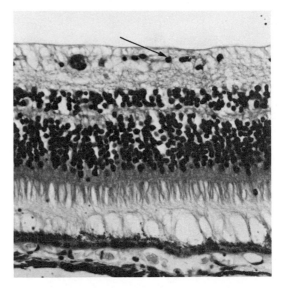

Fig. 20.106 The retina in glaucoma. The nerve fibre layer is atrophic and the ganglion cells are replaced by microglial cells (*arrow*). (Compare with normal retina, Fig. 20.97.) × 240.

defect which has a characteristic arcuate shape. By light microscopy the outflow apparatus in the early stages appears normal, but examination by electron microscopy has shown an accumulation of abnormal collagen in the trabeculae (which narrows the intertrabecular spaces) and in the extracellular spaces of the outer part of the trabecular meshwork, where it impedes aqueous outflow.

In *secondary open-angle glaucoma*, the outflow apparatus is obstructed mechanically by exogenous material, either particulate or cellular. In acute or chronic inflammatory disease, inflammatory cells accumulate within the intertrabecular spaces, while obstruction by macrophages occurs after haemorrhage or traumatic release of lens substance into the anterior chamber. The outflow apparatus can also be obstructed by tumour cell infiltration, e.g. by a primary malignant melanoma of the iris or ciliary body.

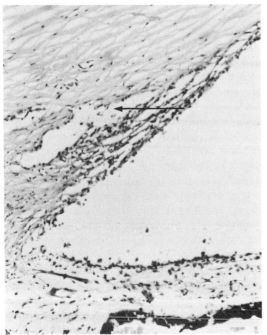

Fig. 20.105 The chamber angle in closed-angle glaucoma (*above*) and open-angle glaucoma (*below*). Note the secondary hyalinisation in closed-angle glaucoma and the preservation of the intertrabecular spaces in open-angle glaucoma. The canal of Schlemm is indicated by arrows. × 100.

elderly in which a slowly progressive increase in intra-ocular pressure leads to an ischaemic sectorial destruction of the nerve fibres in the optic disc (Fig. 20.107) and this is manifest as a field

The effects of increased intra-ocular pressure

The most serious effects on visual function are due to pressure-flow imbalance in the small vessels of the optic disc, so that there is ischaemic atrophy of the axons in the nerve fibres of the disc and secondary atrophy in the nerve fibre layer of the retina. Excavation or cupping of

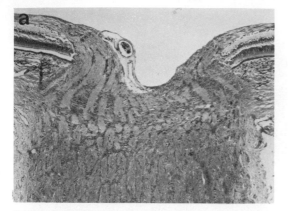

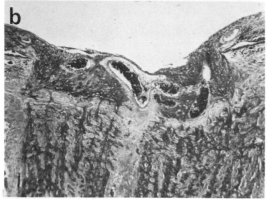

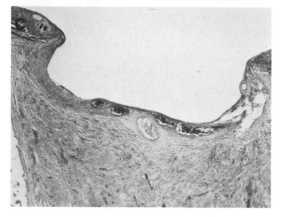

Fig. 20.107   a The normal optic disc: **b** the disc in early glaucoma, showing atrophy of the neural tissue: **c** the disc in advanced glaucoma in which the neural tissue is absent and the lamina cribrosa is bowed posteriorly. × 30.

the disc may become so advanced that it extends into the optic nerve.

The function of the corneal endothelium in maintaining dehydration is disturbed by the high pressure, so that the cornea becomes oedematous and the epithelium separates with the formation of bullae (*bullous keratopathy*). At this advanced stage the uveal tissues become atrophic and fibrosis occurs in ischaemic areas of the iris and choroid; the scleral tissues may stretch to form localised bulges or *staphylomas*.

In infants and children, glaucoma can result from developmental abnormalities in which there is a failure in the separation of the primitive mesodermal tissue which is found in the iridocorneal angle in the early stages of intra-uterine life. Increasing intra-ocular pressure causes the weaker eye of the child to expand uniformly, and it may become so large that it resembles an ox-eye, hence the clinical term '*buphthalmos*'.

Tumours

The tumours of the eyelid, conjunctiva and orbital tissues do not differ significantly in morphology and behaviour from those occurring elsewhere. Intra-ocular tumours are rare, but are important because of their serious effect on vision and their unusual patterns of behaviour.

Melanoma. *Malignant melanomas* and *benign naevi* are tumours of adult life and occur particularly in elderly white-skinned individuals. They are derived from the spindle-shaped melanocytes of the uveal tract. **Benign naevi** are common and clinically unimportant, but there is some evidence that occasionally they may undergo malignant transformation. **Malignant melanomas** are unilateral and solitary and are most commonly situated in the posterior choroid. The tumour expands the choroid, penetrates Bruch's membrane and initially adopts a characteristic collar-stud shape: later it becomes ovoid (Fig. 20.108). Plasma leaks from the tumour surface, and from the disturbed choroidal circulation, into the subretinal space and causes secondary retinal detachment which is often so extensive that visual loss is out of proportion to the size of the tumour. Microscopically the tumour cells are either spindle-shaped (Fig. 20.108) or round ('epithelioid'); predominantly round-cell tumours have a much worse prognosis than mainly spindle-celled tumours; the latter carry a 60% 15-year-survival rate. Growth within the eye leads to disorganisation and often to secondary glaucoma, while

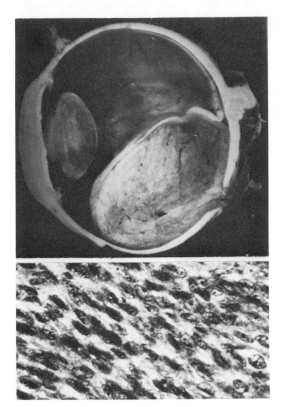

familial cases, the tumour is bilateral and often it is multifocal within the retina.

On gross examination, the retinoblastoma forms a solid pale-grey, partially calcified and partially necrotic mass within the retina. When the tumour fills the vitreous and destroys and detaches the retina, a white mass is seen behind the lens, so that reflected light produces a reflex similar to that in the cat's eye. Blindness in the affected eye causes the child to squint. The tumour is composed of small round or oval cells with scanty cytoplasm and a high rate of

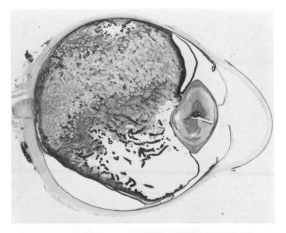

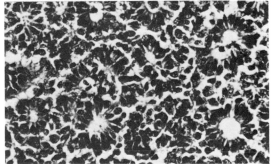

Fig. 20.108 Malignant melanoma of the choroid. *Above*, the gross appearances: the tumour has extended through the sclera. × 2·5. *Below*, the tumour is seen microscopically to be of spindle-cell type. × 410.

extension usually takes place through the intrascleral nerve channels. The choroidal and vortex veins are commonly invaded with consequent blood spread and distant metastasis, especially in the liver. This tumour is notorious for producing multiple rapidly-enlarging liver metastases as long as 20 (symptom-free) years after enucleation of the affected eye (the big liver and glass-eye syndrome). What happens to the tumour cell in the latent interval is a matter for speculation, but current theories invoke an immunological suppression mechanism.

Retinoblastoma. This is a tumour of infancy, the incidence of which is gradually rising and is now 1 in 20 000 live births in this country. Six per cent of the cases are familial and the genetic transmission is considered to be an autosomal dominant with poor penetration, although there is also an association with the D chromosome deletion syndrome in a few cases. In approximately half of the spontaneous and

Fig. 20.109 Extensive growth of retinoblastoma within the posterior part of the eye (*above*). × 2·5. The microscopic features include the typical rosettes (*below*). × 410

mitosis. A relatively common feature, which represents a tendency to differentiation and carries a better prognosis, is the 'rosette' which is a circular arrangement of the tumour cells (Fig. 20.109). Extraocular extension occurs either by spread along the optic nerve into the brain or through the sclera into the orbit. Metastases to visceral organs are a late and unusual event.

Glioma of the optic nerve. Gliomas occur in children and adults, but the behaviour differs remarkably between the two age groups. In children, proliferation of glial cells within the optic nerve causes proptosis and papilloedema when the nerve becomes thickened and vascular perfusion in the disc is disturbed. Nevertheless nerve conduction survives and tumour growth declines, so that some authorities consider childhood gliomas to be hamartomatous tumours. By contrast, the adult glioma resembles the glioblastoma multiforme (p. 723) in its morphology and behaviour.

21

Urinary System

The Kidneys

Fine structure and function

The kidneys are each composed of about one million nephrons, the major functions of which are to remove from the plasma various waste products of metabolism, and to maintain fluid and acid–base balances and normal levels of electrolytes. This is achieved by production of a very large volume of glomerular filtrate, which is subject to selective reabsorption as it passes

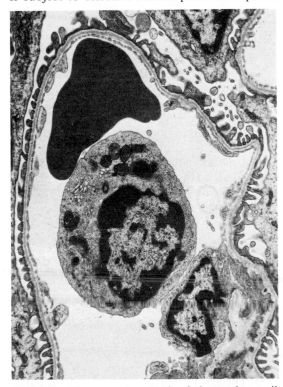

Fig. 21.1 Electron micrograph of glomerular capillary containing a lymphocyte and red cell. Note, from within outwards, the endothelial cytoplasm with fenestrations, the continuous basement membrane, and the foot processes of the epithelium. × 12 000.

down the tubules, urine representing what must be discarded for homoeostasis. Compared with most other organs, the blood flow of the kidneys is enormous; nearly all of this passes through the glomeruli, where 22% of the plasma volume (550 ml/min; 800 litres/day) is filtered off, giving a glomerular filtration rate (GFR) of 180 litres per day (120 ml/min). The process of filtration is doubtless aided by the unusually high pressure in the **glomerular capillaries**. The capillary walls (Fig. 21.1) consist of the vascular endothelium, which is unusual in having cytoplasmic fenestrations where the capillary basement membrane is lined only by an extremely thin endothelial membrane. Outside the basement membrane is a layer of visceral epithelial cells, termed *podocytes*, cytoplasmic processes (*foot processes* or *pedicels*) of which are in contact with the basement membrane: in

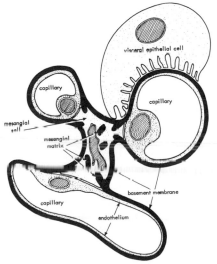

Fig. 21.2 Diagram of a glomerular lobule in cross section. (The fenestrations in the endothelial cytoplasm are not shown.)

the spaces (*slit pores*) between the foot processes the epithelial lining (*slit membrane*) is also extremely thin. Each glomerulus is composed of several lobules, the structure of which is depicted in Fig. 21.2. The capillary loops lie at the periphery of the lobules, while the core is made up of *mesangial cells*, which are capable of collagen production: it contains also basement membrane-like material.

In its passage along the tubules, all but approximately 1·5 litres of the daily 180 litres of glomerular filtrate, and most of its contained solutes, are reabsorbed. This is a process in which the tubule cells exhibit a high degree of selectivity, and some of the fine structural features of the epithelial cells can be related to their special functions. The epithelial cells of the **proximal convoluted tubule** have a prominent brush border, which is seen by electron microscopy to consist of numerous fine, relatively long microvilli (Fig. 21.3): this feature provides a very large surface area for absorption, and

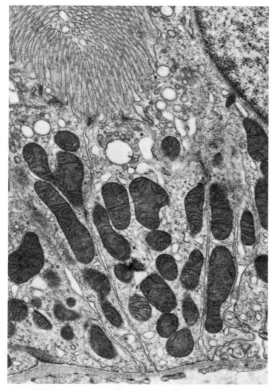

Fig. 21.3 Electron micrograph of parts of two epithelial cells of the proximal convoluted tubule, showing the microvilli (*upper left*) and numerous mitochondria. The basal part of the epithelium rests on a thin basement membrane. × 11 000.

four fifths of the fluid in the glomerular filtrate, together with most of its contained glucose, amino acids, and much of its sodium, potassium and phosphate are reabsorbed here. Reabsorption of these solutes is an active process, requiring energy and this may account for the large number of mitochondria in the epithelial cells. A third feature of these cells is the presence of pinocytic vesicles, which form on the luminal surface of the cells between the bases of the microvilli: there is normally some leakage of plasma proteins into the glomerular filtrate, and this is apparently taken up into these by pinocytosis and presumably metabolised by lysosomal enzymes. When, owing to various glomerular lesions, there is increased leakage of protein into the glomerular filtrate, the cells of the proximal tubules come to contain protein-rich droplets—*hyaline droplets* (Fig. 21.23, p. 764)—due to excessive protein absorption. Finally, the plasma membrane of the basal surface of the cells of the proximal convoluted tubule shows complicated infoldings which have the effect of increasing the surface area, and are probably important in the passage of reabsorbed fluid into the interstitial tissue, whence it enters the peritubular capillaries.

The cells of the **descending limb of Henle's loop**, and of the thin part of the ascending limb, are relatively simple, and their role in reabsorption is probably largely passive, and dependent on the constitutions of the tubular and interstitial fluids. By contrast, the cells of the **thick part of the ascending limb** have abundant large mitochondria (Fig. 21.4), and it is probable that these cells actively remove sodium chloride from the tubular fluid and pass it into the interstitial fluid. This has two effects; firstly, it provides a hypertonic interstitial fluid in the renal medulla, and this allows passive reabsorption of water from the descending and thin ascending parts of Henle's limb; secondly, it renders the tubular fluid hypotonic and facilitates further concentration in the distal convoluted tubule. It is probable that *aldosterone* exerts its sodium-retaining effect by stimulating reabsorption of Na^+ by the cells of the thick part of the ascending limb of Henle's loop. There is evidence that, like sodium chloride, urea undergoes partial recirculation in this counter-current system, thus aiding in passive reabsorption of water. This ingenious concentrating mechanism was suggested by Wirz (see

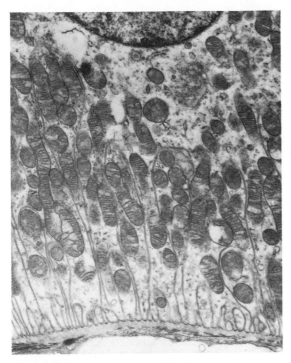

Fig. 21.4 Electron micrograph of the basal part of an epithelial cell of the thick part of Henle's loop. Note large elongated mitochondria situated between the complex infoldings of the basal cytoplasmic membrane. Portion of cell nucleus at top of picture. × 10 000.

Black, 1967) and has since received increasing support. The cells of the thick part of Henle's loop, and of the **distal convoluted tubule**, contain numerous microvesicles, and these may be related to their important functions of deaminating amino acids to produce ammonia, and of providing free hydrogen ion: secretion of NH_4^+ into the lumen by these cells plays an important role in maintaining acid–base balance, and results in an acid urine. Fluid entering the distal convoluted tubule is hypotonic, and isotonicity is restored here by passive reabsorption of water. As the fluid passes through the medulla in the collecting tubules, passive reabsorption of more water is again possible because the concentrations of sodium chloride and urea in the medullary interstitial fluid are high (see above). It is probable that these final adjustments in concentration are mediated largely by *antidiuretic hormone*, which presumably renders the cells of the distal convoluted and collecting tubules more permeable to water.

In addition to these complex tubular func-

tions, there is evidence that some substances are removed from the blood and actively secreted by the tubular epithelium. For example, creatinine and K^+ are reabsorbed in the proximal convoluted tubule, and the amounts appearing in the urine are dependent largely on their secretion, probably by the cells of the thick part of the ascending limb of Henle's loop and of the distal convoluted tubule. Excretion of administered diodone by the kidneys is dependent mainly on tubular secretion, and it may be used to assess tubular function.

In addition to their homoeostatic and excretory roles, the kidneys secrete renin, an enzyme which acts on a substrate in the plasma to produce angiotensin. The site of renin secretion is located in the granular cells of the afferent glomerular arterioles, which, together with the macula densa and the lacis, constitute the **juxtaglomerular apparatus** (Fig. 8.31, p. 221). Angiotensin has a direct effect on peripheral vascular resistance, and hence on blood pressure, and also stimulates the secretion of aldosterone by the adrenal cortex. These phenomena, and the fine structure of the juxtaglomerular apparatus, are described on pp. 221–3.

Another function of the kidneys is the production of **erythropoietin**, a factor stimulating the production of red cells.

Renal clearances. The renal clearance of a substance is an estimation of the volume of plasma completely cleared of that substance by the kidneys in one minute. It is calculated by measuring its concentration in the plasma (P), in the urine (U), and the volume of the urine (V) in ml per minute, and applying the formula

$$\text{Clearance} = \frac{U \times V}{P} \, \text{ml}$$

In the case of a substance which passes freely into the glomerular filtrate, and which is neither reabsorbed nor secreted by the tubules, renal clearance is a measure of glomerular filtration rate. This is approximately the case for inulin, which may be administered for the purpose of measuring the renal clearance. Of endogenous substances, clearance of urea is commonly measured, but 30–50% of the urea in the glomerular filtrate is normally reabsorbed, and accordingly the renal urea clearance (approx. 70 ml) is appreciably below that of inulin (approx. 120 ml). The clearance of creatinine is similar to that of inulin, but this results from a combination of reabsorption by the proximal tubule and secretion by the distal tubule, and is therefore not always a true indication of glomerular filtration rate in pathological states of the kidney.

Heterogeneity of nephrons. It has long been known that individual nephrons show morphological and circulatory differences—for example, in the length of Henle's loop. Thurau and his colleagues (see Horster and Thurau, 1968) have shown important functional differences between the majority of nephrons and the one-fifth of nephrons originating in glomeruli close to the cortico-medullary junction. By micropuncture of individual tubules, they showed differences in glomerular filtration rates, and differences in responses to low and high sodium loading. These findings, based on work on rat kidneys, are likely to apply to the kidneys of other mammals, including man, in which case they will necessitate a reconsideration of various aspects of renal function, both normal and in pathological states, since our present views are based largely on the assumption of a functionally homogeneous population of nephrons.

Important renal diseases

The kidneys are subject to the various general pathological processes which are considered in the earlier chapters of this book. Some of these are without serious effect, e.g. chronic venous congestion or deposition of pigments. Others, such as atrophy and hypertrophy, are of importance, but can be understood from the preceding accounts, and do not require further comment. Some of the general conditions are of particular significance when they affect the kidneys, for example amyloid disease and the various grades of cellular degeneration resulting from injury: these are considered more fully in appropriate sections of this chapter. **Inflammatory changes** of the kidneys are also of great importance: they include some types of glomerulonephritis, which are of special interest not only because of their serious effects on renal function, but also because the glomerular injury is known to result from antigen–antibody reactions, and this knowledge provides a logical basis for treatment and hope of prevention. Bacterial-induced inflammation—*pyelonephritis*—is also a common and important

condition, and will be described in some detail. Because of their excretory and concentrating role, the kidneys are susceptible to various **toxic chemicals**, and the brunt of toxic injury usually falls on the tubular epithelium, necrosis of which is a potentially fatal, but often treatable condition. **Renal tumours** are relatively uncommon, but the commonest malignant tumour—clear-cell renal carcinoma—is important clinically, for early diagnosis and removal carry a fair chance of cure. Finally, **renal homotransplantation**, now practised widely, is meeting with a high success rate, at least for some years following transplantation; one of the major hazards is immunological rejection of the transplanted kidney by the host (p. 138).

Pathological physiology of renal disease

Many of the diseases described in this chapter result in disturbances of renal function, and these are considered in more detail later. The three major disturbances which are responsible for most of the clinical features of renal diseases are as follows.

(1) Impairment of blood flow through the kidneys can result in **arterial hypertension** (**secondary** or **renal hypertension**): this is encountered commonly in glomerular disease, but can result from extensive renal scarring from various causes, and also from an extrarenal lesion, e.g. narrowing of the main renal artery by an atheromatous patch in the aorta.

(2) **Renal failure** ('uraemia') with accumulation in the body of urea and other nitrogenous waste products, disturbances of water and acid–base balances and of electrolyte levels, can result from a reduced glomerular filtration rate, from tubular injury, or from a combination of both. Since lesions which impair renal blood flow reduce the glomerular filtration rate, it is not surprising that renal failure and hypertension are commonly associated.

(3) There are a number of diseases which injure the glomerular capillaries and render them abnormally permeable to plasma proteins; heavy and prolonged albuminuria results in fall of the level of plasma albumin, and this can set in motion a train of events leading to generalised oedema. The combination of proteinuria, hypoalbuminaemia and oedema is known as the **nephrotic syndrome**.

Urinary casts. Increased leakage of plasma proteins into the glomerular filtrate results in proteinuria, most of the escaping protein being albumin. This is accompanied by the formation in the distal tubules of solid, cylindrical-shaped bodies, termed casts (Fig. 21.5), the presence of which in the urine indicates that the proteinuria is attributable to a renal lesion. When the proteinuria is unaccompanied by escape of cells

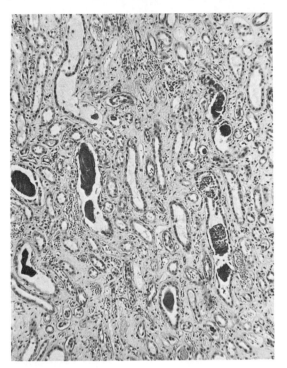

Fig. 21.5 Casts in the distal and collecting tubules. × 90.

in the urine, the casts are transparent and are termed *hyaline, colloid* or *protein* casts; their solid component consists largely of a protein—*Tamm Horsfall protein*—which is probably secreted normally by the epithelium of the distal convoluted tubule, and is precipitated to form casts by the presence of plasma albumin in the tubular fluid. When proteinuria is accompanied by escape of inflammatory cells into the tubular fluid, or desquamation of tubular epithelial cells, these become incorporated into the casts, giving *cellular casts* when the cells are largely intact and *granular casts* when the cells are disrupted. Similarly *blood casts* result from incorporation of red cells escaping into the glomerular filtrate or tubule, and *pigmented casts* from

incorporation of bilirubin when proteinuria accompanies obstructive jaundice, or haemoglobin or myoglobin in conditions giving rise to haemolysis or breakdown of skeletal muscle respectively.

Renal changes in hypertension

The general features of hypertension and the associated vascular changes, namely arteriosclerosis and arteriolosclerosis, have already been described (pp. 319–23). The latter are usually more pronounced in the blood vessels of the kidneys than in other organs, and result in various grades of renal injury. In chronic ('benign') essential hypertension, the renal injury is generally slight, and renal failure does not usually occur, but quite commonly there is some scarring of the kidneys. By contrast, the renal vascular lesions in accelerated (malignant) essential hypertension are severe, and renal failure is a common termination unless the blood pressure can be reduced.

Chronic glomerulonephritis and certain other diseases of the kidneys can result in hypertension—secondary hypertension—and when this occurs further renal injury ensues, indistinguishable from that seen in benign or malignant essential (i.e. primary) hypertension. A complex picture results, and it is advantageous to consider first the pure lesions of essential hypertension before proceeding to the pathology of the various renal diseases which are complicated by secondary hypertension.

Chronic ('benign') essential hypertension

Pathological changes. The renal changes in this disease are attributable to ischaemia resulting from arteriosclerosis and arteriolosclerosis (pp. 319–21).

The larger arteries in the kidneys, as elsewhere, become rigid and thickened, but their lumina are not seriously reduced, and may be enlarged. Similar changes occur in the arcuate arteries, but owing to their smaller calibre, thickening of the wall may result in reduction of the lumen: this is not uniform, and since the arcuates are, in effect, end arteries, ischaemia of patches of cortical tissue, seen as coarse depressed scars, may result. More commonly, ischaemia results from changes in the smaller vessels: the interlobular arteries become elongated and tortuous, with medial fibrosis and fibro-elastic thickening of the intima resulting in significant narrowing of the lumen. The afferent glomerular arterioles are also tortuous and show patchy hyaline thickening, the wall being acellular, homogeneous, eosinophilic, rather refractile and with various degrees of luminal narrowing (Figs. 21.6 and 13.17, p. 321). Regarding the nature of hyaline arteriolar

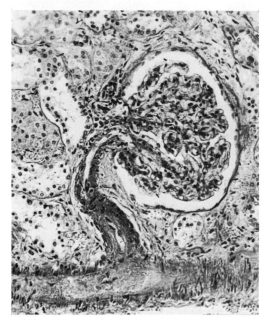

Fig. 21.6 Benign essential hypertension, showing great hyaline thickening of an afferent arteriole. × 180.

thickening, Lendrum (1969) has shown that at an early stage the hyaline material has the staining reactions of fibrin, and that as it ages the staining reactions come to resemble those of collagen. He has suggested that increased permeability of the vascular endothelium allows exudation of plasma constituents and that these form the hyaline material. He has termed the process *plasmatic vasculosis* and the older hyaline material *pseudocollagen*. This interpretation is now supported by histochemical, immunofluorescence, and electron microscopic studies, and provides a satisfactory explanation of the observed changes. These changes result in glomerular ischaemia, the glomerular tuft becoming shrunken and the capillaries gradually replaced by pale-staining homogen-

eous material, also believed to result from plasmatic vasculosis: eventually the whole tuft is converted to an acellular hyaline sphere (Fig. 21.7). This change is often accompanied by obliteration of the capsular space. The related tubules become atrophic and inconspicuous, and fibrous tissue, often infiltrated by lymphocytes, develops between the affected tubules

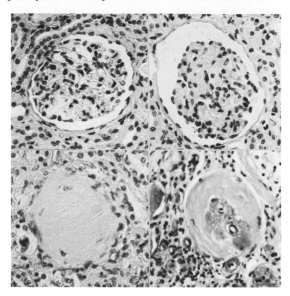

Fig. 21.7 Ischaemic changes in the glomeruli in chronic essential hypertension. The two glomeruli above show partial hyalinisation. The lower left is completely hyalinised and the lower right is collapsed, extensively hyalinised, and encased in fibrous tissue which has formed inside Bowman's capsule. Note its hyalinised afferent arteriole (seen *below*, containing a leukocyte). × 160.

and glomeruli. These changes in the small vessels, and consequent loss of nephrons and scarring, are distributed randomly throughout the cortex of both kidneys. It is probable that the arteriolar changes are more important than those in the interlobular arteries, for the destruction of nephrons does not follow a lobular pattern, but affects single scattered nephrons, while those around may appear healthy.

The destruction of nephrons described above proceeds very slowly, and at necropsy the kidneys may appear macroscopically normal apart from thickening of the arteries on the cut surface. However, enough nephrons are commonly lost to cause a slight or moderate reduction in size and diffuse thinning of the cortex: the capsule may be somewhat adherent, and the subcapsular surface diffusely and finely irregular (*granular*), contraction of scarred areas resulting in fine depressions (Fig. 21.8). In some long-

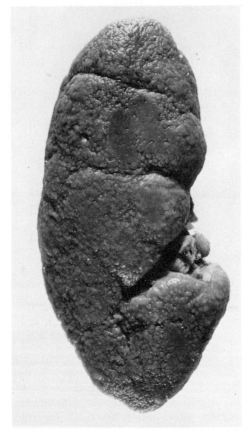

Fig. 21.8 Kidney in longstanding benign essential hypertension, showing slight reduction in size and granularity of the subcapsular surface. × 1.

standing cases, a sufficient number of nephrons may be lost to stimulate hypertrophy in those remaining, and the enlarged, hypertrophied tubules then contribute to the surface granularity (Fig. 21.9), but the kidneys are seldom very small, and renal function is not significantly impaired. In those patients who develop heart failure, the blood urea often rises, but this is attributable to inadequate renal blood flow, and is reversible if cardiac output again improves.

Accelerated (malignant) essential hypertension

This may arise *de novo*, usually at 35–45 years of age, or may supervene on benign essential hypertension. In the former case, the kidneys

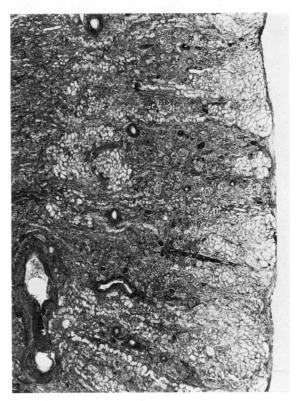

Fig. 21.9 Kidney in benign essential hypertension, showing foci of fine cortical scarring, with enlargement of the tubules in the unaffected cortical areas. Note also the arterial thickening. × 12·5.

are of normal size, and the subcapsular surface is smooth and spotted with dark red areas due to patches of congestion and haemorrhage. The main renal, segmental and arcuate arteries show the usual arteriosclerotic changes of hypertension. The interlobular arteries display great intimal thickening, due to formation of fine concentric layers of connective tissue and smooth muscle cells, with very severe reduction of the lumen (Fig. 21.10). They may also show fibrinoid necrosis of the wall, especially at their distal end. The afferent arterioles show fibrinoid necrosis, the wall being thickened, brightly eosinophilic, granular or homogeneous, and containing few or no living cells, but often pyknotic nuclei and red cells (Fig. 21.11): the necrotic material gives the staining reactions of fibrin, and the lumen is often completely obliterated, or occupied by thrombus which merges with the necrotic wall. The conspicuous fibrinoid necrosis may extend into the glomerulus, where it may involve parts or all of the

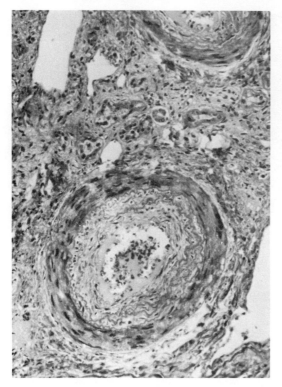

Fig. 21.10 Interlobular artery in malignant hypertension, showing gross intimal fibro-cellular thickening. × 100.

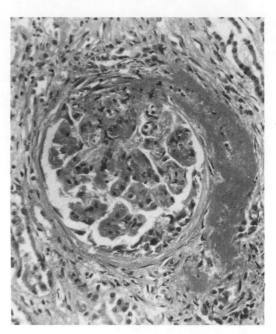

Fig. 21.11 Malignant hypertension. Fibrinoid necrosis of an afferent arteriole and of most of the glomerular tuft. Note also the aggregation of cells in the capsular space (*lower right*) to form a small crescent.

tuft. Other glomeruli are less severely damaged, and show intense capillary dilatation and congestion. There is often blood or exudate in the capsular space, and occasionally proliferation of the capsular epithelium to form a crescent (p. 762). The glomerular changes are the direct result of acute ischaemia resulting from fibrinoid necrosis of the afferent arterioles: this affects one arteriole after another, and even when death has resulted from renal failure, some are still unaffected and their corresponding glomeruli show little or no change. Some tubules show atrophy particularly of the proximal convoluted regions; others are of normal size or enlarged and hyaline droplets (p. 764) are conspicuous in the epithelial lining. Eosinophilic casts and sometimes red cells are seen throughout the length of some of the tubules.

Where malignant hypertension has supervened on benign essential hypertension, the changes corresponding to both conditions are seen in the kidneys. In recent years, the rapid downhill course of many patients with malignant hypertension has been arrested by antihypertensive drugs. Maintenance of the blood pressure below the very high levels of malignant hypertension prevents the severe lesions of the interlobular arteries, fibrinoid necrosis of the afferent arterioles, and the consequent rapid destruction of nephrons. Accordingly the prognosis has improved, particularly if treatment is begun before there is extensive renal damage. This suggests that fibrinoid necrosis of the arterioles is attributable to severe hypertension, and this is supported by various experimental observations; for example, partial clamping of one renal artery prevents fibrinoid necrosis in the clamped kidney in animals with severe hypertension (p. 324).

The vascular changes of malignant hypertension occur also in the other viscera, although the effect is not usually so devastating as in the kidneys: an example of a lesion in the intestine is illustrated in Fig. 13.18, p. 322.

Secondary hypertension

As already indicated, the vascular changes and consequent renal injury observed in essential hypertension occur also in hypertension secondary to other conditions. Various grades of persistent hypertension result from certain renal diseases, and depending on the height of the blood pressure and the rate of rise, the renal changes described above for benign or malignant essential hypertension become superadded to those of the renal disease which has caused the hypertension. Such secondary hypertensive lesions are an important factor in hastening failure of the already damaged kidneys.

Other vascular diseases

Senile arteriosclerosis. Although arteriosclerosis and arteriolosclerosis, and their associated renal changes, are seen particularly in hypertensives, they occur also in some normotensive old people, and the kidneys present the same features as in benign essential hypertension. Here also, the changes do not seriously impair renal function.

Atheroma occurs in the main renal arteries and their segmental branches, but is much less common than in other arteries of comparable size, and, except in diabetes mellitus, is rarely severe enough to interfere with the renal circulation: superadded occlusion by thrombosis is also rare. Disturbances arise more commonly from involvement and narrowing of the origins of one or rarely both renal arteries by aortic atheromatous plaques. This can lead to hypertension, presumably from ischaemia of one or both kidneys. Compared with essential hypertension, this is a rarity, but it is important to diagnose, for in some cases relief of the stenosis by a bypass operation, or removal of the ischaemic kidney, has resulted in cure of the hypertension. Such cases require careful investigation, including bilateral renal biopsy, for the non-ischaemic kidney may be damaged by hypertension or concomitant disease, e.g. pyelonephritis, and removal of the ischaemic kidney may then do more harm than good. The mechanism of hypertension in renal artery stenosis is discussed on pp. 222, 323.

Fibromuscular dysplasia of the renal arteries. This term includes several distinct abnormalities of the main renal arteries, affecting mostly the media, and including irregularities in thickness and in arrangement of the smooth muscle fibres, and irregular fibrosis. The changes are rare, and occur predominantly in women over a wide age range. They can give rise to renal artery stenosis or to dissecting or true aneurysms: we have observed a case in which an aneurysm of 3 cm. diameter compressed the renal pelvis and resulted in hydronephrosis.

The renal changes in *diabetes mellitus* are described on p. 779, and those of *polyarteritis nodosa* on p. 771.

Glomerulonephritis

The term glomerulonephritis embraces a group of diseases in which the renal lesions are primarily glomerular, other changes in the kidneys resulting from the glomerular injury. Lesions due to infection of the kidneys (pyelonephritis) are not included in the group, and although no type of glomerulonephritis is fully understood, there is now very strong evidence that most types are due to injury caused by antigen–antibody complexes deposited in the walls of the glomerular capillaries. Much of this evidence is based on work with animals, and some of the more important experimental findings will be described before turning to human glomerulonephritis.

Experimental immunological glomerular injury

This is of two main types, one due to deposition, in the glomerular capillary walls, of antigen–antibody complexes formed in the plasma (immune-complex glomerulonephritis), the other to the reaction of antibody with the glomerular capillary basement membrane (nephrotoxic-antibody glomerulonephritis).

Immune-complex glomerulonephritis

A basic knowledge of the features of immune-complex disease (pp. 123–27) is necessary to the understanding of the following account, which concentrates on the nature and pathogenesis of the glomerular lesions of experimental immune-complex disease.

When a single large injection of a suitable antigen is administered to an animal (e.g. bovine serum albumin to rabbits), antibody appears after a week or so and reacts with antigen still present in the plasma to form immune complexes. At first these are formed in gross antigen excess and consist of only 2–4 molecules: such small complexes remain in the circulation and do not appear to cause glomerular lesions. As antibody production increases, larger complexes are formed until, at antigen–antibody equivalence, the complexes form large insoluble aggregates (Fig. 4.3, p. 90) which are rapidly removed from the circulation by phagocytes and are not deposited in the walls of vessels. Between these two extremes there is a period of a few days during which **complexes of intermediate size** are formed (Fig. 5.7, p. 125): these are deposited in the walls of blood vessels, especially the glomerular capillaries, where they induce lesions. In chronic immune-complex disease, in which multiple injections of antigen are administered at frequent, e.g. daily, intervals, chronic glomerular injury results in those animals in which the antibody levels and amounts of antigen injected are such that there is intermittent or continuous formation of intermediate-sized immune complexes in antigen excess over a long period.

The mechanism of immune-complex deposition has not been fully elucidated. For complexes to penetrate into the walls of capillaries and other vessels there must be an increase in endothelial permeability: this may be brought about by activation of complement by circulating complexes, with consequent formation of anaphylatoxins (p. 124), or a type I hypersensitivity reaction, mediated in the rabbit via basophils and platelets (p. 125), may be involved.

Why are the glomeruli involved? Not only are the glomeruli an important and sometimes the sole site of deposition of circulating immune complexes, but complexes deposited in this site persist much longer than those deposited elsewhere in the walls of blood vessels. It is likely that the predilection of the glomeruli for deposition is due, at least in part, to the unusually high filtration pressure in glomerular capillaries and to the relative thickness of the glomerular

capillary basement membrane and its special function of filtering large volumes of plasma fluid.

The types and pathogenesis of glomerular injury. Three major types of glomerular lesion are seen in immune-complex disease. The first is a **diffuse inflammatory lesion** affecting all the glomerular capillaries. It consists of swelling and proliferation of endothelial and mesangial cells and variable infiltration of the capillary walls by polymorphs. It is accompanied by increased permeability of the capillary basement membrane with leakage of plasma proteins and escape of red cells and polymorphs into the urinary space: these abnormal constituents appear in the urine. The second type of lesion is a **focal inflammation**, affecting only parts of some glomeruli. Both types of inflammatory lesion may occur in acute or in chronic immune-complex disease: both vary in severity from mild inflammation to necrosis. The acute diffuse lesion, unless unduly severe, will resolve. The focal lesions tend to result in scarring, as do chronic diffuse lesions. The third type of glomerular injury is termed **membranous change**. It occurs only in chronic immune-complex disease and consists of diffuse thickening of the glomerular capillary basement membrane but without associated inflammatory change. It is accompanied by increased permeability and proteinuria but usually without escape of cells.

Among the many factors which probably influence the nature and severity of the glomerular lesions, Germuth and Rodriguez (1973) have emphasised the importance of the size of the circulating immune complexes and the rate of their deposition in the glomerular capillaries. **The acute diffuse inflammatory lesion** develops when relatively small intermediate complexes are present in the plasma in high concentration. Immunofluorescence shows granular or irregular deposits of immune complex distributed diffusely in the capillary walls: at first they are scanty and sometimes even undetectable; later they may become more prominent and persist for some weeks before finally disappearing. Electron microscopy usually shows no more than occasional discrete deposits of immune complex on the epithelial side of the capillary basement membrane. If, as most workers believe, immune complexes are responsible for the acute inflammatory lesion, then it is likely that they are pathogenic when deposited in relatively small amounts in the inner part of the capillary wall, i.e. subendothelially. At this site the products of complement fixation are likely to cause direct injury to the capillary wall and also, by chemotactic activity, attract polymorphs which phagocytose the complexes but in doing so release lysosomal enzymes and so cause tissue injury. There may well be other, as yet unknown, pathogenic mechanisms of the inflammatory lesion. The small complexes diffuse through the basement membrane and form aggregates which, as noted above, may be visible in electron micrographs, and which account for the granular pattern on immunofluorescence microscopy.

Focal inflammatory lesions appear to result from deposition of relatively large intermediate complexes subendothelially. Such complexes tend to be phagocytosed rapidly and so removed from this site by the mesangial cells and it is only when this clearance mechanism is overwhelmed that capillary lesions appear: failure of a mesangium is thus followed by an inflammatory focus in that lobule. This explanation is supported by the demonstration of immune complexes and complement in the mesangial cells and, when focal lesions are present,

also in the adjacent parts of the capillary walls. These sites of complex deposition are confirmed by electron microscopy. Being relatively large, the complexes do not diffuse into the basement membrane.

In chronic immune-complex disease, diffuse inflammatory lesions usually occur in those animals in which high plasma concentrations of relatively small complexes are formed. Low concentrations of small complexes are associated with gradual development of the **membranous change**. Immunofluorescence shows very heavy discrete, 'granular' deposits of immune complexes and complement scattered diffusely along the capillary walls (Fig. 21.12), and electron microscopy shows these deposits to lie in the outer part of the capillary basement membrane (Fig. 21.13). This results from

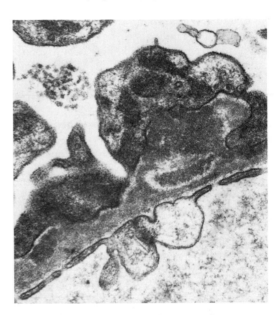

Fig. 21.13 Electron micrograph of segment of glomerular capillary wall in experimental immune complex glomerulonephritis, showing dense nodular deposits in outer part of basement membrane (capillary lumen below; urinary space above). × 25 000.

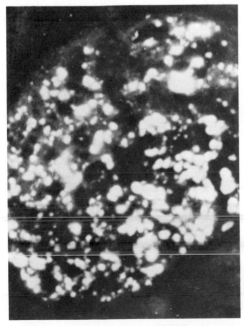

Fig. 21.12 Experimental foreign-protein glomerulonephritis. Irregular deposition of immune complexes in the capillary walls, shown by fluorescent antibody to IgG. (Professor R. Lannigan.)

prolonged but slow deposition of small complexes. At no time are they present in the inner part of the capillary wall in sufficient concentration to induce inflammatory change. The complexes gradually diffuse through the basement membrane and become arrested in its outer part. Although they appear to activate complement in this site, the activation products are liable to be carried away by the filtrate into the urinary space and thus do not cause inflammatory change.

Virus-induced immune-complex glomerulonephritis is of interest because it can occur naturally in animals and is a possible cause of human glomerulonephritis. A good example is provided by infection of mice with the virus of lymphocytic choriomeningitis (p. 694). When the infection is acquired *in utero*, immune tolerance to the virus develops and although the mouse remains infected, lesions do not develop until, in adult life, tolerance declines and antibody to the virus develops. This forms complexes with virus antigen in the plasma, with consequent development of chronic immune-complex glomerulonephritis.

Auto-immune-complex glomerulonephritis is also of possible relevance to human disease. The classical example was provided by Heymann and his colleagues, who administered to rats injections of rat kidney homogenate together with Freund's adjuvant. The animals developed chronic membranous glomerulonephritis which was subsequently shown to be of immune-complex nature and resulted from development of antibody to a constituent of the brush border of epithelial cells of the renal proximal convoluted tubule. This epithelial constituent is apparently released in very small quantities into the blood. It does not normally stimulate antibody production but when antibody production is stimulated artificially, low concentrations of immune complex are formed continuously in the plasma and are deposited in the glomeruli. This experimental condition illustrates the formation of small soluble pathogenic immune complexes in the plasma *in antibody excess*. This is likely to happen with small antigenic molecules possessing few determinant sites or when antibody develops against very few types of antigenic determinant: the latter situation is liable to arise in auto-immune responses, as in this example. Auto-immune-complex glomerulonephritis has also been observed to result in rabbits from immunisation with heterologous thyroglobulin: The antibodies react with the rabbit's own thyroglobulin, which is present in the plasma in low concentration, and immune-complex glomerulonephritis results.

Another important example is provided by 'New Zealand' hybrid (NZB/NZW) mice, which develop spontaneously an illness closely resembling human systemic lupus erythematosus. It is characterised by the production of auto-antibodies to various cellular constituents, including DNA, and by various lesions including immune-complex glomerulonephritis. A chronic virus infection may be involved in the aetiology of this condition.

Nephrotoxic-antibody glomerulonephritis

This condition was first described by Lindemann in 1900 although it is commonly known as 'Masugi-type' nephritis. The experimental disease is produced by immunising an animal, e.g. a duck or rabbit, by injection of crude kidney homogenate, or more purified glomerular basement membrane, from an animal of another species, e.g. a rat. The duck or rabbit develops antibody which, when injected into a rat, reacts with the glomerular capillary basement membrane and induces an acute diffuse glomerulonephritis. The antibody bound to the basement membrane can be seen by the immunofluorescence technique as a continuous, or 'linear' pattern (Fig. 21.14). Both complement and polymorphs appear to play a pathogenic role, for the severity of the glomerular injury can be reduced by lowering the level of plasma complement (e.g. by injection of cobra venom factor, which inactivates C3), or by inducing neutropenia (e.g. by injection of

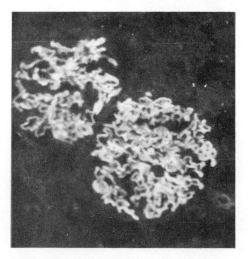

Fig. 21.14 Nephrotoxic-antibody nephritis; linear deposition of nephrotoxic antibody in the glomerular capillary walls, demonstrated by the immunofluorescence technique. (Professor R. Lannigan.)

nitrogen mustard). Injection of doses of nephrotoxic antibody too low to cause direct injury is followed, after some days, by glomerulonephritis which is due to the development of antibody which reacts with the foreign (duck or rabbit) IgG bound to the basement membrane. This delayed injury is now known to differ basically in its pathogenesis from post-streptococcal glomerulonephritis in man, but interest in the experimental disease has been revived by the demonstration by Steblay that injection of sheep with homologous or heterologous basement membrane material results in the development of auto-antibody, some of which reacts with the sheep's own glomerular basement membrane and produces a severe and rapidly progressive glomerulonephritis. The experimental auto-immune condition has since been produced in rabbits and rats and nephrotoxic auto-antibody to basement membrane has been shown to be responsible for some cases of a very severe, rapidly progressive form of human glomerulonephritis.

Glomerulonephritis in man

Classification

The widespread practice of renal biopsy is now providing much information about the histological changes of glomerulonephritis and particularly about the early stages, while immunological studies are providing important aetiological clues. However, there is still much to be learned, and classifications of glomerulonephritis must be regarded as provisional, in the knowledge that modifications will be necessary in the coming years.

As regards the recognition of different types of glomerulonephritis, a major contribution was made by Volhard and Fahr (1914) and has since formed the basis of most classifications of this group of diseases. More recent classifications by Longcope and by Ellis have proved useful, but are now known to be oversimplifications and have fallen into disuse.

In the classification of glomerulonephritis proposed overleaf, we have selected, from the terms in common usage, those which seem to us to indicate best the major glomerular changes.

It must be emphasised that this classification is not intended to be comprehensive. Moreover, some of the types probably include more than one disease entity. Certain other conditions, e.g. systemic lupus erythematosus, diabetes mellitus and amyloidosis, can give rise to glomerular lesions resulting in clinical syndromes resembling one or other types of glomerulonephritis, and it seems appropriate to discuss them together with or immediately after glomerulonephritis.

Acute diffuse proliferative glomerulonephritis

General features. This relatively common type of glomerulonephritis occurs at all ages, but particularly in children and young adults. It affects males more often than females and usually follows an acute infection with Group A haemolytic streptococci—most often pharyngitis (including scarlet fever), but sometimes infections of the middle ear or skin. In many cases, the disease develops 1–4 weeks after the onset of the streptococcal infection, and very often this has settled down and there is a latent period of apparent well-being before glomerulonephritis becomes apparent.

The presenting clinical feature is usually puffiness of the face or discoloration of the urine. Puffiness is due to oedema and affects especially the lax tissues of the eyelids: it is most noticeable in the morning and tends to subside during the ambulatory day. Oedema may affect other parts of the body: in some cases it is more severe and is then seen to be generalised. The blood pressure is commonly raised, and in most cases the rise is slight or moderate.

Biochemical changes. There is usually a mild or moderate rise in the level of blood urea. The urine is diminished in volume, of high specific gravity, and commonly brownish and turbid ('smoky') from the presence of altered red cells. There is moderate proteinuria and, as in all types of glomerulonephritis, the protein is mainly plasma albumin. Quantitative analysis reveals that larger protein molecules, e.g. IgG, are also usually present in appreciable amounts and the proteinuria is thus not a highly selective albuminuria. Microscopy of the urine shows many red cells, moderate or large numbers of neutrophil polymorphs, and hyaline, granular or cellular casts (p. 749).

Course of the disease. Ninety-five per cent of children who develop acute diffuse glomerulonephritis recover completely after an illness lasting a week or two. In adults the condition

CLASSIFICATION OF GLOMERULONEPHRITIS

Recommended	*Alternatives*
Acute diffuse proliferative	Acute post-streptococcal; acute; acute diffuse
Rapidly progressive	Subacute; subacute azotaemic; subacute extracapillary
Membranous (*a*) Nephrotic stage (*b*) Chronic stage	Idiopathic membranous (*a*) Subacute; hydraemic stage; subacute intracapillary (*b*) Chronic or azotaemic stage
Membranoproliferative	Mixed; mesangiocapillary
Lobular (*a*) Nephrotic stage (*b*) Chronic stage	—
Minimal-change	Lipoid nephrosis; light-negative
Focal	
Chronic	Chronic azotaemic

tends to be more severe or persistent and only about 60–70% of patients make a complete and permanent recovery.

Some patients die in the acute stage from the effects of hypertension, e.g. acute heart failure, or from acute renal failure. In others the glomerular lesions and clinical features persist and get progressively worse, causing death from hypertension and renal failure within two years: these patients are correctly classified as *rapidly progressive glomerulonephritis* (p. 761). In a small proportion of patients proteinuria persists long after apparent recovery from the acute attack: proteinuria for several months is consistent with complete recovery but when it continues for over a year, and particularly when there are also some red cells and leukocytes in the urine, it is very likely that the glomerular injury, although clinically silent, is progressing; such patients are liable to develop *chronic glomerulonephritis*, with hypertension and renal failure, at any time within the next twenty years or so.

Pathological features. In acute diffuse proliferative glomerulonephritis the cortex is pale and distinctly enlarged due to oedema. In fatal cases the cortex is up to twice the normal thickness, pale, and the glomeruli may be just visible with a hand lens as light grey dots projecting from the cut surface.

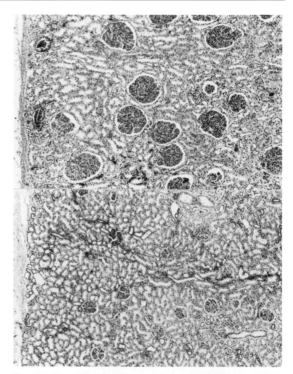

Fig. 21.15   The renal cortex in acute diffuse proliferative glomerulonephritis (*above*) compared with the cortex of a normal kidney (*below*). Note the gross enlargement and hypercellularity of the glomeruli. × 30.

Microscopically, the appearances are similar in biopsy and necropsy material. The most conspicuous changes are diffuse enlargement and increased cellularity of the glomeruli (Fig. 21.15). The enlargement results in narrowing or obliteration of the capsular space. When a glomerulus happens to have been cut in the appropriate plane, part of the glomerular tuft can often be seen to have herniated into the lumen of the first part of the tubule (Fig. 21.16). The capillary lumina appear narrowed, and the endothelial and probably mesangial cells are swollen and increased in number. Neutrophil polymorphs are seen in the glomeruli but vary considerably in number from case to case.

An additional change in the glomerular tufts is an increase in the number of strands of basement-membrane-like material demonstrable by electron microscopy in the mesangial regions. These strands are normally present between mesangial cells and are made more conspicuous by oedema. In cases which fail to resolve the material apparently increases considerably and contributes to the hyaline appearance of the glomeruli in the chronic stage of glomerulonephritis.

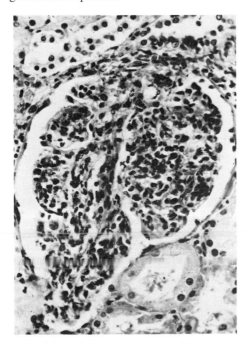

Fig. 21.16 Glomerulus in acute diffuse proliferative glomerulonephritis, showing swelling and increased cellularity of the glomerular tuft, which has herniated into the proximal tubule. × 200.

Electron microscopy shows localised deposits of granular material, mostly projecting from the outer surface of the basement membrane (Fig. 21.17), while in some cases there are deposits also on the inner surface of the basement membrane.

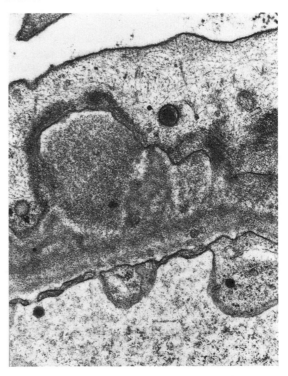

Fig. 21.17 Electron micrograph of part of glomerular capillary wall in acute diffuse glomerulonephritis, showing a large granular sub-epithelial deposit. Note also fusion of the foot processes (lumen below, urinary space above). × 50 000.

The podocytes (p. 745) do not show widespread fusion of foot processes, although this may occur focally. Some proteinous debris, and occasionally red cells, may be seen in the narrowed capsular spaces. In most cases, the epithelium of Bowman's capsule appears normal, but here and there some proliferation may be seen. Epithelial crescents (p. 762) are few or absent in typical cases.

Changes in the rest of the kidney are secondary to the glomerular lesion: there is diffuse oedema, seen as an increase in the loose interstitial tissue between the tubules, and often accompanied by a light scattering of polymorphs or mononuclear cells. The tubules contain proteinous and cellular casts, including red cells, and the epithelial cells of the proximal convoluted tubules contain hyaline droplets (p. 764). Occasionally there are foci of disruption of tubular epithelial cells, possibly attributable to ischaemia secondary to the glomerular changes. Hypertension is not usually sufficiently severe or prolonged to produce changes in the heart and blood vessels.

With recovery from the disease the glomeruli return to normal, although increased numbers of cells in the mesangial zones of the glomerular lobules may persist for months, and are regarded as a retrospective diagnostic feature.

Clinico-pathological correlation. In acute diffuse glomerulonephritis, light- and electron-microscopy show narrowing of the glomerular capillary lumina attributable to increase in number and size of glomerular cells. Some impairment of blood flow through the kidneys might be expected, and indeed the renal plasma flow has been shown to be reduced in some cases, but is normal in others. However, the fraction of plasma filtered off by the glomeruli (the glomerular filtration fraction) is reduced, and hence the total *glomerular filtration rate* (GFR) is also less than normal. This largely explains the usual rise in the blood urea level, although ischaemic injury of the tubular epithelium may play a part by impairing the functional selectivity of reabsorption.

The factors concerned in the production of oedema and oliguria in acute diffuse glomerulonephritis are not yet fully understood. The point is made several times in this chapter that the *volume* of urine produced, and its *concentration*, are dependent mainly on tubular reabsorption and not on the GFR. Two important factors in tubular reabsorption are, firstly the concentration of solutes remaining in the lumen (i.e. not reabsorbed)—a high concentration of solute, e.g. urea, produces an osmotic diuresis by interfering with reabsorption of water (p. 766); secondly, the pituitary antidiuretic hormone, which increases reabsorption of water. It is not clear what part these and other factors play in the oliguria and oedema of acute diffuse glomerulonephritis: the subject is discussed more fully on p. 219. The transient hypertension of this disease is presumed to result from decreased renal blood flow (p. 324).

Urine. It seems reasonable to assume that the appearance of protein, red cells and leukocytes in the urine is attributable directly to the glomerular lesion. It must be admitted, however, that the severity of the glomerular changes does not correlate closely with the amount of protein or numbers of cells escaping in the urine. It is probable that the basement membrane is the main crude filter in the glomerular capillary wall, in which case the glomerular lesion must result in increased permeability of the capillary basement membrane, the pathogenesis of which is discussed below.

In a small proportion of patients with acute diffuse glomerulonephritis, proteinuria is unusually heavy and the nephrotic syndrome results. At the other extreme are patients with the usual clinical and histological changes of acute diffuse glomerulonephritis but little or no proteinuria.

Unfavourable histological features. Thrombosis and necrosis of individual glomerular capillaries, glomerular haemorrhages, deposition of fibrin and the development of numerous large epithelial crescents are all indications of unusually severe glomerular injury and carry the risk of death in the acute disease. There is no sharp dividing line between such severe cases and rapidly progressive glomerulonephritis (p. 761).

Following acute diffuse glomerulonephritis, increase in the size and number of mesangial cells may persist for weeks or even months without serious sequelae. Increase in basement-membrane-like material in the mesangial areas is, however, a more serious feature; it is seen, together with persistent cellular increase, in those few cases which, after a latent period, develop chronic glomerulonephritis.

Aetiology. Immunofluorescence microscopy of renal biopsy material in cases of acute diffuse glomerulonephritis typically reveals granular deposition of immunoglobulin (usually mainly IgG) and components of complement in the glomerular capillary walls (Fig. 21.18). These findings, together with the detection by electron microscopy of dense sub-epithelial deposits (Fig. 21.17), are strongly suggestive of the deposition of immune complexes, and the diffuse inflammatory glomerular changes also resemble those of experimental acute 'small-complex' glomerulonephritis (p. 754). As acute glomerulonephritis usually follows a streptococcal infection it is likely that antibodies to streptococcal products, appearing a week or so after the infection, combine with streptococcal antigens still present in the plasma, thus providing immune complexes which would, at first, be formed in the presence of antigen excess. Attempts to demonstrate streptococcal antigen in the glomerular deposits have provided conflicting results: in general, detection of antigen has been reported mostly in biopsy material obtained early in the course of the disease, and it is likely that, later on, the deposited antigen

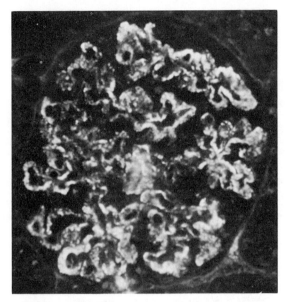

Fig. 21.18 Renal biopsy in acute diffuse glomerulonephritis. Immunofluorescence technique, showing granular and ill-defined deposition of IgG in the glomerular capillary walls. × 350.

becomes coated, and thus obscured, by an excess of antibody. Still later, immunofluorescence microscopy may reveal complement components alone, the antibody, in turn, having apparently been obscured by complement. The difficulty in demonstrating streptococcal antigen in the glomeruli is not surprising because similar difficulty has been experienced in demonstrating antigen in experimental acute immune-complex glomerulonephritis, in which not only is the antigen known, but powerful antibodies are usually available to facilitate its detection by immunofluorescence microscopy. It is not understood why certain types of Group A streptococci, notably Griffiths types 12, 4, 1, 25 and 49, are nephritogenic, whereas other types and other micro-organisms are not.

As in the experimental condition, the mechanisms by which deposited immune complexes cause glomerular injury are not fully elucidated. The acute injury is probably due to the presence of complexes in relatively small amounts in the inner part of the capillary wall: the sub-epithelial aggregates appear at a relatively late stage of the disease and are unlikely to be of early pathogenic importance, as explained on p. 755. At an early stage, there is a fall in the level of serum complement (which is further evidence consistent with the presence of circulating immune complexes), and it is likely that local complement activation, polymorph activity and perhaps the clotting mechanism, all contribute to the acute capillary injury.

Rapidly progressive glomerulonephritis

This usually fatal condition may develop without known predisposing cause, or may follow a streptococcal infection. It can supervene also in patients with the focal glomerulonephritis associated with certain diseases (p. 770). It can occur at any age, and is commoner in males than females. The clinical features and urinary changes may be indistinguishable at first from those of acute diffuse glomerulonephritis (p. 757), but instead of regressing after a week or two, become progressively more severe, and without haemodialysis death usually results from uraemia and hypertension after a period of a few weeks to a year or so. Rarely, proteinuria may be severe enough to give rise to the nephrotic syndrome. In other cases, severe oliguria or even anuria lead to early death.

Rapidly progressive glomerulonephritis is much less common than acute diffuse glomerulonephritis, but because of its severity it makes an important contribution to the number of individuals dying of renal failure.

Pathological changes. The kidneys are normal in size or enlarged due to oedema: on section the cortex is pale, but may show petechial haemorrhages, and the glomeruli stand out conspicuously as grey dots, visible with a lens on the cut surface. In most cases, there is little or no gross scarring and the surface of the kidneys is smooth.

Microscopy shows the most important changes to be glomerular. As in acute diffuse glomerulonephritis, there is proliferation of endothelial and probably mesangial cells with narrowing of the capillary lumina, and variable polymorph infiltration of the tuft (Fig. 21.19). Although all the glomeruli are affected, some glomerular lobules may be more severely involved than others, and there may be necrosis and thrombosis of capillaries or lobules.

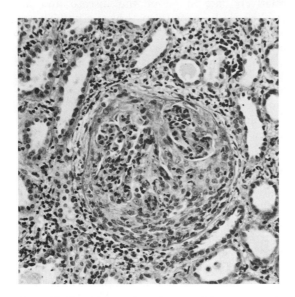

Fig. 21.19 Glomerulus in rapidly progressive glomerulonephritis, showing destruction and fibrosis of parts of the tuft, hypercellularity of the remainder, and formation of a large crescent around the tuft. × 200.

A surprising feature of the disease is the rapidity with which glomerular scarring may occur: thus in cases with a history of only 2 weeks or so, biopsy may reveal sclerosis of lobules or whole glomeruli, and also fibrous adhesions between the tuft and Bowman's capsule (Fig. 21.20). There is thus a combination of glomerular proliferation, necrosis, thrombosis and scarring, amounting to very severe glomerular injury.

A most characteristic histological feature is proliferation of the parietal epithelium of Bowman's capsule to form '*epithelial crescents*' (Figs. 21.19, 21.20) which occupy the capsular space and surround the tuft. (This change used to be known as *extracapillary glomerulitis* to distinguish it from changes in the glomerular tuft, which were termed *intracapillary*: the terms have now largely lost their usefulness). Formation of epithelial crescents occurs in other diseases, for example in subacute bacterial endocarditis, malignant hypertension, and in some cases of acute diffuse glomerulonephritis, but the crescents are neither so numerous nor so large as in rapidly progressive glomerulonephritis, in which they may fill and distend the capsular space of most glomeruli. Crescent formation is not understood, but fibrin deposits are usually demonstrable by immunofluorescence in the crescents, and they are generally

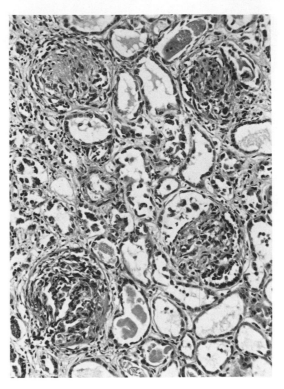

Fig. 21.20 Rapidly progressive glomerulonephritis. The four glomeruli show severe destruction; the lowest one shows crescent formation and the upper two have undergone rapid scarring. The tubules are dilated and there is extensive loss of epithelium. × 110.

associated with severe glomerular injury. In time, the epithelial crescents are usually replaced by fibrous tissue. Study of glomerular explants in tissue culture has led to a recent suggestion that the crescents are composed of macrophages.

The tubules may be dilated (Fig. 21.20), and usually contain hyaline and cellular casts and red cells, and proteinous droplets are present in the cells of the proximal convoluted tubules. There may be focal necrosis or irregular tubular atrophy and increase of intertubular connective tissue, presumably due to ischaemia resulting from the glomerular changes.

In some cases hypertension is severe, and the changes of malignant hypertension (p. 751) become superadded. There may also be left ventricular hypertrophy, and changes associated with uraemia, e.g. fibrinous pericarditis, anaemia and superadded infections.

The glomerular changes result in severely impaired renal blood flow and consequent reduction in GFR: the clinical and biochemical changes are similar to those in acute diffuse glomerulonephritis, but becoming progressively more severe.

Aetiology. This is a heterogeneous group. Some cases, including those with a preceding streptococcal infection, are unusually severe examples of immune-complex glomerulonephritis, as indicated by granular deposition of IgG and complement in the glomerular capillary walls and dense sub-epithelial deposits seen by electron microscopy. The prognosis appears to be rather less grave in such cases, particularly when post-streptococcal. Some other cases show good evidence of nephrotoxic auto-antibody glomerulonephritis similar to the experimental condition (p. 757): there is linear deposition of IgG and complement on the capillary basement membrane, antibody to basement membrane can be eluted from the excised kidneys, and may become detectable in the serum following bilateral nephrectomy (performed prior to renal transplantation). Such eluted or serum antibody has been shown to be capable of inducing nephrotoxic-antibody glomerulonephritis in monkeys, and the disease has sometimes recurred in kidneys transplanted into patients. These observations confirm the view that failure to detect nephrotoxic antibody in the serum (before nephrectomy) is attributable to its absorption by glomerular basement membrane *in vivo*. Nephrotoxic antibody has been observed especially, but not exclusively, in those patients with Goodpasture's syndrome (p. 772).

The nephrotic syndrome

This is described here because it is an important feature of some of the types of glomerulonephritis dealt with below.

The·syndrome occurs when prolonged and severe proteinuria results in **hypoalbuminaemia** and consequently in **generalised oedema**. The proteinuria is virtually always due to increased glomerular capillary permeability and amounts in adults to the daily loss of 10 g or more of plasma protein. As indicated below, it can be brought about by the glomerular lesions of many different diseases and diagnosis of the cause of the condition often requires renal biopsy. Conditions other than the renal disease which bring about hypoalbuminaemia, e.g. chronic malnutrition or protein-losing enteropathy, are similarly accompanied by generalised oedema.

The nature of the oedema and factors involved in its development have been discussed on p. 219. Another common feature of the syndrome is **hyperlipidaemia**, increase in levels of lipoproteins of lower density often being considerable. This biochemical change is unexplained and the evidence on its causation is conflicting.

Pathological changes. In addition to generalised oedema, including free fluid in the body cavities, there is a high risk of infections, and before the introduction of sulphonamides and antibiotics a high proportion of patients used to die of pneumonia, peritonitis or meningitis.

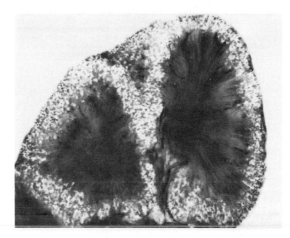

Fig. 21.21 Kidney in nephrotic syndrome, showing abundant cortical deposits of neutral fat and anisotropic lipids. (Photographed through crossed iodide films.) × ⅘.

The kidneys show striking changes in the nephrotic syndrome. These include generalised enlargement and pallor due to oedema, and frequently a yellow, radial streaking of the cortex due to deposition of lipids (Fig. 21.21). The combination of increased glomerular capillary permeability (responsible for the heavy proteinuria) and hyperlipidaemia results in leakage of relatively large amounts of lipoprotein into the glomerular filtrate: some of this is reabsorbed and deposited in the tubular epithelial cells or in the interstitial tissue of the cortex (Fig. 21.22). There may be accumulation of 'foamy' lipid-laden macrophages and also giant-cell

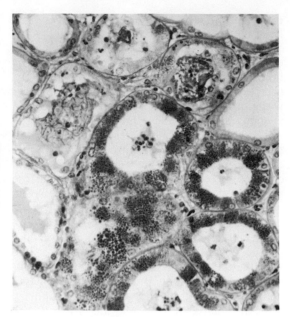

Fig. 21.23 Hyaline droplets in renal tubular epithelium resulting from reabsorption of protein from the filtrate.

Causes of the nephrotic syndrome are numerous. In children, minimal-change glomerulonephritis is much the commonest cause, followed by acute diffuse glomerulonephritis. In adults, the acute diffuse, membranous and minimal-change types of glomerulonephritis are about equally common, followed by membranoproliferative glomerulonephritis, renal amyloidosis, diabetes, systemic lupus erythematosus and increased renal venous pressure, as in renal vein thrombosis or congestive heart failure.

In some reports, chronic glomerulonephritis is regarded as a relatively common cause of the nephrotic syndrome. This is probably a matter of nomenclature, for some forms of glomerulonephritis and other renal lesions manifest as the nephrotic syndrome, which may persist for years, and then progress to glomerulosclerosis with reduced renal blood flow and so diminished GFR, leading to renal failure: frequently the proteinuria diminishes as this stage develops and the nephrotic syndrome subsides, but in some cases there is a combination of nephrotic syndrome and chronic renal failure.

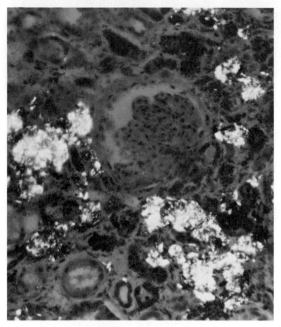

Fig. 21.22 Kidney in nephrotic syndrome, showing abundant anisotropic lipid with some sudanophil neutral fat (dark) in the interstitial tissue and tubules. (Polarised light with crossed Nicol prisms.)

granulomas around crystals of cholesterol. Hyaline droplets due to reabsorption of protein are abundant, along with globules of lipid, in the cytoplasm of the lining cells of the proximal convoluted tubules (Fig. 21.23) and protein casts are present in the distal tubules.

The glomeruli in patients with the nephrotic syndrome show the pathological features of the causal disease. The only feature common to most cases is seen by electron microscopy and consists of loss of the foot processes of the epithelial cells, the cytoplasm of which is closely applied to the outer part of the glomerular basement membrane (Fig. 21.32): this is not specific for the nephrotic syndrome and experimental work suggests that it is a *result* of proteinuria and not its cause.

Idiopathic membranous glomerulonephritis

Clinical features. This disease is commoner in males than females, and occurs over a wide age range, but more often in adults than in children. It presents as *the nephrotic syndrome*, i.e. heavy proteinuria, generalised oedema and hyperlipidaemia (see above). The oedema develops gradually, often being first noticed in the face, and only partly influenced by gravity. It eventually becomes severe and generalised, with free fluid in the pleural and pericardial cavities. Proteinuria is marked, and as a result the plasma albumin level falls, usually to below 16 g per litre. The urine often contains small numbers of red cells, and analysis of the protein reveals significant quantities of globulins in addition to the high concentration of albumin: the urine tends to be concentrated and reduced in volume, but can still vary considerably to accommodate fluid intake.

With effective antibiotic therapy for infections (a common and formerly fatal complication of the nephrotic syndrome), the nephrotic stage may fluctuate for months or years, eventually tending to subside and to be replaced by the chronic stage which presents as chronic renal failure (p. 775) and is clinically indistinguishable from other forms of chronic glomerulonephritis.

Remissions may be prolonged, and probably about half the patients are alive, and some are in remission, 10 years after the onset. Because of the fluctuating course, it is not known whether steroids or other immunosuppressive drugs affect the ultimate prognosis: their immediate effect is disappointing.

Pathological changes. The essential change is in the glomeruli, and consists of a diffuse hyaline thickening of the walls of all the glomerular capillaries. In the early stages this is minimal and hard to detect, but it becomes increasingly obvious as the disease progresses. There is no obvious swelling or proliferation of endothelial or mesangial cells, and no leukocytic infiltration. By light microscopy the capillary walls appear thickened, eosinophilic and hyaline (Fig. 21.24) and silver staining techniques give an appearance of spikiness of the basement membrane (Fig. 21.25). Electron microscopy shows irregular deposition of dense amorphous material in the outer part of the capillary basement membrane, and thickening of the basement membrane between the deposits (Fig. 21.26) corresponding to the spikes seen by light microscopy of silver preparations. There may also be deposits of dense

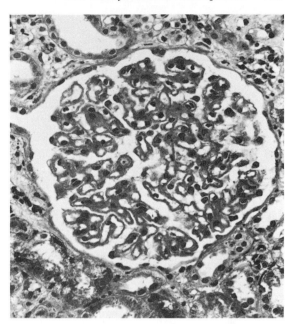

Fig. 21.24 Idiopathic membranous glomerulonephritis. The capillary basement membrane is diffusely and uniformly thickened. × 350.

material between the basement membrane and capillary endothelium, but this is not usually conspicuous and is often absent. At first, the glomerular capillary lumina do not appear to

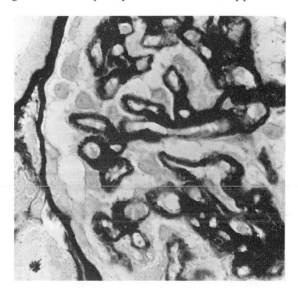

Fig. 21.25 Part of a glomerulus in idiopathic membranous glomerulonephritis, stained by silver impregnation technique and showing, in places, the characteristic spiky appearance of the capillary basement membrane. × 1200.

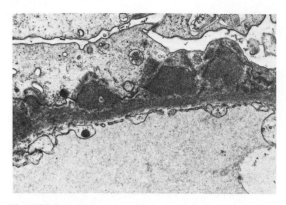

Fig. 21.26 Electron micrograph of segment of glomerular capillary wall in membranous glomerulonephritis (lumen below, urinary space above). The basement membrane is thickened and there are multiple, almost confluent dense deposits on its outer surface. × 16 000.

be narrowed, and ischaemic tubular changes are not seen. Eventually the electron-dense deposits are incorporated in the basement membrane which then shows considerable thickening. The other changes seen in the kidneys at this stage are common to the nephrotic syndrome from all causes (p. 763).

In the chronic stage of the disease, the thickening of the glomerular capillary walls results in narrowing of the lumina; renal blood flow and GFR are seriously diminished, and uraemia and hypertension develop. Proteinuria diminishes, polyuria often develops, and the oedema tends to subside and may disappear.

Microscopy of the kidneys at this stage shows

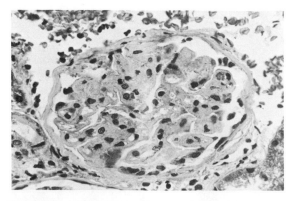

Fig. 21.27 The glomerular change in idiopathic membranous glomerulonephritis which has progressed to the stage of chronic renal failure. The thickening of the basement membrane has resulted in severe narrowing of some glomerular capillaries and obliteration of others.

gross diffuse thickening of glomerular capillary walls, some glomeruli being almost solid eosinophilic hyaline material, while others are less severely affected and still have some patent capillary lumina (Fig. 21.27). Tubular atrophy from ischaemia accompanies the glomerular hyalinisation, and interstitial fibrosis occurs, but lipid deposits, indicative of the preceding nephrotic stage, may persist. The kidneys may be slightly shrunken, and may show the superadded changes of hypertension. The pathological features of the chronic stage are compared with those of other forms of chronic glomerulonephritis on p. 775.

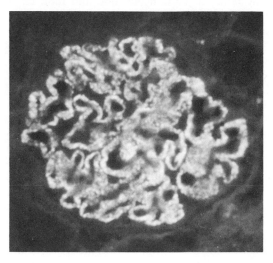

Fig. 21.28 Renal biopsy in membranous glomerulonephritis. Immunofluorescence technique, showing granular deposition of IgG in the glomerular capillary walls. × 250.

Aetiology. Examination of renal biopsies by immunofluorescence microscopy shows deposition of immunoglobulin, usually mainly IgG, along the walls of the glomerular capillaries (Fig. 21.28). The deposition is diffuse throughout all the capillaries and, at an early stage, appears granular. As the disease progresses the deposits increase in size and number and tend to become confluent. Deposition of complement is also usually demonstrable by immunofluorescence: its distribution is the same as that of immunoglobulin but it is deposited in smaller amounts and in some cases is not detectable. These features, together with the dense deposits in the outer part of the basement membrane seen by electron microscopy and the gradual uniform thickening of the capillary basement membrane, provide a close parallel to experimental immune-complex glomerular injury of the chronic 'small-complex' type (p. 755) and the nephrotic syndrome is a major feature of both conditions. The common termination of the human disease in a stage of glomerulosclerosis with chronic renal failure is seen also in those forms of the experimental condition which are progressive, i.e. when foreign protein injections are continued over a long period or in the auto-immune form of the disease in rats.

Although the evidence for immune-complex deposition in membranous glomerulonephritis is strong, the disease is still idiopathic in the sense that the nature of the antigen is unknown. In a few cases 'Australia antigen' has been detected in the blood and in the glomerular deposits. Membranous glomerulonephritis can also result from immune responses to microbial infections, e.g. in quartan malaria and syphilis, while the auto-immune reactions involving DNA, etc., in systemic lupus erythematosus sometimes produce a closely similar condition (p. 772). Identification of the antigen(s) involved in the idiopathic condition might open the way to specific immunotherapy and is thus of practical importance.

Membranoproliferative glomerulonephritis

This condition occurs at all ages but particularly in older children. Its presenting features may resemble closely those of acute diffuse proliferative glomerulonephritis, or there may be symptomless proteinuria or development of the nephrotic syndrome.

In general the outlook is poor, although some patients may recover. The course extends over a variable number of years. At some stage the nephrotic syndrome is likely to develop and many cases terminate in chronic renal failure. Response to steroids, etc., has so far not been very encouraging.

Pathological changes. At an early stage the glomeruli show diffuse proliferative change with increase in size and number of mesangial and endothelial cells; the mesangia in particular show increased cellularity and the lobular pattern of the glomeruli is accentuated (Fig. 21.29). The capillary lumina are reduced and there is irregular thickening of their walls. Silver stains

show, here and there, a double basement membrane, and electron microscopy shows that the cytoplasm of mesangial cells has extended into the capillary walls along the endothelial side of the basement membrane and that, in places, a second layer of basement-membrane-like material has formed between the mesangial and

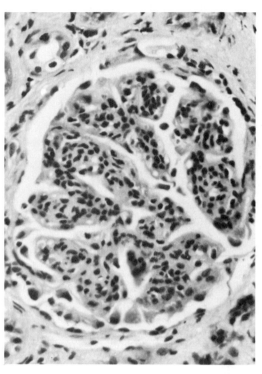

Fig. 21.29 Membranoproliferative glomerulonephritis. The glomerular lobulation is accentuated, there is increased cellularity, and thickening of capillary walls. × 350. (This would formerly have been regarded as lobular glomerulonephritis.)

endothelial cells. Electron microscopy may also show dense, discrete deposits on the outer side of the original basement membrane and more diffuse deposits between the two layers.

As the disease progresses the mesangial cells diminish in number and hyaline material accumulates, while the capillaries become progressively thickened so that glomerulosclerosis and chronic renal failure usually result.

The aetiology of this condition is unknown. In many cases there is granular deposition of complement components in those parts of the capillary walls outlining the lobules: there may also be deposition of IgG with a similar distribution (Fig. 21.30) but this is not always found. In some cases there appears to be good evidence of a preceding streptococcal infection and the disease could be an unusual form of immune-complex injury. In many cases the level of serum complement is low. There is, however, some evidence that complement activation may be proceeding by the alternate pathway (p. 116): the plasma levels of C3 and subsequent complement components tend to be reduced

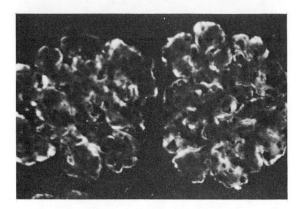

Fig. 21.30 Immunofluorescence staining of two glomeruli in a case of membranoproliferative glomerulonephritis, showing deposition of IgG at the margins of the lobules. × 200. (Dr. J. M. Vetters.)

and a factor which activates C3 (*the nephritic factor*) has been detected in the serum in some cases. Also, deposits of properdin, which is involved in activation by the alternate pathway, have been reported in the glomeruli in some cases.

Lobular glomerulonephritis

This condition resembles membranoproliferative glomerulonephritis in its clinical features. The main histological difference is that there is much greater deposition of eosinophilic hyaline material in the mesangial areas, which are relatively acellular. Immunofluorescence staining usually shows deposition of IgG and complement at the periphery of the lobules, as in membranoproliferative glomerulonephritis, and the two conditions are probably closely related.

Minimal-change glomerulonephritis

While this name is not altogether satisfactory, it is preferable to the more commonly used *lipoid nephrosis* because it indicates that the essential lesion is glomerular and that the structural changes are inconspicuous.

General features. The disease has a peak incidence in children between 1 and 4 years old, but occurs in children and adults of all ages. It is by far the commonest cause of the nephrotic syndrome in children. The oedema and proteinuria tend to fluctuate, spontaneous remission and recurrences being common. The blood pressure and blood urea are usually normal and tests of inulin clearance have confirmed that, in most cases, there is no detectable fall in glomerular filtration rate. As usual in the nephrotic syndrome (p. 763), there is a rise in the level of blood lipids, including cholesterol.

Formerly, there was a high mortality from superadded infections developing in the severely oedematous patient, but the outlook has been improved greatly by the use first of sulphonamides and later of antibiotics. Glucocorticoid therapy has also improved the prognosis, for it cuts short the disease by suppressing the proteinuria. Steroid therapy usually takes 2–3 weeks to show an effect, and the mechanism is quite unknown: there is a risk of relapse on stopping therapy, and at present there is no way of predicting the cases in which this will occur. The progress of large series of children has been observed for some years by Arneil and Lam (1967) and by others, and it appears that the prognosis is good, although a minority of patients eventually develop renal failure with uraemia and hypertension (see below).

The long-term prognosis in adults developing this disease is uncertain. The eventual development of chronic renal failure appears to be more common than in children.

The proteinuria is due to increased glomerular capillary permeability, and is usually highly selective, albumin being accompanied by only very small amounts of the plasma proteins of larger molecular size; this contrasts with the less highly selective proteinuria observed in most other renal diseases, with or without the nephrotic syndrome. The urine contains lipid-rich protein casts and in some cases microscopic, or occasionally macroscopic, haematuria.

Pathological changes. Some patients still die from infection supervening on the nephrotic syndrome and the kidneys show the usual features of this syndrome (p. 763).

Microscopically, the glomeruli look normal apart from an appearance of fixed dilatation of the capillaries; there is no thickening of the capillary walls and no increased cellularity of the glomerular tufts (Fig. 21.31). The most conspicuous glomerular change on electron microscopy is fusion of the foot processes of the

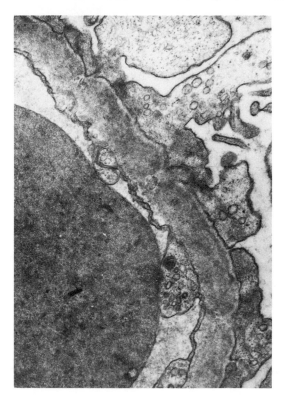

Fig. 21.32 Electron micrograph of glomerular capillary wall in minimal-change glomerulonephritis. The only abnormality is fusion of the foot processes. × 18 000.

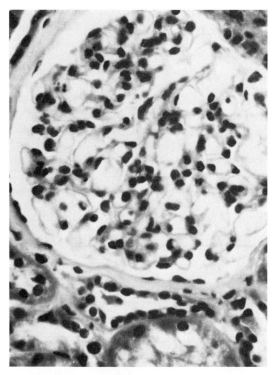

Fig. 21.31 Minimal-change glomerulonephritis. The glomerulus shows no obvious abnormality apart from dilatation of many of the capillaries. × 560.

epithelial cells, the basement membrane being covered externally by a layer of epithelial cell cytoplasm (Fig. 21.32): the epithelial cells also show increased vacuolation and in some cases the basement membrane is slightly thickened with loss of definition of the junction between its inner margin and the cytoplasm of the adjacent endothelial cells. As already explained (p. 764), fusion of the foot processes is probably a result, rather than the cause, of proteinuria. It appears that a reversible increase in the permeability of the capillary basement membrane, not reflected in any obvious structural change, is responsible for the heavy proteinuria and consequent changes in this disease.

Aetiology. The nature of this disease remains unknown. It may follow immediately on a respiratory infection, but does not show a definite relationship to any particular micro-organism. Immunofluorescence studies have failed to demonstrate deposition of immunoglobulin or complement in the glomerular capillary walls, and the aetiology is quite obscure, as is the mechanism of the beneficial effect of steroid therapy in curtailing the albuminuria.

Focal glomerulosclerosis. It is not yet known whether this condition, which was described by Rich in 1957, is a variant of minimal-change glomerulonephritis or a distinct entity. The clinical features are similar to those of minimal-change glomerulonephritis, but proteinuria is less selective and red cells are more commonly present in the urine. Although most of the glomeruli appear normal, those close to the medulla show sclerosis, consisting of deposition of hyaline material with consequent obliteration of capillaries: this change is at first focal but gradually destroys whole glomeruli and extends peripherally to involve more glomeruli.

There is associated tubular atrophy. Renal biopsy is only diagnostic if it includes some of the deeper, affected glomeruli. The condition is resistant to steroid therapy and, although most series of cases are small, it is clear that the prognosis is relatively poor, there being a high risk of chronic renal failure. It is not clear whether those patients diagnosed as minimal-change glomerulonephritis who eventually develop chronic renal failure are really missed cases of focal glomerulosclerosis.

Congenital nephrotic syndrome is a rare familial condition which develops within a few weeks of birth, does not respond to steriods, and has a bad prognosis. The glomeruli may be mostly normal or show various abnormalities and there is usually marked dilatation of the proximal convoluted tubules. Immunological changes have been reported, but the nature of the abnormality is unknown.

Focal glomerulonephritis

This may be defined as a glomerulitis affecting only a proportion of the glomeruli. The lesions usually involve only part of the glomerular tuft,

e.g. one or more lobules. In most cases the condition is 'idiopathic', i.e. of unknown cause, although sometimes the onset is associated with acute respiratory infections. It occurs also as a feature of certain specific diseases, notably subacute bacterial endocarditis, in which the glomerular lesions may be embolic, and also systemic lupus erythematosus, anaphylactoid (Henoch–Schönlein) purpura, the microangiopathic form of polyarteritis nodosa, and the rare Goodpasture's syndrome. It must be emphasised that focal glomerulonephritis is not the only renal lesion which occurs in these conditions: rapidly progressive glomerulonephritis may develop in any of them, and is the common lesion in Goodpasture's syndrome.

Haematuria is the usual presenting feature of focal glomerulonephritis, but in some patients it gives rise to heavy proteinuria and the nephrotic syndrome.

Pathological changes. The glomerular lesion consists of a cellular proliferation, probably of mesangial cells, affecting the peripheral part of one or more lobules (Fig. 21.33), and in some cases accompanied by fibrinoid necrosis of capillary loops: within the lesions, individual

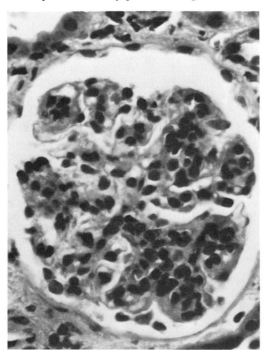

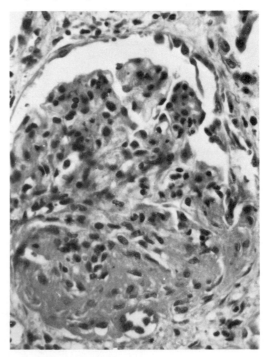

Fig. 21.33 Idiopathic focal glomerulonephritis: early lesion. Note the hypercellularity of the affected part of the tuft on the right. × 350.

Fig. 21.34 Focal glomerulonephritis: late lesion. The lower part of the tuft is scarred and adherent to the capsule. × 350.

capillary lumina may be obliterated by eosino-philic thrombus which blends with the necrotic capillary walls. Red cells may be present in the capsular space and in the tubules, and there may also be some proliferation of the epith-elium lining Bowman's capsule. Lesions may occur in only a small proportion of glomeruli, or may involve the majority. In patients with a long history, old scarred glomerular lesions are usually seen (Fig. 21.34), often adherent to the capsule. In cases developing the nephrotic syn-drome, the renal changes consequent upon this condition (p. 763) may also be evident.

While this account is concerned mainly with focal glomerulonephritis, opportunity is taken below to outline also the additional renal lesions which occur in those diseases of which focal glomerulonephritis is a feature.

Idiopathic focal glomerulonephritis. When it occurs apart from specific diseases, focal glomerulonephritis is usually related to ill-defined respiratory infections, including pharyngitis, 'colds' and 'flu'. In contrast to acute diffuse glomerulonephritis, there is no special relationship with Group A streptococcal infections, and the interval between the respiratory infection and the onset of renal disease is only a day or so. Haematuria is often the presenting feature and is usually of not more than a few days' duration. In most cases, there is only mild proteinuria and the illness subsides with no evidence of residual impair-ment of renal function. Some patients are subject to recurrences, each associated with a respiratory infec-tion, and these may occur over many years: there is evidence that chronic renal failure eventually super-venes in a minority of cases. Patients presenting with the nephrotic syndrome have been observed to recover without evidence of residual impaired renal function. The condition is not common: it occurs particularly in children and young adults, more often males than females. Its aetiology is discussed below.

Subacute bacterial endocarditis. Renal lesions are commonly present in this condition, but in most cases they do not lead to serious impairment of renal function and their practical importance lies mainly in the resulting haematuria, either gross or microscopic, which is of diagnostic value.

As in other organs, infarcts are common in the kidneys in subacute bacterial endocarditis and are usually non-suppurative. Focal glomerulonephritis occurs in about 50% of cases, and tends to develop after some months. Most of the cases have been caused by *Streptococcus viridans* or *Haemophilus influenzae*. Macroscopically, the kidneys are usually of normal size, and show petechial haemorrhages visible on the subcapsular surface and scattered throughout the cortex. Microscopically, a minority

of the glomeruli are usually affected, and the focal lesions show capillary thrombosis, fibrinoid necrosis and proliferative changes (Fig. 21.35). Blood is often seen in the capsular space and tubules, and there may be epithelial crescents. Bacteria cannot usually be seen in the glomerular lesions, but have been recovered in some cases.

In a minority of patients with subacute bacterial endocarditis, diffuse proliferative glomerulonephritis develops, and may progress to renal failure.

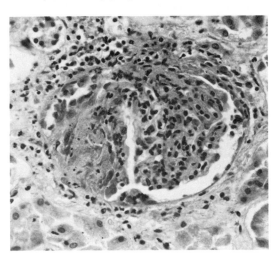

Fig. 21.35 Glomerulus in subacute bacterial endocarditis, showing a large focal necrotic glomer-ular lesion, with inflammatory infiltration around. × 200.

Polyarteritis nodosa. The necrotising arteritis which is the essential lesion of this condition usually involves the larger arteries in the kidneys, with aneurysm formation and/or thrombosis, and renal infarcts are commonly present (Fig. 13.31, p. 330). In about one-third of cases, death results from renal failure with hypertension. In the *micro-angiopathic variant* of polyarteritis, the vascular lesions show the same features—fibrinoid necrosis and inflammatory changes—but involve mainly the interlobular arteries (Fig. 13.29, p. 330), afferent glomerular arterioles, and also the glomerular capillaries, giving rise to focal glomerulonephritis. As the disease progresses, most of the glomeruli may be involved and renal failure may develop, although hypertension is less common than in the classic form of the disease.

Anaphylactoid purpura occurs mainly in children, and gives rise to a skin rash, joint pains and colic with bloody diarrhoea due to a haemorrhagic exudate into the gut. In some cases there is a focal glomerulonephritis, with haematuria and proteinuria, but renal failure is either absent or mild and transient, and the kidneys usually recover completely, even after recurrent at-tacks. Rapidly progressive glomerulonephritis may, however, supervene, and in some other cases chronic renal failure develops after some years.

Goodpasture's syndrome. In this rare condition, haemorrhage from the alveolar capillaries gives rise to haemoptysis, accompanied by haematuria and proteinuria attributable to focal glomerulonephritis. The outlook is poor: pulmonary haemorrhage may become increasingly severe and the renal lesion usually develops into rapidly progressive glomerulonephritis. The glomerular injury is caused by auto-antibody to basement membrane (see below).

Systemic lupus erythematosus (SLE). Clinically apparent renal disease occurs in over 50% of patients with this disease, and carries a poor prognosis. The nephrotic syndrome may develop when proteinuria is heavy, and uraemia, with or without hypertension, is an important cause of death. The essential changes are in the glomeruli, which show a great variety of lesions. These include (1) focal glomerulonephritis which is indistinguishable from the proliferative and necrotising lesions described above except that haematoxyphil bodies (p. 878) are sometimes apparent; (2) a focal thickening of the capillary walls with a refractile eosinophilic appearance, known as the wire-loop lesion (Fig. 21.36); (3) hyaline thrombi in individual glomerular capillaries; (4) various combinations of diffuse proliferative and irregular membranous change; (5) diffuse membranous change resembling that seen in idiopathic membranous

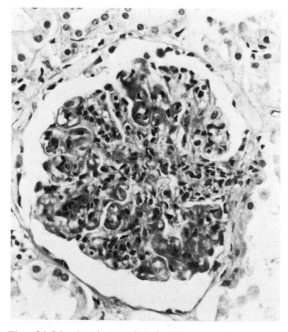

Fig. 21.36 A glomerulus in systemic lupus erythematosus, showing hyaline thickening of some of the capillaries—the 'wire-loop' lesion, and a more diffuse increase in cellularity. × 300.

glomerulonephritis. The duration of these various lesions, and thus the degree of glomerular sclerosis, also vary greatly. Immunofluorescence and electron microscopy provide strong evidence that these glomerular changes represent the spectrum of immune-complex injury as described on pp. 754–6. For example, the focal lesion is accompanied by deposition of immunoglobulin and complement in the mesangia and focally in the inner parts of the capillary walls: more extensive deposition of complexes in the inner parts of the capillary walls is seen in the combination of diffuse proliferative and patchy membranous change, while the diffuse granular pattern of deposition, much of it along the outer part of the basement membrane, is seen in the diffuse membranous lesion. Antibody to DNA has been eluted from the kidney tissue in SLE and there is good evidence that DNA is an important antigenic constituent of the pathogenic complexes. Curious bodies, which may be of viral origin, have also been reported with increasing frequency in the endothelial cells in SLE.

Depending on whether or not the nephrotic syndrome has been present and on the nature and duration of the renal lesions, the kidneys in SLE may be enlarged and pale, of normal size, or small and scarred. The degree of tubular atrophy and interstitial fibrosis will depend upon the nature of the glomerular lesions and there may also be changes resulting from hypertension.

Renal failure is the most important cause of death in SLE and attempts to arrest the glomerular lesions by corticosteroids, cytotoxic drugs and other agents have so far been only partially successful.

Aetiology of focal glomerulonephritis. Idiopathic focal glomerulonephritis is probably not a single entity. In some cases aggregates of immunoglobulin and complement are detectable by immunofluorescence microscopy in the mesangia and in the walls of occasional capillaries. These features are similar to the findings in the experimental focal glomerulonephritis associated with deposition of relatively large immune complexes (p. 755). In occasional cases the immunoglobulin is predominantly IgA and the significance of this is obscure: in others, immunofluorescence tests for Ig and complement are negative.

The available evidence suggests that the diseases which focal glomerulonephritis accompanies are attributable to abnormal immunological reactions. The evidence is strongest in the case of systemic lupus erythematosus (see above). Anaphylactoid purpura, as its name suggests, is widely regarded as a hypersensitivity disease, and the antigens which may be concerned include streptococci and certain foods. Deposition of IgG and C3 is commonly demonstrable in the mesangia and focally in the glomerular capillary walls. Lesions resembling those of polyarteritis nodosa occur in serum sickness, and fixed immunoglobulins have been observed in the early vascular lesions, although evidence for immune-complex deposition in the glomeruli is not convincing.

In subacute bacterial endocarditis the prolonged infection provides a possible basis for immunological injury from circulating antigen–antibody complexes, and the long-held view that the focal glomerular lesions of this

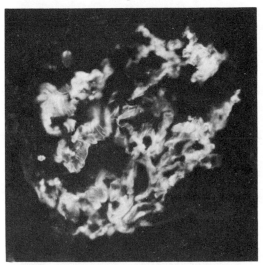

Fig. 21.37 Antibody to glomerular capillary basement membrane showing the characteristic linear pattern of staining by the immunofluorescence technique. Necropsy specimen in Goodpasture's syndrome.

condition are embolic is no longer widely accepted. Antibody to capillary basement membrane is demonstrable in Goodpasture's syndrome (Fig. 21.37).

While the above immunological findings suggest a possible common basis for focal glomerulonephritis, the pathogenesis of the lesions is still largely obscure.

Chronic glomerulonephritis

It is apparent, from the foregoing descriptions of the various types of glomerulonephritis, that an end stage may be reached in which total glomerular function is so reduced that chronic

renal failure develops: this is characterised by uraemia and usually by hypertension. The time taken to reach this stage, and the rate of progression once it has developed, vary with the type of preceding glomerulonephritis, and also in individual cases. Hypertension, sometimes of the accelerated (malignant) type, usually develops and aggravates the renal tissue destruction, leading, if untreated, to end-stage renal failure which progresses rapidly to death. In cases where hypertension is absent or less severe, renal failure may progress more slowly, and the end stage may last for several years.

In over 70% of patients with chronic glomerulonephritis, there is no history to suggest preceding renal disease, and the renal lesions have progressed silently until chronic renal failure develops. In such cases, it is often not possible to decide, even by histological examination of the kidneys, what type of glomerulonephritis has led up to the chronic stage. In other cases, there is a history of previous glomerulonephritis: this may have been an acute attack of post-streptococcal glomerulo-

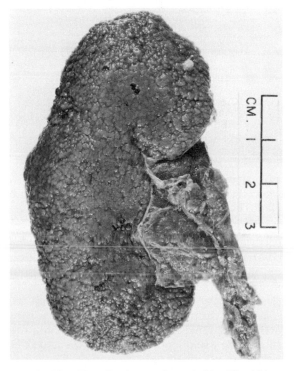

Fig. 21.38 Chronic glomerulonephritis. The kidney is uniformly shrunken, in this case to about half the normal size, and the surface is diffusely granular.

nephritis years before, or the patient may have had membranous, membranoproliferative or recurrent focal glomerulonephritis, which has progressed to the stage of chronic renal failure.

Pathological changes and pathogenesis. Both the kidneys are uniformly and equally reduced in size, sometimes only slightly so, but often to about one-third of normal (Fig. 21.38). In those kidneys which are greatly shrunken, the capsule is often firmly adherent and the sub-capsular

tical mottling and haemorrhages of this condition are superimposed on the changes described above. The other organs and tissues show the changes of chronic renal failure (p. 778).

Microscopically, in the small granular kidneys, it is common to find all degrees of hyalinisation of glomeruli; a small percentage are normal, or nearly so, and may be hypertrophic (Fig. 21.41). Many are completely hyalinised (Fig. 21.40) and some show partial destruction.

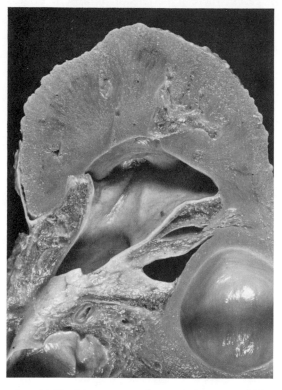

Fig. 21.39 The cut surface of the same kidney shown in Fig. 21.38, showing diffuse cortical thinning. The cyst is incidental. × 2.

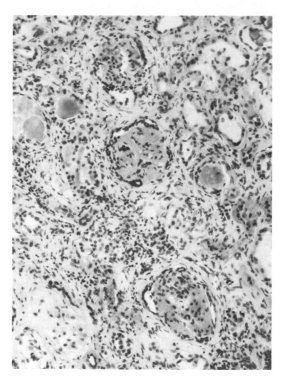

Fig. 21.40 Chronic glomerulonephritis, showing hyalinisation of glomeruli; the tubular epithelium is atrophic and there is interstitial fibrosis. × 100.

surface uniformly and finely irregular ('*granular contracted kidney*'). There is diffuse thinning of the cortex (Fig. 21.39), which accounts largely for the reduction in kidney size, while the medullary pyramids are also, although less markedly, shrunken. The amount of fatty tissue around the renal pelvis is increased. In contrast to chronic pyelonephritis, the calyces and renal pelvis are not distorted.

The renal arteries and their major branches show arteriosclerotic thickening, and in cases complicated by malignant hypertension the cor-

In cases in which the kidneys are not greatly shrunken the glomeruli are usually more uniformly damaged: this is seen in the chronic end stages of membranous and membranoproliferative glomerulonephritis.

The arcuate and interlobular arteries and the afferent arterioles show hypertensive changes which are likely, by causing ischaemia, to have contributed to the glomerular scarring. When malignant hypertension has supervened the consequent changes (Fig. 21.11, p. 752) are seen in those glomeruli which have not been destroyed already by the glomerulonephritic process.

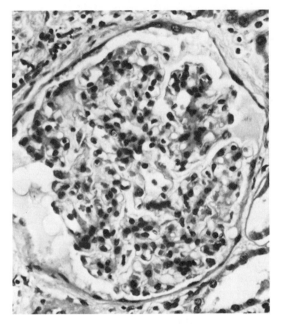

Fig. 21.41 A relatively healthy, hypertrophied glomerulus in chronic glomerulonephritis. × 250.

The tubules show extensive atrophy, many being completely lost, and there is an increase in the intertubular connective tissue and irregular interstitial aggregation of lymphocytes and usually small numbers of plasma cells. In cases with some near-normal hypertrophied glomeruli, the corresponding tubules are enlarged and conspicuous, and account for the

elevations which give the sub-capsular surface its granular appearance. These surviving functioning tubules may show hyaline droplets in the epithelial cytoplasm, and frequently contain protein casts (p. 749), features which relate to the proteinuria: when malignant hypertension has supervened, there may be blood in the capsular spaces and in functioning tubules.

In cases of chronic glomerulonephritis preceded by the nephrotic syndrome, the kidneys may still be enlarged, and lipid deposits may still be visible in the cortex by the naked eye. Although the glomeruli show advanced sclerosis, their appearance may still suggest the type of glomerulonephritis responsible, e.g. membranous (see Fig. 21.27). All the glomeruli are affected to some extent, and the tubular atrophy is accordingly more uniform, without prominent enlarged tubules: for this reason, the surface of the kidney is often smooth and does not exhibit the granularity usual in chronic glomerulonephritis.

Clinical features. Most patients developing chronic glomerulonephritis are between 10 and 50 years old. The clinical features and changes in other organs and tissues are those of *chronic renal failure* and are attributable to *uraemia*, usually accompanied by *hypertension*. Since chronic renal failure results also from various other diseases of the kidneys, a description common to all causes seems appropriate, and is given below.

Chronic Renal Failure

Chronic renal failure results when the functions of the kidneys have been so reduced by a chronic disease process that there is retention of nitrogenous waste products normally excreted mainly in the urine, and loss of the capacity of the kidneys to maintain homoeostasis of fluid and electrolytes and acid–base balance in the face of the normal variations of fluid and dietary intake and of physical activity. In most cases, hypertension is superadded, and may be of the malignant type. Chronic pyelonephritis and chronic glomerulonephritis account for the majority of cases, but there are many other causes, including essential (primary) malignant hypertension, polycystic disease of the kidneys,

systemic lupus erythematosus, diabetes mellitus, amyloid disease, nephrocalcinosis, gout, irradiation injury and analgesic nephropathy. The pathological changes characteristic of these diseases are described in the appropriate sections. In all of them, severe chronic renal injury may occur, but the resulting chronic renal failure presents biochemical, clinical and morphological changes which are sufficiently similar to warrant a common description.

Biochemical disturbances

Non-protein nitrogen retention. As only a small proportion of functioning renal tissue remains in patients with chronic renal failure, it follows that renal blood flow and total glomerular filtration rate (GFR) are considerably reduced. When GFR falls below normal, the amount of urea removed from the blood falls below the normal level of urea production, and the level in the blood rises. If kidney function remains steady, the blood urea will stabilise at a level at which the normal amount is removed in the glomerular filtrate. To give an example, the normal GFR may be taken as 120 ml per minute and the blood urea level as approximately 30 mg per 100 ml (5 mmol/l). Since urea is very highly diffusible, the concentration in the glomerular filtrate will also be 30 mg per 100 ml, and the total amount of urea filtered off from the blood will thus be $120/100 \times 30$ mg, i.e. 36 mg per minute. Some re-absorption of urea takes place from the tubule, and the amount excreted is about 25 mg per minute (36 g daily). Consider now the patient with chronic renal failure and sufficient functioning nephrons to provide a GFR of, say, 12 ml per minute. Obviously, this will result in urea retention, which will be reflected in a high blood urea: when the level reaches 300 mg per 100 ml, the 12 ml of filtrate per minute will then contain 36 mg, i.e. the amount normally filtered, and provided that tubular reabsorption is not altered, the normal amount will be excreted. In fact, this is an over-simplification, for urea production varies with dietary protein intake, and there are also variations in the amount reabsorbed from the tubules. In chronic renal failure there is usually distinct polyuria and, as explained below, less reabsorption occurs from the tubules. In spite of these complicating factors, the level of the blood urea gives useful information in chronic renal failure, and is easy to estimate: provided certain precautions are taken, changes in the level reflect changes in renal function. The level of blood creatinine is less influenced by dietary factors and tubular reabsorption and provides a better indication of renal function, but its estimation is less simple.

Urea itself has little or no toxicity, but its retention is an indication of retention of various other non-protein nitrogenous metabolites, some of which are toxic.

Excretion of water. In normal circumstances, the kidneys play the major role in adjusting water loss to suit intake. This is effected by varying the volume of urine from approximately 400 ml to several litres daily. Within these limits, the excretion of urinary solutes is not affected significantly, and the specific gravity of the urine is inversely proportional to the volume, varying between 1·002 and 1·040. In chronic renal failure, the variability of urine volume is commonly lost, and provided sufficient water is taken in, the kidneys excrete daily approximately 2·5 litres of dilute urine of specific gravity approximately 1·010. If water intake is inadequate in this condition, production of dilute urine continues and dehydration results, with consequent fall in blood volume and blood pressure: renal blood flow and GFR are consequently diminished, the volume of urine falls and uraemia increases. If water intake is excessive, the urine volume is little affected, and the patient develops water intoxication and pulmonary oedema. The supervention of heart failure, a common complication of chronic renal failure with hypertension, results in further impairment of renal blood flow and fall in GFR, with consequent oliguria, increase in uraemia, and cardiac oedema (p. 218).

The **polyuria** of chronic renal failure is at first sight surprising in view of the small amount of glomerular filtrate produced, but it will be recalled that in the healthy individual, the volume of urine is controlled mainly by the degree of concentration taking place in the tubules, and not by variations in the glomerular filtrate. Obviously, in chronic renal failure the polyuria results from failure of the tubules to effect the normal variations in concentration, and the most likely explanation is that the high concentration of urea in the glomerular filtrate exerts an osmotic diuretic effect similar to that which occurs when a large amount of urea is administered to a normal individual. The effect is not peculiar to urea, and can be induced by giving any substance which diffuses readily into the glomerular filtrate and which is largely unabsorbed in the tubules, e.g. inulin. Normally, 80% of the volume of the glomerular filtrate is reabsorbed in the proximal part of the tubule, but the fluid remaining in the lumen does not exceed isotonicity. In chronic renal failure, the high concentration of urea in the glomerular filtrate results in isotonicity being reached when much less than 80% of the volume has been reabsorbed, and further concentration cannot be achieved in this part of the nephron. In the distal part of the tubule and the collecting tubule, the 'sodium pump' normally results in a high concentration of Na$^+$ in the adjacent medullary interstitial tissue, and this facilitates further concentration of the tubular fluid and production of a hypertonic urine. In chronic renal failure (and osmotic diuresis induced in a normal individual) failure to achieve the normal five-fold concentration in the proximal tubule results in a large volume of fluid passing into the distal tubule, and rapid absorption of water here dilutes the Na$^+$ in the interstitial fluid and so interferes with further urinary concentration.

Electrolyte disturbances. It is a remarkable fact that, in contrast to the blood urea, the plasma concentrations of sodium and potassium are virtually unaltered until the terminal stages of chronic renal failure. In the normal individual, the amounts of Na$^+$ and K$^+$ excreted in the urine vary considerably, depending on intake. In chronic renal failure, the range of excretion is limited, and extremes of intake are not well tolerated: nevertheless, considering that, in some cases, few functioning nephrons remain, it is apparent that, to maintain homoeostasis, considerably more Na$^+$ and K$^+$ must be excreted per nephron than normally. This is brought about by the continuous state of osmotic diuresis, referred to above, which pertains in chronic renal failure, for diuresis is accompanied by decreased reabsorption of various solutes, including Na$^+$ and K$^+$. **Deficiency of Na$^+$** is a common late effect, for the urinary loss is somewhat inflexible, and deficiency may result from restricted intake of salt, or from vomiting and diarrhoea, attacks of which are common in uraemia. Na$^+$ deficiency in time leads to fall in plasma volume and blood pressure, and to oliguria: nitrogen retention increases and acidosis (see below) supervenes. In some cases of chronic renal failure due to pyelonephritis, sodium loss is severe, and the clinical features may be similar to those of adrenocortical insufficiency (Addison's disease). Correction of Na$^+$ deficiency in chronic renal failure must be carefully controlled, for administration of too much Na$^+$ and water can readily induce systemic or pulmonary oedema.

In chronic renal failure, **potassium retention** may arise from excessive intake or as a complication of dehydration and acidosis; in this state, dehydration results in oliguria and reduced K$^+$ excretion, while acidosis results in exchange of some intracellular K$^+$ for H$^+$; both effects raise the level of plasma K$^+$, and there is a risk of cardiac arrest. **Potassium deficiency** is uncommon in chronic renal failure, but can occur in certain cases of chronic pyelonephritis, where excessive loss of K$^+$ in the urine can result from secondary aldosteronism attributable, in turn, to excessive Na$^+$ loss, and producing a picture like Conn's syndrome (p. 975).

Another effect of chronic renal failure is **acidosis**. To conserve acid–base balance, the kidneys must excrete 40–60 mEq of acid (H$^+$) daily. This is excreted in combination with urinary phosphate and organic acid radicles (e.g. creatinine), and by combination with ammonia as NH$_4^+$. For homoeostasis, therefore, the glomerular filtrate must provide sufficient dibasic phosphate and other available anions, and the cells of the distal convoluted tubules must produce and secrete an adequate amount of ammonia, which is normally derived by deamination of amino acids. In chronic renal failure, the diminished volume of glomerular filtrate does not contain the normal amount of dibasic phosphate, but tubular reabsorption is also reduced as a result of the continuous osmotic diuresis, and the net amount available for excretion of acid is not very much less than normal until the late stages. Because relatively few functioning nephrons remain, total ammonia production and secretion into the tubules is reduced. There is also some loss of bicarbonate in the urine, whereas normally it is almost completely reabsorbed. As a result of these changes, the patient with chronic renal failure is prone to develop acidosis. In most cases, the **plasma phosphate** level is normal except in the late stages, but if lack of water or salt arises, either from deficient intake or from vomiting or diarrhoea, or if the glomerular filtration rate falls even further as a result of heart failure, phosphate excretion is diminished, the blood level rises and acidosis develops.

The level of **plasma calcium** tends to be slightly low in chronic renal failure, and is further depressed if the level of phosphate rises. In this state, however, acidosis is also likely, and this increases the proportion of plasma calcium in ionic form, with the result that frank tetany does not usually develop, although muscle twitching is common.

Hypertension

This develops in most cases of chronic renal failure, often before there is nitrogen retention, and is sometimes of the malignant type. The renal changes resulting from hypertension cause further injury to the already damaged kidneys, and progress of renal failure is hastened. Life can be prolonged by amelioration of severe hypertension by antihypertensive drugs and this is now an important aspect of treatment.

The cause of hypertension in chronic renal failure (and indeed in renal disease in general) is not well understood (pp. 222 and 323).

Pathological changes

The disease processes most commonly responsible for chronic renal failure are listed on p. 775, and their pathological features are described in the appropriate sections. It remains to describe the pathological changes throughout the body which *result from* chronic renal failure, whatever the cause. These changes are neither constant nor specific. **Fibrinous pericarditis**, accompanied by little or no effusion, is common in the late stages, and also 'uraemic **pneumonitis**', consisting of a sero-fibrinous exudate into the alveolar spaces, sometimes fanning out from the hila, and giving a butterfly shadow on x-ray. The changes resemble those of neonatal hyaline membrane disease (p. 400), but there is often partial organisation of the exudate. Inflammatory changes occur also in the **gastro-intestinal tract**, including haemorrhagic ulceration and also a pseudomembranous enterocolitis. The cause of these various inflammatory lesions has not been established. **Immunological depression**, with a tendency to infections, is known to occur in uraemia, but the fibrinous pericarditis is usually sterile, and cannot be explained thus. In some cases, the fibrinoid necrosis of arterioles resulting from malignant hypertension may be responsible for some of the lesions (e.g. Fig. 13.18, p. 322). The **cardiovascular features of hypertension** are usually obvious in such cases, although cerebral haemorrhage is less common than in essential hypertension. The commonest lesion found in the brain at necropsy is **cerebral oedema**. Changes have also been described in the pancreas (p. 653).

Bone changes. Various bone changes may occur, and are termed collectively *uraemic osteodystrophy* (p. 826). In some cases, the plasma levels of ionised calcium and phosphate are sufficiently changed to induce increased function and hyperplasia of the parathyroid glands, with consequent bone changes (secondary hyperparathyroidism). In children, a condition bearing some resemblance to rickets, and termed *renal dwarfism* or *renal rickets*, may develop.

Haematological changes in chronic renal failure include a normochromic normocytic anaemia which is due to depressed erythropoiesis and is roughly proportional to the degree of uraemia. There may also be a micro-angiopathic haemolytic anaemia (p. 477) in those patients who develop malignant hypertension, this being one form of the haemolytic-uraemic syndrome (p. 789).

Clinico-pathological correlations

Many of the clinical features of chronic renal failure can be surmised from the foregoing account of the biochemical and structural changes. Polyuria may be the presenting symptom, and is most noticeable at night when it replaces the low volume of concentrated urine normally produced. Any of the clinical features of severe hypertension may be present, including heart failure, visual disturbances due to retinal involvement, and convulsions followed by fatal coma from hypertensive encephalopathy. If heart failure supervenes, the volume of urine diminishes and oedema of cardiac type develops (p. 218).

Urea itself is without serious toxic properties, but the retention of other, ill-defined nitrogenous compounds in uraemia gives rise to toxic effects characterised by vomiting and anorexia and by mental dullness: coma often supervenes, but may be long delayed. As already explained, the impairment of renal function renders the patient liable to dehydration and acidosis, with their corresponding clinical features, and in this state there is also a danger of muscular irritability due to fall in plasma calcium, and of hyponatraemia and hyperkalaemia. Excessive fluid and sodium loss, e.g. from vomiting and diarrhoea, must be corrected in order to avoid these serious biochemical disturbances, but care must also be taken to avoid therapeutic overloading with sodium and water, as this leads rapidly to pulmonary oedema.

When uraemia is advanced, severe anaemia is commonly present, and contributes to the clinical picture. Hypertensive encephalopathy may accompany uraemia, with generalised convulsions which are believed to result from cerebral oedema due to vascular spasm (p. 323).

In most instances, the changes in the kidneys which have brought about chronic renal failure are irreversible, and the prognosis depends on the rate of progression and on the availability of, and suitability of the patient for, chronic dialysis or renal transplantation. In some cases of chronic pyelonephritis, however, renal function can improve, at least for a time, if the infection is active and can be suppressed, and while it is therefore important to search for evidence of chronic pyelonephritis, it is even more important that this condition should be detected and eliminated before it has caused sufficient renal injury to result in chronic renal failure.

Miscellaneous Renal Diseases

Diabetes mellitus

Renal failure is an important complication of diabetes. It causes death in more than 10 per cent of all diabetics, and in over 50 per cent of those developing diabetes in childhood. The most important contribution to this high mortality is *diabetic glomerulosclerosis*, which can also give rise to the nephrotic syndrome. Hyaline thickening of the afferent glomerular arterioles is also very common in diabetes: it is similar to that already described in hypertensives and old people, but is more often very severe in diabetics, both with and without hypertension, and affects also the efferent arterioles much more severely than in non-diabetics (Fig. 21.42). Acute pyelonephritis is also unduly common in diabetics, and is particularly prone to be accompanied by papillary necrosis (p. 783).

Diabetic glomerulosclerosis. This consists of deposition of eosinophilic hyaline material in

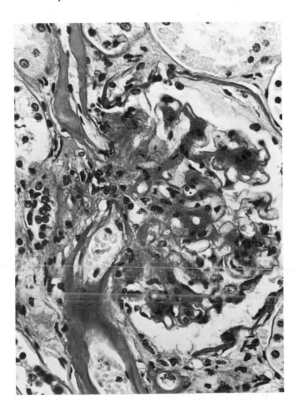

Fig. 21.42 Hyaline change in the afferent and efferent glomerular arterioles in diabetes. Note also the diffuse glomerulosclerosis. × 250.

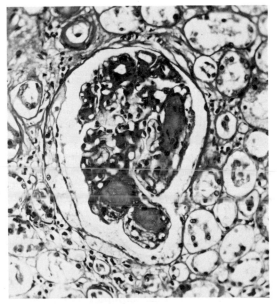

Fig. 21.43 Nodular glomerulosclerosis in diabetes (Kimmelstiel–Wilson lesion). × 205.

the mesangium of the glomerular lobules. The deposits may be discrete rounded nodules, sometimes laminated, situated near the tip of the lobule and therefore appearing peripheral in the glomerulus (Kimmelstiel–Wilson lesion). Such *nodular* deposition affects lobules and glomeruli unequally, and one or more nodules, of various sizes, may be seen in affected glomeruli (Fig. 21.43). The glomerular capillaries are seen around the margin of the nodules, and may long remain unaffected, but nodular glomerulosclerosis is usually accompanied by more diffuse deposition of hyaline material in the mesangium of all the glomerular lobules, with associated thickening of the glomerular capillary basement membranes (Fig. 21.42). This *diffuse* glomerulosclerosis may resemble membranous glomerulonephritis, but shows less uniform basement membrane thickening: it occurs together with the nodular lesion, and may eventually progress to obliteration of most of the capillaries and severe hyalinisation of the glomeruli. Ischaemic changes, including obliteration of the capsular space by collagen and glomerular collapse (Fig. 21.7, p. 750) occur, and are presumably related to hyaline thickening of the afferent arterioles. As a result of glomerulosclerosis, secondary atrophy occurs in the tubules, and the kidneys may be reduced in size with thinning of the cortex and a granular surface.

The pathogenesis of diabetic glomerulosclerosis is not understood, and electron microscopy has so far not contributed much to its elucidation. The deposited hyaline material is PAS-positive and has an electron-microscopic appearance similar to basement membrane. At present, Lendrum's suggestion that the material originates from exudation of plasma constituents (p. 750) seems the most likely explanation, both for the glomerulosclerosis and for the hyaline material deposited in the glomerular arterioles. The observed differences in staining reactions of these two lesions may be due to differences in their age. It has also been suggested that glomerulosclerosis in diabetes may result from an immunological reaction. Beef insulin is antigenic to man, and most diabetics receiving it develop circulating antibody; there is thus the possibility of circulating insulin–antibody complexes and of immune-complex nephritis (p. 753). In support of this possibility, Berns *et al.* (1962) have reported immunofluorescence studies which suggest that beef insulin and antibody to beef insulin are deposited in the glomerular capillary walls. However, this cannot be the sole cause, for diabetic glomerulosclerosis occurs in some diabetics not treated with insulin, and was recognised before the introduction of treatment by insulin. The possibility remains of auto-antibody, i.e. to autologous insulin, with consequent immune-complex deposition, but the evidence for this is not strong.

Diabetic glomerulosclerosis has been reported in 25–50% of diabetics at necropsy. In most instances, the nodular and diffuse forms are combined, but in some the diffuse form occurs alone. It is worth while distinguishing between the two forms, for while the nodular lesion is highly characteristic of diabetes, the diffuse lesion is related much more closely with disturbances of renal function. In many cases, diabetic glomerulosclerosis is unsuspected during life, and may be clinically silent. It is commonly associated with proteinuria, and when severe this may result in the nephrotic syndrome. It may also lead to chronic renal failure with the usual features of uraemia and hypertension. As already mentioned, glomerulosclerosis is especially common in early-onset diabetes; its incidence and severity increase with the duration of diabetes, and there is some evidence that poor control of the diabetic state is a contributory cause.

Other renal changes in diabetes. Atheroma is very common and often severe in diabetics. In non-diabetics the renal arteries rarely show severe narrowing from atheroma unless they are involved at their origins by aortic atheromatous plaques. In diabetes, however, severe atheroma does occur in the main renal arteries and their segmental branches and probably contributes to the high incidence of hypertension.

Other renal lesions occurring in diabetes have been referred to above, and include hyaline arteriolar thickening, pyelonephritis and papillary necrosis. The evidence for a high incidence of chronic pyelonephritis is not entirely convincing, but acute pyelonephritis, often with papillary necrosis, is common at necropsy in diabetics.

Amyloid

The kidneys are involved in nearly all cases of amyloidosis secondary to chronic infections, rheumatoid arthritis, etc., and are also commonly affected in primary amyloidosis. The most important site of deposition is around the glomerular capillary basement membrane (Fig. 21.44): this is accompanied by increased permeability, and proteinuria may be sufficiently heavy to cause the nephrotic syndrome. As the

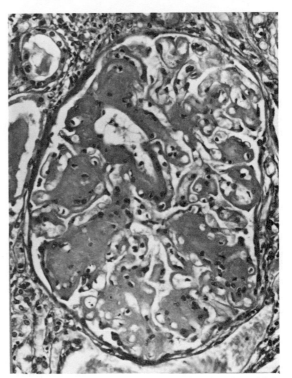

Fig. 21.45 Glomerular amyloidosis, showing thickening and hyaline appearance of capillary walls. × 350.

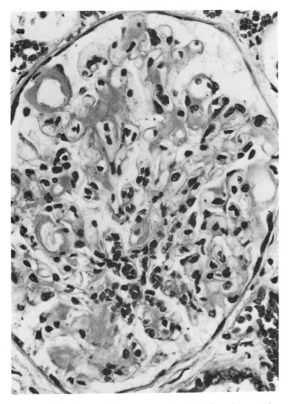

Fig. 21.44 Deposition of amyloid in the glomerular capillaries at a relatively early stage as compared with Fig. 21.45. × 250.

deposits increase, capillary narrowing and obliteration ensue, and the glomeruli may be largely replaced by amyloid (Fig. 21.45). Secondary atrophy of the tubules and interstitial fibrosis result from the glomerular lesion, and chronic renal failure gradually supervenes. The kidneys are firm and pale, may be of normal size, enlarged, or shrunken and granular, and the glomeruli are usually visible by naked eye after treating a slice of kidney with Lugol's iodine (Fig. 21.46). In cases with the nephrotic syndrome, the usual accompanying features are seen in the kidneys (p. 763).

Amyloid is deposited also in the walls of the small blood vessels of the kidneys and upon the tubular basement membranes. The careful studies of Lendrum (1969) have revealed similarities in the pattern of amyloid deposition and hyaline change, e.g. in diabetes (p. 750), which have led him to suggest that amyloid may originate from an exudative process.

There is a tendency to thrombosis of the intrarenal veins in renal amyloidosis, sometimes

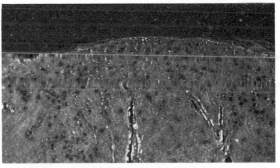

Fig. 21.46 Amyloidosis. A slice of the renal cortex has been treated with Lugol's iodine. The glomeruli contain sufficient amyloid material to be visible as darkly stained spots.

extending to the main renal veins, and causing acute renal failure.

Gout

The main features of gout are described on p. 861. The excretion of increased amounts of urates by the kidneys may result in crystal formation in the medulla. The crystals are deposited mainly in the collecting tubules where they cause local destruction of the tubular wall and become surrounded by a giant-cell reaction and eventually by fibrous tissue. They are usually at first needle-shaped, but tend to become amorphous. The destructive changes in the collecting tubules result in atrophy of the corresponding nephrons and the kidney may be reduced in size with a granular surface and scarring of the medulla. Urate stones may develop in the renal pelves and may cause renal colic, haematuria and obstruction.

A moderate degree of hypertension is common in gout and is accompanied by the usual renal changes. Features suggestive of chronic pyelonephritis are also common at necropsy; polymorphs are often seen in the tubules, but do not necessarily indicate an infection, for it has been shown experimentally that acute inflammation, including polymorph aggregates, can occur around injected urate crystals without superadded infection, and this happens around urate deposits in the acute attack of gout.

In spite of the high frequency and variety of renal changes in gout, renal failure supervenes in only a small proportion of cases.

Kidney lesions in pregnancy

There is no doubt that the incidence of renal disease is increased during pregnancy. A factor which contributes to this is the tendency to dilatation of the ureters, attributable to the relaxation of smooth muscle which is a feature of pregnancy, and also to pressure effects of the enlarged uterus: it is probably as a consequence of these effects that urinary infection, including pyelonephritis, is a common complication of pregnancy.

Secondly, acute tubular necrosis (p. 785), and rarely renal cortical necrosis (p. 789), are encountered as complications of pregnancy, particularly in cases of retroplacental haemor-rhage, infected abortion, and post-partum haemorrhage.

Lastly, pregnancy increases the functional demands on the kidneys, and latent chronic renal disease (e.g. chronic glomerulonephritis) may first become clinically apparent during pregnancy. Essential hypertension may also be aggravated by pregnancy, during which the blood pressure may increase temporarily.

Toxaemia of pregnancy. Albuminuria is a common occurrence in pregnancy, particularly in the last trimester, and may be accompanied by some oedema of the ankles: these disturbances are not of serious significance unless there is also a rise in the blood pressure, when the combination of features is termed *pre-eclampsia* or *pre-eclamptic toxaemia*. This also may be mild, and the changes—oedema, proteinuria and hypertension—do not usually increase to alarming degrees, and subside usually within a few days after parturition. In other cases, the features become progressively more severe during late pregnancy, and impaired renal function is reflected in a rise in the levels of blood urea. In such cases, hypertensive convulsions may occur, the condition then being termed *eclampsia*. Death may result from uraemia or hypertensive encephalopathy, and considerable judgement is sometimes required to decide whether pregnancy should be allowed to continue to term.

In patients dying from eclampsia, the kidneys are of normal size or slightly enlarged due to oedema: the cortex is pale and the glomeruli may be visible with a hand lens as grey dots projecting from the cut surface. Microscopy (of biopsy or necropsy material) shows diffuse enlargement of all the glomeruli, but without obvious increase in cellularity. The glomerular capillaries contain very few red cells: their walls appear diffusely thickened, eosinophilic and refractile, and special staining techniques show the thickening to be due to enlargement of the endothelial cells. Electron microscopy shows the endothelial cell cytoplasm to be increased in amount and vacuolated: the capillary basement membrane is usually normal, but in severe cases may show some thickening. The epithelial cells may also be enlarged, but do not show fusion of foot processes.

The clinical and histological features of pre-eclampsia indicate impaired renal blood flow with narrowing of the glomerular capillary lumina. The hypertensive convulsions of eclampsia are probably attributable to cerebral vascular spasm (seen also in the retinal arteries) and there is evidence also of a reduced uterine blood flow in pre-eclampsia, probably due to arterial spasm, and sometimes resulting in retro-placental ischaemia. The causes of the glomerular changes, and of the vascular spasm, are not known, but the urinary output of aldosterone has been shown to be greatly increased.

Hypertension from any cause during pregnancy increases the risks of abortion, premature labour and retroplacental haemorrhage.

Interstitial nephritis

This term is applied to any acute or chronic inflammatory change involving mainly the interstitial tissue of the kidney. *Pyelonephritis* is mainly an interstitial infection, and inflammatory cellular infiltration of the kidneys is sometimes observed with acute infections elsewhere in the body. *Hypersensitivity reactions* to certain drugs can result in peritubular inflammation and acute tubular injury. The renal lesions of irradiation, of analgesic abuse, and a form of chronic renal disease known as *Balkan nephritis* can all be described as interstitial nephritis, the term being thus applicable to an obviously heterogeneous group of conditions.

Drugs, chemicals and renal disease

Many drugs are excreted predominantly in the urine, and in patients with impaired renal function conventional dosage may result in toxic levels being attained. It is therefore necessary to modify the dosage of many types of drug in patients with acute or chronic renal failure.

Various drugs can cause renal lesions, either by a direct cytotoxic effect, or because the patient has developed a hypersensitivity to the drug. The production of acute tubular necrosis by drugs and chemicals is dealt with on pp. 786–9, and chronic renal disease due to analgesics on p. 784.

Lead poisoning is contracted most often in industry from inhalation of dust or fumes, or ingestion of lead compounds. In Queensland, Australia, lead paint was used up to 1930 for painting the wooden verandas of houses, and children playing on the verandas ingested paint powdered by the strong sunlight: acute lead poisoning was common, and follow-

up studies have shown a high incidence of chronic renal failure, appearing often many years later and progressing very slowly. The kidneys are uniformly reduced in size with a finely granular surface, uniform cortical thinning and hypertensive changes—in fact, closely similar to the changes in chronic glomerulonephritis. Microscopically, the lesion differs from glomerulonephritis; there is marked tubular atrophy with interstitial fibrosis, and the glomeruli are spared for a long time. However, as in granular contracted kidneys from any cause, the specific diagnosis is often difficult. Characteristic inclusion bodies are seen in the nuclei of the tubular and other cells.

The relationship to excessive intake of lead many years before is convincing in the Queensland studies, and the incidence has fallen considerably since the introduction of legislation against lead paints. The use of lead paint for cots and toys has also been responsible for lead poisoning in childhood.

The renal lesion of potassium deficiency

In conditions of potassium depletion and lowering of the plasma potassium level, the kidneys exhibit a striking morphological change consisting of intense hydropic vacuolation of the cells of the proximal tubules (Fig. 21.47), chiefly in the descending straight portion. The lesion is associated with marked loss of concentrating power, but only trivial albuminuria and absence of urea retention.

It occurs most frequently in conditions which cause severe and prolonged diarrhoea, e.g. in ulcerative colitis, or induced by excessive purgation. It occurs also in primary hyperaldosteronism (p. 975) and sometimes in Cushing's syndrome or during glucocorticoid therapy. It is a feature of some disorders of the renal tubules including the diuretic stage of acute tubular necrosis and can result from administration of diuretics. It is also seen in the stage of recovery from diabetic coma under insulin therapy, when the plasma potassium is lowered in the resynthesis and intracellular storage of glycogen. Serial biopsies of the kidney have shown the renal lesions to be completely reversible by restoration of normal potassium levels, and there is no evidence of permanent ill effects.

Papillary necrosis

This consists of necrosis of the distal parts of some or all of the papillae in one or both kidneys. It occurs acutely as a complication of *urinary tract obstruction*

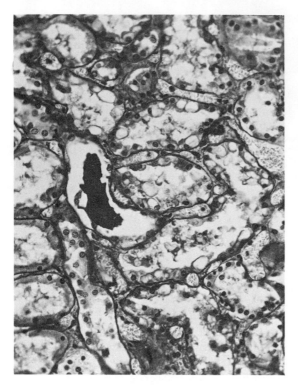

Fig. 21.47 The kidney in severe potassium depletion following prolonged diarrhoea in ulcerative colitis. The cells of the proximal convoluted tubules show gross cytoplasmic vacuolation. × 230.

and *diabetes*, particularly when there is superadded *acute pyelonephritis*. It also occurs in more chronic form as the major renal lesion of *analgesic abuse*.

In acute papillary necrosis, the kidneys frequently show changes of urinary tract obstruction or diabetes, commonly with superadded acute pyelonephritis. The necrotic distal parts of the papillae are usually yellowish-white and demarcated from the living tissue by a red line of congestion. Microscopy shows loss of cells in the necrotic tissue. The junctional zone with living tissue is congested and usually infiltrated with polymorphs. One or more necrotic papillae may have sloughed off, leaving an irregular ulcerated surface.

The clinical features are often dominated by urinary tract obstruction, pyelonephritis, etc. However, if necrosis occurs in most or all of the papillae in both kidneys, acute renal failure supervenes. There may also be haematuria and renal colic due to passage of a sloughed papilla.

Analgesic abuse. Chronic renal failure is now a well recognised cause of death in subjects taking large amounts of analgesic drug mixtures, usually containing aspirin and phenacetin, over a number of years. It seems likely that phenacetin is the important path-

ogenic constituent but this is unproved. Curiously, the incidence of renal failure from this cause is especially high in Australia, Switzerland and the Scandinavian countries, and relatively low in other West European countries and in North America. In Australia, the incidence is greater in Queensland with its warm climate and relatively high urine concentration than in the cooler Victoria. In most cases 0·5–1 kg of analgesic mixture has been taken annually for some years, either for painful chronic disease such as rheumatoid arthritis or for vague subjective illness.

Symptoms may arise from the hypertension and uraemia of chronic renal failure or there may be recurrent urinary infection, polyuria or renal colic due to the passage of sloughed papillae or phosphatic concretions. The urine may contain polymorphs and/or red cells.

Papillary necrosis appears to occur more gradually than in mechanical obstruction or diabetes and the necrotic papillae may remain attached or may sequestrate: frequently they become calcified. Atrophy of the overlying cortex ensues, so that the gross appearances of the kidneys come to resemble those of chronic pyelonephritis with large patches of cortical thinning and surface depression alternating with raised patches of more normal, sometimes hypertrophied renal tissue. The junction between the living and dead papillary tissue may be indistinct and microscopy may show a zone of partial necrosis. The cortex shows atrophy and loss of tubules, interstitial fibrosis and later, glomerular sclerosis.

Diagnosis is important, for striking improvement may result from stopping analgesics. Characteristic changes are sometimes seen in pyelograms.

Pathogenesis. The mechanism of papillary necrosis is not understood. The appearances, particularly in the acute form, are suggestive of infarction and the lesion tends to occur in middle-aged and old people with advanced arterial disease. The renal vascular lesions common in diabetes may be a contributory factor. The rise in pressure in urinary tract obstruction may also interfere with blood flow through the papillae. So far however, there is no good experimental model of this condition and the pathogenesis remains in doubt.

Renal tubular acidosis

Deficient tubular function is partly responsible for the acidosis which complicates chronic renal failure (p. 777). The term 'renal tubular acidosis' is, however, usually restricted to acidosis resulting from a tubular deficiency in the absence of chronic renal failure. It occurs in many conditions and traditionally is divided into two types.

In type I, function of the distal part of the tubule is impaired, with reduced capacity to produce urine of a low pH. This may occur as an inherited tubular defect, or as a result of tubular injury from pyelo-nephritis, hypercalcaemia, urinary tract obstruction or an auto-immune reaction.

In type II, there is impaired secretion of H$^+$ by the proximal tubule. This occurs in association with other tubular defects, e.g. amino-aciduria, renal gly-cosuria, cystinosis, hypophosphataemia.

In both types of tubular acidosis, there is hyper-chloraemia, osteomalacia or rickets which is resistant to vitamin D, and a danger of deposition of calcium salts in the renal medulla (nephrocalcinosis) which may cause further renal damage. In type I cases, oral administration of alkali is effective, but in type II this is of little value.

Acute Renal Failure

Renal function is impaired by any acute condi-tion causing severe reduction in glomerular filtration. This occurs during the circulatory failure of shock following severe trauma and haemorrhage, and also as a result of marked dehydration (*pre-renal uraemia*). Complete obstruction of the urethra also causes fatal acute renal failure unless relieved in time: this condition is termed *post-renal uraemia*. Impair-ment of renal blood flow and glomerular filtra-tion occurs in some degree in most cases of acute diffuse proliferative glomerulonephritis; in some cases, acute renal failure is severe with virtual anuria, particularly in the rapidly pro-gressive variant of the disease.

The commonest form of acute renal failure is however the condition which, for want of a bet-ter name, is termed '*acute tubular necrosis*'. This has a number of causal agents, two of the most important being a state of shock and various toxic chemicals. Other causes of acute renal failure include renal cortical necrosis, renal papillary necrosis, and hypersensitivity reac-tions to certain drugs, but these are less common.

The functional disturbances of acute renal failure are described in the section on the clinico-pathological correlations of acute tubular necrosis (p. 787).

'Acute tubular necrosis'

In this condition there is a sudden onset of *anuria* or *severe oliguria* with consequent ac-cumulation of fluid and urinary waste products and disturbances of electrolyte and pH balance. If it is not fatal, this phase is followed by a *diuretic phase* and, in favourable cases, by *recovery* of renal function.

Causal factors

The mechanism of renal failure in acute tubular necrosis is not fully understood, and will be discussed later. At this point it is useful to note the main predisposing factors.

(a) Shock. During an acute state of shock from whatever cause there is a considerable reduction of blood flow through the kidneys and so impaired renal function. In 'acute tub-ular necrosis', acute renal failure with anuria or severe oliguria persists after the state of shock has passed off. This is liable to occur in cases of severe and prolonged shock, for example in as-sociation with major injury, prolonged and complicated surgical operations or extensive burns. Severe bacterial infection with endotoxic shock, the trauma of unskilled abortion, retro-placental haemorrhage and postpartum haemor-rhage all carry a special risk of acute renal failure. In the bombing of cities in the 1939–45 war, individuals were commonly trapped for some hours under fallen masonry and developed traumatic and ischaemic necrosis of skeletal muscle, particularly in crushed limbs. After rescue, myoglobin and other constituents of muscle from the areas of crush injury dif-fused into the blood, and myoglobinuria developed. The high incidence of acute tubular necrosis in such cases (*crush syndrome*), and also in the rare condition of acute paroxysmal myoglobinuria, suggests that products of muscle breakdown have a special predisposing effect. Acute haemolysis, as in transfusion of incompatible blood, is also followed, although much less commonly, by 'acute tubular necrosis'. Operations on the liver and biliary tract are particularly likely to be complicated by 'acute tubular necrosis' (*hepatorenal syn-drome*), and although it is likely that shock and disturbance of fluid and electrolytes are at least partly responsible, there may be a special relationship between hepatic trauma and the renal lesion. The prognosis is appreciably worse in cases associated with severe trauma or surgery than in those following incompatible transfusion, complications of pregnancy or chemical poisoning (see below).

(b) Various chemicals are nephrotoxic to the tubular epithelium and cause acute renal failure, often together with acute injury to the liver and other organs. Some of the more important examples include carbon tetrachloride, used extensively in the dry-cleaning of fabrics, trilene, ethylene glycol (antifreeze), carbolic acid (phenol), and organic mercurials used as diuretics. Metallic poisons are also important causes, including mercuric chloride and compounds of uranium, arsenic and chromium. Many other compounds have been implicated.

Pathological changes

In fatal cases, the kidneys are usually enlarged and the cut surface bulges, due mainly to dilatation of tubules and interstitial oedema. The cortical vessels contain little blood, and the cortex appears pale, with blurring of the normal radial pattern, while the medulla is often dark and congested. Occasionally there are petechial haemorrhages in the cortex.

Microscopically, the glomerular tufts appear normal. Usually there is some granular debris in the capsular space and the parietal cells lining Bowman's capsule may be unduly prominent and cuboidal. The tubular changes are variable and depend on the severity and duration, and on the particular causal agents involved. In many cases, however, the causation is complex, and specific changes cannot readily be attributed to particular causal agents. Also, it is often difficult to identify, in histological sections, which parts of the tubules have been damaged. At necropsy, the lesion is often obscured by terminal ischaemic changes and post-mortem autolysis.

In cases resulting from shock, etc. (group **a** above), both the proximal and distal convoluted tubules are commonly dilated and the epithelial lining is flattened with basophilia of the cytoplasm and mitotic activity. These changes, which are seen as early as three days after the onset, appear to be a sequel to loss of tubular epithelium; the remaining cells become flattened and undergo proliferation, thus restoring epithelial continuity. In the distal convoluted and collecting tubules epithelial proliferation may be pronounced, the cells sometimes forming syncytial masses, particularly around casts (see below).

Tubular epithelial necrosis is not conspicuous and in many cases cannot be seen. In a minority there are foci of necrosis, most numerous in the distal convoluted tubule but also occurring in the proximal tubule. This change, which was described by Oliver *et al.* (1951) as *tubulorrhexis*, may be accompanied by disruption of the tubular basement membrane and an inflammatory reaction in the adjacent interstitial tissue. This may progress to scarring and in the event of recovery lead to tubular obstruction and so loss of function of the affected nephrons. The tubulorrhexic lesion and its site in the tubule were demonstrated by Oliver *et al.* by dissection of nephrons. The epithelial necrosis is not conspicuous and is readily obscured by post-mortem autolysis.

From the ascending limb of Henle's loop onwards, the tubules contain proteinous and brown granular casts, and in cases associated with haemoglobinuria or myoglobinuria brown pigment casts and rounded granules of pigmented material are particularly prominent (Fig. 21.48).

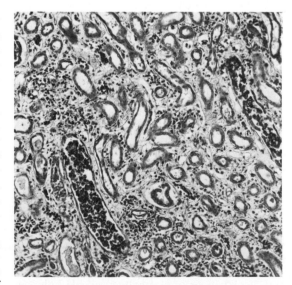

Fig. 21.48   Acute renal failure following incompatible transfusion, showing oedema, cellular infiltration and granular pigmented casts in the renal medulla. × 95.

Distension of the intertubular connective tissue by oedema fluid is conspicuous in some cases, but almost absent in others. The vasa recta of the medulla usually contain groups of nucleated cells which appear to represent erythropoietic foci, a feature which is sometimes seen in the hepatic sinusoids in liver cell necrosis.

The changes described above are seen in acute renal failure resulting from shock, trauma, etc. They occur also in those cases

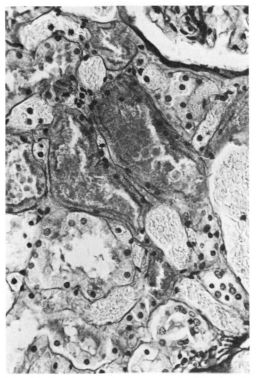

Fig. 21.49 Acute tubular necrosis. The tubule cells show extensive necrosis with nuclear pyknosis. From a case of methyl bromide poisoning. × 300. (Dr. G. Harvey Smith.)

resulting from administration of the nephrotoxic poisons listed above, but in the poisoning cases there is, in addition, more extensive necrosis (Fig. 21.49) affecting mainly the proximal convoluted tubule of all or most of the nephrons and resulting from the direct effect of the toxic compounds or their metabolites. This *nephrotoxic change* is often conspicuous but, unlike tubulorrhexis, it does not involve rupture of the tubular basement membrane, and provided the patient can be kept alive, it is often repaired by epithelial regeneration without leaving any residual damage or scarring.

Some variation is observed in the nephrotoxic lesions brought about by different chemicals. For example, mercuric chloride tends to affect the whole of the proximal convoluted tubule, and in some instances the necrotic part of the tubule rapidly becomes calcified, resulting in permanent injury. Carbon tetrachloride causes necrosis especially of the terminal part of the proximal tubule, and also centrilobular hepatic necrosis (p. 608); if ethylene glycol is ingested, a small proportion of it is converted into oxalate, crystals of which form in the tubular lumina: in addition to tubular necrosis it may cause death from liver or brain injury or from acute heart failure.

Clinico-pathological correlations. Oliguria or anuria lasts from a day or two to about 4 weeks, and is followed by a diuretic phase of roughly the same period. **During the anuric phase**, renal blood flow and GFR are reduced (see below). Tubular function is also disturbed, so that most of the diminished amount of glomerular filtrate produced is re-absorbed non-selectively across the injured tubular epithelium or denuded basement membrane. Consequently there is oliguria (defined as less than 400 ml urine per day in adults) or anuria (less than 100 ml daily), and the urine comes to resemble in composition a protein-poor filtrate of the plasma. There is thus a progressive rise in urea and other nitrogenous metabolites, and unless fluid and electrolyte intake is carefully regulated, death will result from a combination of uraemia, generalised and pulmonary oedema, and electrolyte disturbances. Acidosis may result from breakdown of endogenous fat and protein, particularly in the crush syndrome or other severe injury. Protein catabolism will aggravate the uraemia and accordingly the most appropriate diet is one which is low in protein and provides sufficient calories to avoid excessive endogenous protein catabolism. One of the most important electrolyte disturbances is retention of potassium, particularly in cases with severe injury and tissue breakdown, and dietary potassium should be carefully controlled. The level of plasma Na^+ is often low, usually due to its dilution by fluid retention, but the urine, even though markedly reduced in volume, may contain excess Na^+, and Na^+ administration may become necessary. Plasma Cl^- is similarly lowered, and this may be aggravated by vomiting. The plasma level of phosphate tends to rise, with an associated fall of Ca^{++}, although this is rarely severe. Experience has shown that carefully controlled conservative therapy, including the use of osmotic diuretics such as mannitol, can prolong life in acute renal failure, and where the lesion is reversible, as in acute tubular necrosis, the prognosis has been greatly improved.

However, in some cases haemodialysis is necessary. The blood pressure is commonly raised during the anuric phase.

A factor which has been suggested as contributing towards acute renal failure is leakage of tubular fluid into the interstitial tissue in tubulorrhexic lesions, with subsequent reabsorption into the blood. Obliteration of vessels by interstitial fluid is unlikely to be of importance, as oedema is sometimes minimal, and blockage of tubules by casts cannot always be a major factor, for casts are not always present. **During the diuretic phase**, large volumes of urine are produced but it continues to be very dilute, resembling a plasma filtrate and the levels of blood urea and creatinine may remain raised. There is a great danger of dehydration and loss of electrolytes and death may occur in this stage unless the urinary losses are made good. Renal concentrating power and homoeostatic mechanisms are gradually restored, sometimes over many months, but full renal function may not be achieved.

Aetiology

Two factors are of known importance in the aetiology of acute tubular necrosis. Firstly, the shock associated with trauma, incompatible transfusion, etc., and secondly, nephrotoxic chemicals. The part played by shock is by no means clearly defined: the most obvious possibility is ischaemic injury resulting from impaired renal blood flow, but experimental acute ischaemia of the kidney results in lesions particularly in the proximal convoluted tubules, whereas in those cases attributable mainly to trauma and shock the lesion in man (tubulorrhexis) is focal, and usually affects the distal convoluted tubules most severely. Because of this, and because tubulorrhexis is seen also in cases attributable to nephrotoxic chemicals, it may be that the lesion is produced by some endogenous mechanism which can be set in motion by various causal factors.

Although acute renal failure following the shock of severe injury, haemorrhage, or surgical operations, has long been attributed to tubular injury, there are unexplained discrepancies. For example, the extent of tubular necrosis does not correlate with the degree of renal failure (see Sevitt, 1959). Accordingly, it has been suggested that reduced glomerular filtration rate, attributable to diminished renal blood flow, is an important factor. There is no doubt that the renal blood flow is greatly diminished during the period of shock which precedes acute renal failure, but there is also evidence that the reduc-

tion in flow persists during the period of renal failure, and is largely responsible for it. Tubular injury, which is to be regarded as a consequence of the ischaemia of reduced renal blood flow, would thus be relegated to a secondary role in acute renal failure. These views have been advanced by Lever and his colleagues and other workers, who have provided strong evidence that persistent over-activity of the renin-angiotensin system is responsible for acute renal failure induced experimentally by administration of globin, glycerol or dichromate. By inducing arteriolar spasm, angiotensin impairs renal blood flow and glomerular filtration, and acute renal failure develops. It is of particular interest that antibody to angiotensin II minimised glycerol-induced acute renal failure although it did not prevent tubular necrosis.

Acceptance that increased activity of the renin-angiotensin system plays an important pathogenic role in acute tubular necrosis does not necessarily imply that the renal failure is due to reduced glomerular filtration. Recent investigations suggest that renal blood flow is reduced to about one-third of normal, which is no less than is encountered in heart failure *without* acute renal failure. Although tubular necrosis does not correlate well with acute renal failure, there is no doubt that the tubules are profoundly changed (see above), and it remains likely that their function is impaired. It seems most unlikely that the extensive tubular necrosis caused by various cytotoxic chemicals does not greatly impair renal function, and it is also very difficult to explain the diuretic phase of acute tubular necrosis on any basis other than impaired tubular function.

The part played by haemoglobin and myoglobin in acute renal failure is also obscure. In experimental studies, haemoglobin has not been shown to be nephrotoxic in otherwise healthy animals, although it has been shown to cause injury in conditions of dehydration, acidosis and renal ischaemia. Myoglobinuria has been shown to be more prone than haemoglobinuria to be accompanied by acute renal failure, particularly in crush injuries, and it may be that other products of muscle breakdown, in addition to myoglobin, are involved. The more extensive necrosis of the proximal tubules which occurs in cases attributable to various chemicals is more uniform, and is explicable as a direct toxic effect upon the tubular epithelium.

The haemolytic-uraemic syndrome

This includes a number of conditions in which fibrin thrombi form in the small vessels, especially in the kidneys, and result in renal failure often accompanied by hypertension, and micro-angiopathic haemolytic anaemia (p. 477) often accompanied by thrombocytopenic purpura. These features may be overwhelmingly acute or more gradual.

In early childhood, the syndrome may follow respiratory or alimentary infections. It occurs also in thrombotic thrombocytopenic purpura, mainly in adults, and also in malignant hypertension, toxaemia of pregnancy and following apparently normal pregnancies. In all these forms, the renal vascular changes resemble those of malignant hypertension (p. 751), and include fibrinoid necrosis in the afferent arterioles and glomerular capillaries and fibrous thickening of the larger arteries. When the changes are very severe and acute there may be cortical necrosis (Fig. 21.50). Vascular lesions in other organs may produce a large variety of additional clinical features.

The important pathogenic role of fibrin deposition is indicated by the reduction of mortality effected by heparin. In cases following infections the clotting system may possibly be triggered by antigen–antibody complexes or by endotoxin. (Two spaced injections of endotoxin induce in animals thrombotic micro-angiopathy

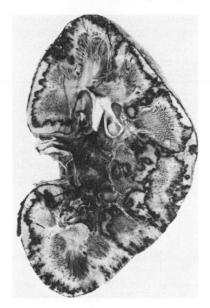

Fig. 21.50 Renal cortical necrosis from a case of eclampsia; the pale necrotic areas with haemorrhagic margins are well shown. × ⅔.

with severe renal injury—**the Schwartzman reaction**—which is more readily induced during pregnancy.) Malignant hypertension can both predispose to the syndrome or develop as one of its features, and is then accompanied by high levels of plasma renin. Localisation of the lesions largely in the kidneys may result from α-receptor stimulation (p. 980).

Pyelonephritis

Introduction

Pyelonephritis is a bacterial-induced inflammation of the renal pelvis, the calyces and renal parenchyma. It can occur in acute and chronic form and affects one or both kidneys, usually in a quite irregular, patchy fashion. Most cases are due to ascending infection of the urinary tract by *Escherichia coli* or less commonly other faecal bacteria, and for this reason urinary tract infection in general will be considered in the present account. Urinary tract infections, including pyelonephritis, are commoner in females at all ages than in males. Acute pyelonephritis causes death only when bilateral and very extensive. In less severe form, and par-

ticularly when recurrent, it may progress to chronic pyelonephritis, which is an important cause of chronic renal failure. In many instances of chronic pyelonephritis, however, there is no previous history indicative of acute attacks, nor indeed of urinary infection at all. There is evidence that asymptomatic bacteriuria in childhood is followed in some instances by chronic pyelonephritis. Any structural abnormality of the urinary tract, but particularly lesions which cause chronic or intermittent obstruction, predispose to infection and in these circumstances the infection tends to be severe, to extend to the kidneys causing pyelonephritis, and to be difficult to eradicate.

Causal organisms. Initial acute episodes of

urinary tract infection are usually caused by *Escherichia coli* or, less commonly, other faecal bacteria (Enterococcus, Pseudomonas, *Strep. faecalis*, etc.), any of which is often obtained in the urine in pure culture. Patients with re-current urinary infections, who have usually received previous antibiotic therapy and who may have been subjected to instrumentation of the lower urinary tract, commonly have a mixed infection of these various faecal bacteria.

Bacteriuria. This is not synonymous with urinary tract infection, for the normal distal urethral mucosa is populated by coliform bacilli, *Proteus*, staphylococci, *Strep. faecalis*, etc. These may be washed off the mucosa by the stream of urine and thus be detectable in the collected sample; alternatively they may be carried into the bladder by a catheter or cysto-scope and the 'catheter specimen' of urine may similarly contain bacteria. In neither instance is there a urinary tract infection although bacter-ial cultures of the urine will be positive. It is therefore necessary to assess the importance of bacteriuric states. Experience has shown that bacterial counts of over 100 000 organisms per ml. of urine usually indicate urinary tract infec-tion but that counts of less than this number can result from contamination.

Asymptomatic bacteriuria. This implies sig-nificant bacteriuria in the absence of symptoms of urinary tract infection. It is encountered in approximately 1% of healthy schoolgirls, only about one-quarter of whom has a history sug-gestive of a previous urinary tract infection. Tests on younger children suggest that bacteri-uria often develops before the age of 3 years. Follow-up studies indicate that some children with symptomless bacteriuria eventually develop chronic pyelonephritis. Symptomless bacteriuria is especially frequent (about 5%) in pregnant women, but fears that it is commonly followed by chronic pyelonephritis appear to be largely unfounded.

Recurrent or persistent infection. The number of individuals who die from acute pyeloneph-ritis in this country is very small, and the chief danger now is the recurrent or smouldering chronic types of infection, for these are often related to the development of chronic pyelo-nephritis with ultimate renal failure. Serial studies have usually shown that repeated attacks of urinary tract infection in subjects without any obvious predisposing cause are due to different strains of bacteria, suggesting an abnormal susceptibility to re-infection. There is no doubt that urinary tract infections are more liable to arise when there is obstruction of the urinary tract, and unless the obstruction can be relieved the infection is often difficult to eradicate and liable to recur. However, in-vestigation of patients with recurrent urinary tract infection has failed to demonstrate an obstructive lesion in most of them.

Pathogenesis

Pyelonephritis may result from bacteria reach-ing the kidney either by the bloodstream or by an ascending infection of the urinary tract.

Blood-borne infection occurs in acute pyaemia or septicaemia (Figs. 7.9, p. 168 and 7.10, p. 169), and this is seen as a complication of staphylococcal infections, e.g. boils and car-buncles. The bacteria normally present in the distal urethra can also gain entrance to the blood during surgical procedures upon the urethra: in these circumstances, the possibility of blood-borne infection of the kidneys is increased if the lesion which has required ureth-ral surgery has also brought about urinary obstruction, e.g. urethral stricture or enlarged prostate (see below). Blood-borne infection is not, however, the cause of the majority of cases of pyelonephritis.

Ascending urinary tract infection. The com-monest site of infection of the urinary tract is the bladder, and it is likely that cystitis is the predisposing factor in most cases of pyeloneph-ritis. As already explained, most attacks of 'spontaneous' cystitis are caused by *Esch. coli*, whereas cystitis following catheterisation is commonly a mixed infection. In normal circum-stances, the uretero-vesical valves are com-petent, and radiological studies have shown that **vesico-ureteric reflux**, i.e. reflux of urine from the bladder to the ureters, is rare. How-ever, there is evidence that cystitis may impair the competence of the valves, perhaps by inflammatory swelling and distortion of the mucosa of the terminal parts of the ureters and adjacent parts of the bladder; in these circum-stances vesico-ureteric reflux during micturi-tion, with consequent pyelitis, is not unusual. It is demonstrable by urography during micturi-tion, which shows that bladder urine may pass into the renal pelves, and explains how infections ascend the urinary tract.

When pyelitis has developed, the bacteria may spread into the kidney directly by the lumina of the collecting tubules, or by passing from the submucosa of the inflamed calyces into the interstitial tissue of the renal papillae. Here they proliferate, and an acute inflammatory response occurs, often with abscess formation, eventually involving the adjacent tubular lumina. From here, infection can spread peripherally to the cortex (Fig. 21.51) via both

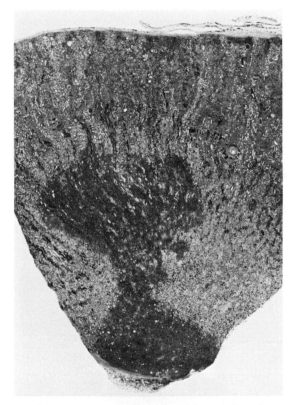

Fig. 21.51 Acute papillitis in pyelonephritis showing severe inflammatory infiltration of the renal papilla extending to the boundary zone. × 5.

the tubular lumina and the intertubular connective tissue spaces. Thus there develop linear streaks of suppuration with considerable tubular destruction. Since there is haphazard spread of bacteria from variably infected calyces, the renal lesion is not uniform and diffuse, but irregular and patchy. Significant bacteriuria can reflect inflammation at any level of the urinary tract and exact localisation is often clinically difficult. It is particularly important to

determine whether or not bacterial inflammation has involved the renal parenchyma and two factors are often helpful in reaching such a conclusion. The first is the presence of a high titre of serum antibody to the bacterium cultured from the urine. If this is present renal involvement is highly probable. The second is the presence of cellular casts in the urine: pus cells in the urine (*pyuria*) can result from infection anywhere in the urinary tract, but their aggregation into cylindrical casts can only have happened in the renal tubules, thus indicating pyelonephritis.

Predisposing factors. *Urinary tract obstruction.* Patients with an obstruction of the urinary tract are particularly liable to develop pyelonephritis, and this is attributable to four factors. Firstly, stagnant urine is a suitable culture medium for coliform and certain other bacteria which in normal circumstances would be washed out. Secondly, obstruction facilitates the upward spread of infection in the urinary tract by predisposing to vesico-ureteric reflux: this can occur intermittently even without gross structural change in the ureters, but in prolonged partial obstruction the ureters become permanently thickened and dilated, allowing free reflux to occur. Thirdly, there is convincing evidence that obstruction impairs the capacity of the kidneys to resist infection. Lastly, chronic urinary obstruction may cause uraemia, and thus lower the resistance to infections in general (p. 778).

Structural abnormalities of the urinary tract without obstruction also appear to predispose to infection. In *diabetes mellitus*, there is a general susceptibility to infections, including cystitis, pyelitis and pyelonephritis (see p. 152).

Age and sex. At all ages, the incidence of pyelonephritis, like urinary tract infections in general, is greater in females than in males. This may be due to the shorter, wider urethra and the turbulence of urethral flow, with peripheral eddying, in the female. As regards age, there is increasing evidence that urinary tract infections, including symptomless bacteriuria, are more likely to be followed by chronic pyelonephritis when they occur in childhood than in adult life.

Pregnancy produces a degree of ureteric dilatation and urinary stasis by virtue of the effect of the hormonal climate upon the musculature of the urinary tract and latterly the mechanical pressure of the enlarged uterus. Symptomless bacteriuria in early *pregnancy* is often followed by acute pyelonephritis later in pregnancy, but there is little evidence that it predisposes to chronic pyelonephritis. *Hypokalaemia, gout*, and the ingestion of excessive amounts of *analgesics* (p. 784) over a long period can all produce renal histopathology similar to bacterial-induced chronic pyelonephritis. Accordingly, these conditions should be kept in mind in the differential diagnosis of chronic pyelonephritis in renal biopsy material.

Incidence

Acute pyelonephritis is a not uncommon disease in young females, including children, and is especially liable to occur during pregnancy. It is less frequent in the male unless there is a pre-existing urinary tract obstruction. The frequency of chronic pyelonephritis is very difficult to assess. Incidences as high as 15% have been reported in general hospital necropsies, but this usually includes cases in which a few cortical scars are present as an incidental finding in otherwise normal kidneys. If the necropsy diagnosis is limited to those cases with severe chronic pyelonephritis, likely to have been of clinical significance, then the incidence is of the order of 1%.

Pathological changes

Acute pyelonephritis

This consists of acute suppurative inflammation of the pelvis, calyces and parts of the kidneys, with pale linear streaks of suppuration bordered by a red rim of congestion, extending radially from the tips of the papillae to the surface of the cortex (Figs. 21.52, 21.53) where adjacent lesions may fuse to produce extensive abscesses. Microscopically, all the features typical of acute inflammation are present in the pelvis, calyces and kidney. Within the kidney the suppurating lesions cause very extensive but focal tubular destruction. In the cortex there is remarkable sparing of glomeruli and large blood vessels, even when these structures are directly surrounded by intense acute interstitial inflammation. All of these changes tend to be

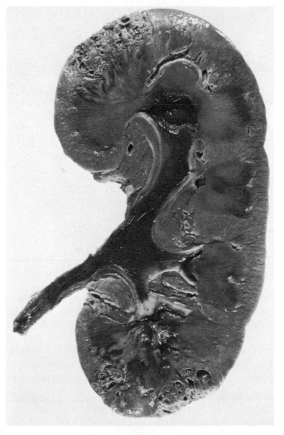

Fig. 21.53 Acute pyelonephritis. In this case the lesions are at the upper and lower poles. Note the cortical abscesses and the streaks of suppuration in the medulla.

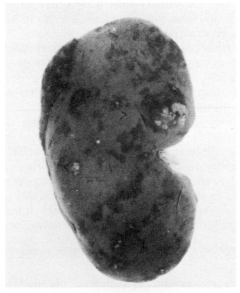

Fig. 21.52 Surface view of child's kidney in acute pyelonephritis, showing small abscesses and areas of haemorrhage. × 1.

more florid and more extensive if there is obstruction in the lower urinary tract. Obstructed cases often, and very intensely inflamed non-obstructed cases sometimes, develop papillary necrosis (p. 783).

Chronic pyelonephritis

The naked eye appearances of the kidney, calyces, and renal pelvis are of paramount importance in the differentiation of chronic pyelonephritic shrinkage from other varieties of scarred kidneys. The pelvic and calyceal walls are usually thickened and their mucosa may be either granular or atrophic: they are always distorted by scarring of the pyramids and the calyces are usually dilated (Fig. 21.54). Pyelography is therefore of great diagnostic value. The kidney is reduced in size and shows irregular patchy contraction in which the pyelonephritic process has largely destroyed the parenchyma and led to focal scarring and shrinkage. The intervening parenchyma may be

normal or may show the changes of hypertension. The cortical surface is depressed over the contracted areas, the cortex and medulla both being consistently narrowed. The cortical surface depressions tend in most instances to be shallower than those produced by ischaemia but they may be very similar, and the single most important diagnostic feature of the pyelonephritic scar is its close relationship to a deformed calyx. Microscopically the pelvic and calyceal mucosa may be thickened by granulation tissue and infiltrated by lymphocytes, plasma cells and polymorphs; lymphoid follicles sometimes form and are often responsible for the surface granularity of the mucosa. When the inflammation is florid, the surface epithelium may be lost, the pelves and calyces then being lined by granulation tissue. In cases where the inflammation has subsided, the walls of the pelvis and calyces are atrophic with some scarring.

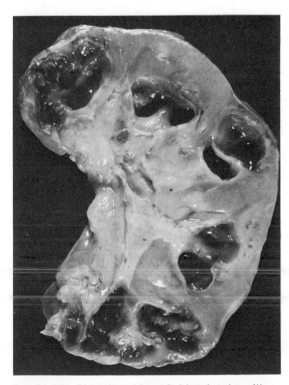

Fig. 21.54 Chronic pyelonephritis, showing dilatation and distortion of the calyces, over some of which the kidney tissue has been largely destroyed and now consists of a thin fibrous layer.

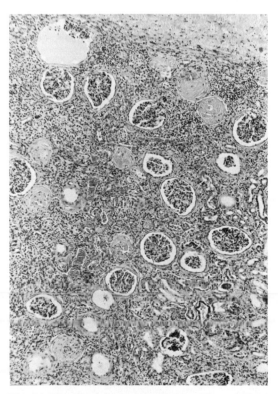

Fig. 21.55 Chronic pyelonephritis. The tubules are greatly atrophied and there is a marked interstitial inflammatory cell infiltrate. Many of the glomeruli still appear normal, but others are completely hyalinised. × 38.

As explained later, chronic pyelonephritic scarring may vary in extent from involvement of only a small proportion of the renal tissue to extensive renal destruction. When of lesser extent, it is usually an incidental finding at necropsy.

The scarred areas. There is extensive atrophy and loss of tubules, especially the proximal segments (Fig. 21.55), and this is a most important histological feature of chronic pyelonephritis. Tubular atrophy is often accompanied by gross thickening of the tubular basement membranes, and there is increase in fibrous tissue between the tubules. Commonly partial destruction of tubules results in survival of isolated segments; these become distended with inspissated eosinophilic secretion (presumably produced by the lining epithelium), and the epithelium becomes flattened: these changes occur in groups of adjacent tubules which come to resemble superficially thyroid acini (Fig. 21.56). The interstitial tissue is densely packed with lymphocytes, plasma cells and sometimes neutrophil and eosinophil polymorphs: in the late stages of the disease the inflammatory cell infiltrate is replaced by dense scar tissue. In such 'burnt out' pyelonephritis, there may be little evidence of active inflammation. The glomeruli are preserved for a very long time but eventually a spectrum of glomerular abnormalities appears, the most specific of which is concentric periglomerular fibrosis around a thickened Bowman's capsule (Fig. 21.57). Other changes

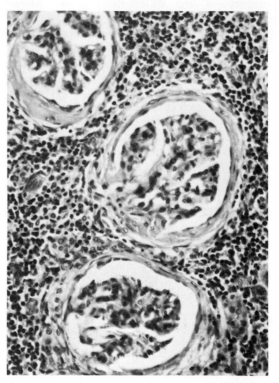

Fig. 21.57 Chronic pyelonephritis. There is periglomerular fibrosis, a heavy chronic inflammatory infiltrate, and almost complete loss of tubules. × 150.

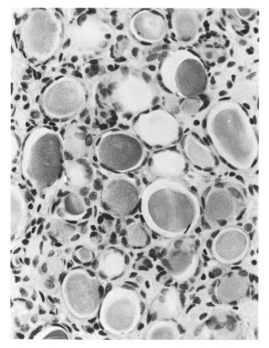

Fig. 21.56 Chronic pyelonephritis. Inspissated colloid-like material in sequestrated portions of renal tubules, presenting an appearance resembling superficially that of thyroid tissue. × 250.

are ischaemic and resemble those in essential hypertension: they include gradual hyalinisation of the glomerular tuft and fibrosis within Bowman's capsule (p. 750 and Fig. 21.55). At an earlier stage some capillary tufts may show irregular proliferation of endothelial and mesangial cells. Arteriolar and glomerular capillary necrosis occurs only if malignant hypertension has supervened. The arteries show variable degrees of medial and intimal fibrous thickening.

The non-scarred areas. The glomeruli may show compensatory hypertrophy. Other glomerular and vascular changes often develop as a result of arterial hypertension.

The pyelonephritic nature of small, irregularly scarred kidneys, which histologically show no evidence of active bacterial infection, is doubtful, and this doubt is increased by the frequent absence of any history suggestive of previous urinary tract infection.

Clinical features

Acute pyelonephritis is usually accompanied by acute infection of the lower urinary tract, i.e. cystitis, so that there is frequency of micturition and dysuria. The features of pyelonephritis itself include fever, often with rigors, and pain and tenderness in the lumbar regions. The urine is heavily infected and contains large numbers of pus cells and often red cells. Microscopy may reveal cellular casts in which most of the cells are polymorphs: this finding is of particular diagnostic importance, indicating pyelonephritis and not just lower urinary tract infection.

In chronic pyelonephritis there is, in most cases, no preceding history suggestive of urinary tract infection. There may be a long history of vague ill-health with, in children, reduced rate of growth. Commonly, however, the presenting features are attributable to the hypertension or uraemia of chronic renal failure. Depending on whether or not the infection is still active, the urine may contain significant numbers of bacteria (see above), pus cells and cellular casts. There is usually mild proteinuria. Perhaps because destruction of the tubules precedes that of the glomeruli, the urine tends to be of greater volume and more dilute than in chronic glomerulonephritis. Demonstration by intravenous pyelography of irregular coarse scarring and distortion of the calyces is particularly helpful in the diagnosis of chronic pyelonephritis.

Hypertension in chronic pyelonephritis. Approximately 70% of patients with extensive chronic pyelonephritis develop hypertension, and in 15–20% of these the hypertension is of the malignant type. There has been some controversy over the nature of the relationship between the two conditions, and it has been suggested that the association might result from a predisposition of individuals with essential hypertension to develop pyelonephritis. We do not consider this a likely explanation, for it would not account for the occurrence of hypertension in young patients with chronic pyelonephritis. The obvious explanation is that chronic pyelonephritis, like other conditions giving rise to extensive scarring of the kidneys, commonly leads to hypertension of secondary (renal) type. Admittedly, the mechanism of production of the hypertension of chronic renal disease is not well understood (p. 323) but this seems no reason for doubting that it occurs in chronic pyelonephritis.

Tuberculous pyelonephritis

This results from blood spread of tubercle bacilli, e.g. from pulmonary lesions. Like other organs, the kidneys are studded with minute tubercles in acute miliary tuberculosis, but of more importance are the localised renal lesions of tuberculous pyelonephritis which may slowly extend to destroy the kidney(s). Other common sites of blood-borne metastatic tuberculous lesions in the genito-urinary tract are the epididymis in the male and the Fallopian tube in the female, and spread from these sites can give rise to tuberculosis of the bladder and ascending infection to involve the kidneys. Conversely, renal tuberculosis can spread to involve the ureters, bladder and other pelvic viscera.

Clinical features. Renal tuberculosis may produce vague illness, with weight loss and fever, or may present with local features such as lumbar pain, dysuria, haematuria or pyuria. *Myco. tuberculosis* can usually be detected in the urine, and pyelography may show distortion of one or more calyces. In most cases, there is neither evidence nor history of tuberculosis elsewhere in the body (although this must, of course, have been present), and even at necropsy active pulmonary tuberculosis is present in only a minority of cases. Renal tuberculosis occurs usually in adult life, and it may be that, as in the lungs, it can remain latent for many years and then flare up: this would account for its occurrence long after any primary lung lesion has healed.

The incidence of renal tuberculosis in Europe has declined along with tuberculosis in general, and it is now a rather uncommon condition: its main danger is the involvement of both kidneys to such an extent as to cause renal failure.

Pathological changes. The initial renal lesion results usually from blood-borne infection, mycobacteria becoming arrested in the cortex, with development of one or more tubercles: these enlarge, caseate and coalesce, while lymphatic and tubular spread leads to tubercles

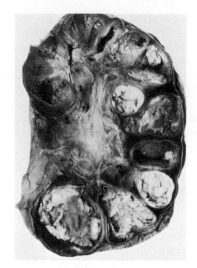

Fig. 21.59 Old tuberculosis of kidney, which has been largely replaced by caseous lesions enclosed by fibrous tissue.

often results in haematuria and the renal lesions tend also to suppurate, giving pyuria.

Cytomegalic virus disease

This occurs in newborn infants as a localised or generalised condition, and also as an opportunistic infection at all ages in subjects with various forms of immunodeficiency or being treated

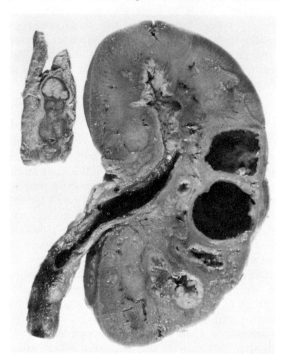

Fig. 21.58 Renal tuberculosis. The kidney contains several caseous lesions, which have discharged into the pelvis. The wall of the uppermost calyx is also caseous and the ureter and seminal vesicle (*inset*) are also involved.

round about, and so the lesion grows as an enlarging patch of caseation. Spread through the adjacent papilla is common, and on reaching the renal pelvis the lesion may soften and discharge its contents, leaving a ragged cavity. Further tubercles develop in the walls of the renal pelvis caseate and ulcerate; from here infection spreads into other parts of the kidney, which may then develop multiple caseous lesions (Figs. 21.58, 21.59). The ureter or renal pelvis may become obstructed by tuberculous lesions in their walls, or by plugging with caseous material, and the urine (coming solely from the other kidney) may then be normal. Apart from this, renal pelvic involvement

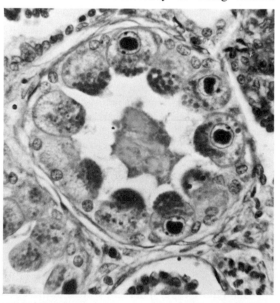

Fig. 21.60 Renal tubules, showing intranuclear and cytoplasmic inclusion bodies in the lining cells in cytomegalic virus disease in an infant. × 400.

with immunosuppressive drugs. Involvement of the liver and bone marrow in infants may cause changes resembling those of erythroblastosis fetalis. Serological evidence of infection has been reported in over 50% of renal transplant patients. Colonised cells become greatly enlarged and often show nuclear or cytoplasmic inclusions (Fig. 21.60). Involvement of the renal tubules does not appear to have much affect on function but may allow the diagnosis to be made by detection of colonised cells in the urine.

Congenital Lesions

Congenital cystic kidneys

This occurs in two main forms, one of which does not usually cause illness until middle-age, while the other is usually fatal in infancy.

Adult polycystic disease is the least rare form of congenital cystic renal disease. The kidneys contain large numbers of cysts which enlarge throughout life. Rarely death from renal failure occurs in infancy or childhood, but more than 50% of patients present in the 3rd to 5th decades with symptoms due to hypertension or uraemia, and most of the remainder die of unrelated causes.

In adult patients, the kidneys are greatly enlarged and occupied by numerous cysts of various sizes, while little kidney substance may be recognisable between the cysts. Prolonged survival presupposes, of course, the presence of enough functioning renal tissue, but as the cysts enlarge they compress, and impair the functional efficiency of the renal tissue, so that various ill-effects follow. Each kidney may weigh 1 kg or even more (Fig. 21.61) and be easily palpable. The cysts may be of any size up to 4–6 cm in diameter; they contain usually serous fluid, colourless or brownish, though it may be mucoid, especially in the smaller cysts. Occasionally the cystic change is practically restricted to one kidney. The condition may be the result of disturbance of normal development due to imperfect fusion between the kidney tubules proper and the collecting tubules, which grow up from the extremity of the ureter to meet them, but other embryological explanations have been proposed. The condition is inherited as an autosomal dominant trait, and there may be accompanying cystic change in the liver, although not sufficient to disturb hepatic function. There is also an association with aneurysms of the cerebral arteries, and about 15% of patients with polycystic kidneys die from subarachnoid haemorrhage.

Lesser degrees of cystic change are common in the kidneys, ranging from a few to many cysts, but with sufficient tissue remaining to avert renal failure. Occasionally a single cyst

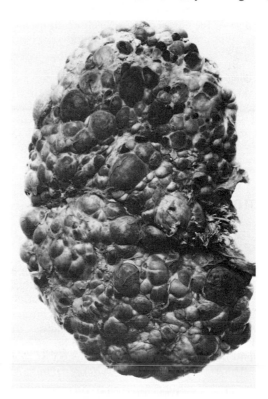

Fig. 21.61 Surface view of congenital cystic kidney, which weighed 1·5 kg.

may reach such a size as to be palpable during life.

Infantile polycystic disease is rare and usually causes death shortly after birth. It may be due to an autosomal recessive trait. The kidneys contain multiple elongated radially arranged cysts lined by cuboidal or columnar epithelium. Renal enlargement may be sufficient to interfere with birth, or in live-born infants with respiration. Occasional patients survive longer and develop fatal hypertension in childhood. The condition is associated with multiple hepatic cysts or abnormalities of the small bile ducts in the portal areas.

Sponge kidney (medullary cystic) disease consists of cystic dilatation of the collecting ducts in the papillae. It is usually bilateral and may affect any or all of the papillae in each kidney. Symptoms usually develop after the age of 30, and are due to the formation of stones composed of calcium salts in the cysts or to superadded pyelonephritis. The cysts are usually less than 5 mm in diameter and their epithelial lining may be single layered or squamous. The diagnosis may be apparent from intravenous pyelograms. The cause of this condition is unknown and its congenital nature uncertain.

There is a similar condition in which small cysts occur also in the cortex and in which death usually results from uraemia in late childhood or young adult life.

Other congenital defects

These are numerous and some are comparatively common. Occasionally one kidney, usually the left, is absent—*agenesia*—and there is generally an absence of the ureter also. In such cases, the surviving kidney undergoes compensatory hypertrophy, and its weight may sometimes double: this occurs also in *hypoplasia* of one kidney, which appears usually as an irregular atrophic structure around the upper end of its ureter. Hypoplasia of both kidneys may occur to such a degree as to be incompatible with life; minor degrees of the condition may possibly lead to renal dwarfism. Sometimes the two kidneys are fused, and this most frequently occurs at the lower pole, so that the '*horseshoe kidney*' results: the pelves are directed somewhat forward and the two ureters pass in front of the connecting bridge. In rarer forms the fusion of the kidneys is more complete and an oval or somewhat irregular kidney results, which varies in position. Occasionally a kidney, more rarely both, may lie in front of the sacrum: its ureter is correspondingly short and the arterial blood supply comes from the lower end of the aorta or an adjacent large branch. In these various renal abnormalities the position of the adrenals is usually quite normal. The kidney is originally composed of five lobules and ordinarily their fusion is complete. Sometimes slight grooves on the surface mark the original lobules and the term *fetal lobulation* is applied; the condition is of no importance. It is more marked in the child than in the adult. The arrangement of the renal arteries is very variable and the so-called aberrant arteries are not accessory vessels but are the segmental renal arteries taking separate origin. Division of such an artery is likely to be followed by infarction of the tissue supplied by it.

Tumours

Benign tumours

These are not very rare, the commonest being a small *fibroma* in the medulla; it rarely reaches 1 cm in diameter. *Adenoma* occasionally occurs, usually in the cortex, and some have a characteristic appearance with narrow bands of stroma and papilliform ingrowths (Fig. 21.62). It is usually benign, but carcinoma may supervene. In the renal pelvis *villous papillary tumours* are sometimes seen; they correspond to the papillary tumours of the bladder (p. 807) and are sometimes associated with them. *Angioma* is another uncommon benign tumour. It may occur in the pyramids or just underneath the lining of the pelvis, and, even when small, may lead to severe haematuria.

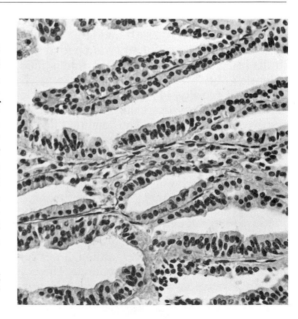

Fig. 21.62 Papillary adenoma of kidney, showing the delicate stroma and the appearances of the epithelium. × 140.

Malignant tumours

Malignant tumours are much less common in the kidneys than in several other organs, but two are of some importance—*renal carcinoma* and *nephroblastoma*.

Renal carcinoma

Clear-cell carcinoma is the commonest type. It was formerly called *Grawitz tumour* or *hypernephroma*. This last term was based on a superficial resemblance of this type of tumour to adrenal tissue, which led Grawitz to suggest that it arose from adrenocortical tissue misplaced within the kidneys. However, it is now widely accepted that it originates from renal tubular epithelium, and accordingly the term hypernephroma is a misnomer.

Clear-cell carcinoma is often large, and may occasionally form an enormous mass. It may occur in any part of the kidney. On section,

there are usually large areas of dull yellowish tissue (presenting a superficial resemblance to the adrenal cortex), interspersed with vascular, haemorrhagic and necrotic areas, and also broad bands and patches of connective tissue, somewhat mucoid or translucent in appearance (Fig. 21.63). Although the tumour may often appear to be encapsulated, like a benign tumour, it shows distinctly malignant properties. It commonly grows into the tributaries of the renal vein and forms thrombus-like masses within them; metastases may follow, especially in the lungs and bones. It may also burst through the capsule of the kidney or into the pelvis. Haematuria is common and often a prominent symptom.

On microscopic examination, such a tumour has, as a rule, a distinctly acinous arrangement in many parts, the spaces being lined by tall columnar epithelial cells: a papilliform type of growth also is sometimes present, and in other parts the arrangement of the epithelium is in solid masses. The tumour cells are large and

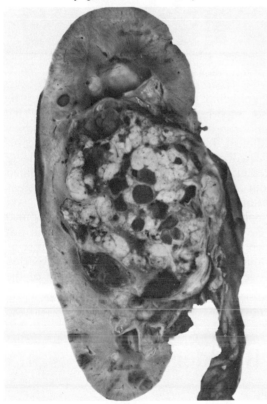

Fig. 21.63 Clear-cell carcinoma of kidney, growing from the central part of the kidney and compressing the renal pelvis. Note the haemorrhagic and gelatinous areas and rounded nodules of whitish tumour.

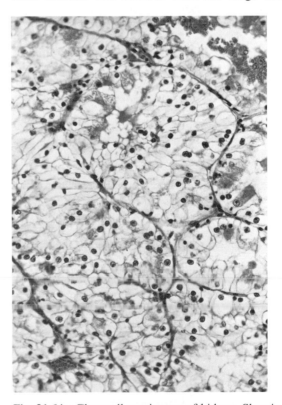

Fig. 21.64 Clear-cell carcinoma of kidney. Showing typical empty-looking cells with well-defined walls and delicate stroma. × 205.

often remarkably uniform, with abundant clear cytoplasm (Fig. 21.64) rich in glycogen and doubly-refracting lipid, and a relatively small round nucleus. There may, however, be greater variation in the cells, which may have an eosinophilic cytoplasm, or may be smaller and more anaplastic. As in other tumours, the prognosis depends on the degree of anaplasia, and invasion of the renal vein is not incompatible with long survival.

Tumours of purely adenocarcinomatous pattern occasionally occur in the kidney and papillary adenocarcinoma may arise both in the renal substance and in the pelvis, the two types being, however, quite distinct. In some renal carcinomas the cytoplasm of the tumour cells contains large homogeneous acidophil inclusions.

Papillary cystadenocarcinoma. This is a rather uncommon type of renal carcinoma: it consists of numerous cysts containing papillary processes, the stroma of which is often packed with foamy lipid-rich macrophages. It tends to invade the regional lymph nodes, and carries a prognosis similar to that of clear-cell carcinoma.

Nephroblastoma is an embryonic tumour, which has the general appearance of a rapidly growing sarcoma. It may reach a large size and, though fairly well enclosed within the kidney capsule, rapidly invades blood vessels and so produces metastases, chiefly in the lungs. It occurs especially in the first three years of life, and is known also as 'embryoma', 'mixed tumour' or 'Wilms' tumour' of the kidney. Although rare, it is one of the commonest malignant tumours in childhood.

Microscopically, the tumour is composed of a spindle-celled tissue, with formation of acini and tubular structures, and apparent transitions may be seen between the spindle cells and those

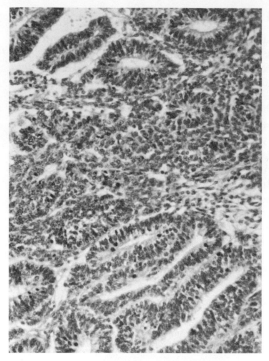

Fig. 21.65 Nephroblastoma, showing cellular tissue with formation of acini by columnar cells. × 200.

of epithelial type (Fig. 21.65). There may be also imperfect formation of glomeruli. This tumour is derived from the cells of the kidney rudiment. In some instances it has a more complicated structure, striped muscle fibres being present, and the tumour may have originated from cells of the mesoderm before the differentiation of the myotomes.

Spindle-cell sarcoma is a rare renal tumour.

Secondary carcinoma in the kidneys is not uncommon, although metastases are neither as frequent nor as numerous as might be expected in view of the very large blood supply of the kidneys.

Renal Pelves, Ureters and Bladder

The lesions of these structures are considered together, as they are so often involved in the same pathological process. Three main factors are concerned in the majority of these lesions, viz. (*a*) *obstruction to urinary flow*, (*b*) *infections* and (*c*) the *formation of stones*. Two or even all three of these conditions may be present at the same time. *Epithelial tumours* of the urinary tract are not uncommon and are mostly malignant, although often low grade.

Effects of obstruction

Serious mechanical obstruction to outflow of urine from the bladder is practically confined to the male sex, and is commonly produced by enlargement of the prostate or stricture of the urethra: occasionally severe phimosis, tumour or calculus are responsible. The chief effect on the bladder is the production of variable degrees of hypertrophy and dilatation. When the outstanding feature is hypertrophy, the muscular part of the wall is thickened and the bands of muscle, which have an interlacing arrangement under the mucosa, enlarge and form prominent ridges or bands with depressions between (Fig. 23.11, p. 890). Occasionally one of these depressions may become enlarged and form a large projecting diverticulum. When infection occurs, as is so often the case, pus may collect in such diverticula, and ulceration and even perforation may follow. Obstruction to the outflow from the bladder ultimately leads to dilatation of the ureters and pelves of the kidneys. The former may undergo considerable dilatation and their walls become somewhat thickened, and the pelves also become enlarged, so that there is a condition of bilateral hydronephrosis. The dilatation is sometimes more marked on one side than on the other.

Hydronephrosis

This means a dilatation of the renal pelvis and may occur on one or both sides.

Causation. Urethral obstruction, referred to above, is the commonest cause of **bilateral hydronephrosis**. It can result also from pressure of a tumour, or neoplastic infiltration, affecting both ureters. Such infiltration occurs commonly, for example, in cancer of the cervix uteri. Occasionally dilatation of the ureters and hydronephrosis are due to congenital abnormality in the posterior urethra, the mucosa of which forms valve-like folds; the resulting renal atrophy may be accompanied by renal dwarfism (p. 778). Another cause of hydroureters and bilateral hydronephrosis is neurogenic disturbance of bladder control due to lesions of the spinal cord. In all these conditions of bilateral hydronephrosis the dilatation of the ureters and pelves is usually moderate. The most striking degree of dilatation is seen, however, in **unilateral hydronephrosis**. This can

result from impaction of a calculus, usually at the upper end of the ureter, at the level of the brim of the pelvis, or at the entrance to the bladder. It may be produced also by a scar, which sometimes follows ulceration due to the passage of a stone, by a tumour of the ureter itself, or pressure of a tumour from outside. It occasionally results when the ureter is attached at an abnormally high level to the pelvis, so that it leaves it at an acute angle, and a valve-like obstruction results. This may cause intermittent accumulation of urine, and ultimately marked

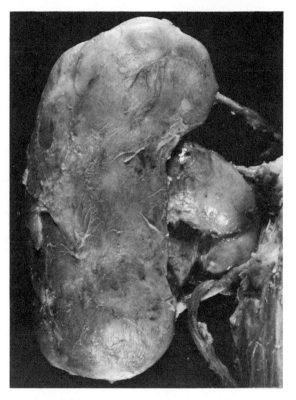

Fig. 21.66 Hydronephrosis due to bending of the ureter around an accessory renal artery to the lower pole of the kidney.

hydronephrosis may develop. Hydronephrosis may result when the ureter is kinked over an aberrant renal artery supplying the lower pole of the kidney (Fig. 21.66). It is also encountered rarely in congenitally misplaced kidneys. In some cases there is pronounced ureteric narrowing just below the uretero-pelvic junction, and while this is occasionally related to an abnormal renal artery, often no cause of the stricture is apparent.

Structural changes. The effects of obstruction vary greatly. Sometimes a calculus may be firmly impacted, and there may be obvious distension of the pelvis and calyces (Fig. 21.67), or the whole pelvis and calyces may be distended by a branching calculus, though this is more common when infection has been superadded

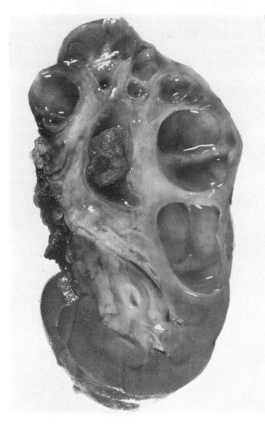

Fig. 21.67 An impacted stone in the renal pelvis, which has caused hydronephrosis and consequent atrophy of the renal tissue. The stone was in such a position that the lower part of the pelvis was not obstructed, and the lower pole of the kidney appears normal.

(p. 805). In such cases, fibrosis and atrophy of the kidney follow. In other cases, distension is so great that the dilated pelvis may become palpable. As the distension progresses, the calyces become flattened, the kidney substance becomes stretched over the dilated pelvis, and ultimately may form a mere rind (*intrarenal hydronephrosis*), the surface of the kidney usually develops a lobulated appearance. Atrophy of the kidney substance may be regular or irregular, so that parts of consider-

able thickness may be left while the rest is much thinned; the latter result apparently depends on the degree to which the vascular supply is impaired, and the microscopic appearances resemble those resulting from major artery stenosis, i.e. the glomeruli are relatively spared, but the tubules are atrophied. Sometimes the dilatation is mainly in the form of a sac projecting medial to the kidney and there is little effect on the appearance of the kidney—*extrarenal hydronephrosis*.

The results of obstruction of a ureter vary greatly. If it is sudden, complete and persistent, production of urine ceases almost immediately and the pelvis does not dilate very much. This may result from impaction of a stone. If, however, obstruction develops gradually, or is partial or intermittent, the kidney continues to produce urine and the urinary tract above the obstruction becomes greatly dilated. This may result from pressure of, or infiltration by, a tumour, from movement of a stone or stricture or from kinking of the ureter over a renal artery. When the kidney becomes greatly stretched and thinned, the tubules, and ultimately the glomeruli, become atrophied, and there ensues general overgrowth of the connective tissue. The contents of a dilated pelvis are, of course, at first urine; but, as the condition becomes chronic, the urinary constituents disappear, while proteins are added to the fluid by transudation from the wall of the sac.

Urinary tract infection

The commonest serious complication of urinary tract infection is extension to the kidneys, and accordingly the subject has already been discussed in the account of pyelonephritis (pp. 789–97). The main features of urinary tract infection are as follows:

(1) Normal urine is often contaminated by bacteria living in the lower urethra: normally, there are fewer than 10^5 bacteria per ml of urine, and greater numbers are suggestive of infection.

(2) Infection is much commoner in females of all ages than in males, possibly due to the shorter, wide female urethra.

(3) Infection is especially common in pregnancy because of the hormonal relaxation of smooth muscle and the pressure of the uterus on the urinary tract.

(4) Most infections are caused by bacteria gaining entrance to the bladder via the urethra, and the renal pelves may be involved, spread being either intra-luminal or in the interstitial tissue of the urinary tract.

(5) In the presence of cystitis, reflux of urine from bladder to ureters is a common occurrence, and is likely to promote ascending infection.

(6) In patients without urinary tract obstruction, who have not been subjected to catheterisation or other instrumentation, urinary tract infections are usually caused by *Escherichia coli*. With obstruction or following instrumentation, mixed infections, including coliform bacilli, *Proteus* and staphylococci, are common.

(7) Urinary tract obstruction, including neurogenic disturbances of bladder control, is of major importance in predisposing to, enhancing and prolonging infection, and promoting its spread. This is especially so when the obstruction is chronic and has resulted in ureteric dilatation.

(8) Once infection has involved the renal pelves and calyces (pyelitis), direct spread into the renal papillae can occur, leading to pyelonephritis.

(9) Chronic infection, especially with *Proteus*, predisposes to formation of phosphate deposits in the urinary tract by splitting urea and thus rendering the urine alkaline: the deposits can both obstruct the flow of urine and enhance the infection.

(10) Symptomless bacteriuria in childhood is followed, in some instances, by the development of chronic pyelonephritis.

In the early stages of an acute urinary infection, the urine may contain a heavy concentration of bacteria with few cells, but pus cells soon appear; in some instances there may be sufficient haemorrhage from the inflamed mucosa to present clinically as haematuria.

The morbid anatomical changes in **cystitis** are usually classified as catarrhal, purulent and pseudo-membranous. In pseudo-membranous, which is found chiefly when there is chronic obstruction and hypertrophy of the bladder, there occurs superficial necrosis of the mucosa with fibrinous exudate, especially over the muscular ridges, and the necrotic mucosa is sloughed off in decomposing shreds. The most severe changes are usually observed where there is alkaline decomposition of the urine. Haemor-

rhages into the mucosa are common, and these may become greenish and almost black, while the surface is covered with pus and often a deposit of phosphates. Such an infection may ascend the dilated ureters, and produce a pyelitis with similar features, and the dilated pelvis may become ulcerated or filled with an accumulation of pus—**pyonephrosis**. Here also secondary deposit of phosphates may occur. Inevitably the infection extends to the kidneys and gives rise to pyelonephritis. Often only one pelvis is affected in this way, but both may be involved.

Pyonephrosis also arises when a hydronephrosis due to a calculus in the renal pelvis becomes infected. The presence of a renal calculus seems to predispose the pelvis to infection, and this leads in turn to alkaline decomposition of the urine. Phosphates are precipitated in the dilated pelvis and calyces and particularly on the pre-existing calculus, which develops into an irregular branching mass with bulbous ends extending into the calyces, the whole forming a rough cast of the pyonephrotic sac. This is known as a *staghorn calculus* (Fig. 21.69).

The urinary tract is not infrequently infected from the kidney by *typhoid bacilli* in the course of typhoid fever. Usually only a mild catarrhal inflammation is the result, and the condition may be almost a pure bacilluria. The bacilli may persist indefinitely, the patient becoming a 'urinary carrier' (p. 574); the establishment of the carrier state is facilitated by almost any anatomical abnormality in the urinary tract. In some cases of coliform infection also, there may be comparatively little inflammatory reaction. Cystitis may rarely be produced by the gonococcus in cases of *gonorrhoea*, and has usually the features of purulent catarrh. Coliform bacilli and the gonococcus do not render the urine alkaline, but infection by *Proteus* is quickly followed by ammoniacal decomposition owing to splitting of urea.

Malakoplakia. This is a rare condition found in some cases of chronic cystitis, and is characterised by the formation of numerous soft rounded elevations or plaques in the bladder wall, varying up to 1–2 cm. They have a pale, sometimes yellowish appearance surrounded by vascular areas, and tend to ulcerate on the surface and be invaded by bacteria. They are essentially composed of cellular granulation tissue in which there are numerous large cells which contain droplets of various kinds and small hyaline spheres with concentric marking known as Michaelis–Gutmann bodies, also inclusions of red cells and leukocytes. The rounded structures may become free by disintegration of the cells. Calcium salts may be deposited in them and they have also an affinity for iron, as can be shown by the usual tests. The lesion is a granuloma of unknown cause.

Tuberculosis. Tuberculous disease of the bladder is, as a rule, the result of direct infection of its mucosa by tubercle bacilli in the urine. It occurs most often in cases of renal tuberculosis, though also in tuberculosis of the genital tract. The bacilli invade the mucosa and give rise to tubercles which then undergo ulceration. In this way, multiple small ulcers are formed, especially at the base of the bladder, and sometimes the orifices of the ureters are specially involved. The ulcers increase in size and form large areas by confluence. Sometimes there is a considerable amount of caseous thickening of the lining. Secondary invasion by other organisms sometimes occurs, and more acute inflammatory change is superadded.

Schistosomiasis (bilharziasis). The bladder is the most frequent site of lesions in this condition, which is produced by *Schistosoma haematobium*. It is very common in many hot countries, notably in Egypt. The adult parasites lie in the veins of the bladder, and the eggs laid by the female pass into the surrounding tissues, where their presence in large numbers induces the formation of abundant vascular granulation tissue which causes great thickening of the mucosa and submucosa. Nodular projections appear, and the interior of the bladder may be beset with rounded and somewhat pedunculated vascular polypi, which tend to become ulcerated. Haematuria is a common feature and the ova are readily found in the urine. Pyogenic infections may become superadded, and carcinoma develops in a proportion of cases in Egyptians, but very rarely in infected Europeans. Schistosomal lesions sometimes occur also in the ureters and renal pelves.

Schistosoma haematobium is a dioecious trematode. The adult male is about 13 mm long, the female about 20 mm; the female is thinner, and lies enclosed in the gynaecophoric canal of the male. The eggs are oval in form, about 130μm in length, and the shell has a distinct terminal spine; the embryo is visible within. When the urine becomes diluted on being mixed with water, the investing shell swells and bursts and a ciliated embryo or miracidium escapes. Further developmental stages take place within fresh-water snails, from which the free-swimming cercariae emerge: these enter the human host,

chiefly through the skin but also through the mucous membrane of the mouth and pharynx. They pass by systemic veins to the lungs, through the pulmonary capillaries, and thence to the systemic arteries via the heart. Those reaching the liver mature into adult worms within the portal vessels. The young adults then pass against the blood stream to the portal radicles, especially those of the inferior mesenteric vein, and thence they reach the vesical plexus, where they settle and pair as described above. Occasionally the parasite remains in the liver and the eggs are discharged into the peri-portal connective tissue and give rise to hepatic fibrosis (p. 635). There are two other pathogenic species of schistosoma, *S. mansoni* and *S. japonicum*: they have similar life cycles to *S. haematobium*. The adult *S. mansoni* colonises the veins of the colon (p. 579), and *S. japonicum*, which

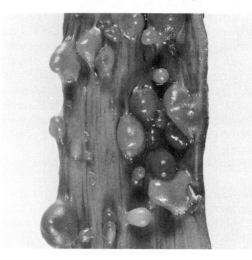

Fig. 21.68   Ureteritis cystica. The thin-walled cysts have formed in sequestered epithelium, but as they enlarged have come to project into the lumen. × 3.

occurs in the Far East, the veins of the small intestine. The ova of both species cause granulomatous reactions in the gut, with ulceration and melaena, and they may also colonise the liver, producing peri-portal fibrosis: the ova are found in the faeces.

Ureteritis cystica. Inflammation of the urinary tract may be followed by formation of multiple small cysts which contain clear fluid and project into the lumen (Fig. 21.68). Apparently foci of epithelium become sequestrated deep to the surface and form these cysts. The change occurs also in the renal pelves and bladder (*pyelitis* and *cystitis cystica*).

Calculi

Urinary calculi are formed by precipitation of urinary constituents, a small amount of organic material also being incorporated. Deposition is favoured by a highly concentrated urine, and by secretion of excessive amounts of one or other constituents (oxalate, urate, etc.). Calculi occur in the renal pelvis or ureter, or in the bladder, although some of the latter originate in the kidneys, and subsequently enlarge in the bladder.

There are 3 main types of urinary calculus composed respectively of (*a*) a mixture of uric acid and urates—uric acid stones, (*b*) calcium oxalate; both (*a*) and (*b*) are laid down in acid urines and stones may contain a mixture of both substances; (*c*) calcium carbonate and phosphate combined in the complex forms of carbonate-apatite and hydroxyapatite; these are laid down in alkaline urines and often form an outer laminated deposit upon other stones.

The commonest pure type of stone consists of calcium oxalate whereas only 6% are of uric acid. Most stones consist principally of the apatites but contain also some oxalate and urate. It has long been supposed that calculi begin as minute deposits in the collecting tubules of the kidney and then pass to the pelvis where further increase in size takes place. Randall has shown that some stones develop by enlargement of plaque-like deposits attached to the apices of the pyramids. Carr has suggested from radiographic evidence that the primary site of deposition is in the lymphatics of the renal papillae that normally remove particulate matter from this region. If this mechanism is overloaded or if the lymphatic pathway is obstructed by inflammation of the papilla, microliths accumulate and are extruded through the lymphatic lining into the calyx where they grow into small concretions by further deposition of urinary solids. The part in stone formation played by organic matter is uncertain, but Boyce and his co-workers have suggested that urinary mucoproteins attract and fix calcium ions which later, as a result of alterations of pH, are precipitated as crystalline salts to form the nuclei of stones. all the calcium-rich calculi except pure oxalate stones have a mucopolysaccharide binding agent. In the formation of calculi, excess of a particular substance is usually an important factor, as, for example, in hyperparathyroidism, where the increased excretion of calcium and phosphate in the urine very frequently leads to the formation of urinary calculi of the apatite variety.

Renal calculi. Stones in the renal pelvis may be single or multiple. They are sometimes particularly numerous when there is partial obstruction and dilatation. A single calculus may, however, grow to the size and shape of the dilated pelvis (Fig. 21.69).

A small calculus may pass along the ureter to the bladder, giving rise to renal colic with haematuria. It may be arrested temporarily, usually at the narrow lower end of the ureter. Permanent impaction, usually at the upper or

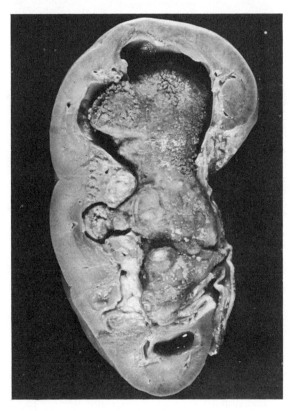

Fig. 21.69 A large 'staghorn' calculus occupying the dilated renal pelvis and calyces.

lower ends of the ureter or at the level of the pelvic brim, produces hydronephrosis as already described, and when the obstruction is intermittent, the hydronephrosis may be extreme. When the urine is infected with urea-splitting bacteria (e.g. *Proteus*) ammonia is produced and calculi or softer deposits composed of phosphates form in the alkaline urine and are precipitated in the inflamed pelvis. The condition may be accompanied by suppuration and ulceration. The large branching 'staghorn' calculi arise in this way and are composed largely of complex hydrated phosphates. A calculus in the renal pelvis, especially when it is movable, may give rise to metaplasia of the lining of the pelvis to stratified squamous epithelium. As a further result of the irritation, squamous carcinoma has occasionally been found to arise, as is illustrated in Fig. 21.70.

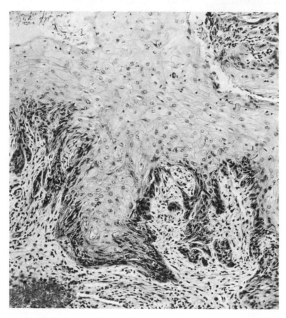

Fig. 21.70 Section through the renal pelvis in nephrolithiasis, showing squamous metaplasia of epithelium and early squamous carcinoma. × 65.

Precipitation of sulphonamide drugs may occur in the renal tubules and pelvis unless the fluid intake is maintained at a high level to promote diuresis. If this is neglected, actual obstruction of tubules, pelves and ureters may result from masses of crystals of the drug or its acetylated form. Acute renal failure from this cause was encountered in the early days of sulphonamide therapy.

Bladder calculi may be single or multiple: they are sometimes numerous and like coarse sand. They are now relatively uncommon in Europe. In many cases calculi form first in the renal pelvis, especially uric-acid and oxalate calculi, and pass to the bladder where they increase in size; in other cases they are formed locally. The larger calculi vary greatly in composition and structure, but as a rule there is a nucleus or primary stone surrounded by concentric laminae. The primary stones are composed of urates and uric acid, or of calcium oxalate or calcium phosphate, rarely of cystine or xanthine. The primary urate stone, seldom larger than a few mm, and often formed first in the renal pelvis, is round, hard and brown. The primary oxalate stone is small and very hard with irregular outline, and is often dark brown from altered blood pigment. Primary phosphatic stones are whitish, often friable, but sometimes hard. They occur in conditions causing hypercalciuria, e.g. hyperparathyroidism, chronic resorptive bone disease, immobilisation in bed, sarcoidosis and the milk-alkali syndrome. In many cases, however, hypercalciuria occurs without known cause. Any of these primary stones may have *secondary* deposits formed on their surface, and thus compound or laminated stones arise. The particular substance secondarily deposited, which need not be in a saturated state in the urine, depends not only on the composition of the urine but also on its pH. Examples of stones are shown in Fig. 21.71. As the state of the urine varies from time to time, the great variations in the composition of stones can be readily understood. Bladder stones sometimes grow to measure several centimetres, and may weigh over 300 g.

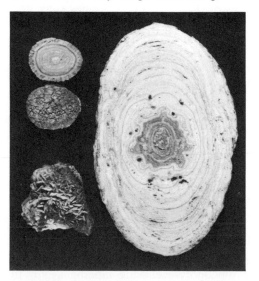

Fig. 21.71 Urinary calculi. *Upper left*, a renal calculus composed of uric acid and calcium oxalate, showing the inner lamellae and rough surface. *Lower left*, a renal calculus composed mainly of calcium oxalate. *Right*, a large bladder stone, which started as a urate stone, probably in the renal pelvis, and subsequently gained layers of phosphates while in the bladder. × 1.

Stones may form without the presence of bacterial infection or inflammation, and lead to mechanical effects—pain and irritation with haematuria, intermittent obstruction, damage to the bladder mucosa with ulceration, etc. When, however, there is secondary bacterial invasion, and ammoniacal decomposition of the urine occurs, then triple phosphates and ammonium urate separate out, often in large amount, and form a further deposit on calculi already formed. Deposits of these substances may occur also in cases of purulent cystitis (p. 803) apart from the previous occurrence of calculi, and form primary inflammatory calculi or irregular deposits.

Tumours

Nearly all tumours of the urinary tract arise from the transitional epithelial lining. There is evidence that chemical carcinogenesis is of aetiological importance, and, in accordance with this, it is not uncommon to encounter two or more tumours in the same individual, either simultaneously or over a period. It is not surprising that, having a relatively large surface area, the bladder should be a commoner site of tumours than the ureters or renal pelves, but the trigone appears to be particularly often involved.

It is difficult to adopt the usual classification of benign and malignant for urinary tract tumours, and the following classification takes into consideration the reported experience of the Institute of Urology of the University of London.

Benign papilloma. This is a pedunculated tumour, often less than 1 cm. in diameter, which projects into the lumen from a narrow stalk and is composed of fine branching fronds, each of which has a thin central core of vascular connective tissue and a lining which is 3–4 cells thick and resembles very closely the normal transitional epithelium of the urinary tract (Fig. 21.72). The cells are regular, and mitoses are few. Tumours showing this very high degree of differentiation are rare, and are benign.

Well-differentiated transitional cell carcinoma. These tumours may be papillary (Fig. 21.73) or solid, or may contain both types of structure. They comprise the majority of urinary tract tumours.

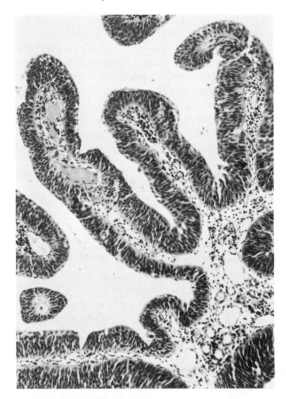

Fig. 21.72 Papilloma of bladder. Part of the tumour, showing the frond-like processes. Where the epithelium has been cut perpendicularly, it is 3–4 cells thick: in other places, oblique section gives a false impression of more cell layers. × 85.

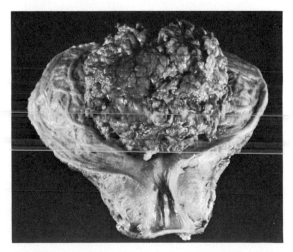

Fig. 21.73 A large papillary carcinoma of the bladder.

(*a*) *Papillary*. Tumours of this type have a structure similar to the benign papilloma; they differ, however, in having a thicker epithelial lining composed of more layers of cells. Mitoses are more numerous, and the epithelial cell nuclei show variations in size, but tend to be larger and more deeply staining, giving the impression of crowding of cells. In spite of these appearances, the cells are sufficiently differentiated to be recognisably of transitional type.

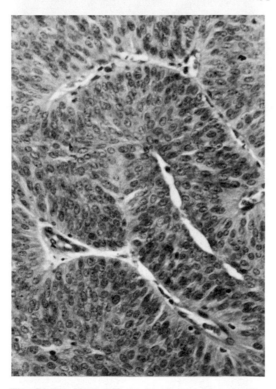

Fig. 21.74   Well-differentiated transitional-cell carcinoma of the urinary bladder. × 350.

The base of the epithelium is not so regular as in the benign papilloma, and it extends more deeply into the underlying connective tissue. Careful search must be made for foci of invasion, and extension into lymphatics or venules. Even in the apparent absence of such changes, some of these tumours recur or behave as carcinomas, but the presence of invasion greatly worsens the prognosis.

(*b*) *Solid*. This has the appearance of a raised plaque attached to the surface by a broad base, and sometimes appearing lobulated or nodular, Microscopy shows solid sheets of epithelial cells with appearances similar to the cells of the

papillary tumours (Fig. 21.74), but enclosed by bands of vascular connective tissue. The prognosis is similar to the papillary type, and the detection of invasion is again of great importance.

Some tumours are papillary in their superficial parts, but have a broad base of attachment and deeper solid elements.

Anaplastic carcinoma. This also presents as a plaque raised above the surface, but usually shows central necrosis and sloughing and thus appears as a sloughing ulcer with raised edges. The epithelium is in solid masses, and may have some resemblance to transitional cells but with obvious cell aberration and

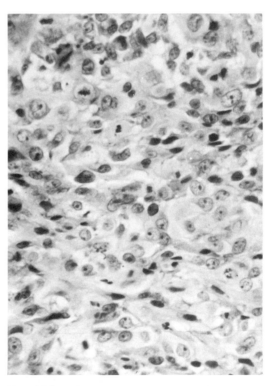

Fig. 21.75   Anaplastic carcinoma of the urinary bladder. × 350.

numerous and abnormal mitoses (Fig. 21.75). Foci of poorly differentiated squamous epithelium are often present. There is frank invasion into the underlying muscle, and lymphatic and venous extensions are often apparent. The prognosis is poor.

Squamous carcinoma also occurs in the urinary tract: in some instances it arises from squamous metaplasia attributable to the presence of calculi and chronic inflammation. In other cases, squamous cancer arises directly from transitional epithelium.

Adenocarcinoma is relatively uncommon. It may arise from transitional epithelium and occurs particularly in congenital extroversion of the bladder, when the epithelium undergoes metaplasia to mucus-secreting type. Another possible origin is from remnants of the urachus around the apex of the bladder.

Clinical features. Both benign and malignant tumours of the urinary tract tend to bleed, and haematuria is the common complaint. In some instances, infection is superadded, and recurrent cystitis is not unusual, particularly with ulcerated malignant tumours. Symptoms may also arise from local invasion or distant metastases.

Aetiology. Bladder tumours, and particularly the transitional cell types, are a well known industrial hazard in workers in the aniline dye industry, in which 2-naphthylamine has been incriminated (p. 256). There is also an increased incidence in workers in the rubber industry, and more recently there is evidence incriminating benzidine. The incidence is also increased in cigarette smokers. A high incidence of bladder tumours has been observed in Egypt, and is attributable to chronic schistosomiasis.

Other tumours. Myxoma and leiomyoma are occasionally encountered, and both leio- and rhabdo-myosarcomas, the last appearing as raised blunt processes.

Congenital abnormalities

Renal pelves and ureters. The ureter may be double in its upper part or in its whole length; in either case, a partial doubling of the pelvis is usually present. When the duplication is complete, the ureter from the upper part of the kidney opens separately into the bladder, or sometimes into the urethra or a seminal vesicle. Such a condition may be present on one or both sides. Congenital narrowing or *atresia* of a ureter may give rise to dilatation proximally; an abnormally high origin of the ureter from the pelvis may lead to hydronephrosis (p. 801). Such abnormalities appear to favour the occurrence of infection and also its persistence when established.

The bladder. The most important abnormality is a defect of its anterior wall, accompanied by a corresponding median defect of the abdominal wall, the condition being known as *extroversion* of the bladder. The posterior wall of the bladder is thus exposed, and appears as an area of vascular mucous membrane, on which the ureters open. The epithelium of the exposed mucosa undergoes metaplastic alteration, in part into squamous epithelium and in part into a columnar mucus-secreting epithelium resembling that of the intestine. In the male, the urethra remains open on its dorsal aspect, the condition being known as *epispadias*; in the female there is usually a split clitoris. The symphysis pubis is also usually deficient, though this may occur apart from extroversion of the bladder.

In the posterior **urethra** valve-like folds of the mucosa may cause obstruction with consequent hypertrophy of the bladder and bilateral hydronephrosis. Other abnormalities of the male urethra include epispadias (see above), and *hypospadias* in which it opens on the ventral surface of the penis.

Locomotor System

Diseases of Bone

Normal bone structure

Bone is a specialised form of connective tissue and certain fundamental concepts of its normal anatomy and physiology are essential to an understanding of its pathology. *Normal bone* consists of cells (osteocytes) lying in small spaces (lacunae) in a matrix formed of collagen fibres, amorphous ground substance and mineral complexes. The mineral consists of calcium and magnesium in combination with phosphate and carbonate, in the complex known as bone apatite.

Bone formation and resorption. Bone may be formed through the intermediate stage of cartilage (endochondral ossification) or directly from collagen (membranous ossification) but in both these circumstances the production of bone is thought to occur in two stages. Firstly, an uncalcified matrix, *osteoid*, is formed and secondly, under normal conditions, this is rapidly mineralised. The removal of bone (resorption) is generally believed to occur in one stage, mineral and matrix disappearing together. The terms decalcification and demineralisation are therefore to be avoided as they give a false picture of the process in living bone. At sites of bone resorption the bone surface has scalloped edges, *Howship's lacunae*, and these often contain multinucleated giant cells (osteoclasts). Bone is not a static tissue and throughout life the two processes of bone formation and bone resorption continue actively though at a slower rate in adult life than in childhood.

Types of bone. While all bone consists of cells, collagen fibres, ground substance and mineral, different types of bone may be formed depending on the arrangement of fibres and cells. Two main types are found in the human skeleton, woven bone and lamellar bone.

Woven bone consists of coarse fibre bundles running in an irregular, interlacing pattern

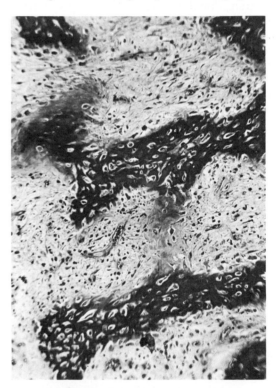

Fig. 22.1 Woven bone, from fracture callus, showing large, closely packed lacunae. × 190.

through a matrix rich in ground substance. The cells are large and closely packed (Fig. 22.1). It is formed whenever bone is rapidly laid down as in the embryonic skeleton, subperiosteally in a growing bone, in fracture callus, as reactive bone in relation to tumours, in Paget's disease, osteitis fibrosa and also in fibrous dysplasia. It is, however, an impermanent structure and, given time, is usually replaced by lamellar bone which is mechanically stronger.

Lamellar bone. The fibre bundles are fine and

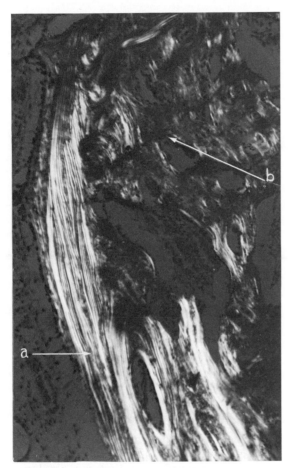

Fig. 22.2 Lamellar bone in polarised light showing **a** the orderly orientation of the bone lamellae. On the surface are some new formed trabeculae of woven bone, **b** showing lack of lamellar orientation, × 190.

run in parallel sheets (Fig. 22.2), different sheets having different fibre directions and so giving the whole a stratified appearance. The cells are smaller and less numerous than in woven bone and have more frequent and delicate processes. The histological differences are most clearly demonstrated either by silver stains or by viewing the sections in polarised light. Lamellar bone usually replaces pre-existing cartilage or woven bone.

Transplantation of bone (bone grafting)

Bone grafting is a relatively common surgical procedure. Grafts may be used to bridge a bony gap, e.g. in a fracture with much bone loss such as may occur following a gunshot wound, or in reconstructive plastic surgery; to fill a space within a bone, e.g. following curettage of a benign intraosseous tumour; and to promote bony union whether of an un-united fracture or across a diseased joint (arthrodesis). The bone used may come from the patient himself, an *autograft*; from another human, an *allograft or homograft* or from another animal species, a *xenograft or heterograft* (see p. 87). It may consist of cancellous or cortical bone and may be fresh, or in the case of allografts or xenografts may have been stored under sterile conditions following a variety of treatments.

Autogenous compact bone is used chiefly when strength and rigidity are required. The removal of the graft cuts off its blood supply and due to the difficulty of transmission of nutrition from tissue fluid through the canalicular system only a few superficially placed osteocytes survive along with some periosteal and endosteal cells. These surviving cells may proliferate and form some new bone but the major contribution is made by invading 'host' osteoblasts which accompany blood vessels from the tissue bed in which the graft is implanted. These vessels grow into the marrow spaces, Haversian canals, and along the surfaces of the graft; osteoclasts resorb some of the dead bone and new bone also forms so that the dead graft is first united with the 'host' bone and then gradually replaced over a period of months by new living bone (Fig. 22.3). At first the new bone is woven and forms an open meshwork; later it is remodelled to become lamellar and compact. The osteocytes in *autogenous cancellous bone* almost all die following transplantation but there is a much larger surface area of bone so that more endosteal cells are available for proliferation, and more importantly there is a greater stimulation of new bone formation by 'host' cells. This type of graft is *par excellence* a stimulator of osteogenesis although the dead graft bone is, as in the compact type, resorbed.

In fresh bone allografts in animals there is, as in the fresh autograft, necrosis of most of the

Fig. 22.3 Incorporation of a bone graft (after Ham). **a** The graft, seen in the centre, consists of cortex with some attached spongy bone trabeculae and marrow. Both the graft and the margins of the bony bed into which it is laid are dead (hatched). New living bone (black) is forming under the 'host' periosteum and around living (white) endosteal trabeculae.

b The amount of new living bone has increased and the graft bone is now attached to the 'host' bone by new trabeculae which have formed partly on the surface of dead bone. Haversian canals in the dead 'host' bone have been revascularised and widened by osteoclastic resorption. Some living bone is also proliferating around the margins of the canals. Union has occurred between the 'host' bone and the graft.

c The remaining amount of dead graft bone is much diminished by osteoclastic resorption and there is also some resorption of the remaining dead bone of the 'host' bed. The dead graft is being replaced by living new bone.

The type of reaction illustrated occurs no matter the type of graft used. There tends to be rather more graft osteoblast contribution to the final amount of new bone when fresh autograft bone is used.

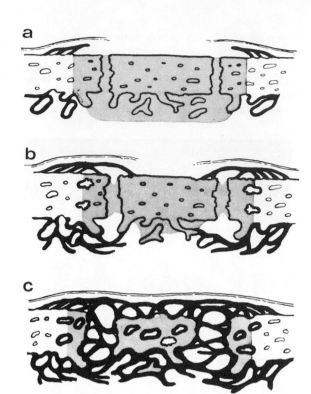

transplant, invasion by host capillaries and some proliferation of surviving graft osteoblasts with new bone formation. About 7 to 10 days after transplantation, however, lymphocytes appear around blood vessels which become obliterated and any surviving transplanted cells and new bone which has proliferated die. The dead graft is then either completely resorbed or acts as a scaffolding for 'host' cells and is slowly replaced by living bone. Second grafts from the same donor undergo accelerated rejection. The rejection process is a delayed hypersensitivity reaction (p. 136). The strongest antigen in the foreign bone seems to be the haemopoietic marrow cells. *Allografts used therapeutically in man are not fresh, they do not contain living cells but have been treated, sterilised and stored.* The aim in selecting methods of treatment, sterilisation and storage is to provide a graft which has low antigenicity, high powers of induction of new bone formation by the 'host' cells and the ability to be actively remodelled. The 'host' response to grafting is enhanced by the removal of soft tissue from Haversian systems and intertrabecular spaces leaving open channels for the ingrowth of vessels and cells, and by implantation of the graft at sites of maximum osteogen-

esis, e.g. in cancellous bone or haemopoietic marrow.

The clinical use of *xenografts* has been abandoned. Autografts, especially of cancellous bone, remain the first choice for transplantation.

Transplantation of cartilage

The clinical use of autogenous cartilage grafts is hindered by variation in composition of the different types of cartilage so that possible donor sites are very limited. A major difficulty in the use of stored allografts is in the preservation of living chondrocytes, for death of the graft is often followed by resorption. Rejection of allografts is not a problem as cartilage appears to be a weak antigen, the graft chondrocytes being protected by the matrix from the host cells.

Aseptic necrosis of bone

The processes of revascularisation, laying down of new bone and gradual resorption of dead bone involved in the replacement of bone grafts also come into play in the replacement of aseptic necrotic bone whether this follows fracture (p. 71), caisson disease (p. 717), sickle-cell anaemia (p. 469), Gaucher's disease, the long-term administration of steroids or is of unknown aetiology. Necrosis involving the medullary cavity is symptomless. However in juxta-articular sites such as the femoral and humeral heads if revascularisation and reossification is incomplete or fails to occur, necrotic trabeculae may eventually collapse with resultant deformity of the joint surface and disabling secondary degenerative changes. Aseptic necrosis is thought to be the cause of a number of eponymous conditions affecting the epiphyses of children (*osteochondritis juvenilis*), the most important of which is Perthes' disease of the femoral head.

Pyogenic infections of Bone

Acute osteomyelitis

Different terms are applied to inflammation of bone according to the site—periostitis, osteitis proper, and osteomyelitis—but these should not be taken as indicating separate conditions; one may lead to another, and sometimes all three are present together. Acute osteomyelitis is seen most often in childhood though it occurs also in neonates and less frequently in adults. The metaphyses adjacent to the more actively growing epiphyses of long tubular bones, i.e. lower end of femur, upper end of tibia, upper end of humerus and lower end of radius, are the sites usually involved, though vertebrae, pubis, clavicle and indeed any bone may be affected.

Aetiology

Bone infection may result from bacterial contamination of a compound fracture, from surgical operation or, in the jaw, by direct spread from an adjacent focus of infection such as an apical tooth abscess, but in most cases it arises as a result of haematogenous spread of organisms and is initially an *osteomyelitis*, the organisms having settled first in haemopoietic marrow. In about half the cases there has been recent trauma at the site. Sometimes there is an obvious inflammatory lesion elsewhere such as a boil or paronychia, but frequently the path of entry cannot be traced and is probably some slight lesion of the skin or mucous membrane. While suppurative osteomyelitis may be produced by various organisms, by far the commonest cause is the *Staphylococcus aureus* (Fig. 22.4); streptococci and *Haemophilus influenzae* produce occasional infections especially in infants, while other pyogenic organisms are uncommon as causal agents. In the tropics an attack of typhoid fever may be followed, sometimes many years later, by osteomyelitis,

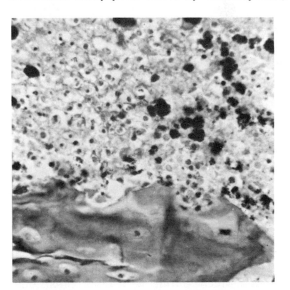

Fig. 22.4 Acute osteomyelitis, showing masses of staphylococci. × 250.

usually in the long bones or spine. Sickle cell anaemia in children and Gaucher's disease may be associated with salmonella osteomyelitis.

In about two-thirds of patients, organisms may be recovered by blood culture at an early stage in the disease but treatment should not be delayed either for the result of the culture or for the appearance of radiological changes, lest fatal septicaemia or irreparable damage to the bone results.

Macroscopic appearances

From the vascular spongy bone of the metaphysis the suppuration may spread widely, so that the medullary cavity becomes largely occupied by pus (Fig. 22.5). In children, because of the presence of the epiphyseal cartilage plate, extension occurs more readily in a transverse direction than onwards into the

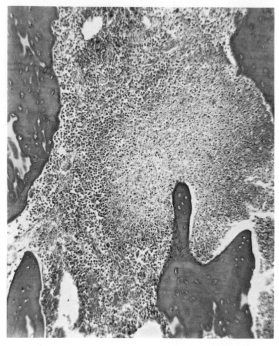

Fig. 22.5 Acute osteomyelitis showing necrosis of bone and marrow and an intense polymorph reaction. × 95.

epiphysis. The infection, after breaking through the thin metaphyseal cortex, may reach the periosteum which during growth is often only loosely attached to the underlying shaft though more firmly anchored at the epiphyseal plate. A *subperiosteal abscess* thus forms which may spread extensively, bathing a large part or even the whole diaphysis in pus but usually sparing the epiphysis. The abscess may burst through the periosteum and lead to diffuse suppuration in the muscles and other soft tissues, and later, if the condition is not treated, may discharge externally. Suppuration leads to thrombosis in blood vessels, which in turn leads to bone necrosis. Suppurative periostitis by itself results in necrosis of only a superficial layer of bone

owing to the anastomoses with the endosteal vessels, while in the case of medullary suppuration also, the resulting necrosis, though varying in degree according to the amount of vascular involvement, may be limited. If, however, both lesions are extensive at the same time, the affected bone tissue is completely deprived of its blood supply and undergoes necrosis (Fig. 22.6). This is especially the case when, as may happen with a large accumulation of pus under

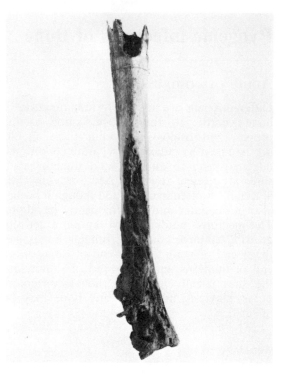

Fig. 22.6 Sequestrum of shaft of tibia from a case of acute suppurative osteomyelitis. Note the partial resorption of the bone at its ends.

the periosteum, the nutrient artery becomes involved and occluded by thrombus. In extreme cases, death of the whole diaphysis may result, and then the dead bone becomes separated from the epiphysis and forms a large *sequestrum* (Fig. 22.6). Towards its ends, the dead bone may become eroded by granulation tissue, and irregular resorption results; but the part actually bathed in pus undergoes little change and the surface remains smooth. As the process becomes less acute, new bone is usually produced under the periosteum and this may form an encasing sheath to the dead bone, known as an *involucrum* (Fig. 22.7). This new bone is irregular and is often perforated by openings or *cloacae* by which the pus may collect locally or may drain to the skin surface, forming a discharging sinus. The above description applies to the severer forms of the disease

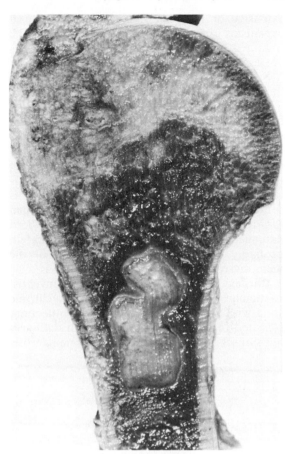

Fig. 22.8 A localised pyogenic bone abscess is seen in the upper end of the humerus of an elderly patient with rheumatoid arthritis treated with steroids. The abscess cavity is surrounded by a rim of granulation tissue. Proximally, the marrow is more diffusely involved.

and of abscesses requiring drainage (Fig. 22.8). Sometimes infection is aborted before any radiological change becomes apparent.

Complications

Septicaemia or pyaemia. These complications are especially likely to arise in haematogenous osteomyelitis due to staphylococci, where, owing to the production of coagulase by these organisms, the delicate vascular channels in the marrow commonly become thrombosed and suppurative softening of the thrombi allows the organisms to invade the blood. Pyaemia with abscesses in the lungs, kidneys and myocardium and acute ulcerative endocarditis may be produced even when the osteomyelitis is not

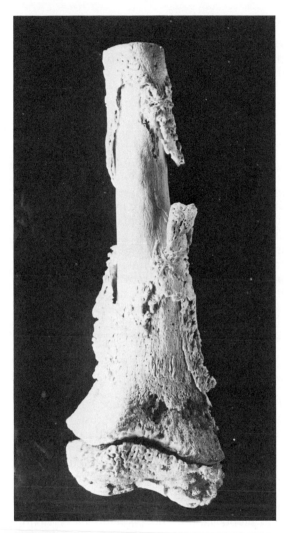

Fig. 22.7 Femur from a case of long-standing suppurative osteomyelitis and periostitis in a child, showing the irregular formation of an involucrum of new bone round the sequestrum.

which are still commonly seen in tropical countries where delay in treatment and mixed bacterial infections tend to lead to large sequestra and sinus formation. In developed countries, however, good host resistance and the early administration of appropriate antibiotics have reduced the incidence both of large sequestra extensive or is at an early stage. The causal organisms are present in the blood and may be obtained from it by culture. Pyaemic abscesses are less frequent in infections with other bacteria.

Septic arthritis occurs more commonly when the metaphysis is within the joint capsule (see p. 852) and although rare in children is more frequent in infants especially when the osteomyelitis involves the femoral neck. Metastatic arthritis involving several joints may complicate infantile streptococcal or pneumococcal osteomyelitis.

Alteration in growth rate. Growth is sometimes retarded especially in infants when the epiphyseal cartilage plate has been damaged, but occasionally is accelerated, probably due to increased vascularity of the metaphyseal side of the growth apparatus.

Chronic osteomyelitis. Acute osteomyelitis, particularly in adults, may progress to a chronic state with recurrent exacerbations of infection, repeated formation of abscesses with discharging sinuses and increasing patchy bone sclerosis

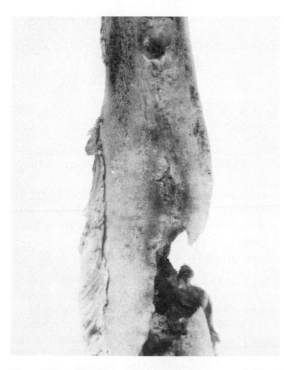

Fig. 22.9 Chronic suppurative osteomyelitis of femur. The lower part of the medullary cavity contains pus and granulation tissue; there is sclerosis of surrounding bone and the medullary cavity above is obliterated. Opening on right is surgical.

(Fig. 22.9). Long continuing osteomyelitis with the discharge of pus may be followed by *amyloid disease* or occasionally by the development of *squamous carcinoma* in the epithelial-lined wall of a sinus.

Neonatal osteomyelitis

Haematogenous osteomyelitis in the newborn presents a rather different picture from the disease in the older child. It may involve one bone only, often the maxilla, or many bones may be affected, so-called *generalised osteomyelitis of the newborn*. It arises sometimes in association with umbilical or other sepsis and is most commonly caused by *Staphylococcus aureus*, often of a penicillin-resistant strain and occasionally by *β-haemolytic streptococcus* or *pneumococcus*. In the more severe cases associated with septicaemia there may be accompanying symptoms of pneumonia or gastroenteritis and the infant is desperately ill. The osteomyelitis itself is characterised by the tendency to form a massive involucrum which may be completely resorbed after recovery, by damage to the epiphyseal cartilage causing growth retardation, and by septic arthritis. The involvement of the cartilaginous epiphysis and the joint may be facilitated by the vascular pattern in which metaphyseal vessels penetrate the epiphysis.

Osteomyelitis in the adult

This condition is relatively rare but may complicate injury or debilitating disease. There is a tendency for the diaphysis of the bone to be involved rather than the metaphysis or epiphysis. The periosteum in the adult is more fibrous and adheres more firmly to the bone; this tends to minimise the formation of subperiosteal abscesses, thereby retaining the cortical blood supply and preventing the separation of large sequestra. However, cortical erosion is common and chronic marrow infection almost invariable in the adult.

Subacute pyogenic infection

An increasing number of patients now seem to develop a subacute pyogenic infection often with an insidious onset and relatively little constitutional upset. This may give rise to localised abscess formation of which Brodie's is one type (see below). Vertebral osteomyelitis, sometimes due to coliform organisms associated with urinary or pelvic organ infection, usually has a good prognosis, since bone destruction is soon followed by sclerosis and bony bridging between affected vertebrae.

Brodie's abscess. This is a form of localised, subacute or chronic pyogenic osteomyelitis which arises insidiously without an acute attack and is usually situated in the metaphysis of a long bone, especially the upper end of the tibia. The central cavity contains pus, which may be sterile, is lined by granulation tissue and surrounded by reactive bone sclerosis.

Acute periostitis

Acute periostitis may occur as the result of trauma, there being inflammatory oedema with swelling and little accompanying leukocytic infiltration. Apart from this, it is produced by bacterial invasion and is sometimes suppurative. It may result from an external wound or from the spread of organisms from a skin ulcer, or, in the jaws, from a carious tooth. Haematogenous infection of the periosteum is rare but is a well-known complication of *typhoid fever*, when it may appear long after the primary illness has subsided.

Tuberculosis of Bone

With the virtual eradication of bovine infection in Britain, the human type of bacillus is the chief cause of tuberculosis of bone. This condition is decreasing in frequency but broadening its age incidence so that fewer children and an increasing proportion of adults are affected. The disease most commonly involves the vertebrae, the metaphyses and epiphyses of long bones such as femur and tibia (in which it is often accompanied by tuberculous arthritis (p. 853)) and the small tubular bones of the hands and feet. Infection usually arises as a result of haematogenous spread of bacilli from a tuberculous lesion in lung, lymph nodes or elsewhere; occasionally there is direct or lymphatic spread to bone from an adjacent focus, e.g. to ribs from pulmonary lesions, to the spine from adjacent lymph nodes and, very rarely nowadays, to the petrous bone from the middle ear.

Structural changes. When tubercle bacilli settle in the spongy bone marrow, tuberculous follicles form and the disease process may then extend either as tuberculous granulation tissue with little caseation or form a frankly caseating mass. In both cases bone destruction results (Fig. 22.10). In contrast to pyogenic osteitis the disease is usually more slowly progressive and new bone formation is scanty in the active stage. The formation of large sequestra as the result of thrombotic infarction is rare although occasionally wedge-shaped areas of necrosis under the articular cartilage may result from

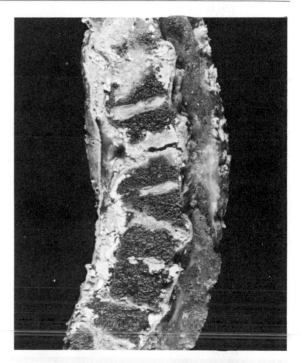

Fig. 22.10 Many thoracic vertebrae are affected by old caseating tuberculosis. Partially calcified caseating material is seen beneath the anterior longitudinal ligament (*on the left*). There is destruction of disc spaces and some vertebral body collapse.

interference with the blood supply, probably due to endarteritis. When healing does occur it is by fibrosis and at this stage some new bone formation may be seen. Tubercle bacilli may remain in these healed foci for a long time and the disease may later recrudesce.

Tuberculosis in different sites

Pott's disease of the spine. Tuberculosis of the spine is commonest in children and young adults. The thoracic, lumbar and cervical vertebrae are affected in that order of frequency. Often more than one vertebra is involved; they are usually adjacent (Fig. 22.10) but occasionally widely separated. The disease most commonly arises near the intervertebral disc, the disc itself being involved early. When the infection arises in or spreads to the periosteum, the caseous material is invaded by polymorphonuclear leukocytes and converted into pus. This tends to accumulate to form a *paraverte-*

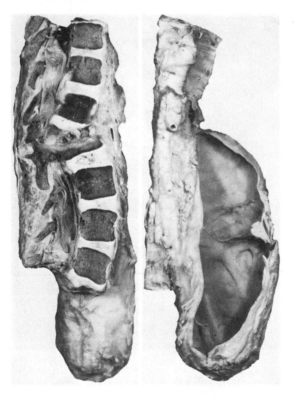

Fig. 22.11 Tuberculosis of spine (Pott's disease). Loss of intervertebral disc and collapse of T.12 and L.1 with paraplegia and formation of psoas abscess.

bral abscess at the front and sides of the vertebra which may spread, especially under the anterior vertebral ligament, to infect other vertebrae. Later the pus sometimes penetrates the sheaths of muscles and extends in their substance (Fig. 22.11). In this way when the lumbar vertebrae are involved a *psoas* or *lumbar 'cold' abscess* may be produced, and the tuberculous pus tracks along the psoas sheath to point in the inner aspect of the thigh. When the cervical vertebrae are affected, a large collection of pus may form behind the pharynx— *retropharyngeal abscess*. The cold abscess may burst through the skin with the formation of a sinus which tends to become secondarily infected. Such patients are especially liable to develop *amyloid disease*. As the vertebral bodies are weakened by bone destruction they collapse anteriorly, and, especially when two adjacent vertebrae are involved, angulation of the spinal column results (Fig. 22.11).

Pott's paraplegia follows in about a quarter of patients in Britain. Usually it is caused by active disease when an extradural abscess, granulation tissue, sequestrated bone or disc material compresses the cord. Only very occasionally does tuberculosis penetrate the dura to produce an intradural abscess or to involve the cord directly. Paraplegia arising years after the original infection may result from recrudescence of infection or, in the absence of active disease, be associated with stretching of the cord over the apex of a severe kyphosis when the prognosis is less good.

Tuberculous dactylitis may involve a single phalanx or rarely several phalanges of a hand or foot. The infection occurs in the medullary cavity and there is abundant formation of tuberculous granulation tissue which leads to resorption and also expansion of the bone, so that it may be reduced to a shell.

Tuberculous trochanteric bursitis. In this condition which usually arises in young adults the bursa is replaced by a mass of tuberculous granulation tissue and caseating material which ramifies in the surrounding tissue planes. This is usually associated with tuberculous disease of the trochanter but the hip joint is not involved.

Other Bone Infections

Syphilis of bone

Bone lesions may occur in both congenital and acquired syphilis but are now rare in Britain.

Congenital syphilis. The commonest form of bone disease in congenital syphilis is *osteochondritis*. The metaphyseal surface of the growth plate is marked by a broad irregular yellowish band which consists of a trellis of unresorbed, patchily calcified cartilage (Fig. 22.12*b*). Bone formation is inhibited and the marrow spaces of the adjacent metaphysis contain fibrous

the skin, ulcerate and discharge; secondary infection with pyogenic organisms follows with further destruction. The bone beneath the gumma may be resorbed producing a rough-floored depression with a raised irregular margin of reactive bone. *Periostitis* is often associated with osteitis; the lesions may be multiple and widespread and great thickening and sclerosis of the bone may occur, the medullary cavity being reduced and the surface becoming extremely irregular (Fig. 22.13).

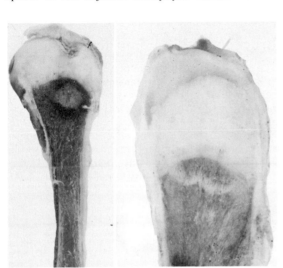

a   b

Fig. 22.12 Lesions of bones in congenital syphilis. **a** shows gummatous epiphysitis and **b** shows the irregularity of the epiphyseal line at an earlier stage. (J. W. S. B.).

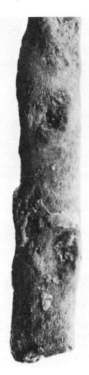

Fig. 22.13 Syphilitic disease of periosteum of tibia, showing nodular thickenings and eroded areas in the bone.

and granulation tissue. In severe cases there may be separation of the epiphysis due to fracture through the delicate cartilage trellis at the metaphysis. Separation sometimes also occurs following gummatous softening which usually starts near the centre of the plate and may spread to the periphery (Fig. 22.12*a*). *Periostitis*, with the formation of subperiosteal new bone, is seen. *Dactylitis* in the hand and foot may involve several bones. *Saddle nose* results from perforation, destruction and collapse of the nasal septum.

Acquired syphilis. Transient periostitis involving especially the tibia and skull bones occurs occasionally in the secondary stage. The bone changes of tertiary syphilis are also seen in congenital syphilis in older children and adults. *Gummas* may form in the periosteum. The lesions may become adherent to

Periostitis may also be associated with actual necrosis with formation of sequestra; this is common when the lesions are extensive, and the vascular supply is interfered with. In the skull large areas of bone may die and sequestra separate, gummas may form both outside and inside the skull, giving rise to apertures with thickened and irregular bony margins (Fig. 22.14). These striking appearances are rarely seen nowadays outside museums. In the palate and nasal bones gummatous periostitis may be followed by ulceration, which penetrates deeply and leads to perforation of the nasal septum and hard palate.

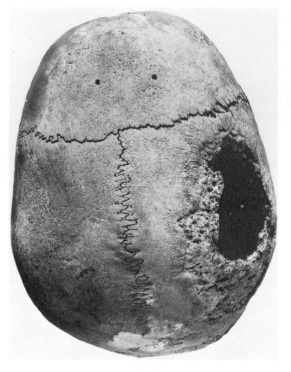

Fig. 22.14 Syphilitic disease of skull. Note the large aperture with irregular margins resulting from a gumma.

Actinomycosis

The bones usually become involved as a result of extension of soft tissue suppuration (p. 187). The jaw may be affected by spread from an oral focus; the cervical vertebrae from a pharyngeal one; the ribs, sternum or thoracic vertebrae from pulmonary actinomycosis; and the pelvis from an abdominal lesion. The infection is characterised by bone destruction and suppuration with the formation of multiple inter-connected abscesses. There is usually little attempt at new bone formation. In *Madura disease*, which may be caused by an allied actinomycete, the prominent feature is extensive destruction of the bones of the foot.

Brucellosis (Undulant fever)

The commonest skeletal symptom in brucellosis is of back pain due to involvement of the thoracic or lumbar spine. As in tuberculosis, bone is eroded with early involvement of the adjacent intervertebral disc and sometimes small paravertebral abscesses form. However, in brucellosis, reactive bone formation is earlier and more abundant: the disease may be self-limiting, healing occurring by bony fusion. Osteomyelitis of long bones is rare (see also pp. 508, 854).

Effects of Radiation on Bone

For a general description of the effects of radiation see pp. 23–9.

Radiation osteitis (Radiation osteodysplasia)

The term radiation osteitis was first used by Ewing to describe pathological changes in bone following external radiation, and later by Martland in his investigations of the bones of watch-dial painters who had ingested radium and mesothorium. While the condition is not inflammatory, the term is widely accepted. The radiation, whether external or internal, probably produces its effect by direct action on cartilage and bone cells as well as indirectly by its effect on blood vessels. A 'safe' dosage cannot be stated with certainty as there is great variation in the individual response to radiation, but in general it is thought unlikely that bone damage will be caused in adults by doses of less than 3000 rads of external radiation though in children smaller doses may be incriminated. Some of the patients with internal radiation developed bone changes after quite small total body dosage; others with much larger dosage escaped injury.

External radiation

Growth. In children inclusion of the epiphyseal cartilage plate in the radiation field may result in retardation of growth due to cessation of division of the cartilage cells and their swelling and degeneration. Sometimes in severely damaged plates there is also premature closure of the epiphysis leading to further stunting of growth.

Aseptic bone necrosis may occur and is accompanied by necrosis and fibrosis of the bone marrow sometimes followed by calcification and the formation of abnormal, basophilic woven bone (Fig. 22.15). There may be some bone resorption and the radiological appearances are of patchy radiolucency and sclerosis.

Pathological fracture has been found in the femoral necks of women who were irradiated for carcinoma of the cervix or other pelvic organ malignancy and less frequently in the ribs or clavicle following postmastectomy irradiation. There is commonly a time interval of many years between irradiation and the fracture, which is often slow to heal.

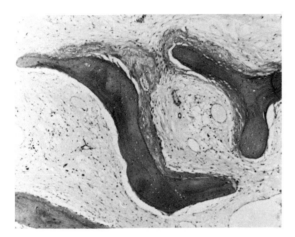

Fig. 22.15 Following irradiation there has been formation of coarsely fibred woven bone on the trabecular surfaces. The marrow is oedematous and shows some fine fibrosis. × 40.

Acute osteomyelitis. Any necrotic bone resulting from irradiation damage to the jaw is very susceptible to infection especially if the teeth are carious. The bone infection usually starts as a spreading periostitis. A rather similar picture of some historic interest was the jaw necrosis followed by osteomyelitis which used to be found in phosphorus poisoning of match workers—so-called *phossy jaw*.

Internal radiation

Radioactive fallout from the explosion of nuclear devices gives rise to increased ^{90}Sr in the soil and vegetation. Cows eat the contaminated grass and excrete some of the radionuclide in their milk. The amount of ^{90}Sr in the human skeleton has risen in the last 20 years but although this has given rise to considerable concern the levels remain low. From animal experiments ^{90}Sr is also thought to be less toxic than radium.

Accidents at atomic reactors tend chiefly to involve contamination with the radioactive element plutonium. ^{239}Pu is concentrated mainly on endosteal surfaces of bone and in marrow macrophages. It,

like radium, has a long half life, emits high energy α-rays and is found experimentally to produce bone tumours in animals and possibly, unlike radium, to have a leukaemogenic effect. Since, however, very little is known about the effect of these substances in man it is the effect of radium which is discussed below.

Bone damage has occurred both as a result of therapeutic administration of radium salts and of accidental intake as in the case of the watch-dial painters. Almost all radium salts which are not excreted are stored in bone, being initially deposited both diffusely and in a patchy manner in areas of active growth or bone remodelling where calcification is incomplete (*hot spots*). Later, when bone resorption takes place, the radioactive material may be laid down again in new sites of active bone formation. With large doses death of the patient is likely to occur at an early stage from blood dyscrasia, and here the only bone abnormality is likely to be necrosis of the mandible with secondary sepsis. With smaller doses the bone marrow may be unaffected and the patient may live long enough to develop aseptic bone necrosis with complicating pathological fractures or acute osteomyelitis in sites other than the jaw.

Neoplasia following irradiation

Leukaemia. External radiation of the skeleton tends to affect most severely the haemopoietic cells of the marrow. There is an increased incidence of myeloid leukaemia in the survivors of the atomic bombs, irradiated patients with ankylosing spondylitis and pioneer radiologists. Leukaemia, however, does not seem a common complication of ingested radium.

Bone sarcoma has occurred in as many as 20% of survivors of those who ingested doses of radium or its salts, but is rare following external radiation. Where radioactive salts have been deposited in bone there is often recognisable radiation osteitis in the skeleton but it is rarely recognisable in association with the tumours produced by external radiation. It is now thought that injury and repair are not necessary accompaniments of sarcomatous change. The latent period before development of bone sarcomas is usually from 5–20 years and may be even longer following internal radiation when the tumours may be found anywhere in the skeleton and are sometimes multiple. Post-radiation tumours are usually osteosarcomas or fibrosarcomas and often rapidly fatal from pulmonary metastases.

Nasal carcinoma. A high incidence of carcinoma of the nose and nasal sinuses has been found up to 50 years after radium ingestion. This is thought to be due partly to the close proximity of the epithelium to the underlying bone and partly to an excess retention of radon in the air sinuses.

Bone Changes Associated with Vitamin Deficiency or Excess

Vitamin C deficiency

Scurvy

Scurvy results from vitamin C deficiency and is now a rare disease in Britain. It is characterised by a generalised defective deposition of fibrous proteins, including bone matrix, dentine and collagen, and results in abnormalities in growing bones and teeth. Also there is a tendency to haemorrhage because of capillary wall weakness and an impairment of healing of bone and soft tissues following injury. Scurvy is most common in infants and young children where bone and other connective tissues are being rapidly formed, but also occurs in old people taking a restricted diet.

Bone changes in infants precede haemorrhage and are due to failure to lay down bony matrix, associated with the persistence of an unabsorbed calcified cartilage lattice. There is no failure of calcification (cf. rickets). The cartilage cells of the epiphyseal plate multiply and orientate themselves normally and the intervening matrix becomes calcified but osteoblasts fail to lay down osteoid and the calcified cartilaginous matrix is only slightly and patchily resorbed (*scorbutic lattice*) so that the epiphyseal plate becomes widened and irregular. Fracture of spicules of the calcified cartilage occurs and a very irregular, radiologically dense zone arises at the junction of epiphysis and shaft. The metaphysis itself is weak because of failure of bone deposition, the marrow spaces contain much loose fibrous tissue, and separation of the epiphysis through this site is not uncommon. The pre-existing bony trabeculae in the shaft are thin and delicate (osteoporosis) probably because of continuing normal resorption without bone deposition.

Haemorrhagic tendency. There is a tendency to bleed spontaneously or from trivial injury. The gums are spongy and bleed readily and the teeth may be loosened. There may be haemorrhage into the skin, mucous membranes, joints or subperiosteally.

Subperiosteal haemorrhages cause the severely affected child to lie immobile and to be apprehensive of movement which causes pain. Nothing may be seen radiologically until subperiosteal new bone is laid down on the surface of the haematoma. Bleeding into the kidney, orbit, brain or adrenals occasionally complicates the picture. The exact cause of capillary haemorrhage in scurvy is not clear even on electron-microscopy.

Failure of healing. In scorbutic patients, skin and flesh wounds and fractures either fail to heal or do so more slowly than normal, and occasionally there have been reports of old wounds breaking down. The administration of extra Vitamin C to non-scorbutic individuals does not however increase the rate of healing.

Anaemia. Nutritional anaemia tends to occur. In some patients there is an associated deficiency of folic acid (p. 502).

'Battered baby' syndrome

This syndrome may be confused clinically with scurvy and accordingly, although it does not arise from vitamin deficiency, is conveniently discussed here.

Subperiosteal haemorrhage with subsequent formation of an involucrum of new bone may be seen as a result of epiphyseal damage in the 'battered baby' syndrome, where an infant has been repeatedly assaulted, usually by the parents. Several bones may be involved, the subperiosteal new bone formation being at different stages in different bones. The epiphyseal damage may be associated with multiple bruises, fractures of limb bones or more commonly of ribs or clavicle and with subdural haematoma or a head injury which may prove fatal. In this condition the bones are normal radiologically apart from the effects of trauma and there is no haemorrhagic tendency. It is important to make the diagnosis since if the infant is returned to his home further assault, sometimes fatal, may occur.

Vitamin D deficiency

Osteomalacia and rickets

Definition. Dietary osteomalacia in adults and rickets in infants and children are due to a deficiency in vitamin D which results in an

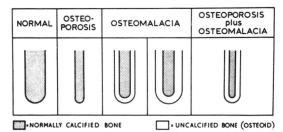

NORMAL	OSTEO-POROSIS	OSTEOMALACIA	OSTEOPOROSIS plus OSTEOMALACIA

☐ = NORMALLY CALCIFIED BONE   ☐ = UNCALCIFIED BONE (OSTEOID)

Fig. 22.16   Diagram of bone changes.

increase in the amount of uncalcified bony matrix (*osteoid*) (Fig. 22.16) and in addition in rickets produces defective mineralisation of the epiphyseal cartilage. These appearances may have other causes than simple vitamin deficiency. It should be noted that the term osteomalacia is applied not only to a disease process but also to the abnormal bone structure.

Introduction. Vitamin D is the name applied to all the sterols with pronounced antirachitic properties. This fat-soluble vitamin exists in two main forms. Vitamin D_2 (calciferol) is produced by irradiation of ergosterol. Vitamin D_3 is present in fish oil and egg yolks, in much smaller amounts in butter and milk and may be synthesised by the action of ultra-violet light on 7-dehydrocholesterol in the human skin. The antirachitic effect of sunlight depends on its angle of incidence so that both latitude and season are important, as is the clarity of the atmosphere. Skin pigmentation may reduce the beneficial effects of ultra-violet rays. Children, particularly those of coloured immigrants, brought up in northern cities with their smoky atmosphere and few hours of winter sunshine are therefore especially liable to be dependent on their dietary intake of vitamin D to prevent rickets. The preventive dose is about 400 international units/day for the fair-skinned infant but there is considerable individual variation both in requirements and in sensitivity to toxic effects of hypervitaminosis. (One international unit has been defined as being equivalent to 0.025 μg of pure crystalline vitamin D.) Since naturally occurring sources of vitamin D are scanty, dried milk and cereals for infants and margarine are fortified either by added calciferol or by irradiation. The dietary requirement of the vitamin in adults is uncertain and probably less than 100 international units/day.

Vitamin D in the presence of bile salts is absorbed from the upper part of the small intestine. It is hydroxylated in the liver to form 25-hydroxycholecalciferol (25-HCC), the main circulating metabolite, which is altered in the kidney to the biologically most highly active form of the vitamin, 1,25-dihydroxycholecalciferol (1,25-DHCC). The production of 1,25-DHCC appears to be stimulated by a low serum calcium, probably working through the parathyroid gland and by a low plasma inorganic phosphate concentration.

The active metabolites of vitamin D are essential for the absorption of calcium from the gut; they probably also have both a direct effect on bone by promoting resorption and an action on the renal tubule to increase phosphate reabsorption. The mechanism by which vitamin D permits bone mineralisation is not clear but whatever the cause, bone laid down after the onset of vitamin D deficiency is poorly calcified and the remains of pre-morbid calcified trabeculae are covered by osteoid borders of varying thickness. Both osteomalacia and osteoporosis may give rise to bone weakness clinically and to decreased bone density radiologically and it is important to grasp the fundamental difference between them. In osteomalacia and rickets a normal or even excessive amount of matrix is produced but it is not calcified. In osteoporosis the matrix is diminished in amount but appears to be normally calcified. Occasionally osteoporosis and osteomalacia may coexist (Fig. 22.16).

Osteomalacia

Osteomalacia, due to a low dietary intake of vitamin D combined with little exposure to sunlight, though rare is now being recognised more often in Britain. Old people, often housebound and living on restricted diets, the coloured immigrant population and food faddists are most often affected. It may develop in pregnancy when there is, in addition to lack of vitamin D, a loss of calcium to the fetus and in the breast milk. The condition is more frequent in India where Moslem women in purdah are particularly at risk. Osteomalacia (vitamin D deficiency) may also arise following gastrectomy, in various forms of intestinal malabsorption and in obstructive jaundice. Excess osteoid may occur with some renal abnormalities (p. 826) and in patients on anticonvulsant drugs (p. 827).

Biochemical findings. Although vitamin D deficiency gives rise to failure of calcium absorption, the plasma calcium is often normal rather than diminished and the plasma phosphate is low. It is thought that the initial tendency to hypocalcaemia stimulates the parathyroids which restore the normal serum level of calcium by release of the mineral from resorbed bone and by reduction of calcium excretion.

The plasma phosphate which may already be slightly lowered by decreased absorption is further lowered by the effect of parathyroid hormone in diminishing the renal tubular reabsorption of phosphate. Some support for this explanation of the biochemical findings is received both from the reports of clear cell hyperplasia of the parathyroids at necropsy in some patients with osteomalacia or rickets and from increased osteoclastic activity and marrow fibrosis in bone biopsies of some osteomalacic patients. The hyperparathyroidism is sometimes sufficiently marked for subperiosteal erosions to be recognisable radiologically (p. 828). Whenever the plasma calcium is low, tetany may occur. The explanation of the failure of the parathyroids to respond to the hypocalcaemia in these cases may be that there is unusually complete coverage of the bone surfaces by osteoid which for some reason inhibits osteoclastic resorption.

The serum alkaline phosphatase is frequently raised, indicating increased osteoblastic activity.

Clinical and radiological features and structural changes. The patient commonly presents with muscular weakness especially noticeable on climbing stairs and with a waddling, penguin gait. Pain is usually vague, aching and poorly localised so that a diagnosis of 'muscular rheumatism' may be suggested. Occasionally attention is first drawn to the condition by a fracture following minimal violence which fails to produce radiological evidence of callus formation although uncalcified callus may be present in abundance. An incomplete or greenstick fracture in an adult may also suggest the diagnosis. Sometimes *Looser's zones* or pseudo-fractures are seen and when present are almost pathognomonic. The radiological picture is of a linear zone of translucency, cutting across at right angles to and usually affecting only one cortex. Looser's zones are painless and are most often found in the pubic rami, ribs, inner scapular borders, neck of humerus and femur, sometimes being bilateral and symmetrical and probably representing bony remodelling at areas of stress. There may be a generalised decrease in bone density, especially noticeable in the peripheral skeleton compared with the spine (c.f. osteoporosis, p. 830). In the more severe cases deformity may occur in the absence of fracture, due to the weakening and softening of the bones. The pubic rami may be buckled and pushed forward into a beak (*triradiate pelvis*) with consequent narrowing of the pelvic outlet; the limb bones may be bowed and the spine kyphotic. These severe deformities are seldom seen nowadays and it must be emphasised that the skeletons of some patients with osteomalacia may show no recognisable radiological abnormality.

Microscopic appearances. The osteoid matrix (uncalcified bone) which is laid down after the onset of vitamin D deficiency fails to calcify (Fig. 22.17). The recognition of the osteoid borders covering the premorbid mineralised bone may be difficult in decalcified material and is best achieved by study of undecalcified sections stained by von Kossa's method (p. 245) in which calcified matrix is stained black and the

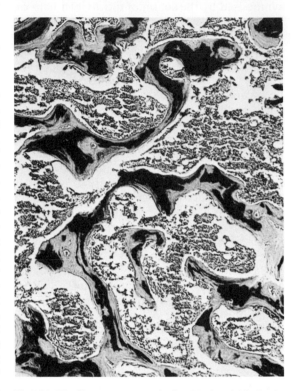

Fig. 22.17 Severe osteomalacia. Undecalcified sections stained by von Kossa's method. Only the bone stained black is calcified. There are wide seams of unstained osteoid. No secondary osteitis fibrosa is seen here. × 40.

osteoid remains unstained (Fig. 22.17). The diagnosis of osteomalacia can be made by bone biopsy and an area containing cancellous bone such as the iliac crest gives least technical difficulty. A word of caution is necessary in the diagnosis of minor degrees of osteomalacia. When bone is being rapidly formed for any reason in normal subjects, a thin border of osteoid may be present on the surface beneath the layer of osteoblasts and even in the slower process of bone turnover in the normal adult skeleton an occasional narrow border of osteoid may be recognisable. Osteomalacia is usually diagnosed either when more than half the trabecular surface is clothed by narrow osteoid seams bare of osteoblasts or, if osteoblasts are present, when osteoid seams are wide. In undecalcified sections of normal bone a haematoxyphilic line, the calcification front, can be seen in most places between calcified bone and any osteoid present. This line tends to be deficient in osteomalacia. The amount of matrix formed in osteomalacia is very variable. It is sometimes markedly increased and the trabeculae are broader than normal probably partly due to an increased amount of formation but also to a decrease in bone resorption, the osteoid for some reason being less readily removed than normal calcified matrix. Occasionally, particularly in the elderly, the total amount of matrix is much diminished and the conditions of osteomalacia and osteoporosis exist together (see Fig. 22.16). Mild changes of osteitis fibrosa may be present (p. 829) with some marrow fibrosis and osteoclasis of bone not covered by osteoid.

The diagnosis of dietary osteomalacia may be difficult sometimes on clinical, radiological or biochemical grounds. In any suspected case bone biopsy should be done and undecalcified sections examined. The diagnosis is very well worth making since the condition rapidly responds to vitamin D administration.

Rickets

Rickets in the infant or child is the equivalent of osteomalacia and also results from deficiency of vitamin D. In addition to the failure of mineralisation of osteoid matrix as seen in osteomalacia there is failure of mineralisation of the cartilage of the epiphyseal growth plate.

Dietary rickets is chiefly a disease of infancy, being commonest from 6 months to 2 years though 'late' rickets is seen especially in immigrant adolescents, perhaps due to an increased demand for vitamin D during the growth spurt. Rickets is present at birth only in infants born to osteomalacic mothers. Prematurity predisposes to rickets since the skeleton is mineralised in the last three months of intra-uterine life. Prolonged breast feeding may also predispose since breast milk provides only about 20 units of vitamin D daily, i.e. about 5% of the infant's requirements. A further group par-

ticularly at risk are infants in large low-income families who are weaned early from fortified dried milk to a share in the vitamin D-poor family diet.

Biochemical findings. As in osteomalacia, the serum calcium level is normal or slightly low, but the serum phosphate is usually between 0·3 and 1 mmol/l (1–3 mg/100 ml) i.e. markedly lower than the normal value for infants (1·3–2·3 mmol/l or 4–7 mg/100 ml). The plasma alkaline phosphatase is frequently raised.

Clinical and radiological features. There are muscular hypotonia, skeletal changes, sometimes anaemia and especially in the early stages, tetany.

The ends of the long bones are swollen and this may be particularly noticeable at the wrists. Radiological examination shows wide, irregular, fuzzy, cupped metaphyses, thin bony cortices and the late appearance of epiphyseal centres which are often indistinct. There may be greenstick fractures with apparent failure of callus formation. Sometimes Looser's zones (pseudo-fractures) are seen (see p. 824). Deformity results from bending of the soft, poorly mineralised bone and antero-lateral bowing of the femur and tibia is characteristic.

The costochondral junctions tend to be swollen (Fig. 22.18) ('rickety rosary') and 'pigeon chest' due to indrawing of the ribs and protrusion of the sternum is sometimes seen. Flattening of the pelvis with constriction of the outlet and

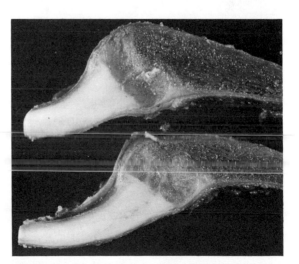

Fig. 22.18 Rickets. Section through two ribs shows marked swelling of the costochondral junctions. The child had a 'rickety rosary' during life.

scoliosis may occur. The skull appears square and box-like with bossing of the frontal bones and the closure of the fontanelles is delayed. Eruption of the teeth may be late.

Microscopic appearances. Under normal conditions proliferation of cartilage cells at the epiphyseal plate is followed by mineralisation of the matrix, hypertrophy of the chondrocytes, vascularisation of the lacunae of these hypertrophic cells by metaphyseal vessels, laying down of osteoid on the surface of the mineralised cartilage and finally brisk calcification of the osteoid followed by metaphyseal remodelling. The primary change at the epiphyseal growth plate in rickets is failure of the normal mineralisation of the cartilage matrix. As a result the hypertrophic cartilage cells persist for

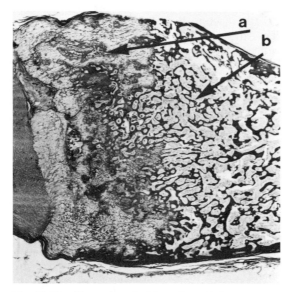

Fig. 22.19 Costochondral junction of rib in rickets. **a** The cartilage plate is thickened and irregular. **b** The spongy bone is partly uncalcified. × 6·5.

an abnormally long time and as proliferation continues at the usual rate the epiphyseal plate becomes thicker. Patchy calcification leads to some irregular ingrowth of blood vessels but long tongues of cartilage remain projecting far down into the metaphysis (Fig. 22.19). The osteoid matrix which is laid down on the surface of the cartilage is not calcified and since osteoid is less readily resorbed by osteoclasts metaphyseal remodelling is also deficient. These microscopic changes account for the gross and radiological appearances of a wide, irregular

growth plate with flared metaphyses. It must be emphasised that if for any reason the infant has ceased to grow the changes in the epiphyseal plate will not be seen though there will of course be osteomalacic change in the bone as in the adult. Osteoid matrix formed by intramembranous bone deposition also fails to calcify.

Administration of vitamin D leads to resumption of calcification which in the epiphyseal plate occurs first in the region of those cartilage cells which have most recently become hypertrophic. Since the amount of osteoid laid down is not usually diminished in rickets and its removal is impaired, the bones may become heavier than normal when calcification does occur. Deformities may become less marked but tend to persist to some extent so that the child with healed rickets may have permanently bent long bones with bow legs, knock knees or other abnormalities.

Non-dietary causes of osteomalacia and rickets

It is unusual to see dietary rickets or osteomalacia in Britain but failure of mineralisation, alone or associated with other bone abnormalities, may accompany a variety of conditions. The structural changes are not different from those described above except that they tend to be less severe and may be modified by other co-existent bone disorders. The more important conditions are as follows.

A. Malabsorption syndromes. The association of rickets and osteomalacia with steatorrhea has been recognised for some time. Osteomalacia has also occasionally been described following gastrectomy, in the blind-loop syndrome and in obstructive jaundice. It probably results from failure of absorption of vitamin D though other factors may contribute. There is sometimes an associated osteoporosis.

B. Uraemic osteodystrophy, renal rickets. Bone changes which, in mild degree, are very common, may result from any renal disease which gives rise to prolonged uraemia, e.g. congenital hypoplasia of the kidneys, valvular obstruction to the urethra with pyelonephritis in infants, and chronic nephritis or pyelonephritis in adults.

In uraemic osteodystrophy the bones may show rickets (osteomalacia) and osteitis fibrosa (p. 829), alone or together and in any degree of severity. The changes of secondary hyperparathyroidism may be very striking (Fig. 22.22) and associated with a diffuse chief-cell or clear-cell hyperplasia of all the parathyroid glands. *In children* growth may be stunted and bony deformities of the rachitic type develop. The changes in the epiphyseal cartilage plates are rachitic but in addition there is often severe osteitis fibrosa, especially in the metaphyses. *In adults* there is usually no deformity though bone pain, decreased skeletal radiodensity, subperiosteal erosions and other abnormalities may be present. Occasionally osteosclerosis may be seen in some bones especially the vertebrae, due to an increase of apparently normal bone or, more commonly, associated with osteitis fibrosa. When osteitis fibrosa is severe, metastatic calcification may occur.

Patients on chronic renal dialysis may develop similar bone changes sometimes with loss of bone volume. The pattern varies from one centre to another and from one patient to another.

Biochemical changes. The serum phosphate is almost always raised, the serum calcium low or normal and if bone disease is marked the alkaline phosphatase is raised.

Osteomalacia may result from failure of conversion of 25-HCC to 1,25-DHCC in the damaged kidney while raised parathormone levels may not only follow hypocalcaemia associated with phosphate retention and poor calcium absorption but be associated with frustrated attempts to increase 1,25-DHCC synthesis. Improvement may be brought about by massive doses of vitamin D, sometimes as much as 200 times the dose given to cure dietary osteomalacia.

C. Renal tubular osteodystrophy.

(1) *Hypophosphataemic vitamin D resistant rickets.* This condition, which is now known to be inherited by a sex-linked dominant gene, is found chiefly in children and is associated with a tubular reabsorption defect of phosphate (and sometimes also glucose) with consequent hypophosphataemia. The condition may be indistinguishable from dietary rickets, leading to stunting and deformity, though muscle weakness is not usually marked. It is relieved by phosphate supplements along with vitamin D. It may regress spontaneously but there is a tendency for recurrence in middle age. Renal failure does not occur.

(2) *Fanconi syndrome.* This disease occurs mostly in children, is due to a recessive gene defect and is associated with impaired tubular reabsorption of phosphate, glucose, various amino acids and sometimes potassium. There may also be inability to form an acid urine and cystinosis—a metabolic defect of cystine metabolism (Lignac–Fanconi syndrome) and patients with these additional defects tend to develop uraemia. Micro-dissection of the kidney has shown a long thin segment at the glomerulo-tubular junction associated with a short proximal tubule. The bone changes, which are initially rachitic and osteomalacic, may later, especially in the uraemic cases, become complicated by osteitis fibrosa.

(3) *Renal tubular acidosis* is another cause of osteomalacia and rickets. This condition can occur at any age and is not usually hereditary. The primary defect is an inability to form an acid urine and the chronic hyperchloraemic acidosis leads to an increased urinary excretion of phosphate and of fixed bases such as calcium and potassium. If treatment with alkali is given there may be little renal damage, but if untreated, nephrocalcinosis and progressive renal failure result. Secondary hyperparathyroidism may then occur.

D. Anticonvulsant drugs. Long-continued high dosage of several anticonvulsant drugs may lead to osteomalacia, probably by stimulating production of liver iso-enzymes which convert vitamin D to inactive metabolites.

Hypophosphatasia

In 1948 a disorder of infancy of rachitic type associated with deficiency in the activity of serum alkaline phosphatase was described. Later it was found also to be accompanied by the presence of phosphoethanolamine in the serum and its excretion in the urine, an observation that is probably significant because this substance can act as a substrate for alkaline phosphatase. The disease is thought to be inherited as an autosomal recessive, the parents being clinically normal but having either or both of the biochemical abnormalities in lesser degree. While the bone changes are similar to rickets in some respects, there is greater severity of defects of intramembranous ossification of skull bones so that the head may become shaped like a water-filled balloon. Vitamin D even in large doses usually fails to improve the condition and when clinical improvement does occur spontaneously, it is commonly not accompanied by any alteration in the serum alkaline phosphatase or the excretion of phosphoethanolamine. At this stage the whole of the cranial suture lines may undergo premature ossification so that further growth is prevented and craniostenosis may result.

Vitamin D excess

Hypervitaminosis D

If doses of vitamin D several thousand times the usual therapeutic dose are administered there is an increase in the blood calcium due partly to increased intestinal absorption and partly to increased bone resorption. Increased excretion of calcium and phosphorus in the urine occurs and renal calculi may form. In addition, there may be widespread metastatic calcification in the kidney, arteries, myocardium and stomach.

Infantile hypercalcaemia

The relatively mild form of this condition is the result of vitamin D poisoning and was fairly common in Britain in the 1950s due to high fortification of many infant foods and of cod liver oil. Individual susceptibility to the toxic effects of the vitamin is a factor since some infants are poisoned by doses which are harmless to others. Although the amount of vitamin D in fortified foods is now reduced, occasional sensitive babies are still affected. Infantile hypercalcaemia is characterised by a raised blood calcium, sometimes over 3·5 mmol/l (14 mg/100 ml), by anorexia, vomiting and failure to thrive. Deposition of calcium in the renal parenchyma (*nephrocalcinosis*), may lead to scarring and uraemia. Radiological examination sometimes shows dense epiphyses. In the severe form of the condition the pathogenesis is not understood and the babies may develop the additional features of mental retardation, cardiovascular abnormalities, goblin facies and osteosclerosis.

Bone Changes in Endocrine Disorders

Primary hyperparathyroidism

This results usually from an adenoma of one of the parathyroid glands (Fig. 24.20, p. 971); occasionally an adenoma may be present in two or more glands and very rarely hyperparathyroidism results from parathyroid carcinoma. Primary hyperplasia of the glands is also a cause of primary hyperparathyroidism but is much less common than an adenoma. Excess hormone may be produced intermittently. It appears to have a direct action on bone, stimulating resorption, as well as inhibiting the reabsorption of urinary phosphate and increasing calcium absorption from the gut perhaps by stimulating the synthesis of 1,25-DHCC (p. 823) in the kidney. The effect of the hormone is to mobilise calcium and raise the blood calcium from the normal level of 2·5 mmol/l (10 mg/100 ml) to 3 mmol/l (12 mg/100 ml) or more. The blood phosphorus falls to 0·7 mmol/l (2 mg/100 ml) or less and the alkaline phosphatase is increased. A rise in the urinary excretion of calcium follows so that these patients tend to develop *renal calculi* (p. 805). Sometimes when the bones are severely affected *metastatic calcification* of the walls of blood vessels, soft tissues, the renal substance and other sites may occur.

Bone changes. Easily recognisable, gross bone changes do not occur in many patients. They tend to be found in the 20% or so with large tumours and high serum levels of parathormone. There is then evidence of increased bone resorption; osteoclasts and Howship's lacunae are prominent on the surface of the trabeculae which become surrounded by delicate, fibrillar fibrous tissue. There may also be 'dissecting resorption' of trabeculae, the central parts being replaced by fibrous tissue. The picture is often one of great activity (Fig. 22.20), with an increase also in osteoblasts; resorption and new bone formation may be seen on opposite sides of the same trabecula. At this stage radiology may demonstrate subperiosteal erosion of the phalanges and of other bones due to patchy

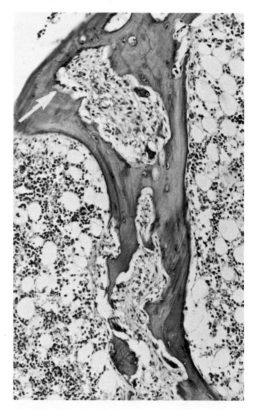

Fig. 22.20 Osteitis fibrosa of hyperparathyroidism. There is osteoclastic resorption of the central part of a bone trabecula with fibrous tissue replacement, so-called dissecting resorption. Some osteoblasts are also seen (*arrow*). × 100.

replacement of subperiosteal bone of the cortex by fibrous tissue. As the condition increases in severity the marrow spaces become filled with fibrous tissue—hence the term *osteitis fibrosa*—and the normal structure of bone in both cortex and medulla is replaced by a meshwork of fine, irregular and delicate trabeculae. These consist chiefly of normally calcified bone; narrow osteoid borders may be present beneath a row of plump osteoblasts as is sometimes observed in fracture callus and indicate only the rapidity of bone formation rather than a real deficiency of mineralisation. Radiology now shows loss of definition between cortex and medullary cavity, the whole bone having a fuzzy, mottled appearance, and because of the loss of normal structure it is more liable to fracture. The loose fibrous tissue is vascular and secondary changes may occur in it as a result of degeneration or haemorrhage. Cystic spaces may form and in areas of haemorrhage the resulting haemo-

siderin and the large numbers of multinucleated giant cells give rise to the '*brown tumour of hyperparathyroidism*' (Fig. 22.21). The differentiation of this lesion from giant-cell tumour of bone may give considerable difficulty and the possibility of brown tumour should always be considered especially in a site unusual for giant-cell tumour such as jaw, skull or phalanges and above all when the lesions are multiple.

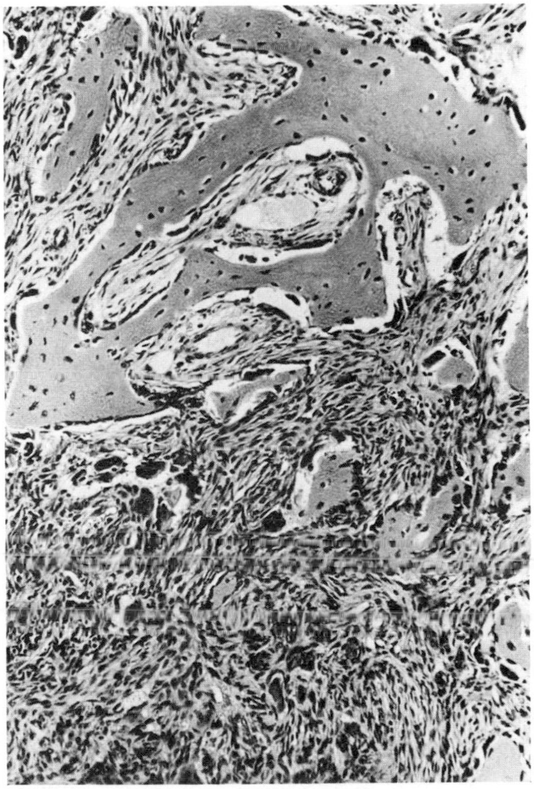

Effect of removal of the parathyroid tumour. Excision of the parathyroid tumour, which may be in the neck or, in some instances, behind the sternum, leads to a fall in the serum calcium level, and within a week bone biopsy may show

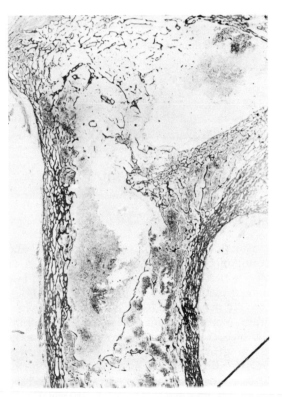

Fig. 22.22   Upper part of femoral shaft from a case of hyperparathyroidism secondary to chronic renal failure. There is osteitis fibrosa and osteoporosis, with severe cancellisation of the cortex. × 1·5.

Fig. 22.21   Bone in hyperparathyroidism. Numerous multinucleated giant cells and spindle cells form a 'brown tumour'. Newly formed bone is seen in the upper part of the photograph. × 120.

diminution of osteoclast activity, the bone structure slowly returning to a more normal appearance. Failure of improvement after operative removal may indicate the presence of a second tumour. In some instances tetany has followed immediately after removal of the affected parathyroid, but function of the remaining parathyroid glands, apparently suppressed by the tumour, soon returns to normal.

Secondary hyperparathyroidism

In dietary rickets, osteomalacia, pregnancy, chronic uraemia and some other conditions, there is a tendency to a fall in serum calcium levels and there may be a compensatory increase in parathyroid activity leading to enlargement of the glands. Of these conditions chronic uraemia especially may give rise to bony changes, slight or severe, mimicking those of primary hyperparathyroidism (Fig. 22.22).

Excess of growth hormone after puberty (acromegaly)

Bone enlargement occurs and is due partly to subperiosteal proliferation but possibly also to re-establishment of endochondral ossification of the articular cartilage and vertebral end plates. The bones of the hands and feet and the jaw are most strikingly affected.

Excess of corticosteroids (Cushing's syndrome)

Cushing's syndrome is associated with osteoporosis and has the usual clinical and morbid anatomical features, the spine and pelvis being especially affected (p. 831). The porosis is thought to be the result of both a reduced rate of bone formation and an increased rate of resorption though osteoclasts are not prominent in histological material. Identical skeletal changes may occur with prolonged cortisone therapy.

Thyroid deficiency in infants (cretinism)

Longstanding hypothyroidism in early life results in severe dwarfing. There is slowing of normal endochondral growth, late appearance of centres of ossification and sometimes delay in closure of epiphyses. The epiphyses may also be irregular, deformed, and radiologically stippled. The bones may become thickened with broad cortices and wide medullary trabeculae.

Excess of thyroid hormone (thyrotoxicosis)

Prolonged hyperthyroidism may cause osteoporosis. There is thought to be an increase of both resorption and bone formation but resorption exceeds formation.

Miscellaneous Bone Conditions

Osteoporosis

In osteoporosis there is a decrease in the amount of bone tissue but the matrix is normally mineralised, at least as judged by histological methods and inorganic analysis (Fig. 22.16). It may result from decreased bone formation, increased bone resorption or a combination of both. Osteoporosis arises in a localised and a generalised form following various unrelated disorders.

Disuse atrophy (immobilisation osteoporosis, disuse osteoporosis, localised osteoporosis). Disuse atrophy is found in immobilised or paralysed limbs, e.g. following poliomyelitis. It may be recognisable within weeks and seems to be associated both with loss of muscle action and with loss of weight bearing. It is striking that in even the most severely affected bones cancellous trabeculae remain prominent along lines of stress. The bones become increasingly radiolucent; the trabeculae of spongy bone are scantier and more slender; the cortical bone becomes thinner due chiefly to opening up of

Haversian spaces on the endosteal surface, so-called *cancellisation*. The changes of osteoporosis may be patchy in distribution and are usually first recognised in cancellous bone especially that in the metaphysis and subchondral articular regions, probably because bone turnover is more rapid in these sites. Focal radiological bone changes due to osteoporosis may be mistaken for other localised osteolytic processes such as tuberculosis.

An initial increase in resorption is thought to cause the porosis (Fig. 22.23) but later bone deposition and resorption may return to equilibrium. Once muscle activity is resumed there is an increase in bone production and the bone slowly returns to normal. Occasionally permanent deformity results from *premature epiphyseal fusion* in children. Generalised immobilisation may be complicated in the early stages by hypercalcaemia and the formation of renal calculi. Similar osteoporosis is said to have been found in the first astronauts, probably due partly to the enforced relative inactivity within the space capsule and partly to the weightless state.

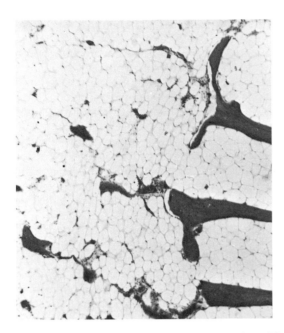

Fig. 22.23 Immobilisation osteoporosis. The articular surface is beyond the left hand border of the picture. The subchondral trabeculae to the left have almost completely disappeared and there is active osteoclasis spreading to involve the normal sized trabeculae on the right. × 45.

Generalised osteoporosis. Only a small proportion of people with osteoporosis suffer from known endocrine abnormalities such as Cushing's syndrome (p. 973), thyrotoxicosis (p. 959) or hypogonadism. There is a much larger group of post-menopausal women and elderly males who have thin bones, vertebral collapse and a tendency to fracture. The cause of the porosis is uncertain. Lack of oestrogens, increased effect of parathyroid hormone, long-standing mild negative calcium balance and minor degrees of vitamin D deficiency with poor calcium absorption from the gut have all been advanced as possible explanations. It is known that skeletal mass decreases in both men and women from about 35 years onwards and it has been suggested that these patients may not lose more bone than normal but have less bone in young adult life. Whatever the cause of the porosis, and many factors may contribute to it, when bone is lost it is not replaced. Search should be made for any treatable hormonal factors, diet should contain adequate amounts of calcium, protein and vitamins D and C and the patient be encouraged to remain as active as possible.

The structural changes associated with osteoporosis, whether they arise in association with known endocrine disorders or with ageing, are essentially the same. Vertebral changes (Fig. 22.24) may be particularly striking with bulging of the intervertebral disc through the weakened

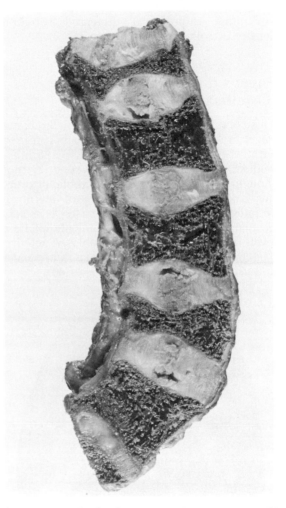

Fig. 22.24 The lumbar spine of this 74-year-old with severe osteoporosis shows bulging of the intervertebral discs and collapse of the vertebral bodies of L1 and L4.

end plate (Schmorl's nodes), increased concavity of the vertebrae (codfish vertebrae), collapse with wedging, or less commonly equal flattening (vertebra plana). These changes give rise to a decrease in stature, development of a thoracic hump or lumbar lordosis, and the compression fractures are frequently accompanied by pain. There is also a tendency to fracture of long bones from trivial trauma, especially at the femoral neck, wrist and ankle and for the production of cough fractures in the ribs. The blood calcium and phosphate levels are usually normal. It is essential to exclude, if necessary by bone biopsy, osteomalacia, osteitis fibrosa, myelomatosis or carcinomatosis before attributing radiological decreased vertebral density or collapse to osteoporosis.

Paget's disease of bone (Osteitis deformans)

This condition was first described by Sir James Paget in 1877. It was for many years confused with the osteitis fibrosa of hyperparathyroidism. Paget's disease, however, is not thought to be a generalised metabolic disorder but a chronic bone dystrophy of unknown aetiology and the blood biochemistry is usually normal apart from a raised alkaline phosphatase level, indicating increased osteoblastic activity. The condition is commoner in males than females and usually appears after the age of 40.

Sites of occurrence. The lumbar vertebrae and sacrum, skull and pelvis are the most frequently affected bones, though limb bones may also be involved. In about 10% of cases a single bone, often a vertebra, or even a part of a bone, is the only area involved. The condition may be widespread but is always multifocal and not diffuse (cf. osteitis fibrosa).

Incidence. Necropsy series show Paget's disease in about 3% of patients over 40 years of age, but in only about a third of these has the disease given rise to symptoms such as bone pain, tenderness, bowing of the lower limbs or increase in skull size.

Macroscopic appearances. In the long bones, the shafts become thickened both subperiosteally and endosteally, so that the bone, as a whole, is enlarged and the medullary cavity is diminished. The femur and the tibia often show forward bowing and the neck of the femur

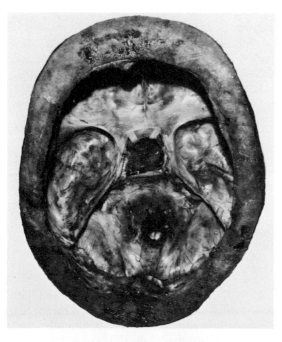

Fig. 22.25 Paget's disease of the skull, showing enormous thickening of the calvarium with loss of distinction of the tables. The sella turcica is much enlarged owing to the fortuitous presence of a chromophobe adenoma of the pituitary.

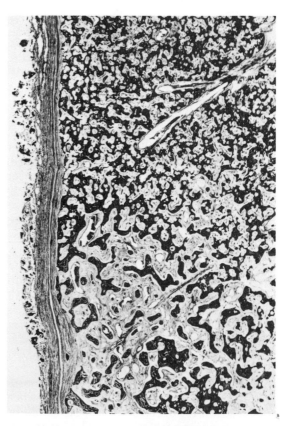

Fig. 22.26 Paget's disease of the skull, showing loss of distinction between the table and the diploë and the variable density of the bone. The marrow is fibrous and highly vascular. × 7·5.

becomes set more nearly at a right angle to the shaft (coxa vara). Cysts and stress fractures may be present. The skull enlarges and the thickness of the calvarium may be three or four times the normal (Fig. 22.25). The distinction between diploë and the tables is gradually lost (Fig. 22.26), and the whole bone becomes fairly uniformly porous and so soft that it may be cut with a knife. (The form of localised rarefaction of the skull known as *osteoporosis circumscripta* is probably a variant of Paget's disease.) Similar less severe changes may be present in the bones of the face. When the vertebrae are involved they tend to collapse anteriorly so that a dorsal kyphus forms and the patient may come to have a crouching attitude.

Microscopic appearances. There is simultaneous and irregular resorption and regeneration of bone with cellular fibrosis and greatly increased vascularity of the intertrabecular marrow. The picture is often, especially in the early stages, one of intense activity, both osteoclasts and osteoblasts being abundant. To begin with, bone resorption is most marked and the bone is lighter than normal with a consequent tendency to fracture and bowing deformities. Later resorption decreases and the trabeculae are often thickened with the formation of a

mosaic pattern of irregular cement lines indicating numerous previous phases of resorption and reconstruction (Fig. 22.27). At this stage the bone may be heavier than normal but because of the destruction of the cortical Haversian systems it remains structurally weaker.

Complications. (1) The weakened bones are liable to *fracture*, which in the long bones is often transverse and due to stress. There may occasionally be sequelae such as cord compression due either to vertebral collapse which is rare or more often to bony overgrowth narrowing the vertebral canal. Occasionally cranial nerves may be compressed.

(2) *Osteoarthritis* (p. 859) may result from the bony deformities throwing unusual stress on joints.

(3) *High output cardiac failure* may stem from the greatly increased bone vascularity which leads to some degree of arteriovenous shunt.

(4) In Paget's disease there is a thirtyfold increase in the risk of developing *bone sarcoma*: more than one bone may be involved. The tumours are almost invariably osteolytic and may be osteosarcomas, fibrosarcomas or occasionally chondrosarcomas, often very pleomorphic and with numerous tumour giant cells. The prognosis is very bad because of early pulmonary metastases. It is interesting that a bone affected with Paget's disease is a common site of *metastatic carcinoma*, probably because of its increased vascularity.

Fibrous dysplasia

Fibrous dysplasia is a benign fibro-osseous abnormality of bone of unknown aetiology. It is sometimes monostotic, less commonly polyostotic and rarely the polyostotic form is associated with patchy skin pigmentation and precocious sexual development (*Albright's syndrome*). In monostotic cases the lesions are commonly found in a rib (often symptomless), jaw bone, femur or tibia, though any bone may be involved. In polyostotic cases the femur and tibia are most frequently affected along with various other bones and often the condition is almost but not entirely unilateral. Attention is often drawn to the lesions in childhood and new foci may continue to appear even after

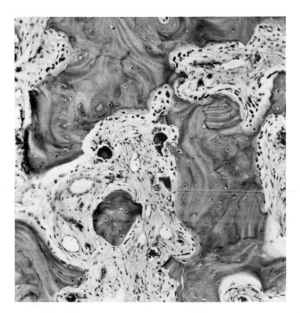

Fig. 22.27 Paget's disease of the femur, showing the typical mosaic structure of the bone, with both active osteoclastic resorption and osteoblastic formation. (Professor J. B. Gibson.) × 90.

puberty. When many bones are affected early in life the condition tends to progress with increasing deformity and multiple fractures. Malignant change to fibrosarcoma is very rare indeed.

Macroscopic appearances. The normal bone is sharply demarcated from the whitish, gritty fibrous tissue, often containing cysts and small nodules of cartilage, which expands the bone. The epiphyses of long bones tend to be spared. The typical focus of fibrous dysplasia shows a ground-glass, finely mottled appearance on x-ray and can sometimes be cut with a knife, but lesions in the skull and jaw tend to be more densely bony and indeed often appear radiologically as areas of increased density.

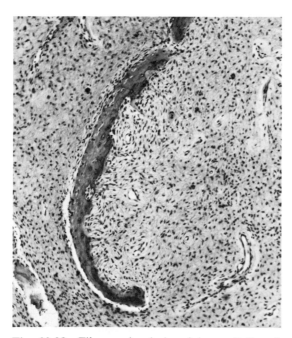

Fig. 22.28 Fibrous dysplasia of bone. Delicately cellular fibrous tissue contains many thin trabeculae of woven bone. × 75.

Microscopic appearances. There is a loose, small spindle-celled fibrous stroma in which curving and lobster-claw trabeculae of non-lamellar woven bone (Fig. 22.28), apparently devoid of osteoblasts, are found irregularly scattered. These trabeculae are characteristic and repeated biopsy has shown that they fail to mature to lamellar bone. Groups of osteoclasts and occasional nodules of cartilage may be present.

Hand–Schüller–Christian disease

This condition, which usually occurs in children, is characterised by the formation of multiple osteolytic lesions, often affecting the skull and consisting of lipid (predominantly cholesterol) filled histiocytes with neutrophil and eosinophil polymorphs, plasma cells and lymphocytes and sometimes small multinucleated cells. As the age of the lesion increases there is a tendency to fibrosis and formation of cholesterol clefts with foreign body giant-cell reaction. Its other features are described on p. 512.

Eosinophil granuloma of bone is usually solitary but sometimes multiple, and affects most often the skull, vertebrae and long bones in children and young adults. The histological picture is that of a granuloma with a preponderance of eosinophils, lipid-containing macrophages and some small multinucleated giant cells. It usually heals but is thought occasionally to progress to a more generalised granulomatosis of the Hand–Schüller–Christian type (see p. 512).

Digital clubbing and hypertrophic osteoarthropathy

Clubbing of the distal phalanges of the fingers and less commonly the toes may be found in association with various chronic lung diseases, e.g. bronchiectasis, fibroid tuberculosis, emphysema, bronchial carcinoma and, more rarely, with other abnormalities such as congenital heart disease, cirrhosis of the liver, ulcerative colitis and Crohn's disease. The phalanges are widened and thickened, whilst the nails are raised, curved, and often fibrous in texture. The clubbing is the result of thickening and fibrosis of the soft tissues particularly under the nailbed, and is thought to be associated with vascular engorgement. Occasionally there is an increase in subperiosteal bone of the terminal phalanges.

Patients with hypertrophic osteoarthropathy develop, in addition to finger clubbing, a periostitis and sometimes also joint disease. Layers of subperiosteal new bone form first in the distal thirds of the shafts of the bones of the forearms and lower legs and later sometimes spread to involve the remainder of these bones and the femora and humeri. The condition is associated most frequently with pleural mesothelioma, bronchial carcinoma of acinar or squamous pattern, sometimes with metastatic lung tumours, rarely with non-neoplastic lung disease and very infrequently with other disorders. Hypertrophic osteoarthropathy may appear early in the course of the pulmonary disease and disappear after surgical resection of the diseased lung. Its cause is not known.

Generalised Developmental Abnormalities of Bone

Osteopetrosis, marble-bone disease (*Albers–Schönberg*). This disorder is characterised by excessive density of all the bones with obliteration of the marrow cavities and development of leuko-erythroblastic anaemia. It is associated with failure of resorption of the cartilaginous spongiosa. Involvement of the skull leads to narrowing of the foramina with deafness and impairment of vision. In spite of the increased density the bones are brittle and fractures occur from slight violence. The disease is a hereditary one, and is transmitted in young severely affected patients as an autosomal recessive character and in its relatively benign form as an autosomal dominant.

Osteogenesis imperfecta. Osteogenesis imperfecta is a hereditary disease characterised by generalised osteoporosis with slender bones and increased fragility. The condition may develop during intrauterine life (*osteogenesis imperfecta congenita*) and is then generally fatal or in later childhood or adult life (*osteogenesis imperfecta tarda*) when the severity varies greatly.

The long bones are thin with narrow, poorly formed cortices. Spontaneous fractures may be numerous and result in short, bowed, deformed bones especially in the lower limbs. Fracture and callus formation may occur *in utero*. Fractures usually heal without trouble but pseudarthrosis sometimes occurs and occasionally callus is very hyperplastic, forming tumour-like masses which may be difficult to distinguish microscopically from osteosarcoma. Severe spinal *osteoporosis* may give rise to markedly biconcave ('codfish') vertebral bodies, to collapse or to scoliosis. Narrowing of the pelvic outlet may occur. Membrane bones are also poorly formed. The skull is thin, bulging, particularly over the ears and with a mosaic pattern due to numerous Wormian bones. It forms little protection to the brain during birth and many affected infants die of intracranial haemorrhage.

Microscopically in bones formed by endochondral ossification there seems to be no defect in the epiphyseal cartilage and invasion of regularly arranged cartilage columns by capillaries is normal but in severe cases little bone is laid down (Fig. 22.29) probably due to inability of osteoblasts to synthesise or organise collagen. The bone which is formed, whether by endochondral or membranous ossification, consists of a spongy, open network of small delicate trabeculae with little production of cortical bone. The bone is thought to show abnormalities of both mineral distribution and fibre pattern with failure of maturation to lamellar bone. There seems to be a defect in maturation and cross-bonding of collagen

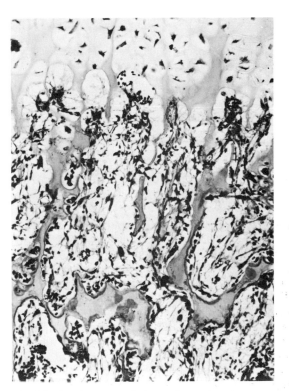

Fig. 22.29   Osteogenesis imperfecta showing poor formation of bone at the epiphyseal line. × 115.

formation beyond the stage of reticulin-like fibres and this may cause other associated abnormalities. The sclerae appear blue because they are so thin that the pigmented choroid shines through and the dentine of the teeth may be poorly formed. Herniae, thin translucent skin and joint hypermobility with lax ligaments may also be present. Patients may become deaf due to defective bone conduction.

Osteogenesis imperfecta tarda is inherited as an autosomal dominant but it is likely that an autosomal recessive form exists, giving rise to the few non-sporadic cases of the congenital type of disease.

Achondroplasia. This remarkable condition, which is known also as *chondrodystrophia fetalis*, is brought about by failure of endochondral ossification. It is present at birth and may be diagnosed radiologically *in utero*. The head appears large, the forehead bulging and the root of the nose is indrawn or sunken; the limbs are short and stumpy, sometimes curved, and as there is more growth of the soft tissues than of the bones, the skin of the limbs is in folds. There are vertebral abnormalities with narrowing of the spinal canal in the lumbar region. Obesity is common, and sometimes there is some oedema. The hands are broad with fingers of equal length (trident hands). While pathological studies have been few it appears that the characteristic changes depend on the failure of the process of bone formation in cartilage. At the epiphyseal line, the cartilage cells form only short rows, or are irregularly arranged, and there is only a little or no ossification, hence the failure of growth. The cartilaginous epiphysis is sometimes considerably broadened, and with the small shaft presents a mushroom-like appearance; there may be also areas of softening in the cartilage. The indraw-

ing of the nose results from a shortening of the base of the skull, and this also is due to imperfect ossification, which is sometimes accompanied by premature union of the basi-sphenoidal and sphenoidal sutures. In fact, all the bones ossified from cartilage are small, whilst intramembranous ossification proceeds normally. There are varying degrees of the condition, and 80% of affected children die within the first year of life, usually of neurological complications such as hydrocephalus due to undue smallness of the skull base and posterior fossa. The less severely affected child may survive to adult life as a dwarf with short thick limbs, but with no other important change. Achondroplasia is due to a dominant gene with a very high mutation rate; thus most cases are the result of a mutation in one or other parent, whose chance of producing a second affected child is no greater than that of other normal persons. Achondroplastic dwarfs who survive to adult life may produce normal and affected children in equal numbers when mated with normal persons.

Multiple osteocartilaginous exostoses (*diaphyseal aclasis*) and **multiple enchondromatosis** (*Ollier's disease*) are discussed with benign cartilage tumours (pp. 842, 843).

Tumours in Bone

Metastatic tumours in bone

Frequency. Metastatic tumours in bone are commoner than primary bone tumours and probably occur in as many as 70% of cases of disseminated malignant disease. Bone, along with lungs and liver, is the most frequent site of secondary spread. An accurate assessment of frequency depends on meticulous post-mortem study. The true incidence of vertebral secondaries, for instance, is higher than suspected from radiological examination, as about one-third of the thickness of a vertebra must be destroyed before any change is evident radiologically.

Sites of occurrence. If metastases are present anywhere in the skeleton the vertebral column will almost certainly be affected, especially the thoracic or lumbar regions. Bony secondaries are commonly found in areas where haemopoietic marrow is normally present, i.e. the axial skeleton and the proximal ends of humerus and femur. Skeletal metastases are uncommon below the knee and very uncom-

mon below the elbow. Tumour usually reaches the bone by arterial emboli but it has been suggested that retrograde spread along the vertebral venous plexus may account for the frequent involvement of lumbar vertebrae by tumours of the pelvic organs.

Common primary sites. Tumours which most often give rise to secondaries in bone are carcinomas of breast, prostate, lung, thyroid, kidney, melanomas and in young children neuroblastomas.

Types of secondary tumours. Bone secondaries are commonly *osteolytic* or destructive, the bone trabeculae being resorbed and pathological fracture often resulting. If the destruction is widespread there may be hypercalcaemia.

Sometimes infiltration of the marrow by carcinoma stimulates marked laying down of new bone by osteoblasts. In these patients especially the serum alkaline phosphatase may be raised due to the increased osteoblastic activity. These *osteoplastic or osteosclerotic* secondaries arise most commonly in association with prostatic

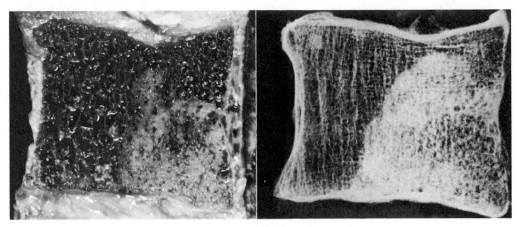

Fig. 22.30 The body of the lumbar vertebra is partially replaced by secondary prostatic carcinoma.

The radiograph of a thin slice shows that this has provoked reactive bone sclerosis.

carcinoma (Fig. 22.30) but carcinoma of breast, lung, stomach and various other sites may infrequently give rise to the same picture. Sometimes both osteosclerotic and osteolytic secondaries are present in the same patient.

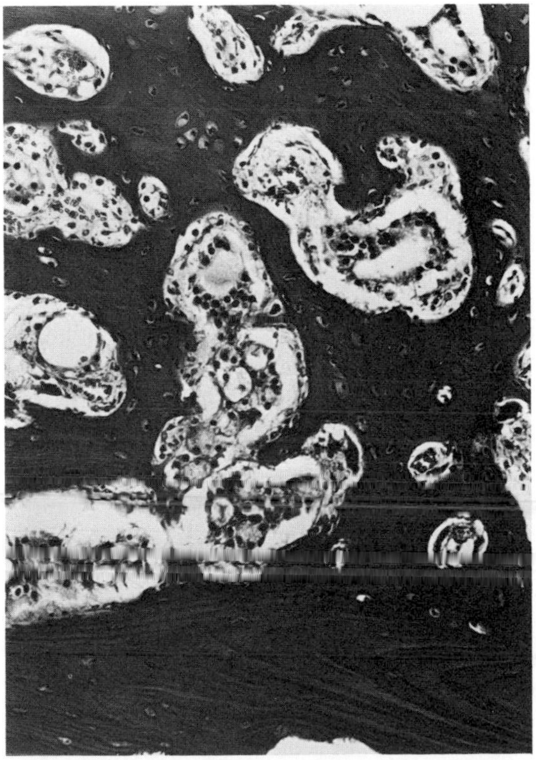

Where much of the bone marrow is encroached on by new bone formation (Fig. 22.31), a progressive anaemia may result. This is often leuko-erythroblastic and is associated with splenomegaly due to extramedullary haemopoiesis (p. 510).

Occasionally there is widespread diffuse marrow replacement with little bony change.

Solitary secondaries. Metastatic tumours in bone sometimes present as solitary lesions and, while this is usually rapidly followed by the appearance of further secondaries, in a very occasional case of renal or thyroid carcinoma, the bony focus may remain the sole metastasis. Only very rarely is surgical resection of both primary and secondary followed by worthwhile remission or by cure.

Primary tumours of bone

The precise diagnosis of certain bone tumours is so difficult that it is essential for the clinical and radiological features to be considered along with the naked-eye and microscopic appearances before a final decision is reached. Classification also is not easy, for in some the histogenesis is obscure and in others the very nature of the lesion is uncertain (see Table 22.1 on p. 838).

Classification. *Firstly,* it may be difficult to decide whether one is dealing with a true tumour or a developmental abnormality, e.g. multiple osteocartilaginous exostoses is clearly a hereditary condition and possibly solitary exostosis is a *forme fruste* of this, but, since

Fig. 22.31 Secondary prostatic carcinoma in bone with reactive new bone formation causing osteosclerosis. × 130.

Table 22.1 Classification of bone tumours

Derivation or type of tumour	Benign	Malignant
Fibrous tissue	Non-ossifying fibroma Desmoplastic fibroma	Fibrosarcoma
Cartilage	Osteocartilaginous exostosis $\longrightarrow$ Enchondroma $\longrightarrow$ Benign chondroblastoma Chondromyxoid fibroma	Chondrosarcoma
Bone	Osteoma Osteoid osteoma Benign osteoblastoma	Osteosarcoma (including some Paget's and post-irradiation sarcomas) Parosteal osteosarcoma
Unknown	Giant-cell tumour $\longrightarrow$	Giant-cell tumour
Vascular tissue	Haemangioma Glomus tumour	Haemangioendothelioma Angiosarcoma
Fat cells	Lipoma	Liposarcoma
Plasma cell precursors	Solitary plasmacytoma $\longrightarrow$	Myelomatosis
Marrow stroma		Malignant lymphoma Ewing's tumour
Neural tissue	Schwannoma Neurofibromatosis $\longrightarrow$ Ganglioneuroma	Neurofibrosarcoma
Notochordal tissue		Chordoma

The arrows indicate that these benign lesions may progress to malignancy

exostoses, whether single or multiple, may progress to malignancy, they are discussed in this section. Similarly, non-ossifying fibroma may or may not arise from a metaphyseal fibrous defect. *Secondly*, in many cases, although the tumour has a distinctive histological appearance, its histogenesis is uncertain; even osteosarcoma is best regarded as a tumour which produces bone or osteoid rather than one which arises from osteoblasts. The number of malignant mesenchymal tissues which may be found in an osteosarcoma points to its origin from a more primitive cell and serves as a reminder that the mesenchymal cell is capable of differentiation in different directions. In spite of these difficulties a classification is worthwhile because when it can be applied to a given tumour it allows a useful prediction of its behaviour.

In this section certain lesions are not discussed but they have been included in the table for the sake of completeness. Lesions of doubtful origin and non-neoplastic lesions simulating bone tumours have been mentioned in relation to the tumours with which they may be confused.

Osteoma

The term 'osteoma' is now almost entirely restricted to bony outgrowths of skull bones which sometimes protrude into the orbit or paranasal sinuses. These lesions may be formed of osteoblastic connective tissue and spongy bone trabeculae or of extremely dense compact bone or a mixture of these components. They are benign but may cause pressure symptoms.

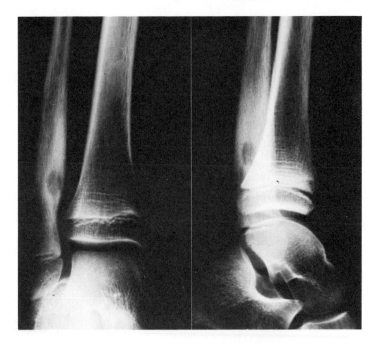

Fig. 22.32 Osteoid osteoma has given rise to an ovoid translucency in the lower end of the fibula. There is a little surrounding reactive bone sclerosis.

Osteoid osteoma

This is a benign osteoblastic lesion which is usually less than 1 cm in diameter. It occurs chiefly in the long bones of the lower limbs of adolescents or young adults although any bone and age may be affected. The clinical history is of increasingly severe and unusually well-localised pain and tenderness, the pain often relieved by salicylates. Radiology shows the lesion itself as a rounded zone of radiolucency (Fig. 22.32). If cortical, there is often massive sclerosis of adjacent bone whereas in cancellous bone sclerosis may be minimal. Macroscopically the osteoid osteoma is usually red and cherry-like and microscopic examination shows a very vascular nidus of osteoblastic tissue with a disorderly mass of irregular small trabeculae of osteoid or bone undergoing active remodelling (Fig. 22.33). Sometimes the central part of the nidus is more solid. If incompletely removed, symptoms may recur.

Osteosarcoma (osteogenic sarcoma)

Osteosarcoma is a malignant tumour in which osteoid or bone is formed directly by sarcoma cells and is thought to arise from cells of the primitive bone-forming mesenchyme. If myeloma is excluded it is the commonest

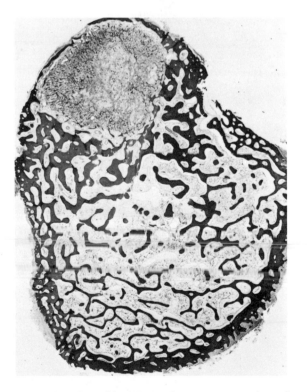

Fig. 22.33 Osteoid osteoma. A transverse section of the fibula shows the radiate small bone trabeculae of the lesion in the cortical bone with slight surrounding reactive sclerosis. × 6.

primary malignant bone tumour and occurs more frequently in males than females.

Age incidence. Osteosarcoma is rare under the age of 5 years and about 75% of patients are between 10 and 25 years old. In more than half of the older patients the tumour is associated with Paget's disease of bone.

Sites of occurrence. The commonest site of osteosarcoma is in the metaphysis of long bones and about half the cases occur around the knee but also frequently at the upper end of femur and humerus. It is sometimes found in vertebrae, pelvis and skull, especially when associated with Paget's disease. Osteosarcoma is very uncommon in the small bones of the hands and feet. Multicentric tumours are occasionally reported usually in association with Paget's disease.

Clinical features. Patients often give a fairly short history of increasingly severe pain, worse at night, and this may be followed by swelling, oedema, increase in local heat and dilated subcutaneous veins. Pathological fracture is relatively rare. The patients are usually in good general health; if they are not, the presence of metastases should be suspected.

Radiological and macroscopic appearances. Osteosarcoma usually arises in the medullary bone in the region of the metaphysis or diaphysis. The epiphyseal cartilage plate may act as a barrier for a while but when this is perforated, the tumour spreads to the epiphysis. The joint cavity is seldom involved. Osteosarcoma may spread quite rapidly through the

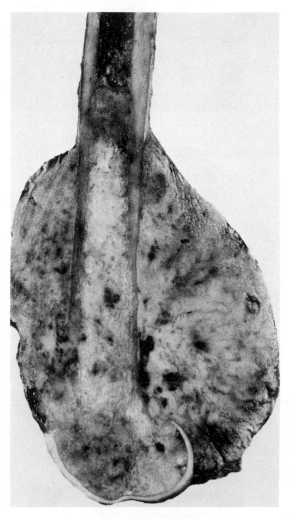

Fig. 22.34 Osteosarcoma of lower end of femur. The medullary tumour has permeated and partly destroyed the cortex, spreading outwards to form a large subperiosteal mass.

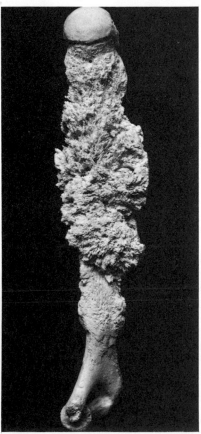

Fig. 22.35 Osteosarcoma of humerus. Macerated specimen to show the characteristic spiculation on the surface of the bone.

bony cortex without either perforating or markedly expanding it and form a subperiosteal mass (Fig. 22.34) which, in its turn, may burst through the periosteum and infiltrate muscles. When the periosteum is raised spicules of new bone are laid down at right angles to the bone shaft (Fig. 22.35) giving rise radiologically to sunray spiculation. At the junction between raised and normal periosteum, Codman's triangle of reactive bone develops. Neither of these appearances is present in all cases of osteosarcoma, nor when present are they specific signs of osteosarcoma; the same appearances may be seen in metastatic carcinoma or even sometimes in infections. Biopsy material should not be taken from an area where reactive bone formation is active as this may greatly increase the difficulty of diagnosis. Apart from spread outside the bone there may be medullary extension of the tumour and this is sometimes greater than is suspected radiologically. The gross appearances of the tumour vary according to the amount of tumour osteoid and bone which has been formed. Some tumours contain little bony matrix (*osteolytic*) and these tend to be soft, friable, vascular destructive lesions with areas of haemorrhage and necrosis. Others may contain much tumour bone (*osteosclerotic*) especially in their central areas, and are dense and of turnip-like consistence in their soft parts. The amount of ossification is not related to the age of the tumour nor does it appear to affect the prognosis.

Microscopic appearances. Though the essential criteria for the diagnosis of osteosarcoma are the presence of a frankly sarcomatous stroma and the direct formation of tumour osteoid or bone from this malignant connective tissue, the histological pattern of osteosarcoma is very variable. In addition to tumour bone, some osteosarcomas contain a large amount of cartilage and others much malignant spindle-celled tissue of fibrosarcomatous type. In the osteolytic type of osteosarcoma the bulk of the tumour is often made up of pleomorphic and giant tumour cells with many aberrant mitoses and irregular vascular channels lined by tumour cells (Fig. 22.36). In the osteosclerotic type, on the other hand, such a mass of tumour bone may be laid down on and between pre-existing trabeculae that malignant cells within the matrix are small and scanty except at the growing edge. Osteosarcomas in Paget's disease are

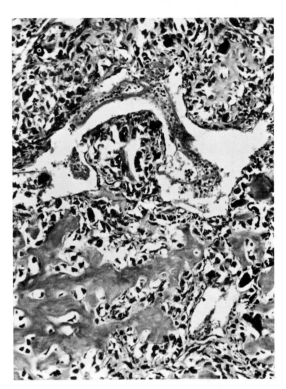

Fig. 22.36 Osteosarcoma. A highly vascular, cellular tumour with osteoid formation well seen in the lower part of the field. × 200.

almost invariably of the osteolytic type (Fig. 22.37) and are characterised by their extreme pleomorphism and by large numbers of tumour giant cells.

Metastatic spread. As in most sarcomas spread of the tumour is almost invariably by the bloodstream to the lungs and sometimes to other bones and viscera, lymph node metastases being rare. Pulmonary metastases occur early and are often thought to have arisen before the patient appears for treatment although at that time they may not be visible radiologically. The prognosis in osteosarcoma is therefore poor and a five-year survival rate of only 5–20% is reported. In some series the outlook is better in tumours of the distal skeleton and of the jaws. Early reports suggest that, following surgery, repeated courses of chemotherapy may increase the life-span. Osteosarcomas arising in Paget's disease may be multicentric and have an even worse prognosis than those arising in normal bone. Local recurrence or seeding of the tumour in the wound is unusual, in contrast with chondrosarcoma (p. 845).

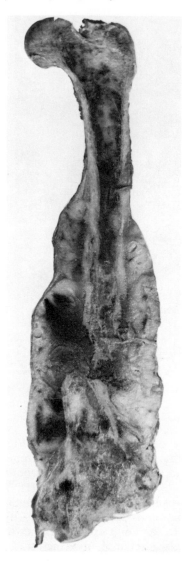

Fig. 22.37 Paget's disease of femur showing osteolytic sarcoma with pathological fracture.

Parosteal (juxtacortical) osteosarcoma. This is a rare tumour but worth distinguishing since it has a much better prognosis than medullary osteosarcoma. In most of the reported cases the tumour has arisen at the metaphysis of the lower end of femur, tibia or humerus. It forms a broad-based swelling arising initially on the surface of the bone and sometimes coming to encircle the shaft, cortical penetration and medullary infiltration being late. Microscopically the tumour usually consists of well-formed bony trabeculae separated by atypical spindle cells; sometimes near the surface the bone is less well formed and there may also be islands of cartilage. The tumour grows slowly and tends to occur in a wider age group

than osteosarcoma. If the lesion is inadequately dealt with it may recur or become frankly malignant and metastasise, sometimes within two years, sometimes not for twenty years. If it is treated by radical surgery initially the outlook is usually good.

Benign cartilage tumours

Osteocartilaginous exostosis (osteochondroma, ecchondroma) is the commonest benign tumour of bone and consists of a bony excrescence. Its outer shell and medulla are continuous with that of the bone from which it arises and it is covered by a cartilage cap from the undersurface of which endochondral ossification occurs (Fig. 22.38). The lesion may be single or multiple; when multiple the condition is familial and may be associated with some failure of bone remodelling (*hereditary multiple exostoses, diaphyseal aclasis*). Exostoses may

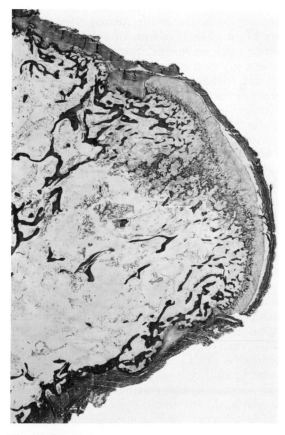

Fig. 22.38 Osteocartilaginous exostosis of humerus consisting of cancellous bone covered by cartilage and perichondrium. Endochondral ossification is occurring. × 8·5.

arise in any bone formed by endochondral ossification but the metaphyses of long bones, especially the femur, humerus and tibia, are the commonest sites. The lesions are usually first noticed in childhood and adolescence and growth commonly ceases in adult life, the cartilaginous cap sometimes completely disappearing. Malignant change is rare in solitary exostoses but between 10–20% of patients with multiple lesions develop chondrosarcoma, usually in adult life. Exostoses of the axial skeleton or proximal limb bones are much more likely to become malignant than those in the peripheral skeleton (see chondrosarcoma for discussion). So-called *subungual exostosis*, which is often painful, is not an exactly comparable lesion. It arises often following infec-

tion or trauma as a result of cartilaginous and osseous metaplasia of the fibrous tissue around the terminal part of the distal phalanx.

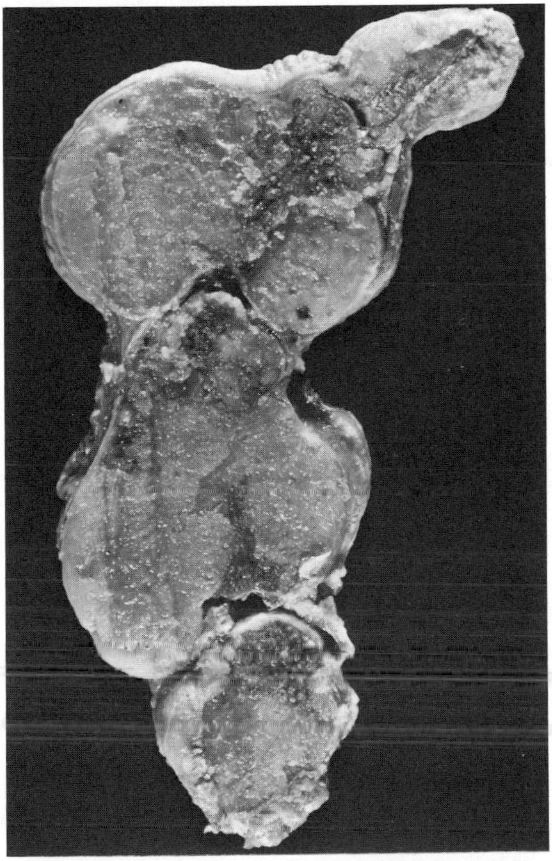

Enchondroma is a benign cartilage tumour arising within the medullary cavity most commonly of the small bones of the hands and feet (Fig. 22.39). The cartilage tumours may be single or multiple and when multiple are thought to arise as a failure of normal endochondral ossification (*multiple enchondromatosis*). In multiple enchondromatosis the hands are almost invariably involved but there may also be lesions in long tubular bones associated with bowing and deformity, especially of the forearm. When the enchondromas are predominantly unilateral the condition is sometimes referred to as *Ollier's disease*. Solitary benign enchondroma may also be found in long tubular bones, particularly the humerus and femur. The tumour arises initially in the metaphysis and may spread into the shaft or occasionally into the epiphysis if the cartilage plate is fused. Radiologically the lesions are radiolucent, sometimes with spotty calcification and naked-

Fig. 22.39 Benign enchondromas of finger. The finger has been amputated just proximal to the metacarpal head. While the joint spaces remain intact each phalanx is replaced by a mass of hyaline cartilage. The cortices have disappeared but periosteum still surrounds the cartilage.

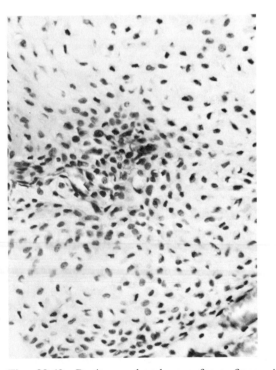

Fig. 22.40 Benign enchondroma from finger in multiple enchondromatosis. The cartilage is highly cellular but the cells are mononuclear and fairly uniform in size. × 250.

eye examination of an enchondroma shows the usual appearance of cartilage though often more gelatinous than normal. Microscopic examination of the benign lesion shows small uniform cells with small and few double nuclei (Fig. 22.40). The lesions of the phalanges and metacarpals, especially in multiple enchondromas, may be unusually cellular without there being any sinister prognostic significance. The common clinical complaints, particularly in the phalangeal lesions, are of swelling or pathological fracture. Malignant transformation in cases of solitary enchondroma is probably rare but the risk is appreciable in patients with multiple enchondromatosis, some authors giving figures as high as 50%. Pain unassociated with fracture, or the onset of enlargement in an enchondroma of the axial skeleton or long tubular bones in an adult, should immediately raise the suspicion of malignant change.

Chondrosarcoma

Chondrosarcoma is a malignant cartilage tumour and may arise *de novo* or, in about 10%

of cases, from a pre-existing benign cartilage tumour. It may be situated within the bone (central) or outwith it (peripheral). The tumour is slightly less common than osteosarcoma and is twice as common in males as in females. In contrast to osteosarcoma, chondrosarcoma is rare under the age of 30 years and most patients are in the 40–70 age group.

Sites of occurrence. About half the lesions arise in the pelvic girdle (Fig. 22.42) and ribs; the proximal femur is another common site. A

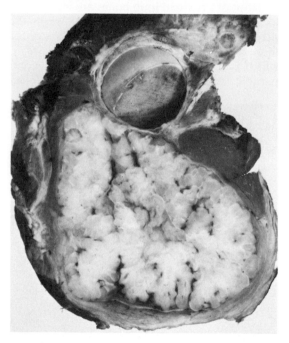

Fig. 22.42 Low-grade chondrosarcoma of pelvis showing the large cartilaginous tumour arising from the ilium.

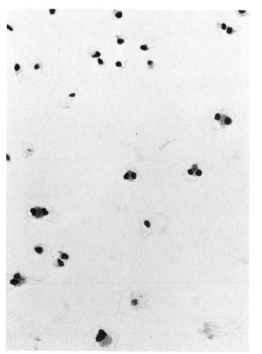

Fig. 22.41 This recurrent low grade chondrosarcoma killed the patient by local spread without metastases. The cartilage matrix is well formed and the tumour is not very cellular but there are numerous foci of chondrocytes with double nuclei. × 250.

careful watch, therefore, should be kept on cartilage tumours of the axial skeleton, particularly in adults and increase in size and pain should arouse the suspicion of malignancy. The incidence of malignant change decreases in the distal part of the skeleton and is very rare in the bones of the hands and feet except for the os calcis and talus.

Macroscopic appearances. *Central tumours.* A central cartilage tumour usually causes slight bone expansion and in slowly growing tumours there is often buttressing of the cortex in response to endosteal erosion. Not uncommonly, however, the cortex is broken through and the tumour is found growing in the adjacent soft tissue. Sometimes, particularly in large tumours which are especially prone to arise in pelvis and ribs, the exact site of origin becomes difficult to identify and the lobulated tumour is soft, slimy and cystic due to mucoid degeneration of the matrix. Spotty calcification may be present and sometimes is extensive, an aid in the radiological diagnosis of these tumours.

Peripheral tumours may arise *de novo* or from previously existing osteocartilaginous exostoses; the cartilage caps are then much thickened and in the early stages the normally smooth surface may be covered with little nodules of proliferating cartilage. Later these tumours may become very large and undergo heavy calcification or myxoid degeneration.

Microscopic appearances. If the cells in a cartilage tumour are pleomorphic with vesicular nuclei and there are abundant multinucleated tumour cells and moderate numbers of mitotic figures, the recognition of malignancy is easy (Fig. 22.43). In slowly growing tumours, however, it may be difficult. The generally accepted criteria of malignancy are the presence, even in

only scattered areas, of many chondrocytes with plump nuclei and of moderate numbers of chondrocytes with two or more nuclei (Fig. 22.41). The absence of mitotic figures does not necessarily indicate that the tumour is benign. The best opportunity of arriving at a correct assessment of the tumour's potentialities is in studying material from the growing edge and every scrap of biopsy tissue must be examined microscopically. Biopsies from heavily calcified or degenerate cartilage are useless. Because of variations in histological malignancy in different parts of the same tumour a microscopic diagnosis of chondroma should be viewed with suspicion if clinical and radiological features suggest malignant change. It is particularly important in this tumour that the pathologist should be aware of the *age* of the patient and the *site* of the tumour. Minor changes from normality which would be alarming in cartilage tumours of the axial skeleton where recurrences may not be resectable may, from experience, be discounted to a large extent in growing cartilage tumours in children, in lesions of the small tubular bones of the hands and feet, in subperiosteal cartilage tumours and synovial chondromatosis.

Implantation. Cartilage cells have low biologic requirements and probably because of this these tumours have a special tendency to implantation and growth in soft tissues. This has great practical importance to the surgeon as it means that the site of biopsy must be carefully planned in a suspected case so that the whole of the tissue planes opened up may be excised at the time of definitive treatment. This characteristic also results in a very marked tendency to local recurrence after excision even when the original operation appeared to be clear of the tumour. In order to prevent this in areas where eradication of a recurrent tumour would be difficult such as chest wall or pelvis, a radical operation is often necessary in the first instance.

Course of the disease and prognosis. Chondrosarcoma runs, in contrast to osteosarcoma, a more prolonged course. The patients have often some years' history when they first come to hospital. The slowly growing tumours may continue with repeated local recurrences for more than twenty years before the patient is finally killed by involvement of some vital structure from local spread rather than by

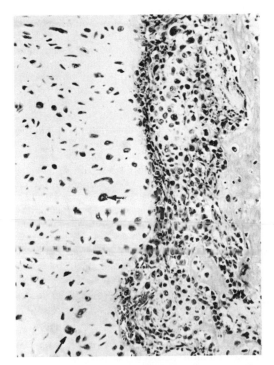

Fig. 22.43 Metastasising chondrosarcoma of ilium. The cartilage cells vary greatly in size and there are several mitoses, two of which are arrowed. × 100.

pulmonary metastases. These are the tumours which respond most successfully to radical treatment in the first instance where this is surgically feasible. More malignant rapidly-growing and metastasising chondrosarcomas may lead to death within a few years but even they may persist for a surprisingly long time. In adolescence primary chondrosarcomas are rare and usually rapidly fatal. Chondrosarcoma metastasises by blood spread, frequently to the lungs and has a tendency to direct retrograde spread along veins. Lymph node metastases are rare. In the past the prognosis has been poor partly as a result of the pathologist's under-diagnosis of the lesion and partly from inadequate initial treatment.

A better prognosis can be anticipated in the light of a fuller understanding of the clinical and pathological features of this tumour.

Chondromyxoid fibroma of bone

This is a rare benign tumour of bone important only because of its tendency to be misdiagnosed as chondrosarcoma. It occurs chiefly in the metaphyses of

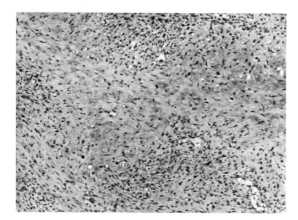

Fig. 22.44 Chondromyxoid fibroma of bone, showing the loose spindle-celled tissue with imperfectly formed cartilage. × 60.

long bones of adolescents or young adults especially in the lower limb. It usually gives rise to a sharply defined, eccentric, osteolytic defect which bulges the periosteum. The tumour is commonly rather firm and rubbery and lacks on naked-eye examination the gelatinous, slimy features that one would expect from the histology. Microscopy shows relatively poorly cellular tissue separated into pseudolobules by curving strands or trabeculae of aggregated cells (Fig. 22.44). The cells of the lobules are spindle-

shaped or stellate and lie in a myxomatous vacuolated matrix. The trabecular cells are similar but may show some hyperchromatism, pleomorphism and occasional mitotic figures—features which may lead to misdiagnosis of malignancy. Small multinucleated giant cells may also be seen. The tumour is benign, and though it may recur, usually responds to simple curettage.

Fibrosarcoma

This is a rare malignant tumour which may arise within the medullary cavity (endosteal) or beneath the periosteum (periosteal), usually in adults. **Endosteal** fibrosarcoma, though other sites are not exempt, affects especially the bones around the knee joint and in long bones commonly involves the metaphysis and sometimes the shaft. While the tumour in general is osteolytic, destructive and may break through the cortex and into the soft tissues, it tends, in some places at least, to infiltrate between pre-existing medullary bone trabeculae without destroying them and sometimes stimulates new bone formation on their surfaces. This gives rise radiologically to a moth-eaten appearance of the bone with irregular areas of translucency and sclerosis. The extent of radiological destruction may thus not indicate the true extent of tumour spread in the medulla. Multiple bones may be involved when the patient is first examined so that a skeletal survey should be carried out in patients with endosteal fibrosarcoma. Microscopically fibrosarcoma varies from a fasciculated spindle-celled tumour producing collagen in its more mature parts, to a highly pleomorphic tumour with little recognisable fibrous tissue. Such variations when present in the same tumour can be misleading. Differentiation histologically from metastatic spindle-celled renal or squamous carcinoma or from malignant melanoma may be difficult.

The 5-year survival rate is around 28% though a few patients develop metastases later. In some series prognosis has been linked to the degree of differentiation of the sarcoma.

Ewing's tumour

In 1921 Ewing described a tumour of bone under the name of diffuse endothelioma and while the endothelial origin has not been accepted there is little doubt that this is a specific variety of tumour. The histogenesis remains unknown and accordingly we prefer to retain the eponymous title.

Age and sex incidence. Ewing's tumour occurs chiefly in young persons; it is rare over the age of 30, and most common between the ages of 5 and 20 years; it is very rare in the first two years of life. Males are slightly more often affected.

Sites of occurrence. The long tubular bones are

most frequently involved, e.g. femur, tibia, humerus and fibula but the pelvis and ribs are also affected.

Naked-eye appearances. The tumour appears to originate within the medullary cavity and in long bones may involve the metaphysis and shaft. It is usually osteolytic and perforation of the cortex with raising of the periosteum may occur early. This subperiosteal elevation may give rise to parallel layers of reactive new bone (onion skin appearance) and less frequently to strands of bone forming at right angles to the cortex (sunray spiculation).

The tumour is usually whitish; some may be rather firm while others are very soft, almost puriform. It is not of very rapid growth, as compared with many other tumours of childhood.

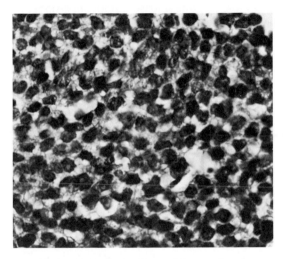

Fig. 22.45 Ewing's tumour of femur showing syncytial structure and uniform cell type. × 450.

Microscopic appearances. Ewing's tumour is composed of fairly uniform rounded, or polyhedral cells, often with pale nuclei due to the fine dispersion of chromatin. The cell boundaries are indistinct and the cells are arranged in syncytial sheets (Fig. 22.45) without a lobular pattern but divided by broad strands of collagen. Reticulin is scanty and there is often much necrosis. Intracellular glycogen may be demonstrated. Here and there the cells may be arranged in clusters resembling rosettes but without clearly defined central fibrils. This very inconstant feature is probably the result of degeneration.

Clinical features. Ewing's tumour usually presents with pain and swelling often of some months' duration. Sometimes fever, anaemia and leukocytosis suggest low-grade osteomyelitis and the patients with these systemic symptoms have the worst prognosis. The tumour is at first radiosensitive, but frequently recurrence takes place later and secondaries appear in other bones, especially the skull, and in the lungs.

The liver is less often involved and lymph nodes only rarely.

Differential diagnosis. While there is no doubt that some alleged examples of Ewing's tumour are metastases from an unrevealed neuroblastoma, the absence of cases in the first two years of life and the paucity of lymph-node and hepatic metastases are features different from those of neuroblastoma. The increased urinary excretion of vanillyl mandelic acid, homovanillic acid and other catecholamine derivatives in many cases of neuroblastoma and their normal values in patients with Ewing's tumour helps to distinguish between these tumours. The lack of clearly distinctive histological features sometimes requires the consideration of leukaemic deposits, lymphoid neoplasms, myelomatosis and secondary carcinoma in the differential diagnosis and occasionally the true diagnosis only becomes apparent at necropsy.

Malignant lymphoma of bone (reticulum-cell sarcoma)

Bone, in contrast to lymphoid and some other tissues, is a relatively uncommon site of primary lymphoma but its true incidence is uncertain because of the difficulty in diagnosis of malignant round cell tumours of bone.

Age, sex incidence and site. Malignant lymphoma is encountered chiefly in adults, with few examples in childhood or early adolescence (cf. Ewing's tumour). It is commoner in males and affects both the metaphysis and the adjacent shaft of long bones, and may arise also in flat bones and the axial skeleton.

Clinical features. Malignant lymphoma of bone presents with pain and swelling but fever is rare. X-ray often shows a fairly widespread, diffuse, moth-eaten area of patchy rarefaction. Periosteal new bone formation is not usually conspicuous but there may be patchy reactive bone sclerosis in the medulla. The radiological appearances may suggest a chronic osteomyelitis, and in small biopsies with much necrosis and secondary inflammatory cell infiltrate, considerable difficulty may also arise in making this histological differentiation. The tumour is radiosensitive, and the prognosis after radiotherapy or amputation is distinctly more favourable than that in Ewing's tumour. About 45% of cases are said to survive for five years and about 30% for ten years. Involvement of regional lymph nodes may occur early or late and may be followed by more extensive infiltration in spleen and liver. The lungs tend only to be affected late in the disease. Occasionally leukaemia develops. In every patient with a presumed primary lymphoma of bone, search should be made for involvement of other bones or of lymph nodes since the relatively good prognosis does not apply if the bone lesion is simply the presenting sign of more generalised disease.

Macroscopic appearances. The tumour tends to affect chiefly the metaphyseal region and adjacent shaft, and it is osteolytic so that the bony cortex becomes mottled and rarefied. The tumour penetrates the cortex usually without eliciting any new reactive periosteal bone, and spreads into the adjacent tissues.

Microscopic appearances. The tumour is composed of round or polyhedral cells often discretely arranged and with large round, oval or reniform nuclei. Between the cells there is sometimes a rich reticulin network, a feature conspicuously absent in Ewing's tumour. Intracellular glycogen is usually absent.

In some cases the distinction between malignant lymphoma and Ewing's tumour may be difficult or even impossible on the initial, often inadequate biopsy. When, however, a group of such cases is surveyed retrospectively with the clinical course, radiological and pathological features fully available, they can often be separated into the two categories.

Giant-cell tumour of bone (osteoclastoma)

Giant-cell tumour is an osteolytic, eccentrically placed tumour arising most commonly in the end of a long bone of an adult.

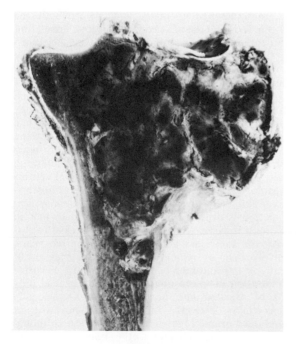

Fig. 22.46 Section of giant-cell tumour of upper end of tibia showing eccentric expansion of the bone end and much haemorrhage within the tumour.

Age. The lesion frequently arises in the 20–40 age group. The diagnosis should be regarded with suspicion at a site where the epiphyseal cartilage plate is still open as there are several benign lesions in children and adolescents which to some extent simulate giant-cell tumour. Some of these are discussed below.

Site of occurrence. Half of all the tumours occur at the knee (Fig. 22.46), in the lower end of femur or upper tibia. The upper end of femur and the lower end of radius are other common sites. Although flat bones may be involved giant-cell tumour is rare in the jaw and in the vertebral column. When giant-cell tumour occurs in a long bone it arises almost invariably in the bone end and the metaphysis is involved only later. Because of this situation symptoms tend to be referable to the joint.

Macroscopic appearances. Giant-cell tumour is usually located eccentrically in the epiphysis and often causes marked expansion of the bone end (Fig. 22.46). It is covered, at least initially, by a thin shell of subperiosteal bone which may be renewed on the surface as expansion goes on but through which it may later break into the soft tissues. Invasion of the joint through the articular cartilage is uncommon. The tumour is entirely destructive and its cells do not form bone. There is none of the subperiosteal sunray bony spiculation seen in an osteosarcoma. As a result of its osteolytic propensities patients often present with a pathological fracture. The tumour is usually reddish-grey and commonly shows areas of haemorrhage and necrosis. If fracture or previous treatment has taken place the picture may be complicated by callus formation, fibrosis and cystic degeneration.

Microscopic appearances. Giant-cell tumour consists of plump spindle or ovoid mononuclear cells abundantly interspersed with giant cells containing many nuclei, sometimes as many as 100 (Fig. 22.47). Fibrous tissue is usually scanty unless the tumour has previously fractured or been treated. Areas of necrosis, haemorrhage, lipid-containing macrophages and cholesterol are sometimes seen.

Prognosis. About half the tumours respond to thorough local removal, about a third recur and the remaining 15–20% are liable to be malignant from the beginning or more often after recurrence, and to metastasise to the lungs. The tumour may recur as a fibrosarcoma. Some help in assessing the prognosis is

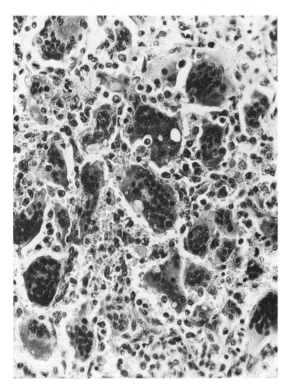

Fig. 22.47 Giant-cell tumour. The mononuclear tumour cells have the same characteristics as the scattered multinucleated cells. × 240.

given by the histology in that tumours which look frankly sarcomatous usually behave badly; however, very rarely, tumours which appear microscopically benign later metastasise.

Lesions likely to be confused with giant-cell tumour

Besides the differentiation of true giant-cell tumour from the benign lesions principally of childhood and adolescence described below, the lesion must be distinguished from brown tumour of hyperparathyroidism (p. 829). Since this may not be possible on histological grounds the blood chemistry should be investigated and a radiological search for subperiosteal erosions made especially if the apparent giant-cell tumour is in the skull or jaw.

Aneurysmal bone cyst. This is probably not a true tumour but has been confused with giant-cell tumour. It is commonest in the long bone *metaphyses* or vertebrae of children or young adults and gives rise to an extremely eccentric osteolytic lesion which may balloon out the periosteum and sometimes involves contiguous bones. On penetrating the thin bony shell the 'cyst' is found to consist of cavernous bloodfilled spaces separated by a brownish spongy meshwork of trabeculae. These are formed of

vascular fibrous tissue, the larger ones reinforced by osteoid or bony strands. Giant cells are smaller and less evenly distributed than in giant-cell tumour (Fig. 22.48). The lesion is benign and is cured by surgery, sometimes even when removal has been incomplete. If untreated it may progressively increase in size, but sometimes appears to be self-limiting.

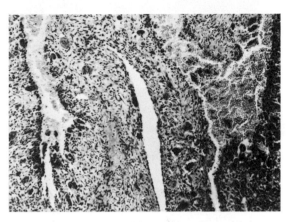

Fig. 22.48 Aneurysmal bone cyst. Vascular spaces lined by fibrous and osteoid tissue with giant cells. × 54.

Benign chondroblastoma. This rare benign bone tumour of uncertain histogenesis is important because it may be mistaken for a malignant giant-cell tumour or occasionally a chondro- or osteosarcoma. Benign chondroblastoma occurs most often in adolescents and is usually located in the epiphysis of long bones, especially around the knee or in the upper humerus. Radiologically there is a well-defined radiolucent area sometimes with mottling due to spotty calcification in the tumour. The tumour may spread across the epiphyseal plate into the metaphysis and rarely into the adjacent joint. Microscopically the lesion consists of fairly uniform small rounded or polygonal cells with a moderate sprinkling of multinucleated giant cells. A characteristic lacy pattern of intercellular calcification may be seen and this is thought to be followed by cellular necrosis and later transformation of necrotic areas to plaques of hyaline chondroid or osteoid like material. The tumour is usually curable by curettage. While it is liable to recurrence, malignant change is very rare.

Non-ossifying fibroma (non-osteogenic fibroma). This doubtfully neoplastic lesion was once thought to be a healing variant of giant-cell tumour. It sometimes appears to arise from a metaphyseal fibrous defect, a developmental lesion which is readily diagnosable radiologically as a small scalloped radiolucent area with a sclerotic edge hugging the metaphyseal cortex in the long bones, particularly the femur, of young children. These

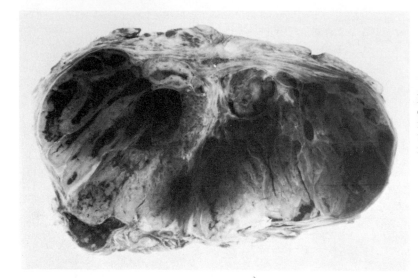

Fig. 22.49 Section of sacral chordoma. Note strands and islets of translucent chordal tissue separated by haemorrhagic areas. × ¾.

developmental abnormalities have the same naked-eye and microscopic appearances as do larger lesions involving the medullary cavity, which are described as non-ossifying fibromas and it seems possible that the larger ones may be derived from the smaller. Macroscopically the tissue is usually orange-yellow and microscopically shows whorled fibrous tissue with moderate numbers of small giant cells, haemosiderin and in some cases large zones of lipid-containing macrophages. These lesions, whatever their derivation, are benign and heal after curettage.

Simple bone cyst. This is a benign non-neoplastic unilocular cystic lesion, probably related to some local disturbance of bone growth and commonly arising in the upper humeral or femoral metaphyses in children and adolescents. As the bone grows the cyst appears to migrate down the shaft away from the epiphyseal line. It is commoner in males. Attention is frequently drawn to the lesion by pathological fracture and occasionally, following this, the cyst fills in. The appearances are of a smooth-walled cavity containing clear fluid and usually slightly expanding and markedly thinning the cortices. The lining consists of a meagre layer of rather acellular collagen. When fracture has occurred the fluid may be bloody and the lining transformed to a thick layer of granulation or fibrous tissue with areas of haemorrhage, cholesterol clefts, calcification, new bone formation and osteoclast aggregates which sometimes have given rise to confusion with giant-cell tumour. The cysts, while perfectly benign, have a strong tendency to recur, particularly if they are near the epiphyseal plate when initially treated.

Chordoma

This tumour arises from notochordal remnants, and usually develops within or in close proximity to the axial skeleton. In post-natal life the notochord persists in the nucleus pulposus of the intervertebral discs. In addition, small remnants are found in the hollow of the sacrum and coccyx and as little gelatinous nodules in the region of the spheno-occipital synchondrosis (*ecchordosis physaliphora*); the latter are, of course, observed as merely incidental findings at necropsy.

Sites of occurrence. Chordoma usually comes to notice in adult life and most commonly involves the sacrococcygeal region (Fig. 22.49) and the spheno-occipital part of the skull base. Cervical, dorsal and lumbar vertebral tumours are much rarer. They, and possibly all chordomas, are thought to arise from ectopic notochordal remnants rather than from the

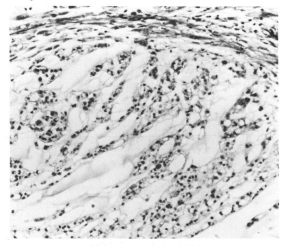

Fig. 22.50 Chordoma from sacrum. Strands of cells, many of them vacuolated, are seen lying in a background of mucinous material. × 140.

nuclei pulposi, for the tumour begins in the bone, the discs at first being spared.

Clinical features. Chordomas are very slow-growing and commonly give rise to pressure on adjacent structures, so that in the sacral region they may attain a large size, causing pressure on the rectum; in the spheno-occipital site the symptoms are chiefly referable to encroachment on cranial nerves or nerve roots but pituitary dysfunction may occur. The latter group are inevitably more quickly fatal. Radiological examination usually shows a lytic bone lesion with a soft tissue shadow and sometimes some patchy calcification. Death usually occurs from local extension of tumour rather than from metastasis.

Macroscopic appearances. The chordoma usually appears well circumscribed in its soft tissue mass but irregularly infiltrates adjacent bone. It is often firm and elastic, lobulated, greyish, semi-translucent and gelatinous with areas of haemorrhage and softening.

Microscopic appearances. The tumour tissue consists of lobules of rounded or polyhedral cells often arranged in alveoli or cords: some of these cells contain numerous intracytoplasmic vacuoles of mucin, *'physaliphorous cells'*. Strands of cells with poorly defined borders may also be present in a sea of extracellular mucin (Fig. 22.50). The differentiation between chordoma and chondrosarcoma or even mucin-secreting carcinoma may be difficult.

A characteristic pattern is that in which long tapering strands of chordoma cells extend inwards from the lobular margin, the central core and space between the strands being filled with gelatinous mucin, which is stained like the connective tissue mucins by the PAS method and gives a very strongly metachromatic reaction with toluidine blue, etc. Staining reactions are, however, of less significance in recognition than careful assessment of the architecture and morphology of the tumour.

Diseases of Joints

Normal joint structure

Joints may be categorised as those without a joint cavity, the non-synovial *synarthroses* and those with a joint cavity, the synovial *diarthroses*. In a diarthrosis the bone ends are almost invariably covered by hyaline articular cartilage and the surfaces lubricated by synovial fluid produced by the synovial membrane which is supported by the fibrous joint capsule.

Articular cartilage. Normal articular cartilage forms a smooth, glistening, slightly elastic covering to the bone ends. It is bluish and translucent in the young, averaging 2–4 mm in thickness; in the old it becomes yellower and more opaque. The matrix consists partly of fine fibrils which run parallel to the surface in the superficial layer, form a meshwork around the cells and elsewhere run as coarse collagen fibres in tight rope-like spirals. This fibre meshwork entraps a gel of proteoaminoglycans consisting of chondroitin and keratan sulphate. These substances give cartilage its metachromatic staining.

The chondrocytes lie in lacunae in the matrix and have branching processes which extend into it. Those cells near the surface are flattened and horizontal, the deeper ones are arranged in columns. In the adult a wavy basophilic line marks the junction between the uncalcified cartilage and the small layer of calcified cartilage which is adjacent to the subchondral bone.

Articular cartilage is avascular and has a relatively low oxygen requirement. Its nourishment is derived from the synovial fluid and probably also, especially in growing animals, from blood vessels of the subchondral marrow. Exchange between the synovial fluid and cartilage is thought to be promoted by joint movement. Hyaline cartilage has little power of regeneration (p. 74).

Synovial membrane forms synovial fluid: it lines tendon sheaths, bursae and it covers all the surfaces of joints except articular cartilage and menisci. The synovium may be smooth or folded and especially at the joint margins may form small villi. It is lined by a layer of ellipsoidal cells, one to four cells thick. These intimal cells are not separated by a basement membrane from the underlying tissues which may be areolar, dense fibrous or fatty in different parts of the joint. Two types of intimal cells are distinguished on electron microscopy. It is thought that Type A, the more numerous, is concerned with absorption while Type B synthesises hyaluronic acid.

The synovial membrane has a rich network of blood vessels, many of which run close to the surface. It is able to regenerate after synovectomy and a lining indistinguishable from synovium may form in adventitious bursae and pseudarthroses, presumably by metaplasia.

Synovial fluid is a dialysate of blood plasma with the addition of hyaluronic acid which gives the fluid its viscous property. The proportion of hyaluronic acid and hence the viscosity is said to diminish with age. The function of the fluid is twofold: to nourish the articular cartilage and to lubricate the joint surfaces. Under normal circumstances human joints contain less than 1 ml of synovial fluid. It is thought that in healthy human joints there are 50–400 nucleated cells per μl with few polymorphs, about 25% lymphocytes, a few synovial cells and a majority of mononuclear phagocytes, perhaps derived from the synovium. In animals and probably in man the number of cells varies in one individual from one joint to another.

Albumin and globulin are present in lower concentration in the fluid than in plasma with a preponderance of albumin in the ratio of about 4:1. Glucose levels are normally much less than those found in the blood.

Joint Inflammation of Known Aetiology

Acute infective arthritis

Acute arthritis formerly sometimes accompanied a generalised infection and occasionally progressed to suppuration, but this is now rare, probably on account of early response to specific chemotherapy. If adequately treated, infection by gonococci, pneumococci or typhoid bacilli seldom causes more than a transient non-suppurative arthritis which leaves little joint damage, at the most some synovial thickening and fibrosis. Accordingly infection by 'pyogenic' organisms does not necessarily lead to suppuration. As an example of suppurative arthritis *acute staphylococcal or streptococcal arthritis* will be described. The disease is commonest in the hip and knee of children and young adults though the debilitated, the aged and those patients on steroid therapy are especially at risk. In children, pneumococci occasionally give rise to a suppurative arthritis.

Path of infection. Acute infective arthritis arises chiefly as a result of haematogenous spread and sometimes a focus of infection such as a staphylococcal boil is identifiable. It may also result from spread from adjacent osteitis especially when the affected metaphysis is within the joint cavity, i.e. upper humeral, upper and lower femoral and all the metaphyses at the elbow. Rarely the organisms gain entrance directly through a penetrating wound or a compound intra-articular fracture.

Clinical features. There are the usual signs of acute inflammation, i.e. local redness, heat, pain, tenderness, oedema, joint effusion and limitation of movement and, associated with this, often pyrexia and a raised white cell count and erythrocyte sedimentation rate. Difficulty in diagnosis may arise when a pyogenic infection complicates pre-existing joint disease such as rheumatoid arthritis.

Early non-suppurative stage. The joint effusion contains a large increase of cells, mostly polymorphs, but may be sterile. Synovial fluid and blood cultures should immediately be obtained in a suspected pyogenic arthritis and antibiotics administered thereafter without delay. The synovium at this stage is intensely red and congested and flecked with yellowish fibrin. Microscopically it shows the features of acute inflammation. If the disease is arrested at this stage the condition resolves with little residual joint damage.

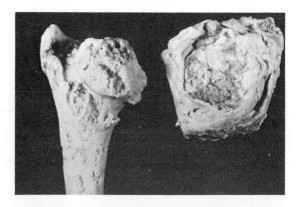

Fig. 22.51 Suppurative arthritis of hip joint. The articular cartilage of both the femoral head and the acetabulum is destroyed and there is erosion of the underlying bone.

Suppurative stage. If, however, suppuration ensues, within a few days there is, particularly over contact points, extensive cartilage destruction due in part to digestion by proteolytic enzymes in the pus. The exposed bone also undergoes necrosis (Fig. 22.51). An acute suppurative arthritis is entirely destructive but once the condition subsides into a subacute or chronic stage there is proliferation of granulation tissue within the joint, which is followed by ossification and bony ankylosis. Bony ankylosis occurs more commonly in untreated suppurative arthritis than in tuberculous or rheumatoid disease.

Gonococcal arthritis. In pre-antibiotic days gonococcal arthritis was a relatively common complication of gonorrhoea, especially in males and often resulted in long-continuing chronic synovitis and in permanent joint damage. Nowadays however it appears to be less common, probably affecting about 1% of patients with gonorrhoea, is seen chiefly in females, responds to systemic penicillin therapy and even when septic arthritis has occurred seldom gives rise to serious joint destruction though occasionally some stiffness may remain. In the more acute form pain, tenderness and soft tissue swelling often affects many joints, especially the knee, wrist, and elbow within a few days of infection. The joint symptoms may be accompanied by chills and fever and by a gonococcaemic skin eruption, but meningitis, bacterial endocarditis and pericarditis are now rare. Tenosynovitis may occur especially around the wrist. Blood cultures are often positive in these patients though the synovial fluid may be sterile.

Sometimes joint symptoms appear relatively late after the original venereal infection; they may then involve only one joint and the infection is usually not septic.

Tuberculous arthritis

Joint tuberculosis is decreasing in incidence. While no age is exempt, the emphasis has slowly changed from children to the elderly: the hip and knee joints are the commonest sites. Since pasteurisation of milk became widespread the disease is usually the result of infection by the human and not the bovine strain of bacillus. Infection occurs almost invariably by blood-spread from a primary or reactivated tuber-

culous focus elsewhere in the body, especially in the lungs or lymph nodes. The synovium is frequently primarily involved but in some cases there may be secondary involvement by spread directly or *via* the periosteum from small or large tuberculous foci in bone.

Macroscopic appearances. There is often a moderate joint effusion, usually of clear or slightly turbid fluid, with 'melon-seed bodies' (see p. 864) and only in the exceptional very late case is there 'tuberculous pus'. The synovial membrane is oedematous, hyperplastic and congested and may be studded by small greyish tubercles with yellowish caseating centres. There may also be an abundant growth of soft

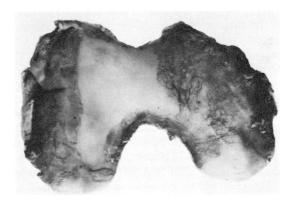

Fig. 22.52 Tuberculous disease of knee-joint. Note the spread of vascular tissue with tubercles over the surface of the cartilage.

gelatinous granulation tissue arising from the synovial membrane and this may grow in from the periphery of the joint to form a *pannus* (Fig. 22.52) creeping over and replacing the articular cartilage where the joint surfaces are not in contact. In addition the articular cartilage may be destroyed by the ingrowth of subchondral granulation tissue which separates it in large flakes from the underlying bone. The cartilage may float free in the joint fluid or retain a tenuous attachment to bone. The exposed bone has an irregular surface with necrosis and exudation. Occasionally caseous foci with suppurative softening form in the capsule of the joint and in the soft tissues outside, and pus may break through the skin surface giving rise to sinuses and allowing secondary infection to occur. Tuberculous arthritis heals by fibrosis, but the fibrous adhesions which form across the joint surfaces may later, if secondary infection occurs, become ossified with complete obliteration of the joint space and the burial in this bony mass of any remaining caseous material.

Microscopic appearances. The histological diagnosis of tuberculosis from synovial biopsy may be made most readily if the synovium is studded with discrete tubercles showing the usual microscopic features of foci of Langhans-type giant cells, epithelioid cells and lymphocytes and sometimes caseation. When the synovium is replaced by gelatinous granulation tissue, however, the condition may appear to be a non-specific inflammation with only a diffuse infiltrate of lymphocytes and plasma cells unless very careful search is made for the scanty and often ill-defined epithelioid follicles. The pannus on the surface of the cartilage and the subchondral granulations are even less fruitful sites for diagnostic examination. The thorough examination of 15 μm thick Ziehl–Neelsen stained tissue sections reveals acid-fast bacilli in rather more than half the cases and bacteriological culture of synovial tissue is positive in about the same number. When bone is also involved the marrow spaces may contain tubercle follicles with caseation and there may be some resorption and necrosis of bone.

The synovial fluid has a raised cell count and half or more of the cells may be lymphocytes. Melon-seed bodies and flakes of articular cartilage may also be present, the melon-seed bodies being formed usually of fibrin and sometimes of necrotic synovial fronds.

In patients with an undiagnosed monarthritis it is advisable to examine a synovial biopsy histologically in order to exclude tuberculosis rather than to rely on synovial fluid culture alone.

Course of the disease. The earlier diagnosis and prompt treatment of tuberculous arthritis with antibiotics now often leads to the disease remaining confined to the synovium and good function returns to the joint. When articular cartilage and bone are involved, function is inevitably impaired and operative arthrodesis may be required. It is unusual in Great Britain now to see cases of joint tuberculosis proceeding to massive joint destruction with discharging sinuses and final spontaneous ankylosis, although these conditions may be seen in countries where tuberculosis is unchecked by specific therapy.

Tuberculous tenosynovitis. Tuberculosis may also affect the tendon sheaths, especially of the flexor tendons at the wrist. There is, as in joint tuberculosis, effusion of fluid into the sheath, the formation of melon-seed bodies and sometimes proliferation of exuberant granulation tissue within the sheath.

Syphilitic arthritis

In contrast to tuberculosis, syphilis comparatively seldom gives rise to important joint lesions.

Acquired syphilis. In the *secondary* stage there may be transient pain and stiffness of joints sometimes accompanied by effusion. Involvement, often bilateral, of the knee joint or of the sternoclavicular joint may be seen.

In *tertiary* syphilis, chronic interstitial inflammation and gumma of the joint capsule may occur. The first may give rise to a mild form of inflammatory arthritis, the latter, whether it arises in the synovium or discharges from intracapsular bone, results in a granulomatous synovitis, which may form a pannus over the articular surfaces. Fibrosis followed by bony ankylosis may result. Patients with tabes dorsalis sometimes develop neuropathic arthritis (p. 861).

Congenital syphilis. There may be joint pain and swelling in infants and young children in association with syphilitic epiphysitis. In older children there is a condition known as *Clutton's joints*, often affecting both knees, characterised by painless effusion with synovial thickening and sometimes associated with interstitial keratitis. It is transient and does not progress to severe joint damage.

Brucellosis (Undulant fever)

Joint symptoms are the presenting feature of about 25% of cases of undulant fever, the joints being involved in the course of the septicaemia. The arthritis is transient and of non-specific inflammatory pattern. Sometimes granulomas similar to those of tuberculosis are seen (p. 508). Bursae may also be involved.

Joint Inflammation of Unknown Aetiology

Arthritis associated with rheumatic fever

Rheumatic fever is a disease of uncertain aetiology characterised by pancarditis, fever and transient arthritis. It is not thought to be related to rheumatoid arthritis. The large joints are usually inflamed, i.e. knees, ankles and wrists, and as the condition subsides in some joints others become affected.

In the acute stage there is usually a sterile joint effusion with a high cell count around $10\ 000/\mu l$ (normal up to $400/\mu l$), most of these being polymorphs.

As the condition subsides the polymorphs diminish in the synovial fluid and lymphocytes become prominent. A diffuse chronic inflammatory cell infiltrate may be seen in the synovium but it lacks both the intensity and the accompanying proliferative changes seen in rheumatoid arthritis. Small granulomas resembling Aschoff bodies (p. 362) may be present in the synovium. The joint usually returns to normal, the inflammatory cell infiltrate disappears and the granulomas fibrose. Occasionally, especially when the capsule has been involved, there may be some residual pain and stiffness with persistent chronic inflammation and synovial thickening. In children small *subcutaneous nodules* up to 10 mm. in diameter may be found in groups at sites of trauma such as around the olecranon and ulnar border of the forearm and about the patella. These granulomas usually consist of small areas of degenerate collagen with histiocytes, chronic inflammatory cells and some proliferation of fibroblasts and capillaries. They become fibrotic and disappear within a few months. (For a discussion of the aetiology of rheumatic fever and its other manifestations see Chapter 14.)

Rheumatoid arthritis

Rheumatoid arthritis is one of the connective tissue diseases (p. 876), and is characterised by a subacute or chronic non-suppurative arthritis usually affecting several joints. Its course is punctuated by spontaneous remissions.

Age and sex incidence. The disease usually begins in the years between 25 and 55 but may affect both older and younger ages. *Still's disease* in children consists of rheumatoid arthritis with associated splenomegaly, lymphadenopathy and occasionally pericarditis. Rheumatoid arthritis is more than twice as common in females as in males.

Sites of occurrence. Any synovial joint may be affected but the joints of the hands and feet are most often involved, the disease often being bilateral and sometimes symmetrical. Temporomandibular, crico-arytenoid joints and those of the cervical spine are occasionally involved. Destructive spinal disease may produce instability and neurological complications.

Course of the disease. The onset is often insidious but sometimes acute. The condition may abate after a single attack but more commonly there are repeated recrudescences and remissions, the joint each time suffering further damage. Involvement of tendons, soft tissue swelling, muscle atrophy, ligamentous and capsular laxity, all contribute to increasing deformity. Sometimes the disease progresses to fibrous, occasionally to bony, ankylosis. The tendency is for the rheumatoid disease eventually to burn itself out but even then the joint disability may increase due to further damage from secondary osteoarthritis. During the active phase of polyarthritis tests for rheumatoid factor are usually positive (p. 857).

Clinical and macroscopic appearances. In the early acute stage or during exacerbations, the joints are hot, swollen and tender; the usual appearances of an acute inflammation. There is often general constitutional upset, the ESR is raised, there is a leukocytosis and sometimes a normocytic, normochromic anaemia. The swelling, which often gives the finger joints a spindle appearance, is partly due to synovial effusion which may be turbid but is sterile. There is an increase in cells, sometimes up to $50\ 000/\mu l$ with about 75% polymorphs, and fibrin flakes may be present. The primary changes are in the synovium which is red and congested, oedematous, markedly frondose and frequently patchily covered by fibrinous exudate (Fig. 22.53). After the early stages it may be heavily pigmented with haemosiderin.

Microscopic appearances. In the florid case

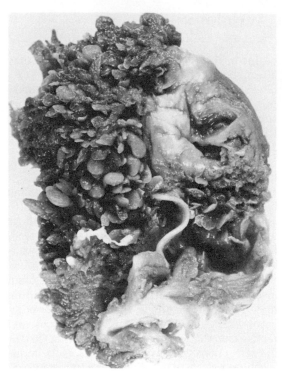

Fig. 22.53 Synovium from a rheumatoid knee joint. The synovial surface is markedly frondose and some of the villi are tipped with white fibrin.

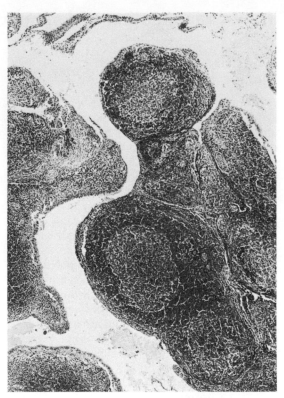

Fig. 22.54 Synovial membrane in chronic rheumatoid arthritis. The synovium shows villous hypertrophy and is extensively infiltrated with lymphocytes, amongst which occur poorly defined germinal centres. Plasma cells also are abundant. × 38.

there is marked villous hypertrophy of the synovium with synovial cell proliferation, fibrinous and polymorph exudate on the surface, lymphocytes in dense focal aggregates, sometimes with germinal centres, accompanied by a heavy and more diffuse plasma cell infiltrate (Fig. 22.54). These appearances may persist for an indefinite period after an acute attack. When these features are all present in a marked degree, the diagnosis of rheumatoid arthritis may be suggested with fair, though not with absolute certainty. However, the synovium has only a limited range of response to different stimuli and less severe degrees of these changes may be seen in a wide variety of conditions, e.g. following trauma, in joints adjacent to tumours, in psoriatic arthritis, in various non-specific arthritides and occasionally even in osteoarthritis. Rarely a typical 'rheumatoid nodule' (see below) may be seen in the subsynovial tissue and clinch the diagnosis.

While the changes in rheumatoid arthritis are confined to the synovium, the functional disability is reversible, but this is often followed by secondary irreversible changes in other joint structures. Subchondral erosions form at the joint margin and a thin layer of vascular granulation tissue (*pannus*) grows over, erodes and destroys the joint cartilage. If the underlying bone is exposed it may become pocketed by chronic granulations. In the later stage this granulation tissue may eventually become fibrosed with resultant adhesions across the joint space and later ossification sometimes converts fibrous to bony ankylosis, especially in the small joints of the carpus and tarsus.

While these changes are going on in the joint, *the bone* at an early stage may become markedly porotic due to hyperaemia and disuse. *The muscles* become atrophic and there is wasting and weakness especially of the interossei and sometimes also of the hand flexors. *Tendons* may also become infiltrated by rheumatoid granulation tissue and this leads to pain and disability and sometimes to rupture of

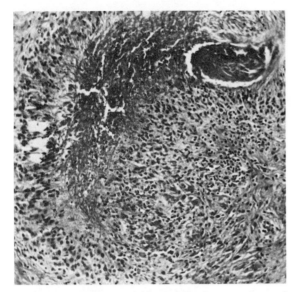

Fig. 22.55a Rheumatoid nodule from region of elbow-joint. × 90.

the tendon with further deformity. As a result of muscle atrophy and tendon destruction, ligamentous and capsular laxity, the hand in particular comes to be greatly deformed with marked ulnar deviation, subluxation and dislocation of joints (Fig. 22.55*b*).

Non-orthopaedic features of rheumatoid disease. Rheumatoid nodules consisting of a central area of fibrinoid necrosis of collagen surrounded by palisaded fibroblasts (Fig. 22.55*a*) occur in the subcutaneous tissues over

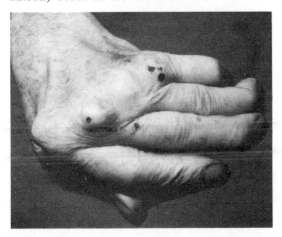

Fig. 22.55b The hand shows the typical severe deformity of rheumatoid arthritis with marked ulnar deviation of the fingers and muscle wasting. Ulcerated rheumatoid nodules are present over the metacarpo-phalangeal joints.

pressure sites in about 20% of cases. These nodules persist throughout life and are a helpful clinical and histological diagnostic aid. They tend to occur in more severely affected patients and to be associated with a worse prognosis (Fig. 22.55*b*).

Similar nodules may be found at other sites, not only in the lungs of coalminers with rheumatoid disease (Caplan's syndrome, p. 436) but also in the pleura, the heart and pericardium, the eye and elsewhere.

Inflammation of arteries and veins may occur and when severe gives rise to skin ulceration and occasionally gangrene, bowel perforation and myocardial infarction. Peripheral neuropathy may also result. The skin is often atrophic, thin and papery.

Reactive and hyperplastic changes occur in lymph nodes and spleen (see p. 877). About 20% of cases of chronic rheumatoid arthritis coming to necropsy have some evidence of amyloid disease affecting the spleen, liver and kidney, although symptoms attributable to amyloid are rare. Sjøgren's syndrome (p. 535) may accompany rheumatoid disease.

Serum factors. The serum of most patients with rheumatoid arthritis contains *rheumatoid factor*, an IgM which behaves like an antibody and reacts with IgG, including the patient's own IgG. The factor is best demonstrated by using as 'antigen' IgG which has been altered by heating or by combination with inert particles, e.g. erythrocytes or latex. In the *Waaler–Rose* test, dilutions of the patient's heat-inactivated serum are tested with sheep erythrocytes sensitised with rabbit IgG. Agglutination in a significantly higher serum dilution than occurs with unsensitised sheep erythrocytes indicates a positive result. The rheumatoid factor may be present at an early stage or appear only later in the disease. Its absence is, in general, associated with less severe cases, although there are many exceptions. The factor is usually absent in cases of polyarthritis associated with psoriasis, with various gastro-intestinal diseases and in ankylosing spondylitis (sero-negative arthritis).

Recent work has demonstrated the complicated nature and heterogeneity of rheumatoid factors. Two factors may be present, one reacting with both rabbit and human IgG, the other only with human IgG. Moreover, rheumatoid factors which react specifically with genetically determined human IgG iso-antigens (termed Gm factors), have been detected, and in some instances the patient's serum has contained such a factor which reacts with an iso-antigen absent from his own IgG. Because of this observation, and the fact that rheumatoid factors react more strongly with altered than with native IgG, it is doubtful whether or not rheumatoid factor should be regarded as an auto-antibody. Although rheumatoid factor has not been implicated as a pathogenic agent, an immunological dyscrasia is suggested by raised incidences of antinuclear factors (p. 134) and of chronic thyroiditis and thyroid antibodies which have been demonstrated in rheumatoid arthritis.

Ankylosing spondylitis

Ankylosing spondylitis is a polyarthritis leading to bony ankylosis of the sacroiliac, intervertebral, and costovertebral joints with ossification of spinal ligaments and the borders of interver-

tebral discs and it results in rigidity of the spine. Sometimes the sternoclavicular and hip joints are similarly involved. The disease is much commoner in males than females and usually the onset is in adolescence or early adult life. It is sometimes familial.

Course of the disease. There is usually an insidious onset of stiffness in the back with clinical and radiological evidence of inflammation of the sacroiliac joints. The condition may be self-limiting or may progress with exacerbations and remissions until the patient is left with an absolutely rigid back showing the radiological appearances of *bamboo spine* (Fig. 22.56a). When the cervical spine is involved there is danger of atlanto-axial dislocation or vertebral fracture and care must be taken in the handling of the anaesthetised patient. During exacerbations the ESR is commonly raised. The hips may be involved transiently, or chronically with final bony ankylosis in the most severely affected patients. Although diminished chest ex-

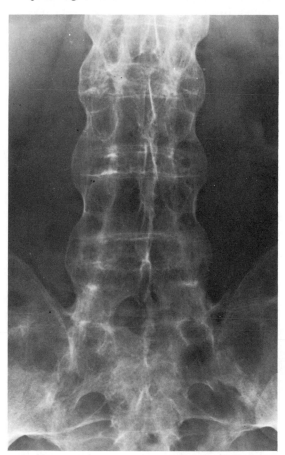

Fig. 22.56a A radiograph shows the typical 'bamboo' spine of late ankylosing spondylitis.

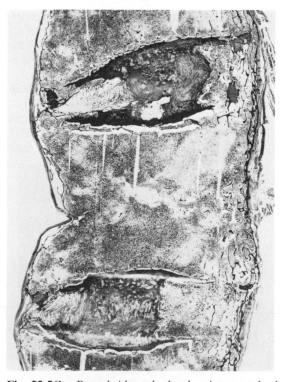

Fig. 22.56b Bone bridges the lumbar intervertebral discs anteriorly (*on the left*). As a result of endochondral ossification much of the disc has been replaced by bone. There is very severe porosis of the vertebral bodies. (Reproduced by permission from Applied Surgical Pathology, Blackwell Scientific Publications.)

pansion is common, respiratory complications are rare. Serological tests for rheumatoid arthritis are usually negative in ankylosing spondylitis. The incidence of HLA–B27 (p. 137) is very high.

Structural changes. The synovial changes resemble those of rheumatoid arthritis. The characteristic extra-articular ossification is thought to result from healing of inflammatory foci at the site of attachment to bone of ligaments, joint capsule or the outer fibres of the annulus fibrosus. This marginal ankylosis may be followed by endochondral ossification of remaining cartilage (Fig. 22.56*b*).

Aortic lesions. A few patients with longstanding ankylosing spondylitis may develop aortic valvular incompetence due to changes in the aorta indistinguishable from those of syphilis, but limited to the immediate vicinity of the aortic valve and sinuses of Valsalva. Serological tests for syphilis have been consistently negative and this appears to be a non-syphilitic lesion associated specifically with ankylosing spondylitis.

Leukaemia. Irradiation of the spine in ankylosing spondylitis includes a large volume of the haemopoietic marrow and this increases tenfold the chance of the patient developing leukaemia.

Psoriatic arthritis

Patients with psoriasis, especially those with in-involvement of the nails, have a tendency to develop a remittent arthritis which has a predilection for the distal joints of the hands and feet. While the microscopic appearances of the synovium show much the same non-specific picture of hyperplasia with lymphocytic and plasma cell infiltrate as is seen in the less florid cases of rheumatoid arthritis, the clinical and radiographic features and the negative test for rheumatoid factor serve to make the distinction. While deformities of the hands and feet may result, the condition is usually less disabling than rheumatoid arthritis.

Reiter's syndrome

This consists of 'abacterial' urethritis, conjunctivitis and arthritis, sometimes following diarrhoea. It may be due to chlamydial infection (p. 188) and occurs most frequently in adult males. The knee, ankle, spine and small joints of the hands and feet are involved in a transient polyarthritis which in contrast to gonococcal arthritis may not respond to penicillin therapy. While often there is no permanent disability there may be recurrences with a tendency to destructive changes in the feet and sacroiliac joints. The incidence of HLA antigen B27 (p. 151) is high in such cases. The mouth may be involved and skin lesions affect especially the soles and palms.

Degenerative Arthropathies

Osteoarthritis or degenerative arthritis

Osteoarthritis is the commonest form of chronic joint disease and is characterised clinically by the insidious but progressive onset of pain and joint stiffness. In spite of the name it is not an inflammatory or systemic disease but results from destructive and degenerative changes in the articular cartilage of joints. While any joint may be affected, disease of the hip or knee is most frequent and most disabling.

Osteoarthritis is found chiefly in the elderly. In younger patients there is usually an obvious predisposing cause. This 'secondary' osteoarthritis may be the result of intra-articular abnormalities such as congenital dis-

location of the hip, of damage to the cartilage by fracture or loose bodies, or by previous inflammation. Extra-articular abnormalities which throw unusual stress on the joint such as malunion of a fracture, bowing of the legs or scoliosis may also predispose to osteoarthritis while obesity is associated with degenerative changes of the knees in women. Osteoarthritis may be associated with certain occupations: it affects the knees and spine in miners working at the coal face, the elbows and shoulders of pneumatic drillers and the feet and ankles of soccer players. The cause of 'primary' osteoarthritis developing in a normal joint is not known though excessive physical activity or misuse may play a part.

Structural changes. *Articular cartilage.* The first abnormality recognised by light microscopy

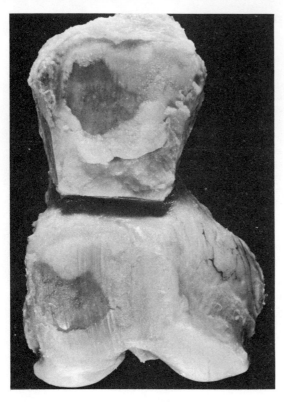

Fig. 22.57 Osteoarthritis of the knee joint has caused complete loss of articular cartilage with exposure of the bone on opposing surfaces of the patella (*above*) and of the femur. There is parallel scoring of the joint surfaces.

is loss of metachromasia in the surface layers. Whether this results from rupture of the superficial collagen network or from increased breakdown following release of enzymes from damaged chondrocytes remains speculative. It is associated with the development of tangential flaking of the surface and this may progress to deeper fissuring or fibrillation. Proliferation of chondrocytes and increased production of ground substance adjacent to the fissures fails to produce healing and loss of the cartilage substance follows so that the subchondral bone may be exposed (Fig. 22.57) with diminution of the width of the joint space radiologically.

The distinction between age changes and osteoarthritis is difficult. Studies of the hip joint suggest that fibrillation in some sites may be a self-limiting age change while in the load bearing area it is the forerunner of progressive destructive changes.

Bone. While these changes are occurring in the articular cartilage the subchondral bone trabeculae become greatly thickened (Fig. 22.58). When this dense bone is exposed it becomes polished and eburnated, sometimes grooved in the direction of joint movement (Figs. 22.57, 22.61). The superficial bone which lines the joint surface is usually necrotic. Fibrocartilaginous metaplasia tends to occur in any exposed marrow spaces.

Marked bone remodelling results in change in the shape of the joint surface. This is particularly obvious in the flattening and mush-

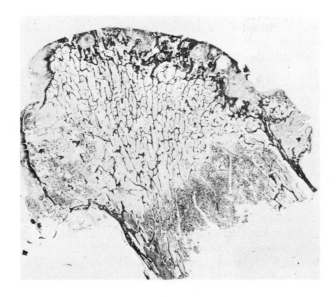

Fig. 22.58 Osteoarthritis of hip joint. The load-bearing surface of the femoral head is flattened and mushroomed and the articular cartilage has largely disappeared. The exposed bone is dense, small osteoarthritic cysts are present and there are peripheral osteophytes.

rooming of the load-bearing surface of the femoral head in osteoarthritis of the hip joint (Fig. 22.58). Another result is the formation of radiological 'cysts' in the subchondral bone. These are areas devoid of bone but filled by fatty marrow or loose rather degenerate fibrous tissue and sometimes surrounded by new bony trabeculae. At the joint margins small excrescences form, giving first an appearance of beading and later of lipping of the joint. These osteophytic outgrowths form by proliferation of cartilage, followed by endochondral ossification (Fig. 22.58), but the stimulus to cartilage production is not fully understood. The osteophytes may give rise to deformity and limitation of movement. Spontaneous ankylosis does not occur in uncomplicated osteoarthritis.

Synovium. In the early stages the synovium is normal but when disintegration of the joint surface takes place there is absorption of abraded fragments of cartilage and bone, associated with villous hypertrophy and followed by subsynovial fibrosis. Chronic inflammatory cell infiltrate is usually minimal. Sometimes fatty villi are prominent in obese patients and occasionally, particularly in the knee joint and sometimes in the elbow, *lipoma arborescens* may be present. In this condition very large numbers of fatty synovial-covered polypi project into the joint. It is thought, however, that these predispose to osteoarthritis rather than result from it.

Synovial fluid. In a small proportion of cases there is synovial effusion and the fluid is thick. The cell count is only slightly raised and only about 15% of cells are polymorphs.

Heberden's nodes. These are small bony elevations on the terminal phalanges of the fingers near the joint line. They may give rise to some deformity and limitation of movement. Some are the result of osteoarthritis; others result from post-traumatic ossification of para-articular tissues.

Primary generalised osteoarthritis sometimes has a familial incidence, affects multiple joints often in relatively young patients and is almost invariably associated with Heberden's nodes.

Chondromalacia patellae is a condition arising in young people and giving rise to pain, effusion, loss of movement and crepitus of the knee joint. A history of trauma to the patella is often given. The naked-eye and microscopic appearances of excised patellae are of localised degenerative changes in the articular cartilage.

Neuropathic arthritis (Charcot's joint)

Neuropathic arthritis is an accelerated form of degenerative arthritis resulting from the progressive disorganisation of an insensitive joint when subjected to trauma. It was first described by Charcot as occurring in tabes dorsalis and has since been found in a wide variety of other neurological conditions. In syphilis the joints commonly affected are the hip, knee, ankle, tarsus, vertebrae and shoulder and in syringomyelia the joints of the upper limb, especially shoulder and elbow. The commonest cause nowadays is probably diabetic neuropathy, the joints of the feet most often being involved. Cases have also been described in leprosy, spina bifida, peripheral nerve injuries, transverse myelitis, subacute combined degeneration of the cord, in the rare condition of congenital universal indifference to pain and following repeated intra-articular injections of cortisone.

The condition can be attributed to continued use of an analgesic joint with associated proprioceptive loss. A cycle of events may occur in, for instance, the knee joint in a case of tabes dorsalis. The ataxia leads readily to some minor or major trauma to the joint which results in effusion, the swelling and muscular hypotonia increase the instability of the joint and its liability to further damage. Because the joint is painless the patient fails to guard it and continued use leads to repetition of the cycle. The morbid anatomical changes in this condition are basically those of an extremely severe, and often rapidly progressive, osteoarthritis. The cartilage is destroyed, the bone ends grossly distorted (Fig. 22.59) partly by remodelling and partly by the early formation of very large osteophytic outgrowths which may fracture and cause further damage. Fracture of the joint surface may also occur and the pathology of neuroarthropathy may be complicated by hyperplastic callus formation. The gross and bizarre radiological changes contrast with the relative lack of pain.

Arthritis associated with gout

Gout is a disease with a hereditary tendency, associated with an incompletely understood disorder of purine metabolism and results in

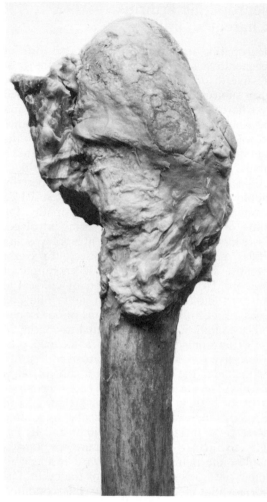

Fig. 22.59 Upper end of femur in neuropathic arthritis of the hip joint in a patient with tabes. Note the irregular absorption of the head and the new formation of bone below.

repeated attacks of acute arthritis which may be followed by chronic degenerative joint changes. Most patients with gout have hyperuricaemia, i.e. a serum urate level of more than 0·4 mmol/l (7 mg/100 ml) in males; 0·34 mmol/l (6 mg/100 ml) in females. Hyperuricaemia is much commoner than clinical gout and the higher the serum urate level the greater the likelihood of the patient eventually developing symptoms.

So-called **secondary gout** may arise in patients with leukaemia, myeloma or polycythaemia vera, especially in the course of treatment with cytotoxic drugs when hyperuricaemia results from the increased nucleoprotein breakdown.

Occasionally secondary gout complicates uraemia, the decreased renal output leading to a raised blood uric acid level.

Age, sex and site incidence. The first attack usually occurs over the age of 40; the disease is much commoner in males, females seldom being affected until after the menopause. In about half the cases the metatarso-phalangeal joint of the great toe is first affected, but the knee, elbow and other toe and finger joints may be involved.

The acute attack. In the susceptible subject an acute attack of gout may be precipitated by many factors such as trauma, over-exertion, alcoholic or dietary excess, certain diuretics and purgation. Some of the drugs given to gouty patients to promote urinary excretion of uric acid may produce an acute attack since they free some of the acid which is bound to plasma proteins and so increase the amount of diffusible uric acid. Acute gout is sometimes ushered in by pyrexia, leukocytosis and a raised erythrocyte sedimentation rate. The onset is sudden, may be nocturnal and there is excruciating pain in the affected joint, often the great toe (podagra) or its associated bursa, which shows all the signs of an acute inflammation. Needle-like strongly negative birefringent crystals, soluble in uricase, may be recognised in the synovial fluid, often within polymorphs (cf. pseudo-gout, p. 863). The polymorphs which have taken up the crystals release a chemotactic substance which attracts other leukocytes. The ingested crystals damage the membrane-limited phagolysosomes in which they lie, hydrolytic enzymes are released into the cytoplasm and the cell dies, releasing the crystal. Cells in the synovial fluid may increase to 14 000/μl with 70% or more polymorphs. The attack lasts usually for a few days or weeks and is followed by remission. The prompt beneficial effect of colchicine which is thought to block the release of, and alter the response to, the chemotactic factors, may be used as a therapeutic test of acute gout.

Chronic gout is associated with the formation of crystalline deposits of sodium biurate often with cholesterol and calcium salts in relatively avascular collagen, hyaline and fibro-cartilage. These deposits are known as **tophi** and may be found in the fibrocartilages of the ear, in bursal walls, especially the olecranon and prepatellar bursae and in the articular cartilage of joints (Fig. 22.60). Tophi are less frequent since drug therapy has become more effective. They may occur at sites of previous acute gouty arthritis or appear insidiously. Tophi are not significantly radio-opaque.

Microscopic examination of alcohol-fixed material from a tophus shows sheaves of biurate crystals, with a surrounding very marked foreign-body giant cell and granulomatous reaction.

In joints the urate deposition occurs first in

middle-aged and elderly. It is characterised clinically by episodes of acute or subacute inflammation of one or more large joints, especially the knees. Involvement of the big toe is rare. During the acute stage rod and tablet crystals of *calcium pyrophosphate* may be identified in the synovial fluid, mostly within polymorphs. The mechanism of production of the acute inflammatory response is similar to that in gout. Calcification may appear in the menisci of the knee, the articular disc of the distal radio-ulnar joint, the annulus fibrosus of

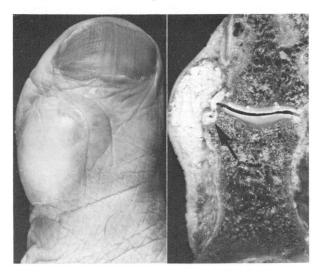

Fig. 22.60 A gouty tophus is seen in the subcutaneous tissue overlying the interphalangeal joint of the great toe. The tophus has produced a little resorption of bone at the joint margin (*arrow*). The articular cartilage is also flecked with white crystalline material.

the superficial articular cartilage where it can be seen as opaque white spots like paint. The crystalline deposits are accompanied by degenerative changes in the articular cartilages which may cause some of the disability of chronic gouty arthritis. Later, urates may be precipitated in the subchondral and subperiosteal bone giving rise to bone destruction and punched out defects which are radiologically diagnosable. Tophi may occur in relation to synovium or para-articular tissues and these may sometimes reach great size and destroy cartilage, bone, synovium and capsule, leaving a totally disorganised joint. (For discussion of renal changes in gout see p. 782 and of aetiology and purine metabolism p. 247.)

the intervertebral discs, the symphysis pubis and also in articular cartilages, ligaments, tendons and joint capsules. Chronic degenerative joint disease may follow. While about a third of patients have hyperuricaemia and an occasional one has clinical gout the condition should be distinguished from true gout by the involvement of large joints, the distinctive radiological findings and the characteristic crystals which exhibit a faint positive birefringence in polarised light. Once the diagnosis of pyrophosphate arthropathy is made predisposing causes such as hyperparathyroidism should be sought.

Pyrophosphate arthropathy (Articular chondrocalcinosis, pseudo-gout)

In recent years a condition with only a slight male preponderance has been described chiefly in the

Haemophilic arthritis

Acute haemarthrosis especially in the knee is a common finding in haemophilia and the joint may become greatly distended by blood which is gradually resorbed. The synovium becomes deeply pigmented with haemosiderin. After repeated haemarthroses there is often some destruction of the articular cartilage, probably partly the result of subchondral haemorrhages. Where damage to cartilage has occurred osteoarthritic changes may supervene.

In addition organisation of intraosseous haemor-rhage may lead to bone resorption and the formation of bone 'cysts', while subperiosteal haematomas may simulate scurvy.

Miscellaneous Joint Conditions

Intra-articular loose bodies

Multiple soft loose bodies are sometimes known as '*rice or melon-seed*' bodies. They are usually formed from fibrin or necrotic synovial tissue and are found in tuberculosis and rheumatoid arthritis. Symptoms are those of the accompanying arthritis.

Hard loose bodies may be caused by:

(1) *Osteochondritis dissecans*. Here the loose body is derived from part of the articular cartilage and underlying bone which for some reason separates from the surrounding tissue. When completely separated, the cartilaginous part of the body remains viable and may proliferate: the bone dies. Usually one, occasionally several, loose bodies may be present, the medial condyle of the femur being most frequently affected.

(2) *Osteoarthritis*. The fracturing of marginal osteophytes is a rare occurrence. This is said to occur more commonly in the severe osteo-arthritis associated with neuroarthropathy.

(3) *Fracture of the articular margins*. Occasionally fracture of the articular margins results in one of the fragments of the fracture entering the joint and acting as a loose body, i.e. in fractures of the lower end of the humerus the medial epicondyle may, in spite of its muscle attachments, form a loose body in the elbow joint.

(4) *Synovial chondromatosis or osteochondromatosis*. In this condition the synovial membrane shows cartilaginous metaplasia. These very numerous cartilaginous nodules may then ossify.

Clinically, hard loose bodies may give rise to episodes of locking of the joint. Damage to the articular cartilage may result in osteoarthritis (Fig. 22.61).

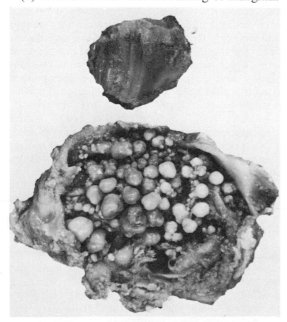

Fig. 22.61 Chondromatosis of synovium of the knee joint. Osteoarthritis of patella.

Pigmented villonodular synovitis

Pigmented villonodular synovitis is an uncommon condition of unknown aetiology, thought to be reactive rather than neoplastic and which may affect joints, bursae or tendon sheaths in a localised or in a diffuse form. Males between the ages of 20–50 years are most commonly affected and the knee or hip joint are often involved. The synovitis gives rise to pain, serosanguineous effusion and sometimes to locking of the joint.

Macroscopic appearances. The diffuse form has a most striking appearance. In the early stages the synovium looks like a tangled reddish-brown beard; matting together of the hyperplastic, pigmented villi later gives rise to a spongy orange and brown pad of great complexity. There may also be firm nodules, sessile or pedunculated and one or several of these may be present in the localised form of the disease. Occasionally adjacent bone is infil-

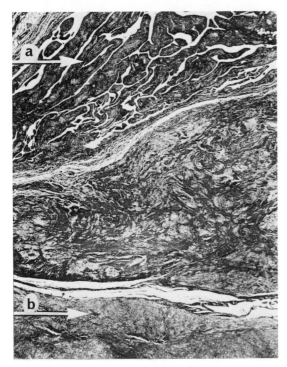

Fig. 22.62 At **a** there is diffuse pigmented villonodular synovitis while at **b** a solid mass containing abundant lipid macrophages and haemosiderin has developed. × 10.

trated by the pigmented tissue and the extra-articular soft tissue may be involved. Regional lymph nodes may become pigmented with haemosiderin.

Microscopic appearances. The villi are enlarged, the synovial lining cells increased and prominent, macrophages and chronic inflammatory cells and sometimes small multinucleated giant cells are abundant (Fig. 22.62). Much haemosiderin is present partly in macrophages and synovial lining cells and also lying free in the tissue. There may also be xanthomatous areas with foamy lipid-laden macrophages. When the villi become matted together clefts lined by synovial cells are seen and may give an appearance alarmingly similar to synovial sarcoma. The nodular projections often are more hyalinised with dense collagen, little pigment and many giant cells and bear a striking resemblance to so-called benign giant-cell tumour of tendon sheath (Fig. 22.63).

Prognosis. This condition in its diffuse form is difficult to eradicate completely and there is a tendency to recurrence. In spite of recurrence, its occasional involvement of bone, its liability to spread into extra-articular tissue and its sometimes alarming histological appearance, no carefully documented case has been known to metastasise and the differentiation between this lesion and synovial sarcoma is of the first importance if needless amputation is to be avoided.

Bursae. The popliteal bursa is the most frequently involved. A tumour-like mass forms, and the gross and histological appearances are the same as in joints.

Tendon sheaths. Very rarely there is diffuse involvement of a tendon sheath but the common finding is of multinodular masses in close proximity to the extensor tendons of the hands

Fig. 22.63 Pigmented villonodular synovitis of tendon sheath. Multiple nodules of pigmented giant-cell tissue are loosely attached to a tendon of the ring finger. × 5·5.

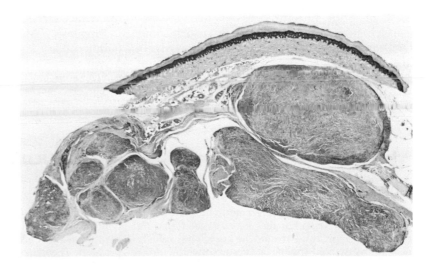

(Fig. 22.63). The histological appearance of these nodules is identical with those of the sessile or pedunculated lumps sometimes seen as part of the diffuse form of the disease. These have formerly been described as benign giant-cell tumours of tendon sheath, and while the aetiology and nature of pigmented villonodular synovitis is still under discussion it is probably immaterial which label is used.

Synovial tumours

Benign giant-cell tumour of tendon sheath

This condition is considered to be analogous to pigmented villonodular synovitis and is discussed above.

Synovial sarcoma (malignant synovioma)

Synovial sarcoma is a rare and highly malignant tumour usually found adjacent to but outside a joint. Though it occurs most often in young adults there is a wide age range. The tumour is most common in the lower limb especially around the knee or ankle.

Macroscopic appearances. This malignant tumour often has, as do many soft tissue sarcomas, a falsely reassuring appearance of encapsulation due to compression of surrounding tissue. It may be white or pinkish-grey, sometimes with areas of haemorrhage and frequently with spotty calcification which may be sufficient to be seen radiologically.

Microscopic appearances. The tumour consists of both fibrosarcomatous and pseudo-epithelial elements, either of which may predominate without altering the prognosis. In the fibrosarcomatous tissue there are clefts or gland-like spaces sometimes containing mucinous material and lined by cuboidal or columnar

cells (Fig. 22.64). Branching strands of hyaline collagen with a superficial resemblance to osteoid are sometimes a feature and may be

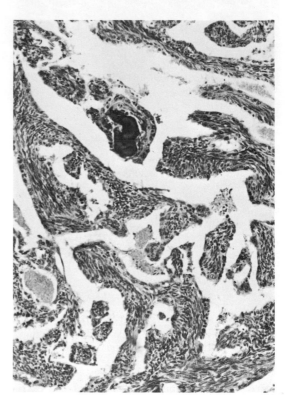

Fig. 22.64 Synovial sarcoma showing fibrosarcoma-like spindle cells and clefts lined by cubical cells. There is a focus of calcification. This tumour metastasised. × 115.

patchily calcified. Invasion of blood vessels is sometimes seen.

Prognosis. Metastases develop in lungs, lymph nodes and other organs. There is a 5-year survival of between 25% and 50% of patients though some die later of their disease.

Miscellaneous Disorders of the Para-articular Tissues

Ganglion. Ganglia occur in the soft tissue around joints or tendon sheaths. The commonest site is the dorsum of the wrist, but they may also be found on the palmar aspect and around the knee. They usually develop by myxoid change and cystic softening of the fibrous tissue of the joint capsule or tendon sheath and occasionally have a direct connection with a joint cavity. Rarely they are found within nerve sheaths and may give rise to symptoms of nerve compression. They consist commonly of a thin, fibrous-walled sac, often rather gelatinous due to the patchy mucoid change, and not lined by synovium. A ganglion contains clear glairy fluid.

Similar lesions occasionally arise in the periosteum particularly of the tibia and also sometimes within bone, beneath a normal articular surface.

Cyst of semilunar cartilage. The cyst arises in relation to the external semilunar cartilage (lateral meniscus) of the knee and has naked-eye and histological features identical with those of a ganglion. Often it appears to arise in the loose fibrous tissue adjacent to, rather than actually within, the fibrocartilage of the meniscus.

Bursitis. A bursa is a synovial-lined sac and is found chiefly over bony prominences. It may communicate with a joint and is subject to many of the same disorders. Inflammation may arise as a result of repeated trauma as, for instance, in prepatellar bursitis (*housemaid's knee*). The bursa becomes distended with fluid, often with much fibrin and the synovial lining may show villous hyperplasia or may be replaced by granulation and later by fibrous tissue. Loose bodies of the melon-seed type may form. *Baker's cyst* arises in the popliteal space by herniation of the synovial membrane through the joint capsule. The connection to the articular cavity may be closed by scarring.

Tumoral calcinosis. In tumoral calcinosis radio-opaque calcium phosphate forms small discrete nodules or larger masses around joints, especially the hip, or in soft tissues. Young Africans are particularly likely to be affected. The condition is usually initially painless though later there may be pressure on nerves. The overlying skin may ulcerate and chalky fluid or granular white material be discharged. Microscopically the deposits of calcium are often surrounded by macrophages, foreign-body giant cells and dense collagen. Plaques of degenerate collagen may be seen near the deposits. The patients are usually healthy and the blood biochemical changes are inconstant. The aetiology remains uncertain. It has been suggested that the deposits may be the result of traumatic fat necrosis or of an abnormality of phosphate metabolism.

Dupuytren's contracture is a painless hereditary condition involving the palmar fascia and resulting in flexion contracture of the fingers. It occurs most commonly in middle-aged males and is often bilateral. The fifth, fourth and third fingers tend to be affected in that order of frequency. The fascia becomes thickened, contracted and sometimes nodular. Microscopy shows, in the active phase, a whorled pattern of very marked fibroblastic proliferation which may give rise to alarm on account of its cellularity (Fig. 22.65). It progresses, however, to extremely dense hyalinised collagen and is entirely benign. Usually a mixture of fibroblastic and hyalinised areas is seen. A similar condition (*plan-tar fibromatosis*) may be present in the sole of the foot, causing nodules in the plantar fascia without contracture. This also is benign though often locally recurrent and difficult to eradicate surgically.

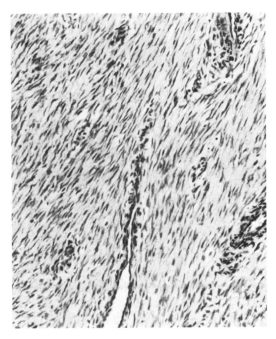

Fig. 22.65 Dupuytren's contracture, showing the highly cellular fascial tissue. × 130.

Fibrositis and panniculitis. The clinical syndrome of muscular pain and localised tenderness may be accounted for by a variety of conditions from cervical spondylosis to Coxsackie virus infection. There is considerable doubt as to whether 'fibrositis' itself exists though tender fibrofatty nodules have been described associated with oedema, a mild chronic inflammatory cell infiltrate and followed by fibrosis. Acute pain of sudden onset may sometimes be due to herniation of a fatty lobule through a small aperture in the investing fibrous tissue and this is termed panniculitis. When associated with obesity the condition may be designated *adiposis dolorosa* or *Dercum's disease*.

Relapsing febrile nodular panniculitis (Weber–Christian syndrome). In this condition successive attacks of weakness and muscular pains are followed by bouts of fever in which tender nodules appear in the subcutaneous and other adipose tissues. These consist of foci of subacute inflammation with areas of secondary fat necrosis and granulomatous reaction. Rarely suppuration may occur and ulceration of the skin then follows, but micro-organisms have not been found in the lesions. The cause is unknown, but it may be associated with focal streptococcal lesions elsewhere, e.g. in the tonsils.

Polymyalgia rheumatica

This clinical syndrome, which usually affects the elderly, consists of pain, stiffness and tenderness of the muscles of the shoulder and pelvic girdles, with a raised erythrocyte sedimentation rate. There is a mild and often transient non-specific synovitis and about half the patients have evidence of giant-cell arteritis (p. 331).

Diseases of Skeletal Muscle

Normal muscle structure

A muscle consists of bundles of muscle fibres bound together by fibrous tissue, the epimysium. This fibrous sheath penetrates between the muscle bundles as the perimysium and each muscle fibre is surrounded by a delicate tenuous sheath of endomysium. Fat cells normally may lie between the muscle bundles but not within them. The muscle or sarcolemmal nuclei in the human lie at the periphery of the fibre under the cell membrane or sarcolemma except in the ocular muscles and at tendinous insertions. Cross-striation, which is recognisable under the light microscope, results from the parallel arrangement of myofibrils with alternating series of interdigitating myosin (thick) and actin (thin) protein filaments. During contraction these filaments are thought to slide into one another.

Each muscle fibre is a single, elongated, multinucleated cell, varying in length and diameter both within a muscle and from one muscle to another. Each fibre has one neuromuscular junction or motor end plate which lies at the midpoint. A motor unit consists of all the muscle fibres which are innervated by a single anterior horn cell and in the human nearly all the fibres in a muscle bundle are included. The number of muscle fibres in a motor unit varies. The more delicate the function to be performed the fewer the fibres in the unit and the smaller the individual fibre diameter. In any one muscle there are two distinct types of muscle fibre, the relative number of each varying from muscle to muscle. Type I fibres, the slow or red fibres, have a high mitochondrial enzyme activity as shown by various histochemical methods, e.g. the succinic dehydrogenase or NADH tetrazolium oxidoreductase techniques. They also contain relatively large amounts of lipid but little glycogen. Type II fibres, the fast or white fibres, have low mitochondrial dehydrogenase activity but a high ATPase activity. They contain little lipid and large quantities of glycogen.

Sensory organs in muscles are numerous, the most common type being the muscle spindle, though other varieties concerned chiefly with stretch and pressure are found in the tendinous insertions. The muscle spindle consists of a long ovoid fibrous capsule containing several thin striated muscle fibres with numerous nuclei in their centres. Sensory endings connected with cells in the posterior root ganglia are present and the fibres receive their motor supply from small cells in the anterior horn. About a third to a half of myelinated fibres in nerves supplying muscle are of sensory origin.

Muscle biopsy. Artefacts produced in the processing of muscle biopsies are common, sometimes confusing and may be minimised by allowing the biopsy to lie unfixed for a minute or two on a piece of card, to which it readily adheres, and then dropping it into fixative. Both longitudinal and cross-sectional blocks should be taken when fixation is complete.

Muscle diseases. Most lesions in skeletal muscle fall into two distinct groups—focal lesions due to trauma, or to inflammatory or circulatory disturbances, and more generalised diseases of muscle. The latter are of three principal types: (i) intrinsic metabolic and often genetically determined diseases of muscle known as the *muscular dystrophies*; (ii) diseases of muscle which are thought to be related to the collagen diseases known as *polymyositis*; and (iii) atrophy of muscle known as *neurogenic atrophy* secondary to disease of the lower motor neuron. Neurogenic atrophy may be a local phenomenon if it is caused by damage to one particular nerve.

General disorders of muscle are characterised by progressive muscular weakness and often pose great clinical problems, special investigations such as electromyography, the measurement of nerve conduction velocity, and muscle biopsy often being required to establish the diagnosis. The examination of a muscle biopsy is now a highly specialised field requiring histological, enzyme histochemical, ultrastructural and often immunopathological techniques. The interpretation of these investigations is beyond the scope of this brief account of diseases of muscle. One particular problem with regard to conventional histological examination is that muscle displays a relatively restricted range of histological abnormalities, and many of these are non-specific. Thus it is often very difficult to distinguish between the early stages of dystrophy and polymyositis while the late stages of dystrophy, polymyositis and neurogenic atrophy may be remarkably similar.

A. Traumatic and circulatory disturbances

Ischaemic necrosis of the flexor muscles of the forearm may follow injuries around the elbow and later give rise to a characteristic deformity with clawing of the fingers (*Volkmann's ischaemic contracture*). Attempts at muscle regeneration are abortive; phagocytosis of dead muscle is followed by the ingrowth of cellular fibrous tissue which later becomes densely collagenous (Fig. 22.66). The inclusion of peripheral nerves, especially the median, in the ischaemic area leads to atrophy of surviving muscle and to sensory changes.

Similar ischaemic necrosis followed by fibrosis sometimes occurs in the anterior tibial muscles following unaccustomed exercise, the swollen muscles being compressed in the relatively unyielding compartment (*anterior tibial syndrome*).

Massive ischaemic necrosis of muscle is seen in cases of 'crush syndrome' where compression of a limb has resulted in prolonged arterial obstruction. On release of pressure and re-establishment of the circulation, large portions of muscle may fail to recover. From these necrotic muscles the myoglobin and other substances are absorbed and excreted in the urine and acute renal tubular necrosis may result (p. 785). The affected muscles become pale and soft—so-called fish-flesh appearance—and if the patient recovers, they undergo fibrous replacement.

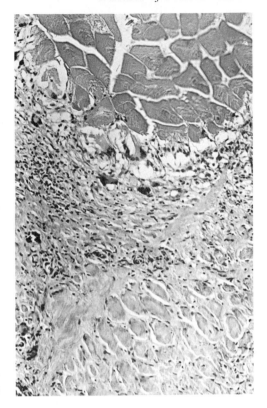

Fig. 22.66 Volkmann's ischaemic contracture. Dead muscle fibres undergoing phagocytosis are seen at the top. In the lower part muscle tubes have been colonised by fibroblasts, and the sarcoplasm replaced by collagen. × 100.

Congenital torticollis. This is a condition of fibrosis and contraction of the sternomastoid muscle which develops in the early years of life. The head tends to be inclined to the affected side, and asymmetry of the face and skull may result.

The torticollis used to be ascribed to the results of fibrous repair of necrotic, ischaemic muscle following a birth injury. However, histological evidence of such a pathogenesis is lacking and the condition is now usually regarded as an example of fibromatosis (p. 291).

Myositis ossificans is a localised benign lesion in which about half the patients have a history of a single injury or of repeated minor trauma. Adolescents and young adults are most often affected and the commonest sites are the muscles of the upper arm and thigh. At first an ill-defined tender mass forms with very active proliferation of undifferentiated and sometimes pleomorphic mesenchymal cells. Then, first at the margin of the lesion, metaplastic cartilage and osteoid are produced. The osteoid usually calcifies and after a few weeks radiographs may show a well-defined ovoid shell of bone within muscle or, if close to a bone surface, a veil-like shadow of bony reaction adjacent to the periosteum; this may be difficult to distinguish from a parosteal osteosarcoma. In the early stages the lesion may readily be misdiagnosed histologically as a sarcoma but the more advanced maturation of the bone at the margins is helpful in arriving at the correct diagnosis (Fig. 22.67).

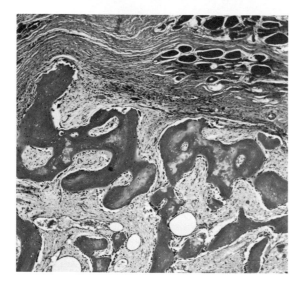

Fig. 22.67   Well-formed bone trabeculae around an area of haemorrhage in muscle

Heterotopic ossification may occur in soft tissues following fracture, dislocation or surgical operation. In paraplegics the hip or knee joint may occasionally become completely fixed by parartiuclar bony bridges.

Progressive myositis ossificans is a very rare disease of unknown aetiology, not hereditary but sometimes associated with congenital abnormalities, in which there is progressive ossification of various muscles in the body, in some cases almost the whole skeleton being immobilised by the newly-formed bone. The affection starts in early life, usually in infancy, and involves the neck, back and shoulders; the disease then extends to other muscles, those of mastication not infrequently being involved. The first indication of the disease is the formation of doughy and sometimes painful swellings in the muscles, and when the swellings subside ossification takes place in the areas of fibrosis. In this way strands and plates of bone of an irregular form are produced in the muscles. The disease advances by a series of attacks rather than by steady progression, and the exacerbations are sometimes accompanied by fever.

B. Inflammatory diseases of muscle

Skeletal muscle becomes secondarily implicated by acute and chronic inflammation of the interstitial tissue. The changes vary according to the nature of the inflammatory lesion. Thus in acute inflammation, oedema and necrosis of the muscle followed by phagocytosis are prominent features, while in chronic inflammation there is fibrosis with atrophy and disappearance of the muscle fibres.

Bacterial myositis

Gas gangrene is an important acute lesion of muscles lacerated by severe trauma and contaminated by soil and often by foreign bodies such as fragments of clothing. If there is suffi-

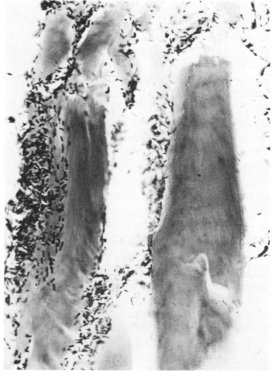

Fig. 22.68   Gas gangrene, showing necrosis and oedema of muscle with numerous *Cl. welchii* but virtually no leukocytes. × 400.

cient deprivation of oxygen in the wound, the muscles are invaded by anaerobic organisms, the commonest of these being *Clostridium welchii*, which spreads within the sarcous sheath, causing oedema and necrosis of the fibres throughout their length and in all the tissues adjacent to the wound through the effects of its α-toxin. The muscle fibres show coagulative necrosis and vacuolation and contain, as do the interstitial tissues, large numbers of Gram+ve bacilli (Fig. 22.68). At the margins of the infection, oedema, haemorrhage and vascular damage are seen, and there is some leukocytic infiltrate which, owing to the leukocidins produced, is abundant only in mild infections and the less severely damaged areas (see p. 170).

Suppuration in muscle is usually the result of direct extension from other suppurative lesions, especially of joints and bones. The metastatic type, due to haematogenous infection associated with *Staphylococcus aureus*, is very uncommon in Great Britain and occurs in the tropics, and particularly in West Africa, when it may have an association with filarial infection.

Zenker's degeneration (pp. 75, 573), a form of focal coagulative necrosis, is sometimes seen in the abdominal muscles in typhoid fever, and occasionally in epidemic influenza. The affected muscles may sometimes be recognised by the naked eye by their pale hyaline appearance.

Viral myositis

Epidemic myalgia (pleurodynia, Bornholm disease) is an acute transient febrile illness due to Coxsackie B virus and involving the muscles in the costal region, back and shoulders. The affected muscles are tender and painful on movement and in some cases biopsy has shown acute myositis. In the CSF there is pleocytosis and a raised globulin level.

Parasitic myositis

Trichinosis. This affection is produced in the human subject usually by the ingestion of uncooked pork containing the embryos of *Trichinella* or *Trichina spiralis*. It is rare in this country, except for an occasional epidemic. When an infested muscle, e.g. a portion of trichinous 'measly' pork, is examined, whitish oval specks may be seen with the naked eye. On microscopic examination, it is found that these represent small oval cysts, containing embryonic trichinellae. A number of the cysts may be calcified, and when the parasites die, they also become calcified. When infested muscle is eaten by another animal, the cyst walls are dissolved by the gastric juice and the embryos are set free. In the bowel they reach full sexual maturity, and the impregnated females bore their way into the wall of the small intestine. The young trichinellae are discharged and migrate by lymphatics to the thoracic duct and circulating blood, from which they penetrate the muscles, especially those of the abdominal and thoracic walls, the diaphragm, muscles of the pharynx, tongue and eye, though the heart and limb muscles may also be affected. The larvae encyst, probably in the interfascicular fibrous tissue, and the adjacent muscle fibres become swollen, lose their striations and are destroyed.

The symptoms which occur during the passage of the young parasites from the intestine to the muscle vary in intensity according to the number of the parasites; when the infestation is heavy there may be fever, muscle pains, difficulty in swallowing and breathing. Oedema of the face, especially around the eyes, is a common symptom. Death occasionally follows due to myocarditis or involvement of respiratory muscles, with bronchopneumonia. There is marked eosinophilia in the acute phase of invasion.

C. Generalised diseases of muscle

1. Muscular dystrophies

The muscular dystrophies are hereditary conditions, usually of insidious onset, characterised by progressive muscular weakness and wasting and due to an intrinsic defect in the muscle itself.

The differentiation between the various types of muscular dystrophy is mainly a clinical problem since the histological findings are similar in each type. Each muscle fibre is affected as an individual unit and this leads to a very intimate admixture of muscle fibres of all sizes, a few of normal size, many in varying stages of atrophy and some of increased diameter. The atrophying fibres lose their polygonal shape on cross-section and become rounded and may be further diminished in size by longitudinal splitting. Degenerative changes such as increased eosinophilia, loss of cross-striation, flocculation and phagocytosis of sarcoplasm are seen, often associated with an interstitial cellular infiltrate (Fig. 22.69). Transverse sections of muscle sometimes show that nuclei, instead of being

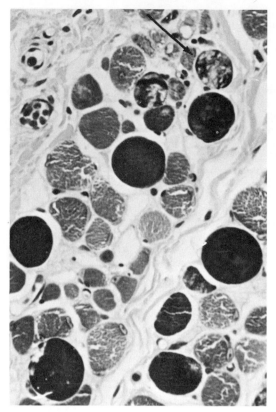

Fig. 22.69   Muscular dystrophy. Muscle fibres of all sizes are intermixed. Enlarged fibres are conspicuous. A group of fibres in the upper right corner (*arrowed*) are undergoing floccular degeneration. × 200. (Dr. A. McQueen.)

confined as normally to the peripheral sheath, are present within the sarcoplasm—*central nuclei*. Infiltration of fat between individual fibres may be notable and endomysial rather than perimysial fibrosis occurs.

Pseudohypertrophic muscular dystrophy (Duchenne type of muscle dystrophy). This form of muscular dystrophy is inherited as a sex-linked recessive, is almost exclusively found in males and usually arises insidiously about the age of 5 years, though occasionally older patients are affected. The wasting and loss of power begin symmetrically in the thighs and pelvic girdle, the calf muscles may be enlarged and the shoulder girdle is sometimes later involved. The child waddles, has difficulty in standing up, rising from sitting and climbing stairs. Tendon reflexes are reduced. The disease progresses inexorably without remission and the patient often dies in adolescence from intercurrent infection. The affected muscles, including the 'hypertrophic' calves, in the terminal stage of the disease are almost entirely replaced by fat, only a few scattered muscle fibres remaining though the muscle spindles are unaffected. The activity of creatine phosphokinase in the serum is usually markedly increased.

Facio-scapulo-humeral dystrophy. The disease, which usually begins in adolescence, may arise earlier or later, the more delayed the onset the better the prognosis. Both males and females are affected and there is often a family history. The initial stage is insidious and asymmetric involvement of the muscles of the shoulder girdle, arms, trunk and face sometimes progresses later to affect the lower limbs. Pseudohypertrophy is not seen. The dystrophy is very chronic, slowly progressive but with long remissions, and seldom gives rise to total disablement. In the later stages there is often some fatty infiltration but not to the same extent as in pseudohypertrophic muscular dystrophy and endomysial fibrosis may be marked.

Dystrophia myotonica. This muscle dystrophy, which occurs in both sexes, usually in adult life, is inherited as a Mendelian dominant. It is associated with premature cataract, gonadal atrophy and sometimes other endocrine disturbances, and is accompanied by myotonia. When a voluntary movement is performed by a patient with myotonia, especially when cold and tired, the muscular contractions take place more slowly and last longer than normal. A similar prolongation of contraction occurs following mechanical or electrical stimulation. The muscles commonly affected by myotonia are those of the tongue, giving rise to dysarthria, and of the hand and forearm resulting in difficulty in releasing any object held in the hand. There is also muscle weakness followed by atrophy of the distal muscles of the upper limb, the face and sternomastoids and sometimes later of the distal muscles of the lower limb. The disease is progressive and disabling, death usually occurring in late middle age.

Microscopically a striking feature may be the presence of long rows of central nuclei.

Other forms of muscular dystrophy are the limb-girdle type which usually begins in adolescence and starts in the shoulder-girdle, and distal myopathy which commonly does not manifest itself until adult life.

2. Polymyositis

This condition presents usually as an acute progressive disease of muscle but subacute and chronic types are also encountered. In acute cases there is often involvement of the skin, the process then being referred to as *dermatomyositis*. The skin shows a diffuse erythema with oedema and sometimes also, in the arteriolar walls, multiple foci of fibrinoid degeneration resembling those lesions found in systemic lupus erythematosus and other connective tissue diseases (p. 998). *Polymyositis* usually begins in adult life and is often rapidly progressive. Unlike muscular dystrophy and the neurogenic atrophies, there may be periods of spontaneous remission. Other cases are more slowly progressive and clinically similar to muscular dystrophy. Muscular weakness, sometimes with tenderness, is an early feature, the proximal muscles being most often affected and in contrast to the dystrophic pattern the bulbar musculature is not infrequently involved with consequent dysarthria and dysphagia. Muscle wasting with diminished tendon jerks follows. The disease may be rapidly fatal due to involvement of the heart or respiratory muscles and in these cases myoglobinuria may result from severe muscle destruction. In less severe cases spontaneous remission may occur at any stage, but is not uncommonly followed by further exacerbation leading to increasing muscle weakness and disability. Occasionally the disease runs a chronic course from the outset.

Microscopic appearances are those of an acute degeneration of muscle fibres with increased eosinophilia, increase in sarcolemmal nuclei, patchy loss of cross-striation and floccular change. In the interstitial tissue a diffuse or focal infiltrate of chronic inflammatory cells, macrophages, neutrophil and eosinophil polymorphs occurs. The muscle fibres show varying degrees of atrophy and some are hypertrophied. There may be attempted muscle regeneration as shown by the presence of thin basophilic muscle fibres sometimes with sarcolemmal giant cells. Even in the later stages endomysial fibrosis is seldom marked. The histological differentiation between dystrophy and polymyositis becomes increasingly difficult the less acute the lesion and in the later stages or in the chronic form of polymyositis may be almost impossible.

3. Neurogenic atrophy

This is secondary to disease of the lower motor neuron and the histological changes in muscle are similar irrespective of whether the abnormality is in the nerve cell body, the spinal nerve root or the peripheral nerve. Probably the commonest cause now of neurogenic atrophy is motor neuron disease. Only those fibres atrophy which have lost their nerve supply and this leads to small or large groups of atrophic fibres lying adjacent to groups of normal unaffected fibres (Fig. 22.70). The atrophied muscle fibres may be 5–10 μm in diameter and there is an apparent increase in sarcolemmal nuclei due to shrinkage of sarcoplasm, which,

however, retains its cross-striations and normal staining reactions. Sometimes the sarcolemmal sheaths are empty but there is little interstitial cellular infiltrate. Later there may be fibrous tissue proliferation around atrophic muscle groups, and a considerable increase in fat. The unaffected muscle fibres usually show little if any compensatory hypertrophy.

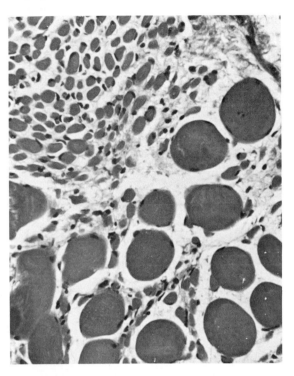

Fig. 22.70 Muscle following neural atrophy. A group of small atrophic fibres in the upper left hand corner is seen adjacent to normally sized fibres. × 320. (Dr. A. McQueen.)

Anterior poliomyelitis is a good example of an acute neural atrophy and here it is common to find, within an atrophic motor unit, between one atrophic unit and another and even in different muscles, that muscle fibres are in much the same stage of atrophy. When there is severe and widespread loss of motor neurons in the spinal cord an entire muscle may atrophy. In diseases of less acute onset, such as motor neuron disease (p. 714) and in the various types of polyneuropathy (p. 717), the fibres show a greater variation of size within the motor unit as though all did not undergo atrophy at the same pace. A particularly characteristic feature in progressive neurogenic atrophy is the occurrence of collateral and ultraterminal axonal sprouting and the formation of new motor end plates (p. 718). Later, groups of muscle fibres may become more uniform in size but there is still variation from one group to another and it is only in longstanding disease that uniform atrophy is seen.

Peroneal muscular atrophy of Charcot-Marie-Tooth. This is a hereditary disease, commoner in boys and usually developing in children or young adults. Weakness and atrophy, often symmetrical, first develop in the extensor and abductor muscles of the feet, giving rise to pes cavus; later all muscles below the middle of the thigh and sometimes the hand and forearm muscles may be involved. The muscular atrophy is thought to be secondary to degeneration of the lower motor neurons, but there may also be changes in the spinal cord similar to those seen in Friedreich's ataxia (see p. 714).

Miscellaneous disorders of muscle

Muscle weakness associated with carcinoma

Muscle weakness and wasting in patients with carcinoma may be due to nutritional factors, to neural atrophy which is sometimes attributable to suitably placed metastases, but sometimes to carcinomatous neuropathy (p. 721), and also possibly to a primary affection of the muscle. In the latter group the weakness, occasionally associated with myasthenia, usually involves the proximal muscles. The condition is most commonly associated with bronchial and pancreatic carcinoma and one of the striking features is that the severity of the myopathy does not parallel the extent of the malignant disease. The myopathy may be striking many months before the carcinoma is diagnosable clinically, or may remit when the patient is dying from the neoplasm.

Histological changes in the muscle may be non-specific, being those of simple atrophy with an increase of sarcolemmal nuclei. In other cases the changes resemble those in polymyositis, with flocculation and vacuolation of the sarcous substance and pronounced cellular infiltration between the fibres, some of which show longitudinal splitting (Fig. 22.71). A clear

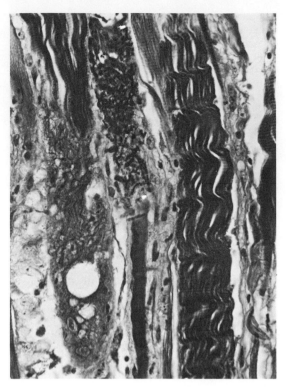

Fig. 22.71 Carcinomatous myopathy showing splitting of muscle fibres, flocculation and loss of striation. × 400.

understanding of this condition has not yet been achieved.

Myasthenia gravis

Definition. This is a disease in which excessive weakness of voluntary muscles develops during prolonged or repeated use, apparently as a result of impaired neuromuscular transmission of motor stimuli.

Neurophysiological considerations. The arrival of a nerve impulse at a neuromuscular junction normally releases acetylcholine, and causes depolarisation of the adjacent, specially modified surface of the muscle fibre: when depolarisation exceeds 15–20 mV, contraction is stimulated. In normal subjects the amount of acetylcholine released is much greater than is required to achieve this degree of depolarisation.

The defect in myasthenia gravis has not been fully elucidated, but the available evidence suggests that there is an inadequate liberation of acetylcholine.

Clinical features. Usually myasthenia gravis begins during adolescence or early adult life and principally affects females. Less often, it presents in middle age and is then commoner in males, rarely it occurs in the babies of myasthenic women—'neonatal myasthenia'. The external ocular muscles and those of the head and neck are most frequently affected, the arm muscles less frequently, and those of the leg and trunk least often. Muscle function may be normal early in the day but with use symptoms develop which are, at least partly, reversed by rest or anticholinesterase drugs. The severity of the disease varies considerably and fluctuations occur in the intensity of the muscle weakness in individual cases. Dramatic accentuation of the myasthenic state—myasthenic crisis—is common, and is sometimes precipitated by infection or trauma. Death may result from weakness of respiratory muscles. Overdosage with anticholinesterase drugs produces a 'cholinergic crisis' due to persisting depolarisation of the motor end plates.

Clinically, myasthenia gravis is frequently associated with various types of thyroid disease, notably thyrotoxicosis.

Pathological features. *Muscles.* Histologically the voluntary muscles are involved in an irregular and patchy fashion. Three distinct types of lesion may occur: (1) patchy coagulative necrosis of individual muscle fibres with an associated inflammatory infiltrate; (2) lymphorrhages, in which there is focal atrophy of a muscle fibre with infiltration of lymphocytes around it; (3) simple focal atrophy without reactive changes affecting single muscle fibres or groups of fibres, especially of type II.

None of these changes is specific for myasthenia gravis. Lymphorrhages occur in Addison's disease, rheumatoid arthritis and Hashimoto's disease, while focal necrosis is seen in various types of myositis, and atrophy in many conditions.

Motor end plates. The motor end plates are elongated and distorted in myasthenia gravis and there is proliferation of subterminal nerve fibres, but it is not clear whether these are primary or compensatory changes. Descriptions of the ultrastructural appearances are somewhat contradictory.

Thymus. Ninety per cent of patients with myasthenia gravis have thymic changes and these are of two kinds: (*a*) Numerous large lymphoid follicles with germinal centres develop in the thymic medulla in over 80% of patients who do not have a thymic tumour and also commonly in the residual thymus gland in patients with a thymoma. In addition to the large germinal centres the glands often show failure of age involution of the cortex. This type of lesion is found predominantly among young female patients. (*b*) Thymic tumours are present in myasthenia gravis in 10% of patients, most of whom are middle-aged and male. The tumour is usually of mixed epithelial and lymphocytic cells, the proportion of the two cell types varying between tumours and in different areas of the same tumour. The epithelial cells are usually plump and rounded. The tumours are locally invasive; they frequently become adherent to the mediastinal blood vessels and may invade the lungs though distant metastases are uncommon. Rarely, myasthenia gravis may develop after removal of a thymic tumour which has presented with other symptoms.

The likelihood of improvement or cure following thymectomy depends on the type of thymic change. In general, response is best in young patients without a thymic tumour, particularly if the symptoms are of short duration, however, there is considerable individual variation and the response in any particular case is not predictable. Removal of a neoplastic thymus is not usually followed by dramatic improvement.

Immunological aspects. It is known that the serum of most normal subjects contains antibodies to the I bands of skeletal muscle. In myasthenia, especially in subjects who have thymic tumours, the titre tends to be higher, and is likely to be a result of muscle damage rather than its cause. Some myasthenic patients with a thymic tumour have antibodies to the A bands of skeletal muscle. There is a significant increase in the incidence of auto-antibodies to thyroid tissue antigens in myasthenic subjects.

Aetiology. Since the thymus is now known to play a major role in immunological responsiveness, the presence of thymic changes in myasthenia gravis, and the response to thymectomy in some cases suggest the possibility that immunological factors might play a part in the aetiology though this still remains obscure. The occurrence of transient neonatal myasthenia raises the possibility of a humoral causal factor but none has been isolated and there is no correlation between neonatal myasthenia and the titre of maternal antibody to muscle. Recently Goldstein has suggested, from immunological studies in guinea-pigs, that the thymus is damaged by an auto-immune reaction and that this leads to the liberation of increased amounts of a substance, 'thymin', which inhibits neuro-muscular transmission. Other workers have so far failed to confirm his findings.

Periodic paralysis

Muscular activity requires that the intracellular potassium concentration be maintained at normal levels but if the plasma potassium is depleted, as in gastro-intestinal fluid loss, in certain renal disturbances, and on recovery from diabetic coma, weakness of the voluntary muscles and cardiac irregularity may develop and the former may amount to temporary muscular paralysis. The rare familial disorder known as *periodic paralysis*, inherited as an autosomal dominant, is associated with inter-mittently low levels in the plasma potassium concentration and attacks of muscle weakness may be precipitated by rest following exercise, and by the ingestion of large amounts of carbo-hydrate. The cardiac irregularity is curiously slight in contrast to the findings in other states of potassium depletion.

Myotonia congenita (Thomsen's disease)

This rare congenital and hereditary disease was de-scribed by Thomsen who suffered from it himself. It is commoner in males and first appears in childhood, muscular contraction either voluntary or on elec-trical stimulation being delayed in onset and slower in performance than is normal. Myotonia may be localised or widespread and the affected muscles are hypertrophied and more powerful than normal. The tendon reflexes are not abnormal. The myotonia may diminish with advancing age and in any case life is not shortened. Occasionally involved muscles may eventually become somewhat atrophic. His-tologically the muscle fibres may be enlarged with some central nuclei, and striation is poorly marked.

The Connective Tissue Diseases

The concept that the connective tissues of the body comprise a system, subject to its own specific diseases, led Klemperer and his col-leagues to introduce the term *diffuse collagen disease*. It has subsequently become apparent that in most types of disease affecting the con-nective tissues, collagen is not solely nor primarily involved, and accordingly the term *connective tissue disease* is to be preferred. The diseases most commonly included under this heading are rheumatoid arthritis (RA), systemic lupus erythematosus (SLE), rheumatic fever, progressive systemic sclerosis, scleroderma, poly-arteritis nodosa and dermatomyositis. The group of diseases is also referred to, somewhat loosely, as the *rheumatic diseases*. They are now classed together not because they are clear-cut examples of diseases affecting primarily the cells or matrix of the connective tissues (which is doubtful), but because they present associa-tions with one another, suggesting common aetiological and pathogenic factors. Many other conditions—mostly rare and of unknown aetiology—could be regarded as connective tissue diseases, but this simply increases the size and heterogeneity of the group.

General features. Little is known of the aetiology of the connective tissue diseases. There are, however, certain features which are generally applicable to the group: these are as follows:

(1) *Sex incidence.* As a group, these diseases affect females more often than males.

(2) *Overlap between diseases.* Although readily distinguishable from one another in typical cases, the connective tissue diseases show considerable overlap. For example, patients presenting mixed features of systemic lupus erythematosus (SLE) and rheumatoid arthritis are not uncommon, while polyarteritis nodosa may complicate either of these condi-tions and develops also in some patients with progressive systemic sclerosis.

(3) *Hereditary factors.* Epidemiological studies suggest that rheumatoid arthritis tends to occur with undue frequency among the

blood relatives of cases. However, this familial tendency is not strong, and moreover it is not known whether it is dependent on genetic pre-disposition, environmental factors (e.g. a trans-missible agent), or both. There is some evidence also that the other diseases tend to occur with undue frequency in the relatives of individuals with rheumatoid arthritis.

(4) *Immunological features.* The serum level of IgG is commonly raised in patients with SLE, less commonly in rheumatoid arthritis and the other diseases. Of more interest is the presence in the serum of various auto-antibodies. The best known of these are rheumatoid factor and antibodies to deoxy-ribonucleoprotein and other constituents of cell nuclei. Rheumatoid factor (p. 135) is present in a high proportion of patients with RA, and a high titre is usually associated with this condi-tion. However, it is by no means always present in RA, and low titres are quite common in ap-parently healthy individuals. The incidence and titres of rheumatoid factor are increased in the other connective tissue diseases. Antinuclear antibodies (p. 134), particularly antibody to deoxyribonucleoprotein, are virtually always present in the serum of patients with active SLE, and are frequently demonstrable in the other diseases. Like rheumatoid factor, anti-body to deoxyribonucleoprotein is not uncom-mon in low titre in apparently normal individuals. Various other auto-antibodies to cellular constituents have been described in the serum of patients with connective tissue diseases: like antinuclear antibodies, they react with antigens common to a wide variety of cells and are not 'organ-specific'.

(5) *Pathological changes.* The lesions of the connective tissue diseases vary considerably in appearance, and the differences are due to the occurrence, in various combinations, of fibrin-oid change, necrosis, acute and chronic inflam-mation and dense fibrosis. The changes occur focally in the connective tissues in various parts of the body, and also in the walls of small blood vessels. Vascular involvement is of particular importance, because it leads to ischaemia and thus to secondary changes, not only in the con-nective tissues, but also in the parenchyma of various organs and in the skin. Since none of these pathological changes is specific, mor-phological diagnosis of the connective tissue diseases depends upon the appearance and site of the individual lesions, e.g. the polyarthritis of RA, the glomerular and skin lesions of SLE, and the necrotising inflammatory arterial lesions of polyarteritis nodosa. The major patho-logical features of the individual diseases are described in the appropriate systematic chap-ters, and the following brief accounts are intended simply to summarise the various mani-festations of each disease.

Rheumatoid arthritis. This disease is de-scribed on pp. 855–8. It usually occurs alone but may accompany overt SLE, or be com-plicated by the incomplete picture of SLE, e.g. a positive LE-cell test (see below). Anaemia is common in RA; usually it is of dyshaemo-poietic nature, but occasionally auto-immune haemolytic anaemia develops.

Polyarthritis resembling RA, but usually relatively mild, complicates some cases of psoriasis, and typical RA is a common feature of Sjøgren's syndrome (p. 535). Pain in the joints, usually without progressive structural changes, is common in rheumatic fever, pro-gressive systemic sclerosis and polyarteritis nodosa.

The aetiology of rheumatoid arthritis remains unknown. Features suggesting an im-munological disturbance include (1) a marked hyperplasia of the cortical germinal centres of lymph nodes, suggestive of an antibody response; (2) the common occurrence of rheumatoid factor and antinuclear antibodies; and (3) the heavy lymphocytic and plasma-cell infiltration of the synovia of affected joints. These features, together with the occurrence of acute arthritis in serum sickness, suggest that the disease is due to a hypersensitivity reaction, but the nature of the hypothetical antigenic stimulus has not been established. A mycoplas-mal disease in pigs resembles RA and there is some inconclusive evidence that *Mycoplasma fermentans* may play a role in RA.

Systemic lupus erythematosus. This is an uncommon condition, affecting mostly adolesc-ent females and young women. It may run an acute course with fever, and if untreated is often fatal in months or years, the commonest cause of death being renal failure. The clinical features and pathological changes show great individual variation. The tissues most often involved are the skin (p. 998), the kidneys (p. 772), the endocardium (p. 371), and the serous membranes, but any organ may be affected.

There may be arthritic pain, pleurisy, albuminuria, haematuria and the nephrotic syndrome. Fibrinoid change is seen in the small vessels—arterioles, capillaries and venules—in the various tissues. This may have important effects by causing ischaemia, but fibrinoid change occurs also in avascular connective tissue, e.g. in the heart valves. Necrosis, a granulomatous reaction and fibrosis are also common features.

Patients with SLE have a strong tendency to develop hypersensitivity to various drugs. Haematological features include leukopenia, sometimes thrombocytopenia, and less commonly auto-immunological reactions. Auto-antibodies to nuclear and other cellular constituents occur with greater frequency in SLE

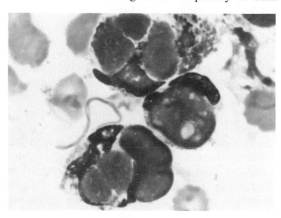

Fig. 22.72 LE cells from a case of disseminated lupus erythematosus. × 600. Three cells are shown with characteristic ingested masses of altered nuclear material. (From a preparation kindly lent by Dr. J. M. Robertson.)

than in the other connective tissue diseases. In the LE-cell test, examination of the patient's leukocytes following incubation of whole blood at 37 °C shows phagocytosis of homogeneous basophilic material by neutrophil polymorphs (Fig. 22.72). These so-called LE cells result from the reaction of auto-antibody to deoxyribonucleoprotein with the nuclei of degenerate leukocytes, with subsequent fixation of complement and phagocytosis of the altered nuclear material. The test is positive in patients with a high plasma level of antibody to deoxyribonucleoprotein ('LE-cell factor'). It is not positive in all cases of SLE, and is positive in a small proportion of patients with RA or other connective tissue diseases. The lesions of SLE commonly exhibit patchy basophilia, the so-called

haematoxyphil bodies, due to deposition of deoxyribonucleoprotein complexed with antibody. Serological tests for syphilis, e.g. the Wassermann reaction, are commonly positive in SLE, and are due to auto-antibodies which cross-react with antigenic constituents of cardiolipin.

There is now good evidence that the glomerular lesions are due to a type III hypersensitivity reaction (p. 772) resulting from deposition of immune complexes composed of auto-antibodies and the corresponding auto-antigens, in the glomerular capillary walls. Fibrinoid lesions in the skin and elsewhere may be of similar nature. The cause of the predisposition to develop auto-antibodies and hypersensitivity to drugs is, however, not known. Investigations on NZB/NZW mice, which develop spontaneously a disease resembling SLE (p. 135) suggest the possibility that virus infection may play a pathogenic role, but virological studies in SLE have so far been inconclusive.

Progressive systemic sclerosis. The main features of this rare chronic disease are intimal thickening of small arteries and arterioles, patchy loss of specialised tissue, and replacement fibrosis. In addition to the skin lesion (p. 999), the gastro-intestinal tract, heart, skeletal muscles, kidneys and lungs are most often affected. Clinical features include dysphagia from fibrosis and loss of smooth muscle of the oesophagus, respiratory insufficiency and repeated infections resulting from progressive pulmonary fibrosis, and disturbances of the gastro-intestinal tract. The interlobular renal arteries are narrowed by severe concentric intimal fibrosis resembling closely that of malignant hypertension: patchy renal ischaemia results, and there may be associated hypertension. Vascular involvement and shrinkage of the skin bring about ischaemia of the extremities, often with Raynaud's phenomenon (p. 332), and sometimes progressing to ulceration and gangrene. There may also be subcutaneous calcification. Cardiac function may be impaired by myocardial fibrosis, hypertension and lung involvement.

The aetiology of progressive systemic sclerosis is quite unknown. Antinuclear auto-antibodies may be present in the serum, and the condition may be accompanied by rheumatoid arthritis or lesions suggestive of SLE.

The major features of *scleroderma* (p. 999), *polyarteritis nodosa* (p. 329) and *dermatomyositis* (p. 872) are described in the appropriate systematic chapters.

Rheumatic fever (p. 360) is characterised by transient polyarthritis, myocardial injury, focal fibrinoid and inflammatory lesions of the connective tissues of the endocardium and of the myocardium, a fibrinous pericarditis and lesions of small vessels. It differs from the other connective tissue diseases in being a complication of a specific infection, namely a pharyngitis due to β-haemolytic streptococci. The pathogenesis is not fully understood, although the cross-reaction of streptococcal antibodies with myocardium, and the demonstration of such antibody attached to myocardium (p. 360) provide strong evidence for the participation of a cytotoxic (type II) immunological reaction (p. 121).

There is little association between the connective tissue diseases and the organ-specific autoimmune diseases (p. 132) except in Sjøgren's disease, in which features of both groups are commonly demonstrable.

23

Reproductive System

I. Male

Inflammatory conditions

Acute inflammations of the male genital tract are due to two main causes, gonorrhoea, and septic infections usually secondary to cystitis. Metastatic infection by the blood stream also may occur, but it is less common.

Gonorrhoea

This is acquired by coitus. It is an acute catarrhal inflammation which ascends from the urethral meatus to the anterior part of the urethra. The discharge, at first thick and glairy, soon becomes purulent, and in it gonococci, mainly in neutrophil polymorphs, are usually numerous. If untreated the disease, after running a course of several weeks, often resolves without residual effects, but not infrequently infection may spread to the posterior urethra and a chronic urethritis is established.

Infection of the prostate may be accompanied by acute inflammatory swelling, while in the chronic stage gonococci often persist in the tubules of the gland and maintain the infection. The organisms may also ascend by the vas deferens and set up acute suppuration in the epididymis, and occasionally extending to the testis, leading to scarring and atrophy. Infection of the bladder by gonococci occasionally causes cystitis. Two other serious complications may occur: firstly, ulceration of the posterior urethra, leading to stricture, dilatation and hypertrophy of the bladder, secondary infection by other organisms and septic cystitis; and secondly, the organisms may be distributed by the bloodstream and give rise to inflammation in other parts of the body. The commonest of these are in the joints and sheaths of tendons,

but occasionally other conditions, such as pleurisy, endocarditis and even septicaemia may develop. Gonococcal infections are usually highly susceptible to treatment with penicillin or the sulphonamide drugs and all these complications have become in consequence much less frequent. However, drug-resistance and changes in social behaviour are probably responsible for the increase in gonorrhoea observed in recent years.

Non-bacterial urethritis

Acute non-bacterial urethritis in males is commonly of venereal origin. The causal agent is unknown, but there is some evidence implicating an organism of the Chlamydia group, apparently identical with the TRIC agent (TR for trachoma and IC for inclusion conjunctivitis of neonates). This form of urethritis, known as Reiter's syndrome (p. 859), is sometimes accompanied by conjunctivitis and followed by arthritis. There is indirect evidence that the same agent may cause infection of the cervix uteri in women as well as conjunctivitis in the newborn.

Orchitis

As mentioned above, epididymitis and orchitis may result from spread of gonococci or coliform bacilli along the vasa deferentia as a complication of gonococcal urethritis or coliform cystitis respectively. The inflammation may progress to suppuration, and result in fibrosis and obliteration of the testicular tubules.

Of infections by the bloodstream, the commonest is that which occurs in mumps, this complication being comparatively common in adults but rare in children. The lesion is a diffuse non-suppurative inflammation of the testis, which may lead to fibrosis with atrophy and, if bilateral, infertility. Orchitis may complicate smallpox and other viral diseases and occasionally also various pyogenic infections.

Strangulation of the testicle* as a result of acute torsion of the spermatic cord leads to infarction, which may be intensely haemorrhagic. Clinically, it may resemble acute orchitis.

Chronic granulomatous orchitis presents clinically as a unilateral painful swelling of the testis; after a few weeks this subsides leaving an indurated organ of diminished sensitivity to pressure. The aetiology is obscure. The lesion is characterised by interstitial inflammatory infiltration of lymphocytes, plasma cells and sometimes eosinophils, together with atrophy of the germinal epithelium and replacement by inflammatory cells including many giant cells. Microscopically it bears a superficial resemblance to tuberculosis because the outlines of the replaced tubules confer a follicular appearance on the lesion, but caseation is absent and tubercle bacilli have not been demonstrated. It is regarded by some as a low-grade infection by coliform bacilli; others have suggested, with little supporting evidence, an auto-immune pathogenesis.

Prostatitis

Acute inflammation of the prostate is usually produced by spread of organisms from the urethra, in either gonorrhoea or septic cystitis. The gonococcus produces an acute catarrhal inflammation in the prostate with swelling of the surrounding tissue and increased secretion. Gonococcal prostatitis may pass into a chronic state in which the organism persists for a long time in the tubules, the secretion of which remains infective. In cases of septic cystitis, acute inflammation of the prostate is often followed by multiple foci of suppuration, or a large abscess may form and the prostate may be extensively destroyed. Similar changes may occur also in the seminal vesicles.

In *chronic interstitial prostatitis* or *prostatic*

fibrosis there is a diffuse scarring of the gland, leading to diminution in size. Like prostatic hypertrophy it may lead to urethral obstruction. Its aetiology is unknown but probably it is the result of a mild infection. A granulomatous prostatitis, with eosinophils, epithelioid cells and giant cells, like that in the testis, has also been observed.

Tuberculosis

Tuberculosis of the male genital tract is now becoming uncommon in most countries. It is usually haematogenous, being secondary to a tuberculous lesion elsewhere; in some instances it results from renal infection with spread of bacilli along the vas deferens from the base of the bladder. In nearly all cases the epididymis is the first part of the genital tract to be affected. Tubercles form in it, enlarge, caseate and

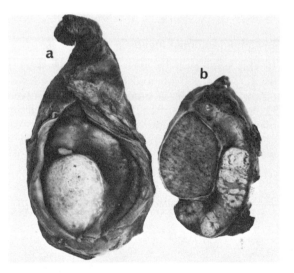

Fig. 23.1 Bilateral epididymal tuberculosis; in **a** the irregularly swollen epididymis is seen above the testis; in **b** caseation in the other epididymis is shown on section. × 0·7.

coalesce, and ultimately the epididymis may be entirely destroyed and caseous. It becomes enlarged and firm, and forms a sausage-shaped structure attached to the testis (Fig. 23.1). Later the tunica vaginalis may become infected with caseation or obliteration by fibrous adhesions: infection may also spread eventually into the testis. In untreated cases there may be involvement of the skin with ulceration and sinus

* By 'testicle' is meant the whole ovoid structure of testis and epididymis together: the 'testis' is the gonad proper.

formation. The vas deferens usually becomes affected, and may be focally obliterated. The infection may spread to the seminal vesicles, prostate and base of the bladder.

Syphilis

Apart from the primary sore, which has been described already (p. 183), the only important site of syphilis in the genital tract is the testis, which is probably the commonest site of tertiary lesions after the aorta. Gumma causes painless enlargement and induration of the testis. Extensive dull yellowish necrotic areas develop with an irregular outline of more translucent granulation tissue which forms a contrast to the rest of the tissue (Fig. 23.2). Syphilitic orchitis without gumma is also seen, with growth of cellular connective tissue and consequent scarring, while the tubules become atrophied and disappear.

Lymphogranuloma inguinale

In this condition (p. 917) the primary sore is usually on the penis and the inguinal nodes on one or both sides are conspicuously involved. Prolonged suppuration, discharge and scarring may occur but rectal stricture and other late complications are much less common than in women.

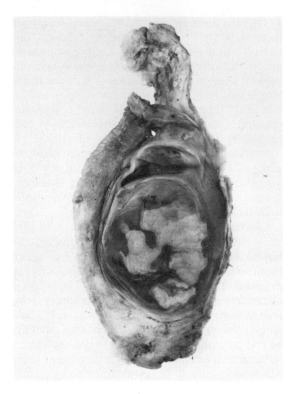

Fig. 23.2   Gumma of testis, showing large irregular central pale areas of necrosis surrounded by darker granulation tissue. The upper pole of the testis is not yet involved. × 0·8.

Functional disorders of the testis

Male fertility depends on the presence of at least one normally functioning testis, and most of the 5% of adult males who are infertile have some testicular disorder.

Sperm count. The ejaculate should be at least 1 ml in volume (normal average 4 ml) and contain at least 50 million spermatozoa per ml (average over 100 million): at least 60% (usually over 80%) of the spermatozoa should be motile and of normal morphology. Total absence of spermatozoa (azoospermia) of course means total infertility if permanent: it is however remarkable that counts consistently under 50 million (oligospermia) also usually mean infertility.

Testicular biopsy. This is usually necessary in the further investigation of azoospermia and persistent oligospermia. (Practical points to note are that the incision should be large enough to allow inspection of the whole testicle, that the biopsy should not be too small, and that ordinary fixation in formalin is unsatisfactory, Davidson's or Bouin's fixatives being recommended.) Findings in biopsies in infertility are usually divided about equally into four categories (*a*) normal (with obstruction), (*b*) scarring, (*c*) diminished spermatogenic activity, (*d*) germ cell aplasia.

Obstructive lesions. A normal testicular biopsy in a case of azoospermia indicates an obstructive lesion of epididymis or vas. Against all expectations based on the behaviour of other glands, obstruction, even life-long, does not affect the testis at all. Instead spermatozoa collect in the epididymis and are reabsorbed there, often causing local inflammatory lesions called sperm granulomas. Obstruction may be post-inflammatory (e.g. old tuberculosis or gonococcal epididymitis), or congenital (e.g. atresia of the vas), or surgical (e.g. accidents during herniorrhaphy, and of course vasectomy). Such lesions can sometimes be corrected surgically.

Scarring. Gross destruction of testicular tissue by granulomatous orchitis, severe mumps orchitis, gumma or torsion, is, of course, followed by extensive scarring and atrophy and, if the lesion is bilateral, azoospermia. None of these is common however, especially in bilateral form, and the fibrosis found in cases of sterility generally consists of multiple scattered small scars, each involving only a few tubules, in an otherwise normal testis. The cause is usually unknown, but is presumably some mild unrecognised infection in early life. The production of azoospermia or severe oligospermia by such inconspicuous scarring may seem surprising but it must be remembered that each of the 700 tubules in the testis is nearly a metre long and without anastomoses. Within each of the dozen or so sectors, the tubules are very intricately coiled together. With numerous small scars scattered through the testis, the chance of any one tubule having any substantial length free from obstruction is therefore small. One is dealing in fact with an intratesticular obstructive lesion.

Diminished spermatogenic activity

Direct damage. As might be expected, the complex activity of the normal tubular epithelium is readily disturbed by a great variety of adverse factors. It may cease temporarily to produce spermatozoa as a result of severe infections, malnutrition, many poisons, uraemia or indeed any major illness. Cadmium, antimitotic drugs and x-rays are particularly inhibitory, and larger doses of the latter agents especially may, by damaging the relatively resistant spermatogonia, produce permanent atrophy.

Spermatogenesis ceases at temperatures above the normal relatively low testicular level, and this is probably a reason for the infertility of an undescended testis (see below) and one

with an increased blood flow due to the vascular disorder of the scrotal vessels called *varicocele*.

Maturation arrest. In some cases of infertility the tubules contain normal numbers of actively dividing cells in the early stages of mitosis, but the process is not completed and no active sperm are formed. No cause can be found usually, and the mechanism remains uncertain. Spontaneous remissions or cures occur occasionally.

Endocrine effects. The testicular epithelium depends both for its original induction in the fetus and its activity in the adult on the local androgens produced by the Leydig cells. These in turn are dependent upon pituitary gonadotrophins. (LH is necessary for Leydig cell activity: it is probable but not certain that FSH is necessary as well as androgens for tubule activity.) Spermatogenesis therefore ceases in most forms of pituitary failure. Often this is caused by oestrogen excess, which acts by suppressing secretion of pituitary LH: the effect is surprisingly rapid and often severe. Oestrogen given in the treatment of prostatic cancer is one example, but the rise of endogenous oestrogen seen in liver disease (p. 631) is also effective, the testes usually showing tubular atrophy in cases of clinically evident cirrhosis.

This type of atrophy is usually readily recognisable. The spermatogenic epithelium is profoundly affected, being often reduced entirely to the stem-cell spermatogonia and the supporting Sertoli cells; the Leydig cells (in contrast to most other tubular atrophies) are greatly reduced in number; and a conspicuous deposit of hyaline forms rapidly between basement membrane and epithelium in the shrunken tubules.

Germ cell defects

Absence or near absence of germ cells is usually congenital. The effect is to produce tubular atrophy without loss of Leydig cells, and a rise of pituitary FSH presumably due to the absence of an unidentified tubular feed-back hormone. Pituitary activity sometimes produced gynaecomastia. This combination was identified by Klinefelter in 1943. His name however is generally used only for the first of the two main forms (below) of germ-cell defect.

(1) Klinefelter's syndrome (of chromosomal

origin). This, one of the commonest of chromosomal disorders, is the result of the presence of a Y chromosome (which ensures the formation of a testis and masculine development generally) together with a second X, which prevents normal development of the testis. The usual abnormal pattern is thus XXY, but variants such as mosaics are not rare and even an apparent pure XX (probably with some part of the Y translocated to another chromosome) may be found. A moderate increase in frequency of mental defect is the only important non-genital consequence. A eunuchoid body-build is frequent and FSH levels are high, but androgens are usually not much below normal. Gynaecomastia is not rare, and carcinoma of the breast is commoner than in normal males. The rare cases with three or four X chromosomes (XXXY, etc.) have a high incidence of congenital defects.

The testis in these cases is very small (5 g or less) and grossly abnormal histologically. The bulk appears to be made up of irregular masses of Leydig cells: among them are occasional tubules lined by Sertoli cells only (similar to those seen in the next group) but most of what tubules are present are inconspicuous and hyalinised 'ghost' tubules. It is probable that the shortage of tubules is not due merely to shrinkage, but that there is a primary defi-

ciency. In a few cases germ cells persist in an occasional tubule, and localised spermatogenesis occurs. A single well authenticated case of a fertile man with XXY presumably represents an extreme example of this.

Diagnosis in these cases is made easy by the sex chromatin test; this is the only condition of any frequency in which it is positive in males (Figs. 23.3 and 23.4). Using this test, it has been shown that 1 in 200 male births are XXY.

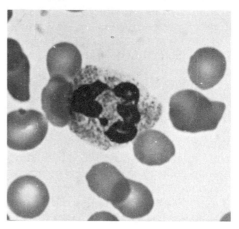

Fig. 23.4 Polymorphonuclear leukocyte showing typical female sex-chromatin drumstick. × 1500.

(2) Germ-cell aplasia (non-chromosomal). (Also called *chromatin-negative Klinefelter's syndrome* or the *del Castillo syndrome*.) Here there is absence or near-absence of the germ cells in the testis, of no known cause but presumed to be congenital. The effects are similar to those of XXY, but are (except for the infertility, which is nearly invariable) less pronounced. There is no associated mental defect and eunuchoidism is less common. The testes are not so small, and the histology is less grossly altered: the tubules are well-preserved but reduced in size, and are lined entirely by tall pale-staining Sertoli cells with no germ cells; between the tubules are what appear to be an excess of Leydig cells. Many cases are partial, with some fertile tubules, producing oligospermia rather than total absence of sperm.

Leydig cells in testicular atrophy. The normal adult has about 0·9 ml of Leydig cells in each testis, and this quantity remains remarkably constant so long as the normal pituitary stimulus is present. If the tubules in both testes

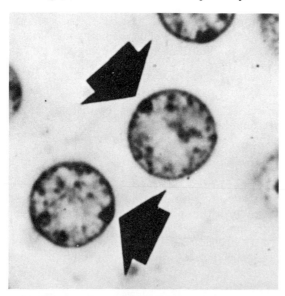

Fig. 23.3 Nuclear sex chromatin, resembling that of normal females, in the Leydig cells of a case of XXY Klinefelter's syndrome. Testicular biopsy. × 1500.

are atrophic, the proportion of the testis occupied by Leydig cells becomes proportionately increased (it may be over 50% in an XXY testis) and it is easy to mistake this for hyperplasia. (True Leydig cell hyperplasia is very rare in man.) When only one testis is atrophic, the Leydig cells appear to be redistributed between the two testes, and little apparent hyperplasia occurs on the affected side. *Hypoplasia* is nearly always a pituitary effect, though a few XXY cases show what may be primary Leydig cell failure.

The undescended testicle

The normal process of descent of the testis from the abdomen through the inguinal ring may be interrupted at any point. Delay up to the age of about five is compatible with a normal testis, but thereafter an increasing proportion show abnormality, indicated before puberty by a lack of germ cells. It is still quite uncertain whether this abnormality is a result of the long sojourn at the abnormal site, or whether there is a primary defect in the testis that interferes with descent. Such defective testes never become fertile, and are probably the chief contributors to the maldescended testes' raised tumour incidence (p. 888). If a testis remains undescended after puberty, spermatogenesis will be defective even where germ cells are present: but of course both sides must be involved for infertility.

Intersexes

It may be worth interjecting a brief note on this subject here. Intersexes are individuals who present some degree of intermingling of the characters of both sexes. Apart from the psychological intersexes, homosexuality and transvestism, with which we are not concerned, the principal varieties are the following.

(a) **Chromosomal intersexes.** The commonest varieties are XXY Klinefelter's syndrome, considered above, and XO Turner's syndrome (p. 925). In both of these, and in contrast to the next group, the general anatomy is far less intersexual than the chromosomal picture.

(b) **Hermaphroditism.** This term is properly confined to the rare individuals who possess both testis and ovary: there may be an ovary on one side and a testis on the other, or various mixtures of the two. Intermediate forms of sexual development are a natural consequence: most often the external genitalia are predominantly male at birth and internal genitalia correspond to the gonad nearest to them. Breast development or other signs of feminisation appear at puberty. In most cases the cause is obscure, but some are true *mosaics*, mixtures of XY and XX cells. There is strong evidence that this can result from double fertilisation, and can be regarded almost as an extreme case of Siamese twinning, with total fusion at the cellular level. These XX/XY mosaics should not be confused with XX/XY *blood cell chimeras*, in which exchange of blood occurs between twins of unlike sex *in utero*: the chimerism in these cases is limited to the blood-forming tissues, and has interesting effects on the blood groups but not on sexual development.

(c) **Adrenal virilism** (p. 975). In this, a defect of steroid hormone synthesis leads to virilisation of the external genitalia in females: the condition is of special importance because, if recognised early, it can be treated effectively.

(d) **Male pseudohermaphroditism.** In this, male external genitalia are imperfectly developed, presumably as a result of temporary failure of testosterone output from the testis *in utero*. In its lesser degrees it fades away into such minor conditions as bifid scrotum and *hypospadias* (in which the urethra opens on the under surface of the penis).

A child of doubtful sex at birth is usually one or other of these last two: the sex chromatin test distinguishes reliably between them.

(e) **Testicular feminisation** is an interesting though rare form of intersex in which there is also apparently a defect of male hormone metabolism which affects target organs rather than Leydig cells: the effect is one of externally complete feminisation, though the patients are XY and possess (undescended) testes. The condition results from a defect of a gene on the X chromosome, heterozygous females acting as asymptomatic carriers.

Tumours of the male reproductive organs

Tumours are much less common than they are in the female genital tract. The following is a summary of the chief types.

Penis

Papillomas may be sessile or pedunculated, reddish lesions, sometimes of considerable size, covering the coronal sulcus and prepuce. These are condylomata acuminata, similar to the commoner vulval growths, and caused by a virus; they are reactive lesions, probably not true tumours (the distinction is not always easy) and may involute rapidly. Giant forms may occur; these are only rarely malignant, but have sometimes been misdiagnosed as squamous carcinoma. The penis is a site of precancerous lesions including Bowen's disease, and a rare variety of uncertain status known as *Queyrat's erythroplasia*, an irregular hyperkeratotic overgrowth with much chronic inflammatory infiltration of the dermis.

Squamous carcinoma is the least rare malignant growth and it usually originates from the glans or prepuce. As in other sites, it varies from an indurated, fissured, ulcerating nodule to a massive fungating cauliflower type of growth. It is an uncommon tumour, occurring mainly in non-circumcised men. Among peoples practising ritual circumcision within a few days of birth, penile carcinoma is virtually unknown, but when circumcision is delayed until about puberty, as in Moslems, the incidence of penile carcinoma is only partly reduced. Apart from this factor, the strong geographical and social-class variations are probably largely related to standards of cleanliness. The smegma which accumulates beneath the prepuce is probably also a factor. *Pigmented naevi* and *malignant melanomas* occur on penile skin; they present the usual features (pp. 1007–14).

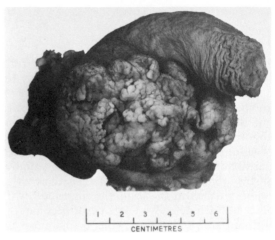

Fig. 23.5 Squamous carcinoma of the scrotum showing ulcerated papillary growth.

Scrotum

In certain occupations, the rugose scrotal skin is prone to retain dirt, and if this is carcinogenic, precancerous papillomas and ultimately squamous carcinoma are apt to develop.

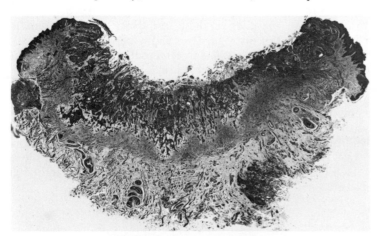

Fig. 23.6 Squamous carcinoma of the scrotum in a foreman in a sheep-dip works who was exposed to powdered arsenic trioxide and failed to wear the prescribed protective clothing. A typical large ulcerated lesion. × 5.

Examples were formerly encountered in the classical chimney sweeps' cancer of the scrotum (Fig. 10.3, p. 255), in the scrotal cancer of machine-tool operators, gas-retort workers and men handling arsenic (Figs. 23.5 and 23.6). Precautions to prevent soiling of the scrotal skin with carcinogenic chemicals have greatly reduced the incidence of the condition, but it still occurs.

Testis

Tumours of the testis are not very common— well under 1% of all cancer deaths, and less than a tenth of the death rate from ovarian tumours. But their unusual peak incidence in early adult life, when they are responsible for one-seventh of all cancer deaths in males in Britain, enhances their importance: the spectacular results of early diagnosis and treatment of the commonest form (seminoma) and the many controversies concerning them also add to their interest.

Classification is much disputed: we use here the Testicular Tumour Panel's version (Collins and Pugh, 1964). The commoner types are *seminoma* (40%), *teratoma* (32%), combined seminoma and teratoma (14%) and *lymphoma* (7%).

Seminoma

This is the commonest malignant tumour of the testis. It occurs particularly in youngish men, with a peak in the thirties, and has a relatively high incidence in maldescended testes, including those in hermaphroditism. The tumour is rounded, has often destroyed the whole testis by the time of removal, and has a white, homogeneous, 'potato-like' cut surface (Fig. 23.8a). It is composed of rounded cells, usually large, which are arranged in sheets with comparatively little stroma, or in smaller groups separated by stroma: the cells may have indistinct margins or may appear to be separate from one another due to a shrinkage artefact. In most cases, the tumour is focally or diffusely infiltrated with lymphocytes (Fig. 23.7). There is some evidence that heavy lymphocytic infiltration improves the prognosis. A granulomatous sarcoid-like reaction is not uncommon. The tumour grows along the spermatic

cord, and metastases frequently occur in the para-aortic lymph nodes. The cells are exceptionally sensitive to radiotherapy, and cure occurs in about 90% of cases without obvious spread beyond the testis, and in over 50% of patients with lymphatic and/or blood spread.

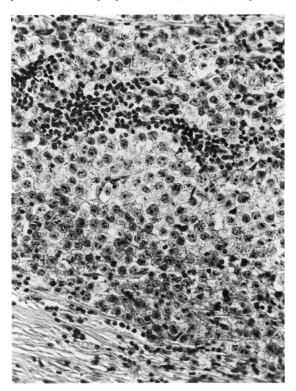

Fig. 23.7 Seminoma of testis. The tumour consists of large round cells with vesicular nuclei. Note also the lymphocytic infiltration. × 210.

Survival is frequent even in cases with lung metastases. If the tumour has not recurred within two years of treatment, it is unlikely to do so.

Teratoma

A general account of these tumours has been given on p. 305. In the testis, they are a little less frequent than seminomas, much more malignant and resistant to treatment (3 year survival about 40%) and occur rather earlier in life (peak age in the twenties, a few cases being seen in early infancy).

They are much more variable in naked-eye appearance than seminomas, the anaplastic ones looking like any anaplastic tumour (Fig.

23.8*b*) but the better differentiated showing signs of the variation in tissues present, most often in the presence of cysts (Fig. 23.8*c*). Histologically they are equally variable (Fig. 23.9). A very few show the same diversity of well-differentiated tissues as the ovarian dermoids (though even these are practically never wholly benign), and some are entirely anaplastic. The

phoblastic tissue are not rare. Gonadotrophic hormone is usually present in the urine in such cases, but it is also present (though usually in lesser amounts) in other teratomas and even in seminomas: the reason for this is not known.

Other elements in the developing ovum which do not form part of the embryo proper,

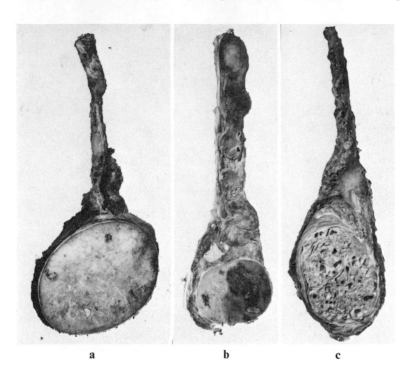

a   b   c

Fig. 23.8 Tumours of the testis. **a** Seminoma: typical 'potato' appearance. × 0·7. **b** Poorly differentiated teratoma; haemorrhagic tumour. × 0·5. **c** Unusually well-differentiated teratoma (but still malignant): multiple cysts. × 0·5.

majority lie between these extremes, showing a variety of tissues, none of which is well enough differentiated for easy identification: often, for instance, they look like a carcinoma (or carcinoma of two or three types) in a sarcomatous stroma. The teratomatous nature of the more anaplastic of these tumours is not obvious, and they have often been treated as a separate group under various names (*embryonal carcinoma* the commonest): but it is increasingly accepted that the whole group has a unity in which no sharp lines of distinction can be drawn. In practice, however, it is of course helpful to distinguish degrees of differentiation, for it affects prognosis.

Trophoblastic   elements.   Choriocarcinoma forms a principal element in a few testicular teratomas (prognosis is particularly bad in these cases), and lesser amounts of tro-

especially of the yolk sac, have been recognised with more or less certainty in teratomas, usually accompanying a high level of malignancy.

The relation of teratoma and seminoma remains uncertain. Indications that a relationship does exist include the following: (*a*) they often occur together (14% of testicular tumours: the mixed tumours have an intermediate behaviour); (*b*) they occur at the same sites, if one accepts the ovarian dysgerminoma as equivalent to a seminoma; (*c*) they both have raised frequency in undescended testes and intersex ovaries. Both appear to arise from the spermatogenic epithelium and probably from germ cells. Evidence for the latter is totipotence in teratomas and resemblance of the seminoma cells to spermatogonia: it is a flaw in this argument (though not a fatal one) that in the undescended testes from which such tumours

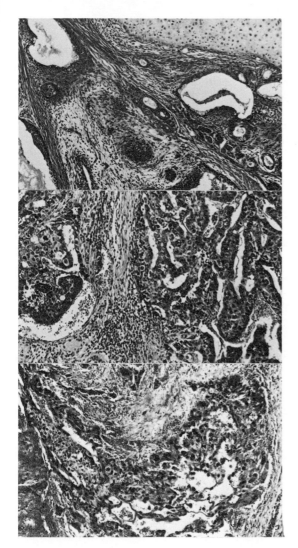

Fig. 23.9 Teratomas of testis. *Top*. Well differentiated, showing cartilage, fibrous tissue, well-formed acini and epithelial-lined spaces. × 45.
Middle. Poorly differentiated, showing papillary adenocarcinoma. × 70.
Bottom. Poorly differentiated anaplastic tumour invading the spermatic cord. × 70.

often arise germ cells are reduced in number and Sertoli cells often appear to be proliferating.

Lymphoma

Malignant lymphoma sometimes presents as a testicular tumour, and may at least appear to be localised there for some time. It is the only testicular tumour outside the seminoma–teratoma group that is at all common. It occurs chiefly in the elderly, and above the age of 65 becomes the commonest tumour at this site. Histologically the tumours are mostly of highly malignant, diffuse type, and the prognosis is even poorer than for teratomas.

Other tumours

These are all rarities, but the following deserve mention.

(a) Orchioblastoma is the least rare testicular tumour of infancy and is of importance in that its prognosis is rather better than that of the slightly rarer teratomas seen at that age. It has a papillary adenocarcinomatous structure with solid areas, the cells being fairly uniformly cuboidal with vacuoles (Fig. 23.10). It has recently been suggested that these are teratomas with predominant yolk-sac differentiation.

(b) Leydig-cell and Sertoli-cell tumours are both rare, and are both usually benign and readily recognisable histologically. They are both often

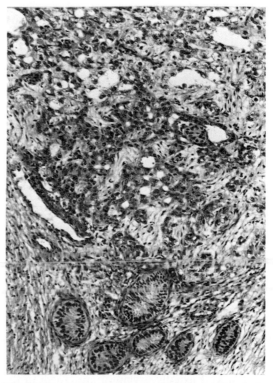

Fig. 23.10 Orchioblastoma of the testis of an infant. Testicular tubules lined by Sertoli cells lie below. The papillary structure of the tumour (*above*) is not prominent here, but the uniform cell type is well seen. × 11·5.

hormonally active, the Sertoli-cell tumours usually secreting oestrogens, and the Leydig-cell tumours surprisingly enough secreting oestrogens at least as often as androgens.

(c) The adenomatoid tumour is benign and arises usually in the epididymis.

Cysts

Cysts are very rare in the testis but relatively common in the epididymis. Commonest is the *spermatocele*. This is usually small, spherical and filled with a clear or opalescent fluid in which spermatozoa can be found. It is lined by epididymal tubular epithelium, and is usually obstructive, being a complication of the obstructive granulomas described in the previous section. Various embryonic remnants also occasionally give rise to cysts.

Distension of the tunica vaginalis with fluid (usually straw-coloured) is common (*hydrocele*). This may be secondary to infection, trauma or tumour of the testicle, but the cause is often obscure. If long-lasting, there may be fibrosis of the lining serosa, or pressure atrophy of the testis. Very much less common are cysts derived from persistent remnants of the processus vaginalis, which may occasionally communicate with the abdominal cavity. Distension of the tunica vaginalis with blood (*haematocele*) is often traumatic but also commonly of uncertain cause. Organisation of blood clot may produce a thickened mass round the testicle, which can imitate a tumour but can also obscure its presence.

Prostate

Benign nodular hyperplasia

This is conveniently considered here, though it is not strictly a tumour, but corresponds to such conditions as nodular goitre and cystic hyperplasia of the breast in which there is irregular overgrowth of many areas of an organ with obvious enlargement, but a lack of the progressive proliferation of single areas that marks the true tumour. This condition is so common in minor and usually asymptomatic form in the elderly as to suggest that it is only an exaggeration of a normal ageing process. In older men there is a tendency to increase in size of the central, peri-urethral glands of the prostate at the expense of those at the periphery, and it is this process that appears to be exaggerated.

There is some evidence that these central glands are stimulated by oestrogens, and the peripheral glands by androgens; hence the drop in androgens in old age, by altering the androgen/oestrogen ratio, might account for the enlargement. But this is far from solidly established. There is, for instance, no good clinical evidence that treatment with androgens prevents, or that treatment with oestrogens promotes, prostatic enlargement, and animal experiments are often contradictory.

The mass of tissue that a surgeon removes by a standard 'prostatectomy' consists almost entirely of the central glands, the remaining

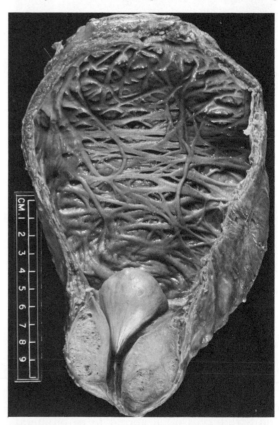

Fig. 23.11 Benign nodular hyperplasia of prostate. The 'middle lobe' is prominent, but the main mass is on each side of the urethra ('lateral lobes'). The compressed peripheral part of the prostate can just be detected as greyer areas in places. Though the urethra is not narrowed, the dilated bladder with prominent muscle bundles gives clear evidence of obstruction. × 0·5.

peripheral tissue being flattened against the capsule and left behind. The mass so removed varies in size, but is rarely less than 30 g, is usually between 50 and 100 g and is not often over 200 g, though 800 g has been recorded. The mass usually has its greatest bulk on each side of the urethra (so-called 'lateral lobes') but in many cases there is a special enlargement of glands just behind the urethra to form a rounded lump (the so-called 'middle lobe') which projects into the bladder just behind the urethral orifice (Fig. 23.11). The tissue is usually firm, and its cut surface is white and more or less nodular. It may occasionally show areas of inflammation, abscess formation, or infarction.

Effects. Though the urethra is much distorted, it is rarely narrowed, and the effects on bladder function are rather the result of a complex disturbance of the bladder sphincter

mechanism by the obtruding prostate than simple obstruction. The pathological consequences, however, are very similar to those of obstruction. These are followed by hypertrophy and dilatation of the bladder, and dilatation of ureters (hydro-ureter) and renal pelves (hydronephrosis). If unrelieved, these changes may impair renal function and chronic uraemia may result. Pyogenic infection of the urinary tract, including pyelonephritis, is often superadded (p. 791), and spread of infection to the prostate may precipitate acute retention, as may also partial infarction of the enlarged gland.

Microscopically there is usually increase of both the glandular elements and stroma (Fig. 23.12). The glands are arranged chiefly in acini lined by columnar cells, and not infrequently

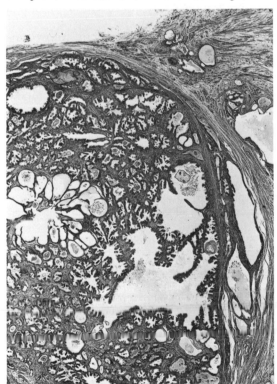

Fig. 23.12 Benign nodular hyperplasia of the prostate. The large adenoma-like nodule that fills most of the field shows predominantly glandular overgrowth, with small cysts. In the less actively growing area at top right, glands are hyperplastic but the stroma, with numerous smooth muscle fibres, is much more prominent. × 10.

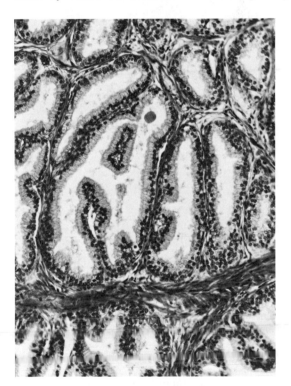

Fig. 23.13 Section of enlarged prostate, showing hyperplasia of the glandular epithelium. × 130.

show small papilliform ingrowths into the lumina (Fig. 23.13). Often some of the acini are dilated and occasionally small cysts are formed; small concentric concretions or 'corpora amylacea' are common. The connective tissue stroma usually contains a substantial proportion of smooth muscle fibres. Muscle hyperplasia is most marked in the earlier stages of the process, and muscle may form a very large proportion of smaller lesions. While the gland acini are usually lined by a single epithelial layer, there may be small foci of more active hyperplasia with the formation of masses of cells, and a cribriform pattern may develop. The relationship between prostatic hyperplasia and carcinoma is considered below.

Carcinoma of the prostate

This is one of the commoner cancers in older men; sometimes it arises in a hyperplastic prostate, but as some degree of hyperplasia is very

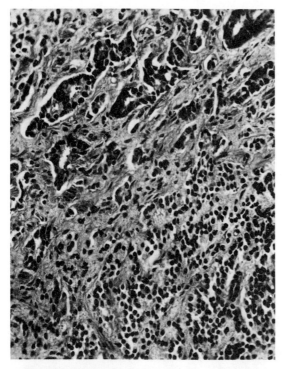

Fig. 23.14 Carcinoma of prostate gland. The growth is of scirrhous type, consisting of poorly formed micro-acini (above) with transitions to a fine permeation of the tissue by rows of small darkly stained cells (below). × 225.

common in old men, the significance of the association is doubtful. Moreover, carcinoma arises most often in the peripheral, i.e. subcapsular, part of the gland, especially on its posterior aspect, in contrast to the predominantly peri-urethral origin of hyperplasia. The tumour

causes urethral obstruction and often pain: it produces general induration of the gland without always causing enlargement, together with adhesions between the gland and its capsule. At first confined to the prostate, the tumour later extends into the neighbouring tissues. The growth may be of scirrhous micro-acinar carcinoma (Fig. 23.14) or a more cellular florid adenocarcinoma. Carcinoma of the prostate has a tendency to give rise to multiple secondary tumours in the bones, often with considerable bony thickening around them—osteosclerosis (p. 836). These osseous metastases may occur without the presence of secondary tumours in the lungs or other organs, and (especially when affecting chiefly the bodies of the lower vertebrae, as they often do) may be due to retrograde venous spread along the veins of Batson, which join the prostatic plexus to the vertebral venous system. Prostatic cancer can often be suppressed by oestrogen therapy for a considerable time.

Acid phosphatase can be demonstrated biochemically in most of these tumours. It is very often liberated from them into the blood, especially once the tumour has metastasised, and its demonstration in the blood is an important means of diagnosis. This should not be confused with the rise in *alkaline phosphatase* which may also occur if bone metastases are extensive, being then a non-specific reaction of the affected bone.

'Latent' carcinoma. Small foci of subcapsular epithelial overgrowth presenting all the histological features of cancer, including local perineural lymphatic invasion, are found with increasing frequency as age advances; they are present in the majority of otherwise normal prostates in men over the age of 90 years. The incidence is lower in glands removed because of benign enlargement, perhaps because the compressed peripheral portion is often left behind in surgical enucleation. The significance of these foci is uncertain, but it is quite apparent from their frequency, and from the relative infrequency of more extensive prostatic cancer, that these small focal 'cancers' are in a latent state, and seldom extend sufficiently to cause symptoms or death. Their presence in a surgically-removed hypertrophic prostate poses a problem to pathologist and surgeon, but for clinical purposes it is probably correct to regard as carcinoma only those tumours which have invaded the capsule of the gland.

Adenomatous nodules—single or multiple—occur in the prostate but are usually part of the picture of prostatic hypertrophy. *Sarcoma* of the prostate is rare but is occasionally observed in children, being then usually a rhabdomyosarcoma.

II. Female Reproductive System

Few regions of the body are so prone to undergo pathological change as the female genital tract. Only a brief account of the more important disorders can be given here, and for detailed information textbooks of gynaecological pathology should be consulted.

The Endometrium

Removal of pieces of endometrium by curettage is a simple procedure of great diagnostic value, and most pathologists acquire considerable experience in the histology of the normal cyclical changes and various abnormalities. Curettage is sometimes also of therapeutic value, for it may cure excessive 'functional' bleeding of uncertain cause.

Before describing the important abnormalities of the endometrium it seems appropriate to give an outline of the normal cyclical changes.

The morphological changes in the endometrial cycle

Light-microscopic changes

The changes which occur in the endometrium during the normal menstrual cycle are of great importance in the study of menstrual disorders. It is essential to be familiar with the morphological appearances in the different phases of the normal cycle; accurate details of the clinical history and menstrual dates are important in assessing the microscopic appearances.

The endometrial cycle consists of three phases—menstrual, proliferative and secretory. Following menstruation, a new Graafian follicle develops and its granulosa cells produce oestrogens which stimulate regeneration of the endometrium producing first a thin surface epithelium, short straight glands and a compact

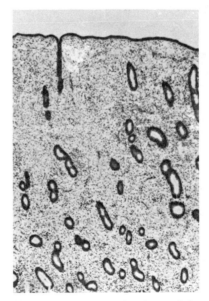

Fig. 23.15 Section of endometrial curetting on 10th day of the cycle. Proliferative phase. The glands are relatively small. × 50.

stroma of spindle cells lying parallel to the surface (Fig. 23.15). Mitotic activity is present in both the endometrial glands and the stroma. This **proliferative phase** continues to develop until ovulation occurs about the 12–14th day, the surface epithelium becomes columnar and the glands tortuous (Fig. 23.16). **The secretory phase** begins after ovulation and is brought about by the combined action of oestrogenic

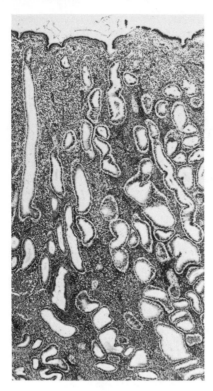

Fig. 23.16 Fifteenth day of cycle. The glands have increased in size and basal vacuolation of glandular epithelium is apparent. × 50.

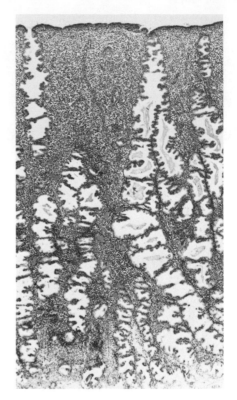

Fig. 23.17 Twenty-fifth day of cycle, showing the secretory phase. × 50.

and progestational hormones produced by the corpus luteum. It is recognised first by basal vacuolation in the gland cells and increasing glandular tortuosity sometimes referred to as the *ovulatory phase*; later, secretion appears in the lumina of the glands which develop papillary ingrowths (Fig. 23.17), and the stroma becomes oedematous. In the premenstrual phase the interstitial cells show a predecidual reaction, their cytoplasm becoming swollen, eosinophilic and appearing continuous, while neutrophil polymorphs and granular cells* appear in the superficial layer. These premenstrual changes take place in the functional layer; i.e. the superficial (luminal) two-thirds. When menstruation ensues, this layer disintegrates and the deeper basal layer remains to give rise to the regenerative phase of the next cycle.

Electron-microscopic changes

Cyclical changes in appearance have been demonstrated at an ultrastructural level by elec-

tron microscopy in the cells of both the endometrial glands and the stroma.

Glandular cells. *The proliferative phase* is characterised by the development of organelles required by the cell later in the cycle. These include well developed rough endoplasmic reticulum, polysomes, smooth endoplasmic reticulum associated at the luminal portion of the cell with the Golgi apparatus, mitochondria scattered throughout the cell, prominent lysosomes and occasionally subnuclear deposits of glycogen.

The ovulatory phase consistently shows abundant glycogen (initially subnuclear), giant digitate mitochondria and the nuclear channel system: these features indicate 'switch on' of specific portions of the genome. Free polysomes disappear and the Golgi apparatus becomes dilated, with consequent apical vacuolation.

The secretory phase is characterised by the accumulation of large amounts of glycogen and glycoproteins, its transference within the cell

---

* These cells are sometimes termed 'granulocytes', but this is obviously unacceptable as the term is already widely used for polymorphonuclear leukocytes.

and release into the glandular lumen. Towards the end of this phase changes of premenstrual involution develop: the giant mitochondria disappear, the Golgi apparatus and rough endoplasmic reticulum become less prominent, the smooth endoplasmic reticulum progressively dilates and becomes empty of secretion and giant autophagosomes appear.

Stromal cells. In the early proliferative phase these contain a largely inactive nucleus and scanty cytoplasmic organelles. The late proliferative phase shows more dispersed, active nuclear chromatin and the appearance of organelles for collagen synthesis (rough endoplasmic reticulum and Golgi apparatus) and for glycogen accumulation (smooth endoplasmic reticulum aggregated in the Golgi apparatus). These features are prominent in the *early secretory phase*. In the *late secretory phase* the stromal cells differentiate either as *decidual* or *granular cells*. Decidual cells contain a large, relatively clear nucleus and abundant cytoplasm with few organelles. Cell to cell contact is established and loss of intercellular space occurs due to the premenstrual loss of extracellular fluid. Granular cells are smaller than decidual cells and have a dense, crenated nucleus, dilated channels in the smooth endoplasmic reticulum and conspicuous granules of uncertain nature.

The effects of oral contraceptives

The use of oral contraceptive pills, consisting usually of mixtures of oestrogenic and progestational steroids, less commonly of the latter alone, interrupts the menstrual cycle and leads to unusual histological appearances in the endometrium. The glands are commonly small and poorly developed (microtubular), and the stroma abundant, but various other bizarre pictures are observed, and in some instances there is a well developed decidual reaction, a reflection of the induced state of 'pseudo-pregnancy'.

Intra-uterine contraceptive devices

The effects on the endometrium vary and depend partly on the type of device used, e.g. plastic or metal. Focal atrophy with fibrosis, infiltration of the stroma with mononuclear leukocytes and plasma cells in the absence of bacterial infection, and squamous metaplasia have all been observed, but most endometria show only slight microscopic changes.

Endometritis

Apart from gonorrhoea, acute pyogenic inflammations of the female reproductive organs are rare except for those which follow pregnancy and parturition, abortion and surgical operations. In most cases the organisms enter by the uterine cavity, and spread to other parts, though infection may occur by the bloodstream and, in the case of tuberculosis, extends from the Fallopian tubes to the endometrium.

Acute endometritis

This is due to bacterial infection following abortion or parturition. In the absence of products of conception, acute endometritis is very rare, but it occurs occasionally in infective fevers. After childbirth or abortion, retention of portions of placenta or decidua, along with lacerations of the cervix, gives an opportunity for invasion by pathogenic organisms. In addition to the usual pyococci, various bacilli of the coliform and proteus types and even clostridia, e.g. *Cl. welchii*, may be present. In some cases the changes are chiefly within the uterus, and the inflammatory process may be severe and may be accompanied by putrefaction of any retained material.

Gonorrhoea leads especially to a *cervical endometritis*, though the condition may spread to the body of the uterus and thence to the tubes. Gonococcal infection is often accompanied by a superficial interstitial metritis, and is apt to become chronic. The endometrium is, however, somewhat resistant to infections, as there is normally free drainage and the regeneration after menstrual shedding facilitates recovery.

Macroscopic appearances. There is swelling and congestion of the mucosa, desquamation of the surface epithelium, sometimes with haemorrhages, and increased secretion from the glands, mucoid from the cervix and more serous from the body. Later the discharge becomes purulent. In severe cases after abortion or parturition with retained gestational fragments, the uterus is bulky and flabby, and there is a fibrinous exudate on the surface of the mucosa, with some superficial necrosis which may be followed by ulceration. In some cases there is a spreading lymphangitis, much inflammatory oedema, and suppuration; spread to the peritoneum readily occurs and peritonitis follows. Acute endometritis may become chronic, and persist until all gestational products have been removed.

Complications. Inflammatory conditions within the uterus are apt to extend into the uterine wall—*myometritis*—and may spread by the lymphatics to the pelvic connective tissue—*parametritis*. The inflammatory exudate may be serous, fibrinous, or even purulent. Some bacteria, including gonococci, may spread along the Fallopian tubes, causing salpingitis and sometimes peritonitis and oöphoritis.

Infection of the placental site, especially by *Staphylococcus aureus*, may lead to septic thrombosis of the veins locally, and from these, thrombosis may spread to the iliac veins, resulting in *phlegmasia alba dolens* or 'white leg'. The thrombi may undergo suppurative softening, and the liberation of septic emboli may cause pyaemia. In cases of infection with haemolytic streptococci, fatal septicaemia may occur. Less acute cases with spreading thrombosis may be caused by anaerobic streptococci. These various infections, singly and combined, were formerly very common and were grouped together as '*puerperal fever*'. After recovery, permanent residual effects were common—thickening of the pelvic connective tissue, peritoneal adhesions, chronic endometritis, subinvolution and displacements of the uterus.

Chronic endometritis

The term 'chronic endometritis' is now limited to a condition in which there is indisputable evidence of a chronic inflammatory process in the endometrium; this is less easily defined than in most organs owing to the normal cyclical changes and also those following disordered endocrine control. In some cases it follows on an acute attack. In many others, however, it is chronic from the onset, the result of mild infection following either pregnancy or gonorrhoea. It is apt to occur along with subinvolution of the uterus after parturition, the size of the uterine cavity being then increased.

True chronic endometritis is characterised by thickening and infiltration of the stroma by chronic inflammatory cells along with failure of the glands to respond to hormonal stimulation (Fig. 23.18). The normal cyclical changes fail to develop and are less advanced than the dates of the menstrual cycle indicate. The presence of numerous plasma cells in the endometrium is diagnostic, as these cells do not normally occur at any stage of the cycle, whereas polymorphonuclear leukocytes are invariably present in the early menstrual breakdown of the endometrium and foci of lymphocytes may also occur

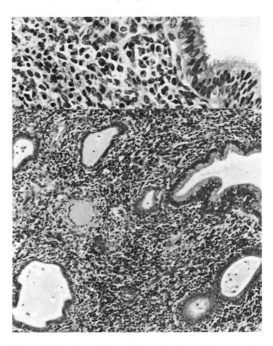

Fig. 23.18 Chronic endometritis. The glands are irregular and there is increased cellularity of the stroma. × 100. The upper strip shows plasma cell infiltration of the stroma. × 250.

normally. In severe and longstanding cases the endometrial stroma may become spindle-celled and almost fibrous, and the glands are then much atrophied. In all such cases the tissue removed by curettage should be carefully examined for products of conception such as degenerate chorionic villi. The possibility of endometrial tuberculosis should also be borne in mind, as this infection is still commoner than is generally realised.

Pyometra. The cervical canal may be obstructed by a tumour or polyp or by cicatricial stenosis following treatment of cervical cancer by irradiation, or occasionally occurs spontaneously in elderly women. Retention of fluid and infection may then result in the accumulation of pus (*pyometra*). This occurs in 4% of cases of cervical carcinoma, and 70% of cases of pyometra are associated with uterine malignancy.

Macroscopic appearance. The uterus is usually distended with pus and the wall is correspondingly thin. In longstanding cases the cavity is lined by a rough pyogenic membrane which may simulate extensive carcinoma. In cases of tuberculous endometritis with cervical stenosis the cavity may be filled with caseous pus.

Microscopically the appearances depend on the duration and severity of the process. There may be marked leukocytic infiltration with atrophy of the endometrium, or even loss and replacement by granulation tissue.

Complications. The condition can be remarkably silent, but eventually rupture may occur, either into the vagina, or rarely into the peritoneum, which is likely to be fatal. Extension to the tubes, producing pyosalpinx, is uncommon.

Tuberculous endometritis is usually due to descending infection from a tuberculous Fallopian tube (p. 909). The bacilli settle in the endometrium, giving rise to microscopic tubercles. It is still seen in uterine curettings from a very small proportion of patients complaining of sterility. It is usually accompanied by non-specific changes such as polymorphonuclear leukocytes in the gland acini and plasma cells in the stroma. During reproductive life, most of the tubercles are shed at menstruation, and extensive caseation is rare. Occasionally, however, obstruction of the lumen may occur, and an accumulation of caseous material may then form. Rarely infection may spread from the uterus to the vagina, and ulcers may be produced in its wall. Tuberculosis of the cervix, which is much rarer than that of the body, may be accompanied by papillary outgrowths. Haematogenous infection of the endometrium occurs in acute miliary tuberculosis.

Endometrial hyperplasia

(a) Cystic glandular hyperplasia

This is a pathological condition of the endometrium associated with irregular uterine hae-morrhage resulting from disordered endocrine control, known clinically as *metropathia haemorrhagica*. It may occur at any time in child-bearing life but its maximum incidence is at about the age of forty; it may also occur, with or without focal adenomatous changes, in the menorrhagia of the pubertal period, before ovulation is fully established. It occasionally occurs in the postmenopausal period, in association with an oestrogen-secreting ovarian tumour, and may also be produced by prolonged oestrogen therapy.

Macroscopic appearances. The hyperplastic endometrium forms a thick, soft and vascular layer with an irregular surface, often showing polypoid projections and sometimes exceeding 10 mm in thickness.

Microscopic appearances. In the deeper parts there is a general hyperplasia of the uterine glands and at a higher level many of these show dilatation with a tendency to cyst formation (Fig. 23.19) and epithelial ingrowths. In the

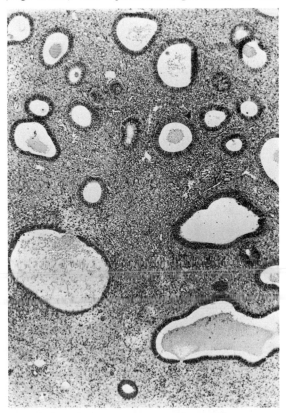

Fig. 23.19 Cystic hyperplasia of the endometrium, showing dilatation of glands and early cyst formation.

superficial parts there are patches of degeneration and necrosis, along with hyaline thromboses in thin-walled vessels and haemorrhage. The interstitial tissue generally is cellular, vascular and oedematous and there may be haemorrhages.

Aetiology. These changes in the endometrium are the result of ovarian dysfunction. Usually a single follicular cyst or several cysts are present in one or both ovaries, and as a rule corpora lutea are absent. The essential factor is failure of ovulation so that the Graafian follicle persists for weeks or months and frequently becomes cystic. It secretes oestrogen, and since there is no corpus luteum to secrete progesterone the phase of endometrial proliferation continues and becomes exaggerated and there is amenorrhoea. Eventually the cystic or abnormal follicle involutes and the supply of oestrogen ceases: areas of localised necrosis and breakdown are then responsible for the irregular bleeding so common in this disorder. In some cases bleeding is severe, and this condition is a common cause of iron-deficiency anaemia. The same changes in the endometrium are brought about also by an ovarian granulosa-cell tumour, which produces oestrogens in excess. In fact, when this endometrial lesion with bleeding occurs after the menopause it should raise the suspicion of this tumour provided that the patient is not on oestrogen therapy.

(b) Atypical or adenomatous hyperplasia

This occurs typically in women approaching the menopause, and is associated with irregular or prolonged menstrual bleeding. Microscopy of the endometrium shows focal areas with increased numbers of glands having tall columnar epithelium and pale eosinophilic cytoplasm. Mitotic activity is brisk and stratification of the glandular epithelium with intraluminal tufting is seen. The stroma is reduced and in places the glands have a 'back to back' arrangement. This picture may be present in an endometrium also showing cystic glandular hyperplasia. Atypical hyperplasia in a diagnostic curettage should be regarded with suspicion, for both prospective and retrospective studies have demonstrated a significant correlation between this appearance and the subsequent development of endometrial carcinoma.

Endometrial polyp

This common lesion is a local proliferation of the endometrium measuring up to 3 cm in diameter (but usually much less), which projects into the uterine cavity and may be sessile or pedunculated. When sessile, it often merges into the adjacent endometrium and resembles a hyperplastic area rather than a discrete tumour. When pedunculated, it may project through the os and acquire a squamous lining, although these features are more typical of endocervical

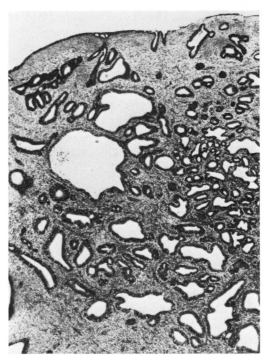

Fig. 23.20 Benign endometrial polyp showing numerous glands, some of which are dilated, in a fibro-cellular stroma. × 25.

polyps (p. 904). The surface is usually smooth and microscopy shows endometrial-type glands which vary in number and size, some often being cystic, set in a fibrocellular stroma (Fig. 23.20).

Endometrial polyps are associated with irregular or excessive menstrual haemorrhage, less commonly with infection and discharge: they occur most commonly towards the menopause and may be multiple. Indeed cystic glandular hyperplasia not uncommonly produces a polypoid endometrium.

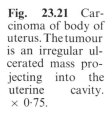

Fig. 23.21 Carcinoma of body of uterus. The tumour is an irregular ulcerated mass projecting into the uterine cavity. × 0·75.

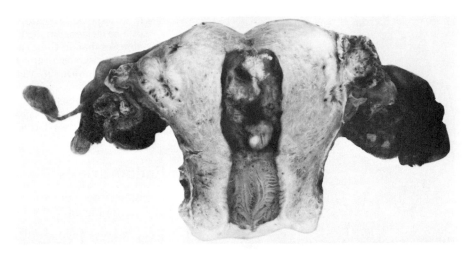

Malignant endometrial tumours

Endometrial carcinoma

Cancer arising from the endometrium is usually an adenocarcinoma but in about 20% squamous metaplasia is also present; in such cases the tumour is termed an adenoacanthoma, but its behaviour is identical with that of endometrial carcinoma in general.

Aetiology. There is increasing evidence that nulliparous women with hypertension, obesity and abnormal bleeding at the menopause are more prone to develop endometrial cancer. An increased frequency has also been reported in patients who have received prolonged oestrogen stimulation either therapeutically or from a feminising ovarian tumour, and this suggests that endocrine dysfunction may play a part in the aetiology of endometrial cancer in general. The presence of focal atypical adenomatous hyperplasia in the endometrium in relation to frank carcinoma also supports this view, and while the evidence is inconclusive, focal adenomatous hyperplasia in a diagnostic curettage should be regarded with suspicion. Endometrial carcinoma is infrequent in women under the age of 45 years and when it occurs in the younger patient some chronic endocrine disturbance has commonly been present; in about 20% of such cases the ovaries have a smooth fibrotic surface beneath which multiple small follicular cysts are present.

Macroscopic appearances. Cancer of the endometrium may be a localised sessile tumour with a broad base, but may become polypoidal, or a diffuse growth involving a large area of the endometrial cavity (Fig. 23.21). The uterus is frequently enlarged but its shape is usually preserved. The tumour invades the uterine muscle and ulceration and infection are inevitable in the later stages. Necrosis and infection in the presence of cervical obstruction results in pyometra. The tumour may extend to the cervix or ovaries. Vaginal metastases occur by lymphatic or venous dissemination. Lymphatic spread via the broad ligament to the para-aortic lymph nodes, or via the lymphatic channels in the round ligaments to the inguinal nodes, occurs in advanced cases.

Microscopic appearances. Cancer of the endometrium is usually a moderately well differentiated adenocarcinoma but more solid areas and a cribriform gland pattern are frequently seen, or the structure may be papillary. An extremely aberrant type of growth is not uncommon, with many enormous multinucleated cells and multipolar mitoses. In *adenoacanthoma*, the adenocarcinoma is well differentiated and the superimposed squamous elements can be readily distinguished (Fig. 23.22), sometimes intimately mingled with the main tumour, sometimes as separate foci; this feature does not influence prognosis or treatment. Carcinoma of the endometrium has a good prognosis if it is well-differentiated and treated while still apparently confined to the body of the uterus: in such cases, over 95% 5-year cure rates have been reported. Even with poorly differentiated tumours or extension to the cervix, the rate is 80% or so. Total

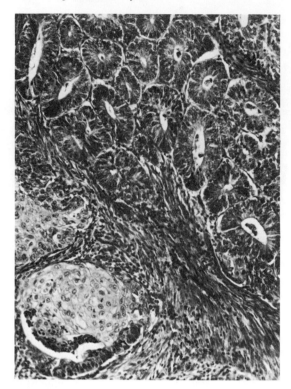

Fig. 23.22 Adenocarcinoma of body of uterus, showing squamous foci (adeno-acanthoma). × 130.

hysterectomy is commonly performed, but there is evidence that radiotherapy is a valuable adjunct.

Endometrial sarcoma and mixed tumours

Endometrial sarcoma is a rare cause of uterine haemorrhage. It rises from the stromal cells, usually in post-menopausal women, and is sometimes called *stromal sarcoma*. It forms polypoid projections and invades the myometrium. The microscopic appearances vary from a resemblance to normal stroma, but with numerous mitoses, to anaplasia and pleomorphism. It tends to metastasise early and has a poor prognosis.

Stromal sarcoma must be distinguished from *stromal endometriosis*, which consists of foci of endometrial stroma of normal appearance in the myometrium. Rarely the stroma grows along lymphatics ('*endolymphatic stromal myosis*') in the myometrium.

Mixed mesodermal tumour also originates from the endometrium usually post-menopausally, and causes haemorrhage and uterine enlargement. It consists of a mixture of adenocarcinoma and sarcoma, the latter sometimes differentiating into osteo-, chondro- or rhabdomyo-sarcomatous elements. It is usually fatal,

due to widespread haematogenous metastases, within a year. The incidence in the USA appears to be higher in Negresses than in Caucasian women.

Rhabdomyosarcoma arising in the cervix uteri or vagina is another rare tumour which can occur at any age, including early childhood. It consists of polypoid projections ('*sarcoma botryoides*'); microscopically it is pleomorphic, and appears to be related to mixed mesodermal tumour.

Endometriosis

Endometriosis may be defined as the presence of functioning endometrial tissue in areas other

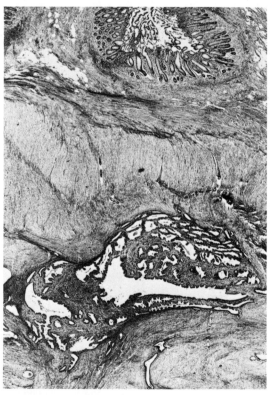

Fig. 23.23 Endometriosis of the appendix and caecum. A focus of endometrial glands and stroma showing cyclical changes is present in the muscular coat of the caecum close to the appendix. × 12.

than the uterine mucosa. The usual sites of pelvic endometriosis are the ovaries, peritoneum and the pouch of Douglas, uterosacral ligaments and serosa of the rectosigmoid region. Endometriosis is also found in the appendix (Fig. 23.23), ileum, rectum, bladder, umbilicus, laparotomy scars and lower genital tract. A few cases are recorded where endo-metrial tissue was found in such unlikely sites as the lung, pleura, breast, arm and thigh.

A feature of endometriosis is that its continued growth depends on oestrogen. It also has the rare characteristic of benign invasion of the supporting tissues.

Aetiology. The histogenesis of endometriosis is unsettled and because of the widely separated sites on which it has been noted, no simple explanation will cover all examples.

Sampson elaborated the theory that during menstruation endometrial fragments are transported via the Fallopian tubes to the pelvic peritoneum and the ovaries with subsequent implantation. There is good evidence that at least some of the desquamated endometrium at menstruation is viable and capable of growth.

Endometriosis is readily induced by implantation of endometrium in a laparotomy wound at Caesarean section or other operations in which the endometrial cavity has been opened, a fact which supports the transplantation theory.

Endometriosis in various unlikely sites (see above) is difficult to explain by haematogenous or lymphatic transport of endometrial fragments, and metaplasia of various tissue cells seems less improbable. The observation that in extra-uterine pregnancy the pelvic mesenchymal tissues may exhibit a pronounced decidual reaction supports this possibility.

Macroscopic appearances. In the pelvis, small puckered, bluish nodules may be found on the serosa of the bowel, uterosacral ligaments, pelvic peritoneum, or ovarian surfaces. Commonly the ovaries are grossly enlarged by cysts containing dark brown 'tarry' material due to haemorrhage at the time of menstruation. These cysts are at first smooth walled and brownish-blue and they are liable to bring about adherence of the ovary to the broad ligament or distal colon. Later they become much distorted by dense fibrosis resulting from organisation of the extravasated blood.

Microscopic appearances. Endometrial glands and stroma are usually evident at first but haemorrhage and resultant pressure atrophy may obscure the ectopic endometrium. The repeatedly shed blood is broken down to haemosiderin and lipids which accumulate in macrophages having a superficial resemblance

to lutein cells; recognition of these may be enough to give a presumptive diagnosis of endometriosis.

Clinical features. The most characteristic symptom is progressive pelvic pain beginning with or just before menstruation, but in 20% of cases pelvic endometriosis is symptomless and is an incidental finding at operation or necropsy. The symptoms of endometriosis improve during pregnancy and during amenorrhoea induced by progestational steroids. Frequent pregnancies, starting in relative youth, appear to prevent the development of endometriosis.

Adenomyoma and adenomyosis

This is a condition in which there is associated growth of endometrial glands and stroma together with non-striped muscle, within the wall of the uterus.

Macroscopic appearances. Adenomyoma may be diffuse or circumscribed. Neither type is a true neoplasm. The *diffuse type* occurs chiefly in the inner part of the myometrium, sometimes in one part, sometimes all round the cavity, the

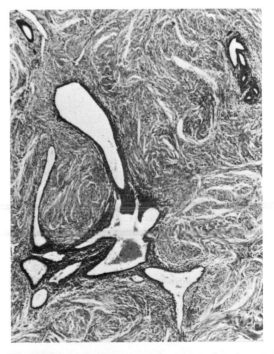

Fig. 23.24 Adenomyoma of uterus, showing multiple foci of endometrial glands and stroma deep in the uterine wall. × 40.

whole uterus being enlarged. The cut surface has the pale, whorled appearance of a uterine leiomyoma, but containing small translucent areas and spaces which represent the glandular tissue. The outer part of the uterine wall is usually unaffected, but the line of the demarcation is not so sharp as in the case of an ordinary myoma. In the *circumscribed type* multiple nodular masses form submucous or subperitoneal projections, especially from the posterior wall. The nodules may become large and develop cystic spaces containing altered blood, due to cyclical changes and menstrual bleeding of the ectopic endometrial tissue. Usually, however, the endometrium is of the basal pattern and fails to undergo cyclical changes. The diffuse type is the commoner and has been called 'adenomyosis', though it appears to be of similar nature to the circumscribed type.

Microscopic appearances. The glandular tissue is seen to be composed of branching slits with tubular and acinar structures, lined with columnar epithelium, and usually surrounded by a cellular tissue like endometrial stroma (Fig. 23.24). The continuity of the glandular tissue with the lining epithelium of the uterus has been established by means of serial sections.

During pregnancy, decidual cells have been observed to have developed in the stroma around the acini.

Myometrium

The myometrium may become infected in acute endometritis, particularly following abortion or childbirth and, as described above, endometriosis may affect the uterine wall (adenomyosis). However, the commonest lesion of the myometrium is the leiomyoma.

Leiomyoma (myoma)

This tumour forms a circumscribed growth of smooth muscle along with supporting connective tissue, which may be abundant—it is thus often incorrectly called a fibromyoma or a 'fibroid'. Uterine myomas are among the commonest of tumours, being said to occur in more than 15% of women over 35, but they often remain quite small and are usually symptomless.

Macroscopic appearances. The tumours may be single or multiple, and one is often much larger than the others. A myoma usually starts in the substance of the wall—it is then described as **interstitial** or **intramural**. But as enlargement takes place it expands either into the cavity of the uterus—**submucous** type—or outwards under the peritoneum—**subserous** type. It may also originate in either of these sites. A submucous myoma expands the uterine cavity, and may project through the os as a pedunculated mass (Fig. 23.25); occasionally it becomes expelled by the hypertrophied uterus. It tends to become infected and ulcerated: severe haemor-rhage is a common result, and if the tumour is not removed, marked anaemia may follow. A subserous myoma passes outwards as it grows, and often comes to have a distinct pedicle. It may reach 10 kg in weight, and may cause great abdominal distension. Also, a superficial

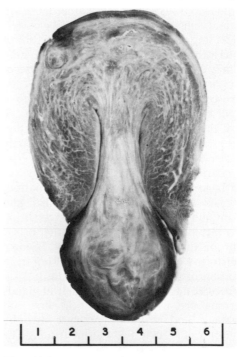

Fig. 23.25 Large submucous myoma of uterus projecting through the cervix. × 0·75.

myoma may pass between, and open out, the layers of the broad ligament.

A myoma is usually of firm and somewhat elastic consistency, with a regular and well-defined outline; the cut surface is, as a rule, paler than the uterine wall and shows a peculiar concentric or whorled marking produced by the bundles of muscle fibres (Fig. 12.13, p. 295). Occasionally the tumour appears to have grown from multiple foci and has a nodular outline. Sometimes a myoma becomes soft and oedematous; or it may be myxomatous in part. It then feels fluctuant and may be mistaken for an ovarian cyst. Infarction also may take place from thrombosis of vessels or from twisting of the pedicle, and softening of the tissue may follow; this may be accompanied by haemorrhage into its substance—the so-called *red degeneration*, which is commoner during pregnancy, and may also occur in patients taking oral contraceptives. **At the menopause**, uterine myomas usually cease to grow, and undergo a process of fibrosis and shrinkage. The muscle cells atrophy and many disappear, while the stroma becomes hyalinised. Deposition of calcium salts often occurs in the hyaline stroma and ultimately the tumour may be changed to a hard stony mass or 'wombstone', in which the characteristic concentric markings may be distinguished. Occasionally the blood vessels in a myoma are telangiectatic, i.e. relatively large but thin-walled, or more rarely, wide lymphatic spaces are formed.

Microscopic appearances. These have already been described (Fig. 12.14, p. 296) but all degrees of cellularity are encountered between tumours composed almost entirely of interlacing bundles of smooth muscle and others in which a high proportion of fibrous stroma is present. Rarely sarcomatous change may arise in a myoma, and the presence of numerous mitotic figures in a myoma should be regarded with suspicion.

Myometrial sarcoma

This is uncommon, and possibly originates in a leiomyoma. The outlook depends on the degree of anaplasia and mitotic activity.

Sarcoma and mixed tumours of the endometrium (p. 900) invade the myometrium at an early stage.

Choriocarcinoma is described below (p. 921).

Cervix

Inflammation

The mucosa of the endocervix and its associated glands are lined by a single layer of tall columnar mucus-secreting epithelium, which at the external os changes abruptly to a stratified squamous type. Acute endocervicitis may result from infection by gonococci or other pyogenic organisms. It also frequently complicates lacerations of the cervix during childbirth, and may then become chronic with failure of the lacerations to heal, and a persistent mucopurulent discharge. In chronic endocervicitis there may be papillary outgrowths of granulation tissue lined by columnar epithelium and heavily infiltrated with inflammatory cells. The appearances must not be mistaken for papillary adenocarcinoma.

Inclusion conjunctivitis in the newborn results from infection of the mother's cervix and vagina with the TRIC agent (p. 880), acquired usually from a sexual partner suffering from non-gonococcal urethritis.

Cervical erosion

This is the term applied to a red area around the external os, spreading on to the exocervix; it is seen on histological examination to be simple replacement of the opaque squamous epithelium by transparent columnar epithelium, and is not a true erosion. It may be present at birth and is frequently noticed during pregnancy; proliferation of the mucosa probably results from stimulation by hormones. Associated mucous discharge and a tendency to become secondarily infected causes the patient to complain of symptoms associated with an erosion, notably vaginal discharge. Clinicians have been tempted to regard cervical erosion as a type of cervicitis, but it is now generally accepted that most erosions are physiological variations of normal. The delicate columnar epithelium is prone to injury and infection when it lines the exocervix, and in the process of healing it may be replaced by squamous epithelium (**'epidermidisation'**), which may also extend into and replace the epithelium of the cervical glands, producing an appearance which has sometimes been mistaken histologically for early invasive carcinomatous change. Another common result of inflammation and healing of the cervix is obstruction of glands causing the formation of small cysts around the os, known as **Nabothian follicles**. They are rarely more than 7 mm in diameter, and are filled with tenacious mucus.

Ectropion

This is an eversion of the lips of the cervix as a result of a fissure of the cervix caused by laceration at parturition. The exposed cervical mucosa is subject to bacterial invasion from the vagina and to irritation, and its columnar epithelium may change to the squamous type. There is persistent mucopurulent discharge, which may give rise to vulvar pruritus.

Cervical or mucous polyp

This is a common lesion, consisting usually of a proliferated portion of endocervical mucosa which has become pedunculated and prolapsed through the external os. Microscopically, it has a glandular pattern. It is usually grey and semi-transparent with a smooth surface, but it frequently becomes ulcerated and inflamed and attracts attention by bleeding. The surface epithelium commonly undergoes squamous metaplasia.

Premalignant changes in the cervix

The invasive stage of carcinoma of the cervix may be preceded for many years by pre-invasive stages termed **dysplasia** and **carcinoma in situ**. This carries the important implication that at least some cases of invasive cervical cancer can be prevented if these preceding changes can be detected and eliminated, and extensive cytological screening programmes have been introduced for this purpose. Dysplasia and car-

cinoma in situ are changes in the squamous epithelium usually arising at or near the squamo-columnar junction of the cervix; they have an undoubted tendency to progress to invasive carcinoma, although this does not occur in all cases. They are symptomless conditions and produce no macroscopically visible change in the cervix. The abnormality is usually first suspected from a positive cervical cytology smear (see below). An adequate 'cone' biopsy of the cervix, including the squamo-columnar junction, is required for the firm diagnosis of these conditions, which must in all cases be histological.

Dysplasia is a disorder in which the epithelial cells fail to mature adequately. In the mild form the nuclei of the cells remain immature but the cytoplasm is better differentiated. Such cells, with relatively large nuclei, are found nearer the surface of the epithelium than normally. There still remains an attempt at orderly stratification, with squames forming on the surface. Distinction between the severe form of dysplasia and carcinoma in situ is largely a matter of opinion—both are sinister findings.

Carcinoma in situ is a condition in which there is complete absence of cellular maturation and stratification, abnormal cells occupying the whole thickness of the epithelium (Fig. 23.26).

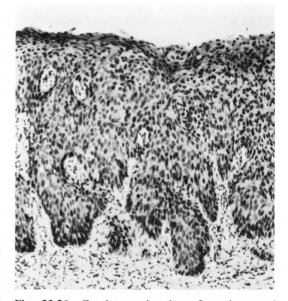

Fig. 23.26 Carcinoma in situ of uterine cervix, showing the typical thickening and alteration of cell type. There is virtually no differentiation into layers, the cells near the surface being similar to those at the base. × 120.

The normal polarity is lost, many cells lying at right angles to their normal axis. Abundant mitotic figures, normally restricted to the deeper layers, are present at all levels and some of them are abnormal. There is also an increased nuclear/cytoplasmic ratio of the individual cells. Carcinoma in situ thus resembles invasive squamous cancer except that it remains within the confines of the epithelium. Extension into endocervical glands is commonly seen, but does not imply invasive carcinoma as long as the basement membrane of the glands is intact. It is important to distinguish carcinoma in situ from squamous metaplasia, epidermidisation and mild dysplasia, none of which have the cytological features of malignancy. Furthermore, it is essential to examine numerous blocks of biopsy material to rule out microscopic invasion since 10% of cases diagnosed as pre-invasive on single biopsy have evidence of invasive carcinoma on further study, and this profoundly influences prognosis and treatment. When the cells penetrate the stroma their staining properties change, and this makes the recognition of micro-invasion fairly simple.

Knowledge of the natural history of these conditions is limited. Mild dysplasia can progress via a stage of carcinoma in situ to invasive squamous carcinoma. However it frequently regresses, especially if associated with a treatable infection. The frequency of progression of severe dysplasia and carcinoma in situ to invasive carcinoma over about 10 years is disputed. The most commonly quoted estimate is that in one-third of cases, carcinoma in situ will progress to invasive carcinoma. It has become the practice to excise these lesions once diagnosed because of the difficulty of foretelling which will progress to invasive cancer. This precludes prospective study of their natural history. On average, the age of diagnosis of carcinoma in situ is 10 years younger than that for invasive carcinoma, suggesting that the latter slowly evolves from the former.

Invasive carcinoma of the cervix

Most carcinomas of the cervix are of the squamous-cell type, only about 5% being adenocarcinomas. The former usually arises in the region of the squamo-columnar junction but 20% appear to arise in the endocervical canal. The exact site of origin, however, often cannot be detected, partly because in many cases the tumour is quite large when first seen, and partly because of the variability in the site of the squamo-columnar epithelial junction due to erosion, metaplasia and epidermidisation.

Macroscopic appearances. Invasive carcinoma is suggested by an irregular induration of the cervix followed by ulceration (Fig. 23.27). It commonly arises in one or other lip of the cervix and may eventually form a huge irregular

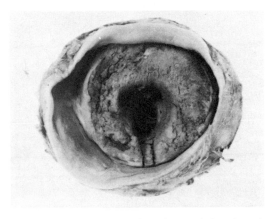

Fig. 23.27 Carcinoma of cervix uteri showing ulceration. × 0.75.

and infected mass with a nodular, often ulcerated grey-green necrotic surface. As the tumour enlarges, it invades the adjacent cervical tissue and upper vagina.

Lymphatic spread is usually early and the regional lymph nodes and parametrial tissues are soon involved, so that partial or complete obstruction of the ureters may follow and death from renal failure is common. The tumour may extend into the bladder or rectum resulting in fistulous communications. Extra pelvic metastases are rare until later and in fact in necropsy studies the disease is localised to the pelvis in two-thirds of cases.

Microscopic appearances. In invasive *squamous carcinoma* large branching solid epithelial masses penetrate the fibromuscular stroma of the cervix (Fig. 23.28). The peripheral cells are cubical and the central cells tend to be polygonal but cell nests and keratinisation are seldom features of cervical carcinoma as the tumour is rarely well enough differentiated. Accordingly, it is usually relatively sensitive to

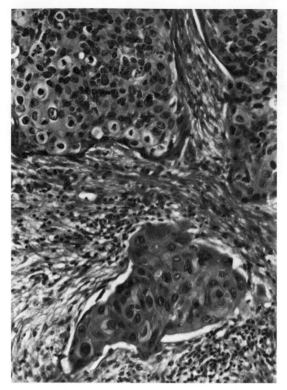

Fig. 23.28 Carcinoma of cervix uteri, showing infiltrating masses of epithelial cells without formation of cell-nests. Note the very numerous mitotic figures. × 165.

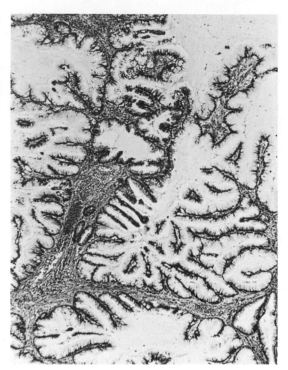

Fig. 23.29 Papilliform mucus-secreting adenocarcinoma of the cervix uteri. × 80. (The late Dr. M. A. Head.)

radiation therapy, which is the most popular method of treatment.

Adenocarcinoma arises from the columnar surface or glandular epithelium of the endocervix; it is usually mucus-secreting and sometimes papillary (Fig. 23.29). It is important to avoid histological mistakes between adenocarcinoma, florid papillary endocervicitis (p. 903) and the polypoid endocervical glandular hyperplasia which results from taking contraceptive pills.

Causes of death. About half the patients die of renal failure. Urinary obstruction may occur due to retroperitoneal spread involving the ureters, or pressure on the bladder and in the pelvis. Fistulas into the bowel and the bladder frequently lead to sepsis. Haemorrhage from the ulcerated tumour may also prove fatal. A combination of cachexia, infection, haemorrhage and renal failure is usual.

Causal factors in cervical carcinoma. The aetiology, like that of other cancers, is not understood but there are certain factors known to influence the development of both invasive carcinoma and the premalignant epithelial abnormalities (dysplasia and carcinoma in situ). Epidemiological surveys have suggested that *early age at first coitus, early marriage, early pregnancy* and *sexual promiscuity* are contributing factors. The low incidence of carcinoma of cervix in Jewesses is interesting. Whether this is genetically determined, due to careful personal hygiene, or to ritual male circumcision, is not known. Venereal transfer of some agent that induces epithelial instability is an attractive theory which has been extensively studied; the transmission of a virus, such as *Herpes simplex* type 2, might fulfil this role (p. 265).

The incidence of cervical cancer seems to be lower in women whose barrier contraceptive method has avoided contact between penis and cervix, and the possibility of a carcinogenic factor in smegma has already been mentioned (p. 886).

In most communities, the disease tends to have a higher incidence in the lower socio-economic classes.

Vaginal and cervical cytology

It is now well established that malignant cells from uterine cancers (both cervical and endometrial) are exfoliated into the vagina. Papanicolaou first realised the potentialities of exfoliative cytology in the early diagnosis of cervical cancer. Aspiration of the posterior vaginal fornix and staining by Papanicolaou's method will detect 10% of endometrial cancers and 80% of cervical cancers. Examination of scrapings from the squamo-columnar junction of the cervix will detect 90% of early cervical cancers. Cytology, however, is not a mode of diagnosing cancer; it is a means of screening apparently healthy and symptom-free women to discover those who require further investigation. In situ and early invasive carcinoma can only be diagnosed by histological examination of tissue.

Cytodiagnosis leads to the occasional discovery and prompt treatment of an early stage of invasive carcinoma of the cervix. The usual lesions found, however, are dysplasia and carcinoma in situ, not all of which, as discussed above, will be the forerunners of invasive carcinoma. A decrease of 30% in the incidence of invasive carcinoma of cervix has been reported over a period of 5–15 years from British Columbia and Ontario where a large section of the female population has had regular cervical cytology screening. Similar falls in the incidence of invasive cancer have been observed in areas where the women have not had this screening procedure, for example in Auckland, New Zealand. Indeed, carcinoma of the cervix is becoming less common, especially in areas where living and educational standards have been raised.

Unfortunately women in the lower socio-economic classes, who have a relatively high incidence of cervical cancer, tend not to take advantage of cytological screening services.

The Fallopian Tubes

The most important disorder of the Fallopian tubes is **bacterial infection** which may lead to two important complications. Firstly, obstruction of the tubes results in **sterility** and secondly, pockets are formed in which the fertilised ovum may embed—**tubal pregnancy**. This latter is described on p. 922.

Salpingitis

Classification. Infections of the Fallopian tubes may be classified as:

(*a*) *Endosalpingitis,* when infection occurs by direct surface spread from the endometrial cavity, as in gonorrhoea, or more rarely from the peritoneum via the abdominal ostia in acute peritonitis.

(*b*) *Interstitial salpingitis,* when infection spreads from the uterine wall via the lymphatics and blood vessels as in post-abortal and puerperal myometritis.

Tuberculosis of the Fallopian tubes is blood-borne and is discussed later.

Endosalpingitis. In acute gonorrhoea the mucosal surface is primarily involved by gono-cocci spreading upwards and a catarrhal and purulent condition, commonly bilateral, results. The tubes are only slightly swollen but greatly congested, and purulent exudate may escape from the fimbrial end; occasionally there is some fibrinous exudate on the fimbrial and peritoneal surface. The inflammation is initially catarrhal, the epithelium is denuded in patches from the surface of the plicae, the stroma of which is engorged and infiltrated with polymorphonuclear leukocytes, while the lumen is filled with exudate.

Interstitial salpingitis. The acute state is mainly the result of spread of pyogenic infection from the uterine wall after inexpert abortion or less commonly other forms of instrumentation. The chief feature is gross enlargement of the tubes due to inflammatory oedema and cellular infiltration of the interstitial tissue of the whole wall and adjacent mesosalpinx, while the mucosal surface may show little involvement.

Both forms of infection can result in chronic salpingitis but interstitial salpingitis is more likely to resolve without serious permanent effects.

Chronic salpingitis. Unless adequately treated, salpingitis may pass into a chronic stage in which the mucosal folds that have lost their epithelium in the acute stage adhere to one another and to the tubal wall. They become permanently fused by growth of the epithelium over them in the process of healing (Fig. 23.30). The plicae thus come to form numerous

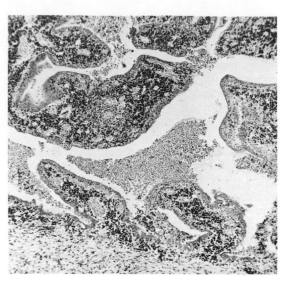

Fig. 23.31 Chronic gonococcal salpingitis. There is pus in the lumen, and the dark staining of the mucosal folds is due to the presence of numerous plasma cells. × 55.

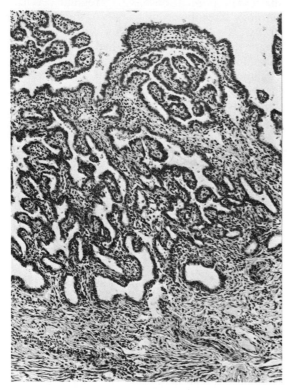

Fig. 23.30 Chronic salpingitis. There is extensive fusion of the plicae, producing blind-ending crypts in the mucosa. × 130.

pockets and depressions which predispose to arrest of the fertilised ovum, and so to tubal pregnancy. The mucosal folds are often heavily infiltrated with lymphocytes and plasma cells and their ends are bulbous (Fig. 23.31). The lumen is irregularly narrowed especially towards the isthmus, where the epithelium grows outwards among the muscle bundles, producing small nodules and crypts beneath the serous coat. The appearances are reminiscent of those in chronic cholecystitis with Aschoff–Rokitansky sinuses. The condition is distinguished from tubal adenomyosis by the absence of endometrial stroma around the gland-like spaces.

Pyosalpinx means distension of a Fallopian tube with pus. It occurs when salpingitis leads to obstruction of the ends of the tube by fusion of the fimbriae together with adhesions to adjacent structures. The lumen of the cornual end is only about 0·5 mm diameter and even mild inflammatory oedema or fibrinous exudation is enough to occlude it.

Macroscopic appearances. The tube becomes distended with pus and is like a bent sausage. The pus may be resorbed, leaving a hydrosalpinx (see below) or it may gradually become inspissated and calcified and the wall greatly thickened as in tuberculosis (see below). Gonococci, other pyococci or *Esch. coli* are sometimes grown from the pus, but frequently cultures remain sterile, particularly in cases with a history of gonorrhoea.

Microscopic appearances. The wall of the tube shows the usual features of chronic pyogenic infection, together with stretching, and flattening of the plicae.

Hydrosalpinx. This usually follows a pyosalpinx. Distension is more marked at the ampulla as the muscle is thinner there and the secretory epithelium is more extensive. The hydrosalpinx is thus usually retort-shaped with a smooth bulbous end that may be fused with the ovary; the wall is thin and semitranslucent and the lining may be as smooth as a serous membrane with only an occasional fold representing the remains of the plicae. The fluid may be discharged into the uterus but may subsequently re-accumulate.

A hydrosalpinx may become twisted, causing some degree of strangulation and consequent haemorrhage into the tube—*haematosalpinx*, but a grossly haemorrhagic tube is more often the result of tubal pregnancy.

Tuberculosis. Like the epididymis in the male, the Fallopian tubes are usually the first part of the genital tract to be involved in tuberculosis. The tubercle bacilli may be blood-borne from a lesion in the lungs or elsewhere, but they may also reach the tubes via the ostia in tuberculous peritonitis. Tubercles form in the tubal mucosa

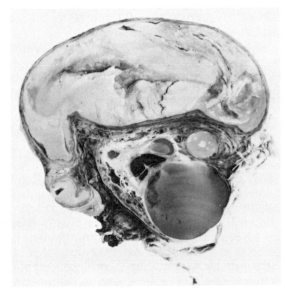

Fig. 23.32 Tuberculous salpingitis. The tube has been sectioned lengthwise, and is full of caseous material. In this instance, the ovary is cystic. × 0·8.

and soon lead to ulceration. Tubercle bacilli may be discharged into the uterus and set up **tuberculous endometritis** (p. 897). Uterine curettage is thus a useful means of detecting tuberculous salpingitis, although in some cases the tube lumen is closed at the ends and the tube becomes greatly distended with caseous material (Fig. 23.32), with a greatly thickened wall. The condition may be bilateral. Adhesions form and the tubes may be grotesquely distorted. Infection may reach the peritoneum by the ostium or through the wall of the tube, the surface of which may be studded with tubercles. Tuberculous salpingitis almost invariably causes sterility. It is possible that early specific therapy may prevent this, but it may also increase the risk of tubal pregnancy.

Talc granuloma of the Fallopian tubes. In some instances of sterility due to tubal obstruction, non-caseating tubercle-like follicles have been found in the tubal mucosa, including giant cells containing birefringent material believed to be talc. This has probably resulted from contamination of the peritoneal cavity, during previous laparotomy, with talc used to lubricate the surgeon's gloves. The lesions may be mistaken for tuberculosis, but the replacement of talc by other lubricants has greatly reduced the risk of its development.

Tumours of the Fallopian tubes

Benign tumours—fibroma, myoma, adenoma—and small cysts sometimes arise from the tubes, and malignant tumours, both carcinoma and sarcoma, are occasionally seen, watery discharge being a diagnostic feature. Choriocarcinoma has been recorded as a sequel to tubal pregnancy. All forms of tumour, however, are extremely rare.

The Ovaries

Oöphoritis

Acute inflammation of the ovaries is rare and is most frequently the result of secondary infection from the Fallopian tube by gonococci or other pyogenic organisms (p. 169). The inflamed end of the tube readily becomes adherent to the ovary, which then becomes involved by the suppurating infection, giving rise to a tubo-ovarian abscess. Infection may occur also from the peritoneal cavity in cases of peritonitis due to appendicitis and other conditions. Occasionally the whole of an ovary may be destroyed by suppuration, and the abscess may reach a large size, and be accompanied by at least local peritonitis.

Chronic oöphoritis may follow on acute pyogenic inflammation.

Non-neoplastic cysts

Cysts of the ovaries form an important group of abnormalities. Some are non-neoplastic, and derived from dilatation of follicles or corpora lutea. Others are cystic tumours.

Some cysts result from dilatation of atretic Graafian follicles, or from corpora lutea—*follicular cysts* and *corpus luteum cysts* respectively. **Follicular cysts** are usually multiple, and the surface of the ovaries may be beset with them. Usually they are small, but occasionally a cyst may reach 5–7 cm in diameter; they are generally bilateral and may cause pressure atrophy of the ovarian tissue. They are unilocular and contain clear watery fluid, although sometimes fresh or altered blood may be present and they may be mistaken macroscopically for endometriosis. Occasionally severe haemorrhage occurs into a large cyst, and the blood may burst into the peritoneal cavity. Follicular cysts have a smooth wall lined by one or more layers of cubical or columnar epithelium; sometimes, however, the epithelial lining is lost. Follicular cysts are sometimes associated with endometrial hyperplasia. **Corpus luteum cysts** are formed by haemorrhage or exudation of fluid into corpora lutea, and their appearances vary according to the age of the latter. The wall is often fibrous or hyaline without a distinct epithelial lining, and sometimes lutein cells derived from the membrana gran-

ulosa are abundant and form a yellowish layer, usually thicker at one side; the term *lutein cyst* is then applied. *Lutein cells* are comparatively large, rounded or polyhedral, and contain abundant lipid and also a yellowish pigment. They may form a broad zone which is surrounded and partly invaded by connective tissue. They may be present in large numbers around true follicular cysts, and are derived from the theca interna. **Theca-lutein cysts** originate from the granulosa cells of atretic follicles which have undergone luteinisation under the influence of chorionic gonadotrophin. Accordingly, such cysts tend to be multiple, causing enlarged polycystic ovaries, in cases of choriocarcinoma and hydatidiform mole (Fig. 23.33) and following the use of exogenous gonadotrophins to induce ovulation.

Ovarian haematomas. These may be formed in two ways; firstly by haemorrhage into a follicular cyst or corpus luteum cyst, and secondly from menstrual haemorrhage in foci of ovarian endometriosis (p. 900), giving the so-called 'chocolate cysts'.

Parovarian cysts. These cysts, which are fairly common, are derived from the epoöphoron or anterior part of the parovarium or Wolffian body, and so they occur in the broad ligament between the ovary and the tube. The cysts are usually single, spherical and unilocular, and contain clear watery fluid. They are usually lined by ciliated columnar epithelium, though in places it may be cubical. As the cyst enlarges, it separates the layers of the broad ligament, and is thus covered by an outer layer of peritoneum.

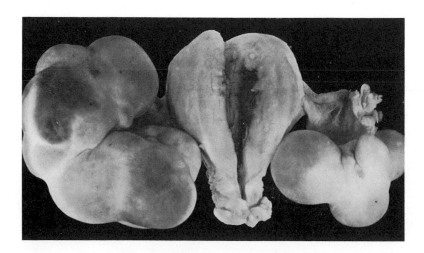

Fig. 23.33 Cystic ovaries, showing large theca-lutein cysts. The patient also had a hydatidiform mole. × 0·5.

The tube is stretched over one side, while the ovary lies on the other and may undergo atrophy. Usually there is no distinct pedicle, but if the cyst is very large it may derive a thick pedicle from the broad ligament.

Cystic tumours

Mucinous cystadenoma or cystoma

This tumour is very common, and unless removed it may become huge.

Macroscopic appearances. It is a rounded mass, usually single but sometimes bilateral, with a smooth surface and 10 cm or more in diameter when removed. Section usually reveals a single large cystic space containing sticky, semi-solid mucus: in one part of the wall there is usually a patch of thickening consisting of numerous smaller cysts lying in a fibrous stroma (Fig. 23.34). Some of these smaller cysts are usually visible by naked-eye, but others are microscopic: they also contain thick mucus.

Microscopic examination shows the cysts to be lined with a layer of tall columnar epithelium; the nuclei of the cells are basally placed,

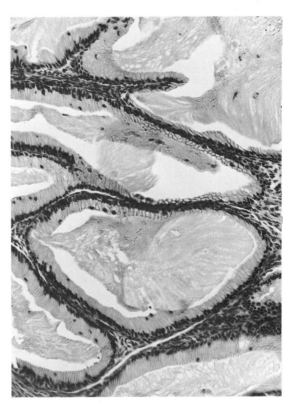

Fig. 23.35 Mucinous cystadenoma of ovary, showing acini filled with mucoid secretion, lined by a tall columnar epithelium. × 130.

while the cytoplasm generally is clear and mucin-containing (Fig. 23.35). The lining of the spaces is thrown into folds, and papillary ingrowths are numerous (Fig. 11.7, p. 276). The stroma between the smaller cysts and in the papillae is scanty and may form merely a thin line. The cysts contain mucoid glyco-protein material, along with desquamated cells and granular debris.

The origin of these cysts is obscure, for the tall mucin-secreting columnar lining epithelium has no normal counterpart in the ovary. The closest resemblance is seen in the endocervical epithelium. In some tumours, argentaffin and argyrophil cells (p. 589) have been detected, providing a resemblance to intestinal epithelium. The possibilities which have been suggested include an origin from metaplasia of ovarian serosa and unilateral development in a teratoma.

Complications. As it increases in size, the cystadenoma rises from the pelvis, and may distend the whole abdomen. It then has a distinct

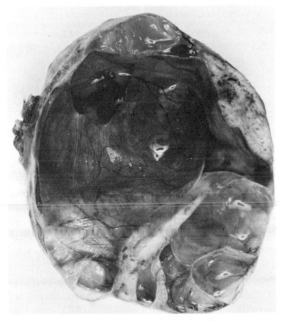

Fig. 23.34 A multilocular ovarian cyst, cut open to show that it contains a number of mucin-filled loculi, one of which is larger than the rest. Note the relatively solid mass in the wall (upper right). × 0·6. (Dr. A. D. Telford Govan.)

pedicle, in which the blood vessels run. Occasionally the pedicle is twisted, obstructing the venous return, i.e. strangulated. The cyst wall becomes dark red from diffuse haemorrhage and blood may escape also into the peritoneal cavity. Rarely a cyst may rupture, and its mucoid contents escape into the peritoneal cavity. Secretion continues to leak from the

diameter, though it is usually considerably smaller. The tumour consists of a single main cyst, but there may also be some small cysts; the contents are usually a clear, watery fluid. The characteristic feature is the presence on the inner surface of the cyst wall of papilliform projections, the surface of which is broken up into numerous outgrowths (Fig. 23.36) covered

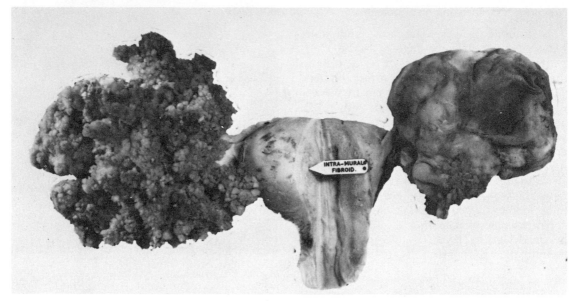

Fig. 23.36   Bilateral papillary cystic tumours of ovary, also an intramural fibroid. The numerous wart-like growths on the external surface of the cyst shown on the left indicate malignant changes. × 0·5.

tumour and in some cases from exfoliated epithelial cells seeded on to the peritoneal surfaces. The mucus acts as a mild irritant, and is invaded by connective tissue cells and young capillaries, i.e. organised. The result is that adhesions form between the coils of intestine and other structures, while the mucoid material still persists. The term *pseudo-myxoma peritonei* (p. 570) is applied to this rare condition which, although not truly malignant, has a poor prognosis. More often adenocarcinoma supervenes in a mucinous cystadenoma and may disseminate throughout the peritoneal cavity. Malignancy should be sought particularly in solid parts of the tumour.

Papillary cystadenoma or cystoma

This form of tumour, known also as **serous cystadenoma**, is also common and is usually bilateral (Fig. 23.36). It may reach 10 cm in

by columnar or cubical, often ciliated epithelium resembling that of the Fallopian tubes (Fig. 23.37). The secretion is non-mucoid and watery. Such cysts grow relatively slowly, and never reach the great size of the mucinous cystadenoma. Not infrequently, however, the cyst wall ruptures, and the contents, along with papillary fragments, escape into the peritoneal cavity, where they may form numerous outgrowths from the peritoneal surface, usually accompanied by marked ascites. After operative removal of the primary tumours, the peritoneal seedlings may undergo atrophy, but usually they continue to grow. Sometimes the surfaces of both ovaries are covered with papillary growths, and there may also be a single cyst or several small cysts in the ovaries. True carcinoma develops much more commonly in a papillary than in a mucinous cystadenoma.

The cell of origin of papillary cystadenoma is unknown.

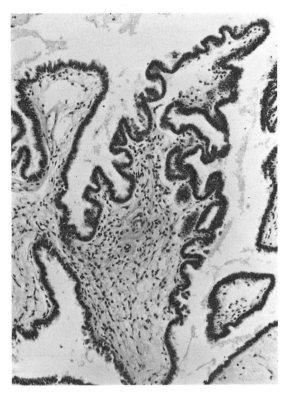

Fig. 23.37 Papillary cystadenoma of ovary, showing the papillae covered by columnar epithelium. × 100.

Ovarian teratomas

(a) Cystic teratomas. The commonest is the tumour which is known as *dermoid cyst* because it usually consists of a large epidermal-lined cyst into which sweat and sebaceous glands open and hairs project. This large cyst contains hairs and desquamated squames and fatty yellow fluid which becomes semi-solid on cooling. The tumour is usually single, but occasionally bilateral and rarely more than one have been present in an ovary. It often forms a rounded swelling which may reach 10 cm in diameter, but is usually smaller. The lining is a stratified epithelium, and the skin structures—hairs, sebaceous and sweat glands—are abundant. At one side there is often a hard protuberance, and on the inner surface several teeth, irregularly arranged, may be present (Fig. 23.38). On section this projection may contain bone and other tissues—cartilage, smooth muscle, various glandular structures representing alimentary and respiratory systems and even nervous tissue. There may be mammary tissue but, in common

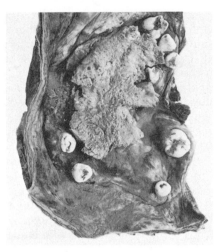

Fig. 23.38 Portion of wall of a cystic teratoma (dermoid cyst) of ovary, showing irregular growth of teeth from inner surface of cyst. × 1·1.

with teratomas in general, gonadal tissue has not been observed. Cystic teratomas vary much in complexity and epidermal structures usually preponderate; occasionally they are composed wholly of thyroid—*struma ovarii*.

These cystic teratomas are nearly always benign, in contrast to 'solid' teratomas of the testes or, more rarely, of the ovary, which are malignant. Very occasionally one element, usually epithelial, undergoes malignant change to produce squamous carcinoma, or less often adenocarcinoma.

(b) Solid teratoma of the ovary is much less common than the cystic type: it usually forms an irregular rounded mass, in which an even greater variety of tissues may be found, and these may give rise to an enormous number of small cysts. Solid ovarian teratomas tend to occur more often in children and young adults, often contain embryonal structures and are essentially malignant. Their origin has been discussed on p. 306.

Ovarian carcinoma and sarcoma

Carcinoma of the ovaries may occur comparatively early in adult life. It is often bilateral but one tumour is often considerably larger than the other. It has the usual invasive properties, but varies in type, being sometimes hard and nodular, sometimes soft and growing very large. It may produce secondary growths in the peritoneum, as well as metastases in the regional lymph nodes and other organs. Microscopically, considerable variations in structure are observed. The cells may be arranged in solid masses as in carcinoma of the breast, they may have an irregular acinous formation, or, in the softer varieties, a more diffuse, anaplastic type of growth may be present. More than 50% of ovarian carcinomas arise from cystadenomas, more often from the papillary than from the mucinous type. The criteria for the diagnosis of malignancy in a cystic ovarian tumour are: (*a*) the presence of nodules on the outer surface of the cyst; (*b*) multiplication and heaping up of the epithelial cells into several layers; (*c*) invasion of the supporting stroma; (*d*) cellular dedifferentiation with many mitoses. A tendency to rupture during removal is often suspicious.

Sarcoma is much less common than carcinoma. It also sometimes affects both ovaries and may occur in association with cysts; the tumour may be large. Usually it is of the spindle-cell type and has a fasciculated appearance on section; forms intermediate between fibroma and sarcoma are observed. Anaplastic and pleomorphic sarcomas also occur. Angiosarcoma, rhabdomyosarcoma and sarcoma combined with carcinoma have been described; these may, however, represent mixed mesodermal tumours.

Primary ovarian tumours with special features

There are a number of ovarian tumours with special features. One of these, the cystic teratoma or 'dermoid cyst' has been described on p. 913. Others include the *granulosa-cell tumour* and *androblastoma*, both of which produce hormonal effects, the *Brenner tumour* and *dysgerminoma*.

Granulosa-cell tumour

The cells of this tumour resemble in appearance, and sometimes in arrangement, the granulosa cells in Graafian follicles. They also secrete oestrogens and commonly show the changes of luteinisation.

Macroscopic appearances. Granulosa-cell tumours are usually unilateral and encapsulated. They vary from a few millimetres to 50 cm in diameter, and are moderately firm, often yellow (due to intracellular lipids), and either solid or containing multiple, usually small, cysts.

Microscopic appearances vary considerably. The cells are often rounded or polyhedral with clear pale-staining cytoplasm, often containing lipids. They are arranged in groups which vary in size and may contain spaces filled with pale eosinophilic fluid, thus resembling the Call–Exner bodies and antrum of the normal

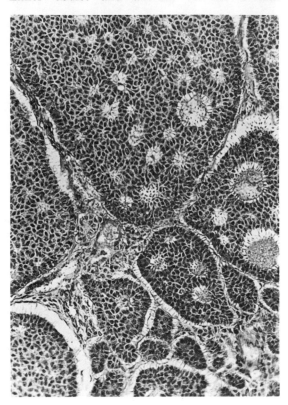

Fig. 23.39 Granulosa-cell tumour of ovary, showing characteristic masses of cells with formation of Call–Exner bodies. × 225.

Graafian follicle (Fig. 23.39). In other instances the cells form irregular strands or glandular acini, or the tumour may in places resemble spindle-celled sarcoma. The histological appearances may vary much in different parts of the same tumour. In most instances, removal is curative, but some granulosa cell tumours are malignant. Although termed granulosa-cell tumours, in many instances the cells resemble thecal cells and show various degrees of luteinisation. These variants are termed **thecomas** and luteomas respectively. The distinction between these various types of tumour is not, however, sharp.

Age distribution and effects. Granulosa-cell tumour is observed most frequently after the menopause, but occurs at all ages. It often secretes large amounts of oestrogens and the occasional cases occurring in childhood cause precocious sexual development, premature closure of the epiphyses, and so short stature. Ovulation does not occur, the endometrium is hyperplastic, and 'menstrual' bleeding is irregular. During reproductive life and after the menopause the effects are endometrial hyperplasia and irregular bleeding. The prolonged and excessive oestrogen stimulation may result in the development of endometrial carcinoma, particularly in post-menopausal cases.

Androblastoma (arrhenoblastoma)

This rare tumour, which occurs chiefly in young women, often secretes masculinising steroids. The explanation for this, and the cell of origin, are unknown. The histological pattern varies from the formation of well-developed tubules (*Sertoli-cell*

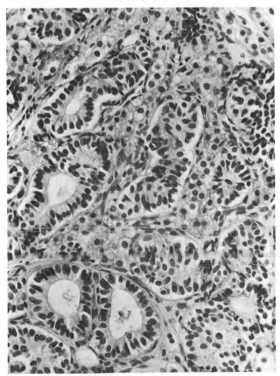

Fig. 23.40 Androblastoma of the ovary, showing tubular structures and Leydig cells. × 220.

tumours) with or without Leydig cells (Fig. 23.40), to poorly differentiated spindle-cells with only occasional acini or tubules. They may be masculinising, feminising or show no hormonal effects. Their masculinising effects include cessation of ovulation and of menstruation, sterility, loss of feminine characters and virilism. In a previously healthy woman there may be atropy of the uterus and breasts, enlargement of the clitoris, growth of facial hair and the appearance of the male secondary sex characters. The degree to which these abnormalities are reversed by removal of the tumour varies; exceptionally fertility has returned. In a minority of cases the tumour is malignant.

Fibroma of the ovary

Benign fibroma is one of the commonest solid ovarian tumours. They are hard, nodular tumours, usually 5–10 cm in diameter but sometimes larger. The cut surface is whitish with the characteristic whorled watered-silk appearance, but when large, the pedicle may undergo torsion, leading to strangulation. In some, there is an admixture of smooth muscle fibres and rarely of other mesenchymal elements. Large fibromas of the ovary and less commonly other ovarian tumours may be accompanied by wasting, ascites and right-sided hydrothorax (Meig's syndrome) which may be mistaken for pleural and peritoneal involvement by a malignant tumour; these disappear when the tumour is removed. It is difficult to distinguish a fibroma from a Brenner tumour or thecoma without microscopic examination.

Brenner tumour

This uncommon ovarian tumour varies in diameter from a few millimetres to over 20 cm. It is firm and resembles a fibroma. Microscopic examination shows an abundant ovarian-type stroma in which are scattered islands or nests of epithelial cells which are rounded or polyhedral and are comparatively uniform and inactive in appearance. The nuclei may show characteristic longitudinal folding. The epithelial islands may be solid or contain a central space (Fig. 23.41) which in some cases is filled with mucin and lined by cells resembling those of mucinous cystadenoma. The tumour is slowly growing and benign. Unlike the gran-

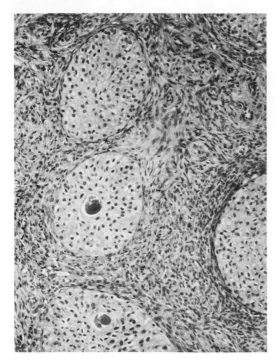

Fig. 23.41   Brenner tumour of ovary. × 150.

ulosa-cell tumour, the Brenner tumour only rarely shows evidence of endocrine activity.

Dysgerminoma

This is another rare ovarian tumour arising from germ-cell precursors and histologically closely resembling seminoma of the testis, including infiltration with lymphocytes and sometimes an epithelioid-cell granulomatous reaction. It can occur at any age, but is least rare around the time of puberty and in young women. It does not produce hormonal effects and causes local symptoms. Like seminoma, it is highly malignant but is also very sensitive to x-irradiation and so has a surprisingly good prognosis in most cases. In many cases it has been associated with retardation of sexual development or with pseudo-hermaphroditism. Its removal, however, has no effect on these abnormalities.

Endodermal sinus tumour

This is a rare and highly malignant tumour of young women. Histologically it resembles the endodermal sinuses of the yolk sac. Similar tumours occur in the testis (orchioblastoma). These tumours secrete α-fetoprotein.

Secondary carcinoma of the ovaries

Metastasis to the ovaries is comparatively frequent in carcinoma of the stomach and colon, and though nodules may also be present over the peritoneum, this is not invariably the case. The secondary tumours sometimes reach a large size. In some instances ovarian metastasis is accompanied by widespread peritoneal in-

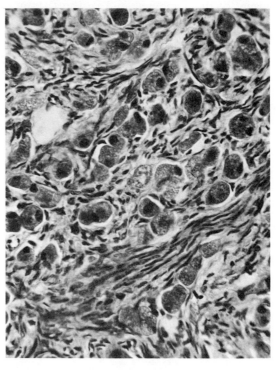

Fig. 23.42   Krukenberg tumour of ovary, secondary to a primary carcinoma of stomach. Note the abundant spindle cell stroma and the large round mucin-containing carcinoma cells. × 315.

volvement and spread to the ovary appears to have been transcoelomic. In other cases, ovarian metastasis occurs without peritoneal involvement and it is uncertain whether this is due to the ovaries providing an especially favourable environment for growth of cancer cells in the peritoneal cavity or whether spread has been by lymphatics.

Krukenberg described a bilateral tumour of the ovaries which now bears his name. It has a very cellular sarcoma-like stroma in which cancer cells are scattered or occur in masses (Fig. 23.42). Many of the cells contain mucin which has pushed the nucleus to one side, giving a signet-ring appearance. Such tumours are metastatic carcinomas, the primary being usually in the stomach, less often in the colon or breasts. Their unusually cellular stroma is only seen when they occur during reproductive life. After the menopause, metastases in the ovaries have the same appearances as elsewhere.

The Vulva and Vagina

The cutaneous tissues of the vulva are comparable to the sex skin of monkeys and so are responsive to sex hormones. Accordingly, the variations in hormonal status throughout life influence the effects of generalised skin diseases on the vulva and predispose vulvar skin to various hypertrophic and atrophic conditions.

The commonest malignant tumour of the vulva is squamous carcinoma, but practically any type of skin tumour can arise in it.

Infections

The glands related to the vulva and vagina are commonly involved in **gonorrhoea**, and another common infection is **moniliasis**, which affects the surface squamous epithelium. The flagellar protozoon *Trichomonas vaginalis* causes an acute inflammation of the vagina: it can be spread venereally, but also by surface contamination of public lavatory seats. In the male, it colonises the urethra and the carrier state is often symptomless.

The vulva, and to a lesser extent the vagina, are subject to bacterial infections as a complication of atrophy. The normal post-menopausal atrophy is sometimes exaggerated and pathological, or in certain conditions atrophy occurs during reproductive life (see below)

The primary chancre of **syphilis** occurs most frequently on the labia but may appear in the vagina or on the cervix uteri; secondary lesions may occur on the portio vaginalis, along with condylomas on the perineum. Apart from these, syphilitic lesions are not common. Gummas and chronic interstitial inflammation in the female genital tract are rare.

Lymphogranuloma inguinale (lymphogranuloma venereum or lymphopathia venereum) is due to a chlamydial infection (p. 188), usually transmitted by sexual contact. It occurs especially where social conditions are poor, e.g. in large seaports and in parts of the tropics. In women the initial lesion is a small ulcer on the external genitalia, the perineum or vagina, which remains small, soon heals, and is often not noticed. Two or three weeks after infection the draining lymph nodes enlarge, i.e. the inguinal nodes draining the external genitalia and/or the pelvic nodes draining the cervix and upper vagina. The nodes enlarge progressively for some weeks, become matted together, fluctuant, and eventually break down and discharge pus. This may continue for many months and result in extensive scarring and sometimes in elephantiasis of the genitalia. When the pelvic nodes are involved they may discharge into any of the hollow pelvic viscera and scarring may cause strictures, e.g. of the rectum.

Histologically the primary ulcer shows inflammatory change with polymorph and macrophage infiltration and fibroblast proliferation. The lesions in the nodes consist initially of macrophage granulomas which, as they enlarge, coalesce and undergo central necrosis and suppuration to form irregular 'stellate' abscesses ringed by a palisade of macrophages admixed with plasma cells and lymphocytes.

A diagnostic skin test (*Frei test*) is performed by injection of the killed organisms but it remains positive for years and so is not much help where infection is widespread in the community. A complement fixation test is also available.

Granuloma inguinale (granuloma venereum). This is a granulomatous disease commonly transmitted sexually and caused by infection with a small pleomorphic bacillus which resembles a Klebsiella and cross-reacts serologically with *Klebsiella rhinoscleromatis*. The lesion starts on the external genitalia, perineum or vagina as a small papule which ulcerates and increases in size. It may gradually become very large and cause extensive destruction. Biopsy shows the base and margins to consist of granulation tissue rich in macrophages but containing also other inflammatory cells. The causal bacteria (*Donovan bodies*) may be seen within macrophages in smears or sections stained by haematoxylin and eosin or preferably by Giemsa. Unless adequately treated, extensive destruction, scarring and sometimes elephantiasis may result.

Leukoplakia

Leukoplakia is a clinical term meaning the presence of white patches. Both in the vulva and elsewhere it can reflect various pathological changes. Indeed, in the vulva any of the chronic dermatoses can be responsible, e.g. neurodermatitis, moniliasis, senile keratosis and *lichen sclerosus et atrophicus*. One form of leukoplakia

Tumours

The only benign epithelial tumour commonly seen on the vulva is the papilloma or condyloma acuminatum—p. 184. A sweat gland tumour with special features—the apocrine hidradenoma (p. 1006)—occurs in the labia.

Malignant tumours are relatively rare; most are squamous carcinomas but adenocarcinoma of Bartholin's gland, basal cell carcinoma, melanoma and sarcoma also occur. Metastases in the vulva occur infrequently from endometrial carcinoma and choriocarcinoma.

Carcinoma of the vulva occurs most commonly after the age of 50 and therefore arises in atrophic tissues. In over 60% of cases the changes of senile keratosis are present in the vulvar skin.

Most vulvar cancers start on the mucocutaneous surface of the anterior half of the labia.

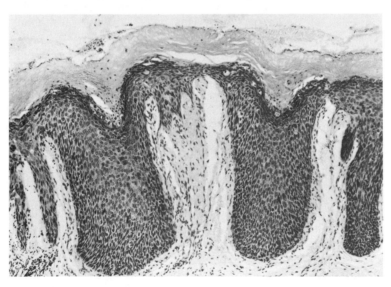

Fig. 23.43 Biopsy from a case of clinical leukoplakia of the vulva, showing hypertrophied rete ridges and hyperkeratosis of the epithelium. × 95.

of the vulva is due to patches of epidermal thickening with hyperkeratosis, parakeratosis and acanthosis in association with hyalinisation of the superficial dermis and evidence of chronic inflammation (Fig. 23.43). Areas of epidermal de-differentiation may occur in hypertrophic lesions and atypical features are present in the basal layer, such as the presence of keratinised cells (dyskeratosis). Some authors restrict the use of the term leukoplakia to this premalignant condition. Between this picture and that of invasive carcinoma is the microscopic pattern of carcinoma in situ.

Naked-eye examination reveals an ulcer with a sloughing surface and a deeply indurated base; less commonly it will appear as a flat plaque or a fungating papillary growth.

The microscopic appearances are those of a typical squamous cell carcinoma (see Fig. 11.22, p. 284), usually moderately well differentiated with keratinisation and cell nests. In about one-third of cases, however, the tumour is anaplastic and very malignant.

The superficial and deep inguinal lymph nodes are involved early and often on both sides because of the bilateral lymphatic drainage. Vulvar cancer may appear to be multifocal. This may indeed be the case or surface growths may appear as a result of lymphatic permeation from the primary tumour.

Carcinoma of the vagina. Squamous carcinoma is uncommon: it occurs usually in the upper part of the vagina in old women and results in fistulas with the bladder, urethra and rectum. Treatment is often unsatisfactory because the tumour is advanced when discovered.

Adenocarcinoma of the vagina in teenage girls is another rare tumour which has been shown to be due to the effect on the fetus of administering diethylstilboestrol during the early months of pregnancy.

Abnormalities Related to Pregnancy

The pathology of pregnancy is too complex to be considered in detail here and an account of only some of the more important abnormalities will be given. The trophoblast possesses the property of invading the maternal tissues to achieve nidation. In normal pregnancy, fragments of chorionic villi enter the uterine veins and pass to the lungs. The factors which prevent trophoblastic growth and invasion in such an abnormal site are poorly understood.

Hydatidiform mole

In this condition the embryo dies but early abortion fails to occur and the terminal branches of the chorionic villi enlarge to form discrete, translucent, tense, grape-like vesicles of 3–15 mm diameter (Fig. 23.44). A true hydatidiform mole occurs in the middle trimester of pregnancy and usually no trace of the fetus is seen. Evidence of hydropic degeneration of the chorionic villi in focal areas is found in 50% of cases of spontaneous abortion where the fetus is abnormal, but there are too few cases intermediate between ordinary abortion and hydatidiform mole to accept a continuous spectrum of transition. The occurrence of cases in which there is an imperfectly developed embryo in its sac, with a partly formed placenta in which hydatidiform villi are embedded, is distinctly uncommon.

Aetiology and pathogenesis. The true cause of hydatidiform mole is unknown but the condition occurs more frequently in mothers under 18 and over 40 years of age. Twin pregnancies have been recorded in which a mole was present along with a normal fetus and placenta, an indication that the defect is in the zygote. It is

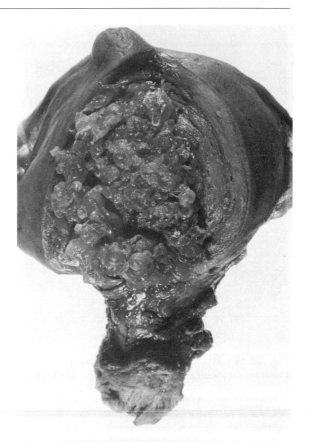

Fig. 23.44 Hydatidiform mole exposed by a longitudinal incision in the body of the uterus. The mole is composed of oedematous grape-like chorionic villi. × 0·7.

not yet agreed whether the defect lies primarily in the death of the embryo or in some abnormality of the trophoblast. The pathological criteria for the diagnosis of hydatidiform mole are (*a*) trophoblastic proliferation of both Langhans layer and syncytium, (*b*) hydropic degeneration of the stroma of the villi, (*c*) virtual absence of fetal blood vessels in the villi. The extent and degree of trophoblastic hyperplasia varies greatly, but the hydropic change in the villi is remarkably constant, the villi merely growing larger with age.

On microscopic examination, the villi are seen to consist of grossly oedematous myxoid tissue. The almost complete absence of capillary blood

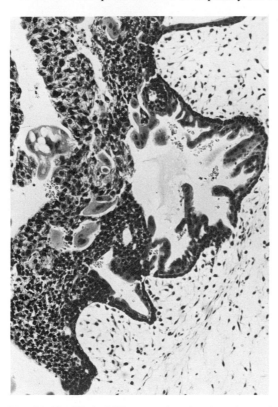

Fig. 23.45 Hydatidiform mole, showing the oedematous avascular villi, covered by hyperplastic Langhans cells and syncytiotrophoblast.

vessels is striking. On the surface the chorionic epithelium shows proliferation. There are several layers of Langhans cells, and the syncytium is correspondingly prominent (Fig. 23.45); the surface in places may, however, be denuded of epithelium. Usually the mole consists almost wholly of altered villi, and there is no trace of fetus or normal placenta; the villi in such cases penetrate irregularly into and destroy the decidual layer. Hydatidiform moles may sometimes reach a weight of 1–1·5 kg, and their presence often causes an abnormally rapid increase in the size of the uterus. They lead to

abortion, which is often preceded by haemorrhage, sometimes severe; the blood may be retained and form a firm clot.

Penetrating (invasive) mole. There are also cases in which the villi of the hydatidiform mole show much more extensive penetration, extending into and destroying the uterine wall (Fig. 23.46), simulating the behaviour of a malignant tumour—the so-called *penetrating* or *invasive*

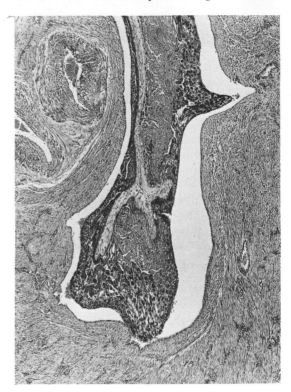

Fig. 23.46 Penetrating mole, showing deep penetration of the myometrium by degenerate villi covered with hyperplastic trophoblast. × 32.

mole. Occasionally 'metastases' of both trophoblast and villi have occurred but the condition is rarely truly malignant and involution of the 'metastases' follows hysterectomy.

Lastly, the chorionic epithelium of the altered villi may become frankly malignant, the tumour then constituting a choriocarcinoma, but, as Park has emphasised, it is not possible to predict on morphological grounds which hydatidiform mole will develop frank malignancy in its trophoblastic epithelium. The hydatidiform mole, like choriocarcinoma, is often associated with theca-lutein cysts in the ovary (Fig. 23.33, p. 910), which appear to arise from the effects of the abundant chorionic gonadotrophin produced by the trophoblastic cells. Chorionic gonadotrophin is usually present in large amounts in the urine, and its detection is of diagnostic value (see below).

Choriocarcinoma

This is a rare malignant tumour of trophoblastic epithelial type in which the tumour cells differentiate into recognisable cyto- and syncytiotrophoblast. It is of special interest as representing an invasion of the maternal tissues by a tumour of fetal origin (p. 307). In half the cases it is a sequel to a hydatidiform mole and, as has been stated, the invasive mole is a transitional form. About 25% of cases of choriocarcinoma follow an abortion, and some of these may have been due to unrecognised hydatidiform degeneration of the chorion. The remainder, excluding those that originate in a teratoma, follow a normal pregnancy, and give rise to symptoms

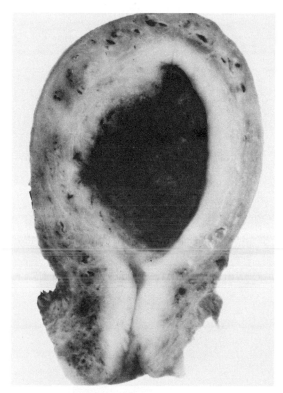

Fig. 23.47 Choriocarcinoma of uterus. The tumour is a large haemorrhagic mass invading the uterine wall and distending the cavity. × 1.

some time, even several years, after delivery: no doubt they arise from portions of retained placenta. Very occasionally choriocarcinoma may develop during a pregnancy and give rise to abortion or premature delivery. It may also occur within a year or so after the menopause.

Macroscopic appearances. The tumour appears as a soft mass within the uterus, often of crumbling texture and dark red owing to haemorrhages (Fig. 23.47) which result from erosion of the blood vessels by the syncytial cells. It invades and destroys the uterine wall, and may penetrate to the peritoneal coat. Dissemination occurs early, mainly by the blood stream, but also by lymphatics, and metastases are seen most commonly in the lungs, vaginal wall and vulva, lymph nodes, liver and brain. The secondary tumours have the same general characters as the primary, and are usually very haemorrhagic and necrotic. Occasionally a secondary nodule in the lungs may undergo complete necrosis, and may become enclosed in fibrous tissue, finishing up as a scar.

Very rarely, choriocarcinoma has been observed to originate in a Fallopian tube or an ovary, and in such cases it apparently develops from an ectopic pregnancy.

Microscopic appearances. The tumour is composed of the two elements of the chorionic epithelium. The Langhans cells, which are rounded or polyhedral with clearly defined margins, often form large masses, on the surface of which are the syncytial cells. The latter present a great variety of shapes, and often have long trailing processes; their cytoplasm is finely granular and more eosinophilic than that of the Langhans cells (Fig. 23.48). There is little stroma, and areas of necrosis and extravasated blood are usually present, even in small metastatic nodules.

In reaching a diagnosis of choriocarcinoma on histological grounds, it must be appreciated that syncytial cells normally penetrate deeply into the myometrium and may persist there for long periods if a portion of placenta is retained.

Hormonal changes. In choriocarcinoma and hydatidiform mole the urine usually contains abundant chorionic gonadotrophin, which is often present in much greater concentration than in a normal pregnancy. The level falls to normal if the tumour is removed completely. Failure to become negative, or the return of a

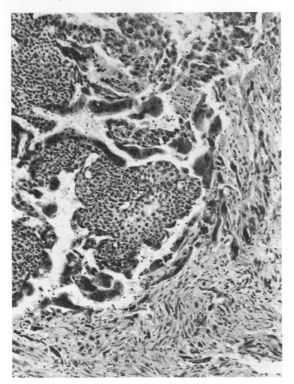

Fig. 23.48 Choriocarcinoma, consisting of masses of Langhans cells and syncytiotrophoblast deep in the uterine wall. × 100.

positive test, indicates the presence of active trophoblastic elements, and the presence of neoplastic chorionic epithelium can be deduced from the hormone titre in the urine. In many cases of choriocarcinoma or hydatidiform mole the ovaries have been found to be replaced by large cysts of the theca-lutein type (p. 910), as a result of this hormonal influence.

Aetiology. The factors that bring about the malignant transformation of the trophoblastic cells are unknown, except that it is commoner late in reproductive life and that age appears to be more important than multiparity. The disease is world-wide in its distribution but has a very much higher incidence in Chinese and other Far Eastern women.

Although choriocarcinoma is a highly malignant tumour, which grows and metastasises very rapidly, these examples arising in the uterus are unusually susceptible to cytotoxic drugs such as methotrexate. This is probably because these tumours are of fetal origin and therefore their cells have 'transplant' antigens incompatible to the maternal host (p. 307).

Choriocarcinoma can arise also in teratomas of the testis, mediastinum, pineal, etc., and these respond relatively poorly to cytotoxic drugs, presumably because they lack foreign transplant antigens.

Ectopic pregnancy

This condition arises when the fertilised ovum becomes implanted and develops before it reaches the uterus. It may occur (*a*) in the Fallopian tube (*tubal pregnancy*), (*b*) between the fimbrial end of the tube and the ovary, when these are adherent (*tubo-ovarian*), (*c*) in the ovary itself (*ovarian*), or (*d*) in the peritoneal cavity (*abdominal*). All these forms, with the exception of the tubal, are rare. Abdominal pregnancy is usually secondary to rupture of a tubal pregnancy, the placenta then becoming attached to the peritoneal surface; but a primary form also is recognised. The commonest site in the tube is the ampullary portion, but

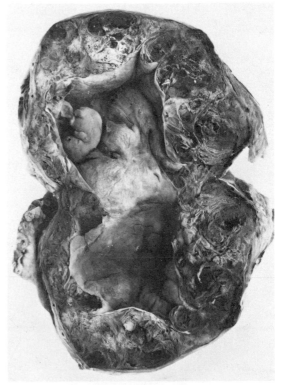

Fig. 23.49 Section through tubal pregnancy, showing the very vascular wall; the embyro is seen in the upper part. × 1.

interstitial pregnancy also occurs, i.e. in the intra-uterine end of the tube. Tubal pregnancy is usually the result of some tubal abnormality —usually scarring from salpingitis, which has resulted in the formation of pockets in which the ovum is trapped. Nidation occurs and the ovum develops in the muscle layer. There is great enlargement of blood vessels (Fig. 23.49), but the formation of decidua is only imperfect. Rupture of the blood vessels is common at a comparatively early stage, and the haemorrhage tends to separate the pregnancy from the surrounding tubal tissues. The relatively thin tube wall is so weakened and stretched that tubal rupture occurs early in the pregnancy, usually with severe haemorrhage. Occasionally the placenta becomes separated from the ruptured tube and then attached to the peritoneum. The fetus may then continue to grow as an abdominal pregnancy. At any stage, it may die, become encapsulated, and eventually heavily calcified (*lithopaedion*). In many instances a live child has been removed by operation from the peritoneal cavity. In extra-uterine pregnancy decidua forms within the uterine cavity. This is an important diagnostic finding in curettage of the uterus in cases of ectopic pregnancy, but it is important to bear in mind that the use of oral contraceptive pills may also induce a decidual reaction in the endometrium.

Inflammation of the placenta

Syphilis. This is now rare. In many undoubted cases of syphilis the placenta is paler, denser and heavier in proportion to the child than normally. The connective tissue of the villi is increased and many villi are fused. This change leads to a diminution in the blood supply and thus of the nourishment of the child. Even when the internal organs of the fetus are swarming with the spirochaetes, it may not be possible to find any in the placenta, and in any given case the presence of syphilis is much more likely to be detected by an examination of the fetus than of the placenta.

Vaccinia. Vaccination during pregnancy should be avoided if possible, for it is likely to cause necrotising inflammatory lesions in the placenta (Fig. 23.50) and also in the fetus. Fetal death is likely to result.

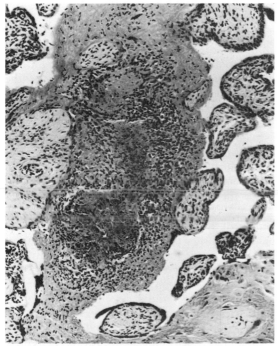

Fig. 23.50 Vaccinial lesion in the placenta, showing necrosis and cellular reaction in the villi. × 112.

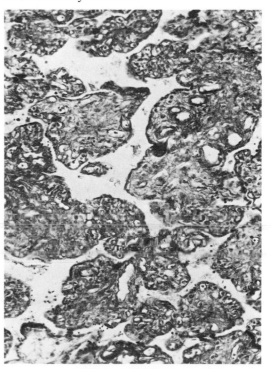

Fig. 23.51 Placenta (full term) in haemolytic disease of the newborn, showing thickening and fibrosis of the villi. × 100.

The placenta in haemolytic disease of the newborn

The placenta is abnormally large and pale in cases of *hydrops fetalis* (p. 474), and when a severely macerated fetus is born, the placental changes may indicate the diagnosis. Microscopically the villi are greatly swollen, fibrous and oedematous (Fig. 23.51), the Langhans cells persist in excessive numbers on their surface and erythroblasts and often haemopoietic foci can be seen in the small blood vessels of the villi. In less severe haemolytic disease, e.g. icterus gravis, the placental changes are usually less conspicuous and the organ may look normal but the cord is often bile-stained.

Congenital Abnormalities of the Female Genitalia

These are due to failure in the normal fusion of parts, to incomplete development or absence of certain structures and to pathological closure or atresia of openings, etc.; there is also the important group of abnormalities due to displacements of cells or portions of tissue, from which certain tumours arise, especially in the ovaries.

Abnormalities of Müllerian ducts. The upper portions of the Müllerian ducts constitute the two Fallopian tubes, while the lower portions coalesce to form the uterus and upper vagina. From imperfect fusion there arise various degrees of duplication, e.g. a double uterus and vagina, a double uterus and single vagina (*uterus bicornis duplex*), or the uterus may be doubled only in its upper part (*uterus bicornis unicollis*). There may also be lesser degrees of failure of fusion resulting, for example, in a uterus with two short cornua (*uterus arcuatus*). Rarely the ducts of Müller have split in their upper part, so that there are two Fallopian tubes on each side; or the splitting may be only partial.

Deficiency of growth or *aplasia* of the Müllerian ducts is likewise of variable degree. Absence of the uterus and tubes is the extreme example, but is very rare, and in such cases it is necessary to determine the true sex of the subject first by examining a buccal smear for sex chromatin followed by chromosome analysis if doubt exists. Absence of the uterus or of its lower part is occasionally observed while the tubes are present. Or the uterus may be well formed but with occlusion or atresia of the os, or less frequently of the isthmus; such lesions may lead to accumulation of the menstrual blood. Occasionally one Müllerian duct has failed to develop, and then there is an absence of one tube, and the uterus is asymmetrical—*uterus unicornis*. In other cases asymmetry is due to a rudimentary cornu on one side, which is sometimes cut off from the uterine cavity. There are also other variations in which a tube or part of a tube is absent.

Persistence of Wolffian duct remnants. The Wolffian (mesonephric) ducts and their associated tubules make no essential contribution to the female genitalia, but persistent remnants may give rise to cysts and possibly tumours. The ducts pass from the vicinity of the lateral ends of the Fallopian tubes across the broad ligaments and laterally adjacent to the uterus: they enter the cervical myometrium and then run in the lateral walls of the vagina to end near the free margin of the hilum. Cysts can occur anywhere along this course, but more commonly in the broad ligaments.

Abnormalities of cloacal division. The normal division of the cloaca, with formation of the septum, may be incomplete resulting in a communication between the vestibulum and the lower end of the rectum—vestibulo-rectal fistula. This condition may be associated with imperforate anus.

Hormonal hypoplasia of the uterus is observed with ovarian defects and may be associated with other abnormalities, e.g. pseudo-hermaphroditism, sometimes due to an abnormality of the adrenal cortex (p. 976). Hypoplasia, or rather the persistence after puberty of the infantile type of uterus, is seen in conditions of infantilism, for example that resulting from deficiency of the thyroid or of the anterior pituitary lobe secretions.

Ovaries. Small congenital ovarian cysts are occasionally encountered. True doubling of the ovaries has been recorded, but is extremely rare; aberrant portions of ovarian tissue are occasionally observed, and one or both ovaries may be in an abnormal situation, for example, one may be present in a patent inguinal canal. The ovaries are sometimes abnormally small, and there is then usually hypoplasia of other parts of the genital system; occasionally pseudo-hermaphroditism is present. For brief descriptions of the gonads in hermaphroditism and the intersexes, see pp. 883–5.

Gonadal dysgenesis (Turner's syndrome). This remarkable condition is the result of a chromosome anomaly, usually XO—i.e. the presence of only one X chromosome and no Y, with only 45 chromosomes in all. The affected individuals are females of normal intelligence, but with ovaries represented only by fibrous streaks and a total lack of sexual development at puberty; they are of very short stature and present a number of other lesser defects of which webbing of neck is particularly characteristic. There are a number of variants depending chiefly upon varying degrees of partial retention of the second sex chromosome.

The Breast

Inflammations

Acute infections

Acute inflammatory conditions of the female breast may be non-suppurative or suppurative, and these have widely different results.

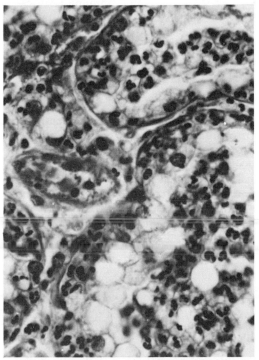

Fig. 23.52 Acute puerperal mastitis showing the secreting mammary acini, heavily infiltrated with polymorphonuclear leukocytes. × 500.

An apparent acute inflammation occurs in connection with lactation, but although accompanied by pyrexia, it is mainly a condition of congestive swelling and oedema, and is essentially hormonal in origin from failure to establish satisfactory lactation. The nipple is a not uncommon site for molluscum contagiosum infection.

Acute pyogenic mastitis. The most important form of suppurative mastitis is also related to lactation and is the result of infection via the ducts or through some abrasion of the nipple. It is usually caused by staphylococci acquired in hospital from the mouth of the suckling infant which has been colonised by the prevalent strain of *Staphylococcus aureus*: less commonly it is due to *Strep. pyogenes* (Fig. 23.52), and a spreading cellulitis may result. Unless effectively treated, staphylococcal mastitis may cause a loculated breast abscess, and extensive destruction and fibrous scarring of the breast may result. Abscess formation may also occur superficial to or deep to the mammary gland.

Chronic inflammatory mastitis

A group of hyperplastic and cystic conditions of the breast was formerly termed 'chronic mastitis'. These are not, however, inflammatory: they are probably hormonal effects and are described on p. 927. True chronic inflammatory mastitis is a localised lesion which usually follows acute mastitis or difficult lactation, when there has been some infection, e.g. from cracked nipples, resulting in chronic low grade infection and granulomatous reaction. It may also develop insidiously, without an obvious acute stage.

Mammary duct ectasia

This condition of progressive dilatation of the mammary ducts commences in the subareolar lactiferous sinuses and extends peripherally to the parenchymal ducts. It is rarely palpable, like a 'bag of worms'. Neutral fat and cellular debris accumulate in the ectatic ducts leading to a pale or coloured nipple discharge which may be confused clinically with that from a duct papilloma; microscopy, however, shows the discharge to contain only foamy macrophages in duct ectasia, while in duct papilloma red blood cells and tumour cells are usually seen.

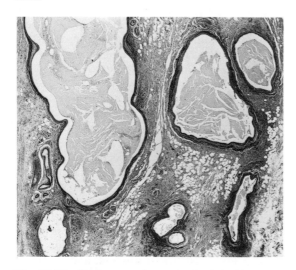

Fig. 23.53 Mammary duct ectasia. The ducts are dilated and filled with fatty material. Their walls show hyperplasia of the elastic tissue. × 13.

Microscopic examination. The dilated ducts show marked elastic hyperplasia with thickening of their walls (Fig. 23.53); there are often many lymphocytes and plasma cells around the ducts. Fibrosis of the ducts may lead to retraction of the nipple and arouse suspicion of malignancy. Low grade infection within the ducts leads to ulceration and liberation of lipids into the surrounding tissue resulting in a

chronic inflammatory reaction (Fig. 23.54) with many giant cells and macrophages. This has sometimes been mistaken for tuberculosis. These changes may be accompanied by a

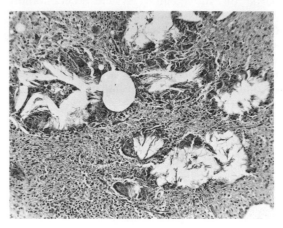

Fig. 23.54 Granulomatous reaction due to duct ectasia. Foreign-body giant cell reaction around fatty material, giving rise to a hard, palpable mass. × 50.

marked plasma cell reaction (*plasma-cell mastitis*) suggesting that some immune response is going on. Plasma-cell mastitis may be mistaken clinically for carcinoma, and frozen-section examination is of value in its diagnosis. It appears to be observed less commonly nowadays.

Recurrent areolar infection

Some women suffer repeated inflammation, scarring and fistulous formation in the subareolar and juxta-areolar tissues; this may be associated with mammary duct ectasia. Sometimes a fistula lined by granulation tissue communicates with a subareolar duct with a squamous lining which may be due to metaplasia but in some cases is congenital, with pilo-sebaceous units in its wall. This is called a *mammillary fistula*.

Traumatic fat necrosis

This lesion in the fatty tissue of an obese and pendulous breast is caused by trauma (often forgotten by the patient). It gives rise to a localised firm or even hard mass which may underlie and be adherent to the skin and has not infrequently been mistaken for carcinoma. The appearances vary at different stages but there is often a central cavity containing brown oily fluid. This is surrounded by a broad zone of dull yellowish-white tissue with scattered areas of similar appearance in the outer part. At the periphery there is a fibrous capsule. Microscopic examination shows the presence of rounded foamy cells containing small fatty globules and multinucleated giant

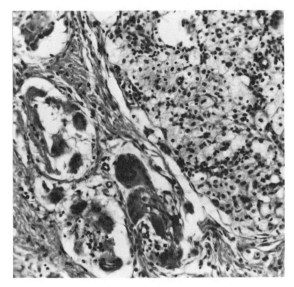

Fig. 23.55 Traumatic fat necrosis of breast, showing lipophages and foreign-body giant cells. × 150.

cells which may form large collections (Fig. 23.55). Many of the giant cells contain crystals of fatty acid and at places a number of them may be arranged around masses of crystals. Macrophages containing iron pigment are usually also present. The lesion represents the result of traumatic rupture of fat cells followed by a slow lipolysis along with phagocytosis and other reactive changes. Similar appearances are sometimes seen after minor surgical operations on the breast.

Tuberculosis

Tuberculosis of the breast is now rare. It may be the result of haematogenous infection, or it may be due to lymphatic or direct spread from caseous axillary lymph nodes or tuberculosis of the pleura or ribs. Sometimes the condition may be localised and lead to a large caseous swelling which may simulate tumour; in other cases, it is a more diffuse infiltration with nodular thickenings, a form of true chronic interstitial mastitis. In untreated cases, the caseous change may spread to the surface of the breast and ulceration with formation of a sinus may result. In view of the histological similarity of various non-tuberculous lesions (e.g. duct ectasia; fat necrosis), the diagnosis of mammary tuberculosis should not be made without proof that tubercle bacilli are present in the lesion.

'Mastopathy'

It is difficult to find a comprehensive term to cover the various pathological changes commonly seen in the breasts that are neither inflammatory nor truly neoplastic. The changes include hyperplasia, metaplasia and cyst formation, and either inflammation or neoplasia may subsequently complicate the picture. The non-committal term 'mastopathy' is a convenient one for this group of changes. The term 'fibro-adenosis' is sometimes applied, but we prefer to restrict its use as described below.

Generalised cystic mastopathy

Generalised mastopathy is commoner in nulliparae and is sometimes associated with menstrual irregularity. The incidence increases towards the menopause, but it may occur in severe form early in the third decade. Although the changes may at first be local they tend to extend progressively and eventually affect much of the parenchyma of one or both breasts.

Structural changes. These are various and complex, but can best be considered under the headings, (a) fibrosis, (b) cyst formation, (c) adenosis and (d) epitheliosis.

The breast tissue is firmer and more nodular than usual and the lobules may be visible on section as groups of small elongated yellowish-brown foci in the white rubbery collagenous stroma. Cysts of 2–10 mm diameter frequently occur in clusters: less commonly one or more larger cysts of bluish appearance, containing a thin mucoid or dark brownish fluid, are present.

Microscopic examination reveals a great variety of structural changes. When the changes are limited to fibrosis, adenosis, sclerosing adenosis and cyst formation, the name **simple cystic disease** is applied; but when epithelial hyperplasia (*epitheliosis*) is marked in ducts and acini the condition is better termed **hyperplastic cystic disease**. This distinction is important since only in the latter condition is there evidence of transition to neoplasia.

Some **fibrosis** accompanies most cases of mastopathy but is difficult to assess; the normally fibrous breast of young women persists even after the menopause in thin women, whereas in obese women the fibrous tissue of the breast may be extensively infiltrated with fat, and as age advances the fibrous mammary stroma becomes hyaline and relatively acellular while the epithelial elements atrophy. It is this collagenisation of pre-existing stroma rather than renewed fibroblastic activity that leads to fibrosis of the breast. Occasionally in heavy pendulous breasts this process leads to the appearance of an indurated mass in the upper outer quadrant.

Local dilatation of ducts, terminal ductules or acini results in **cyst formation**, and is presumably due to duct obstruction. Mammary duct ectasia may also occur (p. 926). Some cysts show metaplasia of the epithelial lining cells; these become large, columnar and eosinophilic with a feathery outline and at their apices may contain granules resembling those seen normally in apocrine gland epithelium. Cyst formation is more frequent at about the time of the menopause or thereafter and tends to affect both breasts. It is probably an involutional effect related to changes in hormone production.

Formation of new breast lobules and/or enlargement of pre-existing lobules occurs and is termed **adenosis**: the lobules retain their usual histological pattern (Fig. 23.56) and there is no intraluminal proliferation of cells to fill the acini, as occurs in pregnancy. A mild degree of adenosis occurs in the second half of each normal menstrual cycle, and the mammary hyperplasia of pregnancy begins as adenosis; during lactation secretory phenomena are superadded.

Adenosis is a feature of some mastopathies, and there it almost certainly results from hormonal stimulation. Adenosis plays no part in the development of carcinoma of the breast but may be prominent in the breast parenchyma around fibro-adenomas.

A perversion of adenosis, termed **sclerosing adenosis**, may occur as an isolated phenomenon producing a palpable rubbery greyish discoid mass in the breasts of young women. Com-

monly it follows incomplete involution after an interrupted pregnancy or lactational failure. Sclerosing adenosis also occurs in microscopic foci in the breasts of women of widely different age groups and may be present along with epithelial proliferative lesions, e.g. papilloma.

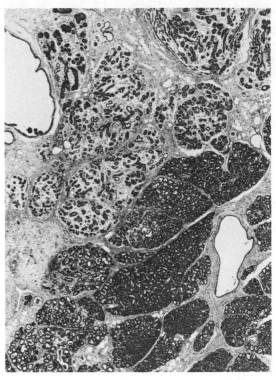

Fig. 23.56 Adenosis. There is a marked increase in the size and number of the lobules. Cystic dilatation of occasional ductules is present. × 22.

As in simple adenosis the changes are always lobular but lack the simple acinar pattern seen in adenosis. Sclerosing adenosis proceeds through a sequence of changes beginning with an early florid, confused picture of proliferation of both epithelial and myo-epithelial elements (Fig. 23.57). Mitotic activity may be high at this stage. Later the true epithelial elements atrophy and the myo-epithelial cells produce a corded appearance which simulates infiltrative carcinoma. Eventually the myo-epithelial elements undergo collagenisation which increases the resemblance to scirrhous carcinoma. Sclerosing adenosis has no significance as a precursor of carcinoma; its importance lies in the possibility of misdiagnosis as cancer, especially on immediate section in the operating theatre. Such errors are best avoided by careful low-power examination which reveals the typical *lobular* nature of the change. It is often accompanied by small papillomata and sometimes by microscopic foci of calcification which may be troublesome in mammography.

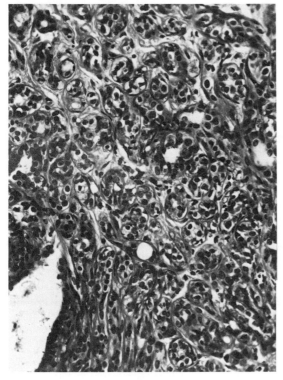

Fig. 23.57 Sclerosing adenosis in the florid phase; many small acini and solid cords of cells with much myo-epithelial hyperplasia. × 200.

The term **epitheliosis** was coined by Mrs. E. K. Dawson to describe the condition in which hyperplasia of the epithelium of ducts and acini results in the heaping up of lining cells which may eventually fill the lumina of ducts and acini more or less completely (Fig. 23.58). This hyperplasia may take three forms (*a*) *a solid type* in which the ducts are solidly filled, (*b*) *a cribriform variety* in which there is a tendency to acinar arrangement without stroma formation, and (*c*) *a papillary arrangement* in which the exuberant epithelial ingrowths are usually less well provided with fibrovascular cores than are true papillomas. Epitheliosis is an important condition and, unlike adenosis and sclerosing adenosis, may be associated with the development of carcinoma, although many

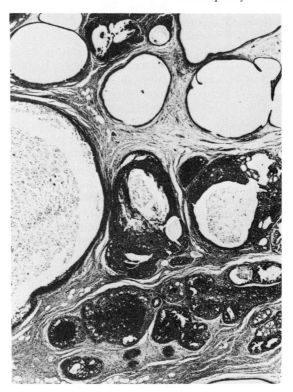

Fig. 23.58 Epitheliosis of breast. Some of the ducts are filled with masses of epithelial cells and others are dilated with granular secretion. × 22.

patients with epitheliosis escape this change. The presence of epitheliosis is the essential feature that distinguishes hyperplastic cystic disease from simple cystic mastopathy.

Localised hyperplastic cystic disease

While all the changes enumerated above may occur in generalised mastopathy it is probable that local areas of epitheliosis more often give rise to a clinically detectable lesion. Localised hyperplastic disease begins during the reproductive period and leads to an irregular induration or discrete swelling of the breast which demands surgical excision for exclusion of malignancy. Pain is not usually a feature and consequently hyperplastic disease often escapes notice. Necropsy studies have shown significant epithelial hyperplasia in about 25% of unselected women. In a similar proportion of breasts presenting with carcinoma, hyperplastic cystic disease is found to coexist with the tumour. In this localised form of disease cyst formation is often slight or absent. The epitheliosis present may be severe and in any combination of patterns, affecting few or many ducts or duct and acinar systems. Examination of a large number of amputated breasts suggests a picture of progressive dedifferentiation of the proliferative cells. Even within the same breast an evolutionary sequence from obviously benign to obviously malignant cells may be traced within the ducts and may, although less frequently, extend to the acini. Ultimately the ducts and acini are filled partially or completely by masses of cells with hyperchromatic and aberrant nuclei to which the terms **intraduct carcinoma**, and **intra-acinar carcinoma** are suitably applied. From either lesion malignant cells may invade the surrounding stroma as an ordinary infiltrative carcinoma.

Nevertheless, in many infiltrative breast cancers, neither epitheliosis nor intraduct cancer can be found. Some authorities do not believe that there is a causal relationship and suggest that epitheliosis and cancer represent different responses to the same aetiological agents.

Aetiology. The cause of hyperplastic cystic disease and its significant component of epitheliosis is still obscure. Inflammation plays no part and the commonly used synonym 'chronic mastitis' is quite unjustified. The changes seem likely to represent an endocrine effect, either from excess of oestrogen, which in certain species has been shown to bring about mammary hyperplasia and neoplasia, or from failure to achieve the normal balanced action of the sex hormones. Hyperplastic cystic disease in adolescents is sometimes accompanied by endometrial hyperplasia and menorrhagia.

'Hypertrophy' of the female breast

This must not be confused with the gross mammary adiposity observed in some obese middle-aged women. It usually develops soon after puberty although occasionally it may follow pregnancy. The breasts enlarge progressively and may eventually weigh several kilograms. The condition is usually bilateral but development may be unequal. The term hypertrophy is not really apt since the breast enlargement is due mainly to increase in soft oedematous connective tissue, and sometimes also of adipose tissue. Glandular tissue is not much increased and often appears scanty. The cause of hypertrophy is quite unknown in most cases. Rarely it accompanies various hormone-secreting tumours.

Tumours of the Breast

Benign tumours

Fibroadenoma

This is by far the commonest benign tumour of the breast and arises from the whole anatomical unit of the lobule. It is a mixed tumour with both stromal and epithelial neoplastic elements, and occurs chiefly in young women. Sometimes in young girls the fibrous component is inconspicuous and the tumour is then termed a simple *adenoma*. Fibroadenomas are small, well-circumscribed, elastic, round or ovoid masses which may occasionally attain a diameter of up to 7 cm. Rarely, they are multiple in one or both breasts. Although apparently encapsulated, they should not be enucleated by the surgeon's finger, for satellite portions of the tumour may be left behind from which recurrence takes place.

Two forms of fibroadenoma are usually distinguished but many tumours show both types of structure in different areas (Fig. 23.59). In young adults the so-called *pericanalicular type* occurs, in which the epithelial arrangement corresponds roughly to that in the normal breast lobule with an investment of loosely fibrillary connective tissue. The predominantly *intracanalicular* type seen usually in older women shows numerous curved and branching clefts lined by epithelium and produced by the pressure of blunt rounded projections of fibrocellular tissue upon ducts and acini. Growth of the lining epithelium merely keeps pace with that of

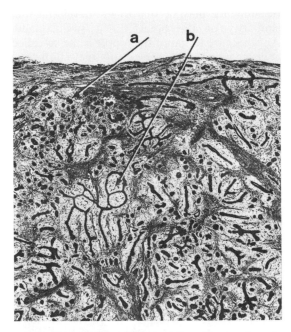

Fig. 23.59 Fibroadenoma of breast, showing the loose periacinar stroma. In places the tumour has a pericanalicular structure **a**, at other parts an intracanalicular arrangement **b**. Transitions are seen between the two types. × 16.

the stroma and the characteristic clefting is produced. When cut across, the surface of an intracanalicular fibroadenoma often appears irregular and nodular.

The site of origin of fibroadenoma is within the ductal elastic tissue; usually this is not obvious on cursory examination but occasional tumours present as intraduct lesions reminiscent of intraduct papilloma. In such cases bleeding from the nipple may occur. Multiple small fibroadenomatous areas sometimes occur in association with cystic disease suggesting an intermediate phenomenon between hyperplasia and neoplasia. Fibroadenomas grow not only by proliferation of the actual tumour but also by incorporating at their periphery altered lobular units showing such fibroadenomatous change. Some intracanalicular tumours contain large amounts of smooth muscle in their stroma: we have seen no convincing evidence that this originates from myo-epithelium and in some cases it appears to be derived from vein walls. During pregnancy a fibroadenoma may show secretory activity.

Giant intracanalicular fibroadenomas. In older women large fibroadenomas tend to recur after

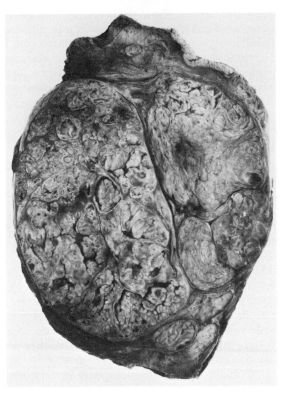

Fig. 23.60 Giant intracanalicular fibroadenoma of the breast. The stroma was very cellular and showed sarcomatous change. × 0·5.

removal (especially if 'shelled out') and the recurrent tumour may show a highly cellular and often a distinctly myxoid stroma. In some cases, especially after repeated recurrence, stromal proliferation is so marked that the epithelial elements may be quite inconspicuous and the tumour merits the designation of **myxo-sarcoma** (Fig. 23.60). The old term *Brodie's serocystic sarcoma* is best avoided. Simple mastectomy or very wide local excision is the treatment of choice. Such tumours should not be designated as sarcoma unless the stromal cells show the morphological changes of unequivocal malignancy; the development of frankly sarcomatous change is discussed further below. Rarely, carcinoma develops in a fibroadenoma.

Papillary cystadenoma

This benign tumour is much less common than fibroadenoma. Cysts of varying size are present and within these there is epithelial proliferation. Often these epithelial tumours have a somewhat papilliform pattern but they are composed of acini and do not show the investment of fibro-vascular cores by epithelium as in a papilloma. Papillary cystadenoma may become large and, if not removed, may ulcerate through the skin and present as papillary masses on the breast surface. Most are benign but occasionally cystadenocarcinoma supervenes. It is usually of low malignancy and careful local excision is adequate.

Duct papilloma

Duct papilloma occurs most often as a rounded pedunculated tumour which forms within and eventually distends a lactiferous sinus, in or close to the nipple (Figs. 11.4, p. 274; 23.61). A papilloma comprises a branching fibrovascular stromal core clothed by a double-layered cuboidal or columnar epithelium (Fig. 23.62), which is sometimes apocrine-like. In time, the epithelium may atrophy and hyalinisation occur. The tumour may be solitary and attain a size of more than 10 mm but sometimes multiple tumours are present throughout the duct system of the breast. The larger tumours are often accompanied by nipple discharge and those in the lactiferous sinus may present with frank bleeding from the nipple. Microscopic examination of such discharges usually shows red blood cells and tumour epithelial cells and often permits distinction from the coloured discharges present in mammary duct ectasia. Some papillomas of the lactiferous sinuses resemble papillary hidradenoma of the vulva. The nipple contains no sweat glands and the

resemblance may be due to the developmental similarity of the breast to a sweat gland. Another rare lesion of the nipple is the so-called adenoma: double-layering of the epithelium helps to identify it as benign despite stromal distortion.

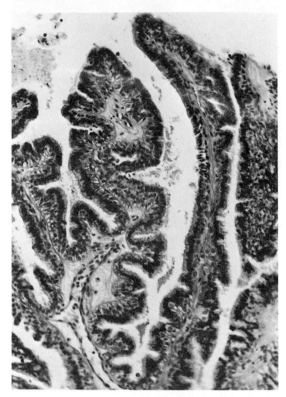

Fig. 23.62 Duct papilloma of breast, showing branching papilliform processes covered by epithelium mainly of columnar type. × 130.

Papillary forms of epitheliosis occur in hyperplastic cystic disease and it is difficult to draw a clear line betwen them and papillomatosis; the presence of well-formed fibrovascular stromal cores suggests multiple neoplasms. When such small papillomas are numerous, multicentric carcinoma occasionally develops. Carcinomatous change is rare in a solitary papilloma, and only local excision is necessary.

Other benign tumours

These are uncommon but fibroma, myxoma, lipoma, angioma and chondroma are recorded. Granular cell myoblastoma (p. 532) occasionally occurs in the breast and clinically may simulate carcinoma.

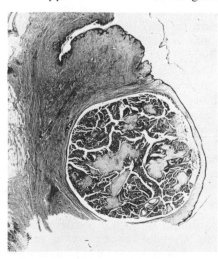

Fig. 23.61 A rounded duct papilloma distending a lactiferous sinus within the nipple. × 9.

Malignant tumours of the breast

Carcinoma

This is among the commonest of human cancers. While it occurs more often in later adult life it is by no means rare in the third and fourth decades: for this reason all lumps in the breast, whatever the age of the patient, must be regarded clinically as possibly malignant until proved otherwise by histological examination. Immediate histological examination of fresh sections at the time of operation is of value in enabling the surgeon to decide upon the type of treatment required. Screening procedures involving clinical examination, mammography, xeroradiography and thermography are being applied to the detection of breast cancer at an early stage, but their value requires further assessment.

Carcinoma of the breast is at least two hundred times more common in women than in men; it is more common in nulliparous than in multiparous women and several successful lactations appear to decrease the risk that it will develop. These observations suggest that endocrine factors may be important in the aetiology of breast cancer.

Varieties of breast cancer

Several types of breast carcinoma are described but this should not obscure the important fact that they are all manifestations of one disease process.

Scirrhous carcinoma. This is the commonest form of breast cancer; it produces an indurated mass of indefinite outline and the resulting fibrosis of the stroma causes contraction and shrinkage rather than obvious enlargement of the breast (Fig. 23.63). Fibrosis is most marked in the atrophic scirrhous carcinoma, which may remain less than 1 cm in diameter. When cut with a knife a scirrhous cancer gives a creaking sensation and the cut surface shows small yellow areas due to degeneration of tumour cells; this 'unripe pear' appearance is very characteristic of a scirrhous cancer. In the late stages distortion or retraction of the nipple or puckering and indrawing of the skin may occur depending on the site of the tumour, which may be in any part of the breast, including the axil-

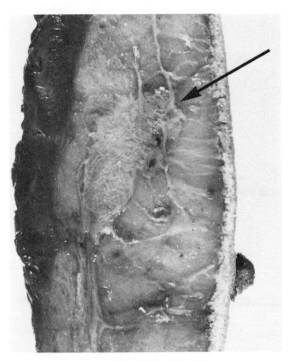

Fig. 23.63 Scirrhous carcinoma of the breast. The skin of the breast, including the nipple, is seen on the right and the pectoral muscles on the left. The cancer is seen on the cut surface (*arrow*) as an irregular paler area, lying in the breast tissue which is mainly fatty.

lary tail, but is most frequent in the upper outer portion. Microscopy shows groups and cords of spheroidal carcinoma cells (Fig. 11.15, p. 281) between bands of fibrous tissue which are more hyaline at the centre while at the periphery this change is less advanced. Recently McGee and his co-workers have provided biochemical and ultrastructural evidence that collagen is produced by the tumour cells, and have cast doubt on the general assumption that the fibrous stroma represents a desmoplastic reaction.

The scirrhous carcinoma of the breast was recognised as early as Hippocratic times and the appearances of a central tumour mass with infiltrating prongs (Fig. 23.64) originally suggested the words *cancer* and *carcinoma* (i.e. crab-like).

Encephaloid carcinoma. This tumour is less common than the scirrhous variety; it forms a large mass or masses, of brain-like softness (hence *encephaloid*) and with ill-defined mar-

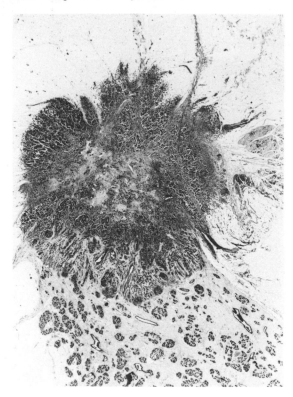

Fig. 23.64 Small scirrhous cancer of breast. The tumour has originated at the periphery and is invading both the breast tissue and the surrounding fat. Note the claw-like extensions. × 5·5.

gins and extensive areas of necrosis and haemorrhage. Sometimes necrosis and ulceration through the skin occurs. Microscopically a comparatively scanty and cellular stroma, often containing many lymphocytes, separates large collections of spheroidal tumour cells among which cellular aberration and frequent, often multipolar mitoses are seen (Fig. 11.16, p. 281).

The tumours with a heavy lymphocytic infiltrate (*medullary carcinomas*) appear to carry a relatively high 5-year survival rate, and the lymphocytes may represent an immunological reaction to the cancer cells.

Mammary carcinoma in pregnancy and lactation may grow very rapidly and be accompanied by hyperaemia, warmth, sometimes pain and fever. The whole picture may thus suggest an acute mastitis. This type of breast cancer is sometimes very diffusely infiltrative, so that the whole breast is swollen, hard and hyperaemic with no discrete lump; consequently it looks more like a cellulitis than a malignant tumour.

Histological appearances of breast carcinoma

In most scirrhous and encephaloid carcinomas the cells are quite anaplastic, spheroidal and arranged in irregular clumps (Fig. 11.13, p. 280). Less commonly the cells retain a certain polarity and a recognisably adenocarcinomatous pattern results. Such adenocarcinomas are said on statistical evidence to have a slightly better prognosis than anaplastic spheroidal cell tumours. Prognosis is also said to be better

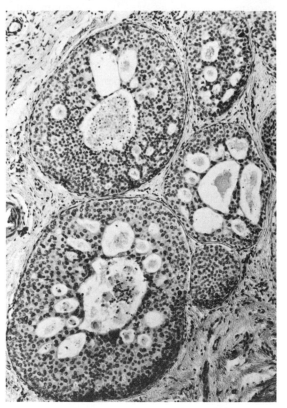

Fig. 23.65 'Cribriform carcinoma', showing masses of carcinoma cells among which are small circular spaces. The growth is still contained within ducts. × 100.

when pronounced elastosis is elicited by breast carcinomas. Rarely breast carcinomas are composed of masses of closely applied cells between which there are small circular spaces, sometimes containing mucoid material (Fig. 23.65): this pattern (*cribriform carcinoma*) is most readily seen in intraduct cancer, and is usually less obvious and often absent in infiltrating parts of the tumour. These observations are of importance in tracing the evolutionary sequences from epitheliosis through intraduct cancer to anaplastic infiltrative tumour.

Mucoid carcinoma (p. 280) is uncommon in the breast. It is usually bulky and often, but not always, less malignant than the commoner varieties, with delay in nodal metastasis.

Focal mucoid change is seen in some breast cancers, and the cells of some spheroidal-cell cancers contain mucin, particularly those in which columns of cancer cells, in 'single file', invade the stroma, often encircling ducts: some of these arise from lobular carcinoma in situ.

Sometimes the stroma of a cancer becomes myxoid (*carcinoma myxomatodes*).

Squamous carcinoma. Areas of squamous metaplasia sometimes occur in anaplastic carcinoma; the two histological variants may infiltrate together through the breast tissue and metastasise to lymph nodes. Occasional carcinomas are apparently entirely of squamous type. A further interesting variant is the fibrosarcoma-like squamous carcinoma in which the bulk of the tumour is spindle-celled; only careful search reveals that these cells are undoubtedly derived from squamous carcinoma which is recognisable in occasional areas. Such tumours are sometimes misdiagnosed as carcinosarcoma.

Spread of infiltrative carcinoma

The axillary lymph nodes are involved at an early stage by lymphatic dissemination and in many cases the internal mammary lymph nodes are also affected. Later the local skin lymphatics may be permeated leading to either focal nodularity or wider-spread involvement known as *cancer-en-cuirasse*. If the skin lymphatics are blocked, lymph-drainage is impaired and the skin becomes oedematous and swollen except where it is tacked down by hair-follicles; this produces the characteristic *peau d'orange* appearance of advanced breast cancer. Further lymphatic spread occurs through the connective tissues to the pectoral fascia and muscles and thence to the pleural cavities. In all of these situations microscopy may be required to reveal collections of malignant cells along the lymphatic pathways. It is upon these observations that the operation of radical mastectomy is based; unfortunately at the time of operation often there is already further spread by lym-

phatics (and possibly by the bloodstream) to other sites. Viscera and the thoraco-lumbar spine are frequently affected, the latter possibly by retrograde venous spread. Oöphorectomy, adrenalectomy and hypophysectomy (p. 936) have also revealed microscopic metastases in these organs. Metastatic spread to the opposite breast is not uncommon. Second primary carcinomas in the other breast also occur and may be identified as such by the presence of intraduct cancer (see below). Lymphatic dissemination of tumour occurs as rapidly in the atrophic scirrhous as in the fast-growing encephaloid variety.

Intraduct carcinoma and its relationship to infiltrative tumour

Intraduct carcinoma is a malignant proliferation of epithelial cells within the ducts of the breasts, i.e. it is a pre-invasive neoplasm which has not yet broken through the walls of the duct system (Fig. 23.66). In the larger ducts it can be recognised macroscopically and is readily seen with a hand-lens. The ducts are filled with cylindrical masses of cells and

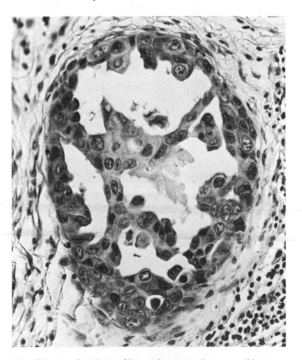

Fig. 23.66 Section of intraduct carcinoma of breast, showing collections of carcinoma cells of characteristic appearance in a duct. × 285.

degenerate fatty material which can sometimes be expressed like toothpaste from a tube; this is termed *comedo carcinoma*. Intraduct cancer may be relatively localised to one area or may affect the duct system extensively. Localised fibrosis (see below) may result in parts of the affected tissue becoming firm and palpable.

Microscopic examination shows rounded or polyhedral cells with a vesicular and often hyperchromatic nucleus, packed closely together or arranged in a cribriform pattern (Fig. 23.65). Both cells and nuclei may show considerable aberration. The condition spreads slowly along the ducts towards the nipple and also deeply into the acini, and may long remain confined within the basement membranes.

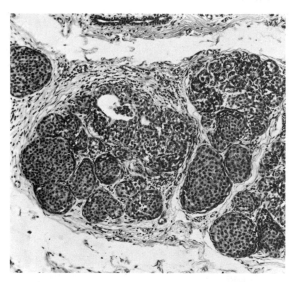

Fig. 23.67 Lobular or intra-acinar carcinoma, showing groups of acini filled with anaplastic carcinoma cells without any break-through into the adjacent stroma. × 75.

Local obliterative changes with fibrosis and elastosis sometimes occur with local healing of the lesion but this sclerosing process is never generalised.

Carcinoma in situ may occur also in the acini (*lobular* or *intra-acinar carcinoma*—Fig. 23.67) either alone or, more commonly, with intraduct carcinoma. Lobular carcinoma is most often found incidentally in a breast biopsy performed because of cystic disease, and empirical biopsies have shown that it is not uncommonly bilateral. The appearances must not be confused with those of lobular adenosis (see p. 928). Lobular carcinoma may long remain confined to the acini, but when infiltration does occur the prognosis is poor.

Endocrine dependence

In 1896 Beatson in Glasgow first showed that bilateral oöphorectomy was followed by prolonged remission in some cases of advanced breast cancer and he postulated that such mammary cancers required for their continuing growth some influence from the ovaries. This original idea has been developed in the light of modern surgery and endocrinology into the concept of hormone-dependent (i.e. oestrogen-dependent) tumours. Some post-menopausal women with breast cancer continue to secrete oestrogens and in an attempt to deprive such patients of all sources of oestrogen, removal of the ovaries was undertaken, followed by adrenalectomy and hypophysectomy when cortisone became available for maintenance treatment. Paradoxically, administration of oestrogens or androgens is sometimes beneficial in cases unsuitable for surgery.

In a small proportion of cases such procedures are successful in relieving symptoms, notably pain from skeletal metastases, but after a variable period the malignant cells resume their uncontrolled growth, i.e. the tumour becomes *hormone-independent*. No histological differences have been demonstrated by which hormone-dependent tumours can be recognised under the microscope and at present therapeutic trial is necessary to determine which cases will respond to endocrine ablation. Hormones other than oestrogen may be implicated, including progesterone, androgens and mammatrophic prolactin. Large-scale prospective studies are being carried out which may throw light on this problem, and the surface receptors of cancer cells are being studied in order to develop techniques of predicting hormone-dependence.

Despite the clinical remission obtained in cases of hormone-dependent cancer by such procedures there is only minimal evidence of tumour-cell destruction in most instances and only temporary arrest of tumour growth, but without doubt these drastic surgical procedures sometimes relieve pain.

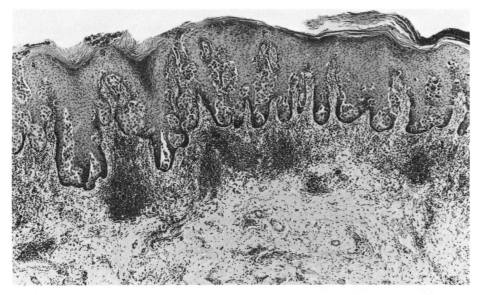

Fig. 23.68 Skin of nipple in Paget's disease, showing scattered Paget cells in deeper part of epidermis. Note marked lymphocytic infiltration of dermis. × 45.

Paget's disease of the breast

In this condition, first described clinically by Sir James Paget in 1874, part or all of the nipple and areola becomes reddened and excoriated and has a florid eczematous appearance with oozing of clear fluid. The tissues of the nipple are often firmer than normal. Paget observed that this state might persist for years but that eventually invasive cancer commonly developed, often deep in the breast parenchyma and separated from the nipple by apparently normal tissue.

Microscopic examination reveals *Paget cells* within the affected epidermis. There has been much debate concerning the nature of these cells, which occur singly or in groups and often most abundantly in the deeper epidermal layers where they may form blunt processes projecting down into the dermis (Fig. 23.68). Paget cells in their active period of growth are large round or oval cells with pale cytoplasm and vesicular, often hyperchromatic nuclei, with prominent nucleoli. Mitotic figures are sometimes seen. The appearance of the cells is reminiscent of those of an undifferentiated carcinoma of glandular origin. They infiltrate and displace the cells of the Malpighian layer which become drawn out or flattened between them (Fig. 23.69). Usually many Paget cells undergo degeneration, i.e. their nuclei become irregular and pyknotic and their cytoplasm has a rather

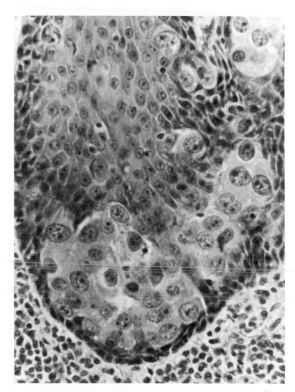

Fig. 23.69 Paget's disease of nipple. Epidermal rete ridge invaded by cancer cells—'Paget cells'. The cells are particularly well preserved and show a marked contrast to the epidermal cells which are being stretched and atrophied. × 345.

shrivelled appearance. When many of the cells show this change their nature may not be clear. Paget cells may take up melanin from adjacent melanoblasts and sometimes they contain a small amount of mucin. The epidermal cells around groups of Paget cells undergo compression atrophy, and may appear to form a dense capsule-like structure. Paget cells never grow down into the underlying dermis but the latter shows reactive changes, e.g. plasma cell infiltration, formation of new capillaries, hyperaemia and serous exudation. It is these changes in the dermis which cause the characteristic clinical appearances of the condition.

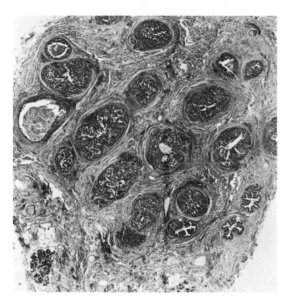

Fig. 23.70 Transverse section through the lactiferous ducts below the nipple in a case of Paget's disease, showing intraduct carcinoma in the ducts. × 12·5.

As Muir showed in convincing fashion, Paget's disease is always accompanied by intraduct carcinoma in the ducts of the nipple (Fig. 23.70) and frequently direct continuity may be traced between the cells in the ducts and those in the epidermis. Statements that Paget's disease is the result of a field change of neoplasia independently but concomitantly affecting the epidermis and the ductal epithelium are not well substantiated. Intraduct carcinoma may be complicated by Paget's disease and/or by infiltrative carcinoma of the breast. Accordingly, Paget's disease indicates the presence of intraduct carcinoma which may invade the breast stroma if it has not already done so. Simple mastectomy is therefore essential. Whether intraduct carcinoma is followed by Paget's disease or by ordinary infiltrative carcinoma depends upon whether the affected ducts are in the nipple or breast parenchyma. Occasional mastectomy specimens show on examination of the apparently normal nipple that Paget's disease is commencing or that intraduct neoplasm is nearing the epidermis. Forms of Paget's disease of the skin may occur in the vulva, perianal region, axilla, etc., by intra-epithelial spread of carcinoma of the sweat glands.

Occasional primary intra-epithelial tumours of the nipple epidermis occur. Bowen's disease of skin and malignant lentigo of the nipple may also produce widespread intra-epithelial growth, but in neither case is there intraduct carcinoma. Squamous carcinoma of the nipple is rare.

Other malignant tumours of the breast

Sarcoma. This is much less common than carcinoma. It may supervene in giant intracanalicular fibroadenoma of middle-aged or elderly women especially after inadequate resection. It is usually well-defined (Fig. 23.71) and spindle-celled, myxomatous or pleomorphic. Cellular aberration and mitotic activity are related to

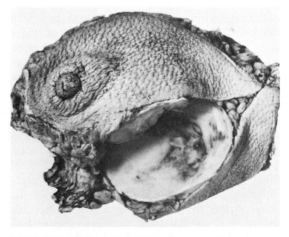

Fig. 23.71 Sarcoma of the breast. The tumour appears sharply circumscribed, and the cut surface shows central necrosis. × 0·6.

the degree of malignancy. Some sarcomas show metaplasia with formation of chondroid and osteoid and may resemble osteosarcoma or giant cell tumour of bone. In these cases the prognosis is bad and death from pulmonary metastases is the rule. The rare malignant haemangio-endothelioma tends to occur especially in the breast and gives rise to very widespread metastases.

Lymphomas. Hodgkin's disease and other lymphomas and leukaemias may all affect the breast. Rarely, enlargement of one or both breasts may be the presenting symptom in leukaemia or Hodgkin's disease. As the axillary lymph nodes are likely also to be affected the clinical diagnosis may be difficult.

Secondary carcinoma in breast. Spread to the contralateral breast may occur from a primary breast cancer. Carcinomas in other organs, e.g. bronchus, may also occasionally metastasise to the breast.

Congenital abnormalities

The absence of one or both of the breasts—*amazia*—is rare; in some instances it has been associated with a corresponding defect of one or both of the ovaries. *Athelia*, or congenital absence of the nipple, is less uncommon and usually bilateral. Hypoplasia of the breasts occurs in association with a similar condition of the ovaries and other parts of the genital system. There may be additional mammary glands (*polymastia*), which are capable of secretion, although they sometimes lack a nipple. They occur anywhere along the mammary line, but most often below the breasts. The term *polythelia* signifies the presence of multiple nipples.

The Male Breast

Hypertrophy (gynaecomastia). The male breast is essentially similar to that of the female until the onset of the secondary sex characters at puberty; in some adolescent males one or both breasts may then enlarge. This is known as *pubertal hypertrophy* and is rarely marked, but may cause pain or discomfort. It is due mainly to increase in stroma and of ducts, but without lobule formation. The hyperplastic duct epithelium may be surrounded by a zone of oedematous, fibrillary stroma. It tends to regress and operative removal is rarely necessary. Similar changes may occur in old age.

Gynaecomastia sometimes complicates cirrhosis of the liver, due to failure of the liver to metabolise and break down oestrogens. Hypertrophy also follows prolonged administration of diethylstilboestrol in the treatment of prostatic cancer, and less commonly other drugs, e.g. digitalis. Occasionally hypertrophy results from an underlying endocrine disease such as a feminising tumour of the adrenal cortex. Less often testicular injury is causal. In chromatin-positive *Klinefelter's syndrome* (p. 883) the enlarged breasts show lobules comparable with those of the normal female breasts. Lobule formation is excessively rare in other forms of enlargement, but is seen occasionally after prolonged administration of oestrogens.

Tumours are rare. Carcinoma may be of anaplastic spheroidal-cell type or adenocarcinomatous. Prognosis is often poor because of early spread to lymph nodes and to the chest wall. Paget's disease of the male breast is very rare. Metastatic carcinoma, e.g. from bronchus, occasionally occurs and the male breast, like that of the female, may be involved in generalised lymphoid neoplasms and the leukaemias.

24

The Endocrine System

The clinical features of most endocrine disorders are attributable to the secretion of too much or too little hormone. Such disturbances can arise in various ways. For example, diminished secretion of thyroid hormone can result from chronic inflammatory destruction of the thyroid, usually due to auto-immune thyroiditis; it can result also from any lesion of the pituitary which interferes with the production and secretion of thyrotrophic hormone (TSH). The secretion of TSH is, in turn, influenced by the secretion of a TSH-releasing hormone (and possibly also by a release-inhibiting hormone) by the hypothalamus. Accordingly, hypothalamic or pituitary-stalk lesions can interfere with thyroid function. This possibility of lesions in various sites having a similar endocrine effect applies also to the functioning of the adrenals and the gonads, which, like the thyroid, are controlled largely by pituitary trophic hormones.

It must also be emphasised that complex functional interrelationships exist between the endocrine glands and between the effects of various hormones. Thus the effects of insulin on sugar metabolism are very largely antagonistic to those of growth hormone, thyroid hormone, glucocorticoids and catecholamines, and the control of glucose metabolism represents a balance between these various factors. Indeed, the normal endocrine status depends on the balanced functioning of the various endocrine glands with their feed-back mechanisms and complex interrelationships.

The relationships between the brain and pituitary are particularly important. The neurohypophysis acts as a store of hormones produced in the basal nuclei, while the release of the hormones synthesised in the adenohypophysis is influenced, as mentioned above, by low molecular weight polypeptide hormones secreted by the hypothalamus.

The pituitary has long been regarded as the 'conductor of the endocrine orchestra': it might now be added that the hypothalamus shares in the selection of the music.

The successful production of antibodies to many hormones in experimental animals has

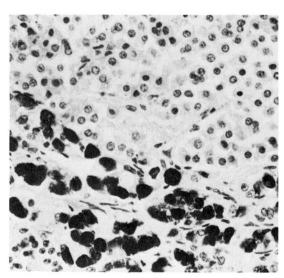

Fig. 24.1 Section of adenohypophysis stained by the immunoperoxidase method, using antibody to growth hormone. The cytoplasm of cells containing growth hormone is stained black. The field includes the edge of a chromophobe adenoma (above), the cells of which are devoid of growth hormone. (Prof. R. B. Goudie.)

allowed the application of two types of immunological technique which are now making major contributions to endocrinology. The first is the use of antibodies to detect the presence of hormones in individual cells, e.g. growth hormone in pituitary cells, by means of fluorescent labels or peroxidase (pp. 91, 92 and Fig. 24.1). Secondly, it is now possible to assay the low concentrations of many hormones in plasma, urine, etc., by radio-immunoassay techniques:

this is of great value both in diagnosis and in endocrinological research.

Most of the endocrine glands have considerable functional reserve, and so can often continue to function apparently normally when partially destroyed by disease. They also have a high capacity for hyperplasia, and can enlarge to meet an increased work load or to overcome some functional defect. For example individuals who are deficient in iodine (an essential component of thyroid hormone) develop thyroid hyperplasia, sometimes visible as enlargement (goitre), and by increasing the rate of iodine turnover the hyperplastic gland may be able to maintain relatively normal function.

In general, endocrine glands are not subject to bacterial infections, an exception being tuberculosis and some other chronic infections of the adrenals. Only a few viral infections are known, e.g. involvement of the gonads, pancreas and sometimes the thyroid in mumps. An important group of endocrine disorders results from the organ-specific auto-immune diseases, which cause destructive inflammation of the thyroid, adrenal and parathyroid glands, and rarely of the endocrine components of the gonads. The common form of hyperthyroidism (Graves' disease) is also of auto-immune nature.

Lastly, all the endocrine glands are subject to neoplasia, the frequency varying for the different glands and in different communities. Endocrine tumours are of special importance because they frequently secrete hormones in uncontrolled fashion: they may also, by compressing or invading the surrounding glandular tissue, lead to hypofunction.

The Pituitary

The adenohypophysis (anterior lobe)

Introduction

The blood supply to the adenohypophysis is peculiar in that, except for the tissue immediately beneath the capsule, there is no direct arterial supply, blood passing from the capillaries in the hypothalamus into venous portal channels which traverse the stalk and break up into the sinusoids of the adenohypophysis. This arrangement allows hormonal factors secreted by the hypothalamus to influence adenohypophyseal function (see below): it also renders the adenohypophysis liable to ischaemic injury, e.g. during the circulatory collapse of shock, and permits almost complete destruction of the gland by deliberate surgical interruption of the stalk.

The adenohypophyseal hormones include (1) *growth hormone* (GH) or *somatotrophin*, a globular protein of molecular weight 44 000, which has been isolated in crystalline form; (2) *lactogenic hormone*, or *prolactin*, also a globular protein; (3) *gonadotrophic hormones* (FSH and LH), which are glycoproteins; (4) *thyroid stimulating hormone* (TSH), also a glycoprotein;

(5) *corticotrophin* (ACTH), a polypeptide; and (6) *melanin-stimulating hormone* (MSH), also a polypeptide.

The hormone-secreting cells

The anterior pituitary hormones listed above are synthesised and secreted by cells of the adenohypophysis. Although different types of cell can be distinguished by their morphological and staining properties, it has proved difficult to determine which cell secretes which hormone(s). Initially, the cells were classified by the presence or absence of basophilic or eosinophilic cytoplasmic granules into basophil (13%), eosinophil (37%) and chromophobe cells (50%), the last containing neither type of granule. Subsequently, it was shown by Pearse's tri-PAS stain that all basophils, some eosinophils and some chromophobes contain PAS-positive granules. Some cells were shown to contain large numbers of these; others were sparsely granular, and were termed *gamma cells*, eosinophils being called *alpha cells* and basophils subdivided into *beta* and *delta cells* on the basis of staining differences. The relationships of eosinophil and basophil cell adenomas with acromegaly (or gigantism) and Cushing's syndrome respectively suggested eosinophil cells as the source of growth hormone and basophils as the source of ACTH. Chromophobe adenomas were usually unaccompanied by evidence of excessive hormone secretion, and accordingly the chromophobe cells were regarded as inactive, possibly precursor cells. These early observations have been largely confirmed, but it is now generally accepted that heavily granular cells are storing hormone, whereas sparsely granular cells, including some of the chromophobes, are actively secreting cells.

Electron-microscopy has contributed to the recognition of cell function. For example, secretory granules of growth hormone are large, spherical, and fairly regular (300–400 nm in diameter), granules of lactogenic hormone are also large and spherical, but vary more in size, and TSH granules are much smaller.

The use of immunofluorescence techniques to detect intracellular hormones has shown that: (1) growth hormone is synthesised by eosinophil cells lying mainly in the lateral parts of the gland; (2) lactogenic hormone is also produced by eosinophilic cells, but they are different from the GH cells; (3) LH is produced by singly-scattered triangular basophil cells, while the source of FSH has not yet been firmly settled owing to the difficulty in developing specific antibody to FSH; (4) TSH is produced by tall polyhedral cells lying mainly centrally in the adenohypophysis; (5) ACTH is produced by basophilic cells which are also situated centrally in the gland and adjacent to the neurohypophysis—it is likely that the same cells also secrete MSH; and (6) approximately 25% of adenohypophyseal cells contain no detectable hormone, and their function is uncertain.

Control of adenohypophyseal function

Secretion of each of the adenohypophyseal trophic hormones—FSH, LH, TSH and ACTH— is controlled by a negative feed-back system in which the hormone secreted by the target organ inhibits secretion of the trophic hormone. For example, TSH secretion is suppressed by a high level of thyroid hormone in the plasma. This control appears to work partly by the direct effect of thyroid hormone, cortisol, etc., on the appropriate cells in the adenohypophysis, but it is also partly under the control of the hypothalamus, which releases from the median eminence oligopeptide hormones which are carried by the hypophyseal portal vascular system to the sinusoids in the anterior pituitary and there influence the secretion of the trophic hormones. Releasing-hormones for TSH (TRH), LH and FSH (LH/FSH–RH) and GH (GRH) have been analysed and synthesised and TRH and LH/FSH–RH are already being used in clinical diagnosis. Release-inhibiting factors have also been detected recently, and growth-hormone release-inhibiting hormone (GHRIH or somatostatin) has been shown to be a tetradecapeptide, produced mainly, but perhaps not only, in the hypothalamus. Unlike the releasing hormones, somatostatin has been shown to affect not only pituitary function, but also to inhibit secretion of insulin and glucagon. It also inhibits secretion of prolactin, but this is not surprising in view of the close association of somatotrophin and prolactin secretion. Some workers, however, claim that there is a specific prolactin release-inhibiting hormone (PRIH).

In view of the number of adenohypophyseal hormones and the complexity of their control and interrelationships, it is not surprising that disorders of the pituitary have complex and varied results. Their complexity is further increased by the situation of the organ in the bony sella, for an adenoma of one cell type may secrete excess hormone and yet lead to compression and destruction of the normal pituitary tissue, with consequent deficiency of the other hormones. Moreover, a lesion in or above the sella may produce various effects on the complex functions of both the pituitary and the hypothalamus.

The adenohypophyseal hormones

Growth hormone (GH) is essential, together with thyroid hormone and insulin, for a normal rate of growth. Its somatotrophic effect has been demonstrated by replacement therapy in dwarf hypophysectomised animals. It may be assayed biologically in hypophysectomised rats by measuring its stimulating effect on the incorporation of [^{35}S]-sulphate into chondroitin sulphate or its effect on the thickness of the epiphyseal plates. One of the effects of GH is to stimulate protein synthesis, although the mechanism is not known. It has, however, been shown to exert its hormonal effects by production of an intermediate factor, **somatomedin**. The human pituitary gland is a surprisingly rich source from which GH has been purified: on injection into patients with hypopituitarism, in doses of up to 10 mg daily, it reverses the negative nitrogen balance, and stimulates growth in hypopituitary dwarfs. Although it has a diabetogenic effect, this is not readily demonstrated in man except in hypophysectomised diabetic patients, in whom it greatly aggravates the diabetes.

Radio-immunoassay of human GH correlates moderately well with bio-assay and has the advantage of much greater sensitivity. By its use, the plasma level in adults is found to be usually below 3 μg/litre. Rapid rise of plasma GH follows exercise, ingestion of amino acids or injection of insulin, and these stimuli are enhanced by oestrogens. Its secretion is also stimulated by the effect of β-adrenergic receptor blockade on the hypothalamus, and by L-dopa.

Lactogenic hormone (prolactin) is concerned in the initiation and maintenance of lactation in breast tissue primed by oestrogen, progesterone, corticosteroids and insulin. It can be assayed by its lactogenic effect on explants of mammary tissue from pregnant mice, but a more rapid, accurate and sensitive method has been provided by radio-immunoassay. The plasma levels of prolactin in normal men and women are not very different, and yet its only known role is in lactation. During pregnancy the plasma level rises progressively but its lactogenic action is held in check by the high levels of oestrogen and progesterone which persist until after delivery. Mammary stimulation is followed by a sharp rise in plasma prolactin, and human TSH-releasing hormone also appears to release prolactin. Prolactin may be concerned in the so-called hormone dependence of some mammary cancers.

Gonadotrophic hormones. Maturation and function of the gonads in both males and females is dependent on the two adenohypophyseal gonadotrophic hormones, **follicle-stimulating hormone (FSH)** and **luteinising** or **interstitial cell stimulating hormone (LH** or **ICSH)**. FSH is essential for the growth of the Graafian follicle and for ovulation, and LH for

luteinisation of the follicle following ovulation. Under the influence of these hormones the Graafian follicle secretes oestrogen, which induces endometrial proliferation, and the corpus luteum secretes progesterone, which inhibits further ovulation and induces endometrial secretory change.

In males, FSH stimulates spermatogenesis and LH stimulates the Leydig cells to secrete testosterone.

Rare cases of infertility in both men and women result from gonadotrophin deficiencies. Excessive production of LH may also give rise to the syndrome of polycystic ovaries and infertility. It is possible that certain abnormalities of the breasts, such as cystic change, may depend upon pituitary abnormality.

Thyrotrophic hormone (TSH) stimulates thyroid epithelium by activating adenyl cyclase. It induces enlargement and proliferation of thyroid epithelium and increases secretion of thyroid hormone into the blood. Thyroxine exerts a negative feed-back on TSH secretion, partly directly and partly via the hypothalamus. Plasma TSH can now be determined by radio-immunoassay: it is undetectable in about 10% of normal subjects, is always elevated in patients with untreated primary hypothyroidism, and is suppressed by administration of thyroxine. As explained later, the form of hyperthyroidism known as Graves' disease is due to an abnormal thyroid stimulator, and TSH secretion is suppressed by the high levels of thyroid hormone.

Adrenocorticotrophic hormone (ACTH) is essential for the secretion of glucocorticoid steroid hormones, e.g. cortisol and cortisone. These steroids operate a negative feed-back effect, partly directly on the adenohypophysis and partly via the hypothalamus, which secretes an ACTH-releasing factor (CRF) and possibly also a release-inhibiting factor. ACTH stimulates adrenocortical cells by activating adenyl cyclase, and hypophysectomy or administration of cortisol results in adrenocortical atrophy.

Reliable radio-immunoassay techniques have now been reported for ACTH and it has been shown that the plasma levels, usually below 50 μg/litre in normal adults, have a circadian rhythm; the level rises in individuals exposed to stress and may exceed 500 μg/litre. High levels are also to be expected, and are observed, in Addison's disease (primary adrenocortical insufficiency) and in patients with 'inappropriate' secretion of ACTH, e.g. by a bronchial carcinoma.

ACTH consists of 39 amino-acid residues of which only the first 24 are necessary for its hormonal effect. It has been synthesised and can be administered repeatedly without development of a refractory state. Its administration causes adrenocortical hyperplasia and increased excretion of glucocorticoid hormones, resulting in gluconeogenesis, atrophy of the thymus and lymph nodes and lymphopenia. The secretion of the adrenal cortical hormone most active in controlling sodium and potassium—aldosterone—does not appear to be under anterior pituitary control; the factors controlling its release are not fully understood, but one of them is renin, produced by the granular cells of the juxta-glomerular apparatus (p. 221).

The importance of ACTH has been emphasised by the therapeutic effects of certain adrenal cortical hormones on various diseases, including some attributable to hypersensitivity reactions, and others of unknown aetiology.

Melanin stimulating hormone (MSH) is a polypeptide with a structure similar to part of the ACTH molecule, and indeed there is some doubt as to whether it is a separate hormone in man, or simply a fragment of ACTH. Most antibodies to human ACTH prepared in animals react also with human MSH, but production of more specific antibodies said to distinguish between the two hormones has now been reported. It is probable, however, that ACTH and MSH are secreted by the same pituitary cells, and their relationship is still obscure.

When the adrenals are destroyed by disease, the output of MSH in the urine is increased, because increased pituitary secretion results from lack of inhibition by adrenal hormones. This is probably responsible for the increased pigmentation in Addison's disease (q.v.), and chloasma of pregnancy is probably also due to increase in MSH secretion.

Adenohypophyseal hyperfunction

Acromegaly and gigantism

These conditions are both due to prolonged and excessive secretion of growth hormone, usually by a pituitary adenoma (Fig. 24.2) but occasionally without a tumour. The adenoma is most commonly of eosinophil-cell type but sometimes chromophobe: electron-microscopy shows the characteristic growth hormone (GH) secretory granules (p. 942), and immunohistology demonstrates the presence of GH in the tumour cells.

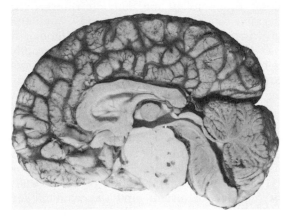

Fig. 24.2 An eosinophil adenoma of the pituitary in a case of acromegaly.

In both conditions there is excessive growth of bone and soft tissues and enlargement of most of the internal organs, e.g. liver, kidneys, heart, thyroid and adrenals. Initially, excessive growth hormone secretion is accompanied by normal or occasionally increased secretion of the other adenohypophyseal hormones. The reason for this latter is not fully understood; there may be great muscularity and abnormal strength, sexual precocity in children and increased libido in adults. Glucose tolerance is diminished and in 10% of cases there is frank diabetes mellitus. The blood pressure is often raised and the heart hypertrophied. As the tumour enlarges, however, it compresses and destroys the surrounding adenohypophysis and lack of the hormones other than GH gradually supervenes. Muscle wasting, weakness and asthenia develop and glucose tolerance increases. In some instances the tumour undergoes infarction, cystic change and fibrosis, ceases to secrete excess of GH, and changes in bone and elsewhere then become inactive. The enlarging tumour may also compress the inner parts of the optic nerves, resulting in bitemporal hemianopia sometimes progressing to blindness. The hypothalamus may also be compressed with various consequences, sometimes including diabetes insipidus.

Acromegaly means enlargement of the extremities. It results when the GH-secreting tumour develops after fusion of the epiphyses so that the bones cannot elongate but can grow thicker by periosteal ossification. The hands and feet are increased in size, especially in width. The increase is at first mainly in the soft tissues though thickening of bone occurs later.

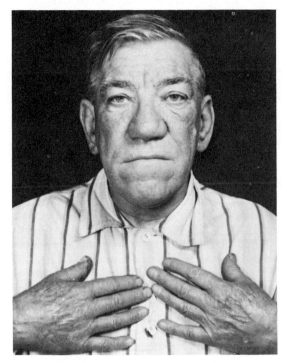

Fig. 24.3 Acromegaly, illustrating the thickening of the nose and enlargement of the lower jaw.

The face is enlarged, especially the nose, which is widened, and the lower jaw is lengthened and its angle widened (Fig. 24.3) so that the teeth project beyond those of the upper jaw. The lips become thickened and there is enlargement of the tongue. The skin is thickened and somewhat warty and the hair is coarse and wiry. In the skeleton generally there tends to be increase of bony prominences and there may be roughening of the surface of the bones. Irregular bone growth distorts the joint surfaces and crippling osteoarthritis commonly results. Kyphosis is often present due to irregular vertebral atrophy and hypertrophy. Pain and paraesthesias may

result from compression of nerves by bone or soft tissue, e.g. the carpal tunnel syndrome. Galactorrhoea due to excessive prolactin secretion sometimes occurs in acromegalic women, even when elderly.

Plasma levels of GH are usually raised, sometimes only slightly, e.g. 5–10 μg/litre, sometimes greatly, e.g. 1 mg/litre. Where the diagnosis is in doubt it may be confirmed by demonstrating failure to induce the normal fall in plasma GH by oral administration of glucose. Gross acromegaly is rare; lesser degrees are more common and sometimes accompany adenomas of chromophobe type. In either case the condition may become inactive due either to infarction of the tumour or in some cases to development of resistance of the various tissue cells to GH. If mild, such 'fugitive' acromegaly may be difficult to diagnose but enlargement of the sella, demonstrable radiographically, will often confirm the diagnosis. There is an increased mortality rate in active acromegaly, mostly from heart failure attributable to hypertension, often extensive atheroma, and sometimes to a form of cardiomyopathy with interstitial fibrosis. Other features of acromegaly occur also in gigantism and are as described above.

Gigantism is much rarer than acromegaly. It results when excessive GH secretion develops before the epiphyses have fused. A considerable increase in height, sometimes to over 8 feet (2·4 m), may result. Growth is proportionate, so that the bones are both long and thick, the thoracic cage enlarged, etc. Epiphyseal fusion is delayed but occurs eventually. If GH secretion is still excessive, the features of acromegaly then become superadded.

The hormonal changes are as described above for both acromegaly and gigantism. The stage of adenohypophyseal compression and insufficiency usually develops around early adult life and unless treated most patients die from infections or various effects of hypopituitarism. As in acromegaly, there is, in most cases, an eosinophil adenoma, but in 10% a chromophobe adenoma. Small eosinophil adenomas are sometimes found at necropsy with no evidence of previous hyperfunction.

The pituitary in Cushing's syndrome

Cushing described a remarkable clinical picture which he attributed to the presence of a small basophil adenoma of the adenohypophysis. It is now known that the condition is due to excessive secretion of glucocorticoids by the adrenal glands, hyperplasia or neoplasia of which is invariably present. A pituitary adenoma, usually of basophil but occasionally of chromophobe cell type, is present in less than 10% of cases. In some cases without evidence of either an adrenal or pituitary tumour, cure has resulted from pituitary ablation. A basophil pituitary adenoma has been reported to develop quite frequently in patients with Cushing's syndrome treated by total adrenalectomy, although such tumours are not seen in patients with Addison's disease (primary adrenocortical insufficiency). Cushing's syndrome may also result from inappropriate secretion of ACTH or an ACTH-like compound by a bronchial carcinoma or, less commonly, tumours of the thymus, pancreas or ovary.

In Cushing's syndrome, Crooke observed cells scattered around the periphery of the adenohypophysis showing a peculiar hyaline change (Fig. 24.4): this was the only pituitary lesion common to all cases. The change, which has since been observed by many workers, is probably a consequence of high levels of glucocorticoids for it is seen not only in associa-

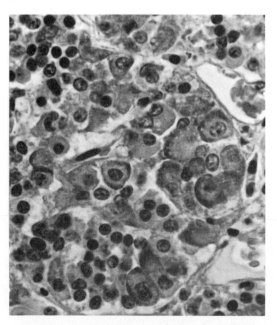

Fig. 24.4 Adenohypophysis in Cushing's syndrome, showing cytoplasmic hyaline change in the basophils. × 500.

tion with adrenal hyperplasia but also in those with autonomously secreting adrenal cortical tumours and also after prolonged therapeutic administration of ACTH or cortisone. Electron-microscopy has shown the hyaline change to be due to increase in micro-tubular material: it does not react with antibody to ACTH and its nature is unknown.

Adenohypophyseal hypofunction

This may occur from an unknown cause, as a result of lesions arising in the pituitary itself, or from pressure and destruction by adjacent lesions. Pituitary lesions include adenomas, post-partum ischaemic necrosis, trauma, various infections and macrophage granulomas of unknown nature. Auto-immune destruction is a possibility and giant-cell granulomas may be present also in the thyroid and adrenals.

The adenohypophysis has large functional reserves and destruction must be extensive to cause deficiencies. In progressive panhypopituitarism, deficiency of growth hormone and gonadotrophins appears first, followed by deficiency of ACTH and of TSH. Occasionally isolated deficiency of any one of the pituitary hormones occurs, the cause being obscure.

The clinical and pathological features of panhypopituitarism are described in the syndromes outlined below. Diagnosis may be confirmed by radio-immunoassay of adenohypophyseal hormones in the plasma. Low plasma corticosteroids with a normal response to ACTH is virtually diagnostic. If the plasma corticosteroid levels are borderline, TSH or growth hormone may be assayed.

The following are the best-known examples of hypofunction of the adenohypophysis.

Simmonds' disease (Sheehan's syndrome)

This is the commonest and most important example of anterior lobe hypofunction. Although first described by Simmonds, Sheehan elucidated the clinical and pathological features, and corrected the misconception that marked wasting was a feature.

Aetiology. The condition occurs in women and is nearly always the result of extensive ischaemic necrosis of the adenohypophysis associated with childbirth. Predisposing factors are the enlargement of the pituitary which occurs during pregnancy, the low-pressure portal vascular supply of the adenohypophysis, and the development of hypotensive shock as a result of difficult labour, often with trauma and excessive haemorrhage.

Clinical features. The first noticeable sign following the causal delivery is failure of lactation, which is due to deficiency of prolactin. Subsequently there is total loss of axillary and pubic hair, amenorrhoea, sterility and absence of libido. Symptoms are sometimes noticed only several years after the childbirth presumably responsible for the pituitary lesion.

Later, hypersensity to cold and other features of hypothyroidism develop, and ACTH deficiency leads to asthenia, hypotension, debility and sometimes fatal collapse. There may be a normochromic anaemia. The fasting blood sugar is usually below normal because the action of insulin is unopposed by growth hormone, corticosteroids and thyroxine, but 'compensatory' fall in insulin secretion usually occurs and averts serious hypoglycaemia. Nevertheless, patients are extremely sensitive to an injection of insulin.

Pigmentation of the skin, as in Addison's disease, does not occur: in fact, the pigment decreases, and the skin has a waxy or alabaster appearance. There is no serious loss of salt and water control, since the secretion of aldosterone is largely independent of the pituitary (p. 972): there does seem to be some mineralocorticoid disturbance, however, for when general metabolism is increased by administration of thyroxine, symptoms of adrenal insufficiency, including water and salt loss, may develop. The neurohypophysis is not usually affected and its function is maintained.

Structural changes. In patients dying soon after the delivery responsible, Sheehan demonstrated extensive necrosis of the adenohypophysis, which he explained by ischaemia resulting from the causal factors noted above. In patients surviving longer, the necrotic tissue is organised and replaced by fibrous tissue.

Other structural changes include atrophy of the thyroid, adrenals, ovaries, uterus and mammary gland tissue.

The diagnosis may be confirmed by assay of the plasma levels of the pituitary hormones, or the demonstration of suppressed adrenal func-

tion and a normal response to ACTH (see above).

Some of Simmonds' cases exhibited generalised wasting and were probably examples of *anorexia nervosa* which is psychogenic and reversible. The distinction is an important one, as adult patients with panhypopituitarism require life-long treatment with thyroxin, corticosteroids and sex hormones.

Fröhlich's syndrome

This condition, described by Fröhlich in 1901 as *dystrophia adiposogenitalis*, occurs in children. Its main features include obesity and failure of sexual maturation. Boys develop a feminine distribution of fat over the breasts and buttocks, and tend to be wide-hipped.

In some cases, lesions are found in the vicinity of the pituitary or hypothalamus, apparently involving both; the least rare is a craniopharyngioma (Fig. 20.89, p. 731) but chromophobe pituitary adenoma, meningioma and glioma have also been found. A condition resembling the syndrome can be induced experimentally in animals by injury to the median eminence and adjacent nuclei: such injury probably interferes with the hypothalamic gonadotrophin-releasing hormone (p. 942) which stimulates release of both FSH and LH.

Cases of Fröhlich's syndrome due to a detectable lesion are much less common than previously believed. Most obese children with delayed maturation have no detectable lesion and eventually attain maturity.

A condition resembling Fröhlich's syndrome also occurs in adults of both sexes, with obesity, particularly of the trunk, sterility and reduced libido. In some cases a causal lesion has been found, least rarely a chromophobe pituitary adenoma, which may have interfered with hypothalamic and adenohypophyseal function. Other pressure effects may include headache and increasing restriction of the field of vision, as with any expanding lesion in this vicinity.

Pituitary dwarfism (Lorain–Levi syndrome)

This results from a severe deficiency of growth hormone in childhood. In most cases, there is deficiency of the other adenohypophyseal hormones, but in some GH alone is deficient: some of these latter cases are familial.

In approximately one-third of cases, the condition is due to a pituitary tumour or a craniopharyngioma, but more often than not the cause is unknown.

Impaired general growth is usually noticed after 1 year of age, sometimes much later: although small, the child shows no disproportion of limbs, etc. (cf. achondroplasia, p. 836) and is not obese (cf. Fröhlich's syndrome). Attacks of hypoglycaemia may occur (cf. adults with hypopituitarism). The mental state is normal for age and so, being small, the child may seem unusually clever.

If GH alone is deficient, puberty is delayed but eventually occurs normally: the majority, however, also lack gonadotrophins, etc., and do not mature. GH is used in treatment, but some children develop resistance to it.

Diagnosis can be confirmed by plasma GH assay before and after provocation by arginine or L-dopa. Conditions which must be distinguished include gonadal dysgenesis (p. 925), cretinism (p. 955) and also simple neglect of a child, which may be reflected in greatly stunted growth. There is also a condition of dwarfism in which plasma GH is high but somatomedin (p. 943) is low.

Adenohypophyseal changes in other diseases

The changes in *Cushing's syndrome* have already been described (p. 945). In untreated *primary myxoedema*, increased functional activity by the TSH-secreting cells is associated with their enlargement, loss of secretory granules, and development of PAS-positive inclusions (Fig. 24.5) seen by electron-microscopy to be in cisternae in the endoplasmic reticulum. There are no characteristic pituitary changes in *hyperthyroidism*. In *Addison's disease*, there is an initial but temporary increase in poorly granulated basophils.

Adenohypophyseal tumours

Minute tumours of the adenohypophysis are often found incidentally at necropsy, but clin-

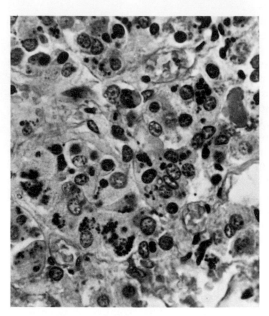

Fig. 24.5 Adenohypophysis in primary myxoedema. The PAS-positive inclusions in the basophil cells show up here as black spheres. × 500.

ically significant tumours are rare. The least uncommon are *adenomas* which may cause symptoms by local pressure effects and/or by secretion of hormone.

Traditionally adenomas are classified into *chromophobe*, *eosinophil* and *basophil* cell types.

Chromophobe adenomas do not usually secrete excessive amounts of hormone, and cause symptoms by pressure effects on the adenohypophysis (progressive panhypopituitarism), the optic chiasma (bitemporal hemianopia which may progress to blindness) and the hypothalamus (diabetes insipidus, fever, etc.). Occasional chromophobe adenomas secrete excess of growth hormone, prolactin or ACTH, with consequent acromegaly (p. 945), etc. During pregnancy, a chromophobe adenoma may enlarge rapidly and become clinically apparent.

Eosinophil adenomas are asymptomatic when small, but when larger cause acromegaly or gigantism (p. 944). Like chromophobe adenomas, they may grow very large and cause extensive local destruction.

Basophil adenomas are rarer than the others, usually remain small, and occasionally cause Cushing's syndrome (p. 945). They tend to develop also in patients with Cushing's syndrome treated by total adrenalectomy.

Pituitary adenomas are soft, brown tumours, usually well-encapsulated, and often showing extensive infarction or fibrosis. They may compress and destroy the surrounding pituitary tissue, enlarge the sella and rupture its diaphragm. Occasionally they may erode into the nasopharynx, but this is more typical of the much rarer **pituitary carcinoma**.

Histologically, adenomas have a solid or occasionally papillary structure: the cells resemble closely one or other of the adenohypophyseal cell types, but some tumours are of mixed cell type, e.g. chromophobe and eosinophil. More precise classification of adenomas depends on the demonstration of intracellular hormones by immunohistological techniques or by testing tumour extracts.

Other tumours and cysts

The commonest tumour outside the pituitary and producing anterior lobe deficiency by pressure is the **craniopharyngioma**, which is derived from Rathke's pouch, *i.e.* from the craniopharyngeal upgrowth from which the hypophysis is developed; it is usually suprasellar in position and is often cystic (Fig. 20.89, p. 731). Cystic tumours or cysts occasionally arise also from the pars intermedia and may contain ciliated epithelium. These are also of Rathke pouch origin and they may cause atrophy of the rest of the gland. **Metastases** from carcinoma of the breast or bronchus are not uncommon, and pericapsular deposits occur in some cases of leukaemia. Extra-pituitary tumours in the suprasellar region may involve the nuclei of the hypothalamus and lead to disturbances of fat metabolism or to polyuria.

The neurohypophysis (posterior lobe)

This is composed of irregular fusiform cells of neural origin, among which are numerous nerve fibres which come from the hypothalamus. Two hormones, *vasopressin* and *oxytocin*, are synthesised in the hypothalamic nuclei and transmitted by modified nerve fibres to the neurohypophysis, where they are stored and released as required. The two molecules are octapeptides and are stored in combination with a common large storage molecule called *neurophysin*.

Vasopressin or antidiuretic hormone (ADH) controls water balance by increasing the permeability of the renal collecting tubules, thus allowing increased re-absorption of water and a more concentrated urine. The name vasopressin is a bad one, for only in very high dosage does it raise the blood pressure. If the plasma osmolarity increases, osmoreceptors in the anterior hypothalamus initiate a neural stimulus which releases neurohypophyseal-stored ADH into the blood. Conversely, ADH secretion is suppressed by hypo-osmolarity of the plasma.

Diabetes insipidus. This is due to deficient secretion of ADH. It is usually caused by a hypothalamic lesion, e.g. head injury, glioma, metastatic cancer or encephalitis. Destruction of the neurohypophysis or high transection of the pituitary stalk do not normally cause diabetes insipidus, as sufficient ADH escapes from the severed neurohypophyseal tract.

The main feature of diabetes insipidus is excretion of a very large volume of dilute urine—often over 10 litres/24 hours. This is accompanied by polydipsia and, if drinking is restricted, concentration of urine increases only slightly and severe dehydration results. Onset of the condition is often surprisingly sudden. Apart from inconvenience, the polyuria has little harmful effect unless drinking is prevented. In *psychogenic polyuria*, withholding of fluid results in a concentrated urine without dehydration. Confirmation of the diagnosis of diabetes insipidus is provided by a response to a dose of ADH or of a recently synthesised analogue which is also valuable in treatment.

Oxytocin causes contraction of uterine smooth muscle and expulsion of milk during lactation. It may play a physiological role in uterine contraction during and after pregnancy, and has been widely used to initiate labour and to contract the uterus in post-partum haemorrhage, etc.

Women with diabetes insipidus, and therefore presumably deficiency of both ADH and oxytocin, can have a normal labour and lactation, and oxytocin has no known function in males.

The Pineal Body

The function of this minute structure, situated above the posterior part of the third ventricle, is very largely obscure. There is evidence that it secretes hormonal factors, one of which, *melatonin*, is derived from serotonin, and appears to antagonise the effects of MSH. Melatonin may also inhibit gonadal maturation and function.

The least rare lesions of the pineal are tumours which occur mainly in childhood. They include gliomas, teratomas and also tumours indistinguishable from seminomas. Effects are produced by pressure on neighbouring structures; thus hydrocephalus, ocular paralyses and deafness from implication of the corpora quadrigemina, also cerebellar effects, giddiness, etc., may result. In young boys precocious puberty may accompany a pineal tumour of any type. In other cases of pineal tumour such effects have been absent, and a similar group of changes has been observed in other lesions in the neighbourhood, such as tumour in the floor of the third ventricle, hydrocephalus, etc. The syndrome is probably not a pineal effect but rather the result of disturbance of nerve tracts possibly related to the pituitary.

The Thyroid Gland

The thyroid gland produces three hormones, thyroxine, tri-iodothyronine and calcitonin. The last is a polypeptide which lowers the concentration of calcium in the blood by causing increased deposition of bone crystal, but its physiological and pathological importance is still uncertain. Calcitonin is secreted by specialised epithelial cells (C cells) which do not form part of the lining of the thyroid vesicles.

Thyroxine (tetra-iodothyronine, or T_4) and tri-iodothyronine (T_3) are iodinated amino acids with a hormonal effect of influencing heat production in the tissues of the body by uncoupling oxidative phosphorylation, i.e. increasing oxygen utilisation relative to the rate of formation of high energy phosphate bonds, two processes which are closely linked in the economy of the cell. T_3 and T_4 are essential in normal physical and mental development and in the metabolism of protein, carbohydrate and fat. Excessive secretion of these thyroid hormones causes the serious disorder known as **thyrotoxicosis** or **hyperthyroidism** while inadequate secretion results in **hypothyroidism** which also has severe pathological consequences. Important physiological mechanisms have evolved to ensure that the amounts of T_3 and T_4 released into the circulation are appropriate to the varying bodily requirements in differing circumstances (e.g. environmental temperature), and, within limits, to compensate for suboptimal intake of dietary iodine.

Iodine metabolism in the thyroid gland. Iodine ions are concentrated in thyroid cells by a special concentrating or *trapping mechanism* which can be inhibited by perchlorate or thiocyanate ions. Iodide within thyroid epithelium is rapidly *oxidised*, probably by a thyroid peroxidase, to an active form which readily enters *organic combination* with the tyrosine present in the glycoprotein, thyroglobulin. This latter is synthesised by thyroid epithelium and stored extracellularly in the colloid within the vesicles. The organic binding of oxidised iodine results in the formation of mono- and di-iodotyrosine within the thyroglobulin molecule and the synthesis of the iodothyronine is accomplished by *coupling* of two appropriate iodotyrosines to give T_3 or T_4. (Both the antithyroid drugs thiouracil and carbimazole inhibit the organic binding of iodine and the coupling reaction.) The hormones, still part of the thyroglobulin molecule, are thought to be stored within the colloid until required in the circulation. Thyroglobulin is then digested by a cathepsin, T_3 and T_4 are released as free amino acids and are transported through the epithelial cells lining the vesicles to the vessels within the stroma of the gland. Hormonally inactive iodotyrosines which have not taken part in iodothyronine formation are also released from digested thyroglobulin but these are deiodinated by a *dehalogenase* enzyme and the released iodide is available for re-oxidation and organification.

Due to inborn errors of metabolism one or other of these steps is sometimes defective and this leads to the condition of **dyshormonogenesis**. Thus failure of the iodide-trapping mechanism, defective organification of iodide, impaired coupling of iodotyrosines, secretion of abnormal iodoprotein, and dehalogenase deficiency each constitutes a different form of dyshormonogenesis and results in a tendency to hypothyroidism.

Control of thyroid secretion. The secretion of thyroid hormone is mainly controlled by TSH. Inadequate plasma levels of T_3 and T_4 cause release of TSH from the pituitary by a feedback mechanism and this stimulates all the processes of thyroid hormone formation and release described above. If prolonged, such stimulation by TSH causes important structural changes in the thyroid: in particular a change of the epithelium from cubical to columnar, proliferation of epithelial cells to form new follicles, and diminution of the volume and concentration of the colloid stored within the vesicles. These changes may result in **goitre**, i.e. enlargement of the thyroid. When the plasma level of thyroid hormone exceeds the physiological requirements of the body, the production of

TSH by the pituitary is suppressed and the thyroid reverts to its resting state with diminished hormone production, diminished secretion and increased storage of hormone within the eosinophilic colloid which accumulates within the vesicles.

Hypothyroidism. The effects of subnormal secretion of T_4 and T_3 vary depending upon the severity of thyroid hormone deficiency and the age of onset of the disorder. Infantile hypothyroidism is called **cretinism** and is described on p. 955.

In the adult the syndrome is called **myxoedema**. In severe cases there is lethargy, slowing of speech and impaired intellectual function sometimes associated with frank psychosis. The hair, brittle and lustreless, tends to fall out. Hydrophilic mucoprotein ground substance accumulates in the dermal connective tissue causing coarsening of the features (Fig. 24.6) and firm non-pitting oedema of the supraclavicular fossae and dorsum of the hands. Similar mucinous deposits around nerves may impair peripheral nerve function and cause, for example, carpal tunnel syndrome or deafness, while involvement of tongue and larynx cause a characteristically slurred croaking voice. Despite a poor appetite the patient gains

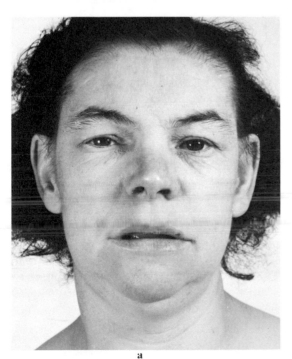
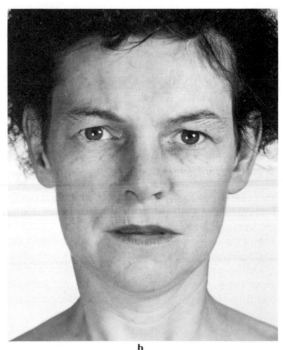

a   b
Fig. 24.6 Myxoedema, (**a**): before treatment, (**b**): the effects of administration of thyroxine.

weight. The pulse is slow, the basal metabolic rate is lowered, and the patient suffers from constipation, feels cold and is unduly prone to develop hypothermia.

Biochemical abnormalities include a raised serum cholesterol level due to reduced rate of catabolism, but most significant is the low thyroid secretion rate of T_4 and T_3, the concentrations of which in the blood can be shown by radio-immunoassay to be abnormally low, while the serum protein-bound iodine is also low.

Secretion of TSH is increased, even in patients with early or subclinical thyroid failure, and this is reflected in the appearance in the anterior pituitary of mucoid cells which contain only a few prominent storage granules (vesiculate mucoid cells—Fig. 24.5). There is diminished sexual function and menorrhagia is common due to failure of ovulation and continued endometrial proliferation. All of the above changes, except the low thyroid hormone secretion rate, are reversed by therapy with T_4 or T_3.

Causes. By far the most common cause of hypothyroidism is primary myxoedema (the atrophic form of auto-immune thyroiditis—see below) but hypothyroidism with goitre is found in Hashimoto's disease, dyshormonogenesis, severe iodine deficiency and as a result of drugs with antithyroid effects. Extensive surgical resection of the thyroid, therapy with radioiodine, and hypopituitarism with diminished TSH secretion are other causes.

Hyperthyroidism (*syn.* **thyrotoxicosis**) results from excessive secretion of thyroid hormone and causes clinical features which are almost the opposite of those found in hypothyroidism. The patient, though weak, is restless, hyperkinetic and emotionally unstable. The appetite is increased but the patient loses weight. There is increased nitrogen excretion, and sometimes impaired glucose tolerance and glycosuria. The skin is warm and sweating, the pulse rapid and bounding and the cardiac output is increased. Cardiac arrhythmia, particularly atrial fibrillation, may occur, especially in older patients and cardiac failure may be the presenting feature.

Osteoporosis affecting cancellous bone may be present, associated with increased calcium excretion in urine and faeces. Many of the above features are attributable to the raised basal metabolic rate which is, in turn, due to the effects of excessive amounts of thyroid hormone on the tissues. The serum levels of T_3, less often T_4, and of protein-bound iodine are raised. Pituitary TSH secretion is inhibited. In the

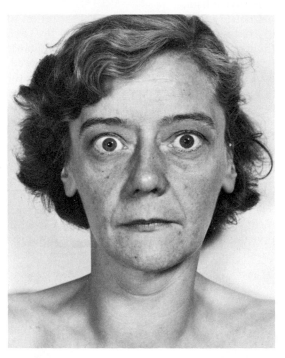

Fig. 24.7 Thyrotoxicosis. Note the prominence of the eyes and the diffuse thyroid enlargement.

common clinical form of hyperthyroidism, **Graves' disease**, there is unexplained prominence of the eyes (*exophthalmos*) (Fig. 24.7) which cannot be attributed to the action of T_3 and T_4.

Most cases of thyrotoxicosis appear to be due to an auto-antibody to thyroid epithelium (p. 961). Less often autonomous hyperfunctioning thyroid nodules are responsible, while in very rare cases, hyperthyroidism is the result of excessive pituitary TSH production in acromegaly.

Nontoxic goitre (simple goitre)

Nontoxic goitre refers to various non-inflammatory conditions which result in enlargement of the thyroid gland without hyperthyroidism. All forms of nontoxic goitre are probably preceded and for a time accompanied by a phase of impaired thyroid hormone synthesis due to inadequate supply of iodide or to impaired thyroid enzyme activity, the result of genetic defect or exogenous toxic substances. To counteract the diminished secretion of thyroid hormone in these circumstances more TSH is produced and there is increased activity of the thyroid epithelium, which becomes hyperplastic. These compensatory changes may increase T_4 and T_3 secretion enough to prevent hypothyroidism, but the defect may be so severe that goitrous hypothyroidism results, a condition which some authors would not include under the heading of simple or nontoxic goitre.

Morphologically, the following varieties of non-toxic goitre are recognised; (*a*) **parenchymatous goitre**, showing hyperplasia of the type illustrated in Fig. 24.8 with little colloid stor-age; (*b*) **colloid goitre**, in which there is marked accumulation of colloid (Fig. 24.10). These varieties may occur in a diffuse form in which the gland is generally involved or in a nodular form in which increase occurs in scattered rounded nodules of various sizes.

Epidemiology. Goitre may occur sporadically in any locality. Before the introduction of iodised salt, it was unduly common in certain districts (**endemic goitre**), notably in the valleys of Switzerland, the Pyrenees, the Himalayas and in New Zealand; in England in the Derbyshire hills; in parts of Southern Ireland, and in North America in the region of the Great Lakes. Where deficiency of iodine was great, as in the mountainous regions, e.g. the Alps, the goitre was usually parenchymatous, diffuse at first and becoming nodular later. Thyroid deficiency and cretinism were common, especially where the disease was very prevalent and of severe type. In goitrous districts in Switzerland the average weight of the thyroid at birth was often double the normal and occa-

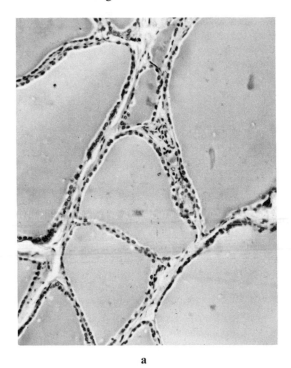

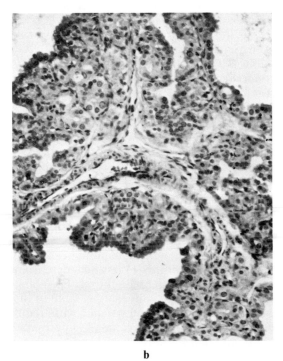

a b

Fig. 24.8 Normal thyroid tissue (**a**) and thyroid showing the effects of chronic stimulation with TSH (**b**). Note the hypertrophy and hyperplasia of the thyroid epithelium and diminished colloid storage. × 185.

sionally a congenital parenchymatous goitre was present. In North America, goitre was usually of the colloid type, either diffuse or nodular.

Aetiology. The causation of endemic goitre is not fully understood, but it is known that deficiency of iodine is the chief factor in its production. In remote communities where little food is imported, lack of iodine in the soil, water, and in locally produced food is the basic defect. There may be contributory factors which render unavailable any iodine present, such as pollution of water supplies by sulphur-containing organic matter or the presence of much calcium or fluoride. In goitrous districts, rats, sheep and other animals are also affected. When iodine deficiency is severe, goitre appears in childhood; when it is moderate, goitre is not only less common but also appears later, occurring especially at puberty and during pregnancy and lactation, when there is a drain on the iodine supply. Males are affected less frequently than females. In the early stages especially, treatment by iodine may arrest the thyroid enlargement or cause it to regress. In the region of the Great Lakes and in Switzerland, the administration of small quantities of iodine to school children has resulted in remarkable diminution in the incidence of goitre. In New Zealand and certain other districts the results have been less striking, perhaps because of the presence of iodine inhibitors.

Sporadic nontoxic goitre, i.e. that occurring in areas where goitre is not endemic, appears to have three main causes: (1) iodine deficiency due to improper dietary habits; (2) dyshormonogenesis due to one of a group of inherited defects of the process of thyroid hormone synthesis or secretion (see pp. 950, 955); (3) the action of substances which interfere with thyroid hormone synthesis. In practice, and excluding antithyroid drugs used in treating thyrotoxicosis, perhaps the most important of these is large doses of iodine given in the form of iodopyrine, or less commonly simply as iodide, as expectorants in asthma or chronic bronchitis. In idiosyncratic subjects this inhibits the iodination of tyrosine; there is a fall in thyroid hormone release, and patients with 'iodide goitre' frequently become hypothyroid. Resorcinol, *para*-aminosalicylic acid and sulphonylureas are other drugs which occasionally cause nontoxic goitre.

Parenchymatous goitre. The initial changes are enlargement of the acinar cells to colum-nar type and new formation of many small colloid-deficient vesicles. The enlarged gland lacks normal thyroid translucency and resembles pancreas to the naked eye. The changes are at first diffuse, affecting the entire gland, but if the iodine lack persists, foci of excessive activity in iodine uptake appear, while other parts of the gland become refractory and fail to take up and store iodine; this can be shown by autoradiography of thyroids excised after a dose of radioactive iodine. The hyperactive foci enlarge and compress the adjacent parenchyma so that the gland becomes nodular.

In the nodular type of goitre a great variety of structure may be encountered. There may be only one or two nodular masses, or the gland may be studded with them, the parenchyma between becoming atrophied. Following the initially diffuse parenchymatous hyperplasia, the subsequent development of hyperplastic nodules probably depends on the severity of the continuing iodine deficiency, however brought about.

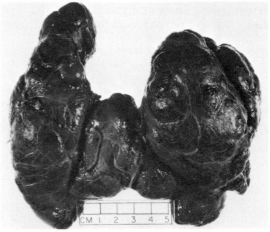

Fig. 24.9 Diffuse colloid goitre, showing general thyroid enlargement.

Colloid goitre. In diffuse colloid goitre the whole gland may be affected (Fig. 24.9), or one lobe may be chiefly involved. The affected tissue is tense and firm, and on section presents a translucent brownish appearance due to the accumulation of dense, firm colloid. Indeed, colloid-filled spaces of considerable size may be present. Dark red or brown areas due to haemorrhage may be seen, and in places there may be fibrosis, sometimes with calcification of the stroma. On microscopic examination, the acini are large and distended with deeply-

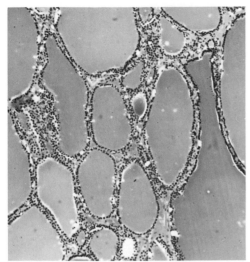

Fig. 24.10 Colloid goitre, showing accumulation of colloid in vesicles with flattened epithelium. × 40.

staining colloid, and the epithelium may be flattened (Fig. 24.10). Cysts may be formed by the confluence of acini. Colloid goitre is much commoner in women than in men, usually appears first at puberty or in pregnancy, and may be dependent on a less severe degree of iodine lack than that associated with parenchymatous goitre. This seems to hold generally with regard to the disease in low-lying countries.

Effects. In nontoxic goitre, thyroid function often appears clinically normal, though minor disturbances are not so rare as was once supposed. The enlarged gland may occasionally cause pressure effects on a recurrent laryngeal nerve, the oesophagus, or on the trachea, and even death by suffocation. Pressure effects are more common when the goitre extends retrosternally. In mountainous regions the thyroid enlargement in children, usually of the nodular type, may be associated with cretinism, the result of severe deficiency of the thyroid hormone. In America, colloid goitre has been associated with some degree of thyrotoxicosis.

Despite much study, it is uncertain whether nontoxic goitre predisposes to the development of carcinoma.

Cretinism

Severe hypothyroidism beginning in infancy is called *cretinism*. Cretins usually seem normal at birth, having received maternal thyroid hormone while *in utero*, but within a few weeks or months it becomes apparent that mental and physical development is retarded. The characteristic cretin is a dwarf with severe mental defect, disproportionately short limbs, coarse dry skin, deficient hair and teeth, a large protruding tongue (Fig. 24.11) and pot belly with umbilical hernia. The skeletal changes of cretinism are mentioned on p. 830. Unless replacement therapy with T_3 or T_4 commences early, the changes, especially the mental defect, become irreversible, though there may be some improvement in physical appearance.

Endemic cretinism occurred almost exclusively in mountainous districts such as Switzerland, where iodine deficiency was severe and endemic goitre common. It is said rarely to appear in a goitrous family until the second or third generation, and cretins of this type are nearly always the offspring of goitrous mothers. Unexplained deaf-mutism is very often present as an additional condition.

The thyroid. In most cases of endemic cretinism a goitre is present, although in some instances the thyroid is atrophic and fibrous. The goitre is nearly always nodular, the parenchyma between the nodules being compressed and atrophic. The appearances are similar to those seen in the nodular goitres of long-standing iodine deficiency.

Sporadic cretinism. This condition, due to congenital absence or hypoplasia of the thyroid tissue, is encountered from time to time in all localities and the causation is unknown. In some cases no trace of thyroid may be found, although in some instances there are small nodules of atrophied thyroid tissue near the foramen caecum at the root of the tongue. In other cases the thyroid is small and shrunken, sometimes containing cysts. The thymus is usually atrophic, but the parathyroids are not affected and occupy their usual position.

Dyshormonogenesis. Goitre in sporadic cretinism is very rare, but it occurs as a familial recessive abnormality manifested by congenital absence of some essential enzyme system. In

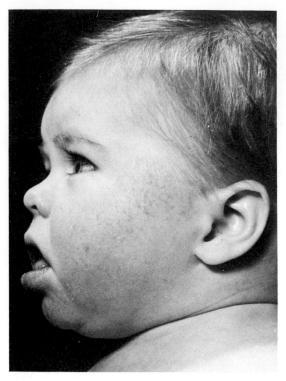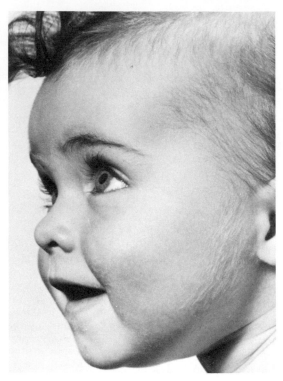

Fig. 24.11   A cretin aged 17 months (**a**), showing the enlarged, protruding tongue, coarse dry skin and dull expression. (**b**), showing the effects of thyroxine treatment for two months. (Prof. J. H. Hutchison.)

one variety, studied by McGirr and Hutchison in a family of Scottish tinkers, absence of the dehalogenase enzyme, which normally removes iodine from iodotyrosine, allows mono- and di-iodotyrosine to escape from the thyroid into the blood, from which they are excreted in the urine, thus leading to gross iodine deficiency. In another type the coupling of iodotyrosines to form T3 and T4 is impaired and hormone synthesis is therefore incomplete. In a third type iodide accumulates in the gland but there is

enzymatic failure to oxidise iodide to free iodine which is therefore not available in the thyroid to combine with tyrosine. Accordingly iodinated hormone synthesis fails. In some of these congenital goitrous cretins deaf-mutism is present, an interesting finding in view of its unexplained frequency in endemic goitrous cretinism.

The thyroid is often greatly enlarged and nodular, and on microscopic examination the epithelial hyperplasia of parenchymatous goitre is found.

Auto-immune thyroiditis

In this condition there is infiltration of the thyroid by lymphocytes and plasma cells associated with abnormalities of the thyroid epithelium and, in many cases, thyroid-specific auto-antibodies in the serum.

Three main variants are encountered: (1) **Hashimoto's disease (lymphadenoid goitre)**—a diffuse and massive lesion causing goitre; (2)

primary myxoedema, in which the thyroid is shrunken and the epithelium atrophic; (3) **focal thyroiditis** in which patchy lesions occur in an otherwise normal or hyperplastic gland.

Gross appearance. Areas of thyroid affected by anto-immune thyroiditis appear solid and white or peach coloured, lacking the translucent appearance normally presented by colloid stored in the vesicles. In Hashimoto's disease the gland is firm and there is enlargement, usually symmetrical and of moderate degree; the cut surface has a solid lobulated appearance resembling pancreas on section, and in most cases the capsule is not adherent to surrounding

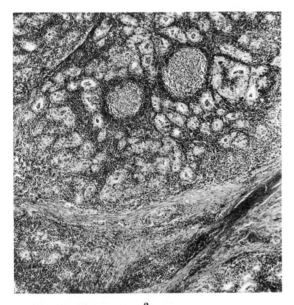

a

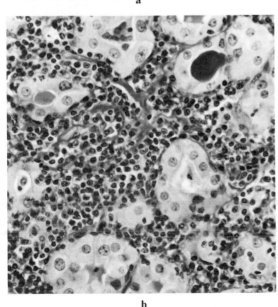

b

Fig. 24.12 Hashimoto's thyroiditis. (**a**), showing the diffuse lymphoid cell infiltrate, germinal centres, fibrosis and small thyroid acini. × 50. (**b**), showing the lymphocytic and plasma cell infiltrate and change in the epithelium to Askanazy-cell type. × 320.

tissues. The shrunken thyroid of primary myxoedema is firm and white while in focal auto-immune thyroiditis ill-defined white patches of about 1 mm in diameter are seen on the cut surface of the gland.

Microscopic appearance (Fig. 24.12). The basic lesion common to all forms is the presence of small follicles lined by large cubical epithelial cells with granular cytoplasm and large nuclei which are frequently bizarre in shape. These cells, known variously as Askanazy cells, Hürthle cells, oxyphil cells or oncocytes, owe their eosinophilic (pale pink to bright red) cytoplasmic granularity to the presence of numerous large mitochondria.

The colloid is scanty, usually densely eosinophilic and may contain macrophages or multinucleated giant cells. Surrounding the abnormal follicles, and sometimes invading them, is an infiltrate of plasma cells and/or lymphocytes, accompanied by a variable amount of fibrous tissue.

In *Hashimoto's disease* (Fig. 24.12) the epithelium is all abnormal and increased in amount. The lymphoid infiltrate is massive and true germinal centres may be present. Mitotic figures are very infrequent. The amount of fibrous tissue is variable. Most of the gland in *primary myxoedema* consists of fibrous tissue (Fig. 24.13)

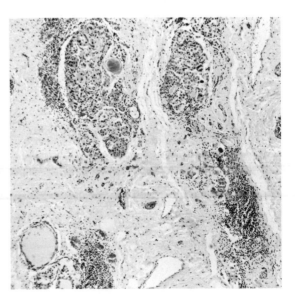

Fig. 24.13 The thyroid in primary myxoedema. Islands of thyroid tissue, showing the changes of chronic thyroiditis, are embedded in fibrous tissue containing wide vascular channels. × 50.

containing sparse clusters of small follicles lined by Askanazy cells and islets or cysts of epithelium sometimes of squamous type (a feature also seen occasionally in Hashimoto's disease). The lymphocytic and plasma cell infiltration is usually slight and situated mainly around the surviving epithelium. *Focal auto-immune thyroiditis* (Fig. 24.14) differs from both these conditions by the presence of greater or smaller areas of normal or hyperplastic thyroid tissue. The more severe examples, however, approach Hashimoto's disease in extent. It is very common in middle-aged women.

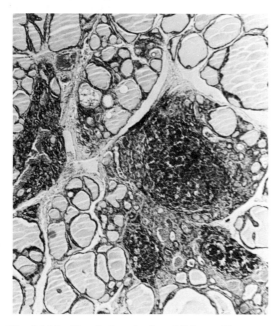

Fig. 24.14   Focal chronic thyroiditis. × 20.

Clinical features. In *Hashimoto's disease* the patient, usually a middle-aged female, has a firm goitre of moderate size. Hypothyroidism is present in about half the cases, and is the rule if partial thyroidectomy is undertaken. The thyroidal uptake of iodine is reduced and organification is impaired. An abnormal iodinated thyroprotein, which differs from serum protein-bound T_4 in being insoluble in butanol, is sometimes found in the serum.

Primary myxoedema is characterised by hypothyroidism in the absence of goitre. *Chronic focal thyroiditis* is usually asymptomatic, but if partial thyroidectomy is performed

hypothyroidism may develop in the more severe cases.

Aetiology. Auto-antibody against thyroglobulin and antibody against a lipoprotein of the membrane of the endoplasmic reticulum ('microsomes') of thyroid epithelial cells are found in high titre in the serum of most, but not all, patients with Hashimoto's disease. The frequency and titre of such antibodies is lower in primary myxoedema and lower still in focal thyroiditis. There is evidence that most of the auto-antibody is formed by the plasma cells which are usually a conspicuous feature of the inflammatory infiltrate of the gland.

Experimental auto-immune thyroiditis can be produced in various animals, including primates, by injecting thyroglobulin in Freund's adjuvant emulsion (p. 94) which enhances immunological responsiveness. The experimental thyroid lesions closely parallel the development of cell-mediated immunity to thyroglobulin, but transfer of the disease to normal animals has been accomplished only with very large numbers of lymphoid cells. Unlike human thyroiditis, the experimentally-induced disease is usually self-limiting and regresses. Although of great interest, these findings have not established the aetiology of human 'auto-immune' thyroiditis. Defective function of suppressor T cells may help to explain auto-immunisation, but the pathogenic importance of delayed auto-hypersensitivity and/or auto-antibodies is not yet firmly established (see pp. 133–4).

Patients with auto-immune thyroiditis are unduly prone to have in addition auto-immune gastritis (p. 548) (sometimes accompanied by pernicious anaemia), or auto-immune adrenalitis (idiopathic Addison's disease, p. 977) and this suggests that the predisposition to organ specific auto-immunity is due to a disorder of the lymphoid tissue rather than to primary abnormalities in these various organs. Furthermore, the occurrence of all these diseases within certain families suggests that the basic predisposition is inherited.

It remains to be discovered what event triggers the auto-immune process, why the disease occurs mainly in females, and what factors determine whether the lesion is focal or diffuse and whether the epithelium becomes hyperplastic as in Hashimoto's disease or atrophic as in primary myxoedema.

Other forms of thyroiditis

Thyroiditis due to causes other than auto-immunity is very rare in Britain. Multiple small abscesses may be found in the thyroid in pyaemia and acute thyroiditis is said sometimes to complicate influenza and typhoid fever.

Giant-cell (de Quervain's) thyroiditis. This variety of subacute thyroiditis begins with the distinctive features of fever and pain in the neck with tenderness. There is a neutrophil leukocytosis and a raised ESR. Elevation of the protein-bound iodine with reduced thyroid iodide uptake is said to be pathognomonic of the disorder. Microscopically, there is polymorphonuclear infiltration followed by lymphocytes and plasma cells; destruction of acini with formation of epithelioid cells and giant cells gives a pseudotuberculous appearance. Israeli workers have recovered a virus having the characters of mumps virus from two cases and have shown the presence of neutralising and complement-fixing antibodies to mumps virus in others.

Riedel's thyroiditis. This very rare disease is characterised by enlargement of the thyroid by fibrous tissue of extremely hard consistency; the condition usually affects only one lobe and involves adjacent muscles. Microscopically, the fibrous tissue may be more or less cellular, and in the affected part the vesicles become atrophic and disappear. Hypothyroidism is unusual. The nature of the disease is unknown; a few cases have been associated with retroperitoneal fibrosis (p. 598); other supposed cases may be more properly classified as sclerotic thyroid adenomas or as fibrous variants of Hashimoto's disease.

Hyperthyroidism (thyrotoxicosis)

Excessive secretion, by the thyroid, of T_3 and usually T_4, occurs in three conditions. (1) **Graves' disease**, the most common, is characterised by diffuse thyroid hyperplasia apparently due to the presence of an inappropriate thyroid stimulator in the blood. Protrusion of the eyeballs (exophthalmos) and certain other features of the disease cannot be ascribed to thyroid hormone excess alone. (2) **Toxic adenoma** is a relatively uncommon condition, in which an autonomous thyroid tumour produces thyroid hormone in excess of the requirements of the body. (3) **Toxic nodular goitre**, in which excessive hormone is produced in multiple discrete foci within the thyroid, occurs in older patients who already have a simple nodular goitre. The main features of hyperthyroidism have already been outlined on p. 952.

Graves' disease (exophthalmic goitre)

In this disease the **thyroid** shows hyperplasia which is characteristically diffuse though sometimes one lobe is larger than the other. On section the parenchyma is less brown and less translucent than normal owing to diminished colloid storage and the gland resembles salivary tissue, being dull greyish-pink in colour and lobulated. However, even in untreated cases some parts may contain a considerable amount of colloid and the surface may be slightly nodular. The gland is moderately firm and succulent, though if thyroiditis is marked (see below) there may be some fibrosis. The surface veins and arteries may be enlarged but the organ as a whole does not look specially vascular after surgical removal or at necropsy. The appearances may be much modified by treatment.

On microscopic examination, hyperplasia of the epithelium and diminution in the amount of the colloid stored are constant (Fig. 24.15). The epithelial cells of the acini are increased in size and more columnar in type. Numerous small acini are formed, while in the larger ones papilliform ingrowths are often present; both of these factors lead to a great increase in the epithelial surface area. What little colloid remains stains palely and appears watery. These changes reflect increased formation of hormones, which are, however, not stored in thyroglobulin but passed on to the bloodstream. In many cases there is focal auto-immune thyroiditis with lymphocytic infiltration (Fig. 24.14), and sometimes the formation of lymphoid follicles. When such infiltration is widespread, the lesion comes to resemble Hashimoto's disease (p. 956), and in such cases hypothyroidism commonly follows partial thyroidectomy.

The alterations described are usually fairly uniform throughout the gland but in places there may be quiescent acini which contain a considerable amount of colloid, especially when, at a later period, the acute symptoms are beginning to subside. The picture may thus be one of hyperplasia and subsequent involution irregularly distributed, even with fibrosis in places.

amount. There may also be some enlargement of the lymph nodes. Some observers consider that such changes are in proportion to the severity of the disease; they may reflect the auto-immune response concerned in the focal thyroiditis which is present in many cases, or may be due to lowered adrenal cortical function resulting from the accelerated inactivation of cortisol found in thyrotoxicosis. Hypertrophy of the heart occurs in most cases of thyrotoxicosis. There may be neutropenia with relative

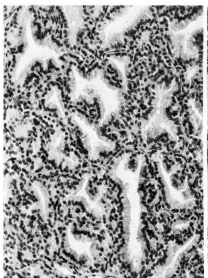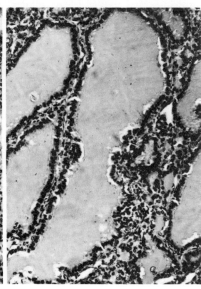

Fig. 24.15 The thyroid in Graves' disease. *Left*, untreated: the epithelial cells are columnar and there is virtually no colloid. *Right*, after treatment with iodine for 10 days. The epithelial cells are cuboidal and some colloid has accumulated. × 125.

The administration of iodine tends to reverse the hyperplastic changes in the thyroid; the epithelium becomes more cubical, and colloid accumulates in the acini (Fig. 24.15). These changes after iodine therapy bring about only temporary improvement in the symptoms, and the mode of action of iodine is uncertain. The anti-thyroid drugs derived from thiourea used in the treatment of hyperthyroidism prevent the synthesis of thyroxine and this leads to a striking reduction in the thyrotoxicosis although the epithelial hyperplasia is undiminished or even exaggerated. The histological effects of iodine and of thiouracil on the thyroid are thus antagonistic and when both are administered before thyroidectomy the histological picture in the excised gland is complex.

Other organs. The thymus shows distinct enlargement in three-quarters of the cases, and the thymic lymphoid tissue (which contains medullary lymphoid follicles) is increased in

lymphocytosis. Occasionally, however, there is an absolute lymphocytosis, and this is thought by some to occur in the more severe cases.

Occasionally bilateral patches of myxoedematous thickening appear on the anterior (pretibial) aspects of the lower leg, even while thyrotoxicosis is active. Before partial thyroidectomy was rendered relatively safe by premedication with antithyroid drugs, it was recognised that in a few cases thyroid involution might culminate in hypothyroidism.

Orbital changes. Exophthalmos in mild cases is attributable to fatty infiltration of the extrinsic muscles of the eye. When proptosis is severe there is, in addition, increase in amount and oedema of the orbital tissue, and marked lymphocytic infiltration of the extrinsic eye muscles and perivascular connective tissue.

Aetiology. The disease is most common in females, particularly during the reproductive period, and sometimes runs in families, especially in those in which there is an abnormally high incidence of organ-specific auto-immune diseases, e.g. Hashimoto's disease and pernicious anaemia.

It is now apparent, largely from the work of Dr. Duncan Adams, that Graves' disease is due to an auto-antibody which reacts with the thyroid epithelial cell surface receptor for TSH. This thyroid-stimulating immunoglobulin is detectable in the blood of most untreated patients by an *in vitro* test in which the binding of labelled TSH by human thyroid cell membrane preparations is competitively inhibited by the patient's serum. In some cases, the thyroid-stimulating antibody can cross-react with mouse or guinea-pig thyroid epithelium and causes thyroid stimulation in these animals *in vivo*. In fact this is how the antibody (termed *long-acting thyroid stimulator* or *LATS*) was first demonstrated. Thyroid-stimulating antibody has been shown to be quite distinct from TSH.

The auto-immune nature of Graves' disease is supported also by the frequent presence of focal auto-immune thyroiditis and other organ-specific auto-immune diseases (p. 132), such as pernicious anaemia. Thyroid-stimulating antibody explains the failure to demonstrate TSH in the serum of patients with Graves' disease, and the failure of administered T_3 to suppress thyroid activity in these patients—findings which indicate that pituitary TSH production in Graves' disease is fully suppressed by the inappropriately high blood levels of thyroid hormone. Further support is obtained from the correlation between the presence of maternal thyroid-stimulating antibody and the occurrence of temporary thyrotoxicosis in the neonate.

Thyroid-stimulating antibody correlates also with pretibial myxoedema and, to some extent, with exophthalmos. The pathogenesis of exophthalmos in Graves' disease is unknown. According to Kriss, thyroglobulin–antithyroglobulin complexes bind preferentially to the membranes of the extrinsic muscles of the eye, which they may reach by the lymphatic drainage of the thyroid and which they may damage by an antibody-dependent lymphocytotoxic reaction (p. 123).

Toxic adenoma

Approximately 1% of thyroid adenomas give rise to hyperthyroidism, usually mild and not accompanied by exophthalmos or thyroid-stimulating antibody in the serum.

The tumours are usually single adenomas more than 3 cm in diameter and are composed of small vesicles resembling those seen in Graves' disease. Towards the centre of the adenoma stromal oedema and fibrosis may separate the vesicles. Haemorrhage may occur into the tumour and destroy so much of the epithelium that the hyperthyroidism subsides.

Scanning of the neck following administration of radio-iodine shows marked radio-iodine uptake by the tumour, and, because of the autonomous nature of the growth, this cannot be suppressed by T_3. The remainder of the gland does not concentrate iodine since the hormone produced by the tumour results in diminished secretion of TSH by the pituitary.

Toxic nodular goitre

This disorder usually affects patients over 50 years of age who have had nontoxic goitre for many years. The thyrotoxicosis which subsequently develops is usually mild as judged by thyroid iodine uptake studies and hormone levels in the blood. Cardiac arrhythmias and failure may be the presenting symptom. Exophthalmos is uncommon.

The macroscopic and histological features are similar to those described in nontoxic nodular goitre (p. 953). Autoradiography shows in some cases one or two hyperfunctioning nodules (in effect, and perhaps in fact, toxic adenomas) with complete suppression of radio-iodine uptake by the remainder of the goitre. In other cases multiple small groups of hyperplastic follicles concentrate radioactive iodine though much of the gland is inactive, the appearances suggesting the effect of some extrinsic thyroid stimulator on a gland part of whose tissue is refractory. Thyroid microsomal antibody is found in the serum of such cases with the same frequency as in Graves' disease, but it remains to be seen whether thyroid-stimulating antibody is also demonstrable.

Tumours of the thyroid

Thyroid adenomas are comparatively common. They are enclosed by a fibrous capsule, compress the surrounding gland, are more often multiple than single, and present varying appearances depending on the extent of degenerative change and the amount of colloid storage. Thus they may be haemorrhagic or cystic and, in the absence of degeneration, they may have the brown honeycomb appearance of colloid goitre on section or be composed of pale, fawn, soft, fleshy tissue. Microscopically some are composed of strands and cylinders of epithelium without acinar structure, others consist of very small acini containing little colloid—

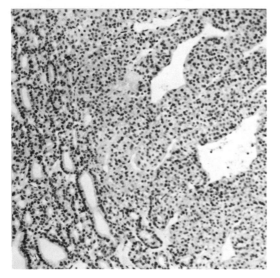

Fig. 24.16 Adenoma of thyroid, showing two types of growth—acinar type on left side of field and more solid type of growth on right. × 120.

such tumours have been called '*fetal adenomas*', but they do not seem to be due to developmental errors (Fig. 24.16). In yet others there may be considerable colloid storage. It is not possible to draw a line between circumscribed hyperplastic changes constituting the nodules in nodular goitres and true adenomatous tumours. Thyroid adenomas usually present clinically merely as localised swellings in the gland; those of the more cellular type are sometimes associated with hyperthyroidism. Some adenomas may possibly become malignant in the later years of life. A point of importance is the clinical difficulty of distinguishing benign adenoma from carcinoma in the absence of metastases; solitary tumours of the thyroid in children and young adults should be regarded with suspicion.

Parathyroid adenomas occasionally occur in the substance of the thyroid. Simple connective tissue tumours such as fibromas and osteochondromas are rare.

Malignant tumours

Carcinoma of thyroid causes about 0·5% of all deaths from cancer in this country. It invades surrounding structures, including the trachea and recurrent laryngeal nerves and death is commonly due to asphyxia. Its incidence is said to be higher in regions with endemic goitre but this is doubtful. It is known to result in some cases from x-irradiation of the neck in childhood, which was formerly used to treat haemangioma or supposed thymic enlargement. Some of the better differentiated human carcinomas may be TSH-dependent for there are records of rapid growth of metastases following total thyroidectomy or the administration of anti-thyroid drugs; and treatment with thyroxine, which suppresses TSH production, seems to have resulted in regression of established metastases in some cases and is thought to have prevented metastases in others. A noteworthy feature of well-differentiated thyroid carcinomas, especially in young patients, is the prolonged survival and well-being of the patient despite the presence of metastases.

Papillary adenocarcinoma is the form most commonly encountered and is sometimes seen in children and young adults, in whom there is often a history of local x-irradiation (see above). The tumour is not well encapsulated, is sometimes only a few millimetres in diameter, and despite its relatively innocuous microscopical appearance it frequently spreads to the cervical lymph nodes, particularly of the side affected (Fig. 24.17). Indeed all papillary tumours of the thyroid should be regarded as potentially malignant. It was previously erroneously thought that cervical lymph-node metastases of this tumour were 'lateral aberrant thyroid'. Pulmonary and skeletal metastases are rarely found.

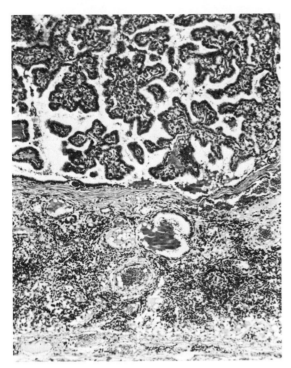

Fig. 24.17   Papillary cystadenocarcinoma of the thyroid in the cervical lymph nodes—so-called lateral aberrant thyroid. × 65.

Follicular adenocarcinoma. Certain encapsulated tumours, with the gross appearance of adenomas, are carcinomas composed of glandular acini. The best differentiated examples closely resemble normal thyroid but more often there are mitotic figures and aberrant cells; in many cases solid sheets of tumour cells are also present, sometimes of eosinophilic 'Hürthle' type. Malignancy is recognised by invasion of the fibrous capsule and blood vessels, and metastasis is particularly common to bone and lung. Some of these tumours take up ^{131}I, which can be used therapeutically.

Occasionally squamous carcinoma is seen, possibly arising from the thyroglossal duct.

Anaplastic tumours. Anaplastic tumours of various types—round-cell, spindle-cell and giant-cell—are relatively common and the majority are probably anaplastic carcinomas rather than sarcomas. They cause respiratory obstruction from rapid enlargement of the gland. Tumours having the general appearance of poorly-differentiated lymphomas are sometimes difficult to distinguish from the more extreme examples of Hashimoto's disease, a difficulty accentuated by the fact that some have responded to radiotherapy and have not recurred, whereas others, histologically indistinguishable, behave as unequivocal malignant tumours. Brewer and Orr proposed the term *struma reticulosa* for this group and drew attention to the frequency of multiple growths of similar structure in the lymphoid tissue of the small intestine.

Medullary carcinoma. This tumour consists of solid masses of neoplastic C cells set in a hyaline stroma which in places contains amyloid and is sometimes calcified. Despite its rather anaplastic appearance the mitotic rate is usually low and survival for many years is common. The blood calcitonin level is usually abnormally high (especially after calcium infusion), making diagnosis possible in familial cases even before the tumour is palpable. No clinical syndrome of calcitonin excess has been recognised but medullary carcinoma, being a tumour of apud cells (p. 967), is sometimes associated with diarrhoea, carcinoid syndrome or Cushing's syndrome. In a familial form of the disease there may be associated bilateral adrenal phaeochromocytoma and parathyroid adenoma (i.e. a special form of multiple endocrine adenoma syndrome) sometimes associated with neuromas of the buccal and conjunctival mucosae.

Other thyroid disorders

Degenerative changes. Excluding changes in nodular goitre and tumours, degenerative changes in the thyroid are comparatively rare and of little importance. Evidence of damage produced by toxins is found in infections, and there may be actual necrosis of the epithelium.

Amyloid degeneration sometimes occurs as an isolated finding or as part of widespread amyloidosis. When well marked, it causes thyroid enlargement (*amyloid goitre*). Amyloid is found in the stroma of medullary carcinoma of the thyroid (see above). Hyaline change, calcification, etc., are often present in the stroma of chronic goitres.

Congenital abnormalities. The isthmus of the thyroid is formed by a downgrowth of a tube of epithelium from the base of the tongue (foramen caecum). The upper portion of this tube above the hyoid bone is lined by squamous epithelium. If this persists and if the buccal end is obstructed, it may give rise to a 'lingual dermoid'. The lower part of the duct below the hyoid bone is lined by columnar ciliated epithelium. Thyroglossal cysts may take origin from this part when it does not undergo involution. Such a cyst may rupture on the skin surface, forming a median cervical fistula. In the walls of these cysts portions of thyroid tissue are sometimes found. Occasionally a mass of thyroid tissue is found in the base of the tongue, the so-called 'lingual thyroid', and the thyroid may be then absent from its normal site. Congenital absence and hypoplasia of the thyroid are among the causes of sporadic cretinism.

The Endocrine Pancreas

The lesions of the exocrine pancreas have already been described (p. 652) leaving for consideration here the disorders of the endocrine pancreas, i.e. the islets of Langerhans. The islets are more abundant in the body and tail than in the head. They consist of small cuboidal cells with a large vesicular nucleus, arranged in cords separated by a fibrovascular stroma. There are three cell types—the β-cell producing insulin, the α-cell producing glucagon, and the δ-cell which probably secretes gastrin but may represent a resting or transitional stage of the other two cell types. Insulin and glucagon are important in the intermediate metabolism of carbohydrates, fats and proteins; insulin increases the storage of these dietary components, whereas glucagon promotes their catabolism, and thus the two hormones have reciprocal functions. Insulin lack, either absolute or relative, causes diabetes mellitus, but in this disease and in normal carbohydrate intermediate metabolism, complex interrelationships exist involving a number of different hormones. Hyperfunction of the islets produces a spectrum of disorders dependent on which cell type is involved.

Diabetes mellitus

In diabetes there are varying degrees of failure to store and metabolise carbohydrates, with consequent hyperglycaemia and glycosuria. Insulin lack results in a failure of transport of glucose into muscle and adipose tissue; in the liver, insulin lack results in a failure to convert glucose to glycogen and in a failure to inhibit normal hepatic glucogenesis. Consequently the blood sugar rises. Normally, the fasting blood glucose level is 80–100 mg/100 ml (4·5–5·5 mmol/litre), and the level does not rise above 180 mg/100 ml (10 mmol/litre) after oral glucose or a meal. In diabetes there is always hyperglycaemia after ingestion of carbohydrate, the glucose level reaching 400 mg/100 ml (22 mmol/litre) or more, and glycosuria results; the fasting blood sugar is usually raised but in mild diabetics may be within the normal range.

Glucose tolerance tests. When 50 g of glucose is given to a fasting normal person the blood sugar rises to a maximum level of about 150 mg/100 ml (8.3 mmol/l) in about half an hour. In spite of continuing absorption from the gut, a comparatively rapid fall then occurs and the blood sugar reaches a normal level again within two hours. The rapid fall is due to stimulation of the β-cells of the pancreatic islets by the rise in the level of glucose; secretion of insulin is increased, and this enhances the utilisation of glucose.

The blood sugar curve of a diabetic patient after 50 g of glucose is quite different. It is absorbed normally from the gut and the blood level rises rapidly as before, and continues to do so for three or four hours, though the curve becomes less steep, and then there is a gradual fall which may go on for some hours. This shows that there is a deficiency in the normal metabolism of glucose. When the blood sugar rises above 180 mg/100 ml (10 mmol/l) or so, glycosuria occurs, but in established cases the renal threshold is raised and glycosuria does not occur until the blood sugar is substantially above the level at which spill-over into the urine normally occurs.

Glucose tolerance tests are not required for diagnosis in frank diabetes, but are of great service in the diagnosis of doubtful cases, where slight or transient glycosuria is found on routine examination in the absence of overt symptoms. Diabetes is excluded by a normal rise followed by the normal fall. In some such cases, the glycosuria is due to the renal threshold value being abnormally low, e.g. about 130 mg/100 ml (7·2 mmol/l), so that when glucose or much carbohydrate is administered and the blood sugar rises above this level, glucose is excreted by the kidneys. Such a condition is usually known as *renal glycosuria*. The condition is without serious effects. The result of a glucose tolerance test in which the 30 and 60 minute specimens show marked elevation of the blood sugar, often with glycosuria but with a normal 2-hour value, the so-called *lag curve*, is usually due to over-rapid absorption of glucose from the intestine without impairment of ability to metabolise glucose. Occasionally this type of curve is seen in persons who show a mild degree of impairment of glucose metabolism, and a few come to give a diabetic type of curve even in the continued absence of symptoms—the *pre-diabetic state*.

Clinical and biochemical changes

The disease is characterised by polyuria, polydipsia, polyphagia and weight loss. The principal biochemical manifestation is hyperglycaemia. When the normal renal capacity for glucose reabsorption is exceeded there is glycosuria and an osmotic diuresis with an accompanying loss of Na^+ and K^+. An increase in serum osmolarity occurs, causing thirst and polydipsia. The loss of weight in spite of polyphagia results from the failure to utilise glucose, and from a compensatory increase in catabolism of proteins and fats.

Insulin normally stimulates the transport of amino acids into muscle and their synthesis into proteins. In insulin lack this protein synthesis is impaired, there is an accelerated rate of amino acid catabolism to CO_2 and H_2O via the citric acid cycle, and in addition there is a marked increase in the rate of conversion of amino acids to glucose in the liver—gluconeogenesis. Glucagon, which is relatively increased in diabetes, helps to stimulate gluconeogenesis thus adding to the hepatic glucose which cannot be converted to glycogen, and so contributing to the hyperglycaemia.

In diabetes there is also an acceleration of fat catabolism. Increased amounts of free fatty acids are released from fat deposits. Normally they are catabolised to acetyl-CoA, which may be synthesised into new fatty acids, converted into ketone bodies, or completely catabolised via the citric acid cycle to CO_2 and H_2O. In insulin lack, increased amounts of acetyl-CoA are formed, and cannot be adequately catabolised because of the intracellular depletion of the carbohydrate components of the cycle. They are therefore preferentially converted into ketone bodies: two acetyl-CoA moieties are formed and in turn are converted into acetoacetic acid, which, together with its metabolites, acetone and β-hydroxybutyric acid, enter the circulation to produce ketosis. These 'ketone bodies' dissociate to yield hydrogen ions, and produce a metabolic acidosis (*ketoacidosis*) with a fall in plasma pH.

The metabolic acidosis (i) stimulates the respiratory centre, resulting in hyperventilation (Kussmaul breathing) which reduces the plasma HCO^-_3; (ii) results in acidification of the urine, excretion of the acidic ions of acetoacetate and β-hydroxybutyrate being accompanied by an increased excretion of NH^+_4 and later of Na^+ and K^+; this further aggravates the cationic loss which accompanies the glucose-induced osmotic diuresis. The total body Na^+ and K^+ are thus depleted; the serum Na^+ level falls, but the serum K^+ level is maintained at the expense of intracellular K^+, in part due to the acidosis and in part due to the lack of insulin, the movement of K^+ into cells being dependent on insulin and glucose.

This complex of metabolic disturbances produces hyperosmolarity, hypovolaemia, acidosis and electrolyte imbalance which have serious effects on the functions of neurons and result in **keto-acidotic coma**. In addition to this type of diabetic coma it has become recognised recently that there are two others. Firstly, **hyperosmolar non-ketotic coma**—approximately 15% of diabetic coma admissions are of this type—in which there is massive dehydration and profound hyperglycaemia (usually in excess of 1000 mg/100 ml (56 mmol/litre) but with minimal or no keto-acidosis: this tends to develop slowly over a period of some weeks or months, usually in mild diabetics. The mechanism is not clear, but it is postulated that there is insufficient insulin for normal intracellular transport but sufficient to inhibit the increased lipolysis necessary to produce ketosis. Secondly, **lactic acidosis**, due to tissue anoxia, usually accompanies diabetic keto-acidosis: in a very small percentage of (usually mild) diabetics, severe lactic acidosis may *per se* produce coma. Some of the oral hypoglycaemic agents, notably phenformin, may produce this pattern, but the mechanisms are uncertain.

In addition to these forms of diabetic coma, **hypoglycaemic coma** is liable to occur when insulin therapy is not accompanied by adequate calorie intake.

Aetiology

The aetiology of diabetes remains unknown. Clinically, two 'primary' forms are recognised.

(1) Juvenile or early-onset diabetes. This appears to have a hereditary tendency of complex and probably multifactorial type. The onset is usually acute, there is a failure of insulin output, and replacement therapy is mandatory. There tends to be a seasonal variation in onset, which is high in autumn and winter. This has suggested a possible environmental factor in pathogenesis, but although a virus has been suggested, the evidence for this is circumstantial and inconclusive. Antibodies to islet cells have been demonstrated in the serum of 50% of patients examined shortly after the onset of juvenile diabetes, but this incidence subsequently falls to 10%. In this 10% there is an increased incidence of other auto-antibodies—gastric parietal cell, thyroid and adrenal—indicating an association with the organ-specific auto-immune diseases. The 50% with no serum

antibodies do not differ clinically or biochemically from the others. The disappearance of islet cell antibodies may reflect a reduction in the appropriate, as yet unidentified, antigen. Morphometric studies have demonstrated that the β-cell mass is reduced in early-onset diabetes, and histological examination shows β-cell degranulation, the degree of which correlates with a reduction in extractable insulin. Extracellular deposition of hyaline, amyloid-like material (Fig. 24.18), fibrosis, lymphocytic infiltration, and, in untreated cases, hydropic degeneration due to glycogen accumulation in the islet cells, have all been observed, but are often inconspicuous at necropsy.

(2) Maturity or late-onset diabetes usually develops insidiously. There is a female preponderance, and the patients are frequently overweight. The hyperglycaemia can be controlled either by diet alone or by diet together with oral hypoglycaemic agents. In some of these patients there is apparent over-secretion of insulin, and the disease is thought to result from 'target cell' resistance, of unknown nature, to the hormone.

Other causes of diabetes. Secondary diabetes may complicate chronic pancreatitis, haemochromatosis, acromegaly, hypercortisolism (Cushing's syndrome or corticosteroid or ACTH therapy), glucagon-secreting tumours and phaeochromocytoma. Lesions of the brain can also cause hyperglycaemia and glycosuria, possibly by hypothalamic disturbance. Acute hyperglycaemia can also occur in acute pancreatitis.

Glycosuria in the absence of hyperglycaemia can result from an abnormally low renal threshold, which is a rare familial condition. Glycosuria can also be induced by phloridzin.

Of theoretical interest is Shaw Dunn's discovery in 1942 of the diabetogenic properties of alloxan. This compound causes a highly selective necrosis of the β-cells, which then liberate insulin so that death in hypoglycaemic coma results. If the animals are kept alive by administration of glucose, the hypoglycaemia is later succeeded by hyperglycaemia and a permanent state of diabetes is produced. This remarkable discovery provided a new experimental approach to diabetes. Alloxan appears to work through attacking certain sulphydryl compounds and a rapid fall in the glutathione content of the blood follows. Injection of glutathione or cysteine before the injection of

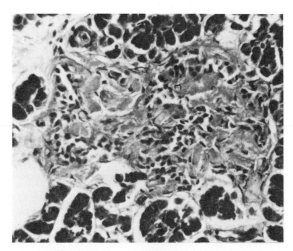

Fig. 24.18 Islet of Langerhans showing hyaline degeneration in a case of diabetes. × 240.

alloxan prevents the selective necrosis of islet cells.

Pathological changes

Apart from the changes in the pancreas discussed above, diabetes predisposes to cardiovascular disease, infections and various other complications.

Cardiovascular and renal complications. Combined cardiovascular and renal disease account for most deaths in diabetic patients. The characteristic features of diabetic glomerulosclerosis are described elsewhere (p. 779). The two diseases of major vessels which occur more frequently in diabetes are **atheroma** and **Monckeberg's sclerosis.** In general, atheroma has been found to develop earlier and to become severe in diabetes, and consequently myocardial infarction and ischaemia are unduly common.

Much recent and current interest has been focused on the occurrence of microvascular pathology in diabetes—the so-called 'diabetic microangiopathy'. In this, two types of lesion have been described: (*a*) a thickening of the basement membrane or an accumulation of basement membrane-like material in capillaries, and (*b*) endothelial cell proliferation together with basement membrane thickening affecting small arteries, arterioles and occasionally venules. The cause of the microangiopathy is uncertain. It is, however, of considerable importance in producing and contributing to peripheral vascular disease, diabetic retinopathy (p. 740), diabetic glomerulosclerosis, and possibly diabetic neuropathy secondary to involvement of the vasa nervorum. Hypophyseal ablation sometimes arrests diabetic retinopathy, and there is some evidence that growth hormone may be implicated.

Infections. There is an increased susceptibility to bacterial and fungal infections, possibly due to glycogen deficiency in polymorphs (p. 152). Boils, carbuncles, urinary tract infections with pyelonephritis and renal papillary necrosis are of frequent occurrence and may precipitate diabetic coma. Diabetics have an increased incidence of tuberculosis, especially of the lungs, and unless treated the disease tends to progress rapidly.

Other pathological effects. Trophic disturbances such as ulceration or Charcot's joints may develop as complications of the diabetic neuropathy. Diabetic mothers show an increased liability to pre-eclamptic toxaemia and pregnancy aggravates the diabetic state. The babies of diabetic mothers are usually much above normal weight, and are flabby and oedematous with a degree of erythroblastosis. A succession of unduly large children is strongly suggestive that the mother is diabetic or will later become so.

Hyperfunction of the endocrine pancreas

This results either from a hormone-secreting adenoma or carcinoma of islet cell type, although in occasional cases hyperplasia of the islets has been reported. The cells of the islets of Langerhans belong to that part of the endocrine system which has been called the **APUD** (**A**mine **P**recursor **U**ptake and **D**ecarboxylation) cell series. This series comprises the cells of the anterior pituitary, the C or parafollicular cells of the thyroid, various endocrine-secreting cells of the gastro-intestinal tract, including the gastrin-secreting G cells of the stomach and those cells which produce secretin and enteroglucagon, and probably also cells of the bronchi. These cells all secrete polypeptide hormones and have similar ultrastructural and histochemical properties. Tumours arising from them have been called **apudomas.**

Islet cell tumour (nesidiocytoma)

This is a discrete, usually solitary mass, most often in the body or tail of the pancreas. There may be more than one such tumour, and sometimes associated tumours in the thyroid, parathyroid or pituitary the *multiple-endocrine-adenoma* or *pluriglandular-adenoma syndrome.* Histologically, the component cells closely resemble normal islet cells, forming cords or clusters, and with a small amount of fibrovascular stroma. In some cases there is local deposition of amyloid material in the stroma (Fig. 24.19). A diagnosis of malignancy can seldom be made histologically, but apparently some 10% of islet cell tumours metastasise.

Islet cell tumours may give rise to a number of syndromes by their secretory activity:

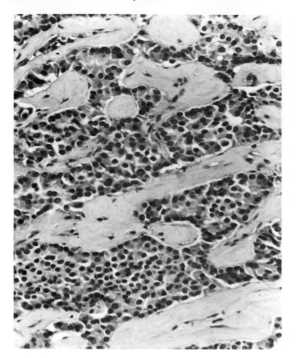

Fig. 24.19 A pancreatic islet-cell tumour showing the cords and clusters of tumour cells. The stroma contains amyloid material. × 230.

these are outlined below. Others are non-functional.

Insulin-secreting tumours are predominantly β-cell tumours and are associated with recurrent attacks of hypoglycemia, which may result in confusion, mania, somnolence, dizziness, loss of consciousness and other nervous symptoms, and can be prevented by taking glucose. Long intervals of freedom from symptoms may occur spontaneously, but prolonged episodes of hypoglycemia may lead to irreversible brain damage (p. 682). These tumours are rarely malignant.

Gastrin-secreting tumours cause persistent hypersecretion of acid gastric juice, producing multiple peptic ulcers which are refractory to medical treatment and may occur even in the jejunum. This combination constitutes the *Zollinger–Ellison syndrome* which tends to be slightly more common in males. More than half of these tumours are malignant. This syndrome may also arise from hyperplasia of gastric G cells, which also secrete gastrin. There may also be severe diarrhoea and also steatorrhoea from inhibition of lipase.

Other functional effects of islet cell tumours include (1) the **Verner–Morrison syndrome** with watery diarrhoea, hypokalaemia and achlorhydria ('WDHA'), in which the active hormone involved is uncertain; (2) a **glucagonoma syndrome**, which presents as diabetes, sometimes with skin manifestations; (3) **inappropriate hormone secretion** (p. 252) which may produce, for example, the carcinoid syndrome, Cushing's syndrome, etc. There is evidence that some tumours may simultaneously secrete a number of hormones.

The Parathyroids

The parathyroids, of branchial pouch origin, usually number four. They are small, yellowish-brown, and difficult to find at necropsy. Usually they are situated in the neck, posterior or postero-lateral to the thyroid but are sometimes in the upper mediastinum. They consist mainly of two cell types, firstly the *chief cells* which appear to be precursors of active cells or 'resting' cells, secondly the *water-clear* cells which appear to be actively secreting. With age, increasing numbers of oxyphil cells appear: their cytoplasm is rich in eosinophilic granules shown by electron-microscopy to be mitochondria.

Parathyroids secrete an essential hormone, *parathormone* (PTH), which is a protein of molecular weight about 9500. The active portion appears to be a peptide at the amino-terminal end of the molecule. The hormone is of major importance, together with vitamin D, in regulating plasma calcium levels: the role of calcitonin (p. 950) in human physiology remains uncertain. The mode of action of parathormone is not completely understood. It is known to stimulate resorption of bone and to decrease reabsorption of phosphate by the renal tubule: it may also promote reabsorption of calcium by the renal tubule and absorption of calcium from the gut. These latter possible effects may be due to enhancement of the synthesis of the most active vitamin D metabolite, 1,25-DHCC (p. 823). There is no evidence of pituitary control of parathyroid function and secretion of parathormone is stimulated by a fall in the level of ionised calcium in the plasma. Alkalosis or a raised plasma phosphate concentration may, by causing a fall in ionised calcium, also stimulate parathormone secretion, and in chronic renal failure phosphate retention may result in hyperplasia of the parathyroid glands.

Parathyroid hyperfunction

This may be classified into *primary* and *secondary hyperparathyroidism*. In primary hyperparathyroidism excessive parathormone secretion occurs in the absence of any known physiological stimulus and various harmful effects result. Secondary hyperparathyroidism occurs when the glands are exposed to increased stimulation, as in the example of chronic renal failure mentioned above.

Primary hyperparathyroidism is usually due to a parathyroid adenoma (p. 970) but occasionally to carcinoma or to primary hyperplasia of the chief or water-clear cells affecting all four glands. It may also result from 'inappropriate' production of parathormone by an unrelated tumour, for example bronchial or renal carcinoma. Primary hyperparathyroidism may occur in as many as 1 in 1000 of the adult population although it is diagnosed much less frequently. It can occur at any age but is commonest in middle age and especially in postmenopausal women.

Presenting features and effects. The presenting features vary considerably depending on whether the symptoms and signs are mainly due to its effects on the kidney or bones or to hypercalcaemia, which may give rise to generalised muscle weakness, tiredness, anorexia, thirst and polyuria. More than half the patients with primary hyperparathyroidism present with symptoms relating to renal stones, which are rich in calcium salts and therefore detectable radiologically. Only a small proportion of patients with urolithiasis have hyperparathyroidism, but nevertheless its detection in this group is important. Metastatic deposition of

calcium salts may occur in the walls of blood vessels, the lungs and gastric mucosa. Deposition in and around the renal tubules (nephrocalcinosis) is of special importance and may be visible radiologically. It leads to fibrosis, tubular injury and loss of nephrons; it is often complicated by pyelonephritis, and is likely to bring about chronic renal failure. Symptoms relating to the bone changes (p. 828) are not frequent and overt radiological changes in the bones are recognisable in only about 10–20% of patients, though most have some minor degree of microscopic abnormality. Obvious bone changes tend to occur in those patients with relatively large and rapidly growing tumours and high levels of calcium and parathormone in the plasma. Patients presenting with renal stones tend to have smaller, slower growing tumours and less obvious increases in plasma calcium and parathormone.

Associated lesions include duodenal ulceration and chronic pancreatitis. Duodenal ulceration occurs in approximately 15% of patients with hyperparathyroidism and is usually due to the enhancing effect of hypercalcaemia on gastrin. In some instances, however, there is more extensive peptic ulceration due to the association of a parathyroid adenoma with an islet-cell gastrin-secreting tumour (pluriglandular adenomatosis—p. 967). The increased incidence of pancreatitis is unexplained.

Diagnosis and sequelae. In suspected cases, repeated plasma calcium assays will usually confirm the diagnosis, but in occasional cases radio-immunoassay of PTH may be necessary. Removal of a functioning parathyroid adenoma is often followed by hypocalcaemia due to suppressed function of the remaining parathyroid glands; this is usually mild and lasts for only a few days. However, in those patients with marked bone changes hypocalcaemia may be more severe and persistent with tetany and psychotic disturbances; this is thought to be due to the avidity of the healing bone for calcium. Treatment with large calcium supplements, vitamin D and restriction of phosphate is necessary. Persistence of hypercalcaemia after removal of a parathyroid adenoma is usually due to the presence of a second, undetected adenoma (approximately 5% of cases) or rarely to metastases from a parathyroid carcinoma. If possible, all four parathyroids should be identified at operation to exclude the possibility of more than one adenoma. In some instances no adenoma is present but all four glands are enlarged and hyperplastic. They may, however, differ considerably in size and an enlarged hyperplastic gland may be mistaken for an adenoma.

Secondary hyperparathyroidism is compensatory to hypocalcaemia and occurs, for example, in chronic renal failure and in untreated malabsorption syndromes with osteomalacia. An additional factor in renal insufficiency may be failure of the kidney to convert vitamin D to its active metabolite (p. 823).

Occasionally in secondary hyperparathyroidism a parathyroid adenoma may develop, presumably in consequence of the hyperplasia. The hyperparathyroidism is then no longer compensatory: it is sometimes called **tertiary hyperparathyroidism**, and is characterised by a rising serum calcium level.

Hypoparathyroidism

Deficiency of parathormone secretion results in a fall in plasma ionised calcium and a rise in plasma phosphate. Hypocalcaemia increases the excitability of sensory and motor nerves, with various effects depending on the severity.

Causes. The commonest cause is *accidental removal of the parathyroid glands* during thyroidectomy. The condition sometimes develops following removal of a functioning parathyroid adenoma and it may then be mild and temporary or more severe and prolonged (see above). Thirdly, there is the so-called *idiopathic hypoparathyroidism* which, in some instances, is one of the organ-specific auto-immune diseases. *Congenital parathyroid deficiency* may also occur, for example in the Di George syndrome (p. 141).

Effects. If severe, hypoparathyroidism results in overt **tetany**. The tone of the skeletal muscles is increased and there may be spasm of the hands and feet in characteristic positions, twitching and jerking movements, and painful cramps of the limb muscles. There may also be generalised convulsions resembling epileptiform fits. These manifestations of motor hypersensitivity are usually accompanied by paraesthesias and there are often psychotic disturbances and sometimes even dementia. In less severe para-

thormone deficiency, muscle tone may be increased but without obvious twitching, spasms or convulsions. Such latent tetany may be demonstrated by increased responsiveness of neuromuscular junctions to electrical stimuli and by various tests depending upon irritability of the nerves to mechanical stimuli. The nails tend to be brittle and there is a high incidence of cataract formation.

Idiopathic hypoparathyroidism. There is a rare acquired form of idiopathic hypoparathyroidism; it is commoner in women than men, and in many cases antibody to a cytoplasmic constituent of parathyroid epithelium is demonstrable in the serum by the immunofluorescence technique. The condition is probably an organ-specific auto-immune disorder (p. 133), and other disorders of this group, notably primary adrenocortical atrophy, pernicious anaemia, chronic thyroiditis or thyrotoxicosis, occur with undue frequency in patients with the parathyroid disorder. Another association is with moniliasis of the fingers and toes.

Pseudo-hypoparathyroidism. A familial hereditary disorder, with the clinical and biochemical features of hypoparathyroidism, skeletal defects and metastatic ossification, has been described and given the above title because the abnormalities are not responsive to parathormone, and the parathyroids are actually hyperplastic. The disorder is therefore not due to lack of secretion but to failure to respond to it.

Other causes of tetany

Tetany used to be seen in children with rickets, in which there is deficient absorption of calcium from the intestine, although in many cases a compensatory hyperplasia and over-activity of the parathyroids is observed and may prevent tetany. Calcium deficiency may also result from the increased loss during pregnancy and lactation and this may lead to tetany. Thirdly, alkalosis may lower the level of ionic calcium in the plasma, and tetany is thus seen occasionally in patients with pyloric stenosis and repeated vomiting of acid gastric juice; indeed, even the alkalosis induced by hyperventilation may bring about or aggravate tetany.

Tumours

The commonest form of tumour is the adenoma, and in most cases this has been associated with hyperfunction as described above. It may exceed 5 cm in diameter but is usually much smaller: it is of yellowish-brown colour, occurring most often in the lower glands. Microscopic examination shows that the cells of the

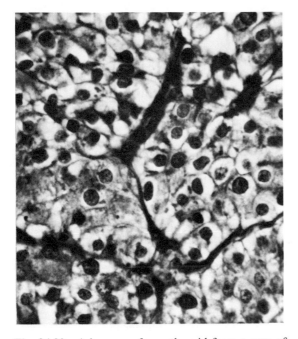

Fig. 24.20 Adenoma of parathyroid from a case of generalised osteitis fibrosa (p. 828). Both pale oxyphil and water-clear cells are present. × 500.

tumour are similar to those of the normal gland—chief, water-clear and oxyphil cells in various proportions (Fig. 24.20). In spite of the richness of oxyphil cells in enzymes and mitochondria, pure oxyphil-cell adenomas seldom

secrete excess of hormone. The cells are often larger than the normal cells and their nuclei may be very large in parts of the tumour; this does not indicate any tendency to malignancy. Also a stretched rim of normal parathyroid is

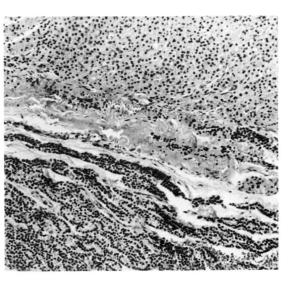

Fig. 24.21 Parathyroid adenoma, showing parathyroid tissue (below) separated by a thin capsule from the adenoma (above). × 100.

often seen at the periphery of the adenoma (Fig. 24.21). These features are not seen in parathyroid hyperplasia. Cells of columnar form may occur and a papillary type of growth may be present in an adenoma, which may be incorporated in the substance of the thyroid. Carcinoma may arise in a parathyroid but is very rare; unless it causes hyperparathyroidism, its histogenesis is usually in doubt.

The Adrenals

Introduction. The adrenal glands are complex organs, the cortex being mesodermal and the medulla of neural origin. The cortex is the site of synthesis and secretion of a large number of steroid hormones termed **corticosteroids**, which have various important effects on water and electrolyte balance, carbohydrate, protein and fat metabolism, immune responses and inflammatory reactions. The

adrenal cortex is essential to life, mainly because of its control of fluid and electrolytes.

The adrenal medulla may be regarded as an effector organ of the sympathetic nervous system, for it secretes the **catecholamines** which are sympathicomimetic. By their secretions, both the cortex and medulla play major roles in the response to mental or physical stress, e.g.

injury, shock, infections, severe illness and emotional disturbances. Also the medullary hormone adrenaline stimulates release of ACTH by the pituitary, which in turn increases the output of cortisol and related steroid hormones by the adrenal cortex.

The adrenal cortex

Adrenocortical hormones

These are all steroids and fall into three physiological groups, the *mineralocorticoids*, *glucocorticoids*, and *cortical sex steroids*.

Mineralocorticoids are so-called because they play a major role in the homeostasis of sodium, potassium and water. The most important one is *aldosterone*, of which, under normal conditions, 80–100 μg is secreted daily into the blood. Aldosterone is synthesised and secreted by the cells of the *zona glomerulosa*, i.e. the peripheral part of the cortex. Its synthesis and release are largely independent of pituitary control, and are stimulated by the renin–angiotensin system (p. 221) so that a low sodium concentration in the renal tubule or low renal perfusion pressure, as in hypovolaemia, leads to secretion of aldosterone which increases renal tubular reabsorption of sodium and chloride and so reduces their loss in the urine. The rise in osmolarity of the blood results in secretion of ADH (p. 949) so that there is oliguria and fluid retention. Aldosterone also increases the tubular secretion of potassium, thus promoting potassium loss in the urine. Conversely, a rise of plasma (or tubular) sodium or increase in blood volume inhibits secretion of renin and so of aldosterone, with the result that renal loss of salt and water increases. Aldosterone also has a very weak glucocorticoid effect.

Glucocorticoids. These, like aldosterone, are C21 steroids. In man, cortisol (hydrocortisone) is the most important, about 20–30 mg being secreted daily; the others of physiological significance are cortisone, corticosterone and 11-dehydrocorticosterone. Synthesis and secretion of glucocorticoids is controlled by ACTH, which, in turn, is regulated by a feed-back mechanism (p. 943).

Glucocorticoids have a number of effects, of which the following are particularly important; (1) they stimulate production of glucose from protein (gluconeogenesis), with consequent rise in blood glucose, and deposition of glycogen in the liver; (2) they inhibit protein synthesis and increase protein catabolism in many tissues, including the muscles; (3) in large dosage, glucocorticoids (*a*) have an anti-inflammatory effect, partly by interfering with emigration of polymorphs and macrophages and by stabilising the lysosomes of these cells, but they probably exert several other anti-inflammatory effects, (*b*) have a cytotoxic effect on lymphocytes, with consequent atrophy of the thymus and other lymphoid tissues and suppression of immune responses, particularly cell-mediated immunity, (*c*) inhibit somatic growth by suppressing secretion of growth hormone, and (*d*) result in deposition of subcutaneous fat in the face and trunk. Glucocorticoids also have mineralocorticoid activity, but this is very much weaker than that of aldosterone.

Glucocorticoids are synthesised and secreted by cells of the wide intermediate *zona fasciculata* and the narrow inner *zona reticularis* of the adrenal cortex. Their output is largely proportional to the concentration of circulating ACTH. In histological and other investigations on necropsy material from patients dying shortly after acute injury, etc., Symington and Currie equated certain changes in the pituitary with ACTH secretion and observed a correlation with loss of lipid from the cells of the zona fasciculata of the adrenals and with increase in RNA and various enzymes in the zona fasciculata and zona reticularis: these adrenal changes, formerly regarded as indicating functional exhaustion, were considered to reflect increased functional activity. As would be expected, destruction of the adenohypophysis is followed by very severe atrophy of the zona fasciculata and reticularis, but persistence of the zona glomerulosa, which continues to secrete aldosterone.

The adrenal sex hormones are *ketosteroids*: their physiological role is obscure, for the amounts of androgen and oestrogen secreted by the adrenals are insignificant compared with the endocrine activity of the gonads. In pathological conditions, excessive secretion of adrenal ketosteroids can, however, cause premature puberty, virilism in females and rarely feminisation in males.

Adrenocortical hyperfunction

As has been stated above adrenal cortical hormones are of three principal types, the mineralocorticoids, controlling electrolyte balance, the glucocorticoids regulating the intermediary metabolism of carbohydrate, fat and protein, and the ketosteroids which have androgenic and oestrogenic effects.

Three corresponding types of adrenal cortical hyperfunction are known to exist.

Cushing's syndrome (chronic hypercortisolism)

Cushing's syndrome results from excessive secretion of cortisol by the adrenal cortex or a cortical tumour. Although its natural occurrence is uncommon, it is important to recognise it as in most cases treatment can relieve an otherwise potentially fatal condition. Closely similar features are observed in patients on prolonged treatment with high doses of glucocorticoids or ACTH.

Clinical features. Cushing's syndrome occurs most often in women over a wide age range but is seen also in men and children. In all instances the main features are due to cortisol excess although there is frequently in addition excessive androgen secretion resulting in virilism.

In a severe case, i.e. with grossly excessive cortisol secretion, the features include: (1) painful adiposity of the face, neck and trunk which contrasts with the relatively thin limbs (Fig. 24.22); (2) increased protein breakdown, with consequent thinning of the skin, generalised osteoporosis and wasting and weakness of the skeletal muscles. The face is highly coloured and the weakened skin becomes stretched along lines of stress, e.g. where fat has accumulated in the abdomen, resulting in purple striae in which the small vessels are visible through the stretched skin. Osteoporosis is particularly important in the spine and may result in collapse of vertebral bodies, with kyphosis, etc. Muscle weakness and wasting are usually prominent

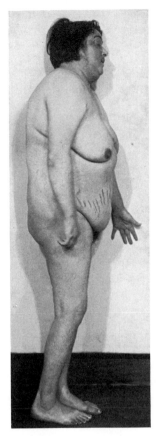

Fig. 24.22 A patient with Cushing's syndrome, subsequently cured by irradiation of the pituitary. Note the characteristic obesity of the face, neck and trunk, dusky cyanosis and facial hair, and striae of the abdominal skin.

features; (3) systemic hypertension in most cases; (4) diminished glucose tolerance, which is usually only apparent following ingestion of carbohydrate, but in approximately 20% of patients is more severe with a high fasting blood glucose level and glycosuria; (5) an increased tendency to bacterial infections and poor healing of wounds, and (6) arrest of growth in affected children. Mental confusion and psychoses are also common.

All the above features are explicable on the basis of excessive cortisol secretion. In addition, women with Cushing's syndrome usually show some features of virilism, e.g. masculine distribution of hair, acne, oligomenorrhoea, and sometimes enlargement of the clitoris and deepening of the voice. The changes in the pituitary resulting from hypercortisolism have already been described (p. 945).

Unless treated, Cushing's syndrome is likely to result in death from the effects of hypertension, from bacterial infections or from suicide. The diagnosis is based on the observation of abnormally high levels of plasma cortisol in evening specimens of blood (when the level is normally lowest), together with excess of 17-hydroxysteroids (excretory products of cortisol) in 24-hour urine specimens.

Causation and types. There are three major types of Cushing's syndrome and effective treatment depends on differentiating between them. Firstly, there may be *an adrenal tumour* which secretes cortisol in uncontrolled fashion. In such cases the high cortisol level suppresses ACTH secretion and so the cortisol hypersecretion is wholly resistant to dexamethasone (which suppresses ACTH secretion). Adrenal adenomas causing Cushing's syndrome are usually 3 cm or more in diameter and excision is curative. In some instances adrenal carcinoma is responsible or there may be *multiple micro-adenomas* necessitating bilateral adrenalectomy. Most cases of Cushing's syndrome in childhood are due to an adrenocortical tumour, but this is a fairly uncommon cause in adults.

Secondly, Cushing's syndrome may be due to *excessive secretion of ACTH by the adenohypophysis*: there may be a pituitary adenoma (as in the condition originally described by Cushing) of basophil or chromophobe type, but unless this is large enough to be shown up by radiography of the sella it cannot be detected. This form of Cushing's syndrome is sometimes confusingly called *Cushing's disease*. The plasma level of ACTH is raised and high doses of dexamethasone will, by suppressing ACTH secretion, reduce the output of cortisol. The adrenals show cortical hyperplasia (Fig. 24.23), although they may be depleted of lipid and so not necessarily enlarged. This is the commonest form of Cushing's syndrome in adults and treatment consists of reducing the excessive secretion of ACTH. This can usually be achieved by irradiation of the pituitary, e.g. by a cyclotron, and it is often possible to relieve the condition without inducing hypopituitarism.

Thirdly, Cushing's syndrome may result from the inappropriate secretion of ACTH by a non-pituitary tumour—the *ectopic ACTH syndrome*. This is most commonly due to an oat-cell bronchial carcinoma but various other tumours

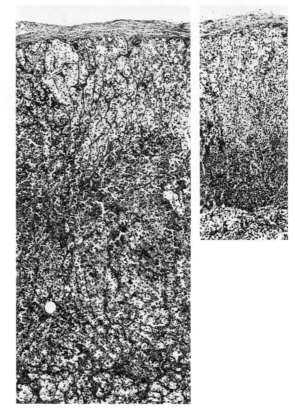

Fig. 24.23 Hyperplasia of the adrenal cortex in Cushing's syndrome (*left*) compared with a normal adrenal (*right*). The zona reticularis is greatly thickened and the cells of the zona fasciculata appear compact. In this instance, the adrenals were appreciably enlarged. × 45.

including carcinoids, thymic, pancreatic and even adrenal tumours may be responsible. The clinical features of this form of Cushing's syndrome are often not conspicuous and wasting and weakness, etc., are likely to be attributed to malignant cachexia. The plasma level of ACTH is high and cortisol secretion is not suppressed by dexamethasone.

Where other methods of treatment are inappropriate there is the possibility of administering drugs which are cytotoxic to adrenal cortical cells.

Iatrogenic Cushing's Syndrome. The prolonged administration of high doses of glucocorticoids or ACTH results in the development of the features of Cushing's syndrome and the decision to use such therapy obviously requires careful judgement. Glucocorticoid therapy and certain forms of

Cushing's syndrome are followed by a period of adrenocortical insufficiency (p. 979).

Primary aldosteronism (Conn's syndrome)

This syndrome, first recognised by Conn in 1954, is due to uncontrolled and excessive secretion of aldosterone usually by an adrenal adenoma. It differs from secondary aldosteronism in which the excessive adrenal activity is in response to angiotensin (p. 222).

Excessive secretion of aldosterone results in retention of sodium, and so of fluid, and increased excretion of potassium. The sodium and water retention result in *hypertension* which is usually moderate but may be severe and even malignant (accelerated). Hypokalaemia is usual but not invariable: if severe it may disturb cardiac rhythm, sometimes causing attacks of syncopy, and there may also be attacks of muscular weakness and hypokalaemic alkalosis associated with tetany, cramps and paraesthesias. Hypokalaemia also impairs renal concentrating capacity, resulting in nocturia and polyuria. The plasma sodium concentration is usually raised or in the upper normal range.

Diagnosis of the syndrome in patients with hypertension depends on the demonstration of an increased rate of secretion (or excretion) of aldosterone during a period of high sodium intake, and a low level of plasma renin during a period of sodium restriction. Both of these criteria are essential as many patients with 'essential' hypertension have a low plasma renin and increased aldosterone secretion occurs commonly as a secondary effect in various conditions. Hypokalaemia can occur from various causes in any type of hypertension.

Primary aldosteronism is usually due to a single adrenal cortical tumour, most commonly an adenoma, rarely a carcinoma. In some cases, however, there is no tumour but bilateral hyperplasia of the zona glomerulosa with or without multiple nodules. Excision of the offending tumour is curative. If no tumour is found removal of one adrenal and part of the other may effect a cure or, if not, facilitate control by drugs, e.g. spironolactone.

Hypersecretion of adrenocortical sex steroids

The adrenals normally secrete much smaller amounts of sex steroids than the gonads, but clinical sexual disturbances can result from adrenocortical hyperfunction. Least rare is the virilism which is usually a feature of *Cushing's syndrome* in women. Secondly, some *adrenal tumours* secrete excess of sex steroids, more commonly androgen than oestrogen, and so may bring about precocious puberty in males

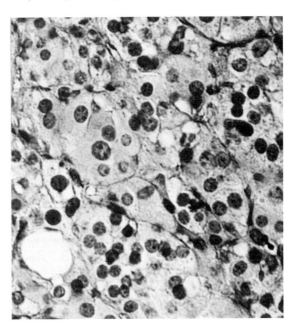

Fig. 24.24 Section of adrenal cortical adenoma associated with virilism, showing trabecular structure with tendency to variation in the size of cells. × 375.

and virilism in girls and women. In such cases, there will be an increase in urinary excretion of 17-ketosteroids unaccompanied by hypercortisolism and resistant to suppression by dexamethasone. An ovarian androblastoma has similar effects. Adrenal virilism may result from an adenoma (Fig. 24.24) or a carcinoma. Feminising adrenal tumours are very rare.

Thirdly, adrenal virilism can arise from *deficiency of 21-hydrolase*, one of a group of enzyme defects described below.

Adrenocortical enzyme defects

There is a group of conditions due to autosomal recessive traits, in each of which there is deficiency of one of the enzymes necessary for steroid hormone biosynthesis.

In one condition, 20-hydrolase is deficient and steroid synthesis in the adrenals and gonads stops at the cholesterol stage. The adrenals become hyperplastic and greatly enlarged due to accumulation of cholesterol. The external genitalia are of female appearance (in both genetic males and females) and the affected infants usually die.

The least rare member of the group is *deficiency of 21-hydrolase*, which is necessary for synthesis of both cortisol and aldosterone. This results in increased secretion of ACTH (and probably also renin), with consequent adrenocortical hyperplasia. The defect varies in severity in different families. In severe cases, deficiency of glucocorticoids and mineralocorticoids results in features resembling those of Addison's disease. There is, however, an increased secretion of precursor steroids, which do not suppress ACTH secretion. They include the androgen dehydroepiandrosterone (DHEA), which causes masculinisation, so that the female infant is born with partially fused labia and clitoral enlargement and resembles a cryptorchid male with hypospadias ('*female pseudohermaphroditism*'), while precocious puberty occurs in affected males. Less severely affected females may present as children with virilism or later because of failure of puberty. In many cases, the defect is not severe, and the adrenal hyperplasia may result in sufficient cortisol and aldosterone production, so that the sex disturbances are the main feature.

Others in this group of enzyme defects include: (i) a condition similar to 21-hydrolase deficiency; (ii) deficiency of sex hormones and of cortisol together with excess mineralocorticoid secretion, resulting in sexual infantilism, and hypertension; (iii) cortisol deficiency with increased secretion of androgens and mineralocorticoids, resulting in virilism and hypertension.

Early diagnosis of these conditions is very important, for it provides the opportunity to administer the deficient steroid(s), thus restoring the functional balance. In 21-hydrolase deficiency, for example, cortisol therapy (with extra salt and fluorocortisone if necessary) suppresses ACTH, and so reverses the adrenal hyperplasia and excessive androgen secretion: affected females treated early are sexually normal and fertile.

Primary adrenocortical hypofunction

The function of the adrenal cortex is partly dependent on normal production and secretion of ACTH and gonadotrophic hormones by the adenohypophysis, and, as already explained, pituitary failure results in depression of cortisol production by the adrenals, thyroxine by the thyroid, etc. In contrast to such *secondary* failure, primary adrenal hypofunction occurs in spite of normal pituitary function, i.e. the defect lies in the adrenals.

Primary adrenocortical hypofunction can occur as an acute condition in states of severe toxaemia, or it can develop from gradual adrenocortical destruction, usually due to an autoimmune reaction or to tuberculosis.

Acute adrenocortical insufficiency

The fatal effects of bilateral adrenalectomy in experimental animals are due to loss of cortical tissue: death can be delayed by giving salt and prevented by corticosteroids. The same applies to man, in whom bilateral adrenalectomy is performed in the treatment of selected cases of breast cancer, cortical hyperfunction or hypertension.

Acute adrenocortical insufficiency occurs

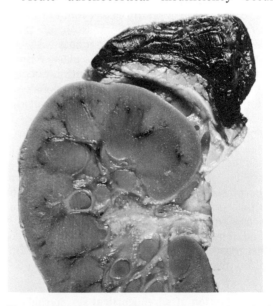

Fig. 24.25 Acute haemorrhagic necrosis of the adrenals in a child who died of meningococcal septicaemia. The adrenal lesion was bilateral.

also in some cases of septicaemia, particularly meningococcal, and in severe endotoxic shock: the adrenals become grossly haemorrhagic—'*adrenal apoplexy*' (Fig. 24.25). The cortex, which in fatal cases is largely necrotic, may be visible as a thin yellow layer stretched over the grossly swollen, haemorrhagic medulla. This condition is known also as the **Waterhouse–Friderichsen syndrome** and requires immediate and vigorous therapy.

Other toxic infections, e.g. diphtheria, may be associated with marked congestion and small haemorrhages in the adrenals, but these changes are now regarded as consistent with increased cortical activity and do not indicate failure.

The symptoms and biochemical changes of acute adrenocortical insufficiency are due mainly to deficiency of mineralocorticoids and glucocorticoids.

Deficiency of mineralocorticoids results in inadequate function of the distal convoluted tubules: there is failure to re-absorb salt and to secrete potassium, so that salt deficiency, hyperkalaemia and dehydration (p. 972) result. Death is due to a combination of hypovolaemic shock and electrolyte disturbances. Loss of medullary function, which is important in adaptation to hypovolaemia (p. 224), is likely to aggravate the condition. These changes can, however, be prevented and reversed by administration of fluid, salt and mineralocorticoid.

Deficiency of glucocorticoids results in failure of gluconeogenesis with consequent hypoglycaemia and greatly increased sensitivity to insulin. Another effect is vomiting which increases the fluid and electrolyte disturbances.

Chronic adrenocortical insufficiency—Addison's disease

Addison's description, in 1855, of this condition and its relationship to lesions of the adrenals provided the first fundamental contribution to the pathology of the adrenals.

Clinical features. The outstanding features of Addison's disease are weakness, loss of appetite and weight, and hypotension. In the absence of these features the diagnosis is unlikely. Libido is usually diminished and the skin pigmented (p. 238), particularly in the exposed parts, in scars, and over the external genitalia; the pigmentation is increased by skin irritants and in

mild cases may be the most noticeable feature. Sometimes, however, it is inconspicuous.

In the absence of high salt intake or steroid therapy, failure of reabsorption of salt in the renal tubules results in hyponatraemia, a finding of diagnostic value, and this is accompanied by chronic dehydration.

These features result from the combined deficiency of mineralocorticoids and glucocorticoids. Mineralocorticoid deficiency, as indicated above, results in loss of salt and water, with consequent hypovolaemia, hypotension, weakness and some weight loss. Chronic glucocorticoid deficiency contributes listlessness, mental confusion, hypoglycaemia, increased secretion of ACTH and MSH, impaired pressor response to catecholamines and poor reaction to stress. Anorexia, nausea, sometimes vomiting, and so weight loss and increased chloride deficiency, are also attributable to lack of glucocorticoids.

In addition to these chronic symptoms and signs there also occur in Addison's disease acute exacerbations or **crises**, which are among the gravest emergencies in medical practice, demanding energetic investigation and therapy to prevent death. In these there occur severe vomiting, which aggravates chloride loss, fall in blood pressure and extreme asthenia with hypoglycaemia terminating in collapse. Such a crisis may be precipitated by even minor infections, indiscretions in diet, or by vomiting or diarrhoea, in fact by anything which depletes still further the blood sodium level. As in acute adrenocortical insufficiency (see above) there is acute salt deficiency, dehydration and pre-renal uraemia, and death is liable to result from hypovalaemic shock and electrolyte disturbances.

Pathological changes. The commonest cause of Addison's disease in Europe was formerly destruction of the adrenals by chronic tuberculosis, which converts both glands into fibrocaseous masses. Where tuberculosis has declined, more cases of Addison's disease are now due to atrophy of the adrenal cortex accompanied by lymphocytic and plasma-cell infiltration (Fig. 24.26). The medulla is relatively unaffected and this shows that loss of the cortex is the main cause of the symptoms of Addison's disease. Antibodies to adrenocortical tissue were first detected in this laboratory (see Anderson *et al.*, 1967), in the serum of two

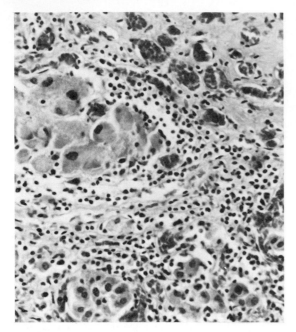

Fig. 24.26 Primary adrenal atrophy (auto-immune adrenalitis) in Addison's disease. Most of the cortical cells have been destroyed and the cortex consists of vascular fibrous tissue. In places there are foci of enlarged cortical cells with associated lymphocytic and plasma cell infiltration. × 320.

patients with non-tuberculous Addison's disease, and their presence in approximately 50% of cases has since been confirmed by various workers. They have been shown to react with lipoprotein of the endoplasmic reticulum of the cortical cells, and are not formed in cases of tuberculous Addison's disease. This finding, and the well-established associations of 'idiopathic' Addison's disease with chronic thyroiditis, thyrotoxicosis, atrophic gastritis and idiopathic hypoparathyroidism, indicate that it is one of the organ-specific auto-immune diseases (p. 132). Less commonly, fungal infections or amyloidosis of the adrenals result in Addison's disease, while rarely destruction of the glands by metastatic tumour is the cause. In all cases the syndrome of Addison's disease depends upon loss of 90% or more of the cortical tissue.

It was also demonstrated in this laboratory that, while the adrenal antibodies of Addison's disease usually react specifically and solely with adrenocortical cells, in occasional cases antibody is present which reacts also with other steroid-producing cells, i.e. the theca-lutein and true lutein cells of the corpus luteum, the theca-interna cells of the Graafian follicle, placental trophoblast, Leydig cells and hilus cells of the ovary. In some female patients with Addison's disease accompanied by amenorrhoea and sterility, Irvine has demonstrated the presence of this steroid-cell antibody, and has shown destructive inflammatory changes in the ovaries.

In tuberculous Addison's disease the adrenals are enlarged, firm and irregular. They are changed into masses of putty-like caseous material, with dense fibrous tissue surrounding it (Fig. 24.27); calcification is frequent and may be detectable radiographically.

In some cases there are no obvious tuberculous lesions in the lungs or lymph nodes.

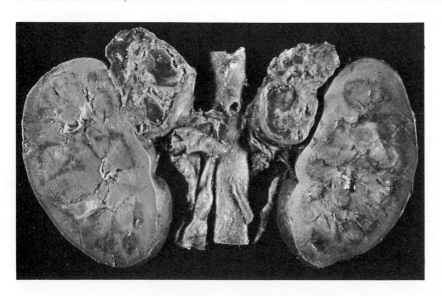

Fig. 24.27 Adrenal glands in tuberculous Addison's disease, showing extensive caseation and enlargement.

Apart from the adrenal lesions the main necropsy finding in Addison's disease is marked wasting of the muscles and adipose tissue. Atrophy of the heart is also striking; it is often more marked than in other wasting diseases, perhaps because of the low blood pressure. The gonads and breasts are also atrophic.

In Addison's disease there is a striking diminution of the basophil cells in the adenohypophysis with increase in sparsely granulated cells, which presumably are actively secreting ACTH. Acidophil cells are also diminished. The disturbance of carbohydrate metabolism results in a marked decrease in liver glycogen, the patients are highly sensitive to insulin and attacks of hypoglycaemia are fairly common.

In mild cases of Addison's disease, oral glucocorticoids and a high salt diet may be satisfactory, but in more severe cases the weak mineralocorticoid activity of glucocorticoids is inadequate and mineralocorticoids must be given.

Diagnosis of Addison's disease is readily confirmed by measuring the plasma levels and urinary output of corticosteroids before and during an infusion of ACTH. The distinction between auto-immune and tuberculous adrenalitis in Addison's disease is based on the history and appropriate tests (see above).

Adrenocortical hypofunction from 'disuse'

The prolonged high dosage of glucocorticoids now used to treat various conditions results in suppression of ACTH secretion and so atrophy of the fasciculate and reticulate zones of the adrenal cortex. This occurs also in Cushing's syndrome due to an adrenal adenoma. Following removal of the tumour or cessation of prolonged glucocorticoid therapy it may take some months for full restoration of cortical function and reserve, and it may be necessary to administer corticosteroids in gradually diminishing dosage, with increased dosage to cover additional stress imposed by infections, surgical operations, etc.

Secondary adrenocortical insufficiency

This results from pituitary failure with diminished secretion of ACTH and consequently of adrenocortical steroids, particularly glucocorticoids. The condition has been considered earlier in relation to hypopituitarism.

Adrenocortical tumours

The commonest cortical tumours are **adenomas**. They occur in the form of comparatively small, rounded nodules, well defined, and usually of yellow colour, owing to the large amount of fat and steroids in the cells; not infrequently they are multiple. In the smaller adenomas the cells are arranged in trabeculae and resemble closely those of the zona fasciculata; but in the larger examples there is a tendency towards alteration in the types of the cells. A cortical adenoma may be associated with abnormal sexual development as described above, causing either precocious puberty or virilism, or Cushing's syndrome, or it may, more rarely, secrete aldosterone in excess (p. 975). It is becoming increasingly apparent that most cortical adenomas synthesise and secrete hormones, although most often in amounts insufficient to give rise to clinical abnormalities. The cells may become large, often contain more than one nucleus, and all transitions to distinctly aberrant forms occur. The tumour rarely becomes carcinomatous. Sometimes carcinoma is bilateral, although one may be a metastasis. Excessive hormone secretion may persist in spite of much cellular aberration.

The adrenal medulla

Sympathetic nerve endings and chromaffin cells (so named because they reduce chrome salts, producing brown reduction products) secrete catecholamines. Sympathetic nerve endings are the main source of the noradrenaline in the blood, while the adrenal medulla is responsible for intermittent secretion of adrenaline. The blood level of both of these catecholamines is increased almost instantaneously by stressful situations, e.g. by emotion, injury or shock. Part of the stimulus is neural, but histamine, bradykinin and various drugs have a direct stimulating effect. Secretion of adrenaline by the adrenal medulla is in some way dependent on a normal functional cortex, the blood from which is rich in corticosteroids and perfuses the medulla. In turn, adrenaline stimulates secretion of ACTH and so indirectly influences cortical function.

The binding of catecholamines to α- and β-receptors has a profound influence on the function of many types of tissue cell, and its elucidation is not only throwing considerable light on control of cellular function, but has also provided opportunity to develop drugs which activate or block α- or β-receptors and thus influence cell functions in various ways. Stimulation via β-receptors activates adenyl cyclase activity and so increases the intracellular cyclic AMP (p. 117) the effect of which depends on the type of cell stimulated and on the additional effects of various other hormones on it. The mechanism by which stimulation via α-receptors influences cells is not known: it may be by altering cyclic guanosine monophosphate (GMP).

This profoundly important aspect of cell physiology cannot be considered here in detail, but it must be emphasised that increased secretion of catecholamines in conditions of shock (p. 224) is of great importance in maintaining the blood pressure by causing vasoconstriction in the skin and splanchnic circulation: noradrenaline has the greater effect, because it causes vasoconstriction also in skeletal muscles.

In spite of these adaptive effects of adrenal medullary function, the most important effects of adrenal failure are due to deficiency of corticosteroids. Hypersecretion of catecholamines is, however, observed in patients with a functioning tumour of the adrenal medulla or of chromaffin cells elsewhere, i.e. a *phaeochromocytoma*, the features of which are described below.

Tumours of the medulla

These are of three types. Two of them take origin from nerve cells, namely the **ganglioneuroma**, a simple growth containing ganglionic nerve cells and nerve fibres, and the **neuroblastoma** or **sympathicoblastoma** composed of embryonic nerve cells or neuroblasts. These tumours are described elsewhere (pp. 726–8). Neuroblastoma is much the commoner growth, in fact it is fairly frequent in children. It may reach a large size, is composed of soft cellular tissue, and is very haemorrhagic. Secondary growths are often widespread and occur both in other organs and in the bones, the skull often being affected. Similar tumours may arise also from other parts of the sympathetic system. Such tumours may secrete catecholamines other than adrenaline and noradrenaline, especially dopamine, which appears in the urine chiefly as vanillin mandelic acid (VMA) and homovanillic acid.

Phaeochromocytoma

This third variety of tumour takes origin from the chromaffin cells. It can arise also from chromaffin cells in other sites (see below) and is then sometimes called a *paraganglioma*. It is composed of polyhedral cells, many of which give the chromaffin reaction, staining a brownish-yellow colour with chrome salts, and rich in glycogen (Fig. 24.28). When placed in

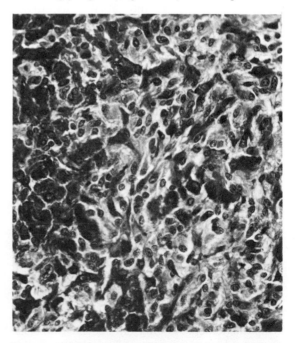

Fig. 24.28 Phaeochromocytoma of the adrenal medulla. The darkly stained elements are cells giving the chromaffin reaction. × 200.

formol-saline it imparts a brown colour to the fixative. The cells are arranged in solid masses which fill alveolar spaces; the stroma is somewhat scanty and vascular. The cells may show aberrant features, but the tumour is usually benign.

Clinical features arise from excessive although usually intermittent secretion of catecholamines. Symptoms include excessive sweating, nervousness, tremors and sometimes psychoses, attacks of blanching or flushing, headache and palpitations; also loss of appetite and weight.

There is hypertension, at first paroxysmal but sometimes becoming continuous; there may also be postural hypotension. The fasting blood sugar is usually raised and the basal metabolic rate increased. Obviously a phaeochromocytoma can mimic various other conditions. In most cases the diagnosis can be confirmed by demonstrating that the daily urinary excretion of vanillin mandelic acid (VMA, a metabolite of catecholamines) is more than doubled. The response to the α-blocking agent phentolamine is also of diagnostic value.

The hypertension is associated with arteriosclerosis even in young subjects. Occasionally death has occurred from cerebral haemorrhage. Neurofibromatosis has been present in 5% of cases. Familial examples of bilateral phaeochromocytoma associated with medullary carcinoma of the thyroid and neurofibromas are encountered. Early surgical removal of the tumour relieves the symptoms. Paragangliomas causing a similar syndrome occur in chromaffin tissues outside the adrenal, e.g. in the organ of Zuckerkandl, but the majority are devoid of excessive hormonal activity. Rarely, phaeochromocytomas are malignant and metastasise.

Other adrenal tumours

These include *lipoma*, *myelolipoma* and *haemangioma*, all of which are rare. *Melanomas* also occur, as a rule bilaterally. *Carcinomatous metastases* are often present in the adrenals, particularly in bronchial carcinoma, in which both glands may be implicated, the ipsilateral gland being first involved and usually the larger.

Congenital abnormalities

Absence of both adrenals is a rare abnormality, incompatible with life; or one (the right only) may be absent. These abnormalities are intimately related to gross defects of the central nervous system, such as micrencephaly or anencephaly; in other cases of such cerebral lesions the adrenals may be hypoplastic.

Accessory adrenals are comparatively common; they are small masses of cortical tissue which can be readily recognised by their brownish-yellow colour. They occur in the surrounding tissues, on the surface or occasionally in the substance of the kidney or liver, and in the region of the ovary or testis, and very frequently at the apex of congenital hernial sacs. Rarely a tumour arises from them.

25

The Skin

Skin pathology is often regarded as so specialised a subject that it is not suitable for inclusion in a general textbook. But the tissue responses in the diseased skin are basically the same as those that occur in other organs, and it is an ideal organ in which to study the correlation of naked-eye changes with microscopic, especially as the evolution of a lesion may be readily followed by repeated biopsy.

As in other tissues, local factors modify the basic responses, and the spectrum of possible changes is less than the number of causes of change. This is particularly true in the case of the inflammatory diseases where topical therapy, particularly with potent fluorinated corticosteroid preparations, may significantly alter the histological picture: here however in making a diagnosis the distribution and naked-eye appearance of the lesion must be considered as well as the histology. The following account is intended only to cover a representative selection of dermatological conditions which have a characteristic pathology. Major omissions are the infective conditions (other than viral) and the granulomas, but some at least of these are dealt with in other chapters.

Some of the reactions peculiar to the epidermis are defined below.

Acanthosis. A generalised thickening of the *stratum malpighii*, which may or may not be associated with hypertrophy of the other layers. It may be closely imitated by oblique section, but this can be obviated by proper orientation of the tissue.

Acantholysis. In this the cells of the epidermis (keratinocytes) lose their cohesive properties, leading to the formation of clefts, vesicles and bullae within the epidermis. It is an important diagnostic feature of several diseases.

Dyskeratosis. Premature, abnormal or individual keratinisation of epidermal cells. These cells lose their prickles and become rounded off, their cytoplasm becomes strongly eosinophilic and the nucleus undergoes pyknosis. While this may be seen in a few rare benign diseases it is most common in malignant and premalignant lesions of the epidermis.

Hyperkeratosis is self-explanatory. It is usually associated with hypertrophy of the granular layer although the rete malpighii may be normal, acanthotic or even atrophic.

Parakeratosis is an abnormal form of keratinisation. The cells of the stratum corneum retain their nuclei and are swollen. This results in a lack of cohesion which is apparent clinically as scaling. It is associated with an absence of the stratum granulosum and is caused by oedema or inflammatory infiltration of the underlying epidermis.

In mucous membranes composed of stratified squamous epithelium it is normal in some areas for the surface cells to retain their nuclei and to have no granular layer. This normal process is often loosely called parakeratosis but it must be differentiated from the pathological parakeratosis which occurs in the skin.

Biopsy. It is of the utmost importance that an early representative lesion be selected for biopsy and that this be taken carefully, with the minimum of trauma, together with a portion of adjacent normal skin. The most satisfactory biopsy is taken by ringing the lesion with local anaesthetic and excising a small ellipse with a scalpel. Forceps should not be used to grasp the tissue and their need is obviated by the use of a Gillies hook to elevate the portion to be removed. High speed punches have been advocated but these cause severe trauma and distortion of the tissues and they are not recommended.

To obtain maximum information it is necessary to orientate the specimen and this is aided by gently pressing the undersurface on to a small square of blotting paper before putting it into the fixative. Failure to do this results in warping of the tissue and may lead to errors in diagnosis.

Hereditary and Congenital Conditions

There are many hereditary disorders in which the skin is involved as part of a general biochemical abnormality: failure to remove ultraviolet light-damaged DNA in xeroderma pigmentosum (p. 254), excess or lack of pigment in haemochromatosis and albinism respectively, and photosensitivity in some forms of porphyria are examples. In others the recognisable disorder appears to be confined to the skin itself. The exact origin of the defect is not known in any of the examples given below, but in the first three it appears self-evident and there is some inherent defect of the epidermal cells.

Ichthyosis or 'fish-skin disease' is not as uncommon as is generally believed. Many individuals suffering from a dry skin are subclinical examples of the condition. In its most severe form the plaque-like scales impede respiratory movement and death ensues. Fortunately this degree of severity is rare.

Two main types of ichthyosis are encountered: (1) an autosomal dominant type and (2) a sex-linked recessive type confined to males. In the former, which is the commoner, the characteristic histological feature is hyperkeratosis with thinning, or often complete absence, of the granular layer. This finding is contrary to the usual hypertrophy of the granular layer when there is hyperkeratosis. The non-keratinised part of the epidermis is thin and the hyperkeratosis at the mouths of the hair follicles may eventually lead to atrophy and disappearance of the hair and its associated sebaceous glands. A mild perivascular infiltrate of chronic inflammatory cells may be present. In one rare variant of this condition, a defect of retinol (vitamin A) metabolism has been demonstrated: it can be treated by oral or topical application of retinoic acid (vitamin A acid). In other types of ichthyosis, treatment is of no avail.

In the sex-linked type there is marked hyperkeratosis, hypertrophy of the granular layer and acanthosis of the epidermis. Sebaceous glands are present in normal numbers and there is a moderate perivascular infiltrate of chronic inflammatory cells.

Darier's disease (Keratosis follicularis). A familial occurrence of this disease is now generally recognised. Though relatively rare, it is included because of its characteristic histological features and its confusion with other conditions. The epidermis shows considerable hyperkeratosis and acanthosis, and is thrown into folds. This causes oblique cuts in the preparation of sections and gives rise to the appearance of a core of dermis surrounded by a single layer of epidermal cells, the so-called papillomatosis. Owing to the process of acantholysis, clefts (lacunae) appear in the epidermis and in properly orientated sections these are found just above the basal layer. The two most striking features are, however, the presence of dyskeratotic cells in the epidermis called *corps*

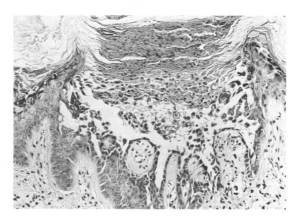

Fig. 25.1 Darier's disease. The corps ronds are seen in the upper layers of the epidermis and the grains underlying the central hyperkeratosis. × 150.

ronds and *grains* (Fig. 25.1). The *corps ronds*, which are enlarged keratinocytes are seen mainly in the upper epidermis in the region of the granular layer. They are easily recognised by their large size (two to three times that of the surrounding keratinocytes) and in haemalum and eosin-stained sections by their hyaline-looking eosinophilic cytoplasm (premature keratinisation). The grains are found in the horny layer and differ only in size and shape from those found in the more usual type of parakeratosis. These changes are focal and may involve only very small areas of the epidermis.

This form of benign dyskeratosis must be differentiated from its malignant counterpart which is seen in some types of intra-epithelial neoplasm.

984   *The skin*

Benign familial pemphigus. This condition resembles Darier's disease in so far as acantholysis and papillomatosis occur (Fig. 25.2). The acantholysis is much more widespread and the epidermis has been aptly likened to a dilapidated brick wall. Dyskeratosis may be seen but is not so severe as in Darier's disease. Areas of grain-like parakeratosis are found overlying the acantholytic epidermis. In cases

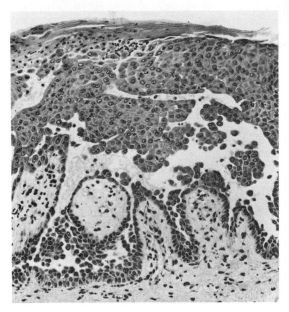

Fig. 25.2 Benign familial pemphigus. Note the extensive acantholysis and 'papillomatosis'. × 175.

lacking dyskeratosis, differentiation from pemphigus vulgaris (see below) may be impossible on purely histological grounds.

Urticaria pigmentosa. This disorder is usually congenital, but may appear first in adult life. No familial background has been established. It usually presents clinically as widespread pigmented macules which urticate, although occasionally the entire cutaneous surface is involved.

Histological examination (Fig. 25.3) reveals a normal epidermis apart from an increase in melanin pigmentation of the basal layer. Depending on the severity of the condition part or all of the dermis contains closely packed mast cells. In routine haemalum and eosin preparations these are seen as polygonal or hex-

agonal cells with abundant eosinophilic cytoplasm and well defined, rather dense nuclei. Staining by toluidine blue or polychrome methylene blue brings out their typical granular appearance. A few eosinophil leukocytes are

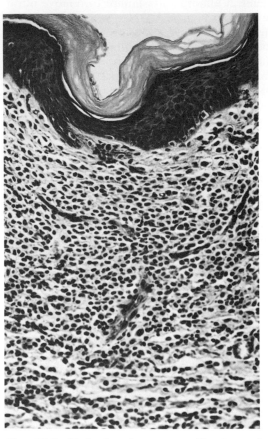

Fig. 25.3 Urticaria pigmentosa. Closely packed mast cells occupy the upper dermis. × 200.

seen. In the urticated phase oedema is evident and may at times be so marked as to cause a subepidermal bulla.

The mast cell infiltration is not confined to the skin and may be seen in lymph nodes, spleen, liver and bone-marrow. Despite the enormous increase of mast cells no significant abnormality of clotting mechanism has been detected. In most cases of urticaria pigmentosa the clinical features regress as the child ages and most cases have completely cleared by puberty.

Virus Diseases

Virus infections of the skin are common, and, as usual with virus infections, have clearly-defined features. They can be divided into the two sharply contrasted groups of those that cause cells to multiply (the tumour viruses) and those that cause necrosis of cells. Of the latter, only the most important infections, caused by the herpes–smallpox group, will be dealt with here.

Warts

These are by far the commonest virus lesions of the skin. The histology of the vulgar wart usually seen on the hands and knees is essentially similar to the plantar wart found on the soles of the feet. The plane wart which is found on the face and dorsum of the hand is also similar histologically. This is not surprising as they are all caused by identical or closely related strains of the same DNA papovavirus.

Verruca vulgaris and verruca plantaris. The epidermis is markedly acanthotic and thrown into folds. The rete ridges are elongated, those at the periphery of the lesion being the longest: they are curved inwards so that if projected they would converge on a central point. There is marked hyperkeratosis alternating with parakeratosis. Scattered throughout the upper layers of the rete malpighii and in the region of the granular layer are large cells with vacuolated nuclei (Fig. 25.4). The cytoplasm contains eosinophilic masses, and the vacuolated nucleus eosinophilic or basophilic inclusions, presumed to be virus aggregations. In older lesions these inclusions may not be prominent: they are usually best seen in plantar warts.

Verruca plana. In contrast to the verruca vulgaris, the acanthosis in this type is a generalised thickening without the formation of folds. There is hyperkeratosis of a peculiar type but no parakeratosis (Fig. 25.5). Numerous

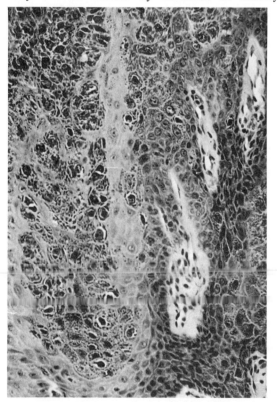

Fig. 25.4 Verruca vulgaris. Margin of a lesion showing the eosinophilic cytoplasmic inclusions. × 200.

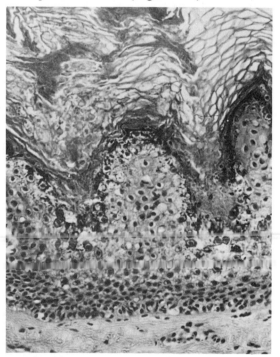

Fig. 25.5 Verruca plana. Vacuolated cells are seen in the upper layers of the acanthotic epidermis. Note the basket weave appearance of the stratum corneum. × 150.

vacuolated cells with pyknotic nuclei are found in the upper layers of the stratum corneum. This gives the stratum corneum an open woven appearance which has been likened to basket weave: this appearance is normal in most parts of the body, where movement and stretching of the skin are of importance. On the palms, soles and other pressure areas, however, the keratin is normally denser and of laminated structure. Intranuclear inclusions or cytoplasmic masses are not usually seen although they have been reported by some observers.

Other virus lesions

Molluscum contagiosum. This relatively common contagious condition, due to a DNA poxvirus, consists of an eruption of waxy skin-coloured papules or nodules with characteristic central umbilication. Pressure on the lesions causes expression of a small quantity of cheese-like material.

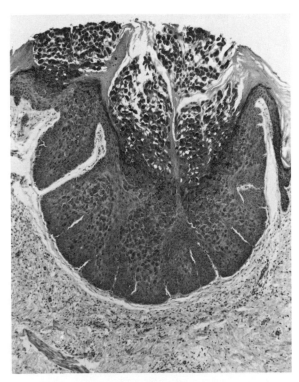

Fig. 25.6 Molluscum contagiosum. The localised over-growth of the epidermis is clearly seen. Numerous molluscum bodies are being extruded at the surface. × 70.

Section through a typical lesion shows a localised overgrowth of the epidermis into the dermis compressing the connective tissue to form a pseudo-capsule (Fig. 25.6). Small oval eosinophilic inclusion bodies are seen in the basal cells. These rapidly increase in size and push the nucleus to one side, the cells at this stage being considerably larger than normal squamous cells. As the degenerated cells approach the surface, the inclusions change their staining reactions and become basophilic. Electron-microscopic examination of these inclusions (molluscum bodies) reveals them to be made up of aggregations of virus particles.

Herpes and Poxvirus infections. Herpes simplex, varicella (chickenpox), zoster, variola (smallpox) and vaccinia are very different diseases, and the DNA viruses which cause them belong to the structurally distinct poxvirus and herpesvirus groups. Despite these differences, the tissue reactions are closely similar in all these conditions, and they may conveniently be considered together.

In all of them excluding vaccination, the original natural infection is probably through the upper respiratory tract or mouth, with a viraemic phase before the definitive localisation to the skin. In all, some minor degree of proliferation of epidermal cells may occur at first. The characteristic skin lesion is, however, a blister, histologically an intra-epidermal vesicle or bulla. The individual epidermal cells attacked by the virus become much enlarged and in the early stage are characterised by a rather homogeneous eosinophilic cytoplasm and one to several enlarged nuclei (Fig. 25.7). Profound degenerative changes with vacuolation then occur (balloon degeneration), the cells lose their adhesion to one another and lie loose in the bulla. Many cells enlarge and rupture so quickly that neighbouring cell walls remain adherent and these may be seen running across various parts of the bulla. This process is known as *reticular degeneration* and gives rise to a multilocular vesicle or bulla.

Inclusion bodies may be seen in the degenerate epidermal cells. In variola these are predominantly cytoplasmic while in herpes simplex, zoster and varicella these are mainly intranuclear. This feature, however, is not reliable enough to differentiate variola from the other three. In spite of their histological similarity, the diseases caused range from the major and frequently fatal variola to the mild and non-disabling herpes simplex. In **variola** the

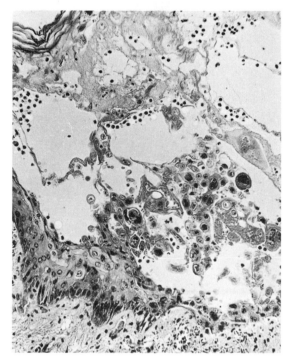

Fig. 25.7 Zoster. Multilocular intra-epidermal bulla, showing large swollen cells (balloon degeneration) and strands of cell walls traversing the bulla (reticular degeneration). × 350.

severity of the disease is due principally to the number and severity of the skin lesions: so much skin is damaged and so much virus produced that, though other tissues may be involved, this alone is enough to cause death. In **vaccinia** the lesions are individually similar, but nearly always remain localised to a small area of the skin, and therefore vaccination produces only a minor illness. Vaccinia virus is, however, sufficiently closely similar antigenically to variola virus to produce cross-immunity against smallpox.

Varicella is a disease remarkably similar to smallpox, but the lesions are smaller and fewer, and serious illness is rare. In spite of this the virus is widely disseminated in the body, producing mild pneumonitis fairly often and widespread visceral lesions in occasional subjects, particularly those with a congenital or acquired defect of cell-mediated immune responses (p. 139). The virus can survive in the body for long periods, for **zoster** is apparently produced by recrudescent activity of the same virus late in life, producing a recurrence of intra-epidermal vesicles within the area of distribution of one sensory nerve, combined with painful lesions of the corresponding posterior root ganglion (p. 696).

Herpes simplex is a ubiquitous infection. Most people acquire it asymptomatically via the oral mucosa when young: thereafter it remains latent, producing skin lesions of the characteristic type, usually around the lips, and often under the stimulus of some incidental febrile illness. Occasionally more severe lesions may occur, usually as part of the original infection, e.g. aphthous stomatitis, keratoconjunctivitis, or meningoencephalitis, the last of which may be fatal (p. 695). Herpes simplex shares with vaccinia virus the ability to colonise areas of dermatitis in children, producing a condition known in both cases as *Kaposi's varicelliform eruption.*

Inflammatory Conditions

Because of the lack of knowledge of the aetiology of skin disease many apparently different conditions are arbitrarily grouped under the heading of inflammatory diseases. This is not so irrational as it may seem because those varied diseases show different degrees and facets of the changes of inflammation.

Dermatitis

Much confusion has been caused by the use of the terms dermatitis and eczema in describing similar conditions but by common usage they are now regarded as synonymous. For the purpose of this discussion dermatitis will be used. The term covers the inflammatory response of the skin to a wide variety of aetiological agents ranging from contact with external primary irritants to a hypersensivity reaction to various antigens, both exogenous and endogenous.

The external primary irritants such as strong acids or alkalis produce an acute inflammatory response similar to that seen in other tissues and the dermatitis is self-limiting once the irritant has been removed.

The hypersensitivity group is however, more complex and as yet imperfectly understood. Most of the chemical substances causing this type of reaction are haptens and need to combine with an epidermal protein, most likely keratin, in order to become antigenic. Once induced the sensitivity, which is of the delayed type (p. 127), tends to be self-perpetuating and overlaps into the field of auto-immune skin disease by way of continued epidermal trauma from scratching or superadded infection.

Drugs which produce a dermatitis-type of skin eruption similarly act as haptens, in this instance combining with one of the plasma proteins to become antigens.

Whatever the causal factor the basic tissue response is similar and for this reason it is better to speak of a dermatitis reaction which, like any inflammatory process, may be classified as acute, subacute or chronic. As this basic reaction occurs in so many named skin diseases the pathologist can only report on the type of dermatitis reaction and is not in a position to give any indication as to the aetiological factors.

Acute dermatitis. The initial lesion is an intercellular oedema which separates the keratinocytes and is followed by lymphocytic infiltration. Then follows degeneration and liquefaction of the cells which leads to the formation of vesicles within the epidermis (Fig. 25.8). In the fully developed lesion the epidermis contains multiple vesicles many of which are separated by thin strands of epithelial cells. At a later stage these may rupture, giving rise to larger vesicles or bullae. The vesicles contain fibrin, degenerated epithelial cells, polymorphonuclear leukocytes and lymphocytes. Overlying these areas the nutrition of the stratum corneum is interfered with and parakeratosis results. Depending on the severity of the reaction the dermis shows varying degrees of oedema, vascular dilatation and congestion, and peri-

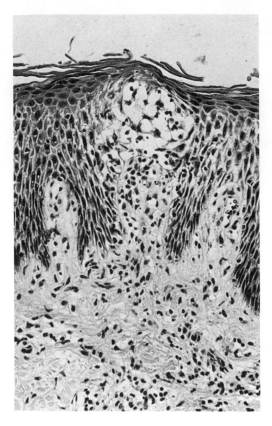

Fig. 25.8 Acute dermatitis, showing an intraepidermal vesicle containing leukocytes and degenerate epithelial cells. × 200.

vascular inflammatory cellular infiltration by lymphocytes, eosinophils and polymorphonuclear leukocytes.

As with other vesicular and bullous diseases of the skin an early typical lesion must be selected for biopsy.

While this histological picture may be seen in the acute phase of any dermatitis it is best observed in an acute contact dermatitis of hypersensitivity type. The margin of the lesion of **pityriasis rosea** shows an acute vesicular reaction in the epidermis.

Subacute dermatitis. As the acute stage subsides the lesions become less vesicular and although oedema and vesiculation may persist, there are fewer and smaller vesicles. The epidermis is acanthotic and parakeratosis is marked. The surface is covered with a mixture of fibrin, degenerating leukocytes and bacteria. Where a vesicle has ruptured on to the surface a naked dermal papilla covered by fibrin and debris is seen (Fig. 25.9), the so-called *dermatitis pit*. There is less oedema and vascular congestion in the dermis, and while the amount of inflammatory infiltrate is greater, this is composed mainly of lymphocytes and macrophages with only an occasional neutrophil leukocyte. **Nummular dermatitis** is the classical example of

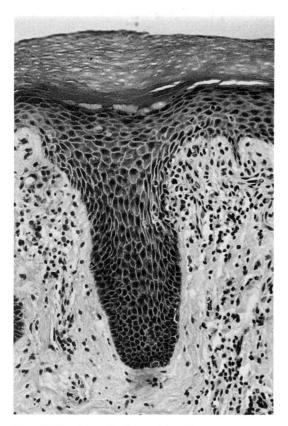

Fig. 25.10 Chronic dermatitis. There is hyperkeratosis, elongation of the rete ridges and a perivascular inflammatory infiltrate in the upper dermis. × 300.

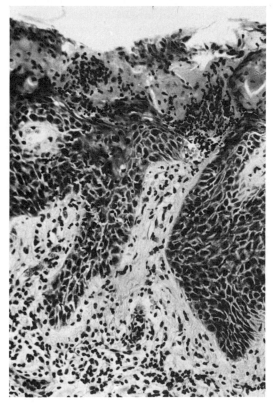

Fig. 25.9 Subacute dermatitis. Note the tip of the dermal papilla in contact with the serous exudate and debris on the surface. × 300.

this stage of dermatitis although it may be seen also as a phase of others, in particular atopic dermatitis. Stasis dermatitis, associated with inadequate venous return from the lower limbs, differs in that, in addition to the changes described, deposits of haemosiderin are found in the dermis.

Chronic dermatitis. The epidermis shows a marked acanthosis with elongation of the rete ridges. There is hyperkeratosis with areas of parakeratosis. Small foci of intercellular oedema may be seen but no vesicles (Fig. 25.10). There is a moderate inflammatory infiltrate in the upper dermis composed of lympho-

cytes, macrophages, fibroblasts and eosinophil leukocytes. The walls of the dermal arterioles and vessels often show a hyaline thickening with reduction in the size of their lumina. This histological picture is seen in the chronic phase of any dermatitic process when the skin is thickened and leathery in appearance (lichenified). The most characteristic clinical condition is, however, that of **neurodermatitis or lichen simplex chronicus**.

The prognosis of dermatitis is variable. Acute and subacute phases can be quickly controlled by the use of appropriate topical treatment, and, in the case of contact and irritant dermatitis, by removing the patient from the source. Chronic dermatitis, particularly those types affecting the hands and feet, is extremely difficult to manage and in many instances persists for life.

Some skin conditions, including parapsoriasis, erythema multiforme and annular erythema, are not clinically examples of dermatitis, and yet show the histological features of dermatitis: this may also be seen at times during the evolution of clinically atypical cases of diseases such as psoriasis or lichen planus, which normally have characteristic changes.

Generalised exfoliative dermatitis, a striking and serious clinical entity, shows a dermatitis reaction in either the subacute or chronic phase. As some 25% of people with this condition develop a malignant reticulosis it is essential to examine repeated biopsies in order to detect any change in the quality of the dermal infiltrate.

Acne vulgaris

This extremely common inflammatory disorder affects adolescent males and females equally. Commencing at or about puberty, it runs a fluctuating course eventually burning itself out sometime in the mid-twenties. The disorder affects mainly the pilosebaceous follicles of the skin of the face, chest and upper back, although in severe cases it may extend over the deltoid region and downwards to involve the buttocks. The initial pathological process consists of a blockage of the pilosebaceous follicle opening by a mass of keratinous debris. This lesion is known as a **comedo** (blackhead) and the black colouration of its tip is due to the deposition of melanin pigment. The pathogenesis of comedo formation is imperfectly understood but it may be related to androgen biosynthesis by the sebaceous glands themselves.

Although the pilosebaceous follicle is blocked the secretion of sebum continues at least for some considerable time. In some cases the pilosebaceous follicle becomes increasingly distended until the pressure within it causes atrophy of the sebaceous gland. At this stage the lesion consists of a cystic dilatation of the follicle which contains a mixture of keratinous debris and sebum (cystic acne). More commonly, however, the contents of the pilosebaceous follicle become infiltrated by polymorphonuclear leukocytes and purulent material is eventually discharged on to the surface (pustular acne). The reason for the development of pustules is obscure. It is thought that the commensal anaerobic diphtheroid organism, *Corynebacterium acnes*, finds the occluded follicle suitable for growth. This organism produces a potent lipase which splits the neutral fat in sebum to free fatty acids, which are extremely irritant to the tissue. Should fatty acids escape from the pilosebaceous follicle, either by spontaneous rupture or aided by pressure caused by the patient trying to express the lesions, an intense inflammatory reaction ensues with subsequent folliculitis and perifolliculitis. Disintegration of the follicular wall allows the altered sebum and keratinous debris into the tissue and this evokes further inflammatory changes, as evidenced by the formation of foreign body granulomas. The healing of the perifolliculitis and the perifollicular granulomas is by granulation tissue with subsequent scar formation. Such scarring is, of course, permanent and may be severe, progressing even to keloid formation. The introduction of long-term, low-dose oral tetracycline therapy for acne has done much to alleviate this distressing disorder. Most cases are completely controlled and the residual scarring reduced to a minimum.

The bullous group

This comprises pemphigus, pemphigoid, dermatitis herpetiformis and erythema multiforme.

It is possible to separate the pemphigus group from the others by histological examination but only if an early representative biopsy is taken. Secondary infection and degenerative changes rapidly alter the histological features. Ideally a small lesion should be taken within 12 hours of its appearance. Pemphigoid, dermatitis herpetiformis and some types of erythema multiforme may all show subepidermal bullae and immunofluorescent studies may be necessary (see below) for accurate diagnosis. Three basic types of pemphigus are recognised, viz. pemphigus vulgaris, pemphigus vegetans and pemphigus foliaceous. In the latter two types bullae may not be in evidence clinically although histological examination will reveal the characteristic changes at the edge of the lesion. Pemphigus is a serious disorder and the vulgaris and vegetans types, if untreated, will cause death. Systemic corticosteroids and immunosuppressant drugs have greatly improved the prognosis. Pemphigus foliaceus is more benign and can often be satisfactorily controlled by one of the more potent topical corticosteroid preparations.

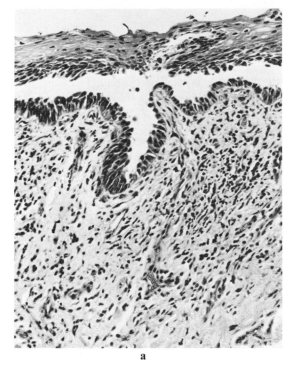

a

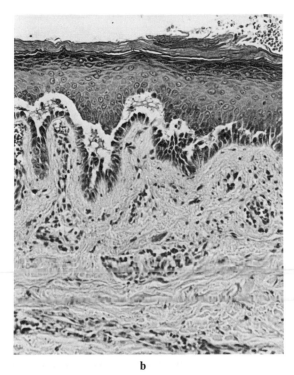

b

The bulla of pemphigus is intra-epidermal and arises as a result of acantholysis of the epidermal cells which produces a horizontal plane of cleavage in the epidermis.

Pemphigus vulgaris. In pemphigus vulgaris (Fig. 25.11) the cleavage takes place above the basal layer, this layer remaining intact due to its attachment to the dermis by cytoplasmic processes. The bulla contains serum and some-what condensed, rounded-off keratinocytes. A few polymorphonuclear leukocytes and eosinophils may also be present within the bulla. The underlying dermis shows slight oedema and a sparse infiltrate of polymorphs and eosinophils.

Pemphigus vegetans. In pemphigus vegetans the early lesion is identical with that of pemphigus vulgaris. As the disease progresses, however, the epithelium proliferates and the characteristic acantholysis is not seen. There is marked acanthosis of a verrucose type and intra-epidermal abscesses composed almost entirely of eosinophil leukocytes (Fig. 25.12).

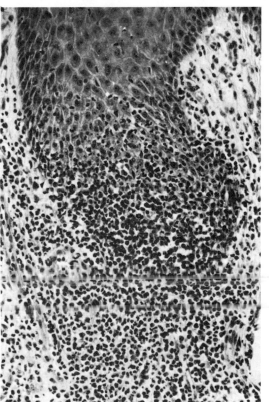

Fig. 25.11 Pemphigus vulgaris. **a** Acantholytic bulla in buccal mucous membrane. × 150. **b** Intra-epidermal bulla containing acantholytic cells, best seen just above the basal layer of the epidermis. × 150.

Fig. 25.12 Pemphigus vegetans. Intra-epidermal abscess composed of eosinophil leukocytes at tip of an elongated rete ridge. × 300.

The inflammatory infiltrate in the upper dermis includes many eosinophil leukocytes and is much more pronounced than in pemphigus vulgaris.

Pemphigus foliaceus. In pemphigus foliaceus the acantholysis occurs high in the epidermis, usually just below the stratum corneum (Fig. 25.13), and if the biopsy is not carefully taken

There is no acantholysis. Difficulty may arise if an older lesion is biopsied as the epithelium regenerates rapidly and may give the impression that the bulla is intra-epidermal. The subepidermal bulla is filled with serous exudate and contains leukocytes, a high percentage of which are eosinophils. The underlying dermis is oedematous and there is a considerable

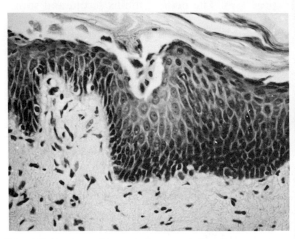

Fig. 25.13 Pemphigus foliaceus. Subcorneal bulla containing occasional acantholytic cells and some leukocytes. × 200.

or the tissue is roughly handled the superficial layer may be lost, making the diagnosis difficult. Careful examination of the surface, however, will reveal acantholytic cells.

Mucosal lesions of pemphigus. While all forms of pemphigus are usually regarded as skin diseases, many cases begin as 'ulcers' of the mouth or genitalia. These may precede the skin lesions by as long as two years. The histological changes in mucous membranes are similar to those in the skin, viz. acantholytic bullae (Fig. 25.11b). Because of the moist conditions within the mouth or on the vulva, maceration occurs rapidly and the roof of the bulla is quickly lost, making histological diagnosis extremely difficult. The recent finding that patients in the active stages of pemphigus have serum antibodies to an intercellular antigen of squamous epithelium, demonstrable by indirect immunofluorescence staining (p. 91), should greatly facilitate the precise diagnosis where histological methods fail (Fig. 25.16a).

Dermatitis herpetiformis. In this chronic condition the early lesion is a subepidermal vesicle (Fig. 25.14) which rapidly enlarges into a bulla.

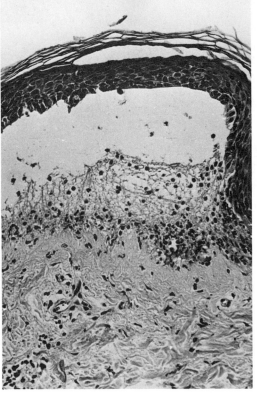

Fig. 25.14 Dermatitis herpetiformis. Subepidermal bulla containing fibrin and leukocytes. × 200.

leukocytic infiltration with a prominent eosinophil content. A useful diagnostic feature is the 'eosinophil abscesses'—oedematous dermal papillae packed with eosinophil leukocytes at the margins of the bullae (Fig. 25.15). These abscesses are not present in all cases but are diagnostic.

It has recently been established that some 60–70% of patients with dermatitis herpetiformis show an abnormality of their jejunal mucosa varying from partial to complete villous atrophy. The precise correlation between these intestinal changes and the skin lesions has not yet been established. Dermatitis herpetiformis is a chronic disorder which causes the patient considerable discomfort. Symptomatic relief can be obtained by administration of small doses of sulphapyridine.

A somewhat similar histological picture is seen in *bullous pemphigoid*; this has hitherto been regarded as a variant of dermatitis herpetiformis seen in the elderly, but the demon-

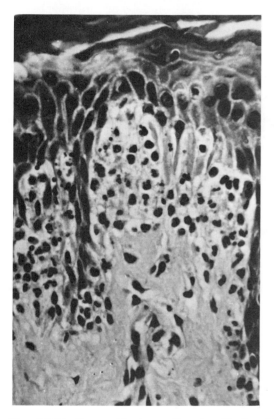

Fig. 25.15 Dermatitis herpetiformis. 'Eosinophil abscess' in an oedematous dermal papilla at the margin of a bulla. × 350.

stration of an antibody reacting with epidermal basement membrane in this condition indicates that it is a distinct entity.

Another condition, *benign mucous membrane pemphigoid*, may be related to bullous pemphigoid. It affects primarily the mucous membranes of the eye, oral cavity and genitalia, and can cause severe scarring of the conjunctiva with adhesions to the globe and eventual blindness. A few bullous skin lesions may occur but are rare. It differs from bullous pemphigoid in that only the direct immunofluorescence test is positive (see below).

Immunofluorescence in the diagnosis of skin disorders

In the **pemphigus group** of disorders, circulating antibodies to some constituent of the intercellular region of keratinocytes may be demonstrated in the serum of patients with active disease. Their titre fluctuates with the severity of the disease, and they may be used to monitor therapeutic response. These antibodies, bound with complement, may be demonstrated either by the direct immunofluorescence test (patient's

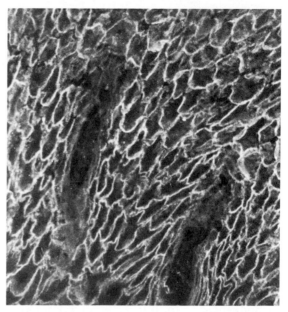

Fig. 25.16 a Pemphigus vulgaris. Intercellular immunofluorescence staining in squamous epithelium. Indirect immunofluorescence technique. × 300.

own skin and serum) or the indirect immunofluorescence test (patient's serum with epithelial substrate, either human vaginal mucosa or monkey oesophagus) (Fig. 25.16a). The antibodies are mainly of the IgG class.

In **dermatitis herpetiformis**, deposits of IgA are found in the dermal papilla adjacent to a blister, using the direct immunofluorescence test.

Patients with **bullous pemphigoid** also have circulating immunoglobulins which bind on to the basement membrane zone of stratified squamous epithelium and fix complement: they can be demonstrated as homogeneous linear deposits of predominantly IgG, by either the direct or indirect immunofluorescence test (Fig. 25.16b). In benign mucous membrane pemphigoid this can only be demonstrated by the direct immunofluorescence method.

Patients with **lupus erythematosus** also have circulating immunoglobulins, predominantly of

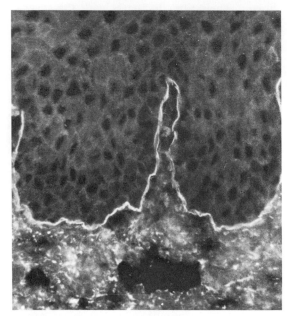

Fig. 25.16 b Bullous pemphigoid. Homogeneous linear immunofluorescence of basement membrane. Direct immunofluorescence technique. × 300.

the IgG class. In both types these can be demonstrated by the direct immunofluorescence test bound to the basement membrane region of diseased skin, together with complement, in the form of a granular linear deposit, thus differing from the homogeneous linear staining of the pemphigoid group. In systemic lupus erythematosus (see below) similar granular deposits can be demonstrated on the clinically normal skin, especially that exposed to light, thus distinguishing systemic lupus erythematosus from the chronic discoid type.

Erythema multiforme. This inflammatory disorder, as its name implies, presents a variety of clinical and histological appearances varying from a dermatitic reaction in the epidermis to subepidermal bullous formation and sometimes to an acute vasculitis. It represents a response in the skin of varying intensity to bacterial toxins and drug sensitivity. In the classical type, of moderate severity, the histological picture is

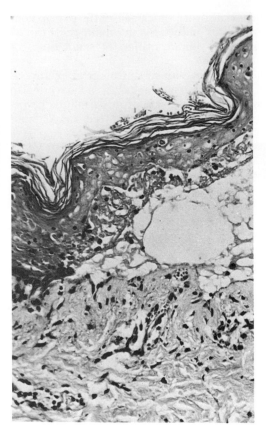

Fig. 25.17 Erythema multiforme. Subepidermal bulla roofed by infarcted epidermis. Regenerating epidermis can be seen at the left of the picture. × 200.

diagnostic and consists of an area of coagulative necrosis of the epidermis, in fact an area of infarction (Fig. 25.17).

Regeneration of the epidermis from the edge is rapid and a single layer of epithelial cells is often seen growing under the necrotic epidermis. The dermis is oedematous and there may be an acute necrotising vasculitis with haemorrhage. More often there is a fairly dense perivascular cellular infiltrate composed of neutrophils, eosinophils, histiocytes and lymphocytes.

The frank bullous forms may be indistinguishable from dermatitis herpetiformis although the eosinophil abscesses, if present, will clarify the diagnosis.

Scaling disorders

Psoriasis. This common, extremely chronic disorder, which is estimated to affect about 2%

of the population, has a characteristic histological picture (Fig. 25.18). There is parakeratosis, the extent and amount of which depends on the chronicity of the lesion. The granular layer is absent. The epidermis shows a peculiar type of acanthosis in which the rete ridges are

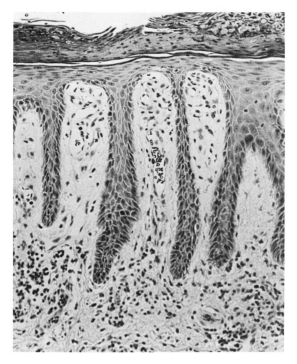

Fig. 25.18 Psoriasis. The surface is covered by a parakeratotic scale containing numerous polymorpho-nuclear leukocytes. The rete ridges are elongated and the suprapapillary epidermis is narrowed. × 150.

greatly elongated. The portions of the epidermis overlying the papillary bodies are, however, narrowed to two or three cells. The papillae are oedematous and broadened at their tips and contain dilated and rather rigid looking capillaries. It is these features which are responsible for the bleeding points which are so easily produced when the psoriasis lesion is scraped. As a rule inflammatory infiltration of the dermis is slight and composed of lymphocytes and macrophages. In early lesions collections of neutrophil leukocytes are found in or just below the parakeratotic stratum corneum (*Munro micro-abscesses*).

Lichen planus. While relatively uncommon this condition is of importance as it may affect mucous membranes and may be misdiagnosed as leukoplakia.

The papule of lichen planus has characteristic diagnostic features (Fig. 25.19). There is marked hyperkeratosis with focal increase in the granular layer. The epidermis is acanthotic

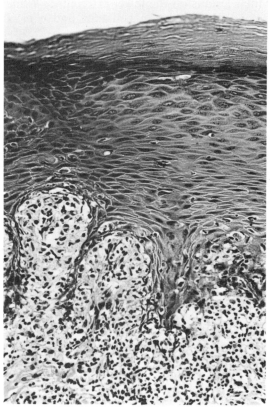

Fig. 25.19 Lichen planus. Note the hypertrophy of the granular layer and the saw-tooth appearance of the rete ridges. × 200.

and the rete ridges assume a pointed outline, giving a sawtooth appearance. There is a dense inflammatory infiltrate composed of lymphocytes with a few macrophages confined to the upper dermis. The upper border of this infiltrate is in contact with the epidermis and may actually invade the basal layers causing the dermo-epidermal junction to be indistinct. Lesions in the mucosa present a similar appearance although the hypertrophied granular layer is not so obvious. Normally there is no granular layer in some areas of mucous membranes.

Vascular Disorders

Erythema nodosum, nodular vasculitis and erythema induratum (Bazin's disease)

These three conditions are all characterised by nodular lesions on the lower extremities. While there are differences in aetiology and clinical course they cannot, in our experience, be clearly separated histologically and the appearances vary with the age of the lesion. The reason for their histological similarity is that they produce areas of inflammation and fat necrosis with subsequent repair. In the early stages there is an infiltrate of polymorphonuclear leukocytes and

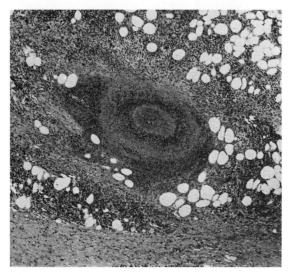

Fig. 25.20 Erythema nodosum. Thrombophlebitis of subcutaneous vein with surrounding inflammatory reaction in adipose tissue. × 30.

lymphocytes in the subcutaneous fat. Inflammatory infiltration of the walls of small veins is seen and in the more severe cases endothelial proliferation and thrombosis may occur. It seems probable that this phlebitis is the basic lesion (Fig. 25.20). As the nutrition of the fat is impaired, foci of epithelioid cells and giant cells appear in response to liberated fat. In severe cases necrosis resembling caseation is seen. These changes gradually resolve and at a later stage the process of healing is observed.

It will be appreciated that the extent of the histological changes will be dependent on the severity or acuteness of the condition. In erythema induratum the fat necrosis may be so extensive that the lesion ulcerates, discharging caseous material on the surface.

Cutaneous Angiitis—anaphylactoid (Henoch–Schönlein) purpura; necrotising or allergic vasculitis

Until recently it was customary to consider such disorders as anaphylactoid purpura and allergic vasculitis, etc., as separate entities. It is, however, now generally accepted that these are all variations on a single theme based on the deposition of immune complexes and complement in or around the vessel walls and the subsequent inflammatory reaction which ensues. The majority of the small dermal vessels involved in this process are venous channels and it therefore seems appropriate to use the term angiitis rather than the previously used term of arteritis.

Small areas of bleeding into the skin (purpura) may be seen in association with increased venous pressure (stasis) or in deficiency states such as scurvy. In such cases histological examination will show merely extravasation of red cells into the dermis with perhaps some swelling of the capillary endothelium. Later the red cells will disintegrate and collections of haemosiderin-laden macrophages will indicate the site of previous haemorrhage.

In true angiitis there are conspicuous changes both in the vessel wall and in the tissues surrounding the vessels. The cutaneous lesions of angiitis tend to occur in dependent parts of the body where there is some slowing of the venous return. The lower limbs are particularly affected where, in addition to a certain amount of slowing of the venous return due to the site, there is further slowing of the blood flow due to cooling which increases the viscosity. The combination of slowing of the circulation and increased viscosity is thought to favour the deposition of immune complexes which initiate the pathological changes. In the early stage of the process the deposition of immune complexes attracts neutrophil leukocytes in and around the walls of the small cutaneous vessels. Many of these neutrophils disintegrate, releasing proteolytic enzymes which further damage the vessel wall. At this stage the endothelium is swollen and there is dense perivascular polymorphonuclear leukocytic infiltration which invades the vessel wall. Much nuclear dust is seen from the disintegrating polymorphs and at

necrosis and becomes surrounded by a mixture of fibrin and polymorphonuclear leukocytes (Fig. 25.22)—*necrotising angiitis*. Despite the extensive involvement of these small cutaneous vessels, ulceration of the overlying epidermis occurs only rarely (*purpura necrotica*). This im-

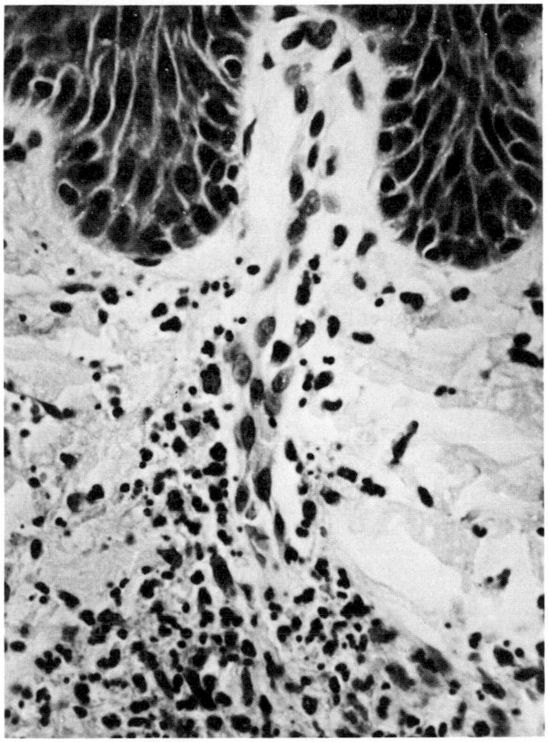

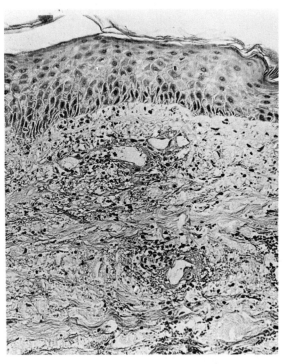

Fig. 25.21 Cutaneous angiitis. Small dermal vessel showing perivascular polymorphonuclear infiltration with invasion of the vessel wall. × 350.

Fig. 25.22 Cutaneous angiitis showing fibrinoid necrosis of dermal vessels. There is haemorrhage under the epidermis and a marked perivascular inflammatory infiltrate. × 200.

this stage the term *leukocytoclastic angiitis* is often used (Fig. 25.21). The damage to the vessel wall allows red cells to escape into the tissue (purpura) and there is more or less deposition of fibrin. The vessel wall finally undergoes

mune complex angiitis may be seen following acute bacterial infections, adverse reactions to drugs, as a manifestation of systemic lupus erythematosus and as a cutaneous manifestation of visceral malignancy.

Connective Tissue Diseases

Lupus erythematosus

Two basic types of this condition are recognised: (1) chronic discoid lupus erythematosus, which is confined to the skin, and (2) systemic lupus erythematosus, in which visceral lesions

predominate (see p. 877) and which may run its entire course without cutaneous manifestations. Intermediate forms between these extremes are encountered and transition from one type to another, although rare, may occur.

Chronic discoid lupus erythematosus. The

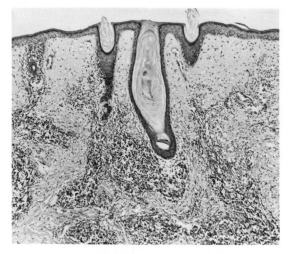

Fig. 25.23 Chronic discoid lupus erythematosus. Flattening of rete ridges, follicular plugging and focal lymphocytic infiltration of the dermis are seen. × 40.

histological changes are usually sufficiently characteristic to permit a firm histological diagnosis (Fig. 25.23). The epidermis is atrophic with loss of the rete ridges. There is moderate to severe hyperkeratosis which is most marked in

relation to the follicular orifices, resulting in dilated orifices filled by keratin (*follicular plugs*). The basal layer of the epidermis and/or the hair follicle epithelium shows degenerative changes causing vacuolation of the cells (*liquefaction degeneration*). This change is focal in nature and is always present (Fig. 25.24). A diagnosis of lupus erythematosus should not be made in its absence.

The dermis shows oedema and there is dense patchy lymphocytic infiltrate in relation to the dermal appendages, in particular to the hair follicles. Eventually dense fibrosis of the dermis occurs. In most cases the disease may be halted by the oral administration of anti-malarial drugs. If untreated, however, the fibrosis may cause considerable deformity such as severe ectropion. Patients with discoid lupus erythematosus should not be given drugs known to cause photosensitivity as these may precipitate the development of the systemic form of the disease.

Systemic lupus erythematosus. The histological appearances of the cutaneous lesions

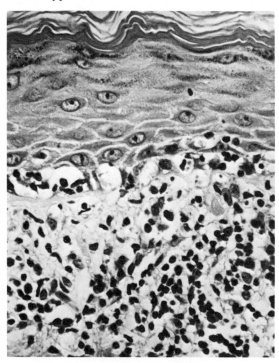

Fig. 25.24 Chronic discoid lupus erythematosus. Liquefaction degeneration of the basal layer of the epidermis. × 300.

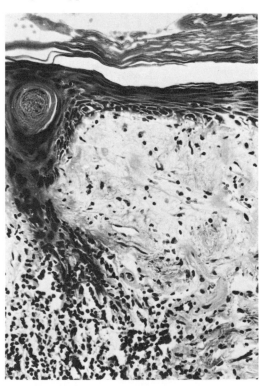

Fig. 25.25 Systemic lupus erythematosus. Liquefaction degeneration of the basal layer with oedema and fibrinoid change in the collagen of the upper dermis. × 200.

are not so striking as in the chronic variety. The epidermis is atrophic and liquefaction degeneration of the basal layer is marked (Fig. 25.25). Small areas of fibrinoid degeneration of the collagen of the upper dermis may be seen and this may also affect the ground substance of the collagenous tissue of the cutaneous vessels, giving an angiitis. Inflammatory infiltrate is minimal. In a proportion of cases, however, there are only mild inflammatory changes of a non-specific nature in the dermis.

It is not possible on histological grounds alone to separate chronic discoid lupus erythematosus from systemic lupus erythematosus, or even to separate these two conditions from certain stages in the evolution of lichen planus. For accurate diagnosis of lupus erythematosus and the separation of the discoid from the systemic type, immunofluorescent staining is extremely valuable (pp. 993–4).

Scleroderma

Much confusion has arisen over the nomenclature of this condition. As its name implies, it is a hardening of the skin and its use should be limited to the cutaneous disease. The condition with which it is confused is **progressive systemic sclerosis**, a generalised disease in which there is sclerosis of the skin of the extremities and which is dealt with on p. 878. The histological features of the skin in these two conditions are quite different.

Clinically scleroderma occurs as localised patches (**morphoea**) or diffuse areas of thickening and hardening of the skin. In the early stages an inflammatory halo is seen at the margin of the lesion. After spreading for an indefinite period, involution occurs with resulting atrophy and depigmentation of the area involved.

In the fully developed lesion (Fig. 25.26) the epidermis is thin and there is loss of the rete ridges due to stretching. The collagen bundles of the dermis are swollen and thickened and lie parallel to the epidermis. The distinction between the papillary and reticular layers of the dermis is lost. Sweat glands and hair follicles disappear but blood vessels remain intact. At the margin of an active lesion there is an inflammatory infiltrate in the dermis composed of lymphocytes and macrophages.

Sections from the sclerosed skin of an extremity in progressive systemic sclerosis show an entirely different picture (Fig. 25.27). Even

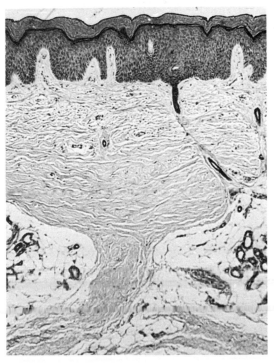

Fig. 25.27 Systemic sclerosis. The general micro-anatomy of the skin is maintained but the sweat glands and subcutaneous fat are much nearer the surface. Although from different regions of the skin, this figure and Fig. 25.26 are taken at the same magnification, illustrating the difference between systemic sclerosis and scleroderma. × 40.

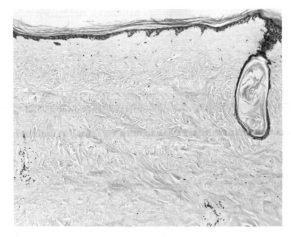

Fig. 25.26 Scleroderma. Note the flattening of the rete ridges and the increase in thickness of the dermal collagen. Dermal appendages are absent. × 40.

in advanced cases the micro-anatomy of the skin is normal with retention of all the dermal appendages. The entire skin has, however, shrunk so that the subcutaneous fat is much nearer the surface. If ulceration or infection supervenes, then some fibrosis will result.

Lymphomas

Lymphomas may involve, and sometimes apparently originate in, the skin. In general, the 'solid lymphomas', particularly those of T-cell origin (p. 523), tend to infiltrate the skin, much more commonly than the leukaemias. Involvement of the skin in Hodgkin's disease is rare. When present, the skin lesions show the histological structure of the parent condition. Pruritic eruptions occur in the leukaemias and Hodgkin's disease but the histological picture is that of a non-specific inflammatory reaction and is not diagnostic.

Mycosis fungoides is a malignant lymphoma peculiar to the skin which has certain clinical and histological characteristics. It has a prolonged course, being preceded for many years by various non-specific pruritic eruptions (premycotic phase) before the characteristic tumour stage is reached.

In the premycotic stage histological diagnosis may be difficult or impossible. The usual histological findings are those of a non-specific dermatitis but certain features should arouse suspicion and call for a repeat biopsy in three to six months' time. These include the presence, in the inflammatory infiltrate, of nuclear pyknosis (provided operative trauma can be excluded), a scattering of plasma cells, and occasionally an aberrant mitosis. Repeated biopsies may be necessary, however, before the diagnosis can be substantiated.

In the tumour stage the upper dermis is infiltrated by a pleomorphic infiltrate composed of macrophages, lymphocytes, reticulum cells, plasma cells and eosinophil leukocytes (Fig. 25.28). The tendency to nuclear pyknosis is more marked and mitotic figures, although not

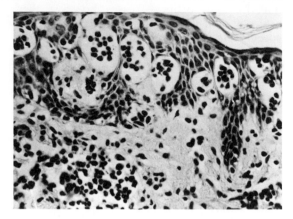

Fig. 25.28 Mycosis fungoides. Several Pautrier 'microabscesses' are seen in the epidermis. In the upper dermis there is a pleomorphic cellular infiltrate. × 265.

numerous, are seen. Of diagnostic importance are the collections of mononuclear cells in the epidermis (Pautrier's 'abscesses'). These are collections of tumour cells, apparently of T-cell nature, which have migrated into the epidermis. Such 'abscesses' are not seen in every case but should be looked for. While not diagnostic of mycosis fungoides (they can be seen in other malignant lymphoid neoplasms affecting the skin), they are of considerable help in differentiating chronic long-standing dermatitis from mycosis fungoides.

There is some confusion in the literature as to whether mycosis fungoides produces lesions in internal organs or not. Our experience is that it remains confined to the skin and that cases reported with visceral manifestations are other varieties of malignant lymphoma.

Tumours of the Skin

The skin is a large and complex organ, and it is directly exposed to many carcinogenic agents in the environment: it is therefore not surprising that tumours are numerous and varied. They are soon detected and easily removed, and the pathologist sees many small and early tumours which would escape attention at less accessible sites. Early diagnosis and relatively early treatment account in part at least for the fact that a much smaller proportion of malignant tumours cause death of the patient than in any other organ.

Skin tumours can be classified readily according to the tissue of origin. Epithelial tumours may arise from the epidermis, the sweat gland or the hair follicle: dermal tumours may arise from the fibrous, vascular, nervous or lympho-reticular elements: and a third

from the surface epidermis, the *squamous group* and the so-called *basal-cell group* which includes rodent ulcer and basal cell papilloma (verruca senilis). Tumours of the sweat glands form a heterogeneous group and are discussed later.

Basal-cell papilloma (verruca senilis) is a fairly common warty growth seen most often on the trunk of older people. It produces a flattened papilloma consisting chiefly of basal-like cells, with relatively little differentiation into keratinocytes unless irritated: keratin is however formed,

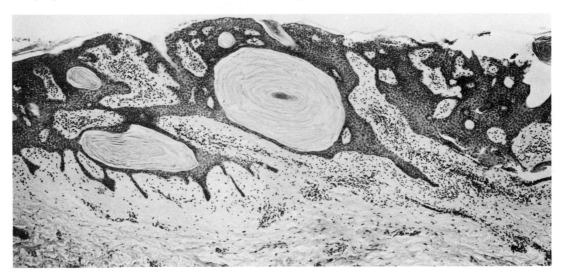

Fig. 25.29 Basal cell papilloma. A flat papillary tumour composed of basal-like epidermal cells. Note the several 'pearls' of keratin formation within the epithelium. × 50.

group arises from melanocytes. Some of the most important tumours, such as squamous carcinoma, have been dealt with already in Chapter 11 as local representatives of more general types, but many are peculiar to the skin.

Epidermal tumours

Embryological studies have revealed that the keratinocytes of the skin undergo specific differentiation at an early stage in development; three distinct cell lines are produced relating to the surface epidermis, the pilo-sebaceous complexes and the sweat apparatus. This probably explains the differing biological behaviour of tumours arising from the epidermis.

Two sharply distinct types of tumour arise

often in fairly large amounts, characteristically in spherical masses (horn cysts) within the epithelium and sometimes reaching the surface (Fig. 25.29). Melanocytes are usually present among the basal-like cells and melanin is often abundant. This may give rise to diagnostic confusion with malignant melanoma. Mitoses are usually absent, growth is slow and malignancy so rare that cases can mostly be explained as coincidences or mistaken diagnoses. The name **seborrhoeic keratosis**, sometimes applied to these tumours, indicates their common occurrence on so-called seborrhoeic sites (forehead, chest and back).

'Squamous' group

These tumours consist of stratified squamous epithelium, and their mode of growth is clearly based on the ordinary process of growth of the epidermis. Normally multiplication occurs in the relatively undifferentiated basal cells, and differentiation occurs through keratinocytes to keratin. In the benign tumours, the undifferentiated basal layer is only one cell thick, and the the aetiology is known, such terms as *actinic* or *arsenical keratoses* are commonly used, and in old people they may be called *senile keratoses*, but the lesions are identical. They are typically dry, rough-surfaced thickenings, arising usually in an area of skin which shows, by its thinness

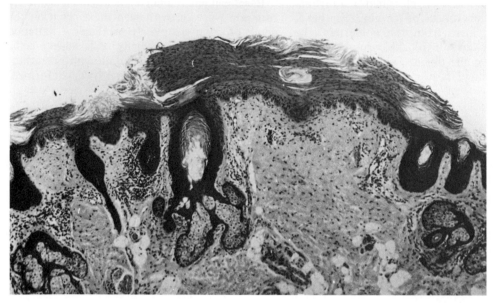

Fig. 25.30   Actinic keratosis, showing a patch of epithelial atrophy with dysplasia, hyperkeratosis and parakeratosis.   × 25.

differentiated cells and the keratin more conspicuous than in normal skin, but with increasing malignancy the undifferentiated cells become more numerous and keratin and keratinocytes diminish, though in skin tumours they hardly ever disappear altogether.

Squamous papilloma is the benign member of this group. It has already been mentioned in Chapter 11 and earlier in this chapter. Most are viral in origin, and seen usually on the hands of children (**juvenile warts**), on the soles of the feet of those who use communal changing-rooms (**plantar warts**), and about the genitalia of those exposed to venereal infection (**condyloma acuminata**). If one excludes viral tumours, and the keratoses dealt with in the next section, the squamous papillomas (Fig. 11.1, p. 273) are probably very rare. Malignant change in a skin papilloma is extremely rare, though occasionally genital tumours show an exuberant growth hard to distinguish from malignancy.

Squamous keratosis. This is the best name for the premalignant lesions of this group. When

(Fig. 25.30), inelasticity and irregular pigmentation, the effects of prolonged exposure to sunlight or other carcinogens: the face and the back of the hands are the usual sites.

Histologically one sees all stages from the slightest thickening and irregularity of the epidermis to large lesions with gross irregular hyperplasia of the epithelium, a massive overlying layer of keratin, and greatly enlarged rete ridges apparently on the brink of invasion. The hallmark of these lesions is the presence of alternating columns of hyperkeratosis and parakeratosis. Nuclear pleomorphism, frequency of mitoses and cellular de-differentiation usually increase in parallel with the above changes. Sometimes, severe cytological changes occur in the presence of relatively minor general hyperplasia, and the term *carcinoma-in-situ* of the skin might reasonably include this condition.

Bowen's disease. This, though also an epidermal hyperplasia which may progress to squamous carcinoma, is a very different lesion.

It may arise anywhere in the skin, but nearly always in non-exposed areas. While the keratosis blends into surrounding skin, which is itself abnormal, Bowen's disease is sharply circumscribed from normal skin forming rounded, reddish patches which spread slowly over a period of years. The epidermis in the affected area shows marked hyperplasia, with deep but fairly

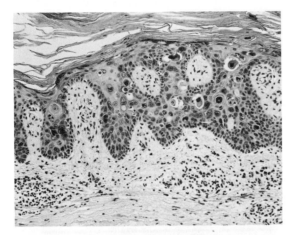

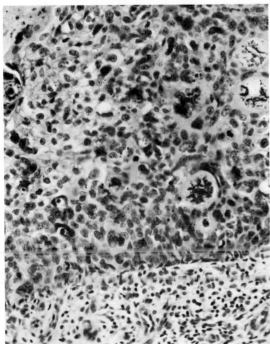

Fig. 25.31 Bowen's disease of the skin. *Above*, showing the large, abnormal cells in the epidermis. × 60. *Below*, showing more cellular detail, including enlarged and clumped nuclei and aberrant mitoses. × 160.

regular rete ridges and usually not much keratin: cellular de-differentiation is prominent, and large cells with multiple large clumped nuclei are a characteristic feature (Fig. 25.31). The importance of recognising Bowen's disease, which is another form of carcinoma-in-situ, is twofold. First, it may look like (and is often treated for years as) a patch of psoriasis or other chronic skin disease. Secondly, a degree of de-differentiation of the epidermis which in a squamous keratosis showing carcinoma-in-situ would mean imminent invasion, in Bowen's disease is compatible with many years of continued limitation to the surface—even though ultimate invasion is usual.

Squamous carcinoma. The description of squamous carcinoma in general in Chapter 11, and the many observations on its aetiology in Chapter 10, make it unnecessary to say much of this important tumour of the skin here. The great majority are better differentiated than the average mucosal squamous carcinoma: this, combined with accessibility, makes for a relatively good prognosis. Dissemination, when it does occur, is by the same routes of local, lymph and blood spread as with other carcinomas. It may arise anywhere on the body surface, but in most countries the face (including the ears) and the backs of the hands are the commonest sites. The muco-cutaneous junctions are also important sites, but the bulk of these arise on the mucosal side of the junction: thus, most lip tumours arise from the red margin, most anal tumours within the canal, and most penile tumours from the glans; however, though some vulvar tumours arise from the modified skin of the labia minora, the majority appear in the true skin of the labia majora.

The tumours of the exposed surfaces presumably arise chiefly from the effect of ultraviolet light in sunlight. Industrial exposure usually produces tumours of the hands and fore arms, but with carcinogens which penetrate the clothes, such as the lighter mineral oils and dusts like soot (Fig. 10.3, p. 255) and powdered arsenic, the scrotum becomes an important site, probably because its rugose surface traps dirt. Some carcinomas may result from prolonged contact with decomposing desquamated keratin: this is suggested by the occurrence of 'dhoti cancer' under the waistbands of Indians living under poor sanitary conditions, and by the fact that early circumcision seems to prevent carcinoma of the glans penis. The relation of circumcision to cancer is a particularly interesting one. Among the Jews who circumcise at birth, cancer of the penis is all but unknown. Among Moslems, who circumcise at puberty, it is rare; but the occasional cases suggest that even before puberty some irreversible change may be induced—a fact that recalls the induction process in experiments on co-carcinogenesis. The majority of penile cancers are associated with an intact foreskin and a low standard of personal hygiene.

There is a small but clinically important group of squamous carcinomas which arise in the edges of long-standing ulcers (the so-called· *Marjolin's ulcer*) and in sinuses, presumably as a result of hyperplasia following prolonged attempts at healing.

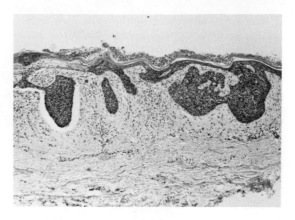

Fig. 25.32 Rodent ulcer. Showing the apparently multicentric origin from the base of the epidermis. × 32.

Rodent ulcer (basal-cell carcinoma)

The typical rodent ulcer begins as a slow-growing, flattened nodule of the skin of the face. The centre breaks down, forming a shallow ulcer, but the periphery of the nodule persists to form a smooth, slightly raised margin to the ulcer which, as the latter spreads, becomes the characteristic rolled edge. If not successfully treated, the ulcer spreads slowly, and ultimately bites deeper and destroys the underlying structures of the face. Death results, if at all (for nowadays treatment is rarely so unsuccessful), from destruction of mouth and nose, or from invasion of the cranial cavity, most often via the orbit.

Neither lymph spread nor blood spread is seen except as the greatest of rarities. This is the only common malignant tumour other than those within the cranial cavity (where conditions are exceptional) which shows this extreme disinclination to metastasise, a finding that remains entirely unexplained.

Histologically, the tumour begins with groups of small, dark, basal-like cells, apparently sprouting from the undersurface of intact epidermis (Fig. 25.32). These cell groups enlarge and grow down into the dermis, forming clumps with an outer layer of columnar cells which resemble the basal layer of the epidermis. Instead, however, of the keratinocytes which one would expect to see arising from this basal layer, the centre of each clump is occupied by a solid mass of darkly-staining spheroidal cells (Fig. 25.33). The term basal-cell carcinoma

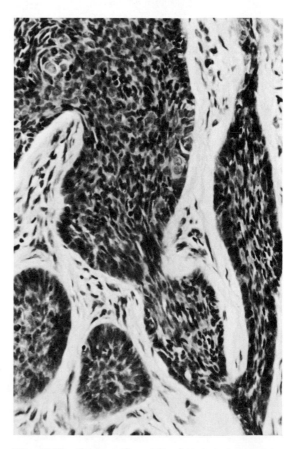

Fig. 25.33 Rodent ulcer. The dermis is invaded by clumps of small, darkly-stained tumour cells resembling basal epidermal cells. The cells at the margin of some of the clumps present a palisaded appearance. × 250.

indicates the similarity of the tumour cells to the basal cell layer of the surface epithelium, but should not be taken to imply that they originate from the basal layer of the surface epidermis.

Continued proliferation of the cell masses beneath the epidermis gives rise to a nodule: breakdown of the overlying epidermis gives rise to the ulcer (Fig. 25.34). The characteristic rolled border is due to lateral invasion of the tumour under the intact epidermis.

tumours consisting of relatively narrow burrowing columns of cells of uniform pattern. Little attention should be paid to the number of mitoses, which can be surprisingly numerous even in slow-growing examples. One variety meriting special mention is the sclerotic type, in which the normal stromal component of the tumour is excessively developed and small thin strands of epithelium are buried in a dense fibrous stroma: this results in the edge being ill-defined and may lead to inadequate excision or irradiation.

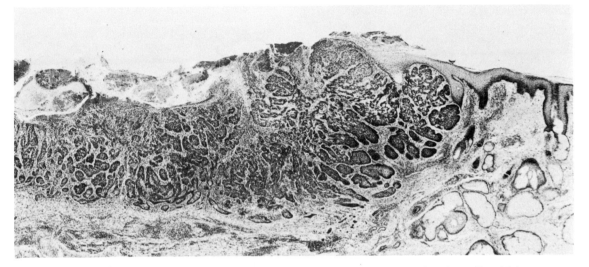

Fig. 25.34 Rodent ulcer, showing the flat, shallow ulceration. Note the extension laterally which accounts for the 'rolled' border. × 24.

The detailed histology of these tumours varies considerably, but the well-defined single peripheral columnar layer ('palisading'—one of several different uses of this word in pathology), and the predominance of 'basal' cells, are constant. The cell masses may be large and uniform, or narrow and ribbon-like. Small patches of squamous differentiation or even keratinisation may cause confusion with squamous carcinoma if one is not aware of their frequency in rodent ulcers. Small cystic spaces form at times, some genuine, some the result of stromal degeneration. Inclusion of a few melanocytes from the original epidermis is common, and rarely so much melanin may be formed that clinical confusion with melanoma may occur.

On the whole, the more complex the histology of the individual tumour, the less malignant; recurrence occurs most often with

Sites. Though they can be found anywhere on the skin (except the palms and soles) the majority of rodent ulcers occur in a relatively restricted area of the face, in front of the ears, above the mouth and below the supra-orbital ridges. In this area, sunlight produces far more rodent ulcers than squamous carcinomas (in some parts of Australia it is the exception for a fair-skinned man to reach the age of 75 without having had at least one rodent ulcer on the face): elsewhere the reverse holds, and a radiation-induced rodent ulcer of the trunk, for instance, or one arising in the margin of a varicose ulcer of the skin is much less often seen than the corresponding squamous carcinoma. However, deep x-ray therapy, for example for ankylosing spondylitis, is sometimes followed many years later by a crop of rodent ulcers distant from the field of irradiation.

Tumours of sweat glands (hidradenomas)

These form a distinct group of varied and often bizarre histological appearances but characteristically they exhibit a two-layered epithelium and show evidence of mucin secretion. Arising from the **eccrine sweat glands** are three main types: (1) from the intra-epidermal portion of the sweat duct, the *eccrine poroma*; (2) from the intradermal portion of the sweat duct, (*a*) the *nodular* and (*b*) the *tubular hidradenoma*. The former is illustrated in Fig. 25.35a and consists

Tumours of pilo-sebaceous follicles

True tumours are even less common than in the sweat glands. True sebaceous adenomas are very rare: the 'tumours' of tuberous sclerosis (p. 722) are fibrous nodules, and 'seborrhoeic keratosis' is a misnomer for the basal cell papilloma. An uncommon tumour which probably arises in the hair matrix is the so-called '*benign calcifying epithelioma*' of Malherbe (pilomatricoma). These form rounded masses lying under the skin, arising anywhere on the body

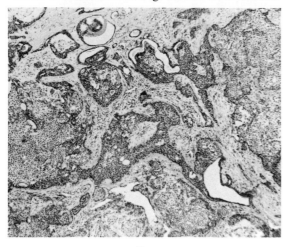
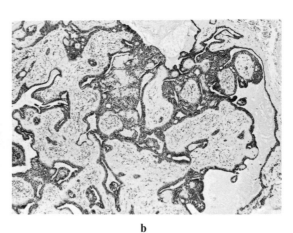

a

b

Fig. 25.35 Hidradenomas of intradermal sweat duct origin. **a.** Nodular hidradenoma, consisting of solid masses of pale-staining cells with occasional duct-like structures (which contain PAS-positive material). **b.** Tubular hidradenoma, showing the typical branching duct-like structures lined by two-layered epithelium and embedded in a hyaline stroma. × 30.

of solid masses and cords of cells containing an occasional duct-like structure which contains mucin. The latter is illustrated in Fig. 25.35b and consists of branching duct-like structures lined by a double layer of epithelium and containing mucin embedded in a prominent fibrous stroma. This type, which bears a resemblance to the pleomorphic salivary adenoma, is sometimes called a mixed tumour of skin; (3) arising from the secretory coils, the *eccrine spiradenoma*. The majority of eccrine sweat gland tumours are benign although nodular hidradenomas may exhibit local invasion and recurrence after removal. True metastasising sweat gland tumours (hidradenocarcinomas) are rare. The **apocrine sweat glands** may also give rise to tumours, the commonest being the benign *apocrine adenoma* of the vulva, the *hidradenoma papilliferum* and the *cylindroma* or turban tumour of the scalp.

surface and at any age, and growing slowly. In spite of the name, only about a quarter show calcification, though when present it may be extensive and spectacular, true bone being sometimes present. The epithelium of the tumours consists of small dark-staining regular cells, which form disproportionately large masses of keratin in which ghosts of the cells that have formed it can often be seen. Foreign body giant cell reaction to the keratin is frequent, and calcification when present seems to be a sequel of this reaction, though sometimes a curious direct calcification of ghost-cell areas of keratin seems to occur.

Molluscum sebaceum (kerato-acanthoma). This tumour-like but self-healing lesion is much commoner than any of the true hair follicle tumours. It occurs predominantly on the face of adults. A nodule in the skin appears and grows rapidly for about eight weeks, forming finally a rounded, slightly umbilicated mass, 10–20 mm in diameter (Fig. 25.36). It stops growing, the central dimple enlarging and becoming dry and scaly, then the central plug is discharged and the lesion heals: the whole process usually takes about six months.

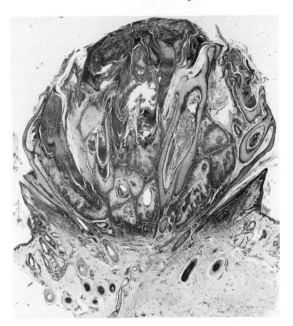

Fig. 25.37 Molluscum sebaceum. A lesion about the same age as Fig. 25.36. Note the resemblance to squamous carcinoma. × 12.

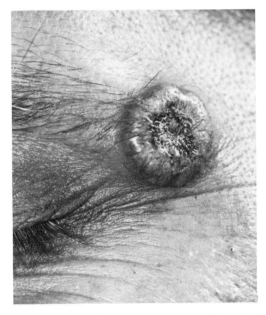

Fig. 25.36 Molluscum sebaceum. Clinical photograph of an eight-week-old lesion near the eye. A firm rounded nodule with epidermis stretched over the edge, and a central crater where the keratin core is exposed. × 1·5.

Histologically, the resemblance to squamous carcinoma is very close during the active phase, so much so that it was only after 1950 that it won general recognition as a distinct lesion that did not require to be treated as a carcinoma. The appearances which mimic invasion are however the result of rapid irregular overgrowth of a group of hair follicles (Fig. 25.37). During the stationary phase, the epithelium so formed is progressively keratinised, and the resulting mass of keratin is finally discharged. The whole appears to be a distortion of the normal cyclical process of growth and regression in the hair follicle: in rabbits, similar lesions can be produced by painting with a carcinogen at the right phase of the hair growth cycle. Recognition of this lesion is obviously of great importance in treatment. However, it is not always possible to differentiate it from squamous carcinoma, even after very careful correlation of the clinical and histological findings.

Self-healing squamous-cell carcinoma of the skin. This is a rare familial disorder, first described by Shaw Dunn and Ferguson Smith. It begins usually in early adult life, and is characterised by the appearance at intervals of tumours of the skin, mostly, but not exclusively, of the exposed parts, which are indistinguishable histologically from squamous-cell carcinomas. After some months of activity, each lesion in succession undergoes involution by keratinisation of the infiltrating columns of cells and discharge of the dead cells leaving shallow depressed pits. We have had the opportunity of studying several such cases and confirm the view of Currie and Ferguson Smith that they are indistinguishable from the ordinary solitary squamous carcinoma until regression sets in. The age and history are therefore very important. It is quite unrelated to molluscum sebaceum.

Melanocytic tumours

The following account attempts to give a clear if somewhat oversimplified explanation of a complex series of phenomena, interpretation of which is still controversial.

Early in fetal life specialised cells migrate from the neural crest to the skin, uveal tract of the eye and the leptomeninges and settle in these sites where they are known as melanocytes. It is in these sites that later in development or in childhood or adult life they may give rise to benign or malignant tumours. Those unit area of skin is constant irrespective of race or skin colouration.

Occasionally some melanocytes fail to reach the epidermis, developing within the dermis to form a Mongolian spot or a more compact mass termed a blue naevus (p. 1014).

In nearly every child at a few or many points the balance between the normal ratio of melanocytes to basal epidermal cells breaks down: the

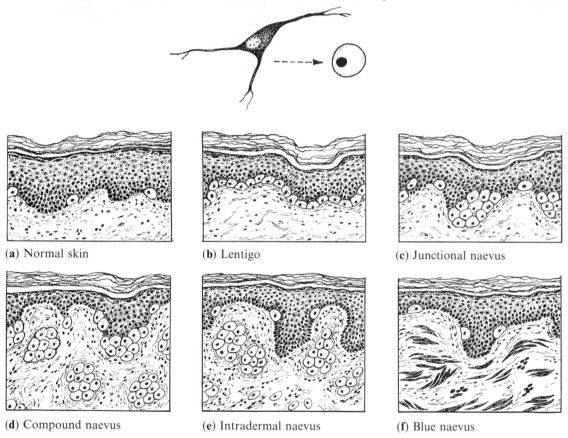

(a) Normal skin   (b) Lentigo   (c) Junctional naevus

(d) Compound naevus   (e) Intradermal naevus   (f) Blue naevus

Fig. 25.38 Diagram of the origin and evolution of the pigmented naevus. At the top of the diagram the dendritic melanocyte, the cell of origin, is seen. Stained by the DOPA reaction, this has a triangular body with long branching processes (dendrites). In fixed tissue sections this cells appears rounded with clear cytoplasm. The distribution of melanocytes in normal skin is seen in (**a**). Replacement of the basal layer of the epidermis by melanocytes is the **lentigo** (**b**). Focal proliferation of melanocytes is the **junctional pigmented naevus** (**c**), and this proliferation at the dermo-epidermal junction is called **junctional change**. Some of these nodules descend into the dermis to become adult naevus cells and the combination of junctional change and intradermal naevus cells is the **compound pigmented naevus** (**d**). Junctional activity ceases and masses of mature naevus cells lie in the dermis, the **intradermal naevus** (**e**). Occasionally melanocytes en route from the neural crest may be arrested in the dermis where they form the **Mongolian spot or blue naevus** (**f**).

melanocytes which migrate to the skin come to lie among the basal cells of the epidermis in the ratio of $1:10$ or $1:5$, depending on the anatomical site. The number of melanocytes per melanocytes multiply too rapidly and become too numerous to be accommodated in their normal position. The lesions resulting from this proliferation of melanocytes are known as pigmented naevi. While precise details of the evolution of these lesions is not known, the probable course is shown in diagrammatic form in Fig. 25.38.

Initially the proliferating melanocytes replace the basal layer of the epidermis over a given area and at this stage the lesion is known as a lentigo (Fig. 25.38b). (This should not be confused with an ephilis or freckle, which terms refer to an increase in melanin pigmentation of the basal layer without an increase in the numbers of melanocytes.) The next stage is more focal proliferation of the melanocytes and the formation of small nodules within the epidermis which bulge downwards towards the dermis: this lesion is known as the junctional naevus (Fig. 25.38c). Eventually the basement membrane is disrupted and some of the nodules or packets of melanocytes pass down into the dermis. At this stage where there is a combination of junctional activity and nests of melanocytes in the dermis, the lesion is known as a compound pigmented naevus (Fig. 25.38d). The melanocytes which reach the dermis soon lose their melanin-synthesising enzymes, become smaller and lose the power to proliferate and are known as naevus cells. At or around puberty, in the

represent the normal evolution of these lesions it should be emphasised that maturation may be arrested at any of the stages described. In addition, similar stages of melanocytic proliferation may occur in adult life, either after exposure to ultraviolet light or from as yet imperfectly understood hormonal changes.

The principal types of pigmented naevus are described below. There are extremely common lesions, few people having none at all and some having large numbers: the mean number per person is said to be 18.

Lentigo. Clinically these present as flat blemishes on any part of the skin surface. They vary in colour from pale brown to deep black. It is not possible to distinguish them with any certainty from junctional naevi. Histologically one sees stretches of the basal layer of the epidermis replaced by melanocytes, which appear in fixed tissue sections as rounded cells with abundant clear cytoplasm. Many of the melanocytes contain varying amounts of fine granular brown melanin pigment. In the underlying dermis, macrophages containing coarser granules of darker melanin pigment are usually seen.

In older persons, on sun-exposed skin, a vari-

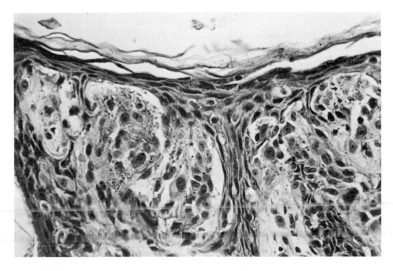

Fig. 25.39 Junctional pigmented naevus. Note the groups of melanocytes lying in the deeper part of the epidermis. × 200.

majority of instances junctional activity ceases, the naevus cells in the dermis undergo further maturation and a certain amount of fibrosis occurs. At this stage the lesion is known as an intradermal naevus and may remain as such for life. (Fig. 25.38e)

While the above account is thought to

ant of the lentigo, the *lentigo maligna*, may be encountered (p. 1013).

Junctional pigmented naevus. As already stated, the clinical appearance of the junctional naevus is virtually indistinguishable from the lentigo. In older lesions, examined with a lens in a good light, small areas of darker speckled pigmentation, corresponding to the nests of junctional activity, can be detected.

Histologically the junctional naevus is composed of rounded aggregates (or packets) of melanocytes which, while occurring at any level

(Fig. 25.40). The cells are often called naevus cells but in order to avoid confusion with other naevi (e.g. angiomas) they should always be referred to as pigmented naevus cells. In the connective tissue of the dermis between the

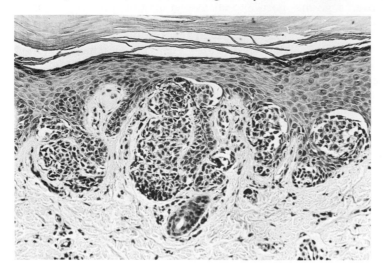

Fig. 25.40 Compound pigmented naevus. Some groups of proliferated melanocytes lie in the deeper part of the epidermis. Other groups have become separated from the epidermis and lie in the superficial dermis. × 100.

of the epidermis, tend to be in the lower layers and bulge down into the underlying dermis, giving the undersurface of the epidermis an irregular configuration (Fig. 25.39). It is this proliferation of melanocytes at the dermo-epidermal junction which gives the junctional naevus its name.

Compound pigmented naevus. This is the commonest type of pigmented naevus in late childhood. Clinically such lesions are usually raised above the surface: they may be papillomatous in appearance and vary in colour from pale brown to black. In some instances there is also an abnormality in the hair follicles, these being increased in number and abnormally large. In such cases variable amounts of coarse dark hair can be seen growing from the surface of the lesion. In rare instances such hairy pigmented naevi may cover an extensive area of the skin surface (giant hairy naevus). Such cases may also be associated with diffuse meningeal melanomatosis and can undergo malignant transformation in childhood (see below).

Histologically compound naevi show junctional activity in the overlying epidermis. In the dermis are loose aggregates of rounded inactive-looking cells, some of which contain granules of melanin pigment. The deeper these cells lie in the dermis, the smaller they tend to be

nests of pigmented naevus cells are found varying numbers of macrophages containing coarser granules of melanin pigment. The gross colour of pigmented naevi depends largely on the numbers and content of these macrophages.

Juvenile melanoma. This variant of the compound pigmented naevus is important because it may easily be mistaken histologically for a malignant melanoma, especially if the age of the patient is not known. They are commonest

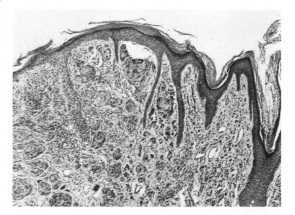

Fig. 25.41 Juvenile melanoma, showing junctional activity and extensive dermal infiltration. Note also the pseudo-epitheliomatous hyperplasia and dilated vascular channels. × 30.

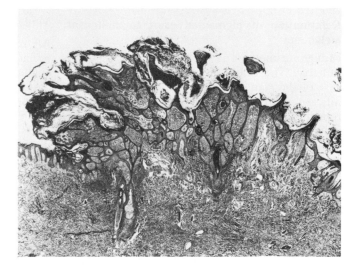

Fig. 25.42 Intradermal pigmented naevus of warty type. The dermal papillae are filled with naevus cells which extend widely in the underlying dermis. × 14.

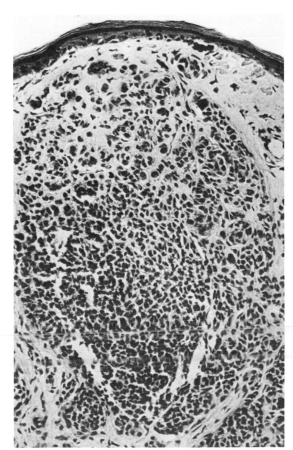

Fig. 25.43 Section through an intradermal naevus, showing collections of so-called 'naevus cells' underneath the epithelium. × 220.

in children although no age group is exempt. There is very extensive, active-looking junctional activity which may be spindle cell in type. This is associated with a more prominent intradermal component which may again contain many active-looking spindle cells. Associated histological features which are of considerable importance for diagnosis are pseudo-epitheliomatous hyperplasia and the presence of numerous large dilated vascular channels (Fig. 25.41). It is this latter feature which accounts for the reddish colour of these lesions to the naked eye.

Intradermal pigmented naevus. The vast majority of pigmented naevi in adults are of the intradermal type. Clinically these are similar in appearance to compound pigmented naevi, being sometimes raised and warty (Fig. 25.42), sometimes flat. Histologically there is no junctional activity in the epidermis although there may be an increase in the number of normal-looking melanocytes. The dermis is occupied by cells similar to those seen in the dermal component of the compound naevus (Fig. 25.43). In older lesions, particularly in the deeper parts, there is often considerable fibrosis and some of the nests of pigmented naevus cells merge imperceptibly into bundles of elongated cells which bear a close resemblance to neurolemmal cells or sensory nerve endings, both of which, like melanocytes, are of neural crest origin. Such appearances are of no practical significance.

Relationship of pigmented naevi to malignant melanoma

Malignant melanoma is exceedingly rare before puberty. The main exception to this is in the case of the giant hairy pigmented naevus, a significant number of cases of which have been reported where death resulted either from metastases from the skin or from diffuse meningeal melanomatosis.

After puberty any pigmented naevus with junctional activity has the potential to undergo malignant change. The proportion of lesions which undergo such change must be extremely small as melanocarcinoma is not a common tumour. Junctional pigmented naevi in certain sites appear to have a higher incidence of malignant change, these being the palms of the hands, soles of the feet and around the genitalia.

The question of prophylactic excision of pigmented naevi is an extremely difficult one as it

Malignant melanoma

All malignant melanomas of the skin are associated with junctional change in the overlying epidermis, although in ulcerated lesions this may be impossible to demonstrate. While the importance of a pre-existing lentigo, junctional naevus, or compound naevus has already been stressed, it should be remembered that any of these lesions with junctional activity can arise in adult life. The crucial event is the invasion of the dermis by pigmented tumour cells streaming down from the junctional nests (Fig. 25.44). Clinically there may be more rapid growth, increase or decrease in pigmentation and sometimes itching or pain, often followed soon by ulceration and bleeding. It should be emphasised, however, that clinical diagnosis of malignant melanoma at the early stage when they can best be treated is often very difficult. An adequate excision biopsy—that is to say excision of the whole lesion with a margin of

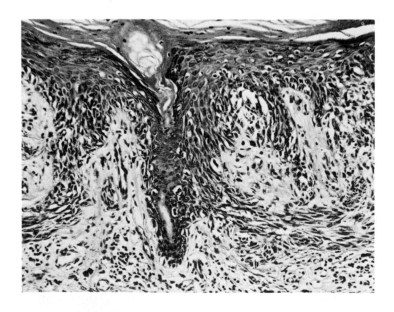

Fig. 25.44 Malignant melanoma. There is junctional change, and the melanoma cells, which in this example are spindle shaped, have streamed into the dermis. Note also the numerous aberrant melanocytes with clear cytoplasm lying singly at various levels in the epidermis. × 100.

would obviously be impossible to excise all such lesions. In the adult, new lesions on the palms, soles and genitalia should be excised. Any pre-existing naevus which is subjected to repeated trauma, e.g. shaving, or friction from clothing, or which changes in colour, bleeds, loses its hair or develops an abnormal sensation such as itching, should be excised completely.

3 mm on all sides—is essential in all cases in which there is any suspicion of this diagnosis: cutting into the tumour as in an ordinary biopsy may aid dissemination.

Microscopically, apart from the highly characteristic epidermal origin, malignant melanomas present a variable and not always characteristic pattern. The presence of melanin may make diagnosis easy, but it may be scanty and hard to see. It may even be totally absent from the area examined, or occasionally absent from all the tumour cells—'amelanotic melanoma'. One must beware also of assuming that brown pigment in a tumour automatically means a melanoma: even if the pigment is melanin one may be dealing with a pigmented epithelial tumour or a blue naevus (see below) or, in the case of apparent metastasis to a lymph node, with melanin drained into the node in the course of a skin disease (*lipo-melanic reticulosis*). The haemosiderin in a very cellular sclerosing angioma has sometimes led to a hasty misdiagnosis of melanoma.

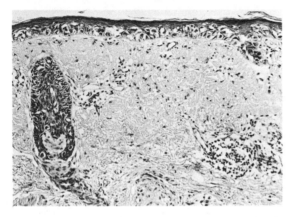

Fig. 25.45 Lentigo maligna. Melanocytes of variable appearance form a continuous deep layer in the epithelium and are seen also in the piloscbaceous unit. The dermis shows pronounced solar elastosis. × 30.

The actual tumour cells vary considerably. They may be spindle-shaped, imitating a cellular fibrosarcoma, but most often they are spheroidal, fairly large, with abundant solid cytoplasm in which there may be a fine dusting of melanin. These cells form clumps such as are seen in carcinoma, but less compact and continuous, and never with any trace of gland formation or squamous differentiation. Cells containing coarse granules of melanin arc usually phagocytes, and their presence should raise the suspicion of melanoma in the adjacent tissue.

Lentigo maligna is the name given to a slowly enlarging flat brown lesion seen on the sun-exposed skin of the older age groups. After many years one or more nodules, usually more heavily pigmented, may appear. Histologically lentigo maligna is essentially similar to the benign lentigo already described except that the melanocytes show variations in size, alterations in nuclear-cytoplasmic ratio, nuclear hyperchromatism and loss of polarity (Fig. 25.45). Eventually all layers of the epidermis may be replaced by aberrant melanocytes and invasive melanocarcinoma develops. This type of melanocarcinoma has a relatively good prognosis and rarely metastasises.

Site and aetiology. Melanomas may occur anywhere in the skin surface, but they have a higher incidence per unit area in the face, the genitalia and the feet than elsewhere. In general, they are less common in dark-skinned races, but in them are particularly often found in the feet. Any carcinogenic agent that increases the incidence of other skin tumours (sunlight in the fair-skinned, x-rays, tar) also increases the incidence of melanomas: of the tumours resulting from these agents, only a small proportion are melanomas, but they have, of course, a disproportionate effect on the mortality.

Metastasis. While *local spread* may include deep invasion, there is a special tendency to superficial spread in the skin itself, producing satellite nodules. This may be the result of spread in dermal lymphatics, but there is sometimes seen a curious intra-epidermal migration of tumour cells similar to that in Paget's disease of the nipple (p. 937). The first distant metastases usually appear in the local *lymph nodes*. Blood spread may be long delayed, but when it occurs is often rapid and extensive, with the spectacular black (or mixed black and white) metastases appearing in large numbers in a short time in many organs.

Prognosis. Malignant melanoma is the most malignant of the skin tumours. It has a curiously sinister reputation, but if properly treated before the appearance of metastases, more than half of all cases are cured. The very long delay that often occurs between excision of the primary melanoma and the appearance of metastases makes exact figures difficult to arrive at. Prognosis is better in females, especially if young, than in males. An attempt has been made in recent years to evaluate the prognosis of melanocarcinoma based on the site of the initial lesion, the depth in the dermis to which the invasion penetrates and the host response as evidenced by the inflammatory reaction at the base of the tumour. Thus a **superficial spreading**

type is described which clinically occurs on light-exposed areas of skin as a flat expanding lesion. A **nodular type** which is found on covered parts of the body presents as a nodular, deeply infiltrated lesion. Histologically in the superficial spreading type one sees invasion of the papillary dermis, lateral spread under the intact normal skin, and a variable amount of lymphocytic and histiocytic infiltration at the base of the tumour. In the nodular type there is invasion down to and including subcutaneous fat and often little or no inflammatory reaction. Unless many areas of the tumour are examined it is impossible to be certain of the precise degree of dermal invasion. On the basis of population statistics it is suggested that the superficial spreading type carries a better prognosis than the nodular type, but so far this has not been of great value in assessing individual cases. In some cases specific antibodies against the surface membrane of tumour cells can be detected but to date there is no clear evidence to suggest that this materially alters the prognosis.

Blue naevus or 'melanophoroma'

In these lesions there are accumulations of deeply pigmented cells in the dermis. (Fig. 25.38f) These are melanocytes in the sense that they produce melanin: they correspond to no normal human cell but have some homology with the frog melanophores—hence the alternative name. The lesions are blue in colour as a result of an optical effect due to their depth beneath the surface. Occasionally elements of blue naevi and ordinary pigmented naevi occur together in one tumour, producing a very confusing histological picture. Malignancy in blue naevi is very rare.

Dermal tumours

With a few exceptions, these are less common and less important than the epithelial tumours. They are, however, too numerous in variety for any systematic treatment here and what follows consists only of notes on some of the more interesting kinds. Reference should be made to Chapter 12 for fibromas (p. 290), lipomas (p. 293) and angiomas (p. 297) and their variants, which include several important skin tumours. Neurofibromas will be found in Chapter 20 (p. 733). Lymphoid tumours and their precursors

have been mentioned earlier in this Chapter (p. 1000).

The sclerosing-angioma/dermatofibroma group

This group contains at least three seemingly distinct tumours (or apparent tumours) which often show transitions and are believed to

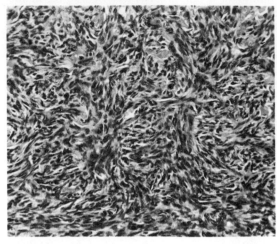

Fig. 25.46   Sclerosing angioma, showing the characteristic whorled pattern, with inconspicuous capillaries. × 154.

represent stages of one process, though this is not certain. The name *subepidermal nodular fibrosis* may be used for the whole group.

The process begins with a hypothetical *angioma*, perhaps too small to be clinically evident. This may undergo, as a result of trauma, a brief phase of haemorrhage and endothelial cell proliferation. The result is a brownish protruding mass, the so-called *sclerosing angioma*, which may reach 25 mm in diameter, though 10–15 mm is more usual, and which may readily be mistaken clinically for a malignant melanoma. Histologically, they show dense masses of proliferating endothelial cells with numerous but inconspicuous angiomatoid vessels (Fig. 25.46) and numerous histiocytes and giant cells containing haemosiderin and lipid, both derived presumably from breaking-down erythrocytes.

Left alone, these lesions regress, most of the endothelial cells and the haemosiderin disappear and one is left with a collagenous nodule in the dermis containing numerous lipid-laden macrophages: this stage is called a *histiocytoma*.

Finally, the macrophages also disappear, and the result is a fibrous nodule, a *dermatofibroma*. Like its predecessors, this is a benign lesion, and commonest on the limbs. They can usually be readily distinguished from true fibromas: in the earlier stages by the persistence of some macrophages, in the later stages by very low cellularity and a general pattern suggesting rather a thickening or distortion of the dermis than new fibroblastic proliferation.

True fibroma of the dermis is very rare, but confusion is possible not only with dermato-fibroma but with neurofibroma.

Dermatofibrosarcoma protuberans

Fibrosarcoma of the skin is represented by this lesion, which arises usually *de novo* from the skin of the trunk. It has the histology of any low-grade fibrosarcoma, and when small a characteristic hour-glass shape, with a base in the dermis and two nodules, one superficial pressing the epidermis outwards (hence 'protuberans') and one larger invading the deeper tissues. It is slow growing and rarely metastasises but recurs persistently after any but the most ruthless excision.

Suggestions for Further Reading and Consultation

The following list consists mainly of textbooks and review articles: their suitability as reading material or for consultation is indicated by the title and length. References to most of the original reports mentioned in the text of this book will be found in the appropriate items listed below, and separate reference to original papers are provided only for a few recent reports of outstanding interest.

General

A History of Medicine. D. Guthrie. pp. 448. Nelson, London, 1945.

An Introduction to Pathology. G. Payling Wright. 3rd ed., pp. 660, Longmans Green, London, 1958. (Still a most instructive and interesting book quite apart from the many historical notes it contains.)

The Pathological Basis of Medicine. Ed. R. C. Curran and D. G. Harnden. pp. 681. Heinemann Medical, London, 1972. (A multiple-author book on general pathology.)

Best and Taylor's Physiological Basis of Medical Practice. Ed. J. R. Brobeck. 9th ed., pp. 1200. Williams and Wilkins, Baltimore, 1973.

Clinical Chemistry in Diagnosis and Treatment. Joan F. Zilva and P. R. Pannall. pp. 430. Lloyd-Luke, London, 1971.

Medical Terms: their Origin and Construction. Ffrangcon Roberts. 5th ed., pp. 102. Heinemann Medical, London, 1971.

Elements of Medical Genetics. A. E. H. Emery. 4th ed., pp. 246. Churchill-Livingstone, Edinburgh, 1975.

Basic Pathology

Chapter 1

The Metabolic Basis of Inherited Disease. J. B. Stanbury, J. B. Wyngaarden and D. S. Fredrickson. 3rd ed., pp. 1778. McGraw Hill, New York and London, 1975.

The Megaloblastic Anaemias. I. Chanarin. pp. 9–39. Blackwell Scientific, Oxford, 1969.

Lysosomes in Biology and Pathology. J. T. Dingle and Dame Honor Fell. 4 vols. North Holland Publishing Co., Amsterdam, 1973 and 1975.

Cellular Injury. Ciba Symposium. Ed. A. V. S. de Deuck and Julie Knight. pp. 403. Churchill, London, 1964.

Chapter 2

Cohnheim's Lectures on General Pathology. Vol. 1, pp. 242 to at least 270. English translation. New Sydenham Society, London, 1889. (The classical account of the microscopic changes of acute inflammation, observed *in vivo*.)

Acute Inflammation. J. V. Hurley. pp. 137. Churchill-Livingstone, Edinburgh, 1972. (A clear, ·readable review, including some of the author's own work and views.)

Chemotaxis and Inflammation. P. C. Wilkinson. pp. 214. Churchill-Livingstone, Edinburgh, 1974. (An authoritative account of chemotaxis, including original observations by the author.)

The Inflammatory Process. Ed. B. W. Zweifach. 3 vols. Academic Press, New York and London, 1973–4. (Accounts of most aspects of the subject by many of the leading workers.)

Inflammation, Mechanisms and Control. Ed. I. H. Lepow and P. A. Ward. pp. 388. Academic Press, New York and London, 1972. (Review articles on selected topics by some leading workers.)

van Firth, R., Cohn, Z. A., Hirsch, J. G., Humphrey, J. H. and Spector, W. G. (1972). The Molecular Phagocyte System: a new Classification of Macrophages, Monocytes and their Precursor Cells. *Bull. Wld Hlth Org.*, **46**, 845.

Chapter 3

Tissue Repair. R. M. H. McMinn. pp. 423. Academic Press, London, 1969.
Sevitt, S. (1970). Bone repair and fracture healing. *Brit. J. hosp. Med.*, **3**, 693–710.
Peacock, E. E., Jr. (1973). Biology of wound repair. Mini-review. *Life Sciences*, **4**, V–IX.

Chapters 4 and 5

Essential Immunology. I. M. Roitt. 2nd ed., pp. 260. Blackwell Scientific, Oxford, 1974. (A clear, concise, well-illustrated account.)
Immunology for Students of Medicine. J. H. Humphrey and R. G. White. 3rd ed., pp. 757. Blackwell Scientific, Oxford, 1970.
Clinical Aspects of Immunology. Ed. P. G. H. Gell, R. R. A. Coombs and P. J. Lachmann. 3rd ed., pp. 1754. Blackwell Scientific, Oxford, 1975. (Extensive reviews by leading workers.)
Autoimmunity, Clinical and Experimental. J. R. Anderson, W. W. Buchanan and R. B. Goudie. pp. 485. Thomas, Springfield, 1967.
Immune Complex Disease in Experimental Animals and Man. C. G. Cochrane and D. Koffler. pp. 186–264 in *Advances in Immunology*. Vol. 16. Academic Press, New York and London, 1973.

Chapters 6 and 7

Medical Microbiology. Vol. 1, *Microbial Infections*. pp. 667, 1973. Vol. 2, *The Practice of Medical Microbiology*. pp. 587, 1975. Ed. R. Cruickshank, J. P. Duguid, B. P. Marmion and R. H. A. Swain. Churchill-Livingstone, Edinburgh.
A Short Textbook of Medical Microbiology. D. C. Turk and I. A. Porter. 3rd ed., pp. 344. English Universities Press, London, 1974.
Principles of Microbiology and Immunology. B. D. Davis, R. Dulbecco, H. N. Eisen, H. S. Ginsberg and W. B. Wood. 2nd ed., pp. 1562. Harper and Rowe, New York, 1973.
The Biology of Animal Viruses. F. Fenner. 2nd ed., pp. 834. Academic Press, New York and London, 1974.
The Pathogenesis of Infectious Disease. C. A. Mims, pp. 246. Academic Press, London: Grune and Stratton; New York, 1976.

Chapter 8

Blood Transfusion in Clinical Medicine. P. L. Mollison. 5th ed., pp. 833. Blackwell Scientific, Oxford, 1972.
Blood Groups in Man. R. R. Race and Ruth Sanger. 6th ed., pp. 659. Blackwell Scientific, Oxford, 1975.
Reactions to Injury and Burns and their Clinical Importance. S. Sevitt. pp. 255. Heinemann Medical, London, 1974.

Chapter 9

Pigments in Pathology. Ed. M. Wolman. pp. 551. Academic Press, New York and London, 1969.
Amyloidosis. G. A. Stirling. In *Recent Advances in Pathology*. pp. 249–69. Ed. C. V. Harrison and K. Weinbren. 9th ed., pp. 279. Churchill-Livingstone, Edinburgh, 1975. (A general review.)
J. A. Boyle (1969). Hyperuricaemia. *Brit. J. hosp. Med*, **2**, 1984–8.
The Validation of Fibrin, and its Significance in the Story of Hyalin. A. C. Lendrum. In *Trends in Clinical Pathology*. pp. 159–83. British Medical Association, London, 1969.

Chapter 10

The Spread of Tumours in the Human Body. R. A. Willis. 3rd ed., pp. 417. Butterworths, London, 1973.
Advances in Cancer Research. Academic Press, New York and London. (A series, published annually.)
Scientific foundations of Oncology. Ed. T. Symington and R. L. Carter. pp. 690. Heinemann, London, 1976. (A large collection of authoritative reviews on the many aspects of neoplasia.)
The Molecular Biology of Tumour Viruses. Ed. J. Tooze. pp. 734. Cold Spring Harbor Laboratory, New York, 1973.

Chapters 11 and 12

Histological Appearances of Tumours. D. Winston Evans. 2nd ed., pp. 1256. Livingstone, Edinburgh, 1966.
Pathology of Tumours. R. A. Willis. 4th ed., pp. 1019. Butterworths, London, 1967.
Atlas of Tumor Pathology. U.S. Armed Forces Institute of Pathology, Washington D.C. (Numerous 'Fascicles' on tumours of particular organs, tissues and regions. A valuable source of detailed information on the histology and behaviour of individual tumours.)

Systematic Pathology

General

Surgical Pathology. L. V. Ackerman. 5th ed., pp. 1394. Mosby, St. Louis, 1974

Applied Surgical Pathology. Ed. A. E. Stuart, A. N. Smith and E. Samuel. pp. 1112. Blackwell Scientific, Oxford, 1976.

Chapters 13 and 14

Cardiovascular Pathology. R. E. B. Hudson. Vols. 1 (pp. 1190) and 2 (pp. 933), 1965; Vol. 3 (Supplement, pp. 1166), 1970. Arnold, London.

Paul Wood's Diseases of the Heart and Circulation. By various authors. 3rd ed., pp. 1164. Eyre and Spottiswoode, London, 1968.

Arterial Disease. J. R. A. Mitchell and C. J. Schwartz. pp. 411. Blackwell Scientific, Oxford, 1965.

Mechanisms in the Development of Early Atheroma. Ciba Symposium. Ed. Ruth Porter and Julie Knight. pp. 288. Associated Scientific Publishers, London, 1972.

Smith, J. P. (1956). Hyaline arteriolosclerosis in spleen, pancreas and other viscera. *J. Path. Bact.*, **72**, 643–56.

Chapter 15

Essentials of Respiratory Disease. R. B. Cole, 2nd ed., pp. 297. Pitman Medical, London, 1975.

Pathology of the Lung. H. Spencer. 3rd ed., pp. 1100. Pergamon Press, Oxford, 1977.

The Human Pulmonary Circulation. P. Harris and D. Heath. 2nd ed. pp. 689. Churchill-Livingstone, Edinburgh, 1977.

The Lung. Ed. A. A. Liebow and D. E. Smith. pp. 400. Williams and Wilkins, Baltimore, 1968.

Chapter 16

Atlas of Haematology. G. A. McDonald, T. C. Dodds and Bruce Cruickshank. 3rd ed., pp. 226. Livingstone, Edinburgh, 1970.

Blood and its Disorders. Ed. R. M. Hardisty and D. J. Weatherall. pp. 1540. Blackwell Scientific, Oxford, 1974. (A comprehensive and authoritative multi-author text.)

Clinical Haematology. M. M. Wintrobe *et al*. 7th ed., pp. 1896. Lea and Febiger, Philadelphia, 1974.

Haematology. A. V. Hoffbrand and S. M. Lewis. pp. 652. Heinemann Medical, London, 1972. (Volume 2 in the series *Tutorials in Postgraduate Medicine*.)

Practical Haematology. J. V. Dacie and S. M. Lewis. 5th ed., pp. 629. Churchill-Livingstone, Edinburgh, 1975.

Short Textbook of Haematology. R. B. Thomson. 3rd ed., pp. 384. Pitman Medical, London, 1969.

Chapter 17

Lymph Node Diseases. C. V. Harrison. In *Recent Advances in Pathology*. Vol. 9, pp. 73–96. Ed. C. V. Harrison and K. Weinbren. Churchill-Livingstone, Edinburgh, 1975.

Lukes, R. J. and Collins, R. D. (1975). New approaches to the classification of the lymphomata. *Brit. J. Cancer*, **31**, Suppl. II, pp. 1–28.

Diseases of the Lymphoid Tissues. C. V. Harrison. In *Recent Advances in Pathology*. Ed. C. V. Harrison. 7th ed., 1960, pp. 35–53. 8th ed., 1966, pp. 207–36. Churchill, London.

Niederman, J. C., McCollum, R. W., Henley, Gertrude and Henle, W. (1968). Infectious mononucleosis. Clinical manifestations in relation to EB virus antibodies. *J. Amer. med. Assoc.*, **203**, 205–9.

Chapter 18

Gastro-intestinal Pathology. B. C. Morson and I. M. P. Dawson. pp. 676. Blackwell Scientific, Oxford, 1972.

Mucosal Biopsy of the Gastro-intestinal Tract. R. Whitehead. pp. 202. (Major Problems in Pathology, Vol. 3.) Saunders, Philadelphia and London, 1973.

Coeliac Disease. Ed. W. T. Cooke and P. Asquith. pp. 238 (Clinics in Gastroenterology. Vol. 3, No. 1). Saunders, Philadelphia and London, 1974.

Morson, B. C. and Price, A. B. (1975). Inflammatory bowel disease. *Human Pathology*, **6**, 7–29.

Glass, G. B. J. and Pitchumoni, C. S. (1975). Atrophic gastritis. *Human Pathology*, **6**, 219–50.

Chapter 19

Diseases of the Liver and Biliary System. Sheila Sherlock. 5th ed., pp. 821. Blackwell Scientific, Oxford, 1975.

Clinics in Gastroenterology. Vol. 2: 1 *Diseases of the Biliary Tract*. pp. 215. Ed. I. A. D. Bouchier. 1973. Vol. 3: 2 *Viral Hepatitis*. pp. 474. Ed. N. Tygstrup. 1974. Vol. 4: 2 *Cirrhosis*. pp. 463. Ed. H. Popper. 1975. Saunders, Philadelphia and London.

Progress in Liver Disease. Ed. H. Popper and F. Schaffner. Vol. 3, pp. 562, 1970. Vol. 4, pp. 640, 1972. Grune and Stratton, New York.

The Liver and its Diseases. Ed. F. Schaffner, S. Sherlock and C. M. Leevy. pp. 353. Intercontinental Med. Book Corp., New York, 1974.

Liver Biopsy Interpretation. P. J. Scheuer. 2nd ed. pp. 171. Baillière, Tindall and Cassell, London, 1973.

Diseases of the Liver. K. Weinbren. In *Recent Advances in Pathology*, Vol. 9. pp. 97–130. Ed. C. V. Harrison and K. Weinbren. Churchill-Livingstone, Edinburgh, 1975.

Modern Trends in Gastroenterology—5. Ed. A. E. Read. pp. 479. Butterworths, London, 1975.

Chapter 20

Greenfield's Neuropathology. Ed. W. Blackwood and J. A. N. Corsellis. 3rd ed., pp. 946. Arnold, London, 1976.

The Nervous System: Structure and Function in Disease. D. M. Robertson and H. B. Dinsdale. pp. 204. Williams and Wilkins, Baltimore, 1972.

Pathology of Tumours of the Nervous System. D. S. Russell and L. J. Rubinstein. 3rd ed., pp. 429. Arnold, London, 1971.

Scientific Foundations of Neurology. Ed. M. Critchley, J. L. O'Leary and B. Jennett. pp. 502. Heinemann, London, 1972.

Tumours of the Central Nervous System. L. J. Rubinstein. pp. 400. Armed Forces Institute of Pathology, Washington, D.C., 1972.

Chapter 21

Pathology of the Kidney. R. T. Heptinstall. 2nd ed., pp. 1171. Little Brown, Boston, 1974.

Renal Disease. D. A. K. Black. 3rd ed., pp. 871. Blackwell Scientific, Oxford, 1972.

Immunopathology of the Renal Glomerulus. F. R. Germuth and E. Rodriguez. pp. 227. Little Brown, Boston, 1973.

Horster, M. and Thurau, K. (1968). Micropuncture studies on the filtration rate of single superficial and juxtamedullary glomeruli in the rat kidney. *Pflüger's Archiv.*, **301**, 162–81.

Lever, 1969. See Brown, J. J. *et al.* (1970). Renin and acute renal failure: studies in man. *Brit. med. J*, **1**, 253–8.

Chapter 22

Metabolic Disorders of Bone. C. R. Paterson. pp. 373. Blackwell Scientific, Oxford, 1974.

Metabolic, Degenerative and Inflammatory Diseases of Bones and Joints. H. L. Jaffe. pp. 1101. Lea and Febiger, Philadelphia, 1972.

Tumours of Bone and Cartilage. H. J. Spjut *et al.* pp. 454. Armed Forces Institute of Pathology, Washington, D.C., 1971.

Muscle Biopsy: A modern approach. V. Dubowitz and M. H. Brooke. pp. 475. Saunders, Philadelphia and London, 1973.

Chapter 23

Novak's Gynaecological and Obstetrical Pathology. E. R. Novak and J. D. Woodruff. 7th ed., pp. 1562. Saunders, Philadelphia and London, 1974.

Gynaecological Pathology. Magnus Haines and C. W. Taylor. 2nd ed., pp. 552. Churchill-Livingstone, Edinburgh, 1975.

Pathology of the Testis. Ed. R. C. B. Pugh, pp. 487. Blackwell Scientific, Oxford, 1976.

Chapter 24

Textbook of Endocrinology. Ed. R. H. Williams. 5th ed., pp. 1138. Saunders, Philadelphia and London, 1974. (An authoritative text by 38 contributors.)

Fundamentals of Clinical Endocrinology. R. Hall, J. Anderson, G. A. Smart and M. Besser. 2nd ed., pp. 494. Pitman Medical, London, 1974. (Deals mainly with the mechanisms and clinical aspects of endocrine disorders.)

Chapter 25

A Guide to Dermatohistopathology. 2nd ed., pp. 724. H. Pinkus and A. H. Mehregan. Appleton-Century-Crofts, New York, 1976.

An Introduction to the Diagnostic Histopathology of the Skin. J. A. Milne. pp. 362. Arnold, London, 1972.

Dermatopathology (2 vols.). H. Montgomery. Hoeber Medical Division, Harper and Row, New York, 1967.

Histopathology of the Skin. W. F. Lever and Gundula Schaumburg-Lever. 5th ed., pp. 793. Lippincott, Philadelphia, 1975.

Index

Page numbers in heavy print indicate the main accounts of topics which also receive attention on the other pages indexed.